The complete mobile solution for nursing professionals and students!

W9-AFZ-263

mynursingapp

MyNursingapp provides easy access to clinical information right in the palm of your hands! Based on trusted nursing resources from Pearson Nursing, this series of mobile products allows you to search across multiple titles seamlessly to find the right information about conditions, nursing management, drugs, labs, skills, and more – all when you need it the most!

Features

- Point and click navigation
- Smart-type searching by topic, disease, drugs, labs, and more
- Book marking capability
- Note-taking and highlighting capabilities
- Navigation history
- Links to the Internet
- And more!

Try any MyNursingapp product free for 30 days!
For more information regarding MyNursingapp, a complete listing of available products,
or to download a FREE 30-day trial version please visit

www.mynursingapp.com

EXPLORE 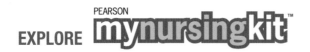 PEARSON mynursingkit™

STEP 1: Register

All you need to get started is a valid email address and the access code below. To register, simply:

1. Go to **www.mynursingkit.com**. Click on the appropriate book cover.

2. In the "First-Time User" column, click "**Register.**"

3. Read the **License Agreement** and **Private Policy**. If you accept, click "**I Accept.**"

4. Under "**Do you have a Pearson account**?" select:

   • "**Yes**" if you have a Pearson account and know your Login Name and Password.

   • "**Not Sure**" if you do not know if you already have an account or do not recall your Login Name and Password.

   • "**No**" if you are sure you do not have a Pearson account.

5. Using a coin, scratch off the silver coating below to reveal your access code. Do not use a knife or other sharp object, which can damage the code.

6. Enter your access code in lowercase or uppercase, without the dashes, then click "**Next**."

7. Follow the on-screen instructions to complete registration.

After completing registration, you will be sent a confirmation email that contains your Login Name and Password. Be sure to save this email for future reference

---

Your Access Code is:

Note: If there is no silver foil covering the access code, it may already have been redeemed, and therefore may no longer be valid. In that case, you can purchase access online using a major credit card. To do so, go to www.mynursingkit.com. Find and click on the cover of your textbook, then click "Get Access," and follow the on-screen instructions.

STEP 2: Log in

1. Go to **www.mynursingkit.com**.

2. Find and click on the appropriate book cover. Cover must match the textbook edition used for your class.

3. Enter the Login Name and Password that you created during registration. If unsure of this information, refer to your registration confirmation email.

4. Click "**Login**."

Got technical questions?

Customer Technical Support: To obtain support, please visit us online anytime at http://247pearsoned.custhelp.com where you can search our knowledgebase for common solutions, view product alerts, and review all options for additional assistance.

SITE REQUIREMENTS
For the latest updates on Site Requirements, go to www.mynursingkit.com. Find and click on the cover of the book you are using. Click on "**Needs help?**" link at bottom of page. Under "**Technical Problems**" select the link "**What do I need on my computer to use this site?**"

Important: Please read the Subscription and End-User License agreement, accessible from the book website's login page, before using the *mynursingkit* website. By using the website, you indicate that you have read, understood, and accepted the terms of this agreement.

0131722166

Success in the Classroom, in Clinicals, and on the NCLEX-RN®

Classroom

- Detailed lecture notes organized by learning outcome
- Suggestions for classroom activities
- Guide to relevant additional resources
- Comprehensive PowerPoint™ presentations integrating lecture, images, animations, and videos
- Classroom Response questions
- Image Gallery
- Video and Animation Gallery
- Online course management systems complete with instructor tools and student activities available in a variety of formats

Clinical

- Suggestions for Clinical Activities and other clinical resources organized by learning outcome

Real Nursing Simulations Facilitator's Guide: Institutional Edition

- 25 simulation scenarios that span the nursing curriculum
- Consistent format includes learning objectives, case flow, instructions for set up, student debriefing questions and more!
- Companion online course cartridge with student exercises, activities, videos, skill checklists, and reflective questions also available for adoption

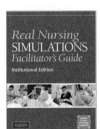

NCLEX-RN®

- Test Item Files with NCLEX®-style questions and complete rationales for correct and incorrect answers mapped to learning outcomes.
  available in TestGen, Par Test, and MS Word

Instructor Resources

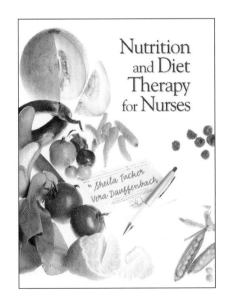

Nutrition and Diet Therapy for Nurses

Sheila Tucker
Vera Dauffenbach

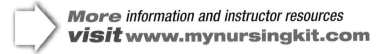

More *information and instructor resources*
visit **www.mynursingkit.com**

Brief Contents

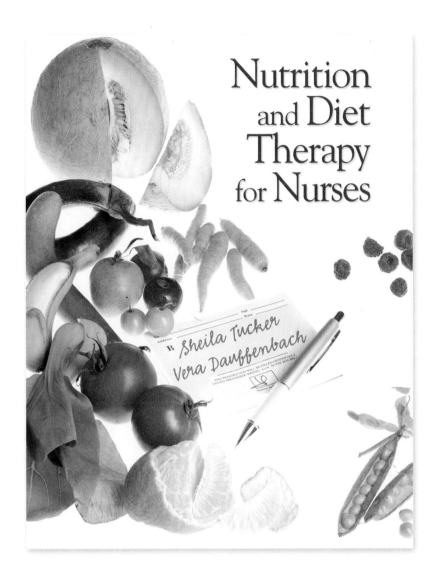

Nutrition and Diet Therapy for Nurses

Sheila Buckley Tucker, MA, RD, CSSD, LDN

Executive Dietitian and Part-Time Faculty, Connell School of Nursing, Boston College

Vera Dauffenbach, EdD, MSN, RN

Associate Professor and Director of the Graduate Program, Bellin College, Green Bay, Wisconsin

Pearson

Boston   Columbus   Indianapolis   New York   San Francisco   Upper Saddle River
Amsterdam   Cape Town   Dubai   London   Madrid   Milan   Munich   Paris   Montreal   Toronto
Delhi   Mexico City   São Paulo   Sydney   Hong Kong   Seoul   Singapore   Taipei   Tokyo

Library of Congress Cataloging-in-Publication Data

Tucker, Sheila.
   Nutrition and diet therapy / Sheila Tucker.—1st ed.
     p. ; cm.
   Includes bibliographical references and index.
   ISBN 978-0-13-172216-3 (alk. paper)
   1. Diet therapy. 2. Nutrition. 3. Nursing. I. Title.
   [DNLM: 1. Diet Therapy—Nurses' Instruction. 2. Nutritional Physiological Phenomena—
Nurses' Instruction. WB 400 T894n 2011]
   RM217.T83 2011
   615.8'54--dc22
                                                  2009041913

Publisher: Julie Levin Alexander
Publisher's Assistant: Regina Bruno
Editor-in-Chief: Maura Connor
Executive Acquisitions Editor: Pamela Fuller
Development Editor: Susan Geraghty
Editorial Assistant: Lisa Pierce
Managing Production Editor: Patrick Walsh
Production Liaison: Cathy O'Connell
Production Editor: Amy Gehl, S4Carlisle Publishing
   Services
Manufacturing Manager: Ilene Sanford

Art Editor: Patricia Gutierrez
Art Director: Christopher Weigand
Cover and Interior Design: Laura Gardner
Director of Marketing: Karen Allman
Marketing Specialist: Michael Sirinides
Marketing Assistant: Crystal Gonzalez
Media Project Manager: Rachel Collett
Composition: S4Carlisle Publishing Services
Printer/Binder: Webcrafters, Inc.
Cover Printer: LeHigh-Phoenix Color/Hagerstown
Cover Photos: Jupiter Images

Section Opener Credits: Page 15: iStockphoto.com; Page 179: Shutterstock; Page 249: iStockphoto.com; Page 349: Shutterstock

Chapter Opener Credits: Page 1: iStockphoto.com; Page 17: iStockphoto.com; Page 39: iStockphoto.com; Page 60: iStockphoto.com; Page 80: iStockphoto.com; Page 111: Shutterstock; Page 143: iStockphoto.com; Page 162: iStockphoto.com; Page 181: iStockphoto.com; Pages 202: iStockphoto.com; Page 225: iStockphoto.com; Pages 251: iStockphoto.com; Page 279: iStockphoto.com; Page 300: iStockphoto.com; Page 327: iStockphoto.com; Page 351: iStockphoto.com; Page 373: iStockphoto.com; Page 401: Letitia Anne Peplau; Page 424: Richard Logan/Pearson Education/PH College; Page 443: iStockphoto.com; Page 472: Michael Hieber/Shutterstock; Page 496: iStockphoto.com; Page 518: iStockphoto.com; Page 539: iStockphoto.com; Page 555: iStockphoto.com

Notice: Care has been taken to confirm the accuracy of information presented in this book. The authors, editors, and the publisher, however, cannot accept any responsibility for errors or omissions or for consequences from application of the information in this book and make no warranty, express or implied, with respect to its contents.

    The authors and publisher have exerted every effort to ensure that drug selections and dosages set forth in this text are in accord with current recommendations and practice at time of publication. However, in view of ongoing research, changes in government regulations, and the constant flow of information relating to drug therapy and drug reactions, the reader is urged to check the package inserts of all drugs for any change in indications of dosage and for added warnings and precautions. This is particularly important when the recommended agent is a new and/or infrequently employed drug.

Copyright © 2011 Pearson Education, Inc., Upper Saddle River, NJ 07458. All rights reserved. Printed in the United States of America. This publication is protected by Copyright, and permission should be obtained from the publisher prior to any prohibited reproduction, storage in a retrieval system, or transmission in any form or by any means, electronic, mechanical, photocopying, recording, or likewise. For information regarding permission(s), write to: Rights and Permission Department, 1 Lake Street, Upper Saddle River, NJ 07458.

Pearson® is a registered trademark of Pearson plc.

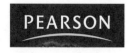

www.pearsonhighered.com

10 9 8 7 6 5 4 3 2 1
ISBN 10:   0-13-172216-6
ISBN 13: 978-0-13-172216-3

About the Authors

Sheila Buckley Tucker graduated with a BS in Food and Nutrition and an MA in Healthcare Administration from Framingham State College in Massachusetts. She is board certified in sports nutrition from the American Dietetic Association. As a registered dietitian for over 25 years, Sheila has provided clinical nutrition care to patients and clients in a variety of settings, including as an in-patient clinical dietitian specializing in critical care, nutrition support, renal nutrition, cancer care, and medical/surgical care. She has also provided nutrition education as a consultant to corporate wellness programs and area colleges. She has over 20 years of teaching experience at the undergraduate and graduate levels in several Boston area colleges and nursing schools. At Boston College, Sheila combines an on-campus clinical nutrition practice, specializing in both sports nutrition and disordered eating, with teaching nutrition in the Connell School of Nursing. She is a contributing author to many nursing textbooks.

Dedication

To Lance, Victoria, and Emma with much love

Vera Dauffenbach has a bachelor's degree from Macalester College and a master's degree in nursing from Pace University. Her doctorate in educational leadership is from Western Michigan University. She has been a faculty member in the baccalaureate nursing programs at Grand View College in Des Moines and Maryville College (now University) in St. Louis. At present, she is an associate professor and director of the graduate program at Bellin College in Green Bay, Wisconsin. She has broad classroom and clinical teaching experience on all levels of the undergraduate curriculum, with a special interest in nutrition and pediatrics. At the graduate level, she teaches courses in nursing theory and leadership. Her research interests relate to critical thinking and leadership development. She has contributed extensive NCLEX®-style test questions for nursing textbooks. She is a past board member of the Wisconsin League for Nursing and president of Kappa Pi-at-Large Chapter of Sigma Theta Tau International.

Dedication

This book is dedicated to my beloved husband, Wil Tabb, and daughter, Hilary Dauffenbach-Tabb, both of whom are the light of my life. They are forever my inspiration and support as I pursue scholarly excellence in my commitment to the profession. This book is also dedicated to my late parents, Laura and George Dauffenbach; they instilled in me the value of education along with the virtues of hard work and persistence.

Thank You...

We extend a heartfelt thanks to the contributors who gave their time, effort, and expertise generously to developing and writing chapters.

Contributors

LeAnne Bloedon, MS, RD
Lecturer, University of Pennsylvania School of Nursing

Cynthia Hoffman, MS, RD
Clinical Specialist in Critical Care Nutrition
Crozer-Chester Medical Center, Pennsylvania

Christie Hust, MS, RD, LD
Director, Texas Tech Diabetes Education Center

Rachael Pohle-Krauza, PhD, RD, CDN/LD
Assistant Professor of Food and Nutrition
Department of Ecology, Youngstown State University

Susan Prion, EdD, RN
Associate Professor, School of Nursing
University of San Francisco

Stacey Schulman, MS, RD, CDN
Nutritionist, CEDAR Associates & Associate
Midtown Nutrition Care, New York

Julie Stefanski, RD, LDN, CDE
Adjunct Professor, York College &
Clinical Dietitian, York Hospital, Pennsylvania

Charlotte Wisnewski, PhD, RN, BC, CDE
Assistant Professor, University of Texas Medical Branch

Supplement Contributor

Angeline Bushy, PhD, RN, FAAN
Professor & Bert Fish Chair
University of Central Florida, College of Nursing
MyNursingKit

Reviewers

We extend sincere thanks to our colleagues from schools of nursing across the country who gave their time generously to help create *Nutrition and Diet Therapy for Nurses*. These professionals helped us plan and shape our book and resources by reviewing the original proposal, chapters, art, and more.

Julie Beck, BSN, MSN, DEd
Department of Nursing
York College of Pennsylvania
York, Pennsylvania

Mary Bell-Braxton, MS, RN
Adjunct Faculty
University of West Georgia
Carrollton, Georgia

Barbara A Britton,
RN, BSN, MSN, NNP-BC
Associate Degree Nursing Instructor
Fayetteville Technical Community College
Fayetteville, North Carolina

Nathania Bush, MSN, APRN, BC
Assistant Professor of Nursing
Morehead State University
Morehead, Kentucky

Angeline Bushy, PhD, RN, FAAN
Professor and Bert Fish Chair
College of Nursing
University of Central Florida
Orlando, Florida

Karen Clark, EdD, RN
Dean of Nursing and Assistant Professor
Indiana University East
Richmond, Indiana

Sherri Comfort, RN, ADN
Practical Nursing Instructor
Department Chair
Holmes Community College
Goodman, Mississippi

Nancy J. Cooley, MSN, CAGS, FNP-BC
Associate Professor of Nursing
University of Maine at Augusta
Augusta, Maine

Vera K. Dauffenbach, RN, MSN, EdD
Associate Professor
Bellin College of Nursing
Green Bay, Wisconsin

Diane Dembicki, PhD, LMT, CYT
Assistant Professor
School of Nursing
Adelphi University
Garden City, New York

Kelly Dempsey, RN, MSN
Assistant Clinical Professor
Indiana University East
Richmond, Indiana

Carol A. DeNysschen,
PhD, RD, MPH, CDN
Assistant Professor
SUNY Buffalo State College
Buffalo, New York

Marian Theresa Doyle, RN, MS, MSN
Associate Professor of Nursing
Northampton Community College
Bethlehem, Pennsylvania

Patricia A. Duclos-Miller, MS, RN, NE-BC
Professor
Capital Community College
Hartford, Connecticut

Denise Eagan, MA, RD, LS
Assistant Professor
Marshall University
Huntington, West Virginia

Patricia L. Franks, MSN, RN
Associate Professor
Louisiana State University Alexandria
Alexandria, Louisiana

Barbara T. Freese, RN, MSN, EdD
Professor of Nursing Emeritus
Lander University
Greenwood, South Carolina

Kevin M. Gulliver, MSN, RN, CNE
Instructor
School of Nursing
University of Nevada, Las Vegas
Las Vegas, Nevada

Laura B. Hammond, MN, RN
Instructor
Seattle Central Community College
Seattle, Washington

William D. Hart, PhD, MPH
Assistant Professor
Rogers State University
Claremore, Oklahoma

Catherine R. Heinlein, EdD, RD, MS, CDE
Assistant Professor, Registered Dietitian
Certified Diabetes Educator
School of Nursing
Azusa Pacific University
Azusa, California

Brenda Hosley, RN, PhD
Associate Professor
Eastern Kentucky University
Richmond, Kentucky

Teresa Johnson, MA, RD, LD
Assistant Professor
Troy University School of Nursing
Troy, Alabama

Mary Justice, MSN, CNE
Associate Professor
University of Cincinnati
   Raymond Walters College
Cincinnati, Ohio

Susan M. Koos, MS, RN, CNE
Professor II, Nursing
Heartland Community College
Normal, Illinois

Jane M. Kufus-Krump, MS, LRD
Professor and Department Chair
North Dakota State College of Science
Wahpeton, North Dakota

Phyllis Magaletto MS, RN, BC
Professor of Nursing
Cochran School of Nursing
Yonkers, New York

Judith M. Malachowski
Associate Professor
Georgia Southwestern State University
Americus, Georgia

Joanne Malenock, PhD, RD
Assistant Professor
School of Nursing
University of Pittsburgh
Pittsburgh, Pennsylvania

Jaimette A. McCulley, MS, RD, LD
Assistant Professor
Fontbonne University
St. Louis, Missouri

Myrtle McCulloch, RD, EdD
Assistant Professor, Nutrition
School of Nursing and Health Studies
Georgetown University
Washington, DC

Jeanie F. Mitchel, RNC, MSN, MA
Nursing Faculty
South Suburban College
South Holland, Illinois

Joseph Molinatti, EdD, RN
Assistant Professor of Nursing
College of Mount St. Vincent
Riverdale, New York

Gene E. Mundie, EdM, MS, RN
Clinical Associate Professor
School of Nursing, Stony Brook University
Stony Brook, New York

Elaine Musselman, RN, MSN/Ed
Instructor
Raritan Valley Community College
Somerville, New Jersey

Patricia J. Neafsey, RD, PhD
Professor
University of Connecticut
Storrs, Connecticut

Jean Nelson, PhD, RN
Clinical Assistant Professor
College of Nursing
University of Missouri-St. Louis
St. Louis, Missouri

Martha Olson, RN, BSN, MS
Assistant Professor
Iowa Lakes Community College
Emmetsburg, Iowa

Cindy Parsons, DNP, ARNP, BC, FAANP
Assistant Professor of Nursing
University of Tampa
Tampa, Florida

Cynthia L. Pins, MS, RN
Nursing Instructor
North Hennepin Community College
Brooklyn Park, Minnesota

Carol Wolin-Riklin, MA, RD, LD
Bariatric Nutrition Coordinator
ASMBS Center of Excellence in Bariatric
   Surgery
University of Texas Medical School
   at Houston
Houston, Texas

Charlene M. Romer, RN, PhD
Associate Professor
Clayton State University
Morrow, Georgia

Karen L. Schmidt, MS, RD, LDN
Instructor
University of Pittsburgh at Titusville
Titusville, Pennsylvania

Julie Stefanski, RD, LDN, CDE
Adjunct Professor
York College of Pennsylvania
York, Pennsylvania

Suzanne E. Tatro, RN, MS
Instructor
York Technical College
Rock Hill, South Carolina

Mary B. Williams, RN, MS
Assistant Professor
School of Nursing
University of West Georgia
Carrollton, Georgia

Janet Willis, RN, BSN, MS
Senior Professor
Harrisburg Area Community College
Harrisburg, Pennsylvania

Charlotte A. Wisnewski, PhD, RN, BC, CDE, CNE
Associate Professor
University of Texas Medical Branch
   at Galveston
Galveston, Texas

Preface

Nutrition and Diet Therapy for Nurses will be a staple in the library of nursing textbooks. It encompasses all aspects of nutrition, building from the foundation of nutrition principles up to the peak that is medical nutrition therapy to construct a solid, evidence-based approach to the practice of nutrition. Nutrition science is an evolving field—having come a long way from simply linking foods to prevention of nutrient deficiencies—and it is often difficult for the client to sift through the media, marketing promotions, the neighbor's advice, and internet information to find the facts. Now, more than ever, it is crucial that nurses possess the knowledge and skills to translate the science of what we know about nutrition and its role in health maintenance and disease prevention and be a reliable resource to the client. Nutrition is not just about vitamins and minerals anymore. Topics such as herbs, sports nutrition supplements, trendy weight loss diets, the effect of specific fatty acids on brain development, and drug interactions with foods or nutrients are examples of the range of topics that are new to nutrition. This book was written because nurses in any field of practice need to understand the role nutrition has in the well-being of the patient or client and be able to apply that knowledge as part of a holistic nursing approach to patient care. *Nutrition and Diet Therapy for Nurses* provides the nurse with the tools and resources to integrate nutrition into the nursing care process and become a reliable source of nutrition information and care over an entire career.

Organization of this book

This textbook is organized in a fashion that allows its use in a variety of nutrition classes or with varying curricula that integrate nutrition in different ways. Section 1, Principles of Nutrition, lays the foundation of normal nutrition, covering the macronutrients, vitamins, minerals, fluids, and energy balance. Section 2, Community Nutrition and Health Promotion, builds upon the principles of nutrition and applies them to population groups, outlining nutrition recommendations and standards and other topics such as sports nutrition, food safety, allergies, and culturally competent nutrition care that are important in many settings. Section 3, Nutrition in the Life Cycle, applies the principles of nutrition to individual patient care and nutrition assessment. Normal nutritional needs are incorporated into the recommendations that are unique for each lifespan group and are presented in a way that encourages the incorporation of this information into the nursing process. Section 4, Clinical Nutrition and Diet Therapy, covers a wide range of therapeutic nutrition topics following an outline that is based on body systems. As in other sections, evidence-based information is presented that can be incorporated into the nursing process. Special features in all sections streamline this approach and provide the nurse with cutting edge information for practice.

Special Features

Special Features are an integral part of the entire text and offer the nurse snapshot views of the latest information on nutrition and nursing along with practical applications. Features include:

EVIDENCE-BASED PRACTICE RESEARCH BOX

Are self-reported height and weight accurate enough for screening purposes with overweight individuals?

Clinical Problem: Many people prefer not to get weighed when visiting a health care provider. This preference is particularly true for overweight and obese individuals. If an accurate body mass index (BMI) could be calculated from self-reported height and weight, the usefulness of screening programs could be increased.

Research Findings: Numerous studies have been conducted using children, adolescents, and adults to determine the accuracy of self-reported height and weight and, therefore, the accuracy of BMI. Because BMI is useful in classifying individuals as underweight, normal, overweight, or obese, knowledge of BMI can be used for determining individuals at risk for disease.

One study of adolescents added an additional variable, body weight perception, in which students were asked if they perceived themselves as underweight, normal weight, or overweight. In the sample of 2,032 youth, 34.8% perceived themselves as underweight, 42.9% saw themselves as about right, and 22.3% perceived themselves as overweight. On the basis of BMI calculated from measured height and weight, only 1.5% of students were classified as underweight, whereas 51.2% were normal weight and 47.4% were overweight (Brener, Eaton, Lowry, & McManus, 2004).

Similar data exist for adults; women tend to understate weight and men tend to overstate height. Self-reported data also led to misclassification of BMI, especially in those who were already overweight or obese (Brunner-Huber, 2007; Engstrom, Paterson, Doherty, Trabulsi, & Speer, 2003; Kuczmarski, Kuczmarski, & Najjar, 2001; Nawaz, Chan, Abdulrahmann, Larson, & Katz, 2001; Nyholm et al., 2007;

- **Evidence-Based Practice Boxes** outline a current nutrition care question, review the available medical evidence on the topic and present a take-away message for the nurse to incorporate into practice. Critical Thinking Questions accompany each Evidence-Based Practice Box to present a scenario for application of the evidence.

NURSING CARE PLAN — Safe Food Handling

CASE STUDY

Alice, 31 years old, comes to the clinic with concerns about intermittent bouts of diarrhea over the last 3 months. She is a single parent who lives with her 8- and 11-year-old daughters in a mobile home park. Her work as a receptionist in a small real estate firm provides a modest income but no health insurance. She makes it clear that she wants as little diagnostic testing as possible because she does not know how she will pay for it. Upon further questioning, she reveals that the diarrhea is accompanied by abdominal discomfort and maybe a low fever, but it always resolves after a few days. She says that her children sometimes have it at the same time as she does, but other times they do not have it. They have all missed occasional days of school and work. When the nurse asks about food preparation and storage, Alice says she tries to be careful but their mobile home is cramped for the three of them and that space is at a premium. She describes the refrigerator as "old and tiny" and she is not sure it keeps things very cold. When she knows she will be using a food soon, she frequently leaves it on the

Applying the Nursing Process

ASSESSMENT

Height: 5 feet 4 inches; Weight: 128 pounds; BMI: 22
T 98.7 P 80 R 16 BP 126/72
Skin warm and dry
Moist mucous membranes
Active bowel sounds

DIAGNOSES

Diarrhea related to possible bacterial contamination from unsafe food storage evidenced by intermittent loose, watery stools
Knowledge, deficient related to lack of information about safe food storage practices evidenced by disclosure of current food storage practices

EXPECTED OUTCOMES

Bowel elimination pattern will return to normal
Alice will discuss causative factors and prevent practices

- **Nursing Care Plans** are included in each chapter to illustrate the nursing process. The case study pulls together key concepts from the chapter and allows the student to follow how the assessment, nursing diagnoses, nursing interventions, and evaluations would be formulated by the nurse.

- **Nursing Process Figures** accompany each Nursing Care Plan to present a visual diagram of the nursing process used in the construction of the case study. This feature helps the visual learner picture the nursing process in addition to learning it through reading the case study.

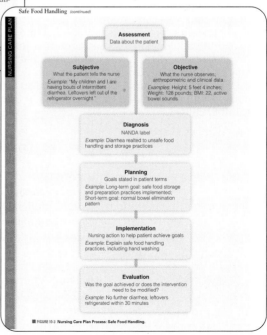

Safe Food Handling *(continued)*

Assessment
Data about the patient

Subjective
What the patient tells the nurse
Example: "My children and I are having bouts of intermittent diarrhea. Leftovers left out of the refrigerator overnight."

Objective
What the nurse observes; anthropometric and clinical data
Examples: Height: 5 feet 4 inches; Weight: 128 pounds; BMI: 22, active bowel sounds.

Diagnosis
NANDA label
Example: Diarrhea realted to unsafe food handling and storage practices

Planning
Goals stated in patient terms
Example: Long-term goal: safe food storage and preparation practices implemented; Short-term goal: normal bowel elimination pattern

Implementation
Nursing action to help patient achieve goals
Example: Explain safe food handling practices, including hand washing

Evaluation
Was the goal achieved or does the intervention need to be modified?
Example: No further diarrhea; leftovers refrigerated within 30 minutes

■ FIGURE 10-3 Nursing Care Plan Process: Safe Food Handling.

Special Features *continued*

- **Critical Thinking Exercises** accompany each Evidence-Based Practice Box and Nursing Care Plan to allow the student to apply the concepts used in those features to actual practice and stimulate further learning. All Critical Thinking Exercises have answers available at the back of the book.

> ## Critical Thinking in the Nursing Process
>
> 1. Why is the nurse particularly concerned about the hydration status of elderly clients?
> 2. What fluids can the nurse recommend to the elderly to maintain adequate hydration?

> ## Cultural Considerations
>
> **Cultural Considerations with a Nutrition Assessment**
> Culture can influence food and health beliefs and practices. The nurse should take into consideration any of these influences when gathering data for a nutritional assessment.
>   Assess for:
> - Core foods in the diet.
> - Food preparation methods and types of ingredients used, such as type of fat for frying.

- **Cultural Considerations** integrate issues of cultural diversity and culturally competent care into each chapter. It is crucial that nurses realize the contribution that cultural beliefs and practices have on nutritional health.

> ## Lifespan
>
> **Anthropometric Measurements across the Lifespan**
> Anthropometric measurements are an important part of a nutritional assessment, but lose their reliability when used incorrectly. Measurements intended for use in the adult, such as waist circumference, have no merit when used to assess nutritional health in a child. Likewise, head circumference should be used only up to age 3 years. Age and gender-specific body composition references are needed when using skinfold calipers or more advanced technology such

- **Lifespan Boxes** discuss the unique nutritional needs of specific age or life cycle groups in all chapters except those already specific to the life cycle. This feature is especially important in the section on Clinical Nutrition and Diet Therapy because of the influence of diseases and medical conditions on nutritional health in pediatrics, pregnancy and lactation, and the older adult.

> ## PRACTICE ♦ PEARL
>
> **Food Safety Myths**
> Many clients hold inaccurate beliefs about food and food safety. The following are the most popular food myths and a short explanation of why it is not true.
> 1. *If it tastes O.K., it's safe to eat.*
>   *Fact:* Your senses can't tell you if the food is contaminated or unsafe to eat. An estimated 75 million Americans experience a foodborne illness each year.
> 2. *"Food poisoning" occurs immediately and goes away quickly.*

- **Practice Pearls** call attention to quick ways that the nurse can apply a nutrition concept directly to patient care.

hot topic

Hair Analysis of Mineral Status

Laboratory Hair Analysis: Fact, Fiction, or Fraud?
Laboratory analysis of hair is used in forensic medicine to detect mineral or heavy metal contamination. The deaths of both President Andrew Jackson and Napoleon Bonaparte have been attributed by some to poisoning, supported by present-day analysis of hair strands indicating that they suffered from lead exposure and arsenic and cyanide poisoning, respectively (Deppisch, Centeno, Gemmel, & Torres, 1999; Kintz, Ginet, Marques, & Cirimele, 2007).

- **Hot Topics** provide the nurse with an overview of trendy nutrition topics and present the latest research. Conclusions are explained that can be used to formulate nursing interventions or serve as a basis for further research.

- **Client Education Checklists** are quick reviews of the major patient teaching points presented in the chapter and serve as a guide to implementing patient education. It is meant as a stand alone tool for patient education. The checklist is presented in steps outlining the intervention with specific examples given. The nurse can use the checklist to structure a teaching session and refer to it during teaching to make sure that all concepts are covered.

CLIENT EDUCATION CHECKLIST ✓	Preventing Foodborne Illness
Intervention	**Example**
Assess knowledge about foodborne illness.	Review how food is purchased, stored, prepared, served, and consumed by the client. Note refrigeration and other food storage practices. Ask about cooking methods and temperatures.
Explain major areas of food handling where foodborne illness risk exists and appropriate practices to prevent illness.	1. Cleanliness: Good personal hygiene when working with food and food products such as proper and frequent hand washing, appropriate dress, covering any open wounds, and staying away from food preparation when sick. Use clean work surfaces and utensils. Keep refrigerator clean, discarding out-of-date food. Rinse fruits and vegetables and scrub those with tough skins. 2. Cross-contamination: Avoid cross-contamination of one food by another from unsanitized cutting boards, kitchen utensils, dirty towels and sponges, unwashed hands, and contact with pets. Avoid contact between raw meats, fish, eggs, and poultry with uncooked produce while shopping and in the refrigerator. 3. Temperature: Time and temperature principles such as using a food thermometer to cook foods to proper temperatures and keeping hot foods hot and cold foods cold during holding periods. Do not leave food at temperatures between 40°F and 140°F for 4 hours or longer. Thaw frozen foods in the refrigerator, not at room temperature.

- **NCLEX® style Questions** are included with each chapter and allow the student to become practiced with this style of testing. The correct answers, rationale, cognition level, nursing process step, and category of client need are outlined for each question. This additional information is found at the back of the book.

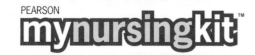

PEARSON
mynursingkit™

- **MyNursingKit** provides interactive activities, case studies, NCLEX®-style questions, and media links to web sites that offer credible nutrition information to further learning on the topic. Many of the sites also feature patient education materials and other teaching tools.

Contents

Vera Dauffenbach

Nursing and Nutrition Care 1

WHAT WILL YOU LEARN?

1. To examine the role of the nurse in individual, family, and community nutrition.
2. To understand nutrition as an aspect of total health care.
3. To use the nursing process as the approach to nutritional care of clients.
4. To formulate relevant nursing diagnoses for individuals with actual or potential nutritional problems.
5. To differentiate between a nutritional screening and a nutritional assessment.
6. To relate the importance of a nutritional screening during each client encounter.
7. To categorize appropriate tools to use as guidelines for nutrient intake and nutritional standards.

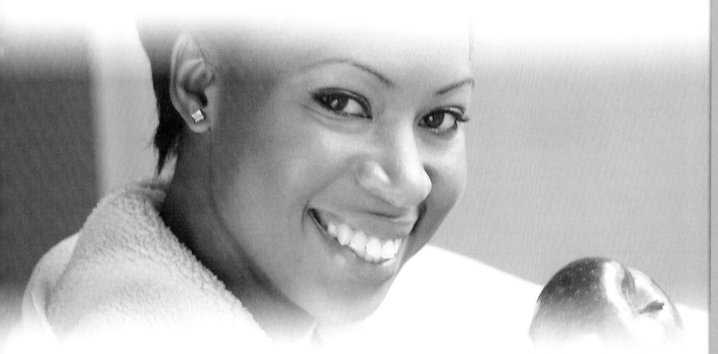

DID YOU KNOW?

▶ People who take five or more prescription or over-the-counter medications are at risk for nutritional problems.

▶ The national government sets standards for adequate nutrient consumption.

▶ The nursing process has five steps and it is different from the medical process.

▶ A nurse may perform a nutritional screening and a dietitian performs a complete nutritional assessment.

▶ Clients who achieve realistic short-term nutritional goals are

more likely to set long-term goals for behavior changes.

▶ There are alternate methods to determine height when the nurse is unable to obtain a standing height.

KEY TERMS

Nutrition and Nursing

Nutrition is a basic human need that remains crucial throughout the lifespan. As providers of holistic care, it is imperative that nurses have more than a passing understanding of the nutritional needs of both healthy individuals and those with chronic conditions or disease. Those nutritional needs are based on life stage, health-illness considerations, cultural and religious preferences, and genetic influences. In today's health care, there is increasing emphasis on wellness and the nurse must be prepared to participate in initiatives that are focused on prevention of problems that have a significant nutritional component.

There is an increasing awareness among health professionals and the public that nutrition plays a key role in disease prevention and health promotion. Nurses are in a position to teach clients about the benefits of a nutritionally sound diet and to advocate for the nutritional needs of clients in the community. They gather data that are used to plan realistic goals in conjunction with clients who are intent on achieving a nutritionally balanced diet. Plans must be age-appropriate and culturally sensitive to have a positive impact on health throughout the life cycle. This chapter presents an introduction to general nutritional guidelines and the role of the nursing process as a means of health promotion. Subsequent chapters expand on these concepts sequentially as they relate to basic nutritional needs across the lifespan as well as those of individuals with chronic conditions or diseases.

Nutrition and Health Promotion

Nutrition is the study or science of how food nourishes the body. It is based on the food requirements of humans for energy, growth, maintenance, reproduction, and lactation. *Nutrients* are chemical substances that the body uses from the foods that are consumed. Some nutrients are essential and must come from the foods that are consumed. Nonessential nutrients are nutrients that the body needs but is able to manufacture. Nutrients include water, **macronutrients** (carbohydrates, proteins, fats), and **micronutrients** (vitamins and minerals). The macronutrients provide energy in the form of **kilocalories** (kcal or cal), whereas micronutrients do not. Micronutrients are essential for other important functions in the body. For example, iron is essential for the oxygen-carrying duties of hemoglobin in the red blood cell. Many of the B vitamins assist in the metabolism of energy.

Good nutrition promotes health and may prevent the onset of conditions like cardiovascular disease, some forms of diabetes mellitus, and cancer. Nutrition also meets the energy needs of the body to allow for basic physiological functions like respiration and any physical activity. Good nutrition promotes a sense of well-being. Well-chosen foods that are consumed in moderation can supply enough of each nutrient to prevent **malnutrition.** Malnutrition includes excess, deficient, or an imbalance of nutrients that lead to disease states.

Nutrition Standards

Nutrition standards exist in most countries for the recommended nutrient intake for healthy individuals across the life span and by gender. Although these standards are not intended as customized recommendations to meet the specific nutrient needs of an individual, they are intended for use by professionals to assist in making decisions about the nutritional health of individuals, groups, and communities. Chapter 9 outlines the nutrition standards in more detail than the overview presented here.

Dietary Reference Intakes

Dietary reference intakes (DRIs) are the standards used in the United States and Canada for the recommended nutrient intake of the population. Within the DRIs are subcategories that are useful to health professionals, such as the recommended dietary allowance (RDA) and guidelines on the upper limits to nutrient intake. The recommendations are outlined by age and gender. They provide recognition of infants, children, adolescents, adults, pregnant and lactating

| BOX 1-1 | **Definitions of Dietary Reference Intakes (DRIs)** |

Estimated Average Requirements (EAR)

The average daily intake expected to satisfy the needs of 50% of the people in that age group.

Recommended Dietary Allowance (RDA)

The average daily dietary intake level of a nutrient considered sufficient to meet the requirements of nearly all (97–98%) healthy individuals in each life-stage and gender group.

Adequate Intake (AI)

The suggested daily intake of a nutrient when there is insufficient research to establish an RDA, but the amount established is believed to be adequate for most everyone in the demographic group.

Tolerable Upper Intake Levels (UL)

The highest amount of a nutrient that can be safely consumed with no risk of toxicity or adverse effects on human health; for example, vitamin D that can be harmful in large amounts.

Source: Institute of Medicine (IOM), Food and Nutrition Board, 2002.

women, and the elderly as having differing nutritional requirements. Box 1-1 includes the definitions of each component of the DRIs. The nurse should know that the DRIs are intended only for use with healthy individuals. Additionally, the recommendations can change when scientific evidence reveals new findings. For example, there is considerable debate that a new recommendation is indicated for vitamin D intake and the research community is addressing this new finding. The nurse should stay up to date on recommendations in order to provide individuals with evidence-based knowledge and care.

Dietary Guidelines

The U.S. Department of Agriculture and the U.S. Department of Health and Human Services jointly publish the *Dietary Guidelines for Americans* every 5 years. The *Guidelines* offer science-based advice for people 2 years and older on how to promote health and reduce the risk of chronic diseases through diet and physical activity (USDA, 2005). They are intended for use by health professionals and the general public to plan healthy, nutritious diets. The *Guidelines* are based on the best evidence that people who balance caloric intake with caloric expenditure; consume diets that are based on variety, balance, and moderation; and engage in regular physical activity are able to enjoy optimum health. Box 1-2 summarizes the recommendations from *Dietary Guidelines for Americans 2005*.

MyPyramid Food Guidance System

MyPyramid was designed to help by following the *Dietary Guidelines for Americans 2005* in providing a pictorial guide to the amounts and kinds of foods that individuals should eat daily to maintain health and to reduce the risk of developing nutrient-related diseases. The overall goals of MyPyramid are to (1) motivate consumers to make healthier food choices

| BOX 1-2 | **Summary of Recommendations from *Dietary Guidelines for Americans 2005*** |

ADEQUATE NUTRIENTS WITHIN CALORIE NEEDS
Key Recommendations

- Consume a variety of nutrient-dense foods and beverages within and among the basic food groups while choosing foods that limit the intake of saturated and *trans* fats, cholesterol, added sugars, salt, and alcohol.
- Meet recommended intakes within energy needs by adopting a balanced eating pattern, such as the USDA Food Guide or the DASH Eating Plan.

WEIGHT MANAGEMENT
Key Recommendations

- To maintain body weight in a healthy range, balance calories from foods and beverages with calories expended.
- To prevent gradual weight gain over time, make small decreases in food and beverage calories and increase physical activity.

PHYSICAL ACTIVITY
Key Recommendations

- Engage in regular physical activity and reduce sedentary activities to promote health, psychological well-being, and a healthy body weight.
  - To reduce the risk of chronic disease in adulthood: Engage in at least 30 minutes of moderate-intensity physical activity, above usual activity, at work or home on most days of the week.
  - For most people, greater health benefits can be obtained by engaging in physical activity of more vigorous intensity or longer duration.
  - To help manage body weight and prevent gradual, unhealthy body weight gain in adulthood: Engage in approximately 60 minutes of moderate- to vigorous-intensity activity on most days of the week while not exceeding caloric intake requirements.
  - To sustain weight loss in adulthood: Participate in at least 60 to 90 minutes of daily moderate-intensity

(continued)

BOX 1-2   **Summary of Recommendations from *Dietary Guidelines for Americans 2005*** (continued)

physical activity while not exceeding caloric intake requirements. Some people may need to consult with a health care provider before participating in this level of activity.
- Achieve physical fitness by including cardiovascular conditioning, stretching exercises for flexibility, and resistance exercises or calisthenics for muscle strength and endurance.

FOOD GROUPS TO ENCOURAGE
Key Recommendations
- Consume a sufficient amount of fruits and vegetables while staying within energy needs. Two cups of fruit and 2½ cups of vegetables per day are recommended for a reference 2,000-calorie intake, with higher or lower amounts depending on the calorie level.
- Choose a variety of fruits and vegetables each day. In particular, select from all five vegetable subgroups (dark green, orange, legumes, starchy vegetables, and other vegetables) several times a week.
- Consume 3 or more ounce-equivalents of whole-grain products per day, with the rest of the recommended grains coming from enriched or whole grain products. In general, at least half the grains should come from whole grains.
- Consume 3 cups per day of fat-free or low-fat milk or equivalent milk products.

FATS
Key Recommendations
- Consume less than 10 percent of calories from saturated fatty acids and less than 300 mg/day of cholesterol, and keep trans-fatty acid consumption as low as possible.
- Keep total fat intake between 20 to 35 percent of calories, with most fats coming from sources of polyunsaturated and monounsaturated fatty acids, such as fish, nuts, and vegetable oils.
- When selecting and preparing meat, poultry, dry beans, and milk or milk products, make choices that are lean, low fat, or fat free.
- Limit intake of fats and oils high in saturated and/or trans-fatty acids, and choose products low in such fats and oils.

CARBOHYDRATES
Key Recommendations
- Choose fiber-rich fruits, vegetables, and whole grains often.

- Choose and prepare foods and beverages with little added sugars or caloric sweeteners, such as amounts suggested by the USDA Food Guide and the DASH Eating Plan.
- Reduce the incidence of dental caries by practicing good oral hygiene and consuming sugar- and starch-containing foods and beverages less frequently.

SODIUM AND POTASSIUM
Key Recommendations
- Consume less than 2,300 mg (approximately 1 tsp of salt) of sodium per day.
- Choose and prepare foods with little salt. At the same time, consume potassium-rich foods, such as fruits and vegetables.

ALCOHOLIC BEVERAGES
Key Recommendations
- Those who choose to drink alcoholic beverages should do so sensibly and in moderation—defined as the consumption of up to one drink per day for women and up to two drinks per day for men.
- Alcoholic beverages should not be consumed by some individuals, including those who cannot restrict their alcohol intake, women of childbearing age who may become pregnant, pregnant and lactating women, children and adolescents, individuals taking medications that can interact with alcohol, and those with specific medical conditions.
- Alcoholic beverages should be avoided by individuals engaging in activities that require attention, skill, or coordination, such as driving or operating machinery.

FOOD SAFETY
Key Recommendations
- To avoid microbial foodborne illness:
  - Clean hands, food contact surfaces, and fruits and vegetables. Meat and poultry should not be washed or rinsed.
  - Separate raw, cooked, and ready-to-eat foods while shopping, preparing, or storing foods.
  - Cook foods to a safe temperature to kill microorganisms.
  - Chill (refrigerate) perishable food promptly and defrost foods properly.
  - Avoid raw (unpasteurized) milk or any products made from unpasteurized milk, raw or partially cooked eggs or foods containing raw eggs, raw or undercooked meat and poultry, unpasteurized juices, and raw sprouts.

and (2) to ensure that the latest nutritional research is reflected in recommendations to consumers (USDA, 2005). Specific goals guide individuals to make healthy food choices as outlined in Box 1-3.

MyPyramid is a comprehensive, interactive system that promotes an individualized approach to physical activity and dietary planning. Figure 1-1 ■ depicts the MyPyramid Physical activity, which is represented by the steps found on the side of the pyramid and reminds individuals to be active every day. The variety of the food

BOX 1-3   **Goals for Individuals from MyPyramid**

- Increase intake of vitamins, minerals, and dietary fiber.
- Lower intake of saturated fats, trans fats, and cholesterol.
- Increase intake of fruits, vegetables, and whole grains.
- Balance nutrient intake with energy needs to prevent weight gain and to promote a healthy weight.

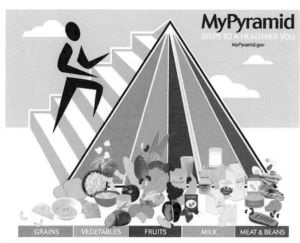

FIGURE 1-1 MyPyramid.

Source: U.S. Department of Agriculture, Center for Nutrition Policy and Promotion, 2005.

groups is symbolized by the six vertical bands that represent the five food groups (grains, vegetables, fruits, milk, and meat/beans) and oils. Foods from all six groups are needed on a daily basis to maintain good health. Moderation is represented by the width of each band (grains the widest, oils the narrowest) and the narrowing of each group from bottom to top.

The Web site for MyPyramid is highly interactive, and individuals of all ages can be taught how to use it so that a personalized recommendation of nutrient intake and physical activity can be made. The site provides educational resources that are useful to nurses, health professionals, and the public for making wise choices from each food group. A particularly helpful feature of MyPyramid is the listing of serving size in household measures. Serving size is often misunderstood by the public and is commonly described as "what I have on my plate," which many times is far larger than a recommended serving size (USDA, 2005). The nurse can use MyPyramid as a teaching tool with groups or individuals to discuss the basic concepts of healthy eating. Chapter 9 outlines MyPyramid in more detail.

Food Labels

The **nutrition facts food label** has been used on food products since 1994. The label format was designed to inform consumers about the serving sizes and nutrient content of foods. The information is not based on the entire contents of the package; it is calculated for the serving size recommended by the manufacturer of that food. It is useful for consumers to compare one product with another. Figure 1-2 ■ depicts a

USE THE NUTRITION FACTS LABEL TO EAT HEALTHIER

Check the serving size and number of servings.

- The Nutrition Facts Label information is based on ONE serving, but many packages contain more. Look at the serving size and how many servings you are actually consuming. If you double the servings you eat, you double the calories and nutrients, including the % DVs.
- When you compare calories and nutrients between brands, check to see if the serving size is the same.

Calories count, so pay attention to the amount.

- This is where you'll find the number of calories per serving and the calories from fat in each serving.
- Fat-free doesn't mean calorie-free. Lower fat items may have as many calories as full-fat versions.
- If the label lists that 1 serving equals 3 cookies and 100 calories, and you eat 6 cookies, you've eaten 2 servings, or twice the number of calories and fat.

Look for foods that are rich in these nutrients.

- Use the label not only to limit fat and sodium, but also to increase nutrients that promote good health and may protect you from disease.
- Some Americans don't get enough vitamins A and C, potassium, calcium, and iron, so choose the brand with the higher % DV for these nutrients.
- Get the most nutrition for your calories—compare the calories to the nutrients you would be getting to make a healthier food choice.

Nutrition Facts

Serving Size 1 cup (228g)
Servings Per Container 2

Amount Per Serving

Calories 250   Calories from Fat 110

	% Daily Value*
Total Fat 12g	18%
Saturated Fat 3g	15%
Trans Fat 3g	
Cholesterol 30mg	10%
Sodium 470mg	20%
Potassium 700mg	20%
Total Carbohydrate 31g	10%
Dietary Fiber 0g	0%
Sugars 5g	
Protein 5g	

Vitamin A	4%
Vitamin C	2%
Calcium	20%
Iron	4%

* Percent Daily Values are based on a 2,000 calorie diet. Your Daily Values may be higher or lower depending on your calorie needs.

	Calories:	2,000	2,500
Total fat	Less than	65g	80g
Sat fat	Less than	20g	25g
Cholesterol	Less than	300mg	300mg
Sodium	Less than	2,400mg	2,400mg
Total Carbohydrate		300g	375g
Dietary Fiber		25g	30g

The % Daily Value is a key to a balanced diet.

The % DV is a general guide to help you link nutrients in a serving of food to their contribution to your total daily diet. It can help you determine if a food is high or low in a nutrient—5% or less is low, 20% or more is high. You can use the % DV to make dietary trade-offs with other foods throughout the day. The * is a reminder that the % DV is based on a 2,000-calorie diet. You may need more or less, but the % DV is still a helpful gauge.

Know your fats and reduce sodium for your health.

- To help reduce your risk of heart disease, use the label to select foods that are lowest in saturated fat, *trans* fat and cholesterol.
- *Trans* fat doesn't have a % DV, but consume as little as possible because it increases your risk of heart disease.
- The % DV for total fat includes all different kinds of fats.
- To help lower blood cholesterol, replace saturated and *trans* fats with monounsaturated and polyunsaturated fats found in fish, nuts, and liquid vegetable oils.
- Limit sodium to help reduce your risk of high blood pressure.

Reach for healthy, wholesome carbohydrates.

- Fiber and sugars are types of carbohydrates. Healthy sources, like fruits, vegetables, beans, and whole grains, can reduce the risk of heart disease and improve digestive functioning.
- Whole grain foods can't always be identified by color or name, such as multi-grain or wheat. Look for the "whole" grain listed first in the ingredient list, such as whole wheat, brown rice, or whole oats.
- There isn't a % DV for sugar, but you can compare the sugar content in grams among products.
- Limit foods with added sugars (sucrose, glucose, fructose, corn or maple syrup), which add calories but not other nutrients, such as vitamins and minerals. Make sure that added sugars are not one of the first few items in the ingredients list.

For protein, choose foods that are lower in fat.

- Most Americans get plenty of protein, but not always from the healthiest sources.
- When choosing a food for its protein content, such as meat, poultry, dry beans, milk and milk products, make choices that are lean, low-fat, or fat free.

FIGURE 1-2 Nutrition Fact Label.

Source: U.S. Department of Health and Human Services, Public Health Service, 2000.

BOX 1-4   Components of the Nutrition Facts Label

Food amount and energy (calorie) content:
The amount of food in the package is listed by serving size, weight, the number of servings that are expected for the container, and the number of calories in each serving. The serving size should be carefully noted because the portion that the individual plans to eat may well exceed the serving size. For example, the label on some ice cream containers lists a serving size of ½ cup, an amount far less than the consumer expects to eat. Remember, the portion size that the consumer expects may be different than the stated serving size.

Macronutrient content:
Fat, carbohydrate, and protein content are listed in grams. The amounts of saturated fat, trans fat, and cholesterol are also listed. Monounsaturated and polyunsaturated fats may also be present.

Carbohydrates have subcategories of dietary fiber and sugars.

Micronutrient content:
The label is required to list sodium, vitamin A, vitamin C, calcium, and iron. The sodium content is listed in milligrams and as a percentage of the upper limit to aid individuals who must watch total sodium intake. The vitamins and minerals are listed as a percentage of the daily reference values.

Daily reference values:
Daily reference values are listed for diets containing 2,000 and 2,500 calories. For individuals who need to consume fewer than 2,000 calories, the percentages of the macronutrients and micronutrients will be higher based on their total caloric intake.

---

nutrition facts label. Food labels are not required on fresh fruits and vegetables.

It is important for the nurse to thoroughly understand the nutrition facts label when working with individuals and families to plan nutritious meals and make healthy food choices. The major components of the nutrition label are the food amount and energy (calorie) content, the macronutrient content, the micronutrient content, and the daily reference values. Because serving sizes on food labels may not always be consistent with those suggested by MyPyramid, the nurse will need to become familiar with the general serving sizes outlined in MyPyramid. See Box 1-4 for specific information about each component of the nutrition label.

Healthy People 2010: Objectives for the Nation

Every decade the U.S. Department of Health and Human Services (USDHHS) sets national objectives related to health and health promotion. The objectives serve as the basis for state and local community health promotion plans and programs. A major subsection of *Healthy People 2010* is related to nutrition and overweight objectives. There are 19 objectives, each of which has measurable outcomes to facilitate data collection and analysis across the decade. The nurse should be aware of the major objectives of *Healthy People* to guide nutritional planning and interventions for individuals and groups. See Box 1-5 for a summary of the goals related to nutrition.

BOX 1-5   *Healthy People 2010* Nutrition and Overweight Objectives

- Increase the proportion of adults who are at a healthy weight
- Reduce the proportion of adults who are obese
- Reduce the proportion of children and adolescents who are overweight or obese
- Reduce growth retardation among low-income children under age 5 years
- Increase the proportion of persons aged 2 years and older who consume at least two daily servings of fruit
- Increase the proportion of persons aged 2 years and older who consume at least three daily servings of vegetables, with at least one-third being dark green or orange vegetables
- Increase the proportion of persons aged 2 years and older who consume at least six daily servings of grain products, with at least three being whole grains
- Increase the proportion of persons aged 2 years and older who consume less than 10 percent of calories from saturated fat
- Increase the proportion of persons aged 2 years and older who consume no more than 30 percent of calories from total fat

- Increase the proportion of persons aged 2 years and older who consume 2,400 mg or less of sodium daily
- Increase the proportion of persons aged 2 years and older who meet dietary recommendations for calcium
- Reduce iron deficiency among young children and females of childbearing age
- Reduce anemia among low-income pregnant females in their third trimester
- Increase the proportion of children and adolescents aged 6 to 19 years whose intake of meals and snacks at school contributes to good overall dietary quality
- Increase the proportion of worksites that offer nutrition or weight management classes or counseling
- Increase the proportion of physician office visits made by patients with a diagnosis of cardiovascular disease, diabetes, or hyperlipidemia that include counseling or education related to diet and nutrition
- Increase food security among U.S. households and in so doing reduce hunger

Source: U.S. Department of Health and Human Services, 2000.

Nursing Process and Nutritional Health

The nurse has a critical role in promoting nutritional health. The nurse works with individuals, families, and groups to identify health needs and develops plans for addressing those needs. See Box 1-6 for examples of how nurses in a variety of settings integrate nutritional knowledge into their practices. Regardless of the practice setting, it is vital that the nurse carefully gather accurate data about the client's nutritional health to aid in the development of a holistic plan of care for the client. The basis for nursing practice is the **nursing process.** The nursing process is the systematic gathering of subjective and objective data, analyzing data for the purpose of establishing nursing diagnoses, planning realistic goals, implementing activities to achieve the goals, and evaluating goal accomplishment. It is important to follow each step of the process to develop an optimum plan of care that is acceptable to the client and meets current standards of nursing practice. Each step of the process and its relationship to nutritional health is outlined next. The nurse should also be aware of the important role of the registered dietitian (RD) in client care. The RD completes comprehensive nutritional assessments, writes nutritional diagnoses, plans interventions, and monitors the client's or family's response to the nutritional plan. The RD should be consulted when the nurse determines that actual or potential nutritional problems exist.

Assessment

Assessment is the first step of the nursing process. This step is lengthy and involves recognition of factors that influence nutrition, activity level, and lifestyle. Typically, assessment data are gathered directly from the client (the history), measurements of the body called *anthropometric data*, and laboratory data. In addition, the client's sociocultural and religious beliefs are important areas to be assessed prior to making a determination of the client's nutritional health. Occasionally, laboratory data may not be available, but the nurse should determine if they are required to formulate an accurate diagnosis. In most health care settings, a registered dietitian is responsible for performing a thorough nutrition assessment. The nurse should collaborate with the dietitian throughout the nursing care process to provide seamless holistic nutritional care to the individual. In some practice settings, there is no registered dietitian on staff, such as in some schools or home care services. The nurse needs to be knowledgeable about the components of a nutrition assessment in such circumstances. See Chapter 12, Nutritional Assessment, for more extensive information about conducting a complete nutritional assessment.

History and Nutritional Screening

A good nursing history will include a dietary intake record. It can be a 24-hour recall in which the client recalls verbally or in writing every food and beverage consumed in the past 24 hours. It may be a food diary in which the client records every food and beverage consumed during a specified time, often 1 week. A food frequency questionnaire asks clients how often they consume specific foods and beverages and the sizes of their usual portions. In addition, data about the timing and location of food consumption along with emotional state will provide valuable information. The history can also include information about physical activity level, including the amount of time spent in sedentary activities. The Evidence-Based Practice Box discusses the link between obesity and

BOX 1-6	Sample Nursing Functions Related to Nutrition in Selected Practice Settings
School nurse	• Classroom teaching about healthy eating, all grade levels • Work with teachers of children with food allergies (e.g., peanuts, eggs, wheat) • Review health forms for nutrition-related diagnoses and any treatments that occur during the school day (e.g., diabetes, use of liquid nutrition supplement)
Home health nurse	• Assess changing nutritional status • Assess the ability of the client and family to acquire foods for healthy eating • Make referrals to community resources for nutrition (e.g., Meals on Wheels) • Reinforce nutrition education or therapeutic diet principles prescribed • Collaborate with team members providing care for individuals on home nutrition support
Long-term care nurse	• Assess for changing nutritional status (e.g., weigh residents, check for properly fitting dentures) • Monitor dietary intake and feeding practices • Provide pleasant environment to allow for a positive dining experience
Postsurgical care nurse	• Check clients for return of gag reflex • Assess for presence of nausea or other side effects • Advance diet as appropriate • Measure and record intake and output • Refer clients at risk for poor nutritional health to registered dietitian for evaluation

STOP ■ Think of additional settings in which nurses practice. Give examples of nursing assessments and interventions that are related to nutrition. For example, what assessments might be used by a nurse or nurse practitioner in a women's health clinic?

EVIDENCE-BASED PRACTICE RESEARCH BOX

Is there an association between television viewing and obesity in children?

Research Problem: Children now spend large amounts of time watching television or using computers and video games, rather than engaging in physical activity. Are children who watch TV more likely to be overweight than those who spend less time watching TV or using computers?

Evidence: Several studies have examined the association between TV viewing in preschool and school-aged children and their weight or body mass index (BMI). Two studies specifically examined whether the presence of a TV in the bedroom was associated with a risk of being overweight (Dennison, Erb, & Jenkins, 2002; Adachi-Mejia et al., 2007). The researchers studied the habits of 2,343 public schoolchildren and found that 48% of children had a TV in their bedroom and that they had a significantly higher BMI ($p < 0.05$) than those without a TV in their bedroom (Adachi-Mejia et al., 2007). A study using data from 2,761 adults of preschoolers had nearly identical findings (Dennison et al., 2002).

Another study of 148 preschoolers enrolled in a Head Start program found that 97% of those with a BMI greater than the 95th percentile watched more than 1 hour of TV per day, compared with less than 80% of those with a BMI less than the 95th percentile (Levin, Martin, & Riner, 2004). In addition, preschoolers who watch TV are found to have greater intake of fast food, although researchers were unable to conclude that TV viewing in itself was responsible for the increased intake of fast food (Taveras et al., 2006). Preschool children's TV habits may also be affected by perceived neighborhood safety, with children in unsafe neighborhoods watching more TV than those in safer neighborhoods (Burdette & Whitaker, 2005), and by eating meals while watching TV (Francis & Birch, 2006). Preschoolers who watch TV were also found to have a higher consumption of sugar-sweetened beverages, red and processed meats, and trans fats (Miller, Taveras, Rifas-Shiman, & Gillman, 2008).

A study of 8,459 school-age children found that those who watched more TV ate fewer meals with the family, and those who lived in neighborhoods perceived as unsafe were more likely to be overweight (Gable, Chang, & Krull, 2007).

Conclusion: The more time children spend watching TV, regardless of age, the greater risk they have of lower quality nutrient intake and of being overweight. Unsafe neighborhoods may contribute to more TV time and, therefore, poorer nutrient intake and greater risk of overweight.

CRITICAL THINKING QUESTION:

1. What suggestions could the nurse offer to the mother who states "I am so tired by the time I get done with work and driving children to activities that all I can do is pick up something from a drive-through and have us eat it while we watch our favorite TV shows. At least we are spending time together." What nursing diagnoses could be used to describe this family or parent?

---

television watching, underscoring the importance of including physical activity patterns in the history.

During a review of systems, the nurse questions the client about each body system and focuses questions about symptoms that may be related to nutritional status. For example, the nurse may ask the client about problems with the frequency of constipation and how the client treats that problem. The nurse also needs a complete list of prescription and nonprescription medications and dietary supplements that the client takes. The client who takes many medications, called **polypharmacy,** is at significantly greater risk of nutritional problems because of possible drug side effects or nutrient interactions.

The nurse may also do a **nutritional screening,** a checklist or brief instrument filled out by the client or nurse, to provide rapid quantifiable data. Numerous instruments that have demonstrated reliability and validity are available for various age groups (Delville, 2008; DiMaria-Ghalili & Guenter, 2008; Gans et al., 2003; Williams & Keir, 2008). In the acute care setting, nutritional screening is particularly important for assessing the client at risk for poor nutrition status because of its effect on medical outcome, including wound healing, length of hospitalization, and mortality (Anderson, 2005; Rodriguez, 2004). A nutritional screening is a pared-down version of a nutritional assessment that does not provide as much in-depth data as an assessment, yet serves to quickly identify individuals who may be at risk for poor nutritional health. When an individual is identified to be at risk for poor nutritional health through nutritional screening, a more thorough nutrition assessment can then be performed.

Anthropometric Measurements

Anthropometric data are physical measurements of the client and include height; weight; and skin fold and circumference measurements such as wrist, waist, and mid-arm circumference. Chapter 12 discusses these measurements in detail. At a minimum, accurate height and weight should be available to the nurse. The stated weight and height provided by the client may differ significantly from the actual weight and height and therefore can provide an inaccurate point of reference for later comparison. **Body mass index (BMI)** assesses the relative weight for body and is easily calculated. The resulting information may be used to classify the client as underweight, healthy weight, overweight, or obese. See Box 1-7 for information on how to calculate the BMI. The numerical value of the BMI must be interpreted with caution because it does not reflect frame size or body composition; individuals with greater muscle mass may appear to be over-

BOX 1-7	Body Mass Index (BMI) Calculation

Body mass index (BMI) is calculated as follows:

$$BMI = weight\ (kg)\ /\ height\ (m)^2\ or$$
$$BMI = weight\ (lb)\ \times\ 703\ /\ height\ (in)^2$$

A BMI of 20–24.9 is considered healthy. Above that is overweight; below is underweight.

weight and yet not have increased body fat. In addition, a number of common disabilities, like strokes, or disease processes, like kyphosis (a curved spine), may make it difficult to accurately measure standing height in clients. Alternate measures may be needed by the nurse for accurate determination of the client's height (Hickson & Frost, 2003). See Lifespan Box: Estimating Height in Bedridden or Disabled Clients for alternate measures that may be used to estimate standing height.

Skin fold and circumference measurements are methods of determining body composition and fat distribution. Overall body fat content and the distribution of body fat are important in assessing health risk potential. Central obesity, increased intra-abdominal fat, is associated with greater risk of cardiovascular disease and type 2 diabetes (American Dietetic Association, 2002). The determination of waist circumference and waist-to-hip ratio correlates with the "apple" or "pear" body types. The ratio is calculated simply by dividing the waist measurement by the hip measurement. An "apple" body type has a waist-to-hip measurement ratio that is close to or exceeds 1.0, meaning the waist and hips measurements are similar. A "pear" body type has a ratio below 0.8, meaning the hips are wider than the waist. Individuals with central obesity are considered to have an "apple" body type and to be at greater risk for cardiovascular disease. The

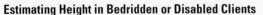

Lifespan

Estimating Height in Bedridden or Disabled Clients
There are three commonly accepted measurements that may be used to calculate standing height. These methods include knee height, forearm length, and demi-span.

- The knee height is measured from the heel of the foot to the top of the knee while the ankle and knee are held at 90-degree angles. A formula must be used to calculate height.
- The forearm length is measured from the elbow to the midpoint of the ulna at the wrist. The result is compared to a standardized height conversion table.
- The demi-span is measured as the distance from the middle of the sterna notch to the tip of the middle finger when the client's arm is held horizontal. A formula is then used to calculate height.

Chapter 12 outlines these techniques in more detail.

actual waist circumference may be a better indicator of healthfulness, with ideal measurements of 35 inches or less in adult males and 30 inches or less in adult females. The results of skin fold measurements provide useful data about overall body fat but are not considered part of the usual nursing assessment.

Clinical Data
Physical signs may give an indication of the client's nutritional status. The nurse should observe the oral cavity for signs of healthy gums, the presence or absence of teeth and their condition, and a smooth red tongue. Lips should be smooth and not cracked or swollen. A curved spine may indicate osteoporosis. Hair and nails should be smooth and shiny. Taken in conjunction with other data that the nurse gathers, data acquired from a physical assessment may be used to form a more complete picture of the nutritional status of a client. In Chapter 12, Table 12-7 outlines these findings in more detail.

Laboratory and Diagnostic Measurements
There is no single laboratory value that accurately measures overall nutritional status. For example, hemoglobin levels reflect the iron intake. A low hemoglobin level may be indicative of decreased available iron, but it may also indicate excess circulating water in the blood. The albumin level may indicate protein status, but it may also be decreased because of inflammation, infection, or liver disease. Laboratory values, when available, should be interpreted cautiously by the nurse and only be considered a part of the assessment data. The use of laboratory data alone to determine nutrition status can limit the accuracy of the assessment on which interventions are formulated.

Cultural Considerations
Cultural and religious practices are important parts of the nursing assessment. The people of the United States come from a multitude of cultural and ethnic backgrounds. Diverse racial, ethnic, and cultural groups now make up approximately one-third of the population, and that percentage is expected to grow (National Center for Health Statistics, 2007). An individual's background influences beliefs about what constitutes healthy eating, acceptable food choices, and eating patterns.

Nurses should become familiar with the favorite foods and eating habits of racial and ethnic groups outside of their own. Although those habits are not inflexible, nurses need to be sensitive to what individuals and groups consider acceptable foods.

In addition to cultural practices, religious practices may influence food selection. Seventh Day Adventists, for example, are vegetarians. Orthodox Jews have strict dietary practices that affect food selection and preparation. For example, animals that can be eaten must either have a cloven hoof and chew their own cud or have fins and scales. This permits cows, sheep, and fish but not pigs, shellfish, and crustaceans, such as lobster and crab. Nurses should be aware of religious practices that influence the acceptability of certain foods. Each chapter of the text addresses cultural practices that relate to nutritional health. In addition, Chapter 10 discusses the cultural aspects of nutrition in more detail.

Nursing Diagnosis

The second step in the nursing process is the identification of the nursing diagnosis or diagnoses. A nursing diagnosis is based on analysis of the subjective and objective data obtained from the nursing assessment. Depending on the client situation, there are numerous nursing diagnoses that have a nutritional focus or may be related to nutrient intake or absence (NANDA International, 2007). These diagnoses are published by the North American Nursing Diagnosis Association (NANDA). Box 1-8 lists many of the NANDA nursing diagnoses that relate to nutrition. Selection of the appropriate diagnosis will depend on the cause of the alteration in nutritional status. For example, *Imbalanced nutrition: Less than body requirements* may be related to decreased nutrient intake, excess energy expenditure, or prolonged anorexia. When stating the nursing diagnosis, the nurse should always include a "related to" statement to link the diagnosis to the assessment data. In addition, the nurse should include the relevant evidence. For example, *Imbalanced nutrition: Less*

PRACTICE PEARL

Establishing Diagnoses

It is important to carefully review the assessment data prior to establishing the nursing diagnoses. NANDA (2007) lists criteria that should be met prior to identification of any specific diagnosis. A diagnosis that is inaccurate, incomplete, or vague will lead to inappropriate goals and ineffective planning.

than body requirements related to decreased nutrient intake as evidenced by unplanned weight loss of 10 pounds in the past 6 weeks. See the Practice Pearl "Establishing Diagnoses" for a discussion of how to formulate a nursing diagnosis.

Planning

Following the establishment of appropriate nursing diagnoses, the third step of the nursing process is to develop a plan of care for the client. Goals, or outcomes, are established jointly by the client and the nurse. Goals must be realistic, achievable, and measurable. They must also arise from the nursing diagnoses and be congruent with them. Goals should also be prioritized by those that require immediate attention and those that are less urgent. Goals may be short term (a few days or less) or long term (a week or longer). For example, a realistic

---

BOX 1-8	Nursing Diagnoses Related to Nutritional Status

The following nursing diagnoses with a nutritional focus approved by NANDA (2007–2008) are frequently used as part of the nursing process. This is not an exclusive list, but these are the diagnoses most frequently used by nursing students when planning client care. Please note that registered dietitians also follow the Nutrition Care Process and have specific language for nutrition diagnoses.

Aspiration, risk for
Blood Glucose, risk for Unstable
Body Image, Disturbed
Breastfeeding,
   Effective
   Ineffective
   Interrupted
Constipation, risk for
Dentition
   Impaired
Development
   Delayed, risk for
Diarrhea
Failure to Thrive
   Adult

Fluid Balance
   Readiness for Enhanced
Fluid volume
   Deficient,
   Excess, risk for Deficient
   Imbalanced, risk for
Infant Feeding Pattern
   Ineffective
Knowledge
   Deficient
   Readiness for Enhanced
Mucous Membrane
   Impaired Oral
Nausea

Nutrition, Imbalanced
   Less than Body Requirements,
   More than Body Requirements,
   Risk for More than Body Requirements
Nutrition,
   Readiness for Enhanced
Sedentary Lifestyle
Self-care Deficit
   Feeding
Swallowing
   Impaired

 ▪ Which diagnosis could be used to describe an individual with weight loss because of an eating disorder? How about the client who lacks knowledge about the influence of diet on blood cholesterol?

Source: NANDA, 2007.

PRACTICE PEARL

Setting Goals
Setting realistic, achievable, and measurable nutritional goals is important for clients. When clients have short-term goals that can be readily achieved, they are more likely to develop confidence in their ability to set long-term goals that can have a lasting impact on their nutritional status.

goal for a client with a nursing diagnosis of *Imbalanced nutrition: Less than body requirements* related to decreased nutrient intake evidenced by unplanned weight loss of 10 pounds in 6 weeks may be to increase caloric intake by 200 calories per day within 1 week. A long-term goal may be to regain the weight within 2 months. A goal that the nurse may consider realistic is "consultation with a dietitian by the client." The planning phase of the nursing process is very important because it sets the stage for the implementation of measures that will assist the client to achieve goals. Practice Pearl "Setting Goals" serves as a reminder when developing goals.

Implementation

The fourth step of the nursing process is the implementation phase. The goals listed in the plan guide the interventions performed by the nurse and/or the client. This is the action step for the plan. While implementing various nursing interventions, the nurse should carefully reflect on what is being done and monitor progress toward goal achievement. It is a challenging step because it often involves considerable effort on the part of the nurse to help motivate a client to make changes in dietary choices or nutritional behavior. The nurse should brainstorm with the client about factors that may assist with achievement of goals as well as those that may be barriers to success. Discussing these factors and any needed solutions early in the process helps improve the collaboration between the nurse and the client when determining the steps needed to achieve a goal. For example, if an overweight client decides that increased exercise is a goal and that it will occur before work every day, the nurse can explore if there have been prior attempts at exercise in the past and if early morning exercise is likely to occur. If rising early to exercise was a barrier to success in the past, the nurse can revisit that goal with the client and formulate one that is more likely to be successful. The initial response of the client to interventions should be monitored. It is appropriate for the nurse to make early corrections to the interventions based on initial client response or the plan may never be fully implemented. During the implementation phase the nurse should carefully document the interventions and the client response.

Evaluation

Evaluation is the final phase of the nursing process. It is related to the planning phase because it focuses on the goals that were established with the client. Assuming the diagnoses were accurate and the goals were realistic, evaluation answers the question, "Were the goals achieved?" It should examine where the client stands in relation to goal achievement. Any changes that occurred that caused the plan to be unworkable must be evaluated and the plan modified. It must further determine if the interventions that were implemented were appropriate and correct. A final part of the evaluation should lead to further assessment of the client and any refinement of the care plan. This provides for the cyclical nature of the nursing process.

NURSING CARE PLAN **Nutrition for Weight Loss**

CASE STUDY
Kay is a 50-year-old school teacher who has come to the clinic for a routine checkup. She has been a regular client for the past 10 years and has had no significant health concerns during that time. She tells the nurse how proud she is of her daughter who has decided to study nutrition science in college. Kay informs the nurse that, given her daughter's major, she feels the need to improve her own nutritional health by losing weight and getting in better shape. She notes that she has developed what she calls "middle-age spread" and wants to keep it from getting worse. She has no other health concerns at this time. Figure 1-3 ■ outlines the nursing process for this case.

Applying the Nursing Process

ASSESSMENT
Height: 5 feet 7 inches Weight: 176 pounds
    BMI: 27.7
BP 128/76 P 76 R 14 Lab Data: Within normal limits
Waist: 39 inches Hips: 46 inches Waist-Hip Ratio: 0.9

DIAGNOSIS
Nutrition: Readiness for enhanced related to stated goals as evidenced by willingness to make lifestyle changes

(continued)

NURSING CARE PLAN

Nutrition for Weight Loss *(continued)*

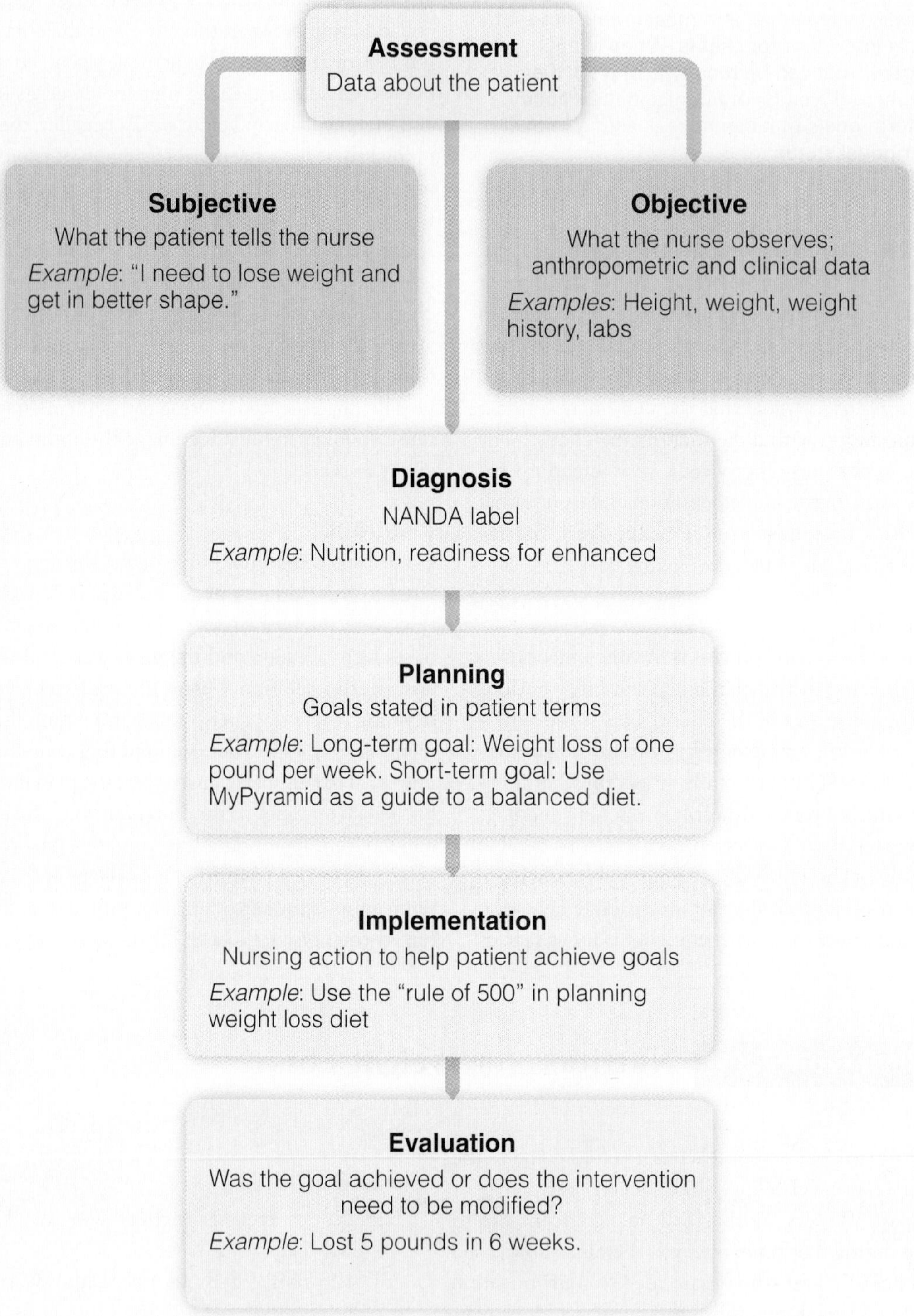

Assessment
Data about the patient

Subjective
What the patient tells the nurse
Example: "I need to lose weight and get in better shape."

Objective
What the nurse observes; anthropometric and clinical data
Examples: Height, weight, weight history, labs

Diagnosis
NANDA label
Example: Nutrition, readiness for enhanced

Planning
Goals stated in patient terms
Example: Long-term goal: Weight loss of one pound per week. Short-term goal: Use MyPyramid as a guide to a balanced diet.

Implementation
Nursing action to help patient achieve goals
Example: Use the "rule of 500" in planning weight loss diet

Evaluation
Was the goal achieved or does the intervention need to be modified?
Example: Lost 5 pounds in 6 weeks.

■ FIGURE 1-3 **Nursing Care Plan Process: Nutrition for Weight Loss.**

Nutrition for Weight Loss *(continued)*

NURSING CARE PLAN

EXPECTED OUTCOMES

Weight loss averaging 1 pound per week for 20 weeks

Increase activity level to 30 minutes a day, four times a week

INTERVENTIONS

24-hour food recall

Food diary for 1 week

Use MyPyramid to introduce a balanced nutritional plan

Collaborate with the client to develop a plan for increased activity with daily and weekly goals

Introduce the "rule of 500" to aid in planning for weight loss where a caloric deficit of 500 kcalories/day leads to a weekly deficit of 3,500 kcalories to foster a 1-pound weight loss. A combination of decreased intake and increased activity can achieve this goal

EVALUATION

After 6 weeks, Kay is excited about the changes in her life. She has been sharing her new knowledge with her daughter, who has also been eager to share what she has learned with her mother. She has started to do some small things like use the steps more at work and park in a more distant parking spot. She has lost 5 pounds and likes using the "rule of 500" because she feels she can make small changes everyday to make progress toward her goal. She plans to stay with her diet and increase her activity by joining the YWCA near her home.

Critical Thinking in the Nursing Process

1. What are some strategies that the nurse can use to assist a client who is otherwise in good health to improve nutritional status?

CHAPTER SUMMARY

- Nutrition plays a key role in health promotion and disease prevention.
- There are several references that serve as guides for promotion of nutritional health, including the *Dietary Guidelines for Americans* and *MyPyramid.*
- Nutrition facts labels are useful for nurses and consumers to assist in planning healthy diets.
- Nurses gather subjective data from clients and combine them with anthropometric, clinical, and laboratory data as part of the assessment process.
- The assessment phase of the nursing process is the longest and most detailed.
- Accurate use of the nursing process is important if client nutritional goals are to be met.

EXPLORE **PEARSON** **mynursingkit™**

MyNursingKit is your one stop for online chapter review materials and resources. Prepare for success with additional NCLEX®-style practice questions, interactive assignments and activities, web links, animations and videos, and more!

Register your access code from the front of your book at
www.mynursingkit.com.

NCLEX® QUESTIONS

1. A school nurse needs to collect anthropometric data for a research project from each elementary classroom. What data will the nurse collect?
   1. Height and weight to calculate body mass index (BMI)
   2. Hemoglobin and hematocrit to assess iron levels
   3. Albumin to assess protein status
   4. Hip circumference to assess growth patterns

2. Which of the following statements by an adult client indicate the need for the nurse to do additional teaching about food fact labels? Select all that apply.
   1. "All ingredients are listed in order of nutritional value."
   2. "State health departments approve all labels."
   3. "The amounts listed on the label are based on a 2,000-calorie diet."
   4. "Major nutrients are included on the label."
   5. "If I select a larger or smaller portion size, I must consider that percentages will differ."

3. The nurse calculates a middle-age client's body mass index (BMI) as 29. Which of the following NANDA nursing diagnoses would be most appropriate?
   1. Knowledge deficit (about nutrition)
   2. Fluid volume excess
   3. Altered nutrition: More than body requirements
   4. Impaired metabolism

4. The nurse needs to assess the nutritional status of an elderly client. Which of the following assessment data will the nurse find most useful?
   1. Height
   2. Socioeconomic level
   3. Wrist circumference
   4. 24-hour diet recall

5. The nurse is writing a care plan for an adult client who has a diagnosis of Imbalanced nutrition: Less than body requirements. What would be a realistic goal for this client?
   1. Limit physical activity to 30 minutes per day
   2. Increase weight by 1 pound per week
   3. Increase consumption of carbohydrates by 10 grams per day
   4. Increase consumption of organic foods

REFERENCES

Adachi-Mejia, A. M., Longacre, M. R., Gibson, J. J., Beach, M. L., Titus-Ernstoff, L. T., & Dalton, M. A. (2007). Children with a TV in their bedroom at a higher risk for being overweight. *International Journal of Obesity (London)*, 31(4), 644–651.

American Dietetic Association. (2002). Position of the American Dietetic Association: Weight management. *Journal of the American Dietetic Association*, 102, 1145–1148.

Anderson, B. (2005). Nutrition and wound healing: The necessity of assessment. *British Journal of Nursing (Tissue Viability Supplement)*, 14(9), S30–S38.

Burdette, H. L., & Whitaker, R. C. (2005). A national study of neighborhood safety, outdoor play, television viewing, and obesity in preschool children. *Pediatrics*, 116(3), 657–662.

Delville, C. L. (2008). Are your patients at nutritional risk? *Nurse Practitioner*, 33(2), 36–39.

Dennison, B. A., Erb, T. A., & Jenkins, P. L. (2002). Television viewing and television in bedroom associated with overweight risk among low-income preschool children. *Pediatrics*, 109(6), 1028–1035.

DiMaria-Ghalili, R. A., & Guenter, P. A. (2008). The Mini Nutritional Assessment. *American Journal of Nursing*, 108(2), 50–59.

Francis, L. A., & Birch, L. L. (2006). Does eating during television viewing affect preschool children's intake? *Journal of the American Dietetic Association*, 106(4), 598–600.

Gable, S., Chang, Y., & Krull, J. L. (2007). Television watching and frequency of family meals are predictive of overweight onset and persistence in a national sample of school-aged children. *Journal of the American Dietetic Association*, 107(1), 53–61.

Gans, K. M., Ross, E., Barner, C. W., Wylie-Rosett, J., McMurray, J., & Eaton, C. (2003). REAP and WAVE: New tools to rapidly assess/discuss nutrition with patients. *The Journal of Nutrition*, 133, 556S–562S.

Hickson, M., & Frost, G. (2003). A comparison of three methods for estimating height in the acutely ill elderly population. *Journal of Human Nutrition and Dietetics*, 16(1), 13–20.

Levin, S., Martin, M. W., & Riner, W. F. (2004). TV viewing habits and body mass index among South Carolina Head Start children. *Ethnicity & Disease*, 14(3), 336–339.

Miller, S. A., Taveras, E. M., Rifas-Shiman, S. L., & Gillman, M. W. (2008). Association between television viewing and poor diet quality in young children. *International Journal of Pediatric Obesity*, 4, 1–9.

NANDA International. (2007). *NANDA-I nursing diagnosis: Definitions & classification 2007–2008*. Philadelphia: Author.

National Center for Health Statistics. (2007). *Health, United States, 2007: With chartbook on trends in the health of Americans*. Hyattsville, MD: U.S. Department of Health and Human Services.

Rodriguez, L. (2004). Nutritional status: Assessing and understanding its value in the critical care setting. *Critical Care Nursing Clinics of North America*, 16(4), 509–514.

Taveras, E. M., Sandora, T. J., Shih, M. C., Ross-Degnan, D., Goldmann, D. A., & Gillman, M. W. (2006). The association of television and video viewing with fast food intake by preschool-age children. *Obesity (Silver Spring)*, 14(11), 2034–2041.

U.S. Department of Agriculture (USDA). (2005). *Dietary guidelines for Americans 2005* (6th ed.). Washington, DC: Author. (www.healthierus.gov/dietaryguidelines)

U.S. Department of Agriculture (USDA), Center for Nutrition Policy and Promotion. (2005). *MyPyramid food guidance system*. Washington, DC: Author. (www.mypyramid.gov)

U.S. Department of Health and Human Services, Public Health Service. (2000). *Healthy people 2010: National health promotion and disease prevention objectives*. Washington, DC: Author.

Williams, G., & Keir, B. (2008). MUST scoring—a 'must' or a waste of nursing time? *British Journal of Nursing (BJN)*, 17(10), 622–624.

Section 1

Principles of Nutrition

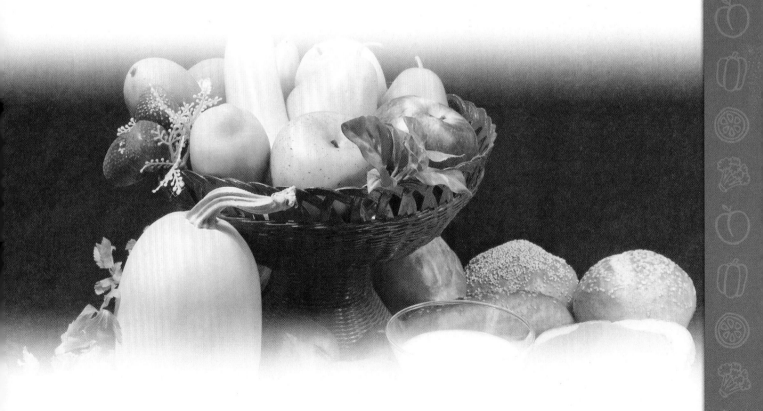

Christie Hust

Carbohydrates 2

WHAT WILL YOU LEARN?

1. To differentiate the types of carbohydrates and list the dietary sources of each.
2. To relate the functions of carbohydrates in the body.
3. To counsel individuals about the dietary recommendations for carbohydrate intake.
4. To examine the appropriateness of the use of nutritive and nonnutritive sweeteners.
5. To formulate nursing interventions that will assist individuals in improving intake of dietary fiber.

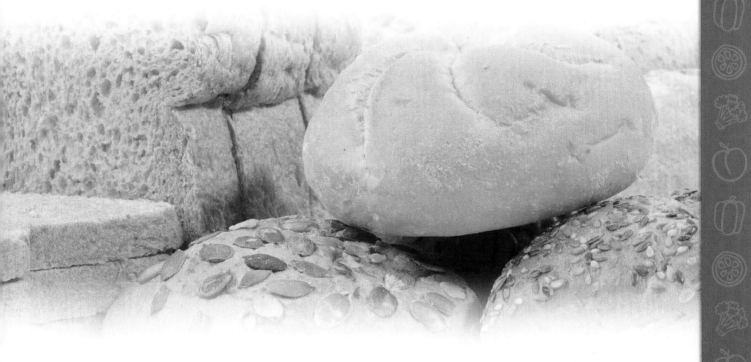

DID YOU KNOW?

▶ Carbohydrates have 4 kcalories/gm, the same as protein.

▶ Some cells in the body, like red blood cells, require glucose as the energy source.

▶ Soluble fiber can help lower blood sugar and blood lipid levels.

▶ Sucralose, an artificial sweetener, is made from sugar molecules but is not absorbed by the intestines.

▶ Whether or not a low-carbohydrate diet is healthy is a matter of ongoing controversy.

KEY TERMS

amylase, *19*

amylopectin, *19*

amylose, *19*

aspartame, *28*

carbohydrate, *18*

complex carbohydrates, *18*

dietary fiber, *27*

disaccharides, *19*

diverticulosis, *33*

enrichment, *25*

fiber, *19*

fortification, *25*

functional fiber, *27*

galactosemia, *19*

glucagon, *21*

gluconeogenesis, *20*

glycemic index (GI), *21*

glycogen, *19*

glycogenolysis, *21*

insoluble fiber, *20*

ketone bodies, *20*

lactose intolerance, *19*

laxation, *20*

monosaccharides, *18*

nonnutritive sweeteners, *28*

nutritive sweeteners, *28*

polysaccharide, *19*

simple carbohydrates, *18*

soluble fiber, *20*

starches, *19*

sugar alcohols, *30*

total fiber, *27*

whole grain, *23*

What Are Carbohydrates?

The complexity of the word or compound **carbohydrate** goes beyond just breads and sugars. Carbohydrates come in many forms, but all start with one molecule. Carbohydrates are molecules that contain a carbon, hydrogen, and oxygen. The general molecular formula is CH_2O. However, this general formulation is more accurate: $C_x(H2O)_y$. This formulation shows just how complex or simple a carbohydrate can be. A simple sugar can be one sugar molecule long, whereas a fiber may have hundreds of sugar molecules.

Carbohydrates are classified into groups by several factors. The length of the carbon chain is the first factor that classifies carbohydrates. Another factor is the number of sugar units. The more sugars, the more complex the substance is. The location of the double bond between the carbon and oxygen molecules will also affect the category of carbohydrate. Although all carbohydrates are formed with a base of at least one sugar molecule, some have two or three molecules and others have hundreds. Some are a straight chain, whereas oth-

ers are branched. These factors are what differentiate the simple and complex carbohydrates from one another.

Simple carbohydrates are those with fewer than three sugar molecules. They are easily broken down in the body to glucose, which is used readily by the body. **Complex carbohydrates** have more than three sugar molecules. The body also breaks these chains down into single glucose molecules to be used by the body.

Simple Carbohydrates

Simple carbohydrates are classified as **monosaccharides** or disaccharides. Monosaccharides have one sugar molecule and disaccharides have two sugar molecules. There are three monosaccharides: glucose, galactose, and fructose. Although all three sugars have the same molecular formula, their structures are very different, as depicted in Figure 2-1 .

Glucose is commonly known as blood sugar and is the form of sugar in intravenous solutions, called dextrose, which is given to clients. It circulates through the bloodstream, pro-

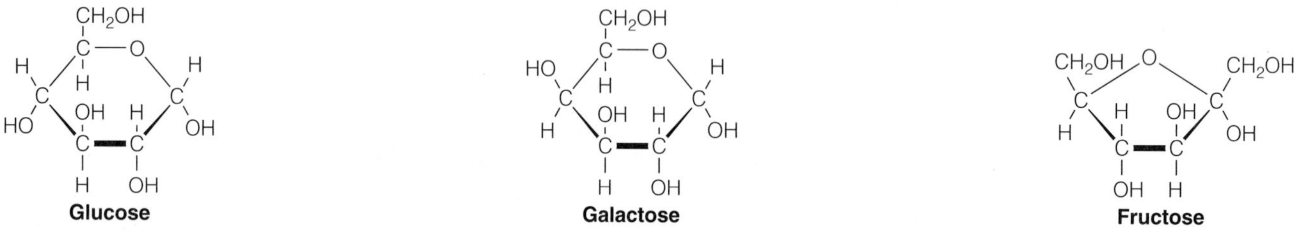

Glucose

Galactose

Fructose

■ **FIGURE 2-1 Chemical Structure of Monosaccharides.**

viding the cells with the fuel to make the energy needed to function. It is also a component of all disaccharides and the single component used to make complex carbohydrates.

Fructose is found in fruit and honey. It is the sweetest of the three monosaccharides, which is why it is used more than glucose or galactose to sweeten foods. It takes less fructose to sweeten a food than any other caloric sweetener. High-fructose corn syrup is commonly used to sweeten processed foods and drinks because of its low cost and easy availability.

Galactose is a monosaccharide that is not found widely in food sources. It is primarily found in milk as a component of the disaccharide lactose but also present in some fruits. In the body, galactose is a component in the formation of glycolipids and glycoproteins. A genetic disease that results from the inability to metabolize galactose is called **galactosemia** and is outlined in the discussion on Wellness Concerns in this chapter.

Disaccharides are double sugars. They are composed of two monosaccharides, one of which is glucose. Disaccharides are broken down into the two monosaccharides before being absorbed by the body. The three most common disaccharides are sucrose, lactose, and maltose. The three disaccharides have different structures due to the different monosaccharides that are used to form them.

- *Sucrose:* common table sugar = glucose + fructose
- *Lactose:* major sugar in milk = glucose + galactose
- *Maltose:* product of starch digestion = glucose + glucose

Sucrose is composed of glucose and fructose monosaccharides. It is most commonly produced from sugarcane or sugar beets. It is refined and then granulated into sugar crystals. It can also be found in some fruit and vegetables. Sucrose is sweeter than glucose but not as sweet as fructose. Table 2-1 compares the sweetness of sugars and other sweeteners to that of sucrose.

Table 2-1   Sweetener Sweetness Comparison*

Sweetener	Sweetness
Lactose	0.16
Galactose	0.32
Maltose	0.33
Sugar Alcohols	0.7–1.0
Sucrose	1.00
Fructose	1.73
Aspartame	180.00
Acesulfame-K	200.00
Saccharin	450.00
Sucralose	600.00
Neotame	7,000.00

*Comparison is made to sucrose or table sugar. For example, acesulfame-K is 200 times sweeter than sucrose.

Lactose is the major sugar found in milk, including human milk. It is comprised of a glucose and galactose and is less sweet tasting than sucrose. Lactose is an important part of calcium absorption and the promotion of beneficial bacteria in the colon. The body produces the enzyme lactase in the brush border of the small intestine to cleave the two monosaccharides apart. Some individuals have insufficient lactase production and thus poorly digest lactose, a condition called **lactose intolerance.** Lactose intolerance is briefly outlined in this chapter in the discussion of Wellness Concerns and in more depth in Chapter 20.

Maltose is the least found disaccharide in nature. Maltose is a preliminary component of starch production. It is found in brewed and fermented drinks such as beer. Maltose is also found as an ingredient in infant formulas and added to baked goods to give a fresh baked aroma and facilitate browning.

Complex Carbohydrates

Complex carbohydrates consist of many sugar molecules. **Polysaccharide** literally means *many sugars.* Complex carbohydrates include starches, glycogen, celluloses, and fibers. One would think that the complex carbohydrates would be sweet because of so many sugar molecules. However, because of the molecular size, they are too large to fit on the taste bud and impart a sweet taste.

Starches are the storage form of energy in plants. Plants convert the excess glucose into starch and store it in places such as the seeds, roots, stems, or tubers. Starches are long chains of glucose that can be up to 4,000 units in length and are found in two forms: **amylose** and **amylopectin.** Amylose is a straight chain, whereas amylopectin is a branched structure and a major component of starch. During digestion, starch is broken down by **amylase,** a pancreatic enzyme. The starch then is digested into glucose and maltose. Potatoes, rice, wheat, and corn are examples of major sources of starch in the diet (Murray, Granner, & Rodwell, 2006).

In animals, including humans, starch is stored as **glycogen.** Glycogen is stored in the liver and muscles. Glycogen is an energy stockpile that can be accessed when glucose falls too low in the body. The body stores approximately 70 to 100 gm of glycogen in the liver and 400 gm in muscle, amounts that can supply the body with a sufficient source of glucose for approximately 2 days before requiring a renewed source of glucose. In some rare instances glycogen cannot be stored, such as the disorder called glycogen storage disease, which results in an enlarged liver and low blood sugar among other problems.

Fiber is a term that refers to polysaccharides that are not digested by the body. They are generally part of the plant cell wall or intercellular structures. Fiber is resistant to mammalian intestinal enzymes and thus moves through the digestive tract until it is partially fermented by bacteria naturally found in the colon. Fiber is classified into two categories, water soluble and insoluble.

Insoluble fiber includes cellulose, hemicelluloses, and lignins. Cellulose is the most abundant polysaccharide in nature. Like starch, cellulose has glucose as its only monosaccharide. Cellulose is composed of long, straight, rigid molecules. There are no branch chains in cellulose, resulting in a compound that can lie close together, creating a rigid fiber. This formation is what provides structure to a plant, such as creating cell walls. All three components of insoluble fiber give plant foods texture. Examples include the skin of fruit, the shell of corn and peas, the covering of seeds, and the bran of the outer layer of a grain. Insoluble fibers add bulk to the stool by increasing stool volume and by absorbing water, which promote **laxation,** or a bowel movement.

Soluble fiber includes gums, pectins, some hemicelluloses, and mucilages. Soluble fiber forms a gel in the intestine that slows digestion. This slower emptying from the stomach diminishes how quickly sugar is absorbed in the intestine. Individuals with diabetes mellitus may benefit from including fiber as a regular component in the diet for this reason. Fiber and the diabetic diet are discussed in Chapter 19. Soluble fiber also binds fatty acids in the intestine, which can lower blood cholesterol by reducing the recycling of bile back to the liver after reabsorption. Chapter 18 outlines the role of soluble fiber in the treatment of high blood lipid levels.

Function

The functions of carbohydrates are varied. Both simple and complex carbohydrates supply energy to the body in the form of glucose, the simple sugar that is the end point of carbohydrate digestion and metabolism. Many cells of the body use both glucose and fat for energy needs. However, red blood cells, the brain, and the central nervous system require glucose as a preferred fuel source. This need is an important reason that carbohydrates are required as part of the human diet. Both simple and complex carbohydrates provide the body with glucose.

Carbohydrates provide 4 kcalories/gm. Protein also provides 4 kcalories/gm. Another function of carbohydrate is to spare protein. If energy needs are not met, the body will turn to protein and fat for energy. Glycogen stores provide a source of stored glucose but the amount is limited. There are functions in the body that only proteins can accomplish. Making hormones, blood cells, antibodies, enzymes, and building new tissue for growth, development, and repair are all dependent on protein. If the body is not provided with an adequate amount of carbohydrate to make glucose, it utilizes proteins as energy through their conversion to glucose. When glucose is synthesized from protein or glycogen, it is called **gluconeogenesis.** If dietary or internal proteins, such as skeletal muscle or blood proteins, are sacrificed for energy, the essential functions that rely on protein substrate become compromised. Carbohydrates spare protein by serving as a source of glucose, allowing protein to be used for its other functions.

In addition to catabolizing protein for energy when there is insufficient glucose supply, fat stores are broken down as well. For the body to metabolize fat for energy some glucose is required. When excessive fat is broken down the result is a large accumulation of **ketone bodies,** which are byproducts of incomplete fat metabolism. Ketone bodies can be used for energy by some parts of the body, but the brain and other tissue that depend on glucose will have compromised function. The ketone bodies are also acidic and change the pH of the blood to an acid medium. *Ketosis* is the term that describes this state of acidosis and elevated ketones in the blood. Dehydration, fatigue, nausea, and lack of appetite are other symptoms of ketosis. One way the nurse can check for ketosis in a client is by using a urine dipstick that detects ketone bodies that are excreted in urine. Ketone bodies also cause the breath to smell fruity or like alcohol because of acetone, a ketone body. Adequate carbohydrate intake prevents ketosis from occurring in a healthy person. Approximately 50 to 100 gm/day of carbohydrate are needed to prevent ketosis.

Carbohydrates are also used to make other compounds, such as ribose, which is an essential part of RNA and DNA; keratin in fingernails; and glycoproteins used for immunological protection and blood clotting.

Carbohydrate intake in excess of the body's need for glucose or synthesis of other compounds is stored as glycogen in muscle and the liver. When glucose needs and the capacity to store glycogen are met, excess glucose is metabolized into triglycerides, a type of fat.

Whereas both simple and complex carbohydrates provide a source of glucose to the body, fiber does not because it is not absorbed in the small intestine. Fiber can be fermented by bacteria in the colon and produce short-chain fatty acids with less than 2.5 kcalories/gm (Institute of Medicine [IOM], 2002). It is this fermentation that can cause the bloating side effect of fiber intake because methane and carbon dioxide are produced as well. The fibers in fruits and vegetables are fermented to a greater extent than are most cereal fibers (IOM, 2002). Fiber has important functions in the maintenance of health. It promotes laxation, and adequate intake is recommended to prevent or treat constipation. Chapter 20 outlines nursing interventions for this condition. Fiber has also received attention for a role in control of blood cholesterol and blood glucose. Its role in prevention of certain cancers is heavily researched but without firm conclusions (American Dietetic Association [ADA], 2008). Functions of fiber and other carbohydrates are outlined in Box 2-1.

Digestion and Metabolism

All foods must be broken down in the gastrointestinal tract in order to be used by the body. The process is orderly and well refined. Carbohydrate digestion is the process of hydrol-

| BOX 2-1 | Functions of Carbohydrates |

Simple and Complex Carbohydrates:

Supply energy from glucose – 4 kcal/gm

Spare protein

Prevent ketosis

Provide substrate to make ribose, keratin, and glycoproteins

Fiber

Promotes laxation

Treats constipation

Soluble fiber absorbs intestinal cholesterol found in bile

Soluble fiber delays gastric emptying and lower postprandial (postmeal) blood glucose

ysis where long chain carbohydrates are broken down by enzymes to shortened chains and, ultimately, monosaccharides.

Carbohydrate digestion begins in the mouth where the enzyme salivary amylase acts on starches to begin the process of hydrolysis. In the brush border of the small intestine, the membrane of the microvilli secretes enzymes responsible for catalyzing the polysaccharides and disaccharides into monosaccharides for absorption. Those enzymes have names such as lactase, dextrinase, isomaltase, maltase, and sucrase. The names are an indicator of what disaccharide they catalyze. For example, sucrase hydrolyzes sucrose into glucose and fructose (Murray et al., 2006).

A deficiency in any brush border enzyme may cause diarrhea, bloating, and flatulence after ingesting the sugar requiring that missing enzyme for digestion. For example, insufficient lactase production causes lactose intolerance, which some people erroneously call "milk allergy." This condition produces intestinal symptoms because of insufficient digestion of lactose, not from an allergy. When the undigested lactose reaches the colon, bacteria there ferment it, producing the symptoms of bloating and diarrhea. Lactose intolerance is very common worldwide and can occur with age or because of a medical condition. Chapter 20 covers lactose intolerance in detail.

Once absorbed, the glucose moves into the capillaries via the GLUT 2 transport system (Murray et al., 2006). This mechanism also transports galactose. Fructose utilizes a different mechanism. Fructose is transported independent of sodium, glucose, or galactose. It is carried via a transporter named the GLUT 5. Then it is transported into the blood by the same GLUT 2 transporter as glucose (Murray et al., 2006).

The capillaries then take the glucose into the hepatic portal vein where it is directed to the liver. The liver then releases the glucose into the bloodstream for the body to use. Fructose and galactose are further metabolized before entering the Kreb's cycle. The level of the blood glucose in the blood is regulated and kept constant by hormones. When a rise in blood glucose occurs, the hormone insulin is released from the pancreas. The insulin then moves the glucose out of the bloodstream and into the cells where it is used for energy via metabolism in the citric acid cycle (Murray et al., 2006). Muscle and liver cells are able to metabolize extra glucose and store it as glycogen. Muscle glycogen is primarily utilized within the muscle, whereas liver glycogen can generate glucose that is carried via the blood to supply the needs of other tissues and to maintain blood glucose level. When glycogen is broken down to generate glucose, it is called **glycogenolysis. Glucagon** is the hormone that stimulates this conversion when blood glucose levels are too low. Cells other than liver and muscle utilize available glucose for energy production but cannot store any extra (Ganong, 2005). The brain has little capacity to store glucose and must rely on a constant supply through the blood.

The term **glycemic index (GI)** refers to a measure of how much blood glucose rises during the 2 hours following ingestion of 50 gm of carbohydrate. The index compares various foods to sucrose or white bread as a reference and categorizes them as low, medium, or high glycemic. For example, white bread, white rice, and corn flakes are considered high GI foods, and a banana is considered medium GI. Examples of low GI foods include lentils and apples. A high glycemic index food would cause a quick elevation in blood glucose following intake, whereas a low glycemic food has a blunted response. Individuals such as those with diabetes who need to monitor blood glucose levels may find it helpful to understand the body's glycemic response to certain foods. However, this tool is cumbersome and not clear cut when foods are consumed as part of a meal instead of singly. Factors such as preparation or cooking method alter glycemic index as does the presence of protein, fat, or fiber in the food itself or other meal components. For example, a baked potato with skin has a different GI than without skin. Generally, foods with higher fiber content have a lower glycemic index than those with little or no fiber because fiber slows gastric emptying. The nurse can give this latter version of glycemic index advice to a client wishing to improve the postmeal blood glucose levels. Examples include using whole wheat pasta or bread instead of the white flour versions and consuming edible skin on fruit instead of peeling it. Those wishing to learn the more complicated use of glycemic index should be referred to a registered dietitian.

Where Are Carbohydrates in the Diet?

Carbohydrates are found in plant-based foods, milk, and yogurt, and in prepared and processed foods that have added sugars.

Simple Sugars

Food sources of simple sugars include both naturally occurring sugars and added sugars and syrups. Fructose is a natural

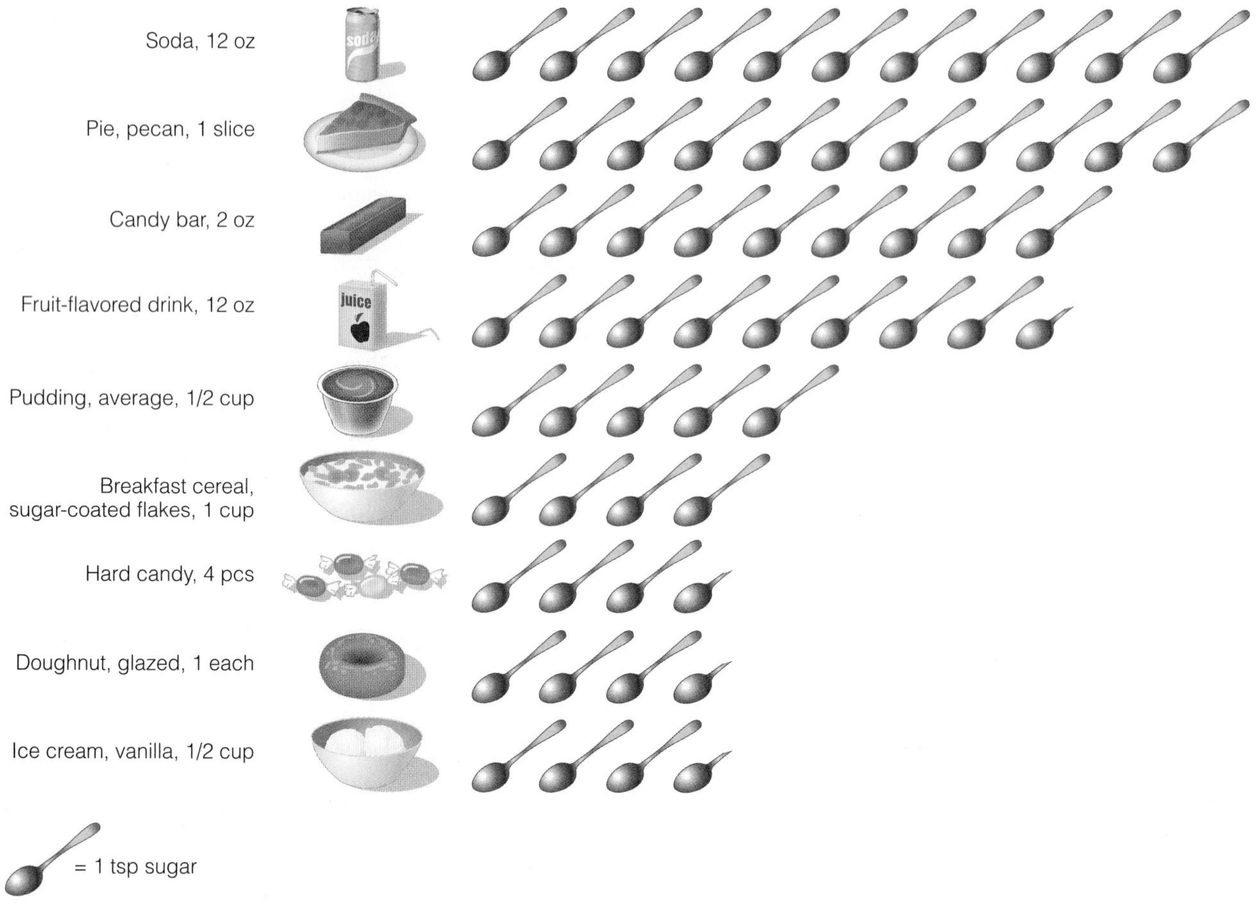

Soda, 12 oz

Pie, pecan, 1 slice

Candy bar, 2 oz

Fruit-flavored drink, 12 oz

Pudding, average, 1/2 cup

Breakfast cereal,
sugar-coated flakes, 1 cup

Hard candy, 4 pcs

Doughnut, glazed, 1 each

Ice cream, vanilla, 1/2 cup

= 1 tsp sugar

FIGURE 2-2 Added Sugar in Common Foods.

part of fruit and imparts the sweetness associated with those foods. Lactose, or milk sugar, is in milk, yogurt, and cheeses and can be found as a filler in some foods and medications. These naturally occurring sugars are also called intrinsic sugars. Added sugars include sucrose, commonly called table sugar, which has 4 gm of carbohydrate in each teaspoon. Sucrose is added in processing or in food preparation, such as with cakes, pies, cookies, ice cream, and other sweet treats. Other added sugars include high-fructose corn syrup, which is added to many processed foods and sweetened drinks. Added sugars are also called extrinsic sugars. Soft drinks are the leading contributor to added sugar intake in the American diet, followed by sweets such as candy, cakes, pies and cookies, sweetened grains, and other sweetened drinks such as fruit punch and fruit ades (IOM, 2002). Figure 2-2 ■ depicts the amount of added sugar in some common foods.

The nutrition facts panel on food labels lists sugars as a component but does not differentiate between added sugars and those naturally occurring in foods. Generally, naturally occurring sugars such as fructose or lactose are found in foods that are nutrient rich, such as fruits and milk, respectively, whereas added sugars are found in foods that have less nutrients. Yet, individuals may be confused when they read the nutrition facts panel and see high amounts of sugar listed for a food they thought nutritious. For example, a whole wheat

flake and raisin cereal might list an equal amount of sugar as a sweetened children's cereal because of the sugar present in the raisins while the overall nutritional value is superior. Practice Pearl: Sugar on the Food Label offers advice that the

PRACTICE ▶ PEARL

Sugar on the Food Label
The nutrition facts panel on a food label lists sugars but does not differentiate between natural and added sugars. The nurse can teach a client to read the ingredient list instead to search for added sugars. By law, ingredients are listed in descending order by weight; those listed first are present in higher amounts than those listed at the end of the list. Here are words that denote added sugar:

Brown sugar	Lactose
Corn sweetener	Malt
Corn syrup	Maltose
Dextrose	Maple sugar or syrup
Fructose	Molasses
Glucose	Raw sugar
Granulated sugar	Sucrose
High-fructose corn syrup	Sugar
Honey	Syrup
Invert sugar	Turbinado sugar

nurse can give to better determine the source of sugar listed on a food label. The nurse should also know that despite the food manufacturer's use of label terms such as "low impact carb" and "net carb" that are sometimes used to market foods, these terms have no recognized definition by the Food and Drug Administration (FDA), which oversees labeling laws.

Complex Carbohydrates

Complex carbohydrates include foods that contain starches and fibers. Grains, starchy vegetables such as potatoes and green peas, and legumes such as black beans, chickpeas, and lentils contain complex carbohydrates. Starches are the form of carbohydrate stored in plants in contrast to glycogen, the stored form of carbohydrate found in animals. Some food sources may contain a combination of simple sugars and complex carbohydrates because of processing; for example, breakfast cereal with added sugar or dried fruit. Box 2-2 lists some examples of food sources of complex carbohydrate with serving sizes that contain equivalent amounts of carbohydrate for comparison.

The term **whole grain** refers to those that have not been overly processed during milling and still retain the outer

BOX 2-2	Food Sources of Complex Carbohydrates

Grains Example Serving Size

		Amount That Counts as 1 Ounce Equivalent of Grains	Common Portions and Ounce Equivalents
Bagels	whole wheat	1 "mini" bagel	1 large bagel = 4 ounce equivalents
Breads	100% whole wheat	1 regular slice	2 regular slices = 2 ounce equivalents
Bulgur	cracked wheat	½ cup cooked	
Crackers	100% whole wheat, rye	5 whole wheat crackers 2 rye crispbreads	
English muffins	whole wheat	½ muffin	1 muffin = 2 ounce equivalents
Muffins	whole wheat	1 small (2½" diameter)	1 large (3½" diameter) = 3 ounce equivalents
Oatmeal		½ cup cooked 1 packet instant 1 ounce dry (regular or quick)	
Pancakes	whole wheat, buckwheat	1 pancake (4½" diameter) 2 small pancakes (3" diameter)	3 pancakes (4½" diameter) = 3 ounce equivalents
Popcorn		3 cups, popped	1 microwave bag, popped = 4 ounce equivalents
Ready-to-eat breakfast cereal	toasted oat, whole wheat flakes	1 cup flakes or rounds	
Rice	brown, wild	½ cup cooked 1 ounce dry	1 cup cooked = 2 ounce equivalents
Pasta—spaghetti, macaroni, noodles	whole wheat	½ cup cooked 1 ounce dry	1 cup cooked = 2 ounce equivalents
Tortillas	whole wheat, whole grain corn	1 small flour tortilla (6" diameter) 1 corn tortilla (6" diameter)	1 large tortilla (12" diameter) = 4 ounce equivalents

Vegetables Serving Size

	Amount That Counts as 1 Cup of Vegetables	Amount That Counts as ½ Cup of Vegetables
Dark-Green Vegetables		
Broccoli	1 cup chopped or florets 3 spears 5" long raw or cooked	
Greens (collards, mustard greens, turnip greens, kale)	1 cup cooked	
Spinach	1 cup, cooked 2 cups raw is equivalent to 1 cup of vegetables	1 cup raw is equivalent to ½ cup of vegetables
Raw leafy greens: Spinach, romaine, watercress, dark green leafy lettuce, endive, escarole	2 cups raw is equivalent to 1 cup of vegetables	1 cup raw is equivalent to ½ cup of vegetables

(continued)

BOX 2-2	**Food Sources of Complex Carbohydrates** *(continued)*

Vegetables Serving Size

	Amount That Counts as 1 Cup of Vegetables	Amount That Counts as ½ Cup of Vegetables
Orange Vegetables		
Carrots	1 cup, strips, slices, or chopped, raw or cooked 2 medium 1 cup baby carrots (about 12)	1 medium carrot About 6 baby carrots
Pumpkin	1 cup mashed, cooked	
Sweet potato	1 large baked (2¼" or more diameter) 1 cup sliced or mashed, cooked	
Winter squash (acorn, butternut, hubbard)	1 cup cubed, cooked	½ acorn squash, baked = ¾ cup
Dry Beans and Peas		
Dry beans and peas (such as black, garbanzo, kidney, pinto, or soy beans, or black-eyed peas or split peas)	1 cup whole or mashed, cooked	
Tofu	1 cup ½" cubes (about 8 ounces)	1 piece 2½" × 2¾" × 1" (about 4 ounces)
Starchy Vegetables		
Corn, yellow or white	1 cup 1 large ear (8" to 9" long)	1 small ear (about 6" long)
Green peas	1 cup	
White potatoes	1 cup diced, mashed 1 medium boiled or baked potato (2½" to 3" diameter) French fried: 20 medium to long strips (2½" to 4" long) (Contains *discretionary calories.*)	
Other Vegetables		
Bean sprouts	1 cup cooked	
Cabbage, green	1 cup, chopped or shredded raw or cooked	
Cauliflower	1 cup pieces or florets raw or cooked	
Celery	1 cup, diced or sliced, raw or cooked 2 large stalks (11" to 12" long)	1 large stalk (11" to 12" long)
Cucumbers	1 cup raw, sliced or chopped	
Green or wax beans	1 cup cooked	
Green or red peppers	1 cup chopped, raw or cooked 1 large pepper (3" diameter, 3¾" long)	1 small pepper
Lettuce, iceberg or head	2 cups raw, shredded or chopped = equivalent to 1 cup of vegetables	1 cup raw, shredded or chopped = equivalent to ½ cup of vegetables
Mushrooms	1 cup raw or cooked	
Onions	1 cup chopped, raw or cooked	
Tomatoes	1 large raw whole (3") 1 cup chopped or sliced, raw, canned, or cooked	1 small raw whole (2¼") 1 medium canned
Tomato or mixed vegetable juice	1 cup	½ cup
Summer squash or zucchini	1 cup cooked, sliced or diced	

Source: United States Department of Agriculture, 2008. Inside the pyramid. Retrieved March 27, 2009, from http://www.mypyramid.gov/pyramid/vegetables_counts_table.html

portions of the grain, called the germ and the bran as depicted in Figure 2-3 ■. Removal of the germ and the bran causes the loss of fiber and nutrients, such as thiamine, riboflavin, niacin, and iron. White flour and white rice are examples of processed or refined grains, and whole wheat or oat flour and brown rice are examples of whole grains. Rye, cornmeal, barley, and bran products are other examples of whole grains. Whole grains can be made into the same type of foods as processed grains but offer a more nutrient-dense profile. Cereals, breads, pastas, baked goods, and any other

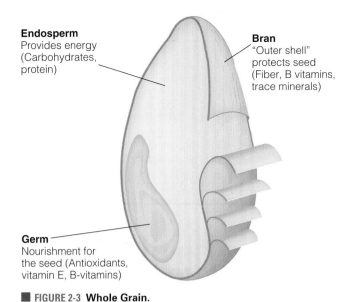

Endosperm
Provides energy
(Carbohydrates,
protein)

Bran
"Outer shell"
protects seed
(Fiber, B vitamins,
trace minerals)

Germ
Nourishment for
the seed (Antioxidants,
vitamin E, B-vitamins)

■ FIGURE 2-3 **Whole Grain.**

product made with flour can be made in a whole grain version or a processed version. The nurse should emphasize the greater nutritional value of whole grains when discussing carbohydrate intake. The ingredient listing can be checked for the word "whole" before the name of the grain. For example, "whole wheat" versus just "wheat" is preferred. The client should look for whole grains listed among the first ingredients and before other grains on the ingredient listing. Table 2-2 compares the fiber content of many foods, including both whole and refined grains. Refined grains have some of the nutrients replaced following processing. It is called **enrichment** when lost nutrients are replaced. When nutrients are added that were not naturally present, it is called **fortification.** In the United States white flour products are enriched with thiamine, riboflavin, niacin, and iron and are fortified with folic acid.

Fiber

Fiber is found in foods that are plant based. Whole grains contain fiber as do fruits, vegetables, legumes, seeds, and nuts. Foods closer to their original form will contain more fiber than those that are processed or prepared. For example, an orange has more fiber than orange juice and an apple eaten with the skin has more fiber than without the skin. Consumption of edible skins or seeds from a fruit or vegetable increases the fiber content. Likewise, whole grains have more fiber than processed grains. Most fiber-containing foods are made up of a mix of fiber types, both soluble and insoluble. Practice Pearl: What Is the Difference between Soluble vs. Insoluble Fiber? contains a quick way to remember the difference between these fibers. However, foods are often classified by the predominant fiber type they contain. Table 2-3 outlines sources of soluble and insoluble fiber.

Table 2-2	Fiber Content of Foods
Amount of Fiber	**Food Sources**
1 gm or less	Apple, orange or tomato juice, 1 cup
	Bread, wheat, 1 slice
	Cantaloupe, ½ cup
	Cereal, puffed rice, 1 cup
	Crackers, saltines, 6
	Lettuce, various, 1 cup
	Muffin, blueberry, avg
	Rice, white, cooked, ¾ cup
	Spaghetti, cooked, ½ cup
2–3 gm	Almonds, peanuts or pistachios, 1 oz
	Apricots, dried, 5
	Blackberries or blueberries, ½ cup
	Bread, rye, 1 slice
	Cereal, o-shaped oats, 1 cup
	Crackers, whole wheat, 6
	Kiwi, 1 med
	Muffin, corn, avg
	Orange, 1 med
	Peach, 1 med
	Potato, baked, no skin, avg
	Rice, brown, ¾ cup
	Spaghetti, whole wheat, cooked, ½ cup
	Tomato, chopped, 1 cup
	Vegetables, broccoli, green beans, winter squashes, cooked, ½ cup
	Vegetables, green leafy, cooked, ½ cup
4–5 gm	Apple with skin, 1 med
	Bulgur, cooked, ½ cup
	Cereal, oatmeal, quick cook, 1 cup
	Cereal, whole wheat flakes, 1 cup
	English muffin, whole wheat, 1
	Figs, dried, 2
	Pear with skin, 1 med
	Potato, baked, with skin, 1 med
	Raspberries, ½ cup
	Sweet potato with skin, 1 med
	Vegetables, green peas, cooked, ½ cup
5–6 gm	Cereal, raisin bran, 1 cup
	Cereal, shredded wheat, 1 cup mini or 2 lg biscuits
	Chickpeas, cooked, ½ cup
	Raisins, seedless, 1 cup
	Soybeans, cooked, ½ cup
7–8 gm	Cereal, bran flakes, ½ cup
	Kidney beans, cooked, ½ cup
	Lentils, cooked, ½ cup
	Split peas, cooked, ½ cup
	Trail mix w/ dried fruit, seeds, nuts, 1 cup
9–10 gm	Cereal, 100% bran, ½ cup
	Navy beans, cooked, ½ cup

C_T? What choices could you make to meet your daily recommended fiber intake?

Table 2-3 Soluble and Insoluble Fiber Sources

Fiber Type	Insoluble	Soluble
Food Sources	• Whole wheat and wheat bran • Corn bran, popcorn • Vegetables such as green beans, onions, broccoli, cabbage, and leafy greens • Skins from fruits and root vegetables • Edible seeds from fruits and vegetables • Seeds and nuts	• Oats and oat bran • Rice, quinoa, and barley • Legumes such as kidney beans, chickpeas, lentils, soybeans, and split peas • Fruits such as citrus (orange, grapefruit), apples, pears, and bananas • Vegetables such as carrots, cucumbers, and zucchini • Flaxseed

PRACTICE PEARL

What Is the Difference between Soluble and Insoluble Fiber?

Insoluble fiber makes up the walls of the plant cells and is considered a structural-type fiber.

Soluble fiber is found inside the cell. This type of fiber forms a gel-like material in the digestive tract that is beneficial for lowering blood cholesterol and glucose levels.

An easy way to remember the difference between the two types is the letter **S**: **S**oluble is **s**oft and **s**pongy, which **s**lows digestion of sugars and **s**oaks up cholesterol.

Carbohydrate Recommendations

The recommended dietary allowance (RDA) for carbohydrate is a minimum of 130 gm (IOM, 2002). This recommendation is applicable to children and adults. This minimum is the amount needed by the brain to function and should not be interpreted as the amount the body will need for other functions, such as overall energy needs. Determining the need for total carbohydrate will differ with every person based on factors such as weight and activity level. Carbohydrate needs are elevated during pregnancy and lactation to 175 gm and 210 gm, respectively, in order to meet the glucose needs of the fetus and to replace the carbohydrate secreted in breast milk (IOM, 2002). Carbohydrate recommendations for athletes are outlined in Chapter 11.

There is no set recommendation for carbohydrate intake for optimal health because this number is unknown. It is recommended that a range of 45% to 65% of total calorie intake should come from carbohydrates each day (IOM, 2002). This recommendation is based on evidence that the risk of cardiovascular disease and obesity is lower at this level of intake when combined with a low-fat diet compared with other ranges of intake (IOM, 2002). Box 2-3 outlines the calculations that the nurse could use to determine carbohydrate needs based on this range. Current intake of carbohydrate by Americans is approximately 50% of kilocalories, well within the recommended range (USDA, 2007a). However, it should be noted that average total kilocalorie intake has risen in this

BOX 2-3	Carbohydrate Calculations

Carbohydrate should comprise 45% to 65% of the total kilocalories per day. The nurse can translate that recommendation into grams of carbohydrate per day for an individual using these steps:

1. Total estimated kcal needs × 45% to 65% (or 0.45 to 0.65) = total kcal/day from carbohydrate
2. Total kcal/day from carbohydrate ÷ 4 kcal/gm = recommended grams of carbohydrate/day

Example: Nellie requires 2,000 kcal/day.

1. 2,000 kcal × 0.45 to 0.65 = 900 to 1,300 total kcal/day from carbohydrate
2. 900 to 1,300 kcal from carbohydrate/day ÷ 4 kcal/gm carbohydrate = 225 to 325 gm carbohydrate/day

After you read Chapter 8, determine your own calorie needs and calculate your personal carbohydrate recommendation.

country and increased carbohydrate intake is the primary contributor (Centers for Disease Control and Prevention [CDC], 2004).

Simple Sugars

Recommendations regarding intake of simple sugars are given specifically for added, or extrinsic, sugars rather than for simple sugars as a whole. No recommendation exists that suggests a range or limit on intake of naturally occurring sugars given the rich nutrients generally present in fruits and milk products. Conversely, it is recommended that daily intake of added sugars not exceed 25% of total calories (IOM, 2002). The World Health Organization suggests an even tighter recommendation of a 10% limit on contribution to total calories (WHO, 2003). These recommendations should not be interpreted as suggested intake, but rather limits. In the United States, intake of total sugars is approximately 23% of kcalories consumed, but differentiation between extrinsic or intrinsic sugars is not reported (USDA, 2007b). It is felt that higher intakes of added sugars result in consumption of a less nutrient dense diet at higher intake levels, contribute to development of dental caries, and may contribute to the intake of excessive calories and therefore obesity (IOM, 2002; Mann, 2003; WHO, 2003). Discussion of whether carbohydrate intake has a link to obesity is outlined in "Wellness Concerns" later in this chapter.

The Dietary Guidelines for Americans and Health Canada both recommend that added sugars be limited in foods and drinks for both dental health and avoidance of excessive calorie intake (Health Canada, 2007; USDA & DHHS, 2005). Both authorities encourage limiting intake of sweetened drinks as well as fruits, vegetables, and grains that have been prepared with added sugars. The dietary guidelines offer specific suggestions regarding added sugar intake as part of an individual's discretionary calorie intake. Discretionary calories are those that remain after intake of all servings of food groups recommended to meet nutrient needs. Discretionary calories are comprised of any combination of calories from added sugars, fats, and alcohol. For example, an individual who requires 2,000 kcalories/day has approximately 270 kcalories of discretionary energy intake. If a diet with 29% fat and no alcohol is consumed, 32 gm of added sugars would remain to arrive at the 270 kcalories. Because there are 4 gm of carbohydrate in each teaspoon of sugar, this 32 gm of added sugar equals 8 teaspoons of sugar, or the amount in one soft drink (USDA & DHHS, 2005). Consuming more fat or alcohol would lower the suggested added sugar limit.

Complex Carbohydrates

Both the Dietary Guidelines for Americans and Health Canada recommend that carbohydrate intake come from a variety of food groups and specifically encourage fiber-rich versions of fruits, vegetables, grains, and legumes (Health Canada, 2007; USDA & DHHS, 2005). Whole fruits versus juices are emphasized. Both authorities specifically recommend that whole grains comprise at least half of the recommended intake of that food group. Increasing intake of whole grains in the diet has been shown to have a positive effect on risk factors for type 2 diabetes and cardiovascular disease (McKeown, Meigs, Liu, Wilson, & Jacques, 2002). The nurse can suggest whole grain alternatives to refined grains such as switching to whole wheat bread from white bread, or trying a new whole grain such as quinoa (pronounced *keen-wah*) or brown rice. Cultural Considerations: Fiber outlines some whole grains that are common in a variety of cultures for the nurse to suggest. Making small changes over time can result in eventual achievement of the goal of consuming more whole grains.

Fiber

The recommendation for daily total fiber intake in adult females and males is 25 gm and 38 gm, respectively, based on 14 gm fiber per 1,000 kcalories consumed (IOM, 2002). The recommendations for children and adolescents are based on those for adults and adjusted for energy intake as outlined in

Cultural Considerations

Fiber
Many cultures have traditional fruits, vegetables, grains, nuts, and legumes that are part of the diet. When people immigrate to a new country, the traditional diet choices are often adapted to the new land and some traditional practices are stopped. Cultures that rely less on meats and refined foods often have higher fiber content than those that are meat based. Various types of rice and bean dishes are an example of foods that are part of many cultures. Although some cultures may favor a certain type of bean, such as black-eyed peas or kidney beans, any type is a good source of fiber. When educating an individual about improving fiber intake, the nurse should explore sources of fiber that are part of both the original and present culture food choices. Ask about use of legumes such as soybeans, split peas, lentils, chickpeas, black beans, and the like. Find out which grains are used and whether a whole grain version can be considered. Corn tortillas, whole wheat noodles, bulgur, and brown rice are examples. Assess what vegetables, fruits, and nuts are included. Root vegetables, tubers, and leafy greens are common in many cultures. Yucca, sweet potato, mustard greens, and kale are examples. Often vegetables are part of a mixed dish, such as a stir-fry, stew, or casserole. Fruits vary according to the region of the world. Cold climate areas have seasonal fruit such as apples and pears, whereas hot weather areas enjoy a variety of tropical fruits. Dried fruits such as figs and apricots are used in the diet in the Middle East and Mediterranean areas. Peanuts are a staple in some African nations, whereas tree nuts are found in temperate areas. The nurse should not assume that all people from an area eat the same type of foods, but rather explore with the individual which high-fiber foods are part of the individual's cultural practices.

Appendix C. The recommendation for fiber intake is based on epidemiological studies that show a link between a decreased risk of coronary heart disease and a diet high in fiber (IOM, 2002). Many studies have found an association between high-fiber intake and lower blood cholesterol levels when compared to lower fiber intake (Wheeler & Pi-Sunyer, 2008). Although fiber has other benefits in the diet, it is this specific benefit that guides the recommendation. **Total fiber** is the sum of **dietary fiber** and **functional fiber,** terms that differentiate between fibers that are merely nondigestible and those that also have a physiological, or functional, benefit (IOM, 2002). For example, functional fibers are those that promote laxation, are associated with normalizing blood lipids, or slow the elevation of blood glucose after a meal. Functional fibers are comprised of both soluble and insoluble fiber types and can include commercially prepared fibers that are added to foods or available for purchase. Dietary fibers are intact in plants and include lignins, the woody portion of the plant cell wall (IOM, 2002). Because there is often confusion over the use of these technical terms, the nurse will find it easier to stick with describing fiber as soluble and insoluble when making suggestions to a client. A variety of fibers from both types is recommended rather than specific amounts from each type (American Dietetic Association [ADA], 2008).

In the United States, intake of fiber falls short of that recommended. Average fiber intake for those age 2 years and over is only 14.8 gm/day, with adult males and females consuming an average 17.5 gm and 13.7 gm, respectively (USDA, 2007b). Lifespan Box: Fiber and Dental Issues outlines issues affecting fiber intake in the older adult. When offering advice on increasing fiber intake, the nurse should suggest a gradual increase in intake to avoid unwanted intestinal side effects from bacterial fermentation of the fiber. A slow increase in intake over time allows the intestine to adapt to the increase (ADA, 2008). Adequate fluid intake should be encouraged as well to improve tolerance. Client Education Checklist: Improving Fiber Intake outlines advice that the nurse can offer to assist an individual in improving fiber intake. Cultural Considerations: Fiber on p. 27 lists some good sources of fiber among the traditional diets of a variety of cultures for the nurse to include when educating a client about fiber in the diet.

Lifespan

Fiber and Dental Issues

For many older adults fiber intake becomes a challenge because of dental issues. Dental caries, improperly fitted dentures, or lack of teeth can make it difficult to consume needed fiber. The following recommendations may be helpful:

- Start the day with high-fiber breakfast cereal such as oatmeal that requires little chewing. Add small pieces of soft fruit if tolerated.
- Add flaxseed, crushed bran, or whole grain flake cereal to casseroles.
- Consume split peas, cooked beans, and lentils in soups, casseroles, or other mixed dishes.
- Use whole grain breads such as whole wheat, oatmeal, and rye.
- Choose whole grain rice and noodles such as brown rice and whole wheat spaghetti.
- Cut raw fruit into small, bite-size pieces. Peel skins if needed. If raw fruit is too difficult to eat, encourage intake of canned fruit.
- Choose raw fruits with soft skins or edible seeds like berries and kiwi.
- Choose vegetables with soft skins or edible seeds like tomatoes and eggplant.

CT? Dental health issues can be a barrier to fiber intake among other population groups, too. What recommendations might the nurse offer to the adolescent who wears orthodontic braces and has trouble with hard fruits and raw vegetables? What food sources can be recommended for the school-age child who does not like vegetables?

Excessive fiber intake was previously believed to be harmful because of potential diminished absorption of some minerals such as zinc, iron, and calcium from the diet. However, research has failed to substantiate this theoretical concern (IOM, 2002). On the other hand, phytate, a component of some plant foods that is not a type of fiber, is known to bind these minerals and make them less available for absorption (IOM, 2002). Phytate is found in leafy greens, such as spinach, among other foods. Excessive intake of fiber is a self-limiting practice because of the uncomfortable side effects of intestinal distention or bloating that can occur. Thus, no upper limit recommendations for fiber intake have been made. Excessive intake of fiber and fiber supplements is known to bind the cardiac medication, digoxin, and render it less effective (Schmidt & Dalhoff, 2002). The nurse should educate clients taking this medication about avoiding excess fiber at the same time as the medication dose. For example, digoxin should not be taken along with a high-fiber breakfast cereal or a high-fiber dietary supplement.

Nonnutritive and Nutritive Sweeteners

Nonnutritive sweeteners are sugar substitutes that contain insignificant or no calories. **Nutritive sweeteners** are those that do contain energy. The food label may tout that a product containing these sugar alternatives is sugar free, but the nurse should remind those who are trying to manage their weight that this term does not equate to calorie free. In the United States, the FDA oversees the approval of sweeteners for use in food as either an ingredient or an additive.

The nurse may be asked about the use of stevia as a sugar alternative. This plant-derived, noncaloric sweetener from South America is not approved in the United States or Canada for use as sweetener or food additive, yet it is available as a dietary supplement because it is a botanical product. Concerns exist regarding a potential link between stevia and infertility and mutagenic risks (Harvard College, 2005; Schardt, 2004). The nurse should advise individuals who inquire about the use of stevia that significant research on its safety is lacking in humans. Conclusions about safe amounts to consume and long-term effects of use are unknown.

Nonnutritive Sweeteners

Five nonnutritive sweeteners are approved for use with guidelines given for Accepted Daily Intake (ADI) based on available evidence on safe levels of consumption. Aspartame, acesulfame-K, Sucralose, and Neotame are approved as general-purpose sweeteners, whereas saccharin is approved for use in beverages and as a tabletop sweetener (ADA, 2004).

Aspartame is marketed as Nutrasweet and Equal. It is over 150 times sweeter than sucrose. Aspartame is made by linking aspartic acid and phenylalanine, two amino acids that are found in proteins. Like other proteins, it contains 4 kcalories/gm, but because it is so powerfully sweet, the amount needed to sweeten a food results in an insignificant

CLIENT EDUCATION CHECKLIST	Improving Fiber Intake
Intervention	**Example**
Assess diet for sources of fiber. Include fiber supplements.	Ask about intake of plant-based foods (grains, vegetables, fruit, legumes, nuts, seeds). Determine whether edible skins are eaten and whether whole grain versions of grains are used. Assess amounts consumed.
Determine reasons that fiber intake may be low.	Assess dental health or intestinal intolerance to fiber. Determine if cost of foods is barrier to intake. Assess for knowledge deficit regarding fiber recommendations and sources.
Educate about the role of fiber in health.	Fiber promotes laxation and can be part of nutrition interventions for weight management and lowering blood cholesterol and glucose.
Outline sources of fiber in the diet.	Plant foods "closest to the original form" will have more fiber than the processed version of the same food. Animal-based foods contain NO fiber. Sources include: whole grains, such as whole wheat, oats, cornmeal, barley, rye, brown rice; fruits and vegetables, especially those with edible skins and seeds; legumes, such as beans, split peas, lentils; nuts and seeds. See Table 2-2 for fiber amounts.
Customize advice to address reasons that fiber intake was low.	Offer ideas for easily chewed fruits, vegetables, grains, and legumes if dental health is an issue (see Lifespan: Fiber and Dental Issues). Add fiber slowly if gastrointestinal side effects are a problem (see next). Many high-fiber foods are low in cost, such as various types of beans, split peas, and lentils. These can be used in place of animal proteins to lower food costs as well. Bran and other whole grain cereals are often less expensive than sweetened, processed cereals. Bulgur, barley, and corn are inexpensive whole grains.
Advise that fiber be added slowly to minimize bloating side effect.	Add only 5 gm fiber/day each week until the goal is reached. Suggestions include: • Swapping refined flour products for whole grains (breads, cereals, crackers) • Consuming plant-based proteins (beans, peas, lentils) • Targeting intake of at least 5 servings of fruits and vegetables a day. Whole fruits and vegetables with edible skin have more fiber than juices and peeled produce. Ingredient labels for grain products should be checked for the word "whole" in the listing (e.g., *whole wheat* vs. *wheat*).

calorie contribution. Products that contain aspartame carry a warning about phenylalanine content for individuals with phenylketonuria (PKU), an inborn error of metabolism that is reviewed in Chapter 3. Those with PKU must limit total daily intake of phenylalanine in the diet. Popular lore has blamed aspartame for a number of illnesses and conditions, none of which have been substantiated with scientific research. A review of safety based on current intake and available studies has not found aspartame to be associated with any negative health effects (Magnusun et al., 2007).

Acesulfame potassium, better known as acesulfame-K, is 200 times sweeter than sucrose. It is often blended with other nonnutritive sweeteners because of its intense sweetening power (ADA, 2004). Acesulfame-K is used as an all-purpose sweetener, including in cooking and baking. Sunette is the trade name for acesulfame-K.

Sucralose is marketed as Splenda and is 60 times sweeter than sucrose (FDA, 2006). This product is a sucrose molecule chemically combined with chlorine. This combination causes the sweetener to be poorly absorbed by the intestines and of no caloric value. Unlike many nonnutritive sweeteners, sucralose can be used successfully in cooking and baking because it is heat stable (ADA, 2004). Anecdotal reports exist that link sucralose with a variety of medical conditions such as migraine, but scientific evidence is lacking to support such associations (Grotz, 2007).

Neotame is 7,000 to 13,000 times sweeter than sucrose (FDA, 2006). This nonnutritive sweetener was approved by the FDA in 2002 but is not yet widely available in foods. Neotame is chemically similar to aspartame because it contains the same two amino acids, aspartic acid and phenylalanine. Although the metabolism of neotame does produce phenylalanine, it is of such insignificant quantity that no warning for PKU is required (FDA, 2006).

Saccharin is an artificial sweetener made from synthetic chemicals that has been on the market for a number of years despite some turbulent times in the 1970s, during which it was challenged as a potential cancer-causing agent. Saccharin was removed from the National Institute for Health's list of potential carcinogens in 2000. The FDA has approved saccharin for use in beverages, as a packaged sugar substitute, and in some processed foods at specifically controlled levels that must be listed on the product label (ADA, 2004). Saccharin is marketed under the trade names Sweet 'N Low and Sugar Twin.

Nutritive Sweeteners

Sugar alcohols, also called polyols, are lower calorie sugar replacements that are derived from sugars. Sorbitol, mannitol, and xylitol are common sugar alcohols. The "ol" suffix indicates that sugar alcohols are an alcohol version of the sugar molecule, but they do not contain ethanol as do alcoholic beverages. These nutritive sweeteners are absorbed more slowly and in lesser amounts than simple sugars, leading to an average energy content of 2 kcalories/gm compared with the 4 kcalories/gm of sugars and other carbohydrates. Manufacturers may voluntarily list sugar alcohol content on the nutrition facts panel on food labels. If the manufacturer makes a label claim touting the decreased risk of dental caries associated with polyols compared with sugars, the sugar alcohol content becomes a mandatory feature on the label (Federal Register, 1997). Hot Topic: Carbohydrates, Diet, and Dental Caries outlines the issue of dental caries and carbohydrates and addresses sugar alcohols in this regard. Excessive intake of sugar alcohols has a laxative effect and may cause diarrhea because of the highly concentrated nature of these products, which draw water into the intestine during digestion. The nurse can warn those who use these products of this undesirable side effect. Additionally, chewable and liquid medications often contain sorbitol as an inactive ingredient. When the amount of sorbitol in the formulation is significant or several medications are taken, each with sorbitol, diarrhea can result. The nurse should consider this effect when caring for a client receiving tube feedings who is prescribed liquid medications and experiences diarrhea.

Wellness Concerns

In addition to the functions of carbohydrates that have been outlined, there exist other potential health effects of carbohydrates. Additionally, some health effects are erroneously blamed on carbohydrates despite scientific evidence to the contrary.

Dental Health

Tooth decay occurs for a number of reasons. Dietary choices, including carbohydrate intake, is one of the components that can increase risk of dental caries. The presence of bacteria in the mouth coupled with the presence of carbohydrate as an energy source begins the decay process. Other factors such as acids and fluoride can increase or decrease risk of decay developing. Hot Topic Box: Carbohydrates, Diet, and Dental Caries discusses the role that carbohydrates have in the development of dental caries.

---

hot Topic

Carbohydrates, Diet, and Dental Caries

Certain aspects of the diet can increase the risk of developing dental caries, or cavities. Sugary foods are associated with cavity development, but these foods are not solely responsible for the multistep process that leads to tooth demineralization. In addition to offering advice about good oral hygiene, including use of a fluoridated toothpaste, the nurse can explain the role of the following dietary components in tooth decay:

- *Sugars:* Sugars, such as sucrose, provide a source of energy for the oral bacteria responsible for demineralizing teeth through production of acid. Sugars that are sticky, slowly dissolving, or that otherwise remain in contact with the teeth worsen the risk of cavity development by prolonging the time that bacteria have access to this energy source.

- *Fermentable carbohydrates:* Salivary amylase is an enzyme present in the mouth that breaks down starchy carbohydrates in an initial step of digestion. The resulting form of carbohydrate is then fermented by oral bacteria to form an acid, which can erode teeth and favor further bacterial growth.

- *Acid:* Exposing the teeth to acid, whether from the diet or an internal source, can lead to tooth erosion. Dietary sources of acid include sodas, sports beverages, citrus fruit, and chewable vitamin C supplements. Tooth exposure to internal (stomach) acid occurs because of vomiting (including bulimia) and gastric reflux, or heartburn. Exposure to acid sources weakens the teeth over time.

- *Saliva flow:* Consuming sugary or acid foods singly may allow longer tooth exposure than when consumed with a meal. Increased saliva production with a meal, along with the buffering effect of other foods, can lessen the exposure by the teeth to bacterial action.

- *Time and frequency of exposure:* The amount of time that a suspect food stays in contact with the tooth is a factor in cavity development. Carbohydrate-containing foods that become lodged between or on teeth until brushing and flossing occur or those that are sipped or nibbled on over an extended time increase the time that bacteria have to metabolize the sugars and produce acid. Limiting consumption of risky foods to a short time span or with meals will limit the time of exposure to offending foods. For example, soda can be consumed along with other foods at a snack rather than sipped over the course of an hour or more. Hard candies or breath mints taken frequently cause similarly long exposure to sugars and should be limited. Putting a child to bed with a bottle or cup of a carbohydrate-containing beverage such as formula, milk, or juice allows the bacteria long exposure to these sugars, a habit that is responsible for much of the tooth decay of young childhood.

- *Sugar-free chewing gum:* Xylitol-sweetened chewing gums have been studied for a possible anticariogenic effect. Xylitol is one of the sugar alcohols used as a sugar substitute and is not metabolized by oral bacteria. Additionally, it may prevent plaque accumulation on the tooth surface. Other sugar alcohols found in chewing gum may have similar effects but to a lesser extent because of differences in bacterial metabolism. Chewing gum increases saliva flow, another beneficial effect for reducing risk of caries. Sugar alcohols as a group are not considered to contribute to the development of cavities.

Sources: Adapted from American Dietetic Association, 2004; American Dietetic Association, 2007; Burt, 2006; Touger-Decker & van Loveren, 2003.

Obesity and Weight Management

Much media attention has focused on blaming carbohydrate intake, or certain types of carbohydrates, for the ever-increasing amount of obesity reported in children and adults. Likewise, low-carbohydrate diets are popular with some as a way of managing weight. The truth about carbohydrates and weight most likely falls somewhere in the middle of these extreme views. Studies have focused on a possible relationship between high-carbohydrate intake and weight gain, specifically blaming sugar-sweetened beverages such as soda and fruit drinks. Daily intake of these beverages has increased over the last decade among children, especially those aged 6 to 11 years, where a 20% increase has been observed (Wang, Bleich, & Gortmaker, 2008). Although consumption of soft drinks and other sweetened beverages is associated with increased energy intake, these beverages in and of themselves have not been found to cause obesity (Forshee, Anderson, & Storey, 2008; Vartanian, Schwartz, & Brownell, 2007). Rather, it is excess energy intake from any source of calories that leads to weight gain. Of note, beverages in general are less satiating than solid foods. Studies have found that individuals do not compensate for the calorie intake of beverages in the same way that occurs with intake of solid food. Liquids cause less lasting fullness compared with solid foods. Additionally, there is less reduction, or compensation, in caloric intake elsewhere in the diet following intake compared with solid foods (Mattes, 2006; Wang et al., 2008). The nurse can advise those trying to manage weight to consume less sweetened beverages as a way of decreasing calorie intake but should correct any misinformation about the high-carbohydrate content causing weight gain at a rate different than excess calories from other sources, such as excess fat or alcohol. Population groups who traditionally consume a high-carbohydrate diet, such as vegetarians, generally weigh less compared with nonvegetarians (ADA, 2003; Berkow & Barnard, 2006). However, overall calorie intake is lower in this same population—a fact the nurse should reinforce when discussing weight management and carbohydrates.

Low-carbohydrate diets have ridden a wave of popularity over many years with a renewed interest in this method of weight management more recently. No one definition exists as to the amount of carbohydrate allowed in a low-carbohydrate diet—some diets are as low as 20 gm, whereas others approach 100 gm of carbohydrate/day. As a result, research results vary and are difficult to compare. Little long-term research exists comparing this category of diet with the more traditional low-calorie or low-calorie, low-fat diet. Short-term studies find that a low-carbohydrate diet for less than 6 months leads to faster weight loss than the traditional low-calorie diet, but this difference is erased when studied for up to 1 year (Adam-Perrot, Clifton, & Brouns, 2006; Gardner, et al., 2007; Nordmann et al., 2006). The use of such diets needs to be evaluated individually because there are potential negative side effects, such as unfavorable changes in blood lipid levels, increased loss of urinary calcium, and insufficient intake of nutrients traditionally found in the fruits, vegetables, whole grains, and milk that are limited by this diet. The Evidence-Based Practice Research Box discusses the use of low-carbohydrate diets. Further discussion on weight management is found in Chapter 17.

EVIDENCE-BASED PRACTICE RESEARCH BOX

Are low-carbohydrate diets a nutritionally sound way to lose weight?

Clinical Problem: Low-carbohydrate and very-low-carbohydrate diets are promoted for their ability to produce weight loss. Is there evidence to support this recommendation due to these diets' effectiveness and safety?

Research Findings: The recommended intake of carbohydrates (CHO) is 45–65% of daily calories or a minimum of 130 grams (or 520 calories) per day. Low-carbohydrate diets (less than 20% carbohydrate intake) and very-low-carbohydrate diets (less than 10% carbohydrate intake) promote weight loss by limiting carbohydrates as the main sources of energy and by increasing the proportion of protein in the diet. Several of the many studies that have looked at the effect of these diets on weight loss in obese individuals, those with diabetes mellitus (DM), and those with elevated lipid levels are reviewed.

A study that included 78 morbidly obese (BMI greater than 40) individuals, 86% of whom had DM or metabolic syndrome, compared the effects of low-carbohydrate and conventional diets on lipid levels over a period of 6 months. The researchers found that the low-carbohydrate diet had a more favorable effect on blood triglyceride and C-reactive protein but similar effects on LDL and HDL cholesterol as a conventional diet (Seshadri et al., 2006). Volek and colleagues (2004) found that a 4-week very-low-carbohydrate diet and a low-fat diet followed by 13 overweight women found that neither the LDL nor the HDL cholesterol, but insulin sensitivity was increased on the very-low-carbohydrate diet, a favorable result. A more recent study lowered the very-low-carbohydrate diet, compared to a low-fat diet, resulted in a significant decline in blood fatty-acid levels (Forsythe et al., 2008).

Individuals with diabetes have special concerns about serum lipid and glucose levels as well as weight management. A study by Dyson, Beatty, and Matthews (2007) followed 13 subjects with type 2 DM and 13 subjects with no DM for 3 months. They were randomized to either a low-carbohydrate (less than 40 grams of CHO per day) or "healthy eating" diet. There was a significantly greater

(continued)

Evidence-Based Practice Research Box *(continued)*

weight loss in the low-carbohydrate group, and there were no adverse effects of HbA(1c), a marker of long-term blood glucose levels, or lipid levels. Another study examined risk factors of DM and cardiovascular disease. Meckling, O'Sullivan, and Saari (2004) compared low-carbohydrate (15% CHO) and low-fat (18%) diets in 31 obese men and women. They found that the low-carbohydrate diet was as effective as the low-fat diet in promoting weight loss and that the low-carbohydrate diet had a significant decrease in circulating insulin.

Several more recent and larger studies explored the effects of low-carbohydrate or very-low-carbohydrate diets on weight loss. Gardner et al. (2007) compared the Atkins, Zone, Ornish, and LEARN diets in a randomized trial with 311 premenopausal overweight women. They found that the subjects on Atkins diet, which has the lowest CHO intake, had the greatest weight loss and most beneficial metabolic effects after 12 weeks on the diet. Another study assigned 88 individuals to either a low- or high-carbohydrate diet. Both diets resulted in weight loss with no significant difference between them (Tay, Brinkworth, Noakes, Keogh, & Clifton, 2008). Low-carbohydrate, Mediterranean, and low-fat diets were compared in a study conducted by Shai et al. (2008). Using 322 obese subjects, they found that the subjects on the low-carbohydrate diet had significantly

more weight loss and reduction in lipid levels over 1 year than those who followed the low-fat diet.

Perhaps most significantly, the American Diabetes Association finds low-carbohydrate and low-fat diets equally effective for up to 1 year for weight loss for individuals with diabetes (American Diabetes Association, 2008). Their position emphasizes the need for the individual to find a diet that is acceptable and one they can adhere to in order to lose weight. Their recommendation is coupled with the emphasis on sustained, moderate weight loss and increased physical activity. Adequate fiber intake and avoidance of excessive protein intake are also encouraged. Long-term use of a low-carbohydrate diet is discouraged because of lack of evidence concerning effects.

Nursing Implications: Current evidence supports the use of low-carbohydrate diets for weight loss in some individuals with positive to neutral effects on lipid levels. Individuals choosing this diet approach should be monitored for metabolic effects.

CRITICAL THINKING QUESTION:

1. How should the nurse respond to the individual who says that low-carbohydrate diets are just a fad and real weight loss can only come with reduction in calories and fat?

Behavior and Neurological Health

A long-held folk belief is that sugar causes hyperactive behavior, especially in children. Long-term research has not established a link between sugar intake and hyperactivity (ADA, 2004; IOM, 2002). Chapter 14 discusses other aspects of diet in hyperactivity and attention-deficit disorders.

An altered carbohydrate diet may be indicated in some children. In rare cases of intractable seizure disorders that do not respond to medications, a low-carbohydrate diet has been found to be effective although not without negative side effects. Hot Topic Box: Low-Carbohydrate Diets for Epilepsy outlines the use of this diet with this population of children.

Altered Digestion or Metabolism

Lactose intolerance occurs because of insufficient production of the enzyme lactase in the small intestine. As discussed, symptoms are a result of the disaccharide reaching the large intestine where it is fermented by bacteria. Treatment of lactose intolerance does not involve the complete elimination of lactose from the diet, but rather customized intake of a tolerable amount of lactose intake to preserve what lactase production does exist. Small amounts of lactose-containing foods, such as yogurt or some cheese, can generally be tolerated, especially when consumed with a meal. Special dairy products that are treated with lactase enzyme are available. Individuals find these to be sweeter tasting than regular milk products because the lactose is already converted to glucose and galactose in the

hot Topic

Low-Carbohydrate Diets for Epilepsy

Although the use of a low-carbohydrate diet for weight loss treatment is a controversial topic, this diet has been used in the treatment of drug-resistant seizure disorders in children since the 1920s with a resurgence in popularity over the last 10 years (Zupec-Kania & Spellman, 2009). Normally, glucose is the preferential fuel for the brain. Decades ago, it was discovered that children who had intractable epilepsy had diminished seizure activity when they fasted. The mechanism for this response was not understood at the time, but is now believed to be related to the production of ketone bodies, metabolic by-products of fat metabolism, that occur in the starved state. Ketone bodies can cross the blood-brain barrier and be used as an alternative fuel source by the brain in the absence of adequate glucose (Hartman, Gasior, Vining, & Rogawski, 2007). It is not clearly understood how the presence of ketone bodies in the brain suppress seizure activity; potential theories include a direct anti-seizure effect and alteration in neurotransmitter concentration, among others (Wiznitzer, 2008). Studies have reported between a 50% to 90% reduction in seizure activity on a low-carbohydrate diet, with some clients becoming seizure free (Zupec-Kania & Spellman, 2009).

Use of a low-carbohydrate diet is not without side effects. Some side effects are of little consequence, whereas others lead to nonadherence to the diet. The majority of children are prescribed the diet for a relatively short time span of months to a few years, after which the benefits of reduced seizure activity persists. Side effects of this treatment in children have included:

- *Growth faltering.* Growth is reported to slow because of a lack of overall calories in the diet when not planned carefully, poor palatability of high-fat foods that replace carbohydrates, and reduced hunger and lack of energy because of elevated ketone bodies in the blood (Peterson et al., 2005; Santoro & O'Flaherty, 2005). The nurse working with this pediatric population should be involved in the ongoing monitoring of growth and development, working closely with the dietitian to ensure adequate dietary intake or supplementation as appropriate. The dietitian is responsible for calculating a diet prescription that meets both nutritional needs and the careful ratio of carbohydrate to fat and protein that is essential to the success of this diet.
- *Kidney stones.* Approximately 5% of children will develop kidney stones on this diet, an outcome believed to be due to the acid pH that develops in the blood and urine from elevated ketone bodies (Freeman, Kossoff, & Hartman, 2007). Medicine, such as potassium citrate, can be given to counter this effect (Sampath, Kossoff, Furth, Pyzik, & Vining, 2007). The nurse should encourage intake of adequate fluid to prevent stone formation. Chapter 21 covers the treatment of kidney stones.
- *Elevated blood lipids.* Cholesterol levels have been reported to increase on this diet, but the long-term risk associated with this side effect in young children is not clear because most children do not stay on the low-carbohydrate diet indefinitely (Freeman et al., 2007).
- *Gastrointestinal complaints.* Nausea, vomiting, and constipation are among the more common complaints and can be cause for nonadherence (Neal et al., 2008). These effects occur early in treatment and are transient (Freeman et al., 2007).
- *Poor bone health.* Decreased bone density and increased risk of skeletal fractures has been reported (Groesbeck, Bluml, & Kossoff, 2006). It is unclear whether this effect can be prevented.

The health care team and client or guardian must weigh the benefits of potentially reducing seizure activity against the known risks associated with the diet. A well-informed nurse can assist the client and family in this decision making and offer supportive intervention if side effects are encountered.

container, giving it the sweeter taste than lactose. Chapter 20 contains a Client Education Checklist to use when educating the individual with lactose intolerance about diet.

Fructose maldigestion or intolerance causes symptoms similar to those of lactose intolerance. Unabsorbed fructose is fermented by colonic bacteria, leading to bloating and diarrhea. It has been postulated that some individuals who are diagnosed with a condition called irritable bowel syndrome may benefit from a modification in fructose intake to alleviate diarrhea and bloating symptoms that could be from fructose intolerance (Shepherd, Parker, Muir, & Gibson, 2008). A modified fructose diet limits intake of certain fruits and juices. Clients suspected of having fructose intolerance should be referred for medical testing to confirm this diagnosis to avoid overly restricting the diet unnecessarily.

Galactosemia is a genetic disorder that affects the metabolism of galactose because of enzyme deficiencies. Elevated blood

galactose levels can lead to life-threatening effects in a young infant. Symptoms appear in the first weeks after birth and include vomiting, diarrhea, enlarged liver, lethargy, cataracts, and excessive bleeding (Bosch, 2006; Kaye & the Committee on Genetics, 2006). Newborn screening for galactosemia is routine to allow for prompt dietary management. Infants are fed a galactose-free formula and later must avoid all sources of lactose because it is comprised of glucose and galactose. This diet devoid of dairy products must be followed indefinitely (Kaye & the Committee on Genetics, 2006). Long-term consequences of this disorder include developmental delay and poor growth despite dietary treatment.

The most commonly known dysfunction of carbohydrate metabolism is diabetes mellitus. Insufficient production of insulin by the pancreas leads to elevated circulating blood glucose levels and its associated symptoms. Diabetes occurs for different reasons as discussed in Chapter 19. Consumption of sugary foods is not one of the reasons diabetes occurs. Prevention of type 2 diabetes, associated with overweight and obesity, does not target limiting sugar intake, but rather encourages lifestyle modifications to manage weight (American Diabetes Association, 2008). Individuals with diabetes monitor and moderate carbohydrate intake as a way of managing blood glucose levels along with medical treatment. Chapter 19 outlines medical nutrition therapy for diabetes.

Fiber and Health

Adequate intake of fiber is associated with many health benefits. Intestinal health, weight management, and regulation of blood lipids and glucose are among the positive effects of a high-fiber diet.

Intestinal Health

Consumption of adequate fiber normalizes the transit time of substances through the intestinal tract and promotes laxation. Many sources of fiber increase stool bulk and weight and can ameliorate constipation (ADA, 2008; IOM, 2002). Herniations, or pockets called diverticula, in the colon wall can develop because of increased intestinal pressure from insufficient stool bulk and constipation. This condition is called **diverticulosis.** If these pockets become inflamed because of trapped bacteria, medical intervention is necessary. A high-fiber diet can prevent further development of diverticula as discussed in Chapter 20.

Whether or not fiber has an effect on the development of colon cancer is unclear. Some research points to the benefit of a quick intestinal transit time associated with a high-fiber diet because it limits exposure to potential carcinogens in the diet. In addition, the bacterial fermentation of fiber in the colon may produce beneficial by-products that have a potential cancer prevention role (IOM, 2002). Most authorities cite the lack of evidence that fiber specifically plays a role and instead encourage intake of a variety of fruits; vegetables; whole grains; and other plant-based, fiber-containing foods for the potential synergy of these components rather than their individual components (Kushi et al., 2006).

Weight Management

A high-fiber diet may benefit weight management in more than one way. High-fiber foods are generally less energy dense, meaning they have fewer calories compared with other foods of equal weight (for example, fatty foods) (ADA, 2008). Additionally, increased consumption of high-fiber foods often replaces higher-calorie foods in the diet when such lifestyle modifications are undertaken. High-fiber foods extend fullness because of the volume of these foods, which can limit intake of other foods. Some fibers delay gastric emptying, furthering the feeling of satiety (IOM, 2002).

Regulation of Blood Lipids and Glucose

Soluble fibers, such as oats, oatbran, barley, and apples, interfere with enterohepatic recycling of bile, a process that causes the reabsorption of bile acids in the small intestine. Bile acids used in fat digestion contain cholesterol and are normally reabsorbed and transported to the liver. By preventing the reabsorption of bile, cholesterol is excreted bound to the fiber and, therefore, some of the body's pool of cholesterol is reduced. The nurse can encourage increased intake of soluble fibers as one dietary intervention for elevated blood cholesterol levels. Chapter 18 outlines this dietary approach in more detail.

Consumption of a high-fiber diet is associated with improved postmeal blood glucose levels in diabetics (American Diabetes Association, 2008). In particular, some types of soluble fibers are known to slow gastric emptying and, therefore, absorption of glucose following a meal. This leads to lower blood glucose compared to after meals with nonfiber carbohydrates (IOM, 2002). The nurse can encourage those with diabetes to include fiber-containing foods regularly in the diet. Current recommendations for total fiber intake by individuals with diabetes are the same as for the general population (American Diabetic Association, 2008).

NURSING CARE PLAN Constipation

CASE STUDY

Brad, 31 years old, has come to the clinic for a general checkup prior to getting married in a month. He is an athletic trainer at a local health club and works out regularly in addition to running half-marathons. He reveals that he is eager to get the wedding over because all the planning is getting quite stressful. He doesn't have any particular concerns but is aware that his dad has hypertension and his mom has diverticulosis. During a review of systems, he confides to the nurse that he has "bad constipation" and has to take a laxative about once a week to "get things going." He says he can't understand why this is a problem because he feels he eats lots of protein to build up his muscles, exercises regularly, and drinks lots of water and sports drinks, including protein shakes. It seems to be getting worse and he wonders if there is something simple that can be done to correct this problem without medication.

Applying the Nursing Process

ASSESSMENT

Height: 6 feet Weight: 218 pounds BMI: 29.6
BP 128/74 P 68 R 14
Skin smooth and clear, moves extremities freely, good muscle tone
Hard, formed stool once or twice per week. Uses laxative once per week to "get cleaned out." Feels like he has to have a bowel movement but cannot. Barely audible bowel sounds

DIAGNOSES

Constipation related to decreased peristalsis evidenced by laxative use and feelings of rectal pressure
Knowledge, readiness for enhanced, related to health concern evidenced by request for information about constipation

EXPECTED OUTCOMES

Soft, formed bowel movement at least three times per week
Increase fiber content of diet to at least 25 grams per day
State high-fiber foods

INTERVENTIONS

Review high-fiber foods
Encourage at least 2,500 mL of water per day
Maintain activity level
Try to use the bathroom at the same time every day
Replace laxative with a stool softener for occasional use if dietary modifications seem ineffective

EVALUATION

A month later, Brad reports that small changes have had big results. He and his fiancée have switched to whole grain breads and muffins. He had been unaware that whole grain pasta was available and has found he likes the taste. He now knows he had been eating meat in large quantities in an effort to build more muscle but was not getting sufficient carbohydrates for energy and fiber. He realizes that this was contributing to his problem, so now he eats less meat and more whole grains, fruits, and veg-

Constipation *(continued)*

Assessment
Data about the patient

Subjective
What the patient tells the nurse
Example: "I need a laxative for a BM."

Objective
What the nurse observes; anthropometric and clinical data
Examples: BMI: 29, but very muscular

Diagnosis
NANDA label
Example: Constipation related to inadequate fiber intake

Planning
Goals stated in patient terms
Example: Long-term goal: soft, formed stool 3x per week; Short-term goal: increase fiber to 25 gm per day

Implementation
Nursing action to help patient achieve goals
Example: Replace some protein with carbohydrates with fiber; drink 2,500 mL water per day

Evaluation
Was the goal achieved or does the intervention need to be modified?
Example: Has soft, formed stool 2-3x per week without taking laxative

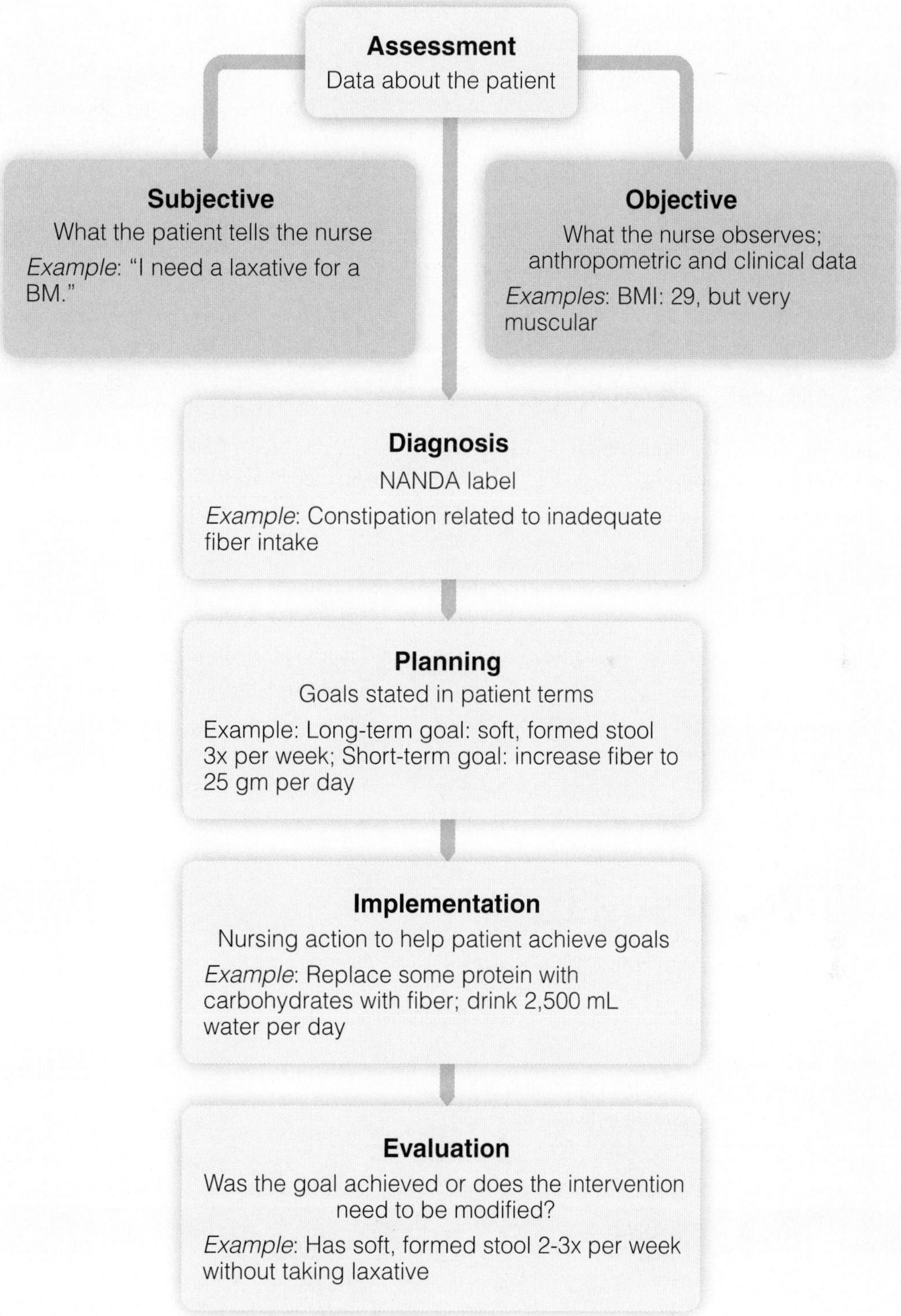

■ FIGURE 2-4 **Nursing Care Plan Process: Constipation.**

(continued)

Constipation *(continued)*

etables. He has stopped peeling the skins off fruits, such as apples and pears, before eating them and eats the skin when he has a baked potato. He said cutting out protein shakes has not been difficult and has saved money. He said it took a couple weeks for him to feel like he didn't need to use a laxative but he has had soft stools two or three times a week. Figure 2-4 ■ shows the nursing process for this case study.

Critical Thinking in the Nursing Process

1. **What are some high-fiber fruits and vegetables that the nurse can suggest for the client who is troubled with constipation?**

CHAPTER SUMMARY

- Carbohydrates are molecules that contain a carbon, hydrogen, and oxygen.

- Simple carbohydrates are less than three sugar molecules long.

- Complex carbohydrates have more than three sugar molecules.

- Carbohydrates are an essential component of the human diet.

- Simple carbohydrates are classified as monosaccharides or disaccharides.

- Complex carbohydrates consist of many sugar molecules.

- *Fiber* is a term that refers to polysaccharides that are not digested by the body.

- Fiber is usually broken down into two subcategories: soluble and insoluble.

- The functions of carbohydrates include provision of glucose for energy, sparing protein, and prevention of ketosis.

- Lactose intolerance and diabetes mellitus are examples of conditions arising from altered carbohydrate digestion or metabolism.

- Sugar substitutes are a way of reducing the amount of simple sugars that a person consumes.

EXPLORE PEARSON **mynursingkit**™

MyNursingKit is your one stop for online chapter review materials and resources. Prepare for success with additional NCLEX®-style practice questions, interactive assignments and activities, web links, animations and videos, and more!

Register your access code from the front of your book at
www.mynursingkit.com.

NCLEX® QUESTIONS

1. A middle-age client has begun a very-low-carbohydrate diet to lose weight. What possible consequences should the nurse be aware might occur with prolonged carbohydrate deficiency?
   1. Iron-deficiency anemia and weight loss
   2. Bleeding gums and muscle weakness
   3. Ketosis and metabolic acidosis
   4. Headaches and muscle weakness

2. The nurse has been teaching a client about low-carbohydrate diets. What response by the client indicates to the nurse that teaching has been effective?
   1. "I can only lose weight by cutting carbohydrate intake in half."
   2. "Each gram of carbohydrate that I eliminate from my diet should be replaced by a gram of protein."
   3. "Any carbohydrates I do eat should be fiber."
   4. "I need over 100 grams of carbohydrate every day to supply my brain with needed energy."

3. Which of the following foods would the nurse suggest for a client who wants to increase consumption of complex carbohydrates?
   1. Celery
   2. English muffins
   3. Whole wheat spaghetti
   4. Peaches

4. A client tells the nurse, "All artificial sweeteners are bad for you." How should the nurse respond?
   1. "Most are bad, but some have no harmful effects."
   2. "Artificial sweeteners have been studied and are approved by the Food and Drug Administration for use in foods and beverages."
   3. "A small amount on a daily basis is not likely to cause any harm to anyone."
   4. "Artificial sweeteners are good for you because they prevent tooth decay."

5. What foods can the nurse suggest to a client who is concerned about preventing diverticulosis?
   1. Peanut butter and bread
   2. Puffed wheat cereal and milk
   3. Apples and pears
   4. Buttered popcorn

REFERENCES

Adam-Perrot, A., Clifton, P., & Brouns, F. (2006). Low-carbohydrate diets: Nutritional and physiological aspects. *Obesity Reviews, 7,* 49–58.

American Diabetes Association. (2008). Nutrition recommendations and interventions for diabetes. A position statement of the American Diabetes Association. *Diabetes Care, 31,* S61–S78.

American Dietetic Association (ADA). (2003). Position of the American Dietetic Association and Dietitians of Canada: Vegetarian diets. *Journal of the American Dietetic Association, 1043,* 748–765.

American Dietetic Association (ADA). (2004). Position of the American Dietetic Association: Use of nutritive and nonnutritive sweeteners. *Journal of the American Dietetic Association, 104,* 255–275.

American Dietetic Association (ADA). (2007). Position of the American Dietetic Association: Oral health and nutrition. *Journal of the American Dietetic Association, 107,* 1418–1428.

American Dietetic Association (ADA). (2008). Position of the American Dietetic Association: Health implications of dietary fiber. *Journal of the American Dietetic Association, 108,* 1716–1731.

Berkow, S. E., & Barnard, N. (2006). Vegetarian diets and weight status. *Nutrition Reviews, 64,* 175–188.

Bosch, A. M. (2006). Classical galactosemia revisited. *Journal of Inherited Metabolic Disorders, 29,* 516–525.

Burt, B. A. (2006). The use of sorbitol and xylitol-sweetened chewing gum in caries control. *Journal of the American Dental Association, 137,* 190–196.

Centers for Disease Control and Prevention (CDC). (2004). Trends in intake of energy and macronutrients: United States, 1971–2000. *Morbidity and Mortality Weekly Review, 53,* 80–82.

Dyson, P. A., Beatty, S., & Matthews, D. R. (2007). A low-carbohydrate diet is more effective in reducing body weight than healthy eating in both diabetic and non-diabetic subjects. *Diabetic Medicine: A Journal of the British Diabetic Association, 24*(12), 1430–1435.

Federal Register. (1997). *Health claims: Dietary sugar alcohols and dental caries.* (Code of Federal Regulations, Title 21, Section CFR101.8). Retrieved October 26, 2008, from http://www.cfsan.fda.gov/~lrd/fr971202.html

Food & Drug Administration (FDA). (2006). Artificial sweeteners: No calories . . . sweet! *FDA Consumer, July–August.* Retrieved June 19, 2008, from http://www.fda.gov/fdac/features/2006/406_sweeteners.html

Forshee, R. A., Anderson, P. A., & Storey, M. L. (2008). Sugar-sweetened beverages and body mass index in children and adolescents: A meta-analysis. *American Journal of Clinical Nutrition, 87,* 1662–1671.

Forsythe, C. E., Phinney, S. D., Fernandez, M. L., Quann, E. E., Wood, R. J., Bibus, D. M., et al. (2008). Comparison of low fat and low carbohydrate diets on circulating fatty acid composition and makers of inflammation. *Lipids, 43*(1), 65–77.

Freeman, J. M., Kossoff, E. H., & Hartman, A. L. (2007). The ketogenic diet: One decade later. *Pediatrics, 119,* 535–543.

Ganong, W. F. (2005). *Review of medical physiology* (22nd ed.). New York: McGraw-Hill.

Gardner, C. D., Kiazand, A., Alhassan, S., Kim, S., Stafford, R. S., Balise, R. R., et al. (2007). Comparison of the Atkins, Zone, Ornish, and LEARN diets for change in weight and related risk factors among overweight premenopausal women. *Journal of the American Medical Association, 297,* 969–977.

Groesbeck, D. K., Bluml, R. M., & Kossoff, E. H. (2006). Long-term use of the ketogenic diet in the treatment of epilepsy. *Developmental Medicine and Child Neurology, 48,* 978–981.

Grotz, V. L. (2007). Sucralose and migraine. *Headache, 47,* 164–165.

Hartman, A. L., Gasior, M., Vining, E. P. G., & Rogawski, M. A. (2007). The neuropharmacology of the ketogenic diet. *Pediatric Neurology, 36,* 281–292.

Harvard College. (2005, June). Response to readers: More about stevia, a nonnutritive sweetener. *Harvard Women's Health Watch,* 6–7.

Health Canada. (2007). Eating well with Canada's Food Guide. Retrieved June 30, 2008, from http://www.hc-sc.gov/fn-an/food-guide-aliment/order-commander/index-eng.php

Institute of Medicine (IOM). (2002). *Dietary reference intakes for energy, carbohydrate, fiber, fat, fatty acids, cholesterol, protein, and amino acids.* Washington, DC: The National Academies Press. Retrieved August 15, 2007, from http://books.nap.edu/openbook.php?isbn=0309085373

Kaye, C. I., & the Committee on Genetics. (2006). Newborn screening fact sheets. *Pediatrics, 118,* e934–e963.

Kushi, L. H., Byers, T., Doyle, C., Courneya, K. S., Demark-Wahnefired, W., Grant, B., et al. (2006). American Cancer Society guidelines on nutrition and physical activity for cancer prevention: Reducing risk of cancer with healthy food choices and physical activity. *CA Cancer Journal for Clinicians, 56,* 254–281.

Magnusun, B. A., Burdock, G. A., Doull, J., Kroes, R. M., Marsh, G. M., Pariza, M. W., et al. (2007). Aspartame: A safety evaluation based on current use levels, regulations, and toxicological and epidemiological studies. *Critical Reviews in Toxicology, 37,* 629–727.

Mann, J. (2003). Sugar revisited—again. *Bulletin of the World Health Organization, 81,* 552.

Mattes, R. D. (2006). Beverages and positive energy balance: The menace is the medium. *International Journal of Obesity, 30,* S60–S65.

McKeown, N. M., Meigs, J. B., Liu, S., Wilson, P. W., & Jacques, P. F. (2002) Whole-grain intake is favorably associated with metabolic risk factors for type 2 diabetes and cardiovascular disease in the Framingham Offspring Study. *American Journal of Clinical Nutrition, 76*, 390–398.

Meckling, K. A., O'Sullivan, C., & Saari, D. (2004). Comparison of a low-fat diet to a low-carbohydrate diet on weight loss, body composition, and risk factors for diabetes and cardiovascular disease in free-living, overweight men and women. *The Journal of Clinical Endocrinology and Metabolism, 89*, 2717–2723.

Murray, R. K., Granner, D. K., & Rodwell, V. W. (2006). *Harper's illustrated biochemistry* (27th ed.). New York: McGraw-Hill.

Neal, E. G., Chaffe, H., Schwartz, R. H., Lawson, M. S., Edwards, N., Fitzsimmons, G., et al. (2008). The ketogenic diet for the treatment of childhood epilepsy: A randomized controlled trial. *Lancet Neurology, 7*, 500–506.

Nordmann, A. J., Nordmann, A., Briel, M., Keller, U., Yancy, W. S., Brehm, B. J., et al. (2006). Effects of low-carbohydrate vs. low-fat diets on weight loss and cardiovascular risk factors. *Archives of Internal Medicine, 166*, 285–293.

Peterson, S. J., Tangney, C. C., Pimental-Zablah, E. M., Hjelmgren, B., Booth, G., & Berry-Kravis, E. (2005). Changes in growth and seizure reduction in children on the ketogenic diet as treatment for intractable epilepsy. *Journal of the American Dietetic Association, 105*, 718–725.

Sampath, A., Kossoff, E. H.,, Furth, S. L., Pyzik, P. L., & Vining, E. P. (2007). Kidney stones and the ketogenic diet: Risk factors and prevention. *Journal of Child Neurology, 22*, 375–378.

Santoro, K. B., & O'Flaherty, T. (2005). Children and the ketogenic diet. *Journal of the American Dietetic Association, 105*, 725–726.

Schardt, D. (2004, May). Sweet nothings: Not all sweeteners are equal. *Nutrition Action Healthletter*, 6–9.

Schmidt, L. E., & Dalhoff, K. (2002). Food-drug interactions. *Drugs, 62*, 1481–1502.

Seshadri, P., Iqbal, N., Stern, L., Williams, M., Chicano, K. L., Daily, D. A., et al. (2004). A randomized study comparing the effects of a low-carbohydrate diet and a conventional diet on lipoprotein subfractions and C-reactive protein levels in patients with severe obesity. *The American Journal of Medicine, 117*(6), 398–405.

Shai, I., Schwarzfuchs, D., Henkin, Y., Shahar, D. R., Witkow, S., Greenberg, I., et al. (2008, July). Weight loss with a low-carbohydrate, Mediterranean, or low-fat diet. *New England Journal of Medicine, 229*–241.

Shepherd, S. J., Parker, F. C., Muir, J. G., & Gibson, P. R. (2008). Dietary triggers of abdominal symptoms in patients with irritable bowel syndrome: Randomized placebo-controlled evidence. *Clinical Gastroenterology and Hepatology, 6*, 765–771.

Tay, J., Brinkworth, G. D., Noakes, M., Keogh, J., & Clifton, P. M. (2008). Metabolic effects of weight loss on a very-low-carbohydrate diet compared with an isocaloric high-carbohydrate diet in abdominally obese subjects. *Journal of the American College of Cardiology, 51*(1), 59–67.

Touger-Decker, R., & van Loveren, C. (2003). Sugar and dental caries. *American Journal of Clinical Nutrition, 78*, 881S–892S.

U.S. Department of Agriculture (USDA). (2007a). *Nutrient intakes from food: Mean amounts and percentages of calories from protein, carbohydrate, fat, and alcohol, one day, 2003–2004.* Retrieved June 23, 2008, from http://www.ars.usda.gov/ba/bhnrc.fsrg

U.S. Department of Agriculture (USDA). (2007b). *Nutrient intakes from food: Mean amounts consumed per individual, one day, 2003–2004.* Retrieved June 23, 2008, from http://www.ars.usda.gov/ba/bhnrc.fsrg

U.S. Department of Agriculture. (2008). *Inside the pyramid.* Retrieved March 27, 2009, from http://www.mypyramid.gov

U.S. Department of Agriculture (USDA), & Department of Health and Human Services. (2005). *Dietary guidelines for Americans* (6th ed.). Washington, DC: U.S. Government Printing Office.

Vartanian, L. R., Schwartz, M. B., & Brownell, K. D. (2007). Effects of soft drink consumption is associated with increased energy intake and body weight. *American Journal of Public Health, 97*, 667–675.

Volek, J. S., Sharman, M. J., Gomez, A. L., DiPasquale, C., Roti, M., Pumerantz, A., et al. (2004). Comparison of a very-low-carbohydrate and low-fat diet on fasting lipids, LDL subclasses, insulin resistance, and postprandial lipemic responses in overweight women. *Journal of the American College of Nutrition, 23*(2), 177–184.

Wang, Y. C., Bleich, S. N., & Gortmaker, S. L. (2008). Increasing caloric contribution from sugar-sweetened beverages and 100% fruit juices among U.S. children and adolescents, 1988–2004. *Pediatrics, 121*, e1604–e1614.

Wheeler, M. L., & Pi-Sunyer, X. (2008). Carbohydrate issues: Type and amount. *Journal of the American Dietetic Association, 108*, S34–S39.

Wiznitzer, M. (2008). From observations to trials: The ketogenic diet and epilepsy. *Lancet Neurology, 7*, 471–472.

World Health Organization (WHO). (2003). *Report of a joint FAO/WHO consultation. Diet, nutrition and the prevention of chronic diseases* (WHO Technical Report Series 916). Geneva: Author.

Zupec-Kania, B. A., & Spellman, E. (2009). An overview of the ketogenic diet for pediatric epilepsy. *Nutrition in Clinical Practice, 23*, 589–596.

Rachael Pohle-Krauza

Protein 3

WHAT WILL YOU LEARN?

1. To relate the way proteins are formed from amino acids.
2. To differentiate the classification of amino acids and proteins.
3. To summarize the physiological functions of protein, including its role in tissue growth and maintenance, synthesis of other proteins, regulation of body processes and immune function, and provision of energy.
4. To illustrate the processes by which proteins are metabolized.
5. To classify the current recommendations for protein consumption and how requirements can change with certain diseases or conditions.
6. To appraise risk factors for protein malnutrition and formulate nursing interventions to reduce risk.

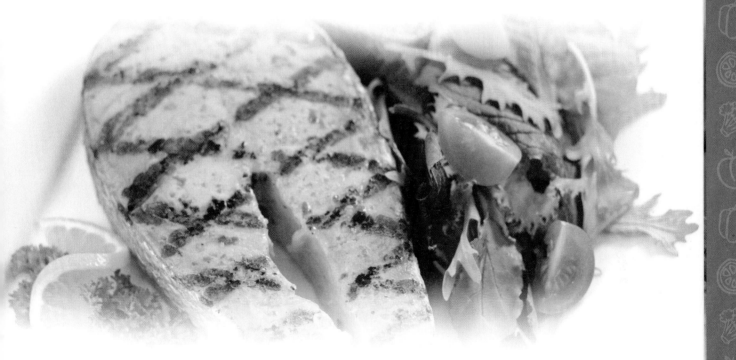

DID YOU KNOW?

▶ Protein provides the material to build our bones, muscles, skin, cartilage, and blood and to make hormones and enzymes that keep our bodies functioning properly.

▶ Most Americans eat approximately twice the recommended amount of protein per day!

▶ Protein that is consumed in excessive amounts can be metabolized and stored as fat.

▶ Foods of animal origin contain the most protein per serving, but beans and other legumes have significant amounts as well.

▶ With careful planning, it is possible to meet the body's requirements for protein without consuming meat.

KEY TERMS

Structure of Proteins

Protein is the major structural component of all cells within the body. Many hormones and membrane components are composed of protein as well as all enzymes, membrane carriers, blood transport molecules, and the intracellular matrices. Structural proteins allow different biological components to retain their shape. For example, connective tissue (cartilage) is composed of the proteins elastin and collagen, whereas keratin, another protein, is a key component of hair and fingernails.

Proteins are unique from carbohydrates or fats because they contain a nitrogen, which is also referred to as an amino group. In addition to nitrogen, proteins are composed of carbon, hydrogen, and oxygen. Some may also contain phosphorus, sulfur, iodine, or iron.

Amino Acids

Proteins are composed of building blocks known as **amino acids.** The basic chemical structure of all amino acids is similar as shown in Figure 3-1 ■. A hydrogen (H), amino group (NH_2), and an acid group are all attached to a central carbon (C). A fourth group, the side chain or functional group, differs between each amino acid and dictates the function of that amino acid. For example, some side chains can carry electrical charges or have **hydrophobic** or **hydrophilic**

properties, meaning that they repel or attract water. The amino acid glycine has the most basic structure with a single hydrogen as its side group, whereas other amino acids have more complex side groups. For example, phenylalanine, tryptophan, and tyrosine are categorized as aromatic amino acids because their chemical structure includes a benzene ring.

Amino acids are linked together by **peptide bonds.** When positioned in a particular order, they create proteins, and the specific sequence of amino acids in each protein is known as the **primary structure.** A **dipeptide** is two amino acids bonded together, whereas a **tripeptide** contains three amino acids. When 10 or more amino acids are joined together, they form a **polypeptide.** Polypeptides can contain more than 100 amino acids; proteins are an example of large polypeptides.

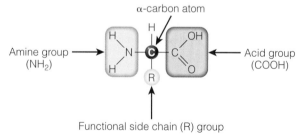

■ FIGURE 3-1 **Basic Chemical Structure of Amino Acids.**

Classification of Amino Acids

Amino acids are commonly classified into two groups: nonessential and essential. The **nonessential** (dispensable) **amino acids** are those that can be synthesized by the body using available simple molecules and are often derived from other amino acids. The **essential** (indispensable) **amino acids** are those that cannot be synthesized by the body and must be provided from dietary sources. For example, the **branched chain amino acids** (valine, leucine, and isoleucine) are classified as essential and are important for maintaining muscle tissue. In foods, the **limiting amino acid** is the essential amino acid found in the smallest quantity. For example, the limiting amino acids in cereals are lysine and threonine and the limiting amino acids in legumes are methionine and cysteine.

Amino acids may also be classified as **conditionally essential,** also called *acquired indispensable*. This means that under most conditions the body is able to synthesize adequate amounts of these amino acids; however, there may be certain physiological conditions when additional dietary sources are necessary in order to meet the needs of the body. For instance, babies who are born prematurely are unable to synthesize the amino acids cysteine and proline and, therefore, must obtain these from dietary sources. Similarly, individuals with severe liver disease are unable to properly metabolize phenylalanine and methionine. As a result, the amino acids tyrosine and cysteine (normally synthesized from phenylalanine and methionine) become essential until liver function returns to normal. In severe kidney disease, serine cannot be synthesized in sufficient quantities, thereby making its provision from outside sources essential. Glutamine is considered conditionally essential under circumstances of severe physiological stress, such as with burns, trauma, and other critical illness (Bongers, Griffiths, & McArdle, 2007). Chapter 22 discusses amino acid needs during physiological stress. Table 3-1 lists amino acids that have been classified as essential, nonessential, and conditionally essential.

Table 3-1 Essential, Nonessential, and Conditionally Essential Amino Acids

Essential (Indispensable)	Nonessential (Dispensable)	Conditionally Essential
Histidine	Alanine	Arginine
Isoleucine	Aspartic Acid	Cysteine
Leucine	Asparagine	Glutamine
Lysine	Glutamic Acid	Glycine
Methionine	Serine	Proline
Phenylalanine		Tyrosine
Threonine		
Tryptophan		
Valine		

Physiological Functions of Protein

Proteins participate in a variety of physiological functions that are vital for an organism to survive. These functions include tissue growth and maintenance, synthesis of other proteins, regulation of body processes and immune function, as well as provision of energy.

Tissue Growth and Maintenance

A primary function of protein is to supply material for the growth and maintenance of various body tissues. The body of an 80-kg (175-pound) man contains approximately 13 kg (29 pounds) of protein. Skeletal muscle accounts for about 43% of this protein, whereas the skin, blood, and other organs account for the remainder (Lenter, 1981).

Anabolism and Catabolism

The term **anabolism** refers to the production of new cellular material. For example, in a growing child, bone is formed from a protein (collagen) matrix along with various minerals. Similarly, the muscle cells in an athlete make new proteins in response to exercise, thereby increasing muscle mass. Proteins are also needed to replace old cells from skin, hair, and the gastrointestinal tract. **Catabolism,** the opposite of anabolism, is the breaking down or destruction of body tissues so that they can be reused or excreted. In the body, anabolism and catabolism are continuous and happen at the same time. Proteins are broken down into their constituent amino acids that are then used to make new proteins for growth or repair.

Nitrogen Balance

Although anabolism and catabolism occur simultaneously, they are not always in balance. Sometimes protein breakdown and excretion can exceed intake or vice versa. Dietary proteins provide about 1 gram of nitrogen for every 6.25 grams of protein consumed. This means that about 10 to 14 grams of nitrogen are excreted every day by a healthy adult consuming 60 to 90 grams of protein. When proteins are degraded, nitrogen is excreted through urine, feces, and sweat. **Nitrogen balance** refers to the difference between the amount of nitrogen taken in and the amount lost as described in Box 3-1. An individual is said to be in **nitrogen equilibrium,** or zero nitrogen balance, when the individual's nitrogen intake is equal to the nitrogen lost. Negative nitrogen balance indicates that a person is consuming less nitrogen and, therefore, protein, than excreted. This can occur as a result of inadequate protein intake or excessive loss. For example, injury from burns is considered to be a severe form of physiological stress and is characterized by an accelerated breakdown of lean body mass (skeletal muscle), resulting in negative nitrogen balance and wasting of these tissues (Prelack, Dylewski, & Sheridan, 2007). Clients who have sustained moderate to severe burns can remain in a state of severe negative nitrogen

BOX 3-1	Assessment of Nitrogen Balance

Although the majority of nitrogen loss occurs through the urine, sweat, and feces, small amounts of nitrogen can be lost in other ways as well. Thus, the calculation of nitrogen balance requires that intake of protein is tightly measured and estimation of nitrogen losses through the urine, feces, skin (sweat and dermal cells), and other miscellaneous means (i.e., hair, toothbrushing, and exhaled ammonia) occurs (Rand, Pellett, & Young, 2003). In a clinical setting, these losses are difficult to quantify. Therefore, in many cases, nitrogen balance is estimated by using laboratory measurements of urinary urea nitrogen (UUN). The nurse plays a crucial role in this careful calculation. Dietary intake of all food and fluids must be accurately recorded for 24 hours for the dietitian to calculate nitrogen intake. Urinary urea nitrogen calculations are obtained from a 24-hour urine collection to calculate nitrogen losses. A factor of 4 grams of nitrogen is added to the nitrogen losses to account for the insensible losses that cannot be directly measured (Chopra & McVay, 2003).

- What effect would it have on nitrogen balance calculations if a client mistakenly did not use the collection jug even once while urinating over the 24-hour collection period? How could the nurse emphasize the importance of adherence to accurate collection?

balance despite intake of adequate calories. Similarly, clients who are critically ill as a result of bacterial or other systemic infections show a catabolic response and negative nitrogen balance (Marik, 2004). Therefore, it is important to provide adequate protein in addition to kilocalories in these clients. Chapter 22 outlines physiological stress and nutritional requirements further. Table 3-2 describes several laboratory studies that may be useful in assessing protein nutritional status in clients. Chapter 12 covers this topic in more detail.

In contrast to negative nitrogen balance, when individuals consume more nitrogen than they excrete, they are in a state of positive nitrogen balance. Young, growing children, pregnant women, and adults who are recovered from an illness are often in this state because their net intake of nitrogen exceeds what is lost through urine, feces, and sweat.

Protein Synthesis

Simply defined, **protein synthesis** is the process by which cells build proteins that are specific to the needs of the body. Protein synthesis occurs in cellular organelles called ribosomes where the structure of the protein is determined by a specific genetic code. This code is contained in a form known as deoxyribonucleic acid (DNA) and is located within the nucleus

of the cell. Messenger ribonucleic acids (mRNA) copy the amino acid code contained in DNA and bring it outside the nucleus where it attaches to ribosomes. Then another form of RNA, transfer RNA (tRNA), is responsible for transporting amino acids from the cellular fluid to the mRNA and ribosomes. Through a series of events, tRNA, mRNA, and the ribosomes all act together to put the amino acids together in the correct sequence to make a new protein. Figure 3-2 ■ shows the sequence of events by which protein synthesis occurs.

The Regulatory Role of Proteins

Proteins are necessary for manufacturing enzymes and hormones, and they play an essential role in the maintenance of fluid balance. These functions are essential for regulating processes in the body.

Enzymes

Enzymes are proteins that exist in all cells of living things. They allow biochemical reactions to accelerate and are necessary for many body functions, including digestion and metabolism. Table 3-3 lists common categories of enzymes. A specific example of an enzyme is salivary amylase in the mouth that helps to break down starches from ingested foods.

Table 3-2	Serum Proteins Used to Assess Protein Nutritional Status				
Laboratory	Normal Value	Mild Malnutrition	Moderate Malnutrition	Severe Malnutrition	Nonnutritional Causes of Altered Value
Albumin	3.5–5 gm/L	2.8–3.4 gm/L	2.1–2.7 gm/L	Less than 2.1 gm/L	Inflammation, infection, liver disease, renal losses
Transferrin	200–400 mg/L	180–200 mg/L	160–180 mg/L	Less than 160 mg/L	Inflammation, infection, iron deficiency, liver disease, renal losses
Prealbumin	150–350 mg/L	110–150 mg/L	50–109 mg/L	Less than 50 mg/L	Inflammation, infection, liver disease, renal losses

Sources: Adapted from Beck & Rosenthal, 2002; Fuhrman, Charney, & Mueller, 2004; Omran & Morley, 2000; Shenkin, Cederblad, Elia, & Isaksson, 1996.

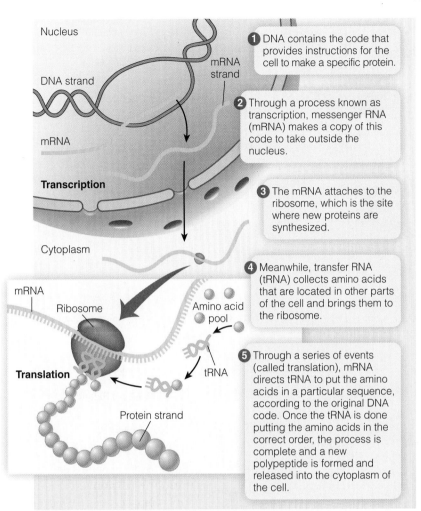

Nucleus

DNA strand

mRNA

Transcription

mRNA strand

Cytoplasm

mRNA

Ribosome

Translation

Amino acid pool

tRNA

Protein strand

❶ DNA contains the code that provides instructions for the cell to make a specific protein.

❷ Through a process known as transcription, messenger RNA (mRNA) makes a copy of this code to take outside the nucleus.

❸ The mRNA attaches to the ribosome, which is the site where new proteins are synthesized.

❹ Meanwhile, transfer RNA (tRNA) collects amino acids that are located in other parts of the cell and brings them to the ribosome.

❺ Through a series of events (called translation), mRNA directs tRNA to put the amino acids in a particular sequence, according to the original DNA code. Once the tRNA is done putting the amino acids in the correct order, the process is complete and a new polypeptide is formed and released into the cytoplasm of the cell.

■ **FIGURE 3-2 Protein Synthesis.**

In the stomach, the enzyme pepsin breaks dietary proteins down into smaller peptide units. Similarly, the pancreatic enzymes trypsin, lipase, and amylase further aid in the digestion of proteins, fats, and carbohydrates, respectively. Enzymes serve as **catalysts** for many biochemical reactions, meaning that they can alter the rate of a reaction without being changed or consumed in the process. Furthermore, enzymes are very specific to their **substrates** (reactants) and reactions that they catalyze. Figure 3-3 ■ demonstrates the way in which an enzyme interacts with its specific substrate.

Table 3-3	Common Categories of Enzymes
Enzyme Type	**Function**
Hydrolase	Cleaves (breaks apart) compounds
Isomerase	Transfers atoms within molecules
Transferase	Moves functional groups
Oxidoreductase	Transfers electrons
Ligase	Joins compounds together

Hormones

Hormones are chemicals released by glands in the body that are carried through the bloodstream to have effects on other parts of the body. Hormones act as messengers or signals to relay instructions to stop or start certain physiological processes. For example, the sex hormones estrogen and progesterone are responsible for controlling a woman's sexual development and reproductive capability. Proteins are a component of some hormones. Thyroid hormones, including thyroxine (T_4) and triiodothyronine (T_3), are responsible for a number of functions, including regulation of metabolic rate and cellular development. Two other hormones, insulin and glucagon, are synthesized in the pancreas and play an integral role in maintaining stability of blood glucose concentrations. Insulin is secreted in response to elevated blood glucose to facilitate entry of glucose into cells. Glucagon is secreted in response to low blood glucose to facilitate the release of glycogen from the liver for gluconeogenesis.

Fluid and pH Balance

Because they contain amino acids, proteins can act as **buffers.** In the body, a buffer is a compound that allows the

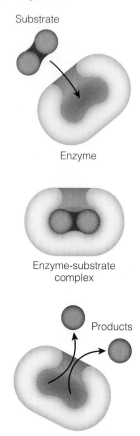

Substrate

Enzyme

Enzyme-substrate
complex

Products

■ FIGURE 3-3 **Mechanism of Enzyme Activity.**

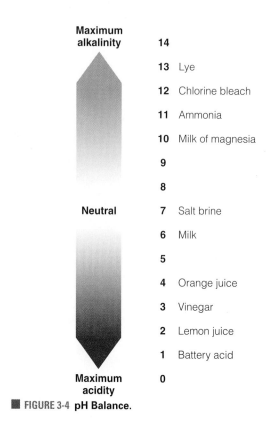

Maximum
alkalinity   **14**

13   Lye

12   Chlorine bleach

11   Ammonia

10   Milk of magnesia

9

8

Neutral   **7**   Salt brine

6   Milk

5

4   Orange juice

3   Vinegar

2   Lemon juice

1   Battery acid

Maximum
acidity   **0**

■ FIGURE 3-4 **pH Balance.**

fluids and tissues to keep a constant pH, even when they are exposed to an acidic or basic substance. Figure 3-4 ■ explains pH in more detail. Amino acids are able to release or accept hydrogen ions, so they are a major contributor to the physiological buffering system.

    Proteins are also essential for maintaining proper fluid balance. Along with fluid in the blood, proteins such as albumins and globulins are present in the capillary beds or thin blood vessels that connect the arteries and veins. The fluid is pushed from inside the capillaries into the extracellular space by blood pressure; however, the proteins stay behind because they are too large to move out. These remaining proteins serve to pull the fluid back inside the capillary, counteracting the pressure of the blood. This effect is referred to as **oncotic pressure** or colloid osmotic pressure. When intake of protein is inadequate, the number of blood proteins in the capillaries is reduced so that insufficient amounts of fluid are pulled back inside. This results in a condition known as **edema** when the fluids accumulate inside the tissue, causing the tissue to swell. Individuals with protein malnutrition or advanced liver disease, where production of plasma proteins diminishes, exhibit this effect. The nurse would notice edema of the extremities or accumulation of fluid in the midsection, called ascites. Figure 3-5 ■ is an example of a child with protein malnutrition with edema.

Immune Function

Proteins are a vital component in cells used during an **immune response.** The immune response is the way the body identifies and defends itself against antigens that are derived from harmful materials, such as viruses, bacteria, or other foreign matter. When the body detects antigens, it

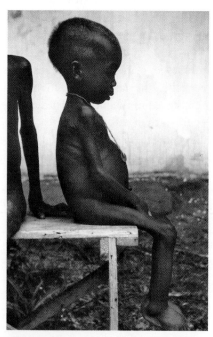

■ FIGURE 3-5 **Protein Malnutrition and Fluid Balance.**
Source: CDC/Dr. Lyle Conrad.

synthesizes **antibodies,** which are large protein molecules that attach to the antigen susceptible to destruction by other immune cells. Each antibody is created in order to attack one specific antigen. Once a specific antibody is manufactured, the body keeps a record of its characteristics so that the next time the antigen appears, the antibodies will be made more quickly and the immune response happens more rapidly.

Energy

Under normal circumstances, the body prefers to use carbohydrates and fats as fuel for working tissues. However, when there is inadequate energy supply, the body will begin to break down its own muscle tissue for conversion to energy. This ultimately results in depletion of lean body tissue. In order to preserve lean body mass, intake of all macronutrients is essential. When protein is utilized for energy, it supplies 4 kcalories/gm, the same as a carbohydrate.

Protein Metabolism

Similar to other macronutrients, proteins have their own unique metabolic pathways. Figure 3-6 ■ depicts a general overview of protein metabolism. Proteins and amino acids can also be reassembled through the process of protein synthesis, discussed in the preceding section.

Protein Digestion

After mastication by the teeth and mouth, proteins from foods are further degraded in the stomach by hydrochloric acid (HCl) through a process known as **denaturation,** which alters the structure of the protein by breaking apart some of the bonds that hold it together. On its own, HCl is unable to break all of the bonds. However, it activates the enzyme pepsin that can then break the remaining bonds. The products of protein digestion in the stomach include polypeptides and some free amino acids, and these end products are emptied into the small intestine for further digestion.

In the small intestine, partially digested proteins elicit the release of regulatory peptides from the intestinal endocrine cells. These regulatory peptides, including cholecystokinin (CCK) and secretin, act as signals to the pancreas to release pancreatic juice and digestive proenzymes. In turn, these proenzymes activate other enzymes that are then able to further degrade polypeptides and amino acids. Table 3-4 lists some of the enzymes responsible for gastric and intestinal protein digestion along with respective proenzyme activators and site of action.

After intestinal degradation, some small peptides and free amino acids are used by intestinal cells for energy and synthesis of other compounds. The remaining amino acids are absorbed through the intestinal brush border into the interstitial

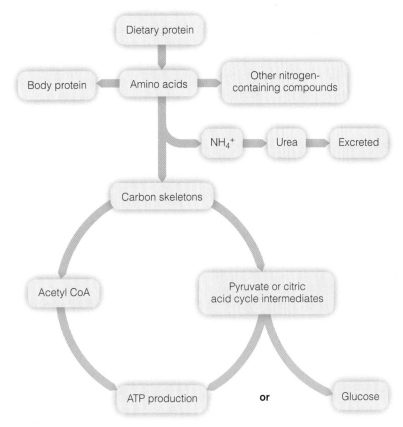

■ **FIGURE 3-6 Summary of Protein Metabolism.**

Table 3-4 Some Enzymes That Participate in Protein Digestion

Enzyme	Activated By (Proenzyme)	Site of Action
Pepsin	Pepsinogen	Stomach
Trypsin	Trypsinogen	Intestine
Chymotrypsin	Chymotrypsinogen	Intestine
Carboxypeptidases	Procarboxypeptidase	Intestine

fluid and capillaries where they are eventually transported to the liver. The liver monitors the amount of amino acids that are absorbed and adjusts the rate of their metabolism according to the needs of the body.

Amino Acid Catabolism

As previously discussed, protein degradation results in the release of free amino acids that are transported to the liver, where they are further degraded as needed by the body. There are several components to amino acid catabolism. **Deamination** is the process by which nitrogen is removed. Nitrogen removal can result in the accumulation of ammonia, which is toxic to the nervous system. For that reason, the body converts ammonia to urea for excretion by the kidneys. The carbon skeleton that remains after deamination can be used for energy or to make other substances. Amino acids can also be modified through **transamination,** or the transfer of the nitrogen from one chemical group to another without the formation of ammonia.

Amino Acid Pool

Within the cells of the body, **protein turnover** refers to the process by which proteins are continuously being synthesized and degraded at the same time. New amino acids, derived from the diet, mix with the amino acids that already exist in the body to form an **amino acid pool** within the tissues and blood. The rate between protein intake and synthesis and that of protein degradation may not be consistent, yet the amounts and types of amino acids within the pool remain relatively stable. A stable amino acid pool allows amino acids to be used to make other compounds as needed regardless of their source.

Protein from Food Sources

In developed countries where dietary protein is abundant, people generally consume adequate quantities in order to meet needs for specific amino acids. However, in countries where food sources are scarce, people may consume much less protein, making its quality become an important factor. The **protein quality** of a food is determined by the types and amounts of amino acids it contains and how well it can be digested. Protein digestibility depends on a variety of factors,

including the source of the protein and the other foods with which it is consumed. The digestibility of proteins from animal sources is high, whereas plant proteins are less digestible. The quality of protein is best quantified by calculating its **protein digestibility-corrected amino acid (PDCAA) score.** The PDCAA score corrects the amino acid composition of a food protein for digestibility, then compares this value to that of the human requirement for the essential amino acids. Some may refer to this as the biological value of a protein. In terms of PDCAA scores, a value of 1 is the highest and 0 the lowest. Examples for values of several common food items include eggs (1.0), milk (1.0), soy protein (1.0), beef (0.92), kidney beans (0.68), lentils (0.52), peanuts (0.52), and wheat (0.25).

Complete and Incomplete Proteins

Protein from food sources can be divided according to quality into two main categories: **complete** (high-quality) **proteins** and **incomplete** (low-quality) **proteins.** A complete protein contains all of the essential amino acids in the correct amounts needed by humans. Animal proteins such as meat, poultry, eggs, dairy, and seafood, along with the plant protein soy, are typically considered to be complete sources of protein with the exception of gelatin. This is because although gelatin is derived from animal protein, it lacks the essential amino acid tryptophan.

Alternatively, incomplete proteins tend to contain too little of one or more of the essential amino acids. Incomplete proteins generally come from plant sources, including beans (other than soy), peas, nuts, seeds, and grain. A small amount of incomplete protein is also found in vegetables. Incomplete proteins from nonanimal sources can be combined to provide all of the essential amino acids. Proteins from different sources that combine to form a complete protein are known as **complementary proteins.** Consumption of complementary proteins at the same meal is not necessary; current recommendations suggest that a variety of protein sources be consumed over the course of a day without concern for matching complementary proteins at a given meal as long as adequate calories are also consumed (American Dietetic Association [ADA], 2003). Examples of combined, complete plant proteins are those contained in peanut butter and wheat bread, in rice and beans, or in milk and wheat cereal. Incomplete proteins from plant sources can usually be combined with small amounts of animal-derived protein to make a complete protein. Macaroni and cheese is an example of one such combination.

Protein and Satiety

In recent years, the role of dietary protein as a factor in controlling **satiety** and **satiation** has been the subject of much interest. Although they are often used interchangeably, satiety and satiation are two separate concepts. Satiation refers to the processes that affect the termination of a meal, whereas satiety refers to the effects of a food or a meal on future food intake. Research has demonstrated a correlation between serum amino acid concentrations and fluctuations in appetite (Potier, Darcel, & Tome, 2009). Dietary protein can limit food intake by stimulating the release of peptide hormones, which subsequently affect food intake (Aziz, Anderson, Giacca, & Cho, 2005). As a macronutrient, protein appears to be more satiating than either carbohydrate or fat, although there is some conflicting evidence (Potier et al., 2009). Additionally, dietary protein digestion can increase total energy expenditure because of increased energy required for protein metabolism compared with carbohydrate or fat metabolism (Soenen & Westerterp-Plantenga, 2008). Further research is needed to demonstrate the immediate effects of dietary protein on food intake, satiety, and satiation as well as the degree to which it participates in the regulation of long-term energy balance.

Requirements for Dietary Protein

The dietary reference intakes (DRIs) provide a summary of estimated protein needs for different groups. Protein requirements may also change when an individual sustains illness or injury. The recommended dietary allowances (RDAs) component of the DRI refers to a level of intake that will meet the requirements for a defined level of adequacy (for protein) for 97.5% of a particular age and sex group. For adults, daily protein recommendation for all adults aged 19 to 70 years is approximately 0.8 gm/kg/day (Box 3-2). Estimations for pregnant women, infants, and children are slightly more than this and are summarized in Table 3-5. The average usual protein intakes for adults aged 19 to 30 years is 91 gm/day (Flugoni, 2008). This amount is likely to exceed estimated require-

Table 3-5 Estimated Protein Requirements for Infants and Children

Group	Dietary Reference Intake	Estimated Protein Need
Pregnant Women	RDA	1.1 gm/kg/day
Infants (0–6 months)	AI*	1.52 gm/kg/day
Older Infants (7–12 months)	RDA	1.5 gm/kg/day
Children (1–3 years)	RDA	1.1 gm/kg/day
Children (4–13 years)	RDA	0.95 gm/kg/day
Adolescents (14–18 years)	RDA	0.85 gm/kg/day

*Based on average volume and protein composition of human milk intake.
Source: Adapted from IOM, 2002.

ments for the majority of people in this age range. Average usual intake in the older adult is 66 gm/day (Flugoni, 2008). The need for total protein is reported by some to be no different than that of a younger adult (Campbell, Johnson, McCabe, & Carnell, 2008). Other researchers point to the fact that recommendations for protein intake in older adults is based on nitrogen balance studies in young adults and that muscle loss in the older adult is not prevented with the recommended intake of protein (Millward, 2008). The nurse working with the older adult should assess the diet for adequate intake of energy and protein to ensure that needs are being met for both nutrients. A lack of adequate energy intake contributes to the use of protein as an energy source rather than its needed role in synthesis of other proteins.

Wellness Concerns

Wellness concerns can arise because of insufficient or excessive protein intake as well as from metabolic errors that are inherited.

Inborn Errors of Protein Metabolism

An **inborn error of metabolism** refers to a disorder caused by an inherited defect in an enzyme pathway that affects the way in which the body metabolizes substrates. There are a number of inborn errors of metabolism that are specific to protein, and the majority of hospitals screen infants at the time of birth. Several of these disorders are described here.

Phenylketonuria

Phenylketonuria (PKU) disease is most often caused by a deficiency of phenylalanine hydroxylase, the enzyme responsible for converting the amino acid phenylalanine to tyrosine.

BOX 3-2	Estimating Daily Protein Needs

The DRIs recommend that adults consume approximately 0.8 gram of protein per kilogram of body weight per day. For example, in a man weighing 70 kg:

$$70 \text{ kg} \times 0.8 \text{ gm/kg} = 56 \text{ gm protein per day}$$

MyNursingKit PKU

MyNursingKit MSUD

In the United States, PKU affects approximately 1 in 25,000 (American College of Medical Genetics, 2005). Left untreated, PKU causes harmful accumulation of phenylalanine, which results in nerve damage that causes mental retardation and other health problems. A person who has PKU disease must follow a diet that contains very little phenylalanine. This restriction means that foods that contain high amounts of protein, such as milk, dairy products, meat, fish, chicken, eggs, beans, and nuts, must be limited (MacDonald & Asplin, 2006). However, if the disease is detected early and treated properly, a normal lifespan can be achieved (Giovannini, Verduci, Salvatici, & Fiori, 2007). In order to meet nutrient needs, people with PKU consume special phenylalanine-free dietary supplements that contain additional protein, micronutrients, and energy. The whole health care team is involved in the care of individuals with PKU. Careful monitoring of plasma phenylalanine levels is done especially in infants, children, and pregnant females. Referral to a registered dietitian for nutrition intervention is essential. Chapter 13 further discusses the importance of adherence to dietary restrictions during pregnancy to avoid negative effects on the fetus.

Branched Chain Ketoaciduria

Branched chain ketoaciduria is caused by a deficiency of the metabolic enzyme branched chain α-keto acid dehydrogenase, whose role is to degrade the branched chain amino acids (BCAAs) leucine, isoleucine, and valine. Deficiency of this enzyme causes a buildup of BCAAs and their toxic byproducts in the blood and urine. The disease is commonly called maple syrup urine disease (MSUD) because of the presence of sweet-smelling urine in infants with this disease. MSUD affects approximately 1 in 200,000 individuals, but the incidence is far higher among those belonging to the Old Order Mennonites, where it affects almost 1 in 350 births (Puffenberger, 2003). Severe neurological damage and death occur if this disease is not treated with timely dietary modification and close monitoring of the blood. Because BCAAs are also classified as essential amino acids, special protein formulas containing substitutes and adjusted levels of the amino acids are available so that clients with MSUD are able to meet nutrient requirements without experiencing harmful effects of the disease (Hallam, Lilburn, & Lee, 2005).

Protein Requirements in Illness or Injury

In situations of severe illness or trauma, adequate provision of protein is vital in order to promote healing and to prevent loss of lean body mass. Critical injury inflicts severe stress to the body, causing accelerated tissue breakdown and resulting in negative nitrogen balance and loss of body mass. Protein requirements are greatly elevated in trauma, sepsis (severe bacterial infection), and brain injury, or when a person has sustained burns or other large wounds or is undergoing certain types of

kidney replacement therapy (dialysis). Providing 1.5 grams of protein per kilogram of ideal body weight per day is usually adequate for those who are critically ill, but in persons with severe burns, even higher intake is appropriate because of excess losses from wounds (Powell-Tuck, 2007). In contrast, in certain types of kidney or liver failure, protein must be reduced because the body's ability to effectively metabolize proteins has been compromised. Further information on protein needs during illness is presented in the respective chapters on clinical nutrition.

The nurse can offer advice about increasing protein intake when indicated. The Client Education Checklist: Tips for Increasing Dietary Protein outlines options for good sources of dietary protein. When an increase in quality or quantity of intake is difficult for a client, the nurse may suggest use of an oral liquid supplement as suggested in Practice Pearl: Nutrition Supplements.

Protein Malnutrition

Protein malnutrition can occur when an individual has insufficient intake of nitrogen-containing foods (protein) in order to maintain nitrogen balance. It also refers to the related conditions kwashiorkor and marasmus. **Kwashiorkor** is a form of malnutrition where the person may have adequate energy (calorie) intake but insufficient intake of protein. Symptoms include edema, hair discoloration, and altered skin pigmentation. **Marasmus,** a type of protein-energy malnutrition (PEM), occurs with inadequate consumption of energy, where protein status also becomes compromised. Common symptoms include abnormally dry or loose skin folds, altered pigmentation of the hair, and severe loss of tissue from normal areas of fat deposits like the buttocks and thighs. Both kinds of malnutrition can make a person more susceptible to infection and disease because of the compromised immunity and micronutrient deficiency that accompany malnutrition. Kwashiorkor usually occurs in children living in underdeveloped countries after they are weaned from breast milk and are no longer consuming a good source

PRACTICE PEARL

Nutrition Supplements
Clients presenting with increased energy needs, decreased oral intake of foods or fluids, or with protein or energy malnutrition will often be prescribed a liquid oral nutrition supplement, such as Boost® or Ensure®. Supplements should be used as an adjunct to meals and snacks, not as meal replacements. Serving liquid supplements with meals can result in diminished intake of food and no overall increase in intake. Nursing staff should promote intake of food items from meals and snacks first, and then administer supplements afterward. Liquid supplements can be used when passing medications in place of other liquids, as long as there is no known food–drug interaction.

Tips for Increasing Dietary Protein

Although the majority of individuals in developed countries consume sufficient amounts of protein, there may be certain populations who have inadequate intakes because of poor diet quality or increased needs (secondary to stress or disease). Uses for the following protein-containing foods may be helpful for those wanting to increase the amount of protein in their diet.

Food	Approximate Protein per Serving (gm)	Use in . . .
Ice Cream, Yogurt or Frozen Yogurt	5–13 gm per 8 oz serving	• Add to cereals, fruits, gelatin desserts, and pies. • Mix with carbonated drinks such as root beer or ginger ale, and to milk drinks such as milkshakes. • Blend or whip with soft or cooked fruits (e.g., smoothie). • Sandwich ice cream or frozen yogurt between cake slices, cookies, or graham crackers.
Nuts and Seeds	5 gm per oz	• Sprinkle on fruit, cereal, ice cream, yogurt, vegetables, and salads. • Use in recipes as substitute for bread crumbs. • Add to casseroles, breads, muffins, pancakes, cookies, and waffles. • Blend with cream and herbs to make sauce for other main/side dishes. • Roll bananas or other cut fruits in chopped nuts.
Legumes	7–9 gm per 1/2 cup	• Use canned or cooked dried peas and beans in soups or add to casseroles, pastas, and grain dishes that also contain meat or cheese. • Use bean curd (tofu) in stir-fried dishes, casseroles, and desserts. • Puree cooked or canned beans with herbs and use as sandwich spread or as a dip for raw vegetables or fruits.
Cheese	3–7 gm per oz	• Melt on sandwiches, bread or other bread products, meats, eggs, and vegetables. • Melt and use as a dip for cut vegetables and/or cubed bread or cooked meat (e.g., fondue). • Add to sauces, soups, casseroles, or other vegetable or starch side dishes. • Use ricotta or cottage cheese in lasagna or to stuff pasta shells or manicotti.
Eggs	6 gm per egg	• Use with cheese, meat, and vegetables to make omelets or scrambled eggs. • Hard-cook eggs and add to salads, vegetables, or starch dishes and casseroles. • Add extra yolks to quiches, puddings, pancake, and french toast batter (before cooking). • Make custard with egg yolks, milk, and sugar. • Use hard-cooked eggs to make deviled eggs and make egg salad sandwich spreads.
Peanut Butter	4 gm per tablespoon	• Use as a spread for sandwiches, crackers, and other bread products. • Use as a dip for raw vegetables and fruits. • Blend with ice cream and milk to make a milkshake. • Blend with ice cream and yogurt/frozen yogurt.
Meats/Fish	7 gm per oz	• Use in omelets, or chop for use in sandwich fillings. • Wrap in pie crust or biscuit dough to make turnovers. • Eat organ meats (e.g., calf liver or chicken liver or heart) because they are especially good sources of protein, vitamins, and minerals.
Milk	8 gm per cup	• Use milk in place of water in beverages and/or in cooking whenever possible (e.g., in preparation of foods such as hot cereal, soups, or cocoa). • Use in pudding or custard. • Use in cream sauces to be added to vegetables and other dishes. • Add nonfat, dry, powdered milk to regular milk, cream soups, and vegetable or meat dishes.

of protein. Marasmus may occur in underdeveloped countries where food sources are scarce, in persons with severe wasting diseases such as acquired immune deficiency syndrome (AIDS) or cancer, or in the elderly population. Lifespan Box: Malnutrition in the Older Adult outlines the important issue of protein malnutrition among older adults.

The treatment of protein malnutrition includes identifying the cause and formulating interventions that address contributing factors. Adequate intake of protein and energy is essential. Without adequate energy intake, protein intake can be sacrificed for energy use instead of as a building block for needed protein synthesis.

High-Protein Diets

The health consequence of chronic consumption of excess protein is the subject of much debate. The on-again, off-again popularity of high-protein diets for weight loss and the tendency for bodybuilders to consume excessive protein has garnered some attention by the scientific community. The Evidence-Based Practice Box discusses the issue of protein and amino acids that are used by some athletes. In addition to the issues outlined in Chapter 2 regarding low-carbohydrate, high-protein diets, concern exists that excess protein intake can negatively affect kidney and bone health. A review of the effects of high-protein intake on kidney health is found in Hot Topic Box: High-Protein Diets and Kidney Health. Cultural

Lifespan

Malnutrition in the Older Adult

Studies have shown that up to 60% of older adults are malnourished (Hickson, 2006) and this condition is often underdiagnosed (Wells & Dumbrell, 2006). Prevalence of malnutrition is highest among the very old and those acutely hospitalized or under dependent care. The etiology of malnutrition in this population is multifactorial and includes changes in body composition associated with age, loss of appetite from medical conditions and medication side effects, and psychosocial issues, among many others. Nursing staff should carefully screen older adults for signs and symptoms of malnourishment. If malnutrition is suspected, the nurse should refer the client to a multidisciplinary health team, so that a more detailed assessment and appropriate care plan can be devised. Chapter 15 outlines the specifics of nursing interventions for the older adult who is malnourished.

Considerations Box: Excess Protein and Bone Health outlines the issue of high-protein intake and bone health.

Vegetarianism

Approximately 2.5% of adults in the United States and 4% of adults in Canada follow vegetarian diets (ADA, 2003). There are several common classifications of vegetarianism.

EVIDENCE-BASED PRACTICE RESEARCH BOX

Is there a relationship between protein or amino acid supplementation and enhanced athletic performance?

Clinical Problem: Athletes of all ages and performance levels frequently seek substances that might give them an "edge" on their competition. Protein or amino acid supplements have often been promoted in health-food stores, popular magazines, and Web sites as being the answers to athletes' dreams. Is there evidence to support such claims?

Research Findings: Numerous studies have been conducted in which amino acids and/or protein supplements have been researched with respect to aerobic and anaerobic exercise, body or muscle composition, strength, and endurance. Some of the more widely studied amino acid supplements contain glycine, beta-alanine, branched chain amino acids (BCAA), glutamine, and leucine. Protein supplements often contain whey or casein, which are milk proteins.

Resistance training has been studied with both amino acid and protein supplements and combinations of each. Findings with adult males in several small studies demonstrated various combinations that resulted in increased muscle mass (Kerksick et al., 2006; Kerksick et al., 2007; Cribb, Williams, & Hayes, 2007). Additional studies showed re-

duced muscle damage (at the cellular level) and maintenance of muscle strength (Kraemer et al., 2006; Nosaka, Sacco, & Mawatari, 2006), as well as muscle anabolism, mass, and strength (Willoughby, Stout, & Wilborn, 2007; Derave et al., 2007). One small study of 18 young adult females showed only that subjects who took the amino acid beta-alanine had a slight delay in neuromuscular fatigue during a high-intensity cycling test (Stout et al., 2007).

Other small studies have failed to demonstrate significance when comparing supplements with placebos. Strength, leg power, and endurance did not change over 6 weeks in highly trained athletes who took either an amino acid supplement or a placebo (O'Connor and Crowe, 2007). A 10-week study of 26 young males failed to show changes in muscle mass, strength, or body mass index (BMI) after using supplements. Smith, Fry, Tschume, & Bloomer (2008) found that the amino acid glycine had no significant effects on aerobic and anaerobic exercise performance over 8 weeks in 32 young males and females. Phillips (2007) found that glutamine failed to increase strength or muscle recovery in athletes. Macdermid and Stannard (2006) actually found a decrease in endurance following a whey-supplemented, high-protein diet in cycling performance over two 7-day periods.

Branched chain amino acid (BCAA) supplements were given to seven males in hopes of increasing exercise per-

Evidence-Based Practice Research Box *(continued)*

formance in high-heat conditions; they failed to show significant benefit (Cheuvront et al., 2004). However, there was some evidence to suggest that BCAA may slow muscle damage during prolonged exercise (Greer, Woodard, White, Arguello, & Haymes, 2007) and improve endurance in select athletes (Crowe, Weatherson, & Bowden, 2006). What is unknown is what specific combination or dosages of amino acids and/or protein, or the timing of their administration, has on athletic performance.

The current RDA for protein is 0.8 gm/kg/day for adults. Whereas some elite athletes need to consume up to twice the recommended amount of protein, the average healthy athlete can easily consume the RDA amount and more by eating even the minimum amount of protein foods found in the government's diet recommendations in MyPyramid. The

use of supplements has not been shown conclusively and across time to have exclusive benefits to athletes.

Nursing Implications: Research is inconclusive. Athletes are likely to gain most benefit from spending money on eating a nutritionally dense diet that emphasizes variety, balance, and moderation. Sufficient intake of protein from dietary sources, along with adequate calories, can meet the needs of an athlete without reliance on any type of amino acid or protein supplement.

CRITICAL THINKING QUESTION:

1. A member of the high school soccer team asks the school nurse about the quickest way to get more protein to build more muscle. How should the nurse respond?

hot Topic

High-Protein Diets and Kidney Health

Many popular weight-loss diet plans promote substituting an increase in protein intake for decreasing carbohydrate intake. This is thought to encourage loss of body fat by decreasing calorie intake (Bravata, Sanders, & Huang, 2003; Dansinger, Gleason, Griffith, Selker, & Schaefer, 2005; Foster et al., 2003; Gardner et al., 2007). Such diets can contain more than 160 gm per day of protein (St. Jeor et al., 2001), an amount that far exceeds dietary recommendations (Institute of Medicine [IOM], 2002). The increasing popularity of high-protein diets has led to a number of research studies investigating the safety of these diets.

In the body, the kidneys are largely responsible for excreting wastes that result from protein metabolism. It is recommended that persons with certain types of kidney disease avoid diets high in protein in order to minimize negative effects that are believed to accelerate a decline in kidney function (Kasiske, Lakatua, Ma, & Louis, 1998). The question remains as to whether high-protein diets are harmful to healthy individuals. In a recent review of the literature, Bernstein, Treyzon, and Li (2007) concluded that in healthy adults, long-term consumption of high-protein diets may cause injury to the kidneys, but these findings conflict with those reached by previous investigations (Manninen, 2004; Manninen, 2005; Matrin, Armstrong, & Rodriques, 2005; Pecoits-Filho, 2007; Walser, 1999). Other research has demonstrated that diets high in protein tend to decrease blood pressure (Manninen, 2004; Matrin et al., 2005; Pecoits-Filho, 2007) and encourage management of body weight (Lejeune, Kovacs, & Westerterp-Plantenga, 2005; Westerterp-Plantenga & LeJeune, 2005). Future research is needed to investigate the effect of different types of protein on kidney health in a well population and the overall health effects of long-term consumption of high-protein diets. In the meantime, the nurse can urge that individuals at risk for kidney disease avoid a high-protein diet. Further, those who choose to follow a high-protein diet should be advised to consume adequate fluids to excrete the metabolic waste products associated with high-protein intake that affect the kidney (Brehm & D'Alessio, 2008).

Cultural Considerations

Excess Protein and Bone Health

Adequate dietary protein is essential for bone health, with protein comprising about one-third of bone mass and playing a crucial role in the cross-linking during collagen formation (Heaney & Layman, 2008). A low-protein diet is believed to have a negative effect on bone health because of a deterioration in bone mass and strength (Bonjour, 2005). In contrast, several worldwide surveys have documented that the countries with highest animal protein intakes are those with highest hip fracture rates (Abelow, Holford, & Insogna, 1992; Frassetto, Todd, Morris, & Sebastian, 2000). Scientists believe that this relationship may be attributed, in part, to the fact that animal proteins contain acids that may compromise the integrity of bone, because the body uses calcium to buffer an aciditic state (Heaney & Layman, 2008). This condition may be counteracted by consumption of foods that oppose the acidic effects of animal protein (vegetables, fruits, nuts, and seeds); however, populations consuming high amounts of animal protein tend to eat lower amounts of these food items. In cultures where high intake of animal protein is typical, dietary intake of fruits, vegetables, and calcium-containing food should be encouraged. When calcium intake is adequate, high-protein intake is associated with greater bone mass and fewer fractures (Heaney & Layman, 2008; Rizzoli, 2008).

Semi-vegetarians (also called flexitarians) eat a mostly vegetarian diet but occasionally consume meat. **Lacto-ovo vegetarians** include people who do not eat beef, pork, poultry, fish, or shellfish but do eat eggs and dairy products. **Pescatarians** are those who abstain from eating all meat and animal flesh with the exception of fish. The most restrictive category of vegetarianism, **vegan,** describes those who do not eat meat of any kind, dairy, eggs, or foods containing these or other ingredients derived from animal sources. Some vegans also abstain from consuming food items that are made using animal products, such as gelatin, or are derived from an animal, even if the food item itself does not contain animal products. Honey is an example.

Vegetarian Diets and Health

Vegetarian diets have a number of nutritional benefits because they contain lower levels of saturated fat and cholesterol as well as higher amounts of fiber, magnesium, potassium, folate, and antioxidants. Some scientific research suggests that vegetarians have lower body mass indices than nonvegetarians as well as decreased mortality from certain heart diseases. In addition, vegetarians show lower blood cholesterol concentrations and blood pressure levels and decreased rates of disease such as diabetes and certain cancers (ADA, 2003). It is important to remember that vegetarians tend to have healthier lifestyles overall, meaning that they are more likely to maintain healthier weights, abstain from tobacco use, and exercise, when compared to nonvegetarians. These differences must be taken into account before relationships between vegetarian diets and health can be determined.

Planning a Vegetarian Diet

The United States Dietary Guidelines state, "Vegetarian diets can be consistent with the Dietary Guidelines for Americans, and meet Recommended Dietary Allowances for nutrients" (USDA, 2005). In conjunction with the Food Guide Pyramid, the United States Department of Agriculture (USDA) provides helpful tips for vegetarian meal planning, which are listed in Box 3-3. These guidelines can help a vegetarian ensure that he or she is consuming adequate intakes of the main nutrients that the diet might otherwise lack, such as iron, zinc, calcium, vitamin B_{12}, and vitamin D. It is recommended that vegetarians follow the USDA food guide with modifications as needed. Those who are lacto-ovo can follow the regular plan (including eggs and dairy products), substituting legumes, nuts, and seeds (and food products made from them such as tofu and peanut butter) in place of meats. Because they do not consume animal products, vegans should consume a variety of complementary proteins from plant sources in order to fulfill amino acid requirements. In addition, they may consider adding a balanced multivitamin and mineral supplement if there is concern that micronutrient needs cannot be provided from dietary sources. Pregnant or lactating female and pediatric clients who are vegan require a carefully planned diet that supports growth and development. Lifespan Box: Vegan Diets during Growth and Development outlines key nutrients that the nurse can emphasize with this population.

BOX 3-3	Vegetarian Nutrition Planning

- Protein has many important functions in the body and is essential for growth and maintenance. Protein needs can easily be met by eating a variety of plant-based foods. Combining different protein sources in the same meal is not necessary. Sources of protein for vegetarians include beans, nuts, nut butters, peas, and soy products (tofu, tempeh, veggie burgers). Milk products and eggs are also good protein sources for lacto-ovo vegetarians.
- Fat is essential in the diet to provide essential fatty acids to the body. However, vegetarians who rely heavily on full-fat dairy products such as milk, yogurt, and cheese for protein sources should be encouraged to choose the low-fat or skim versions to lessen saturated fat and cholesterol intake. Soy-based milk and meat alternatives do not contain

cholesterol and are generally lower in fat than their full-fat dairy or meat counterparts.
- Iron functions primarily as a carrier of oxygen in the blood. Iron sources for vegetarians include iron-fortified breakfast cereals, spinach, kidney beans, black-eyed peas, lentils, turnip greens, molasses, whole wheat breads, peas, and some dried fruits (dried apricots, prunes, raisins). A vitamin C source, such as leafy greens, tomato sauce, or citrus fruit, consumed at the same meal as an iron source will increase iron absorption.
- Calcium is used for building bones and teeth and in maintaining bone strength. Sources of calcium for vegetarians include fortified breakfast cereals, fortified soy products (tofu, soy-based beverages), calcium-fortified orange juice, and some dark green

BOX 3-3   **Vegetarian Nutrition Planning** *(continued)*

leafy vegetables (collard greens, turnip greens, bok choy, mustard greens). Milk products are excellent calcium sources for lacto vegetarians.

- Zinc is necessary for many biochemical reactions and also helps the immune system function properly. Sources of zinc for vegetarians include many types of beans (white beans, kidney beans, and chickpeas), zinc-fortified breakfast cereals, wheat germ, and pumpkin seeds. Milk products are a zinc source for lacto vegetarians.
- Vitamin B_{12} is found in animal products and some fortified foods. Sources of vitamin B_{12} for vegetarians include milk products, eggs, and foods that have been fortified with vitamin B_{12}. These include breakfast cereals, soy-based beverages, veggie burgers, and nutritional yeast. There are no plant

foods that naturally contain a form of vitamin B_{12} that is bioavailable to humans. Vegans must consume vitamin B_{12} from a synthetic source, such as a fortified food or vitamin.

- Vitamin D is found in some fortified foods and can be made in the skin upon exposure to the sun. Because the main natural source of vitamin D is oily fish, vegetarians and especially vegans must ensure intake of good sources of vitamin D-fortified foods, such as fortified milk and soy milk. Margarine is also fortified. There is an increasing array of other vitamin D-fortified products appearing on the market, such as juices and cereals. The food label will list vitamin D content of fortified foods as a percentage of the recommended amount needed each day.

STOP

- What suggestions can the nurse make about protein intake in the client who consumes only dairy sources of protein and no plant-based sources? What nutrients are present in legumes, nuts and seeds, and other plant proteins that are not found in high amounts in dairy proteins?

Source: Adapted from USDA, n.d.

Lifespan

Vegan Diets during Growth and Development

Well-planned vegan diets can provide adequate nutrition to support growth and development across the lifespan. Conversely, lack of attention to specific nutrient needs can lead to poor nutrition status and health risks. The nurse should advise the vegan client of the following:

- The pregnant vegan female requires a reliable source of vitamins B_{12} and D. Supplemental forms or fortified foods are commonly recommended. A lactating mother requires the same two vitamin supplements in order to supply the infant with adequate intake. Reports exist of neurological damage in breastfed infants of vegan mothers with inadequate vitamin B_{12} status.
- Soy-based infant formula is the appropriate choice for the term vegan infant who is not breastfed, because it provides adequate nutrition to meet needs for growth and development. Soy formulas are not recommended for preterm infants because of concerns related to poor bone health associated with such formulas in this population. Homemade infant formulas are not advised for any infants because of insufficient overall nutrients compared

with breast milk or soy formulas. The guidelines for sequencing the introduction of solids, including nuts and nut butters, in a vegan child is no different than for a nonvegan child.

- Toddlers and children may be challenged to consume adequate calories and protein if the diet contains significant high fiber or bulky foods that cause a quick sense of fullness. The nurse can suggest mashed beans, tofu, bean dips or spreads, nut and seed butters, peanut butter, and even some refined starches in place of whole grains to meet calorie and protein needs. Nutrient-dense snacks are also needed. Vegan children are generally slightly smaller than their peers but on average remain within normal range for weight. Careful attention to vitamins B_{12} and D remains because of limited plant-based sources of these nutrients. Calcium- and vitamin D-fortified soy versions of dairy products can be suggested. Vitamin B_{12}-fortified cereals are an easy way for a child to consume this vitamin.

Sources: American Dietetic Association (ADA), 2003; Bhatia, Greer, & the Committee on Nutrition, 2008; Dunham & Kollar, 2006.

NURSING CARE PLAN Protein for Athletic Enhancement

CASE STUDY

Fred, 17 years old, has come to the clinic for a sport's physical prior to his senior year in high school. He has been on the football team all through high school and really wants to have his senior year be the one in which he can be the "play-maker" for the team. The team has had successful seasons but his real goal is to make it to the state championships. He knows he won't be able to play football in college, so it is important for this to be his best year. He has never had a significant injury despite all his playing time and attributes that to being in great shape. His summer job will be over soon, and he confides to the nurse that he has saved most of his money so he could get the best protein supplements. He assures the nurse he will not use steroids but wants to know if there are prescription-strength protein supplements he could get to build muscles faster.

Applying the Nursing Process

ASSESSMENT

Height: 6 feet 1 inch Weight: 220 pounds BMI: 29
BP 122/76 P 64 and regular
Skin smooth and clear, well-developed muscles
Hgb: 16.4 Hct: 46
Eats 3 meals a day and 3 snacks a day; prefers burgers and fries but will eat any kind of meat
Drinks milk, water, or lemonade; no soda

DIAGNOSES

Readiness for enhanced nutrition related to improving performance capabilities evidenced by questions about protein supplements
Nutrition, risk for imbalanced related to plans for excessive protein intake

EXPECTED OUTCOMES

Stable weight and BMI
Identify nonmeat sources of protein
State risks and benefits of protein supplements
Plan dietary intake that accounts for intense physical activity

INTERVENTIONS

Introduce MyPyramid and explain how it can be used to evaluate current dietary intake and to plan future intake
Discuss physiological problems that may develop with excessive protein intake
Discuss relationship of protein intake to intake of saturated and total fat
Discuss how much protein is really needed for adequate functioning as an athlete
Demonstrate calculation of percentages of caloric need for each macronutrient

EVALUATION

A month later, Fred returned to the clinic to share how he was progressing. He had not realized that excessive protein intake did not mean more muscle strength. He had done some reading and confirmed that what the nurse had shared with him was true—that he did need protein to build muscle, but that he needed sufficient energy intake to fuel his workouts and muscle-building. The coach had also told the team to save their money and spend their time in the weight room instead of the nutrition stores. He figured he was eating at least 3,000 kcalories a day with about 20% coming from protein. His mom always had meat at dinner, but he loaded up on carbohydrates at breakfast and lunch along with a low-fat protein source like fat-free milk with the cereal and roast turkey in a sandwich, saving burgers from a fast-food place for snacks with friends. The season was about to begin and he reported feeling better than ever about his team's chances and his opportunities. Figure 3-7 ■ outlines the nursing process for this client.

Critical Thinking in the Nursing Process

1. How can the nurse tactfully explain that protein supplements are not necessary for a healthy teen athlete?

2. What foods could the nurse suggest that are high in protein but low in fat?

Protein for Athletic Enhancement *(continued)*

NURSING CARE PLAN

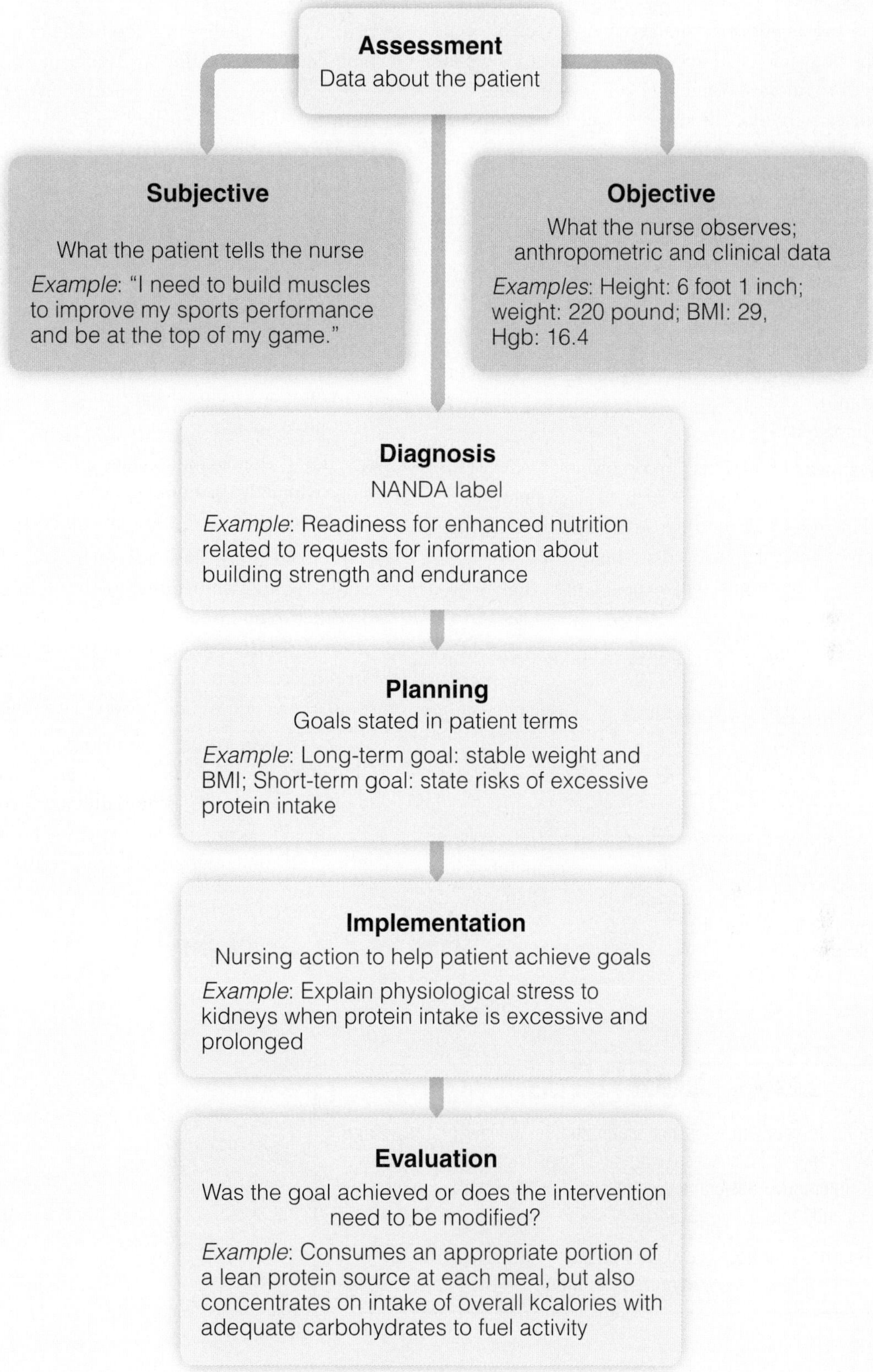

Assessment
Data about the patient

Subjective

What the patient tells the nurse

Example: "I need to build muscles to improve my sports performance and be at the top of my game."

Objective
What the nurse observes; anthropometric and clinical data

Examples: Height: 6 foot 1 inch; weight: 220 pound; BMI: 29, Hgb: 16.4

Diagnosis
NANDA label

Example: Readiness for enhanced nutrition related to requests for information about building strength and endurance

Planning
Goals stated in patient terms

Example: Long-term goal: stable weight and BMI; Short-term goal: state risks of excessive protein intake

Implementation
Nursing action to help patient achieve goals

Example: Explain physiological stress to kidneys when protein intake is excessive and prolonged

Evaluation
Was the goal achieved or does the intervention need to be modified?

Example: Consumes an appropriate portion of a lean protein source at each meal, but also concentrates on intake of overall kcalories with adequate carbohydrates to fuel activity

■ FIGURE 3-7 **Nursing Care Plan Process: Protein for Athletic Enhancement.**

CHAPTER SUMMARY

- Protein is the major structural component of all cells within the body and is an important element in the construction of hormones, membrane components, enzymes, membrane carriers, blood transport molecules, and the intracellular matrices.

- Proteins are composed of amino acids that contain nitrogen, carbon, hydrogen, and oxygen. Some may also contain phosphorus, sulfur, iodine, or iron.

- Amino acids are classified as essential (must be consumed from dietary sources because the body cannot synthesize them), nonessential (the body can make them on its own), or conditionally essential (may need to be consumed from the diet under certain conditions when synthesis is impaired).

- The physiological functions of protein include its role in the growth and maintenance of body tissue, immune function, and in protein synthesis. Proteins also act as enzymes and hormones and help to regulate fluid and pH balance in the body. Under some circumstances, proteins can also be used for energy.

- Amino acids from dietary proteins are broken down through specific metabolic pathways. They can then be reassembled to make new proteins or used to make energy according to the needs of the body.

- Some people are not able to metabolize all amino acids because of a genetic error and may experience health effects after consumption of certain protein sources. These conditions are sometimes called inborn errors of metabolism, and examples include phenylketonuria (PKU) and maple syrup urine disease (MSUD).

- The protein quality of a food is determined by the types and amounts of amino acids it contains and how well it can be digested. It is often quantified by calculating a protein digestibility-corrected amino acid (PDCAA) score that corrects the amino acid composition of a food protein for digestibility and compares this value to that of the human requirement for the amino acid.

- Complete proteins are those that contain all of the essential amino acids in the correct amounts needed by humans and include animal proteins. Incomplete proteins contain too little of one or more of the essential amino acids and are generally derived from plants. Complementary proteins are those that come from incomplete protein sources that are combined to form a complete protein.

- For adults the recommendation for daily protein intake is approximately 0.8 gm/kg/day; however, this value increases when a person sustains illness or injury.

- Protein malnutrition occurs when an individual has insufficient intake of nitrogen-containing foods (protein) in order to maintain nitrogen balance. Populations at increased risk for protein malnutrition include those living in underdeveloped countries where food sources are scarce, the elderly, and persons with severe diseases.

- Vegetarians are those who restrict animal sources of protein. Classifications of vegetarianism include flexitarian (semi-vegetarian), pescatarian, lacto-ovo vegetarian, and vegan. With careful planning, vegetarians can meet dietary recommendations for macronutrient and micronutrient intake.

EXPLORE PEARSON **mynursingkit**™

MyNursingKit is your one stop for online chapter review materials and resources. Prepare for success with additional NCLEX®-style practice questions, interactive assignments and activities, web links, animations and videos, and more!

Register your access code from the front of your book at
www.mynursingkit.com.

NCLEX® QUESTIONS

1. What should the nurse say to a client who expresses interest in beginning a high-protein diet?
   1. "Weigh yourself and use a formula to determine the minimum amount of protein you need and then double that amount."
   2. "Why do you want to start a high-protein diet?"
   3. "A high-protein diet is expensive so you need to make sure you have the resources to continue once you start."
   4. "Make sure you eat only high biologic value protein for best results."

2. The school nurse is teaching a high school class about complete and incomplete proteins. What is the best explanation of complete protein?
   1. It is the best source of protein.
   2. A minimum amount needs to be consumed for good health.
   3. It is the protein necessary to promote positive nitrogen balance.
   4. It contains all of the essential amino acids.

3. The nurse has been teaching a client about complementary proteins. Which of the following statements by the client indicates that teaching has been effective?
   1. "I need to combine specific incomplete proteins each day so that over the course of a day I have adequate protein intake."
   2. "High biologic value proteins are the preferred source of proteins."
   3. "If I consume a variety of incomplete proteins, I will have the amino acids I need."
   4. "Complementary proteins are required for a vegetarian diet."

4. Which of the following individuals is most likely to have a negative nitrogen balance?
   1. An elderly client with an open leg ulcer that is not healing
   2. A teenager who is on the school basketball team
   3. A young adult vegetarian who is a teacher
   4. A preschooler with asthma

5. The nurse has taught a client with renal disease about high biologic value protein. Which of the following statements by the client indicates the need for more teaching?
   1. "Eggs are a good source of high biologic value protein."
   2. "Eating protein at each meal increases its biologic value."
   3. "I can eat only a limited amount of protein so should select those sources with a high biologic value."
   4. "A good vegetarian source of high biologic value is soy protein."

REFERENCES

Abelow, B. J., Holford, T. R., & Insogna, K. L. (1992). Cross-cultural association between dietary animal protein and hip fracture: A hypothesis. *Calcified Tissue International, 50,* 14–18.

American College of Medical Genetics. (2005). *Newborn screening: Toward a uniform screening panel and system.* Retrieved January 6, 2009, from http://mchb.hrsa.gov/screening/

American Dietetic Association (ADA). (2003). Position of the American Dietetic Association and Dietitians of Canada: Vegetarian diets. *Journal of the American Dietetic Association, 103,* 748–765.

Aziz, A., Anderson, G. H., Giacca, A., & Cho, F. (2005). Hyperglycemia after protein ingestion concurrent with injection of a GLP-1 receptor agonist in rats: A possible role for dietary peptides. *American Journal of Physiology, Regulatory, Integrative and Comparative Physiology, 289,* R688–R694.

Beck, F. K., & Rosenthal, T. C. (2002). Prealbumin: A marker for nutritional evaluation. *American Family Physician, 65,* 1575–1578.

Bernstein, A. M., Treyzon, L., & Li, Z. (2007). Are high-protein, vegetable-based diets safe for kidney function? A review of the literature. *Journal of the American Dietetic Association, 107,* 644–650.

Bhatia, J., Greer, F., & the Committee on Nutrition. (2008). Use of soy protein-based formulas in infant feeding. *Pediatrics, 121,* 1062–1068.

Bongers, T., Griffiths, R. D., & McArdle, A. (2007). Exogenous glutamine: The clinical evidence. *Critical Care Medicine, 35,* S545–S552.

Bonjour, J. (2005). Dietary protein: An essential nutrient for bone health. *Journal of the American College of Nutrition, 24,* 526S–536S.

Bravata, D. M., Sanders, L., & Huang, J. (2003). Efficacy and safety of low-carbohydrate diets: A systematic review. *Journal of the American Medical Association, 289,* 1837–1850.

Brehm, B. J., & D'Alessio, D. A. (2008). Benefits of high-protein weight loss diets: Enough evidence for practice? *Current Opinion in Endocrinology, Diabetes & Obesity, 15,* 416–421.

Campbell, W. W., Johnson, C. A., McCabe, G. P., & Carnell, N. S. (2008). Dietary protein requirements of younger and older adults. *American Journal of Clinical Nutrition, 88,* 1322–1329.

Cheuvront, S. N., Carter, R., III, Kolka, M. A., Lieberman, H. R., Kellogg, M. D., & Sawka, M. N. (2004). Branched-chain amino acid supplementation and human performance when hypohydrated in the heat. *Journal of Applied Physiology, 97*(4), 1275–1282.

Chopra, R., & McVay, C. (2003). Nutritional requirements. *Nutrition, 19,* 187–199.

Cribb, P. J., Williams, A. D., & Hayes, A. (2007). A creatine-protein-carbohydrate supplement enhances responses to resistance training. *Medicine and Science in Sports and Exercise, 39*(11), 1960–1968.

Crowe, M. J., Weatherson, J. N., & Bowden, B. F. (2006). Effects of dietary leucine supplementation on exercise performance. *European Journal of Applied Physiology, 97,* 664–672.

Dansinger, M. L., Gleason, J. A., Griffith, J. L., Selker, H. P., & Schaefer, E. J. (2005). Comparison of the Atkins, Ornish, Weight Watchers, and Zone diets for weight loss and heart disease risk reduction. *Journal of the American Medical Association, 293,* 43–53.

Derave, W., Ozdemir, M. S., Harris, R. C., Pottier, A., Reyngoudt, H., Koppo, K., et al. (2007). Beta-alanine supplementation augments muscle carnosine content and attenuates fatigue during repeated isokinetic contraction bouts in trained sprinters. *Journal of Applied Physiology, 103,* 1736–1743.

Dunham, L., & Kollar, L. M. (2006). Vegetarian eating for children and adolescents. *Journal of Pediatric Health Care, 20,* 27–34.

Flugoni, V. L. (2008). Current protein intake in America: Analysis of the National Health and Nutrition Examination Survey, 2003–2004. *American Journal of Clinical Nutrition, 87,* 1554S–1557S.

Foster, G. D., Wyatt, H. R., Hill, J. O., McGuckin, B. G., Brill, C., Mohammed, B. S. et al. (2003). A randomized trial of a low-carbohydrate diet for obesity. *New England Journal of Medicine, 348,* 2082–2090.

Frassetto, L. A., Todd, K. M., Morris, R. C., & Sebastian, A. (2000). Worldwide incidence of hip fracture in elderly women: Relation to consumption of animal and vegetable foods. *Journals of Gerontology: Series A Biological Sciences & Medical Sciences, 55,* M585–M592.

Fuhrman, M. P., Charney, P., & Mueller, C. M. (2004). Hepatic proteins and nutrition assessment. *Journal of the American Dietetic Association, 104,* 1258–1264.

Gardner, C. D., Kiazand, A., Alhassan, S., Kim, S., Stafford, R. S., Balise, R. R., et al. (2007). Comparison of the Atkins, Zone, Ornish, and LEARN diets for change in weight and related risk factors among overweight premenopausal women. *Journal of the American Medical Association, 297,* 969–977.

Giovannini, M., Verduci, E., Salvatici, E., & Fiori, L. (2007). Phenylketonuria: Dietary and therapeutic challenges. *Journal of Inherited Metabolic Disorders, 30,* 145–152.

Greer, B. K., Woodard, J. L., White, J. P., Arguello, E. M., & Haymes, E. M. (2007). Branched-chain amino acid supplementation and indica-

tors of muscle damage after endurance exercise. *International Journal of Sport Nutrition and Exercise Metabolism, 17,* 595–607.

Hallam, P., Lilburn, M., & Lee, P. J. (2005). A new protein substitute for adolescents and adults with maple syrup urine disease (MSUD). *Journal of Inherited Metabolic Diseases, 28,* 665–672.

Heaney, R. P., & Layman, D. K. (2008). Amount and type of protein influence bone health. *American Journal of Clinical Nutrition, 87,* 1567S–1570S.

Hickson, M. (2006). Malnutrition and aging. *Postgraduate Medicine Journal, 82,* 2–8.

Institute of Medicine (IOM). (2002). *Dietary reference intakes for energy, carbohydrate, fat, fatty acids, cholesterol, protein, and amino acids.* Washington, DC: The National Academies Press.

Kasiske, B. L., Lakatua, J. D., Ma, J. Z., & Louis, T. A. (1998). A meta-analysis of the effects of dietary protein restriction on the rate of decline in renal function. *American Journal of Kidney Disease, 31,* 954–961.

Kerksick, C. M., Rasmussen, C., Lancaster, S., Starks, M., Smith, P., Melton, C., et al. (2007). Impact of differing protein sources and a creatine containing nutritional formula after 12 weeks of resistance training. *Nutrition, 23,* 647–656.

Kerksick, C. M., Rasmussen, C. J., Lancaster, S. L., Magu, B., Smith, P., Melton, C., et al. (2006). The effects of protein and amino acid supplementation on performance and training adaptations during ten weeks of resistance training. *Journal of Strength and Conditioning Research, 20,* 643–653.

Kraemer, W. J., Ratamess, N. A., Volek, J. S., Hakkinen, K., Rubin, M. R., French, D. N., et al. (2006). The effects of amino acid supplementation on hormonal responses to resistance training overreaching. *Metabolism: Clinical and Experimental, 55,* 282–291.

Lejeune, M. P., Kovacs, E. M., & Westerterp-Plantenga, M. S. (2005). Additional protein intake limits weight regain after weight loss in humans. *British Journal of Nutrition, 93,* 281–289.

Lenter, C. (1981). *Geigy scientific tables. Units of measurement, body fluids, composition of the body, nutrition* (Vol. 1, 8th ed.). West Caldwell, NJ: Ciba-Geigy Corporation.

Macdermid, P. W., & Stannard, S. R. (2006). A whey-supplemented, high-protein diet versus a high-carbohydrate diet: Effects on endurance cycling performance. *International Journal of Sport Nutrition and Exercise Metabolism, 16*(1), 65–77.

MacDonald, A., & Asplin, D. (2006). Phenylketonuria: Practical dietary management. *Journal of Family Health Care, 16,* 83–85.

Manninen, A. H. (2004). High-protein diets and purported adverse effects: Where is the evidence? *Sports Nutrition Review Journal, 1,* 45–51.

Manninen, A. H. (2005). High-protein diets are not hazardous for the healthy kidneys. *Nephrology Dialysis Transplantation, 20,* 657–658.

Marik, P. E. (2004). Monitoring therapeutic interventions in critically ill septic patients. *Nutrition in Clinical Practice, 19,* 423–432.

Matrin, W. F., Armstrong, L. E., & Rodriques, N. R. (2005). Dietary protein intake and renal function. *Nutrition & Metabolism, 2,* 25.

Millward, D. J. (2008). Sufficient protein for our elders? *American Journal of Clinical Nutrition, 88,* 1187–1188.

Nosaka, K., Sacco, P., & Mawatari, K. (2006). Effects of amino acid supplementation on muscle soreness and damage. *International Journal of Sport Nutrition and Exercise Metabolism, 16*(6), 620–635.

O'Connor, D. M., & Crowe, M. J. (2007). Effects of six weeks of beta-hydroxy-beta-methylbutyrate (HMB) and HMB/creatine supplementation on strength, power, and anthropometry of highly trained athletes. *Journal of Strength and Conditioning Research, 21*(2), 419–423.

Omran, M. L., & Morley, J. E. (2000). Assessment of protein-energy malnutrition in older persons, part II: Laboratory evaluation. *Nutrition, 16,* 131–140.

Pecoits-Filho, R. (2007). Dietary protein intake and kidney disease in Western diet. *Contributions to Nephrology, 155,* 102–112.

Phillips, G. C. (2007). Glutamine: The nonessential amino acid for performance enhancement. *Current Sports Medicine Reports, 6,* 265–268.

Potier, M., Darcel, N., & Tome, D. (2009). Protein, amino acids and the control of food intake. *Current Opinion in Clinical Nutrition and Metabolic Care, 12,* 54–58.

Powell-Tuck, J. (2007). Nutritional interventions in critical illness. *Proceedings of the Nutrition Society, 66,* 16–24.

Prelack, K., Dylewski, M., & Sheridan, R. L. (2007). Practical guidelines for nutritional management of burn injury and recovery. *Burns, 33,* 14–24.

Puffenberger, E. G. (2003). Genetic heritage of the Old Order Mennonites of southeastern Pennsylvania. *American Journal of Medical Genetics, Part C, Seminars in Medical Genetics, 121,* 18–31.

Rand, W. M., Pellett, P. L., & Young, V. R. (2003). Meta-analysis of nitrogen balance studies for estimating protein requirements in healthy adults. *American Journal of Clinical Nutrition, 77,* 109–127.

REFERENCES *(continued)*

Rizzoli, R. (2008). Nutrition: Its role in bone health. *Best Practice & Research Clinical Endocrinology & Metabolism, 22,* 813–829.

Shenkin, A., Cederblad, G., Elia, M., & Isaksson, B. (1996). Laboratory assessment of protein energy status. *Clinica Chimica Acta, 253,* S5–S59.

Smith, W. A., Fry, A. C., Tschume, L. C., & Bloomer, R. J. (2008). Effect of glycine propionyl-L-carnitine on aerobic and anaerobic exercise performance. *International Journal of Sport Nutrition and Exercise Metabolism, 18*(1), 19–36.

Soenen, S., & Westerterp-Plantenga, M. S. (2008). Proteins and satiety: Implications for weight management. *Current Opinion in Clinical Nutrition and Metabolic Care, 11,* 747–751.

St. Jeor, S. T., Howard, B. V., Prewitt, T. E., Bovee, V., Bazzarre, T., & Eckel, R. H. (2001). Dietary protein and weight reduction: A statement for healthcare professionals from the Nutrition Committee of the Council on Nutrition, Physical Activity, and Metabolism of the American Heart Association. *Circulation, 104,* 1869–1874.

Stout, J. R., Cramer, J. T., Zoeller, R. F., Torok, D., Costa, P., Hoffman, J. R., et al. (2007). Effects of beta-alanine supplementation on the onset of neuromuscular fatigue and ventilator threshold in women. *Amino Acids, 32,* 381–386.

United States Department of Agriculture (USDA). (2005). *Dietary Guidelines for Americans* (5th ed.). Washington, DC: U.S. Government Printing Office.

United States Department of Agriculture (USDA). (n.d.). *MyPyramid.gov Tips & resources: Vegetarian diets.* Retrieved January 2, 2008, from http://www.mypyramid.gov/tips_resources/vegetarian_diets_print.html

Walser, M. (1999). Effects of protein intake on renal function and on the development of renal disease. In Committee on Military Nutrition Research, Institute of Medicine (Ed.), *The role of protein and amino acids in sustaining and enhancing performance.* Washington, DC: National Academies Press, 137–154.

Wells, J. L., & Dumbrell, A. C. (2006). Nutrition and aging: Assessment and treatment of compromised nutritional status in frail elderly patients. *Clinical Interventions in Aging 1,* 67–79.

Westerterp-Plantenga, M. S., & Lejeune, M. P. (2005). Protein intake and body-weight regulation. *Appetite, 45,* 187–190.

Willoughby, D. S., Stout, J. R., & Wilborn, C. D. (2007). Effects of resistance training and protein plus amino acid supplementation on muscle anabolism, mass, and strength. *Amino Acids, 32,* 467–477.

Stacey Schulman

4 Fats

WHAT WILL YOU LEARN?

1. To classify the three types of lipids in the body and relate their functions.
2. To differentiate between the classifications of fatty acids.
3. To categorize dietary sources of fat, including saturated and unsaturated fatty acids.

4. To summarize the current recommendations for dietary fat and health.
5. To compare the lifespan-specific recommendations for dietary fat intake.
6. To develop strategies for nursing interventions that target dietary fat intake.

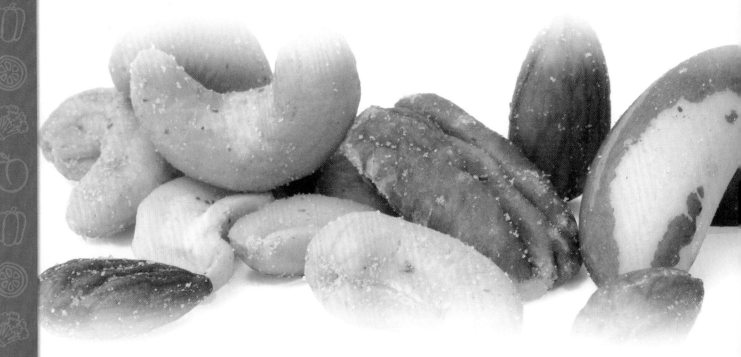

DID YOU KNOW?

► A gram of fat provides more than double the amount of calories as a gram of carbohydrate or protein.
► Fat alone has nothing to do with making you fat! An imbalance of calories from any source is what makes you gain or lose weight.

► A diet too low in fat could lead to a deficiency of essential fats that results in a scaly skin rash and fat-soluble vitamin deficiencies.

► Dietary trans fats and saturated fats raise blood cholesterol and must be listed on a food label.

KEY TERMS

What Are Fats?

Fats, also called *lipids*, are organic compounds that are necessary for good health. Lipids differ in many ways from the other macronutrients—carbohydrates and proteins—despite the fact that they contain the same three elements, carbon, hydrogen, and oxygen. In addition to the different chemical structure, lipids are not water soluble. An example that illustrates this chemistry is how oil and vinegar salad dressing separates after it is made because the fat content does not dissolve in the vinegar solution, which contains water. Lipids are classified according to chemical structure into three categories: triglycerides, phospholipids, and sterols. Each plays different roles, yet all are necessary for the body to function properly.

Triglycerides

Biochemically speaking, a **triglyceride** is a glycerol molecule attached to three fatty acids. Figure 4-1 ■ depicts a triglyceride. A more practical way of looking at triglycerides is as the chief form of fat found in foods and the major storage form of fat in the body.

What Is a Fatty Acid?

Fatty acids are carbon chains with an oxygen-containing carboxyl group at the glycerol end and a hydrogen-containing methyl group at the terminal end as shown in Figure 4-1. Fatty acids come in several forms based on chain length and saturation. The number of carbon atoms determines the length of the fatty acid chain, whereas the degree of saturation refers to the number of double and single bonds between the carbon molecules. Fatty acids can be termed **unsaturated** if there are double bonds on the carbon chain or **saturated** if no double bonds exist. In nature, most triglycerides exist with a mixture of fatty acids, both saturated and unsaturated, though some have

more of one type than another in the mixture. Figure 4-2 ■ depicts both a saturated and unsaturated fat.

Unsaturated Fats

Unsaturated fats include both monounsaturated and polyunsaturated fats. Unsaturated fats have at least one double bond on the carbon chain. These fats tend to be liquid at room temperature because this configuration lowers the melting point of the fat compared to fats with no double bonds. Unsaturated fats are classified according to the length of the carbon chain and the placement of the first double bond between carbons from the terminal, or omega, end of the chain. **Monounsaturated fats** have only one double bond on the carbon chain. The most common dietary monounsaturated fat is called oleic acid, containing 18 carbons (American Dietetic Association and Dietitians of Canada,

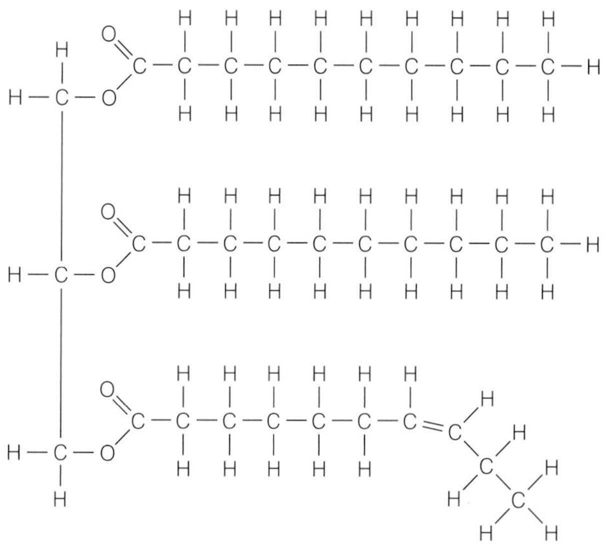

■ **FIGURE 4-1** **Triglyceride.**

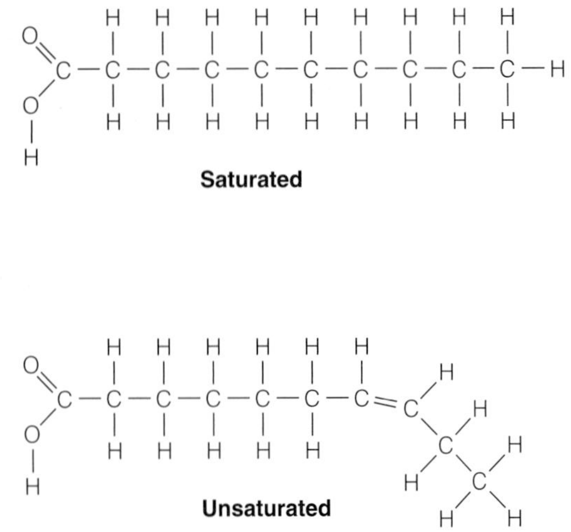

FIGURE 4-2 Saturated and Unsaturated Fat Structure.

2007). As denoted by the name, **polyunsaturated fats** have more than one double bond. Two classifications of polyunsaturated fats are **omega-3** and **omega-6 fatty acids.** The first double bonds on these carbon chains are at the third carbon and sixth carbon, respectively, from the omega end of the fatty acid. The nurse should be familiar with this shorthand system for naming fatty acids because of the rising popularity of referring to fats using this method, coinciding with increasing research on these two categories of fats. Figure 4-3 ■ outlines an example of the chemical structure of omega-6 and omega-3 fats.

Two polyunsaturated fats, **linolenic acid** and **linoleic acid,** are considered essential fatty acids. As the names suggest, **essential fatty acids** are unable to be made by the body and, therefore, must be provided in the diet. Linoleic acid is an omega-6 fatty acid and a common polyunsaturated

fat in the diet. It is considered the parent fatty acid used by the body to synthesize many other omega-6 fats. Linolenic acid is an omega-3 fat and is often more specifically referred to as alpha linolenic acid. Linolenic acid is the parent fatty acid to other omega-3 fats and can be converted by the body to two important omega-3 fatty acids, eicosapentaenoic acid (EPA) and docosahexaenoic acid (DHA) as pictured in Figure 4-4 ■. EPA and DHA have anti-inflammatory properties that may have health benefits. These are discussed in the Wellness Concerns section of this chapter. DHA affects neurodevelopment and visual acuity in infants as outlined in Lifespan Box: DHA and Infants.

Essential fatty acids play a role in maintaining healthy skin and promoting normal growth in children. Essential fatty acids make up part of our cell membranes and are involved in blood clotting and inflammation. Even though the body cannot make essential fatty acids, deficiency is rare due to the abundance in the food supply. Deficiency of essential fatty acids occurs when intake of fat is too low or because of fat malabsorption, such as with cystic fibrosis or inflammatory bowel disease. Premature infants are at risk for essential fatty acid deficiency because of borderline stores of these fats at birth coupled with high-energy needs (Marcason, 2007). Visible symptoms of deficiency include poor growth in children; poor wound healing; and scaly, dry skin. Additionally,

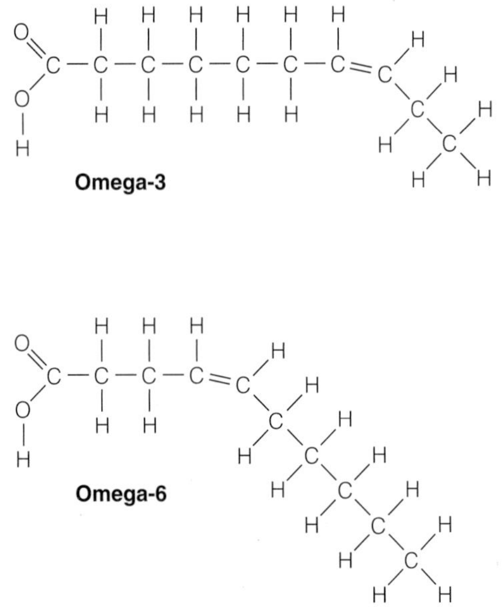

FIGURE 4-3 Omega-3 and Omega-6 Fatty Acids.

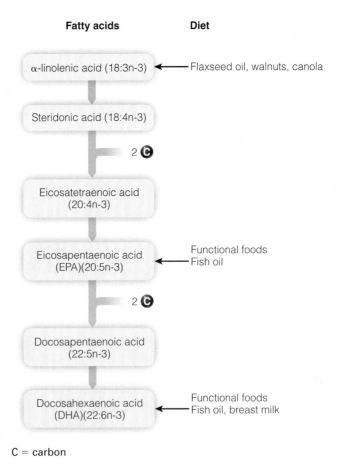

C = carbon

FIGURE 4-4 Linolenic Acid Conversion to EPA and DHA.

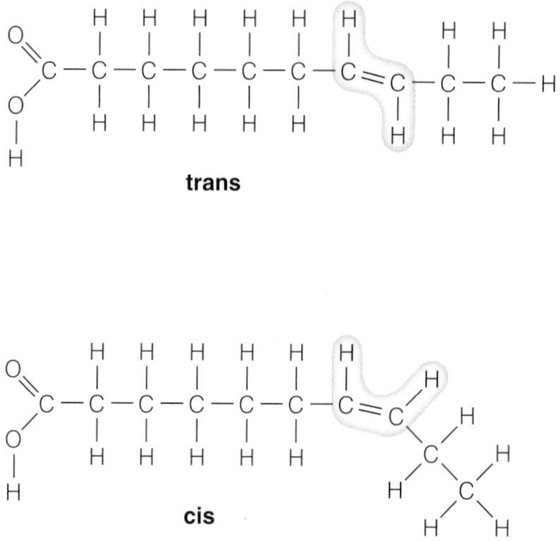

FIGURE 4-5 Cis and Trans-Fatty Acids.

DHA and Infants
Omega-3 fatty acids are essential fats needed throughout life, but especially during growth and development. Of particular interest is docosahexaenoic acid (DHA), which is used for growth and function of nervous tissue. DHA is synthesized from linolenic acid and is also found in the foods we eat; thus, the amount of DHA in a mother's diet determines how much DHA is available to a fetus. Reduced DHA may be associated with impairments in cognitive and behavioral performance, effects that are particularly important during brain development. As a result, much of the research on DHA and infancy has looked at whether supplementation is indicated, both in infants who are bottle fed and breastfed. Some research has shown that supplemental DHA in infants is associated with increased test scores of neurodevelopment and visual acuity (American Dietetic Association and Dietitians of Canada, 2007). Other research has supported the need for increased DHA only in the preterm infant (Makrides, 2008). Preterm infants have less accrued fat stores and less long-chain polyunsaturated fats present in the retina of the eye and the brain cortex to supply adequate DHA for development.

The conversion of linoleic acid to DHA is increased during pregnancy. This change provides DHA to the developing fetus and a supply of the fat for breast milk (Innis, 2005). Breast milk remains the preferred recommendation for infant feeding. More recently, DHA has been added to most infant formulas in amounts that mimic those found in breast milk. It is recommended that DHA comprise at least 0.2% of the fatty acids in infant formula (American Dietetic Association and Dietitians of Canada, 2007).

there can be changes in immune function and blood cells and increased water loss through skin because of decreased production of oil from the sebaceous glands on the skin surface (Institute of Medicine [IOM], 2002).

Saturated Fats and Trans Fats
Saturated fatty acids have no double bonds on the carbon chain and, therefore, each carbon is attached to the maximum number of hydrogen atoms. This structure gives the fatty acid more of a straight-line configuration than is seen with unsaturated fats and results in fats that are usually hard at room temperature. Exceptions are coconut and palm oils. These have short-chain fatty acids that are liquid at room temperature. The chemical structure of saturated fats also causes the fats to be more chemically stable, increasing the shelf life of a food product containing these fats compared to an unsaturated fat.

Trans fats are a type of fatty acid that behave like saturated fats in the body yet are not a fully saturated fat. A process called **hydrogenation**—a chemical process by which hydrogens are added to an unsaturated fat, thereby making it more saturated—creates a trans-fatty acid. "Trans"

means the hydrogen atoms are across the carbon chain from one another, instead of the cis formation generally found in fats. Figure 4-5 ■ depicts a trans and cis fat. Although trans fats behave similarly to saturated fats in the body, they have a greater detrimental effect on health, especially risk of cardiovascular disease. This concern is discussed in the Wellness Concerns section of this chapter. Trans fats became popular in food manufacturing because they are inexpensive and create a longer shelf life for foods by making the fat content more resistant to oxidation. Because of the mounting evidence of negative health consequences linked to trans fats, the Food and Drug Administration has amended its regulations on nutritional labeling to require that the trans fat content be listed on the nutrition facts label of any packaged food (Office of Nutritional Products, Labeling, and Dietary Supplements/CFSAN, 2006). These changes became effective January 1, 2006. For the same reason, some communities have banned the use of trans fats in local restaurants. Figure 4-6 ■ summarizes the classification of fatty acids.

Phospholipids
Like triglycerides, **phospholipids** have a backbone of glycerol, but instead of having three fatty acids attached, they have only two. Instead of the third fatty acid, phospholipids have a phosphate group (Figure 4-7 ■). What makes phospholipids unique is this phosphate group—it allows phospholipids to be soluble in water, while the fatty acids allow solubility in fat. These unique properties benefit the food industry—often phospholipids are used as emulsifiers, substances that mix with both fat and water. Mayonnaise is an example of an emulsifier. In addition to being an important part of the food supply, phospholipids are vital to our bodies. They constitute cell membranes and allow bodily fluids to exist in both fat- and water-soluble environments. Lecithin is the most common phospholipid in

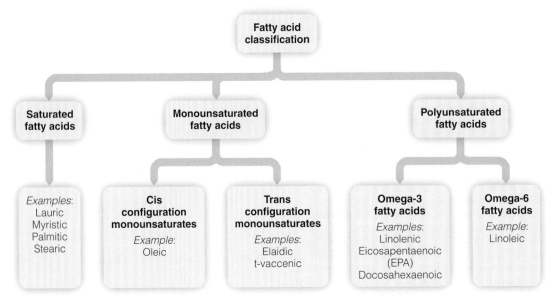

■ **FIGURE 4-6** **Classification of Fatty Acids.**

the body and is found in cell membranes and surrounding nerve fibers. Sphingomyelin is another phospholipid contained in cell membranes and the myelin sheath surrounding nerves. Phospholipids are synthesized by the body and are not required in the diet.

Sterols

Sterols are the third class of lipids and are composed of large, interconnected rings of carbon. Sterols are synthesized by the body and not required in the diet. Cholesterol is the most well-known sterol, whereas vitamin D, testosterone, and estrogen are other familiar examples. Although plant and animal foods contain sterols, only foods that come

from an animal contain cholesterol. See Figure 4-8 ■ for an example of a sterol.

Cholesterol is not an essential nutrient in the diet because it is made in the liver from glucose and saturated fat. After cholesterol is synthesized, it can be made into bile salts and stored in the gallbladder to be used to emulsify fat during digestion, be transported to the body's cells as lipoproteins via the bloodstream, or made into compounds such as steroid hormones and vitamin D. Elevated blood cholesterol can occur because of increased synthesis by the liver owing to dietary or metabolic reasons. The health consequences of excessive cholesterol in the blood are discussed in Wellness Concerns in this chapter.

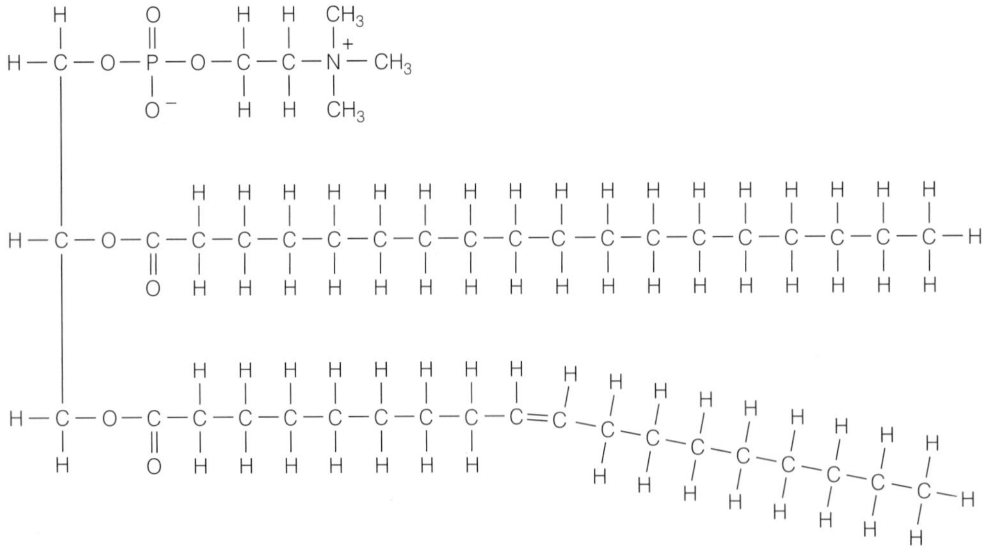

■ **FIGURE 4-7** **Phospholipid.**

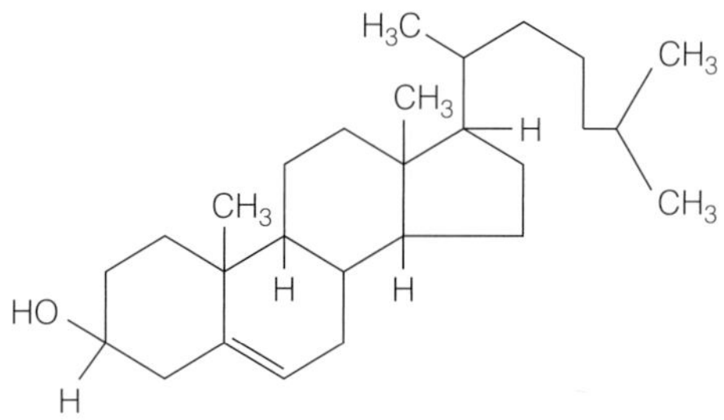

■ FIGURE 4-8 **Cholesterol.**

Functions of Fats

The functions of fats in the body and in foods share some similarities. Fat is a major source of metabolic fuel in foods, containing energy in the form of 9 kcalories/gm in contrast to carbohydrate and protein, which have 4 kcalories/gm. Likewise, fat is the chief form of stored energy in the body, where it is referred to as **adipose tissue.** Fat in adipose tissue is also responsible for helping the body to maintain core body temperature by providing insulation. Organs are cushioned and protected by adipose tissue. Additional functions of fats are summarized in Box 4-1.

Digestion and Absorption

Unlike other macronutrients, fat cannot dissolve in water and, therefore, is not as easily digested as carbohydrates and proteins. Digestion of fat requires that it be processed in a way that allows it to be absorbed into the bloodstream—a water-soluble solution. Lipase is the key enzyme in fat digestion.

BOX 4-1	**Functions of Fat**

Functions of Fat in the Body

Transports fat-soluble vitamins A, D, E, and K
Cushions and protects organs
Insulates body to maintain core temperature
Provides lubrication
Source of stored energy
Component of cell membranes
Component of myelin in the nervous system
Building block for synthesis of other lipid-based
    compounds, such as hormones, vitamin D,
    prostaglandins, and bile

Functions of Fat in Foods

Provides essential fatty acids
Source of energy with 9 kcalories/gm
Emulsifying agent
Taste and aroma
Texture
Transfers heat in cooking
Causes satiety or fullness

Small amounts of lipase are produced in the mouth and the stomach, whereas the majority of fat digestion occurs in the small intestine, especially the duodenum. It is here that bile is secreted from the gallbladder to emulsify fat in response to cholecystokinin secretion in the stomach. Emulsifying fats allows the surface area to increase so that lipase can work effectively. After emulsification, lipase from the pancreas is secreted into the small intestine to break down the fat into glycerol and fatty acids. Most of the fat that we consume is absorbed in the small intestine. Smaller fat particles, called medium- or short-chain fatty acids, are absorbed directly into our circulatory system. Larger fat particles, or long-chain fatty acids, are insoluble in water and, therefore, need to be encapsulated for transportation. The lymphatic system is responsible for the transport of longer chain fatty acids into circulation by delivery to large blood vessels in the trunk of the body. Figure 4-9 ■ depicts fat digestion and absorption.

Once in the bloodstream, fat is transported to the liver for metabolism and to cells in the body for use as energy. The liver can break down fats for use as energy or for synthesis of other compounds, including bile, hormones, or **lipoproteins**—compounds containing lipid and protein that transports fats. Low-density lipoprotein (LDL), "bad cholesterol," and high-density lipoprotein (HDL), "good cholesterol," are associated with risk of coronary artery disease. Lipoproteins are discussed in Chapter 18.

Where Are Fats in the Diet?

Fat is found in all food groups and can be visible or invisible. Table 4-1 outlines common sources of fat in the diet. Fat is not only essential to the body but essential to our food supply because it adds flavor, texture, and appeals to our sense of smell. Olive, canola, and peanut oils are used for cooking and have an effect on how foods taste on our palate. Butters and margarines can alter texture. Fats in food provide a medium for vitamins A, D, E, and K because these vitamins are fat soluble. Without fat in food, the body would be unable to absorb the fat-soluble vitamins.

Saturated fats are generally solid at room temperature. Due to their "straight" formation (no double bonds) they are usually capable of being packed into a solid at room temperature. Food manufacturers prefer to use saturated fats in packaged foods because these fats are less likely to decompose over time into a product that smells and tastes bad. Although saturated fats are prevalent in many foods, they are the predominant fat source in animal-based foods, including dairy products and meats; and tropical oils, such as palm kernel and coconut oils; and cocoa butter. The nurse may note that tropical oils are increasingly present in processed foods, because manufacturers seek a cost-effective replacement for trans fats. Although such a choice lowers trans fat content, it increases saturated fat, which also is not beneficial. Trans

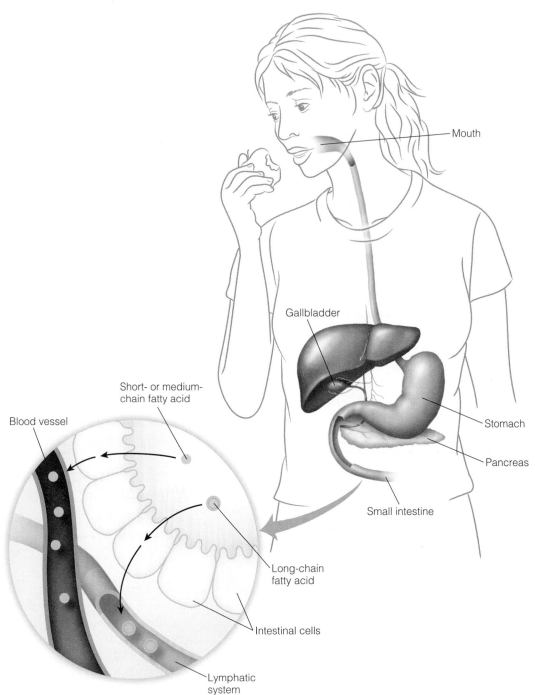

■ **FIGURE 4-9 Fat Digestion and Absorption.**

fats are present in fried foods; bakery goods such as cakes, pies, and cookies; and snack foods. Ruminant animals, such as sheep, lamb, and cattle produce trans fats, but it is debatable whether this form has the same negative health risk as the industrially manufactured form (Willett & Mozaffarian, 2008). The predominant sources of saturated fat in the diet of Americans are cheeses and beef products (USDA and DHHS, 2005).

Foods comprised mainly of unsaturated fatty acids are easy to spot on the supermarket shelves. They are soft or liquid at room temperature and more susceptible to rancidity.

Rancidification is the decomposition of lipids into glycerol and fatty acids that results in a product with an unpleasant and noxious odor and flavor and can also destroy the nutrients and vitamins in the food. Practice Pearl: Type of Fat outlines a quick way to differentiate between unsaturated and saturated fats that the nurse can teach to a client. Monounsaturated fat sources include avocados, olives, canola oil, and peanuts including peanut oil and peanut butter. Polyunsaturated fats include plant oils, such as corn, sunflower, and safflower oils, and wheat germ, nuts, and

Table 4-1 Fat in Foods

Food Group	Examples of Foods	Type of Fat	Lower Fat Alternatives
Fat	Oils, butter, margarine added to food or used in cooking, such as frying; dressings and sauces, such as salad dressing, cream sauces, mayonnaise; lard; salt pork	Saturated, Unsaturated Trans	Use sparingly.
Dairy	Whole milk versions of milk, yogurt, cheese, cream, ice cream, sour cream	Mostly saturated	Fat-free or low-fat versions.
Protein	Fatty cuts of meat such as prime cuts, ground meat; processed meats such as bacon, cold cuts, sausage, and hot dogs; poultry skin; fatty fish; eggs; seeds; nuts and nut butters	Saturated and unsaturated	Leaner cuts of meat (select white meat, beef loin and round, veal and lamb from the loin or leg, and pork tenderloin or center loin chop), egg whites, soy protein and other legumes (dried beans, peas, lentils), wild game, fish. Baked or other dry heat methods of cooking have less fat than frying or sautéing.
Fruits and Vegetables	Olives, avocados	Monounsaturated	Most other fruits and vegetables. Minimize use of sauces and dressings that add fat.
Starches	Baked goods, such as pies, cakes, cookies, muffins, croissants Fried potatoes, rice	Saturated or unsaturated Check label or recipe	Unsaturated fats can be substituted for saturated fats in many recipes. Total fat can be reduced by using fruit or vegetable puree in some recipes, such as muffins. Minimize use of added fat and sauces and dressings to grain-based products, such as cream sauces on pasta or butter on bread or potato.

PRACTICE PEARL

Type of Fat

An easy way to remember whether a fat is saturated or unsaturated is to think about its origin; saturated fat comes from an animal, unsaturated fat from a plant. Be wary of just a few exceptions: Palm and coconut oils and cocoa butter do not come from an animal but are saturated fats!

seeds. Figure 4-10 ■ is helpful when determining sources of unsaturated and saturated oils.

Omega-6 oils are found in plant oils such as safflower, sunflower, corn, soybean, and cottonseed. Omega-3 oils are found in fish oils such as salmon, sardines, trout, herring, swordfish, oysters, and mackerel, as well as plant oils such as canola oil, flaxseeds, walnuts, soybeans, and hazelnuts. The plant sources of omega-3 fats contain linolenic acid, whereas the marine forms contain EPA and DHA. Less than 5% of linolenic acid is converted to EPA and DHA, except during pregnancy when the rate increases to provide for the needs of the developing fetus (Van Horn et al., 2008). Individuals trying to improve EPA and DHA levels because of potential health benefits are generally advised to consume deep, cold-water fish sources of omega-3 fats because the conversion from plant sources is so low. Figure 4-11 ■ outlines the EPA and DHA content of seafood. Vegetarians are advised to choose plenty of linolenic acid from plant sources, such as canola oil, walnuts, flaxseed, and soybean products. The nurse should warn a client that ground whole flaxseed can have a laxative effect, but flaxseed oil does not.

Recommendations for Fat Intake

A dietary reference intake (DRI) for fat has recommended that adults should get 20% to 35% of their calories from fat (IOM, 2002). This recommendation is based on evidence that intakes greater than this amount are associated with risk of cardiovascular disease and obesity. This recommended range of fat intake is not meant for infants and children because of unique needs for fat during growth and development as outlined in Lifespan Box: Recommendations for Fat Intake: Infants and Children and Evidence-Based Practice Box. There are no specific recommendations for essential fatty acid intake based on scientific knowledge of health needs. Instead, amounts are advised for which it is known that essential fat deficiency can be avoided. A daily intake of 17 grams of linoleic acid and 1.6 grams of linolenic acid is advised for adult males (IOM, 2002). Adult females are advised to consume 12 grams of linoleic acid and 1.1 grams of

MyNursingKit Fats 101

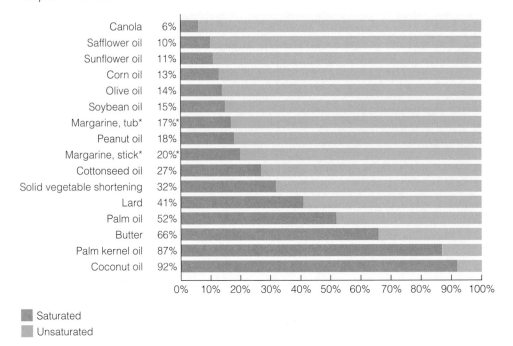

■ Saturated
■ Unsaturated

*An average of margarines listing liquid oil as the first ingredient.

■ **FIGURE 4-10 Saturated Fat Content of Common Dietary Fats.**

Source: National Institutes of Health, National Heart, Lung, and Blood Institute (n.d.).

Considering this graph, why is the practice of dipping bread into a bit of olive oil a better idea than using stick margarine or butter on the bread?

linolenic acid per day (IOM, 2002). The recommended combination of these fats alone comprises approximately 10% of the daily energy intake (IOM, 2002). The nurse can stress the importance of fat in the diet with a client who is overly restricting fat intake and deliberately consuming an extremely low-fat diet.

The American Heart Association (AHA) has made specific recommendations to urge intake of omega-3 fatty acids because of benefit to cardiac health. Two fish meals per week of deep, cold-water fish provide the amount of EPA and DHA associated with decreased risk of heart attack or sudden cardiac death. For individuals with existing heart disease, 1 gram of combined EPA and DHA in capsule form should be considered, as discussed in the Wellness Concerns section (Lichtenstein et al., 2006). Concern exists about the safety of intake of fish on a regular basis by pregnant females

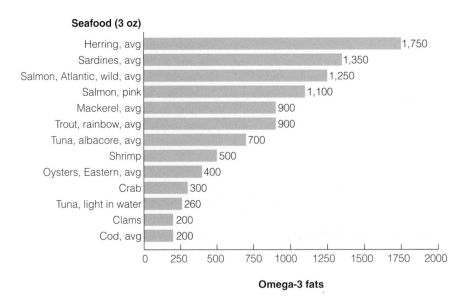

■ **FIGURE 4-11 Omega-3 Fatty Acids in Fish.**

Source: United States Department of Agriculture Nutrient Data Laboratory. Retrieved March 24, 2009, from http://www.nal.usda.gov/fnic/foodcomp/search/

Lifespan

Recommendations for Fat Intake: Infants and Children

Adequate fat in the diet is an essential component to support normal growth and development in infants and children. A normal part of brain development includes the accumulation of fat, which occurs throughout the first 2 years of life and requires adequate fat in the diet. A diet of 30% to 40% fat is recommended for children aged 1 to 3 years to supply needed fat. Specifically, full-fat rather than low-fat milk is recommended for children under age 2 years. From ages 4 to 18 years, children can gradually be transitioned to the recommended fat intake for adults.

CT? What guidance can the nurse offer to the parent who is offering skim milk to an 18-month-old toddler?

Source: IOM, 2002.

and children because of risk of contamination by environmental pollutants, especially mercury. The Environmental Protection Agency (EPA) and the Food and Drug Administration (FDA) have issued a joint statement addressing this issue, which is discussed in Lifespan Box: Fish Intake in At-Risk Populations.

Recommendations for limiting fat intake are found in the Dietary Guidelines for Americans and outlined in Box 4-2. These guidelines are similar to the DRIs, but they provide further guidance on reducing risk of heart disease by recommending that saturated fat intake be limited to less than 10% of total kcalories daily. The AHA provides more specific advice about trans fats, urging an intake of no more than 1% of total energy intake (AHA, 2008). This amounts to less than 3 grams of trans fat per day in the average 2,000 kcalories diet. Health Canada recommends that trans

EVIDENCE-BASED PRACTICE RESEARCH BOX

Are low-fat diets suitable for toddlers?

Clinical Problem: Many adults, by choice or necessity, follow a low-fat diet; children are often part of the household that follows a fat-restricted diet. Young children ages 1 to 3 years are classified as toddlers, a period of growth that is slowed from that of infancy but characterized by a growing sense of self and the development of habits. What evidence exists to guide families in making healthy food and diet choices for their toddlers who are going through a developmental stage that may affect their eating habits and food preferences for the rest of their lives? Are low-fat diets appropriate for this age group?

Research Findings: The average healthy toddler gains about 10 pounds and grows about 10 inches from ages 1 to 3 years. Variations exist, but it is important for this age group to stay on the height/weight trajectory. The current Dietary Reference Intake for fats for children ages 1 to 3 years is 30% to 40% of total caloric intake (IOM, 2002). This increase allows for the energy needs of this age group.

Children easily consume the recommended fat intake and more, with a disproportionate amount of fat coming from saturated fats and trans-fatty acids (Institute of Medicine, 2005; Kaitosaari et al., 2006; Ziegler, Hanson, Ponza, Novak, & Hendricks, 2006). Increasingly, the metabolic syndrome has been identified in children and youth (Harrell, Jessup, & Greene, 2006). Information from the Institute of Medicine (2005) shows that using a BMI of the 95th percentile, 10% of children ages 2 to 5 years are overweight or obese. Given the evidence of obesity and the interest in prevention of cardiovascular disease, hypertension, diabetes, and the metabolic syndrome, a few researchers have studied the effects of low-fat diets (those with 30% of calories from fats) on young children.

A longitudinal study begun with 7-month-old infants measured the effects of dietary counseling with parents to reduce fat intake to 30% of calories and insulin sensitivity. The study lasted 8 years and those in the intervention group

had improved insulin sensitivity that could not be fully explained by the decreased saturated fat consumption (Kaitosaari et al., 2006). The same data were analyzed by Talvia and associates (2004), who found that the diets of the intervention group continued to be favorably influenced over time.

Based on a comprehensive review of the literature, the American Dietetic Association (2008) continues to recommend that children 2 to 3 years old have a total fat intake of 30% to 35% of calories with most fats coming from polyunsaturated and monounsaturated sources, such as fish, poultry, lean meats, and vegetable oils. Children younger than age 2 need slightly more fat but no more than 40% of calories. Fats are a nutrient-dense source of energy for toddlers and are needed for ongoing development of the brain and nervous system at this age. Restricting fat calories means that energy needs must be met by increased protein or carbohydrate consumption and that intake of essential fats could be compromised. Whole milk is recommended for this reason when a child is weaned from breast milk or formula after age 1 year.

Nursing Implications: Toddlers need fats for energy and nervous system development. The restriction of dietary fat at less than 30% of calories has not been extensively researched in young children. The concern exists that if fat calories are restricted in toddlers, the energy needs will be met by increased consumption of carbohydrates in the form of simple sugars, a ready source of calories but little nutritional value.

CRITICAL THINKING QUESTION:

1. What kind of dietary counseling should the nurse do when a couple comes to the clinic with their 2½-year-old daughter who is at the 50th percentile for height and 5th percentile for weight, and they share with the nurse that they use only low-fat or fat-free foods because they do not want their daughter to get fat?

MyNursingKit Fats Translator

MyNursingKit Reading Food Labels

Lifespan

Fish Intake in At-Risk Populations

The cardiovascular benefits of omega-3 fats from fish and fish oil sources are well recognized. As a result, the American Heart Association has made recommendations for consuming two servings of fish per week. However, contamination of some fish with methylmercury is cause for concern, especially in children and pregnant females, because of the negative effects on development of the brain and nervous system. Mercury levels vary among fish species depending on environmental exposure to pollutants and place on the food chain. Larger fish contain more mercury than smaller fish. In response to this concern, the Environmental Protection Agency (EPA) and the Food and Drug Administration (FDA) have issued guidelines for fish consumption by children and pregnant or lactating females. The guidelines advise limiting fish intake to 12 ounces per week, including no more than 6 ounces of albacore tuna, and avoidance of high-mercury fish, such as swordfish, tile fish, king mackerel, and shark (FDA, 2004). The nurse can direct concerned clients to the EPA, where information on local fish advisories for specific bodies of water can be accessed (EPA, 2008). Overall, it still remains safe and beneficial advice for children and pregnant and lactating women to consume fish within these recommended guidelines (Mozaffarian & Rimm, 2006).

fat intake be limited to 2% of fats in oils and soft margarines and 5% of overall fat intake (Health Canada, 2007).

The nurse can educate a client about fat intake by calculating a personalized recommendation based on the calorie needs of the client. Box 4-3 outlines an example of how this can be done. Additionally, the individual can be taught how to use the nutrition facts panel on packaged foods to compare the amount and type of fat in foods. By law, the nutrition facts panel must contain the amounts of total, saturated,

BOX 4-2	Fat Recommendations: Dietary Guidelines for Americans

1. Consume less than 10 percent of calories from saturated fatty acids and less than 300 mg/day of cholesterol, and keep trans-fatty acid consumption as low as possible.
2. Keep total fat intake between 20% and 35% of calories, with most fats coming from sources of polyunsaturated and monounsaturated fatty acids such as fish, nuts, and vegetable oils.
3. When selecting and preparing meat, poultry, dry beans, and milk or milk products, make choices that are lean, low fat, or fat free.
4. Limit intake of fats and oils high in saturated and/or trans-fatty acids, and choose products low in such fats and oils.

Sources: U.S. Department of Agriculture (USDA) and Department of Health and Human Services (HHS), 2005.

BOX 4-3	Calculating Recommended Fat Intake

The recommended range for dietary fat is 25% to 35% of total calories each day. Here is how the nurse can calculate that range for a client:

1. Multiply the daily calorie needs by 25% to 35% (or 0.25 to 0.35) = daily calories from fat.
2. Divide daily calories from fat by 9 kcal/gm = daily grams of fat.
3. To calculate recommended saturated fat limits, use less than 10% of total calories in place of the 25% to 35% range and follow step 2.

Here is an example: Winfred knows his daily caloric needs from using an on-line calculator that estimates energy needs. He is trying to trim down his saturated fat intake to reduce his risk of heart disease but does not know where to begin. He asks the nurse how to figure his recommended saturated fat intake.

1. Winfred needs 2,000 kcalories/day × 0.25 − 0.35 = 500 to 700 kcalories/day from fat
2. 500 to 700 kcalories/day ÷ 9 kcalories/gm = 55 to 78 gm of total fat/day
3. 2,000 kcalorie/day × 10% (or 0.10) = less than 200 kcalories/day from saturated fat maximum
4. 200 kcalories/day ÷ 9 kcalories/gm = less than 22 gm saturated fat/day

- It is more important that Winfred concentrate on saturated fat intake than total fat for heart disease risk. What guidance can the nurse give about how to find this information on food labels?

trans, and polyunsaturated fats. Figure 4-12 ■ depicts the nutrition facts panel and the mandatory fat information. The ingredients listing will reveal the source of fat in the food and allow the individual to make informed choices when grocery shopping. The nurse should encourage clients to consume as little trans fat as possible, while making wise choices to include monounsaturated and polyunsaturated fats that provide needed energy and essential fats.

Strategies for Modifying Fat Intake

Fat is essential and should not be overly restricted in the diet. However, excessive intake of total trans or saturated fat deserves modification to lessen risk of obesity and, potentially, heart disease. High-fat foods can be replaced in the diet by lower-fat counterparts. Alternatively, foods high in saturated or trans fats can be replaced with foods that contain unsaturated fat. Removing high-fat foods from the diet without replacing them with other foods results in decreased energy intake and can lead to weight loss. Although this may be indicated with those who are overweight or obese, it is not the goal of dietary modification with all individuals. By encouraging a diet with whole grains, fruits, vegetables,

Nutrition Facts

Serving Size 1 cup (228g)
Servings Per Container 2

Amount Per Serving

Calories 250	Calories from Fat 110

	% Daily Value*
Total Fat 12g	18%
Saturated Fat 3g	15%
Trans Fat 3g	
Cholesterol 30mg	10%
Sodium 470mg	20%
Potassium 700mg	20%
Total Carbohydrate 31g	10%
Dietary Fiber 0g	0%
Sugars 5g	
Protein 5g	

Vitamin A	4%
Vitamin C	2%
Calcium	20%
Iron	4%

* Percent Daily Values are based on a 2,000 calorie diet.
Your Daily Values may be higher or lower depending on
your calorie needs.

	Calories:	2,000	2,500
Total Fat	Less than	65g	80g
Sat Fat	Less than	20g	25g
Cholesterol	Less than	300mg	300mg
Sodium	Less than	2,400mg	2,400mg
Total Carbohydrate		300g	375g
Dietary Fiber		25g	30g

FIGURE 4-12 Nutrition Facts Panel.
Source: USDA Center for Nutrition Policy and Promotion.

low-fat dairy, and lean protein sources, the nurse can help a client achieve a balanced diet that is also low in total fat and saturated fat. Added fats used in cooking or food preparation that are primarily unsaturated oils will help to avoid excessive intake of saturated or trans fats. For example, olive oil instead of butter can be used to sauté foods. Practice Pearl: Which Is Better for My Heart? is useful for when clients ask about using margarine versus butter. Other advice can include removing the skin on poultry and trimming fat off meats before cooking .When high-fat foods are used, a smaller portion can modify the amount of fat contained in a serving. When working with a client who has immigrated to the United States, the nurse should be aware that often the westernization of an individual's diet can lead to an unhealthy increase in saturated fat compared with traditional dietary practices. Cultural Consideration: The Westernized Diet discusses this effect. Client Education Checklist: Managing Fat in the Diet outlines further advice for modifying fat intake to achieve recommended intake.

PRACTICE PEARL

Which Is Better for My Heart?

There has long been a debate as to whether butter or margarine is a better choice for your heart. This question arises because of the potentially harmful amounts of saturated and trans fat in these foods—but which one is a better choice? Butter contains both saturated fat and cholesterol, whereas margarine contains vegetable fat but no cholesterol. A great rule to remember: The more solid the fat, the more saturated or trans-fatty acids it contains. A soft tub margarine with no trans fats can be a better choice than butter. Conversely, a stick margarine with trans fats and saturated fats might not be as good of a choice. Teach clients to read the nutrition fact panel for the sum of trans and saturated fats to make this assessment.

When fat intake is insufficient to meet recommended needs, the nurse can recommend sources of unsaturated fats that will provide both essential fats and energy. Nuts, nut butters, seeds, olives, or avocados can be incorporated into dishes and snacks. Putting a handful of nuts into oatmeal or avocado in a salad is an example. Added oils can be used in cooking, such as peanut oil in a stir-fry or canola or olive oils

Cultural Considerations

The Westernized Diet

Some cultures are known for the lower disease risks associated with traditional food habits. Traditionally followed in Greece, Crete, southern France, and parts of Italy, the Mediterranean diet emphasizes fruits and vegetables, nuts, grains, olive oil, and grilled or steamed chicken and seafood. Eggs, red meat, and dairy products are rarely eaten, whereas red wine is a regular part of the diet. This diet is high in unsaturated fats and low in saturated fats and is associated with a low incidence of heart attack, stroke, and type 2 diabetes (Willett, 2006). Diets such as this one should be encouraged even when individuals are no longer living in the country of origin. Research on many population groups has shown that when the diet is affected by western influences, whether from industrialization of a country or immigration to the United States, intake of saturated fats increases. Examples include Latinos who have altered traditional dietary practices when moving to the United States and adopting a diet with more processed foods (Mainous, Diaz, & Geesey, 2008). This effect has also been seen within a country when native populations, such as Alaska and Greenland Eskimos, adopt a diet of processed foods rather than the traditional diet with marine sources of dietary fat (Bersamin, Luick, King, Stern, & Zidenberg-Cherr, 2008; Deutch, Dyerberg, Pedersen, Aschlund, & Hansen, 2007). The nurse should explore traditional dietary practices with individuals and encourage preservation of practices that use unsaturated fats from sources such as plant oils, nuts, avocado, and deep, cold-water fish.

CLIENT EDUCATION CHECKLIST	Managing Fat in the Diet
Intervention	**Example**
Assess diet for sources and type of fat intake.	Assess fat intake from food groups and added fat used in food preparation and at the table. Consider sources of saturated fats and unsaturated fats.
Educate about the role of fat in health.	Fats are needed: • To provide essential fats • As sources of energy • To transport fat-soluble vitamins in the body Omega-3 polyunsaturated fats: associated with decreased risk of heart disease. Excess saturated fat intake: increases risk of cardiovascular disease by raising blood cholesterol.
Customize advice to fat modifications needed.	*Decrease total fat:* • Minimize use of fatty methods of food preparation and added fat, such as frying, heavy sauces, and dressings. • Use low-fat alternatives to full-fat dairy products. • Trim fat from meat and poultry. • Use leaner cuts of meat, skinless poultry, fish, and dried beans as protein sources more often. • Use dry-heat methods of cooking such as baking or broiling vs. frying. *Decrease saturated fats:* • Minimize intake of sauces, dressings, and added fats that are hard at room temperature. • Avoid tropical oils. • Substitute plant-based oils for saturated fats in the diet, using monounsaturated fats such as canola oil, peanut oil, soybean oil, and other oils that are liquid at room temperature. • Trim visible fat from meats and poultry and choose lean cuts of meat, poultry, and fish more often. • Try to substitute plant-based proteins such as soy or other beans for meats. • Use dry-heat methods of cooking, such as baking or broiling vs. frying; substitute low-fat dairy alternative for full-fat products. *Decrease trans fat:* • Minimize intake of processed snack and bakery foods unless known to not contain trans fats. • Minimize intake of fried foods in restaurants unless known to not contain trans fats. • Choose soft margarine in place of the stick form. *Increase omega-3 fats:* • Choose deep, cold-water fish such as herring, salmon, tuna, and sardines. • Choose plant foods rich in linolenic acid such as flaxseed, walnuts, hazelnuts, soybeans, canola oil. *Increase essential fats:* • Use plant-based oils, such as corn, safflower, sunflower, soybean, and canola. • Consume nuts and seeds, such as walnuts, almonds, and flaxseed. • Sprinkle wheat germ into cereals or recipes.
Educate about use of the food labels.	Outline the use of the nutrition facts panel and explain how it contains information on total, saturated, trans, and polyunsaturated fats. Keep the sum of trans and saturated fats to recommended levels. Outline the use of the ingredient listing to determine the source of fat contained in a food. Watch for the word *hydrogenated* in the listing. Choose products with plant-based oils that are not hydrogenated. Avoid tropical oils.

in a recipe. Peanut oil can be used with high-temperature cooking because it is less likely to smoke than many other oils. A soft margarine or olive oil can be used on bread. The nurse should stress the importance of fat in overall health when making these suggestions, especially with the client who has been deliberately consuming a very low-fat diet.

Fat Substitutes

Fat substitutes have been developed to lower fat content of some traditionally high-fat foods by replacing some or all of the fat found in the food. There are three general categories of fat substitutes: carbohydrate based, protein based, and fat based. Carbohydrate-based fat substitutes replace fat with a source of carbohydrate such as fiber, gums, or starches. Fruit purees are also considered a replacement for the fat content in some baked goods. Although swapping carbohydrate and fat in a food decreases the fat content, the nurse should advise a client purchasing low-fat foods with these types of substitutes to read the nutrition fact panel for calorie content if weight management is a concern. Some products will have equal or greater calorie content to the original food.

Protein-based fat substitutes replace fat with a protein substance in the product. Examples include Simplesse and Dairy-Lo, products used by manufacturers in processed foods and not available as a single ingredient to the consumer to use.

Fat-based fat substitutes provide from 0 up to 9 kcalories/gm, depending on how the body absorbs the substance. Some act as emulsifiers to mimic the feel of fat in the mouth and give the food a similar texture to the higher-fat counterpart but are either used in small amounts or are only partially digested, leading to an overall lower fat and calorie content. Caprenin and Benefat are examples of this type of fat substitute. The fat substitute olestra, or sucrose polyester, is not absorbed at all because of the size of the molecule (American Dietetic Association [ADA], 2005). It has been reported that olestra also causes small decreases in absorption of the fat-soluble vitamins, A, D, E, and K (Neuhauser et al., 2006). Manufacturers using olestra must fortify the foods with these vitamins for this reason (FDA, 2003).

The food technology industry has been developing alternatives to trans fats for use in processed foods. These products do not qualify as fat substitutes because they are simply a different type of fat. The nurse should be aware of these fats in order to respond to the individual who questions their use as a fat alternative. Newer oils are being developed through genetic engineering and plant breeding to alter the fatty-acid composition mix in the oil. Interesterified fats are chemically blended fats that customize the fatty acids mixed on the triglyceride molecule (Tarrago-Trani, Phillips, Lemar, & Holden, 2006). The nurse can advise that individuals check the nutrition facts panel for total and type of fat, rather than the slick marketing on the label to determine whether any new product is suitable for their dietary goals.

Wellness Concerns

Fat is often implicated when talking about disease progression and prevention, most commonly when discussing risk of heart disease and cancer. Research supports the role that too much fat can play in some disease processes but is less clear with others. Additionally, higher intake of some fats is being recommended for some medical conditions, such as omega-3 fatty acids used to treat high blood triglyceride levels.

Obesity

Regardless of the type of fat, high-fat diets are generally high in calories and can increase the risk for obesity. Obesity occurs as a result of any combination of excess energy intake and decreased energy expenditure. This concept is discussed in Chapter 8. Excess energy intake can occur with excess intake of any macronutrient, carbohydrate, protein, or fat. High-fat foods are often to blame for excess calorie intake because they are generally more calorically dense than high-carbohydrate or protein foods, making it easier to consume extra calories in a serving. The difference is because fat has 9 kcalories/gm compared with 4 kcalories/gm for carbohydrates or proteins. When working with an individual who is seeking weight management advice, the nurse can strategize with the client about sources of excess calories in the diet from high-fat foods and suggest lower-fat, lower-calorie alternatives. Simply replacing high-fat foods with those high in carbohydrate or proteins may not achieve any change in energy intake if total calorie intake is not monitored. Chapter 17 outlines this topic in greater detail and discusses nursing interventions.

Cardiovascular Disease

Cardiovascular disease is a general term that describes all diseases of the heart and blood vessels. The cholesterol levels in our blood can promote or serve as protection against cardiovascular disease. Blood cholesterol level has several components that can be influenced by diet, specifically the amount and types of fat eaten. Blood cholesterol is comprised of several components, including LDL ("bad" cholesterol) and HDL ("good" cholesterol).

Reducing intake of saturated fat is widely recommended for prevention of cardiovascular disease. Whether to replace saturated fat with unsaturated fat, protein, or carbohydrates remains debated (Hodson, Skeaff, & Chisholm, 2001). The evidence is clear that limiting trans fat in the diet is also essential (Lichtenstein et al., 2006). Chapter 18 discusses the role of dietary fats in cardiovascular disease in more detail, including recommendations for intake of saturated and unsaturated fats.

Dietary omega-3 fatty acids are recommended for two distinct purposes in those with lipid disorders and cardiovascular disease. First, increased intake of omega-3 fats in supplemental form is part of the treatment of high blood triglyceride level, a risk factor for cardiovascular disease (Yuan, Al-Shali, & Hegele, 2007). Second, intake of omega-3 fats is associated with a decreased risk of cardiovascular disease and sudden death. Hot Topic: Omega-3 Fatty Acids: Use in Medical Conditions outlines this issue. Both epidemiological and interventional studies have demonstrated beneficial effects of omega-3 fatty acids on many aspects of cardiovascular disease (Psota, Gebauer, & Kris-Etherton, 2006).

hot Topic

Omega-3 Fatty Acids: Use in Medical Conditions

Omega-3 fatty acids are a family of unsaturated fats that are thought to have many health benefits. The most well known of these types of fats are alpha linolenic acid (ALA), eicosapentaenoic acid (EPA), and docosahexaenoic acid (DHA). Omega-3 fatty acids have been implicated as beneficial in anti-inflammatory diseases and coronary heart disease.

Cardiovascular Disease

The research on omega-3 fatty acids and cardiovascular disease has been conducted for decades, and the majority of data have been consistent and conclusive. Epidemiological and interventional studies have shown that EPA and DHA decrease the risk of heart attack and sudden death (Psota et al., 2006). In addition to the anti-inflammatory effect, a decrease in platelet adhesion that normally causes blood clotting and a lessened risk of cardiac arrhythmias are felt to contribute to the positive outcomes from including EPA and DHA in the diet (Van Horn et al., 2008).

As a result of the overwhelming evidence, treatment guidelines for the prevention and treatment of cardiovascular disease encourage that EPA and DHA be incorporated into the diet, preferably in the form of oily fish, but alternatively in the form of supplements. The American Heart Association recommends the consumption of two servings of fish per week, preferably oily, deep, cold-water fish (Lichtenstein et al., 2006). Examples include mackerel, herring, salmon, trout, sardines, and tuna. For individuals with existing coronary artery disease, consumption of 1 gram of EPA + DHA/day is recommended, either in the form of oily fish or dietary supplements under the guidance of a physician (Lichtenstein et al., 2006). Use of omega-3 fatty acid supplements for this purpose is discussed in more detail in Chapter 18.

Inflammatory Diseases and Other Conditions

Omega-3 fatty acids are touted for their anti-inflammatory properties. As a result, their use in inflammatory diseases such as rheumatoid arthritis (RA) has been studied. Research has shown that omega-3 fats benefit treatment of symptoms of RA and improve the effects of anti-inflammatory medications (Galarraga et al., 2008; National Institutes of Health [NIH] Medline Plus, 2008). Omega-3 fats have also been investigated in the treatment of other inflammatory diseases, such as inflammatory bowel disease and asthma, but the evidence has not been strong enough to prove a consistent effect (NIH Medline Plus, 2008). Although most commonly EPA ad DHA are studied, dietary supplementation with other omega-3 fatty acids, such as flaxseed oil, borage oil, and echium oil, has shown to suppress proinflammatory markers in the body (Chilton, Rudel, Parks, Arm, & Seeds, 2008).

The use of omega-3 fats in treatment of neurocognitive conditions and mood disorders, such as depression, is another area of research using dietary supplements. Deficits of omega-3 fatty acids are associated with depression, but it is not proven that a clear benefit exists with use of omega-3 supplementation; therefore, more research is needed (Parker et al., 2006). In the meantime, the American Psychiatric Association has approved use of 1 gm/day of EPA + DHA for depression, but not in place of antidepressant medication (Freeman et al., 2006). Other conditions that may benefit from more research on the effects of omega-3 fats include attention-deficit hyperactivity disorder and dementia-related conditions. Results in this area are inconsistent, but some positive effects have been demonstrated (Kris-Etherton & Hill, 2008; NIH Medline Plus, 2008).

Nursing Implications

The nurse can recommend consumption of at least two servings of deep, cold-water fish per week for its known cardiovascular health effects. Guidelines for avoidance of excessive intake of methylmercury in children and pregnant or lactating females should be heeded. Individuals who follow a vegetarian diet that does not contain fish should be encouraged to consume good sources of linolenic acid on a regular basis. Examples include canola oil, flaxseed, and soy products such as tofu and soybeans. Additionally, algal supplements containing DHA can be considered (Kris-Etherton & Hill, 2008).

Use of omega-3 fatty-acid supplements should be discussed with the primary health care provider because of the increased risk of prolonged bleeding time (NIH Medline Plus, 2008). The nurse should routinely include questions about dietary supplement use as part of the nursing assessment. Clients who are allergic to fish should avoid omega-3 fatty-acid supplements that are derived from fish (NIH Medline Plus, 2008). Clients who are taking supplemental omega-3 fats in doses that exceed the 1 gm/day threshold should be referred to a registered dietitian for assessment of overall omega-3 fatty acid intake from food, fortified foods, and supplements.

Cancer

Although concern exists that high intake of fat is associated with increased risk of some cancers, research results have been inconsistent. Research has encompassed all types of fats, including trans fats and omega-6 and omega-3 fats with varying results. The nature of epidemiological research, where populations are observed over time or asked to recall behaviors that have already occurred, makes it difficult to draw firm conclusions with this type of disease that can take many years to manifest symptoms. A possible link between fat intake and breast cancer has been extensively researched without a definitive conclusion (Thiebaut, Kipnis, Schatzkin, & Freedman, 2008). Obesity, which often accompanies a higher-fat diet, has a positive association with prostate cancer risk, as does saturated fat intake (Thiebaut et al., 2008). The Women's Health Initiative Dietary Modification Randomized Controlled Trial evaluated the effects of a low-fat dietary pattern on several types of cancers; they were able to conclude that a low-fat diet may reduce the incidence of ovarian cancer among postmenopausal women (Prentice et al., 2007). Of particular interest, the ratio of omega-6 to omega-3 fats is being investigated. Omega-6 fats foster an inflammatory response in the body that may cause damage to body tissues, whereas omega-3 fats are considered anti-inflammatory substances that may temper the effects of omega-6 fats (American Dietetic Association and Dietitians of Canada, 2007). More research is needed in this area before advice can be translated to clients.

Inflammatory Diseases and Other Conditions

Many conditions and diseases in the body are caused by an inflammatory response. Rheumatoid arthritis and inflammatory bowel disease are examples. Omega-3 fats are often touted in the popular press for the ability to treat these conditions, but the amount of scientific evidence on this subject varies. The effect of omega-3 fats on neurological and cognitive conditions has also been the subject of research. Mood disorders, such as depression, and attention-deficit hyperactivity disorder are examples.

Fat Malnutrition

Both lack of adequate fat intake and fat malabsorption can have negative health consequences. Regardless of the etiology, these issues can lead to deficiencies of essential fatty acids and the fat-soluble vitamins A, D, E, and K. Additionally, extremely low-fat intake is associated with decreased circulating testosterone levels (Lambert, Frank, & Evans, 2004).

Treatment of fat malnutrition should first address the cause of extremely low-fat intake or fat malabsorption. The nurse can assess the reason that a client may follow an ex-

tremely low-fat diet and provide appropriate education about the recommendations for fat intake. Those who may be trying to lose weight and build muscle can be advised that muscle-building can be negatively affected by the decreased testosterone that results from such a diet. Additionally, some individuals who follow a self-prescribed extremely low-fat diet with the goal of improved health may be surprised to learn that HDL cholesterol can decrease on such a diet, an outcome that is contrary to the desired goal of improved health (Ashen & Blumenthal, 2005).

Fat malabsorption can occur for a number of reasons. Cystic fibrosis, pancreatic disease, and a number of gastrointestinal diseases are risk factors for fat malabsorption. Chapter 20 discusses fat malabsorption. When sufficient fat cannot be absorbed via the gastrointestinal tract to prevent essential fatty-acid deficiency, a small amount of intravenous fat emulsion is often prescribed. A topical cutaneous application of essential fats has also been used with some effect. This method of delivering essential fatty acids with safflower or sunflower oil has been reported to normalize plasma essential fatty-acids levels but not improve tissue stores (Marcason, 2007).

NURSING CARE PLAN ## Client with High Blood Lipid Levels

CASE STUDY

Fred, age 57 years, comes to the occupational nurse at the company where he is a sales manager to discuss dietary interventions for his high blood lipid levels. He recently had a required screening for life insurance and reports that his lipids were found to be "out of whack." He wants to know what he needs to do to get things going in the right direction. His father died at age 61 years from a heart attack and he admits to being concerned, because he is getting near that age. He says that he has not been to a doctor in years and would not have had the blood tests had they not been required this year as part of the insurance plan. Now that he knows the results, he wants to make some changes before he actually goes for a full physical in a few months. He says that his real goal is to avoid being on medication. Fred reveals that he typically stops at a coffee shop for a coffee with cream and a donut to eat in the car on the way to the office. He and his wife eat out a lot since the children left home and they both work late.

Applying the Nursing Process

ASSESSMENT

Height: 6 feet 1 inch Weight: 274 BMI: 36
BP 152/90 P 84 R 22

Labs: Cholesterol: 345 mg/dL Triglyceride: 151 mg/dL
HDL: 27 mg/dL LDL: 280 mg/dL

DIAGNOSES

Nutrition, imbalanced: More than body requirements related to excess nutrient intake evidenced by weight of 274 pounds

Deficient knowledge related to lipid management evidenced by request to begin dietary intervention

EXPECTED OUTCOMES

Differentiate among saturated, unsaturated, polyunsaturated, monounsaturated, and trans fats and foods that are representative of each

Weight loss of 1 to 2 pounds per week

Decrease dietary saturated and trans fat intake

Increase activity level

INTERVENTIONS

24-hour diet recall

Diet journal for 1 week

Referral to a dietitian for specific dietary interventions for high blood lipids

Discuss options for increasing activity level

Teach about each type of fat and significant food sources

(continued)

NURSING CARE PLAN

Client with High Blood Lipid Levels (continued)

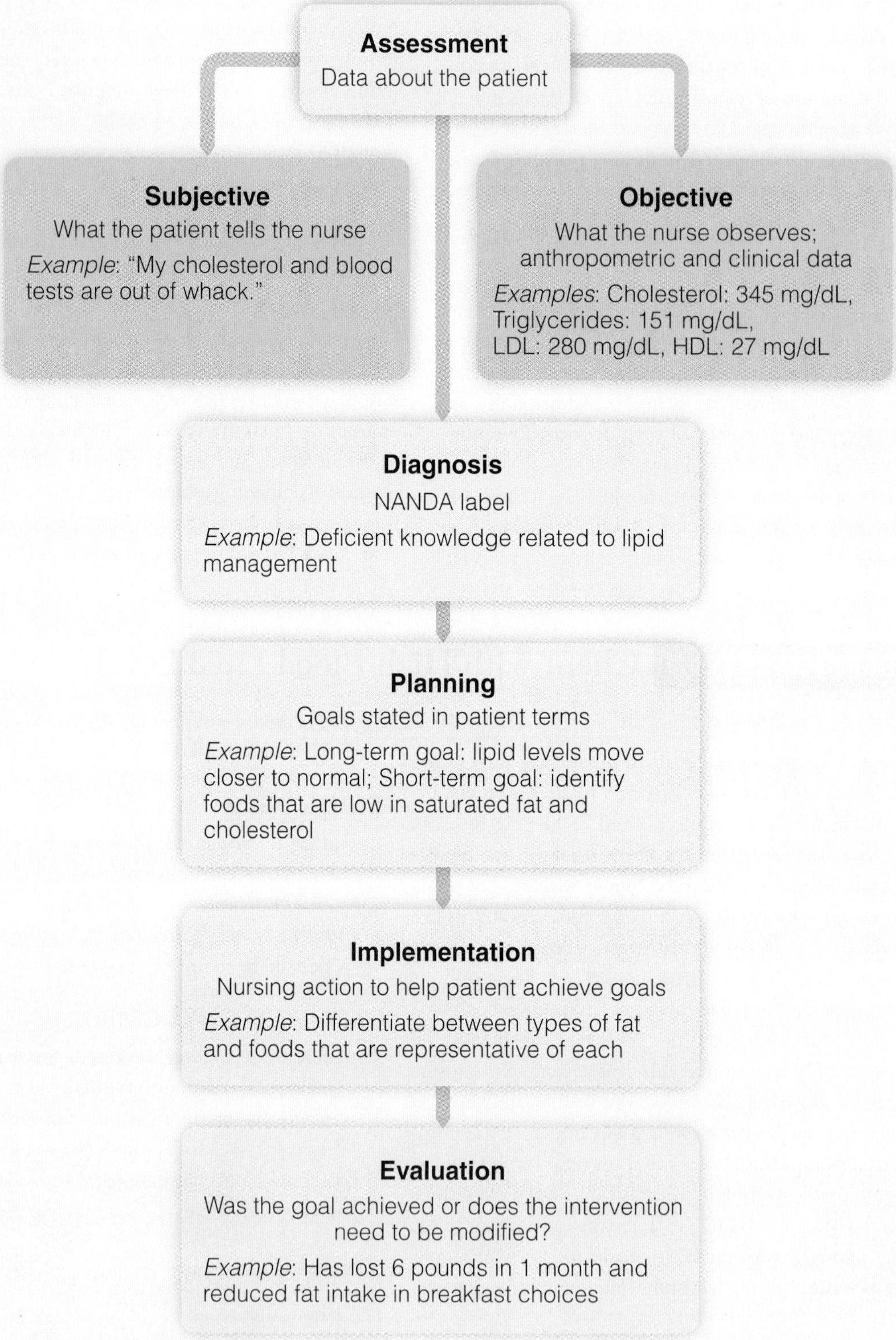

Assessment
Data about the patient

Subjective
What the patient tells the nurse
Example: "My cholesterol and blood tests are out of whack."

Objective
What the nurse observes; anthropometric and clinical data
Examples: Cholesterol: 345 mg/dL, Triglycerides: 151 mg/dL, LDL: 280 mg/dL, HDL: 27 mg/dL

Diagnosis
NANDA label
Example: Deficient knowledge related to lipid management

Planning
Goals stated in patient terms
Example: Long-term goal: lipid levels move closer to normal; Short-term goal: identify foods that are low in saturated fat and cholesterol

Implementation
Nursing action to help patient achieve goals
Example: Differentiate between types of fat and foods that are representative of each

Evaluation
Was the goal achieved or does the intervention need to be modified?
Example: Has lost 6 pounds in 1 month and reduced fat intake in breakfast choices

■ FIGURE 4-13 **Nursing Care Plan Process: Client with High Blood Lipid Levels.**

Client with High Blood Lipid Levels *(continued)*

NURSING CARE PLAN

EVALUATION

Fred stops in every week to be weighed and have his blood pressure checked. His weight is slowly going down, 6 pounds in the first month. He has found the sessions with the dietitian helpful, but he is finding it hard to break old habits and switch to alternative foods when eating out. He has started to have coffee with low-fat milk instead of cream and a bagel on the way to work so looks to that as progress. He knows he has a long way to go but feels that if he can stay with a diet for 2 more months he will have a better report when he has a physical and blood drawn again. Figure 4-13 ■ outlines the Nursing Process for this client.

Critical Thinking in the Nursing Process

1. When a client presents with high serum lipid levels, what are some initial dietary suggestions that the nurse can make?

CHAPTER SUMMARY

- Fats are divided into three main categories: triglycerides, phospholipids, and sterols. Triglycerides make up the largest group and are contained in most of the food that we eat.

- Fatty acids are the building blocks of triglycerides and are divided into three groups: saturated, unsaturated, and trans. The groups vary based on degree of saturation, or the number of double bonds.

- Most of the fat in our diet is nonessential with the exceptions of linoleic and linolenic acids.

- Trans-fatty acids are manufactured by the food industry and appear to be more detrimental on our lipid profile than saturated fat. They now appear on the nutrition facts panel as of January 1, 2006.

- Cholesterol is the most well-known member of the sterol group. Our body manufactures cholesterol in the liver and it is consumed in the diet.

- Fat is found in all of the major food groups and therefore is impossible to avoid completely. Most of the fat eaten is hidden in foods.

- Increased fat intake has been linked to cancer and heart disease, although the type of fat consumed is just as important as our total fat intake. Unsaturated fat clearly has health benefits over saturated and trans.

- Those who need to gain weight may benefit from increasing the fat in their diets due to the increased amount of calories available for absorption. Conversely, those looking to lose weight may want to decrease the amount of fat they eat for the same reason.

PEARSON

EXPLORE **mynursingkit**

MyNursingKit is your one stop for online chapter review materials and resources. Prepare for success with additional NCLEX®-style practice questions, interactive assignments and activities, web links, animations and videos, and more!

Register your access code from the front of your book at
www.mynursingkit.com.

1. How should the nurse respond to the client who already limits trans and saturated fats and now wants to reduce cholesterol in the diet?
   1. "Read the food fact label and select only those foods that have less than 7 grams of total fat per serving."
   2. "Limit the portion of foods from animal sources."
   3. "Eat no more than two eggs a week."
   4. "Eliminate fried foods from the diet."

2. The school nurse is preparing to teach a class of 16-year-olds about cholesterol. Which of the following statements would the nurse use to describe cholesterol?
   1. The body manufactures some of its own cholesterol in the liver.
   2. Cholesterol should be eliminated from the diet of middle-age and older adults.
   3. Red meat is the primary source of cholesterol.
   4. Foods that are high in omega-3 fatty acids do not contain cholesterol.

3. The nurse encourages clients to increase consumption of omega-3 fatty acids. Which foods would the nurse suggest? Select all that apply.
   1. Fresh salmon
   2. Whole grain bread
   3. Whole wheat pasta
   4. Canned tuna
   5. Skinless chicken breast

4. The nurse has taught a client about limiting trans-fatty acids in the diet. Which statement by the client indicates that teaching has been effective?
   1. "I need to eat more fish to reduce trans-fatty acids."
   2. "Eating vegetables at the same meal as meat will limit the absorption of trans-fatty acids from the meat."
   3. "Trans-fatty acids come from the same source as monounsaturated fats."
   4. "I need to limit my intake of processed foods."

5. The nurse has been working with a client about the necessity of limiting intake of total fat. Which diet selection by the client indicates that the client has understood the teaching?
   1. Stir-fried beef with broccoli
   2. Macaroni and cheese
   3. White chicken chili
   4. Shredded beef taco with refried beans

REFERENCES

American Dietetic Association (ADA). (2005). Position of the American Dietetic Association: Fat replacers. *Journal of the American Dietetic Association, 105,* 266–275.

American Dietetic Association (ADA). (2008). Position of the American Dietetic Association: Nutrition guidance for healthy children ages 2 to 11 years. *Journal of the American Dietetic Association, 108,* 1038–1047.

American Dietetic Association and Dietitians of Canada. (2007). Position of the American Dietetic Association and Dietitians of Canada: Dietary fatty acids. *Journal of the American Dietetic Association, 107,* 1599–1611.

American Heart Association (AHA). (2008). *Trans fats.* Retrieved October 18, 2008, from http://www.americanheart.org/presenter.jhtml?identifier=3045792

Ashen, M. D., & Blumenthal, R. S. (2005). Low HDL cholesterol levels. *New England Journal of Medicine, 353,* 1252–1260.

Bersamin, A., Luick, B. R., King, I. B., Stern, J. S., & Zidenberg-Cherr, S. (2008). Westernizing diet influences fat intake, red blood cell fatty acid composition, and health in remote Alaskan Native communities in the Center for Alaska Native Health Study. *Journal of the American Dietetic Association, 108,* 266–273.

Chilton, F. H., Rudel, L. L., Parks, J. S., Arm, J. P., & Seeds, M. C. (2008). Mechanisms by which botanical lipids affect inflammatory disorders. *American Journal of Clinical Nutrition, 87,* 498S–503S.

Deutch, B., Dyerberg, J., Pedersen, H. S., Aschlund, E., & Hansen, J. C. (2007). Traditional and modern Greenlandic food— Dietary composition, nutrients, and contami-

nants. *Science of the Total Environment, 384,* 106–119.

Environmental Protection Agency (EPA). (2008). *The National Listing of Fish Advisories.* Retrieved October 18, 2008, from http://map1.epa.gov/scripts/esrimap.dll?name=Listing&Cmd=Map

Food and Drug Administration (FDA). (2003). *Olestra labeling changes.* Retrieved October 18, 2008, from http://www.fda.gov/fdac/departs/2003/603_upd.html#olestra

Food and Drug Administration (FDA) and Environmental Protection Agency (EPA). (2004). *What you need to know about mercury in fish and shellfish.* Retrieved October 18, 2008, from http://www.cfsan.fda.gov/~dms/admehg3.html

Freeman, M., Hibbeln, J. R., Wisner, K. L., Davis, J. M., Mischoulon, D., Peet, M., et al. (2006). Omega-3 fatty acids: Evidence basis for treatment and future research in psychiatry. *Journal of Clinical Psychiatry, 67,* 1954–1967.

Galarraga, B., Ho, M., Youssef, H. M., Hill, A., McMahon, H., Hall, C., et al. (2008). Cod liver oil (n-3 fatty acids) as a non-steroidal anti-inflammatory drug sparing agent in rheumatoid arthritis. *Rheumatology, 47*(5), 665–669.

Harrell, J. S., Jessup, A., & Greene, N. (2006). Changing our future: Obesity and the metabolic syndrome in children and adolescents. *Journal of Cardiovascular Nursing, 21*(4), 322–330.

Health Canada. (2007).*Trans fats: It's your health.* Retrieved October 18, 2008, from http://www.hc-sc.gc.ca/hl-vs/alt_formats/pacrb-dgapcr/pdf/iyh-vsv/food-aliment/trans-eng.pdf

Hodson, L., Skeaff, C. M., & Chisholm, W. A. (2001). The effect of replacing dietary saturated fat with polyunsaturated or monounsaturated fat on plasma lipids in free-living adults. *European Journal of Clinical Nutrition, 10,* 908–915.

Innis, S.M. (2005). Essential fatty acid transfer and fetal development. *Placenta, 26,* S70–S75.

Institute of Medicine (IOM) Food and Nutrition Board (2002). *Dietary reference intakes for energy, carbohydrate, fiber, fat, fatty acids, cholesterol, protein, and amino acids.* Washington, DC: National Academies Press.

Institute of Medicine (IOM). (2005). *Preventing childhood obesity.* Washington, DC: National Academies Press.

Kaitosaari, T., Ronnemaa, T., Viikari, J., Raitakari, O., Arffman, M., Marniemi, J., et al. (2006). Low-saturated fat dietary counseling starting in infancy improves insulin sensitivity in 9-year-old healthy children: The Special Turku Coronary Risk Factor Intervention Project for Children (STRIP) study. *Diabetes Care, 29*(4), 781–785.

Kris-Etherton, P. M., & Hill, A. M. (2008). N-3 fatty acids: Food or supplements? *Journal of the American Dietetic Association, 108,* 1125–1130.

Lambert, C. P., Frank, L. L., & Evans, W. J. (2004). Macronutrient considerations for the sport of body building. *Sports Medicine, 34,* 317–327.

Lichtenstein, A. H., Appel, L. J., Brands, M., Carnethon, M., Daniels, S., Franch, H. A., et al. (2006). Diet and lifestyle recommendations, revised 2006. *Circulation, 114,* 82–96.

Mainous, A. G., Diaz, V. A., & Geesey, M. E. (2008). Acculturation and healthy lifestyle among Latinos with diabetes. *Annals of Family Medicine, 6,* 131–137.

Makrides, M. (2008). Outcomes for mothers and their babies: Do n-3 long chain polyunsaturated fatty acids and seafoods make a difference? *Journal of the American Dietetic Association, 108,* 1622–1626.

Marcason, W. (2007). Can cutaneous application of vegetable oil prevent an essential fatty acid deficiency? *Journal of the American Dietetic Association, 107,* 1262.

Mozaffarian, D., & Rimm, E. B. (2006). Fish intake, contaminants, and human health: Evaluating risks and benefits. *Journal of the American Medical Association, 296,* 1885–1899.

National Institutes of Health (NIH) Medline Plus. (2008). Omega-3 fatty acids, fish oil, alpha-linolenic acid. Retrieved September 23, 2008, from http://www.nlm.nih.gov/medlineplus/druginfo/natural/patient-fishoil.html

Neuhauser, M. L., Rock, C. L., Kristal, A. R., Patterson, R. E., Neumark-Sztainer, D., Cheskin, L. J., et al. (2006). Olestra is associated with slight reductions in serum carotenoids but does not markedly influence serum fat-soluble vitamin concentrations. *American Journal of Clinical Nutrition, 83,* 624–631.

Office of Nutritional Products, Labeling, and Dietary Supplements/CFSAN. (2006). *Trans fat now listed with saturated fat and cholesterol on nutrition facts panel* Retrieved May 14, 2008, from http://www.cfsan.fda.gov/~dms/transfat.html

Parker, G., Gibson, N. A., Brotchie, H., Heruc, G., Rees, A., & Hadzi-Pavlovic, D. (2006). Omega-3 fatty acids and mood disorders. *American Journal of Psychiatry, 163,* 969–978.

Prentice, R. L., Thomson, C. A., Caan, B., Hubbell, F. A., Anderson, G. L., Beresford, S. A., et al. (2007). Low-fat dietary pattern and cancer incidence in the Women's Health Initiative Dietary Modification Randomized Controlled Trial. *Journal of the National Cancer Institute, 99,* 1534–1543.

Psota, T. L., Gebauer, S. K., & Kris-Etherton, P. (2006). Dietary omega-3 fatty acid intake and cardiovascular disease. *American Journal of Cardiology, 98,* 3i–18i.

Talvia, S., Lagstrom, H., Rasanen, M., Salminen, M., Rasanen, L., Salo, P., et al. (2004). A randomized intervention since infancy to reduce intake of saturated fat: Calorie (energy) and nutrient intakes up to the age of 10 years in the Special Turku Coronary Risk Factor Intervention Project. *Archives of Pediatric and Adolescent Medicine, 158*(1), 41–47.

Tarrago-Trani, M. T., Phillips, K. M., Lemar, L. E., & Holden, J. M.(2006). New and existing oils and fats used in products with reduced trans-fatty acid content. *Journal of the American Dietetic Association, 106,* 867–880.

Thiebaut, A. C., Kipnis, V., Schatzkin, A., & Freedman, L. S. (2008). The role of dietary measurement error in investigating the hypothesized link between dietary fat intake and breast cancer—A story with twists and turns. *Cancer Investigation, 26,* 68–73.

U.S. Department of Agriculture (USDA) and Department of Health and Human Services (DHHS). (2005). *Dietary Guidelines for Americans.* Washington, DC: National Academies Press.

U.S. Department of Health and Human Services. (2005). The report of the dietary guidelines advisory committee on *Dietary Guidelines for Americans.* Retrieved October 30, 2008, from http://www.health.gov/DietaryGuidelines/dga2005/report/

Van Horn, L., McCoin, M., Kris-Etherton, P. M., Burke, F., Carson, J. S., Champagne, C. M., et al. (2008). The evidence for dietary prevention and treatment of cardiovascular disease. *Journal of the American Dietetic Association, 108,* 287–331.

Willett, W. C. (2006). The Mediterranean diet: Science and practice. *Public Health Nutrition, 9,* 105–110.

Willett, W. C., & Mozaffarian, D. (2008). Ruminant or industrial sources of trans fatty acids: Public health issue or food label skirmish? *American Journal of Clinical Nutrition, 87,* 515–516.

Yuan, G., Al-Shali, K. Z., & Hegele, R. A. (2007). Hypertriglyceridemia: Its etiology, effects, and treatment. *Canadian Medical Association Journal, 176,* 1113–1120.

Ziegler, P., Hanson, C., Ponza, M., Novak, T., & Hendricks, K. (2006). Feeding Infants and Toddlers Study: Meal and snack intakes of Hispanic and non-Hispanic infants and toddlers. *Journal of the American Dietetic Association, 106,* S107–S123.

5 Vitamins

WHAT WILL YOU LEARN?

1. To verbalize the connection between vitamins and health maintenance.
2. To summarize good dietary sources of water-soluble and fat-soluble vitamins.
3. To differentiate risk factors for hypovitaminosis and hypervitaminosis.
4. To evaluate signs and symptoms of vitamin deficiency that can be found when conducting a nursing assessment.
5. To examine the role of the nurse in identifying individuals at risk for altered health related to poor vitamin status.

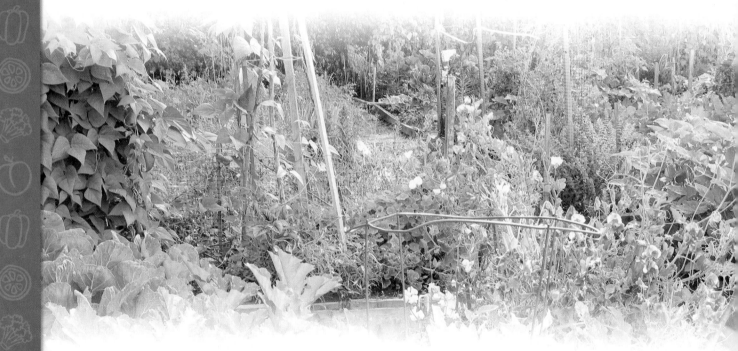

DID YOU KNOW?

▶ Excessive intake of active vitamin A or vitamin A-related acne medication can lead to birth defects in a developing fetus.

▶ Up to half of adolescents and adults have poor vitamin D status. Teen and adult females have the lowest intake of vitamin D compared with other age and gender groups.

▶ Smokers need more vitamin C than nonsmokers to maintain plasma levels of the vitamin.

▶ Folic acid can help prevent neural tube defects, a type of birth defect that occurs during the very early stages of pregnancy before some females even realize that they are pregnant.

▶ A synthetic or supplemental form of vitamin B_{12} is recommended for vegans because plant forms of the vitamin are not biologically available to humans.

KEY TERMS

Vitamins in Health

Before the discovery of specific vitamins, scientists first observed an association between certain foods and health. In the mid-1700s Lind discovered that keeping a supply of limes or lemons on naval ships prevented **scurvy,** a condition that we now know is caused by a vitamin C deficiency. The discovery of specific vitamins did not begin to occur until much later, in the early 1900s, when the B vitamins and eventually others were isolated. Early research focused on vitamin food sources and on understanding the amount of vitamins necessary to prevent deficiency symptoms. National recommendations for vitamin and nutrient intake in healthy individuals, now known as the *dietary reference intakes* (DRI), coincided with this initial research focus on the prevention of nutrient deficiencies. Presently, the role of vitamins in health is emerging into new territory surrounding potential disease prevention at intakes well above the amounts that prevent deficiency states. With this newer focus, scientists are also realizing the potential toxicity of higher doses of vitamins. As a result, the DRIs now include a **tolerable upper intake limit (UL)** for some nutrients when sufficient research exists to establish a safe upper limit for vitamin intake. DRIs are discussed in detail in Chapter 9.

The nurse today faces the challenging task of balancing advice about healthful amounts of vitamin intake from food or supplements while maintaining up-to-date knowledge regarding both positive and negative effects of high doses of vitamin intake.

What Are Vitamins?

Vitamins are organic compounds made up of molecules of elements such as hydrogen, oxygen, carbon, and others. Both vitamins and minerals are referred to as **micronutrients** because only small amounts are required by the body. The human body cannot synthesize sufficient amounts of most vitamins, with the exception of vitamin D when sunlight exposure is adequate. Vitamins play many different biological roles in the body. Vitamins are important components of many cellular activities in the body, including metabolism, growth, and repair. Some vitamins act as cofactors or coenzymes in metabolism, meaning that their presence is essential for specific biochemical reactions to take place. Other vitamins are **antioxidants,** preventing oxidative damage to cells from by-products of metabolism or the environment called **free radicals.** Vitamin D is considered to be a hormone-like vitamin because its active form originates in a different part of the body than that where it exerts its action. More recently, vitamins have been used as pharmaceutical agents, such as with the use of high doses of niacin to treat certain types of hyperlipidemia. Table 5-1 outlines the different roles that vitamins play in the body.

Do All Vitamins Have a Recommended Dietary Allowance?

DRIs are used as reference values in outlining recommendations for vitamin intake for healthy people. Under the umbrella of the DRIs, some vitamins have an established recommended dietary allowance (RDA) if sufficient scientific findings exist to support a specific recommendation. Vitamin A is an example of a vitamin with an RDA. Other vitamins, such as vitamin D, have an adequate intake (AI) recommendation because of insufficient data to set an RDA.

MyNursingKit National Institute for Health, Office of Dietary Supplements

Table 5-1   Vitamin Functions

Function	Vitamin Examples
Cofactor or coenzyme of metabolism	Thiamin: Cofactor in metabolism of carbohydrate and amino acids. Riboflavin: Coenzyme in production of energy
Growth and repair	Vitamin C: Collagen formation Vitamin D: Bone mineralization
Antioxidant	Vitamin C: Prevent oxidation in lung and gastric mucosa Vitamin E: Prevent oxidation of lipids
Hormone	Vitamin D: Maintenance of serum calcium and phosphorus
Medication	Niacin: Treatment of high blood lipids

Table 5-2   Risk Factors for Hypovitaminosis

Risk Factor	Examples
Decreased nutrient intake	Poor appetite Restrictive eating or dieting Fad diets Pain Medication side effects Gastrointestinal symptoms Difficulty chewing or swallowing Food intolerance or allergy Overly restrictive therapeutic diet Food insecurity (lack of finances or access to food) Lack of food preparation skills Knowledge deficit regarding nutrition
Altered absorption or metabolism	Malabsorptive disease Alcohol intake Medication interaction Medical condition
Increased nutrient needs that go unmet	Growth Pregnancy and lactation Excessive or intense physical activity Wound or fracture healing Burns Medical condition (e.g., fever, obstructive pulmonary disease, infection) Excessive nutrient losses (e.g., chronic diarrhea, exudative wound)

The DRIs for all vitamins, including the RDAs, AI, and UL are contained in Appendix C.

Vitamin Deficiency and Toxicity

Alterations in health can occur from either too much or too little vitamin stores. **Hypovitaminosis** is the term used to indicate insufficient vitamin stores and occurs for three primary reasons: decreased intake of the vitamin, altered absorption or metabolism, and unmet increased need for the vitamin. Table 5-2 outlines some examples of hypovitaminosis and its risk factors. Physical signs and symptoms of hypovitaminosis generally do not occur early on in a deficiency. First, vitamin storage or plasma levels are diminished, but there is not always an accurate laboratory value to measure this decrease. Only when vitamin status has been diminished for a longer period are alterations in vitamin function, including physical signs and symptoms, evident. The nurse should be alarmed when physical evidence of poor vitamin status is present because this indicates that the problem has not been a short-term one. Deficiency of water-soluble vitamins occurs in a shorter time span than for fat-soluble vitamins because of the body's limited storage of water-soluble vitamins. When poor vitamin status is suspected but no clinical evidence is obvious, the deficiency is considered a subclinical one.

Hypervitaminosis is the term used to indicate excessive vitamin stores. Most cases of hypervitaminosis occur because of use of supplemental vitamins rather than from foods with naturally occurring vitamins. Additionally, the popularity of fortified foods containing most of a day's worth of vitamins in a single serving presents another avenue for hypervitaminosis, especially when combined with supplemental vitamin use. **Fortified foods** are those with nutrients added that are not naturally found in the food.

Enriched foods are those that have nutrients replaced that may have been lost in processing.

The nurse should be aware of the signs and symptoms of altered vitamin health discussed here that can be found during a nursing assessment. Often, these physical symptoms are difficult to distinguish from other medical symptoms or have shared findings with other vitamin states. A good nursing assessment is a key starting point to determining vitamin status in individuals.

Vitamin Classification

Vitamins are classified according to solubility in solutions. The fat-soluble vitamins are vitamins A, D, E, and K. Fat-soluble vitamins are soluble in fatty substances or fatty tissues in the body. Water-soluble vitamins include vitamin C and all the B vitamins, sometimes referred to as B-complex vitamins: thiamin, riboflavin, niacin, folate, vitamins B_6 and B_{12}, biotin, and pantothenic acid. Water-soluble vitamins dissolve in watery solutions in the body. In general, the water-soluble vitamins are more prone to destruction from excessive heat, air, or light exposure during food storage or cooking than are fat-soluble vitamins. The type of solubility affects the way in which vitamins are absorbed, transported,

Table 5-3   Fat-Soluble and Water-Soluble Vitamin Characteristics

Vitamin Class	Absorption	Transport	Storage and Excretion	Toxicity/Deficiency Issues
Fat soluble A, D, E, and K	Requires bile for absorption in the small intestine. Absorbed into the lymphatic system with fats. Fat malabsorption will compromise absorption of fat-soluble vitamins.	Bound to proteins for transport in the blood.	Stored in fatty tissue, adipose, organs, especially the liver. Some excretion of excesses occurs in feces.	Excessive intake can result in excessive storage and toxicity. Deficiency occurs after long-term inadequate intake and depleted storage.
Water soluble C, B complex	Passively and actively absorbed by the small intestine.	Transported freely or by specific carriers.	Stored in watery solutions in small amounts; regular consumption, therefore, needed. Excesses are generally excreted in urine or feces.	Toxicity possible with some water-soluble vitamins when taken as supplements. Deficiencies occur within weeks because of minimal storage by the body. Vitamins C and B_6 and folate are easily destroyed by prolonged storage, cooking, or chilling.

and stored in the body. Table 5-3 outlines the generic differences between fat-soluble and water-soluble vitamin absorption, transport, and storage in the body.

Vitamins are also classified as **provitamins** and **preformed vitamins.** Preformed vitamins are the metabolically active form of the vitamin, whereas provitamins are the inactive form. For example, retinol is an active form of vitamin A, and beta carotene is an inactive form of vitamin A. Provitamins require conversion by the body to the active form of the vitamin.

Fat-Soluble Vitamins

Vitamins A, D, E, and K share the characteristic of being fat-soluble vitamins, yet their functions in the body vary widely from one another. Deficiencies of vitamins A and D are common worldwide, but deficiencies of E and K are unusual. The body can synthesize vitamin D, and bacteria in the intestine produce some vitamin K, but adequate intake of vitamins A and E is essential because the body does not produce these vitamins.

Vitamin A

Over 125 million children under age 5 years worldwide are affected by a deficiency of vitamin A (Johns Hopkins, 2007). This public health problem primarily affects those living in developing countries in Africa and Southeast Asia where

food sources of vitamin A are scarce (World Health Organization [WHO], 2008). In contrast to this prevalent deficiency, it has been reported that chronically high intake of vitamin A is associated with impaired bone remodeling and potential risk of fracture, especially among those with high intake of retinol, the active form of the vitamin, and low vitamin D intake (Caire-Juvera, Ritenburgh, Wactawski-Wende, Snetselaar, & Chen, 2009).

Function

Vitamin A is critical in maintaining many important functions in the body, including:

- Healthy vision
- Bone growth
- Immune response
- Cell proliferation and differentiation
- Epithelial cell integrity

Dark adaptation by the retina requires retinol, the preformed version of vitamin A, in order to synthesize rhodopsin, or visual purple (Institute of Medicine [IOM], 2001). Each time the eye is exposed to a light source while in the dark (such as when driving on a dark road and oncoming headlights approach) the photo cycle recombines retinol and opsin to form rhodopsin. Box 5-1 outlines the photo cycle containing vitamin A as retinol.

BOX 5-1   **Simplified Photo Cycle Including Vitamin A**

11-cis-retinal + opsin → rhodopsin (visual purple in rods in retina of eye)

　↑ ↓

　↑ ↓ ← ←— Light absorption by eye

　↑ ↓

Retinol (preformed vitamin A) ← ← ← ← ← all-trans retinal

Vitamin A is important to the body's immune response by participating in maintenance of circulating levels of natural killer cells, increasing phagocytic activity, and producing cytokines involved in inflammation (IOM, 2001). By maintaining the integrity of the epithelial cells in the body, such as the surface lining of the intestines, lungs, eyes, skin, and mucous membranes, vitamin A further assists in immunity through the synthesis of these healthy barriers to infection (National Institutes of Health [NIH], 2006).

Gene encoding and embryonic development require vitamin A. Cell proliferation and differentiation require vitamin A for healthy growth and development.

Table 5-4 outlines the functions of vitamin A and all other fat-soluble vitamins.

Recommended Intake

The RDA for vitamin A is 700 mcg retinol activity equivalents (RAE) for women and 900 mcg RAE for men (IOM, 2001). The use of RAE for vitamin A incorporates all its forms, preformed retinoids and provitamin forms, such as the carotenoids beta carotene, lycopene, and lutein. Provitamin A sources have lower RAE than preformed sources because they are not in the active form (IOM, 2001). Retinoids are found in animal foods and some vitamin supplements; carotenoids are found in plant foods and some vitamin supplements. It is essential that the nurse understand the difference between these forms of vitamin A because high intake of retinoids is associated with greater risk of toxicity than from provitamin forms of the vitamin. Vitamin A recommendations for infants, children, and pregnant or lactating females are contained in Appendix C.

Food Sources

Preformed vitamin A in foods is found only in animal sources such as liver, fatty fish, egg yolks, whole milk, and butter. Margarine and low-fat and skim milk are fortified with vitamin A. Preformed vitamin A as retinol can also be present in vitamin supplements, including multivitamins. Provitamin A, called carotenoids, is found in leafy green vegetables and deep orange, yellow, and red fruits and vegetables. Spinach, broccoli, winter squashes, cantaloupe, carrots, tomatoes, and sweet potatoes are examples. Practice Pearl: Plant Sources of Vitamin A provides the nurse with a quick way to explain good sources of plant forms of vitamin A to the client. Provitamin A sources, such as beta carotene, can also be in vitamin supplements. Lycopene, lutein, and zeaxanthin are other carotenoids found in foods and some supplements, but they are not felt to be sources of vitamin A (NIH, 2006). Additionally, vitamin A can be found in fortified foods, such as meal replacement drinks or cereals. Reading the supplement facts label on the vitamin package or the nutrient facts

PRACTICE ☙ PEARL

Plant Sources of Vitamin A
Plant sources of vitamin A are generally green or orange in color. The darker the green or the deeper the orange color, generally the more vitamin A present in the fruit or vegetable. For example, spinach has more vitamin A than iceberg lettuce, and pumpkin has more than a peach. Of course, fruits and vegetables with added food coloring do not qualify for this rule!

Table 5-4 Fat-Soluble Vitamins

Vitamin	Function	Adult DRI	Deficiency Symptoms	Toxicity Symptoms
A	Maintenance of epithelial cell integrity, eye health, immune function	RDA: 700 mcg RAE females; 900 mcg RAE males	Night blindness Corneal ulceration Goose-bump flesh	Nausea and vomiting Blurred vision Birth defects
D	Maintenance of blood calcium and phosphorus levels Bone mineralization Cell growth Immune function	AI: 5 mcg up to age 50 years; 10 mcg age 51–70 years; 15 mcg over age 70 years	Muscle pain Skeletal pain Rickets in children Osteomalacia in adults	Hypercalcemia with resultant: • Calcification of soft tissues (e.g., kidney, heart, blood vessels) • Renal stones • Anorexia, nausea, vomiting • Confusion, depressive symptoms • Heart arrhythmia
E	Antioxidant Immune function Alters platelet aggregation	RDA: 15 mg	Fragile red blood cells in premature infants Peripheral neuropathy Ataxia	Decreased platelet aggregation, bleeding
K	Manufacture of blood clotting factors Bone health	AI: 90 mcg females; 120 mcg males	Altered blood clotting	No adverse effects reported

Table 5-5   Vitamin A Food Sources

Vitamin A Source	Vitamin A Content, RAE mcg*
Beef liver, cooked, 3 oz	6,582
Sweet potato, cooked, 1 potato	1,403
Carrots, cooked, 1 cup	1,341
Spinach, cooked, 1 cup	1,145
Kale, cooked, 1 cup	955
Winter squash, cooked, 1 cup	535
Cantaloupe, 1 cup	270

CT? How do these values compare to the general advice given using Practice Pearl: Plant Sources of Vitamin A?

*Recommendation Reminder: RDA for adult females—700 RAE mcg, adult males—900 RAE mcg.

Source: Adapted from U.S. Department of Agriculture Nutrient Data Lab. Retrieved March 25, 2009, from http://www.nal.usda.gov/fnic/foodcomp

on a food label will delineate the amount of each type of vitamin A present. Regular consumption of a variety of vitamin A sources is recommended to ensure adequate vitamin A storage for periods of low intake (NIH, 2006). Table 5-5 outlines food sources of vitamin A.

Deficiency

Deficiency of vitamin A occurs because of insufficient intake or from intestinal losses with chronic diarrhea from fat malabsorption, such as with pancreatic disease or cystic fibrosis. Excess alcohol intake compromises vitamin A status by depleting liver stores and by potentially diminishing dietary intake with a poor-quality diet (NIH, 2006).

Deficiency of vitamin A leads to changes in eye health called **xerophthalmia.** These changes first include impaired dark adaptation, called night blindness. As the deficiency progresses, xerosis, or dryness of the conjunctiva and cornea, ulceration of the cornea, and scarring occur, leading to blindness. Figure 5-1 ■ illustrates the effects of vitamin A deficiency on the eye.

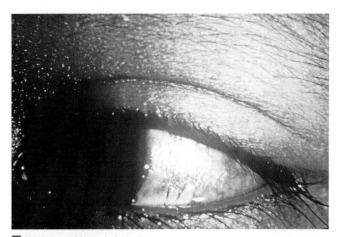

■ **FIGURE 5-1 Xerophthalmia.**

Source: Centers for Disease Control and Prevention.

Vitamin A deficiency causes changes in the integrity of epithelial cells that lead to skin alterations known as **follicular hyperkeratosis,** or "goose-bump flesh," where small raised bumps of skin surround the hair follicles on the body. Immune status can be compromised by poor vitamin A status. Children in developing countries lacking in vitamin A have higher risk of death or severe illness from common infections and measles; for that reason immunization programs in those countries are partnered with vitamin A supplementation efforts (IOM, 2001; WHO, 2008).

Deficiency of vitamin A is often confirmed by measuring plasma retinol levels, but because 80% of vitamin A storage is in the liver, not plasma, and reports of toxicity exist even with normal plasma retinol levels, research is underway to determine a more sensitive indicator of vitamin A status (Penniston & Tanumihardjo, 2006). The nurse should be aware that infection or protein malnutrition can confound plasma retinol levels because the carrier protein for retinol, called retinol-binding protein, is lowered because of these conditions (IOM, 2001). Treatment of clinical vitamin A deficiency or prevention of deficiency in high-risk populations does not follow established recommendations for daily intake, because the DRIs are intended for a well population. Treatment involves high-dose supplementation and medical monitoring.

Toxicity

The UL for vitamin A as retinol in adults is 2,800 mcg for females and 3,000 mcg for males (IOM, 2001). Most cases of excess vitamin A occur from excess intake of vitamin A supplements rather than overconsumption of foods containing the vitamin. About 25% of adults in the United States take a vitamin supplement that contains vitamin A (Sheth, Khurana, & Khurana, 2008). Preformed vitamin A, or retinoids, and not provitamin A forms in food, are associated with toxicity symptoms. Hypervitaminosis A occurs when excess storage of the vitamin occurs. Increased storage can go on to cause toxicity symptoms. Symptoms occur from excessively high intake over a short period or moderately elevated doses over a longer period. Short-term intake of 15 mg (or 50,000 international units) in adults can cause symptoms such as nausea and vomiting, headaches, blurred vision (Allen & Haskell, 2002). In infants, an additional finding is a bulging fontanel (Allen & Haskell, 2002). The nurse should educate the pregnant female client about the negative outcomes associated with high intake of vitamin A during pregnancy as outlined in Lifespan Box: Vitamin A and Pregnancy. Chronic vitamin A toxicity leads to liver damage (Sheth et al., 2008). Individuals with high alcohol intake or preexisting liver damage are advised to avoid excess preformed vitamin A from supplements (IOM, 2001).

Wellness Concerns and Supplement Use

Hypervitaminosis A has been associated with diminished bone mineral density. High intake of vitamin A as retinol

Lifespan

Vitamin A and Pregnancy

High-dose vitamin A intake by pregnant females can lead to birth defects at doses over 10,000 international units per day (Wooltorton, 2003). Medications for acne and other skin conditions can contain synthetic forms of retinoids, such as isotretinoin, that also can lead to birth defects. For this reason, women of childbearing age who are prescribed these medications are advised to use an effective method of birth control (NIH, 2006). Some females with acne symptoms may take vitamin A supplements because of the similarity in chemistry to these acne treatment medications and inadvertently expose a fetus to excess vitamin A. Vitamin A supplementation should only be under medical guidance during pregnancy (IOM, 2000).

from foods, fortified foods, and supplements has been reported to increase the risk of hip fracture in observational studies (Caire-Juvera et al., 2009). Cumulative intake of 1,500 mcg per day up to 3,000 mcg per day has an observed association with reduced bone mineral density, especially in those with poor vitamin D status (NIH, 2006). The nurse should be aware that although this level of intake is above the RDA for vitamin A, it approximates the UL recommendation of 2,800 mcg retinol for women and 3,000 mcg of retinol for men. Further study is needed to understand the association between higher levels of vitamin A intake and poor bone health. In the meantime, the nurse should assess clients for intake of fortified foods with vitamin A and supplements containing retinol. Cautionary advice is needed with pregnant females and clients who approach the UL of vitamin A intake on a chronic basis. The optimal source of vitamin A is from food sources; overuse of dietary supplements containing retinol should be avoided.

Vitamin D

The active form of vitamin D—1,25 dihydroxyvitamin D, or calcitriol—technically is classified as a hormone because it is activated in one tissue and exerts its effect on other tissues in the body. Provitamin forms of vitamin D must first undergo hydroxylation by the liver and then the kidney to become biologically active. Vitamin D is unique among other nutrients because provitamin D_3 can be synthesized in the skin when exposed to sunlight, providing a major source of the vitamin to the body.

Function

Vitamin D is responsible for maintaining blood levels of calcium and phosphorus within narrow normal limits by regulating bone mineralization and the intestinal absorption of these minerals; in this role vitamin D is acting as a hormone. Proper bone mineralization relies on adequate vitamin D to promote calcium absorption. Vitamin D receptors exist in the intestine and bone to support the finely tuned regulation of serum calcium. Receptors also exist in other tissues in the body, suggesting a wider role for vitamin D beyond that of bone mineralization and regulation of calcium and phosphorus. Figure 5-2 ■ illustrates the relationship between vitamin D and maintenance of calcium and phosphorus balance. In addition to the long-associated link between vitamin D, calcium, and bone health, more recent research is investigating new potential functions of vitamin D in health. Epidemiological studies have found an association between low vitamin D levels in the body and risk of certain cancers, type 1 diabetes, and cardiovascular disease, among other chronic diseases (Cannell & Hollis, 2008). Observational studies have noted an inverse relationship between vitamin D levels and risk of prostate, colon, breast, and pancreatic cancers. Evidence is strongest for the association between low vitamin D levels and increased incidence of colon cancer (Davis, 2008). It is known that vitamin D plays an important role in immune function and cell growth and division, but more clinical research is needed before conclusions can be drawn regarding its role in disease prevention. The Evidence-Based Practice Box outlines this new disease-prevention perspective on vitamin D.

Recommended Intake

The DRI for vitamin D exists as a recommendation for AI because sufficient research does not exist to support the establishment of an RDA (NIH, 2008). The AI for vitamin D is (IOM, 1999; Wagner, Greer, & Section on Breastfeeding and Committee on Nutrition, 2008):

- Birth to age 50 years: 5 mcg or 200 international units. This recommendation has not been updated in many years, in contrast to the current American Academy of Pediatrics recommendation that infants, children, and adolescents consume 10 mcg or 400 international units daily.
- Age 51 to 70 years: the AI doubles to 10 mcg or 400 international units.
- After age 70 years: the AI further increases to 15 mcg or 600 international units because of concerns outlined in Lifespan Box: Vitamin D and aging.

Great scientific debate exists surrounding the current DRI for vitamin D for adults because of more current evidence that a substantially greater amount of vitamin D intake is needed for health than is recommended (Cannell & Hollis, 2008). Most experts are recommending 800 to 1,000 international units/day for adults (Holick, 2007).

Sources

Sun exposure is an important source of vitamin D because natural food sources of this vitamin are limited. Oily fish such

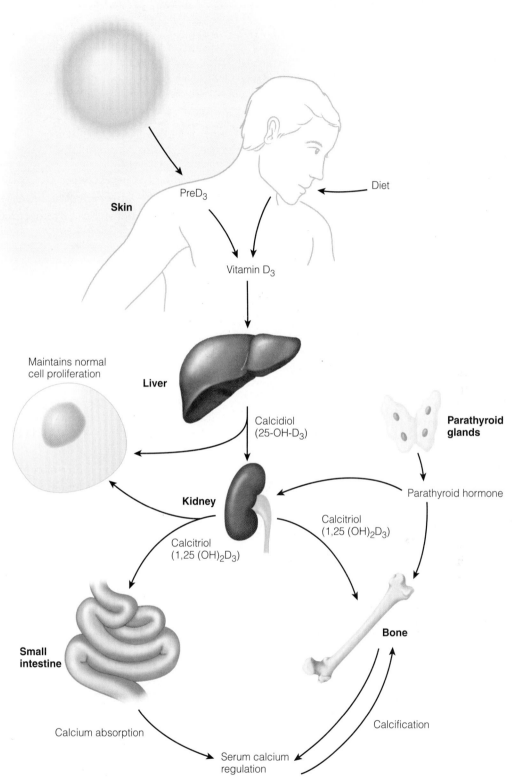

Skin

PreD₃

Diet

Vitamin D₃

Maintains normal
cell proliferation

Liver

Calcidiol
(25-OH-D₃)

Parathyroid
glands

Kidney

Parathyroid hormone

Calcitriol
(1,25 (OH)₂D₃)

Calcitriol
(1,25 (OH)₂D₃)

Small
intestine

Bone

Calcium absorption

Calcification

Serum calcium
regulation

■ FIGURE 5-2 **Vitamin D and Calcium Balance.**

EVIDENCE-BASED PRACTICE RESEARCH BOX

What is the recommendation about taking vitamin D to prevent multiple sclerosis?

Clinical Problem: Vitamin D is being closely scrutinized as a possible way to prevent multiple sclerosis and to ameliorate symptoms in those who have it.

Research Findings: Multiple sclerosis (MS) is a condition in which there is demyelinization of nerves in the brain and spinal cord. It is characterized by varying degrees of disability, ranging from none to difficulty with vision, ambulation, muscle weakness, fatigue, or bladder control. The overall incidence of MS increases with distance north or south of the equator; therefore, researchers believe that there is an association of the disease with vitamin D, which the body produces naturally when skin is exposed to sunlight. People who live closer to the equator are exposed to more sunlight and they tend to have higher blood levels of vitamin D.

Data from the Nurses' Health Study (1980–2000) and the Nurses' Health Study II (1991–2001) were examined for dietary intake of vitamin D and supplement use (Munger et al., 2004). Data from thousands of participants showed that nurses who had the highest intake of vitamin D had the lowest risk of developing MS. This inverse relationship of high intake associated with lower risk of MS suggests a protective effect of vitamin D. A review of current literature and research by Brown (2006) led to the conclusion that most studies have been relatively small but that adequate intake of vitamin D, especially before age 20, may help prevent MS. There is also some evidence that oral supplementation of vitamin D may be a useful addition to medical therapies for MS.

An extensive study of stored blood from U.S. Army and Navy personnel who developed MS was compared to a control group who did not develop MS (Munger, Levin, Hollis, Howard, & Ascherio, 2006). Findings showed a 62% reduced risk of developing MS in Caucasians who had the highest blood levels of vitamin D. No association was found for blacks or Hispanics, perhaps due to small numbers of those groups who developed MS.

Nursing Implications: Health care providers should be aware that vitamin D is often consumed in suboptimal amounts in all age groups. There is increasing evidence that vitamin D from dietary sources and supplements, when consumed in amounts that do not exceed AI, may be useful in decreasing risk of MS.

CRITICAL THINKING QUESTIONS:

1. How should the nurse respond to the 23-year-old client whose 49-year-old father was recently diagnosed with MS and who wants to know the risk of developing it and if the disease can be prevented?

2. What should the nurse suggest to the 23-year-old vegan who wants to ensure adequate intake of vitamin D?

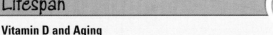

Lifespan

Vitamin D and Aging

Increased intake of vitamin D is recommended in older adults because of a diminished capacity to produce vitamin D through cutaneous synthesis from the sun. When compared with adults age 20 to 30 years, those over age 65 years have a fourfold decrease in ability to produce vitamin D from the skin (IOM, 1999). Additionally, institutionalized or homebound older adults can have decreased exposure to sunlight. Aging can also lessen the ability of the kidney to produce active vitamin D (NIH, 2008).

as salmon, sardines, and mackerel and fish oils are good sources. Food fortification was begun in 1930s to provide improved dietary sources of vitamin D because so few foods naturally contain the vitamin. Milk, margarine, and some orange juices and ready-to-eat cereals are fortified with vitamin D. Table 5-6 outlines food sources of vitamin D.

Cutaneous synthesis of vitamin D occurs in the presence of sunlight when a precursor to cholesterol in the skin reacts with solar ultraviolet B (UV-B) radiation (Holick, 2007). As little as 10 to 15 minutes of midday sun exposure of the face, arms, and legs a few times a week is enough to establish adequate vitamin D synthesis (NIH, 2008). Living at a latitude greater than 35° during winter months (farther north than North Carolina), smog pollution, having darker pigmented skin, and using sunscreen with sunscreen protection factor (SPF) rated 8 or greater reduces UV-B exposure and, therefore, vitamin D synthesis (Cannell & Hollis, 2008; Holick, 2007; NIH, 2008). Individuals who are homebound because of disability, institutionalization, or unsafe environment have decreased sun exposure and are at risk for altered vitamin D status. The effects of culture on vitamin D status should be considered as outlined in Cultural Considerations: The Effects of Dress on Vitamin D.

Table 5-6   Vitamin D Food Sources

Vitamin D Source	Vitamin D Content, International Units*
Cod liver oil, 1 tablespoon	1360
Salmon, cooked, 3½ oz	360
Milk, skim, vitamin D-fortified, 1 cup	98
Egg, 1 whole	20

How could an older adult meet the AI of 600 international units of vitamin D using only food?

*Recommendation Reminder: AI for adults up to age 50 years—200 international units, 51–70 years—400 international units, over 70 years—600 international units.

Source: Adapted from U.S. Department of Agriculture Nutrient Data Lab. Retrieved March 25, 2009, from http://www.nal.usda.gov/fnic/foodcomp

Cultural Considerations

The Effects of Dress on Vitamin D
In cultures where clothing covers most of the body, such as with traditionally dressed Muslim women, sunlight exposure and, therefore, vitamin D synthesis is limited.

Deficiency

Vitamin D insufficiency is reportedly becoming an increasing problem worldwide (Holick, 2007). Serum 25-hydroxy-vitamin D (calcidiol) is measured as an indicator of vitamin D status. Calcidiol levels below 30 to 40 ng/L are considered insufficient (Cannell & Hollis, 2008; Holick, 2007). Poor vitamin D status occurs because of:

- Insufficient intake
- Little exposure to sunlight
- Medical conditions such as malabsorptive disease and liver or kidney disease that impair vitamin activation
- Medications such as anticonvulsants and steroids (glucocorticoids) that can cause deficiency because of drug–nutrient interactions

The prevalence of hypovitaminosis D has been reported to be about one-half or more of healthy adult and adolescent Americans, Canadians, and Europeans, especially during the winter months (Holick, 2007). Poor intake of vitamin D-fortified foods and lack of sunlight exposure are cited as the major contributors to low vitamin D levels. Teenage girls and adult females have the lowest intake of vitamin D from food when compared to other age and gender groups (Moore, Murphy, Keast, & Holick, 2004). Up to 90% of older adults in the United States reportedly do not consume adequate vitamin D (Moore et al., 2004). Older adults are at increased risk of vitamin D deficiency because of poor intake and decreased cutaneous synthesis (Moore et al., 2004; NIH, 2008). Individuals who follow a vegan diet and consume no animal products, or those with intolerance to milk products, can have inadequate vitamin D intake unless specific attention is paid to intake of good sources of the vitamin. Infants who are exclusively breastfed are at risk of poor vitamin D status because human milk is not a good source of the vitamin. Breastfed infants and those not consuming more than 500 mL of vitamin D-fortified infant formula should receive a vitamin D supplement of 400 international units/day (Wagner et al., 2008). Box 5-2 outlines additional populations at risk for poor vitamin D status.

Rickets is the term used to denote myriad symptoms that comprise clinical vitamin D deficiency in children. In adults, the deficiency disease is called **osteomalacia.** Poor vitamin D status exists for months before clinical signs of deficiency become apparent on physical examination. The prevalence of rickets has increased worldwide, especially

---

BOX 5-2 — Risk Factors for Vitamin D Insufficiency

Inadequate intake:
Poor quality diet
Lactose intolerance
Milk allergy
Exclusive intake of breast milk without supplementation
Vegan diet

Limited sun exposure:
Homebound or institutionalized living
Cultural dress traditions
Use of sunscreen
Northern latitude living in winter months
Smog pollution
Dark skin pigmentation

Altered vitamin absorption, activation, or metabolism:
Liver disease
Kidney disease
Fat malabsorption, such as can occur with pancreatitis, celiac sprue, inflammatory bowel disease, cystic fibrosis
Medication interactions, such as with corticosteroid or anticonvulsant use
Aging

Source: Adapted from National Institutes of Health, Office for Dietary Supplements, 2008.

among infants who are exclusively breastfed and those who have dark skin (Wagner et al., 2008). Rickets is the result of poor bone mineralization yielding soft and malformed bones, particularly at the growth plates. Osteomalacia also is a result of poor bone mineralization but occurs in older individuals when bone growth has ceased. Clinical signs and symptoms of rickets are described in Box 5-3 and illustrated in Figure 5-3 ■.

BOX 5-3 — Rickets Signs and Symptoms

Frontal bossing of cranial bones in infants
Delayed closure of fontanelle
Widened wrists and ankles from calcium deposition at the growth plate
Rachitic rosary (beaded appearance at costochondral junction of ribs)
Pigeon breast (forward projection of the breastbone)
Bowed legs or knock-knees
Narrowed pelvis
Spinal curvature
Delayed tooth eruption with increased risk of caries in first dentition
Impaired growth

MyNursingKit University of Nebraska, Lincoln Extension: Nutrition and Osteoporosis

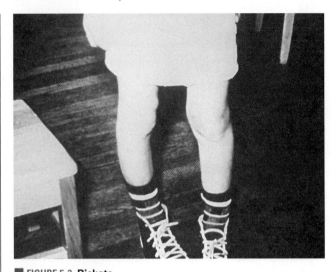

■ FIGURE 5-3 Rickets.

Source: Centers for Disease Control and Prevention.

Vitamin D deficiency is associated with nonspecific musculoskeletal pain that is often misdiagnosed as fibromyalgia or wrongly associated with other disorders (Holick, 2007). Muscular weakness and pain in the older adult with vitamin D deficiency is associated with an increased risk of falls and hip fracture (Cauley et al., 2008; Dawson-Hughes, 2008).

Osteoporosis is a different condition than osteomalacia, but the diseases share a risk factor of poor vitamin D status. Bones become soft and pliable with osteomalacia, whereas osteoporosis is the result of decreased bone mass and porous bones. Osteoporosis occurs when less than optimal peak bone mass is achieved. When bone mass is diminished, but not to the extent that qualifies for a diagnosis of osteoporosis, the condition is referred to as **osteopenia.** Bone health is influenced by the partnership between vitamin D and calcium. Both nutrients are necessary for proper mineralization of bone. Poor nutrition, including diminished intake of calcium and vitamin D, contributes to risk of osteopenia and osteoporosis. Restrictive eating, including dieting and disordered eating, or excessive alcohol intake contribute to poor vitamin D and calcium intake. Medications that interact with calcium or vitamin D absorption or utilization pose a risk as well. Accumulation and preservation of bone mass are also influenced by hormone status. Males and females are at risk for osteoporosis with advancing age because of declining reproductive hormone status (Cashman, 2007). The nurse should include an assessment of vitamin D and calcium status in clients across the lifespan. Poor accumulation of bone during childhood and adolescence can lead to later risk of osteoporosis. In adulthood, preservation of bone is paramount. Appropriate recommendations should be given to improve vitamin D and calcium intake as outlined in Client Education Checklist: Vitamin D. Supplementation may be necessary with some individuals who cannot achieve adequate intake. Calcium nutrition is discussed further in Chapter 6.

Toxicity

Hypervitaminosis D is more likely to occur from oversupplementation than from excess intake of food sources of vitamin D (NIH, 2008). A physiological limit exists to vitamin D synthesized from sun exposure and no reports exist in the literature regarding toxicity from this source (Holick, 2007; NIH, 2008). The UL for vitamin D in children and adults is 50 mcg (2,000 international units) daily, but this recommendation is receiving heavy negative scrutiny for being too conservative (Hathrock, Shao, Vieth, & Heaney, 2007). Critics argue for a

---

CLIENT EDUCATION CHECKLIST ✓ **Vitamin D**

Client Education Checklist: Vitamin D

1. Assess diet for sources of vitamin D. Include fortified foods and supplements.
2. Determine any reasons why vitamin D intake is low. Consider diet and sun exposure.
3. Educate the client on the role of vitamin D in health:
   - Bone and teeth formation
   - Osteomalacia and rickets prevention
   - Fosters absorption of calcium
4. Customize advice based on causes of poor vitamin D intake. Suggestions follow each contributor to low intake.
   a) Lactose intolerance: Milk with lactase added, vitamin D- and calcium-fortified juice or soy products, fish with small bones (sardines, anchovies).
   b) Vegan diet: Vitamin D- and calcium-fortified soy or rice milk, vitamin D- and calcium-fortified juice.
   c) Cost: Fortified breakfast cereals, lower cost cheeses, skim or low-fat milk. Fortified soy milk is a more expensive source of vitamin D.
   d) Dislike plain dairy foods: Make a smoothie with milk and fresh or frozen fruit; cook with milk instead of water, making hot cereal, pancakes, or cocoa; make desserts with milk—like pudding; choose nondairy sources like oily fish.
   e) Knowledge deficit: Explain good sources of vitamin D—like milk; margarine; oily fish such as salmon; and fortified juice, cereals, and soy products.
5. Discuss the ability of the body to synthesize vitamin D from 15 minutes of sun exposure to the upper body a few times a week during warm weather months. Advise against overexposure to UV rays and urge use of sunscreen when in the sun for longer than 15 minutes. Customize this advice to an individual's risk factors for skin cancer.
6. Advise older adults and those unable to improve intake of vitamin D to meet daily vitamin D needs with a supplement.

higher UL given that toxicity symptoms do not occur until much higher intakes and the current UL is thwarting scientific attempts to improve vitamin D fortification of food in the United States. Toxicity causes hypercalcemia and its associated symptoms are outlined in Table 5-4.

Wellness Concerns and Supplement Use

Some individuals require supplementation to meet the daily recommendation for vitamin D. Limited sun exposure, poor intake of vitamin D-containing foods, and malabsorptive conditions may warrant regular supplementation to avoid diminished vitamin D status. The nurse should recommend a multivitamin or single vitamin D supplement with the appropriate AI content for individuals with limited sun exposure, those with inadequate intake of vitamin D, and adults over age 50 years (NIH, 2008). Infants should receive vitamin D to meet the 400-international unit recommendation either in the form of a supplement or fortified infant formula (Wagner et al., 2008). Individuals should be encouraged to improve intake of food sources of vitamin D where tolerated. The nurse should consult with a registered dietitian when considering vitamin D supplementation for any individuals with fat malabsorptive conditions, such as pancreatitis, or following bariatric surgery.

Vitamin E

Vitamin E is a universal name given to a group of eight forms of the vitamin. According to current recommendations, only the form known as α-tocopherol contributes to the body's need for the vitamin (IOM, 2000). Other forms are absorbed from the diet but are not preferentially metabolized by the liver and found in plasma. Another common vitamin E form found in some nuts, soybean, and sesame oils, γ-tocopherol, has begun to receive attention for a potential metabolic or health role in humans, but more research is needed to establish any conclusive finding (Cooney, Franke, Wilkens, & Kolonel, 2008).

Function

Vitamin E functions as an antioxidant in the body. It is specifically involved in preventing oxidation of lipids, especially polyunsaturated fats within membranes and lipoproteins such as low-density lipoprotein (LDL-cholesterol) (IOM, 2000). Additionally, vitamin E is known to alter platelet aggregation and adhesion and to play a role in immune function (IOM, 2000; NIH, 2007a). Theories that link the prevention of oxidative injury with prevention of cardiovascular disease and cancer have fueled much investigation into a possible role for vitamin E in the risk reduction of these conditions. Observational and animal studies have indicated an inverse relationship between vitamin E intake and risk of cardiovascular disease and some cancers, but these findings have not been supported by the outcome of clinical trials (Gaziano et al., 2009; Sesso et al., 2008).

Recommended Intake

The RDA for vitamin E is 15 mg (16.5 international units) for males and females over age 13 years (IOM, 2000). The recommendation is given as α-tocopherol equivalents (ATE) to account for the differing forms of α-tocopherol in foods and supplements. Natural forms of α-tocopherol are more biologically active than are synthetic forms found in some supplements and fortified foods (NIH, 2007a).

Food Sources

Vitamin E is naturally occurring in some vegetable oils, nuts, and seeds. Some fortified foods, such as breakfast cereals or juices, have vitamin E added. Vitamin E is also available in vitamin supplements as part of a multivitamin or as a single supplement in varying doses. Table 5-7 outlines sources of vitamin E.

Deficiency

Deficiency of vitamin E is uncommon and most often linked to an inherited metabolic disease or fat malabsorption (IOM, 2000; NIH, 2007a). Deficiency first manifests itself as **peripheral neuropathy,** or tingling in the hands and feet, and then progresses to ataxia, myopathy, and retinopathy (IOM, 2000). Premature, low birth weight babies can have vitamin E deficiency resulting in fragile red blood cells and anemia (Debier, 2007). Vitamin E supplementation is indicated to correct a deficiency. Chronic supplements can be required when malabsorption or genetic alterations in metabolism exist (Eggermont, 2006). Individuals on chronically low-fat diets can have diminished intake of vitamin E if careful food choices are not made (IOM, 2000). The nurse should advise these clients of good sources of vitamin E as outlined in Table 5-7.

Toxicity

The UL for vitamin E intake is 1,000 mg daily (1,500 international units/day) (IOM, 2000). The UL was established based on a tendency toward increased bleeding or hemorrhaging with high doses (IOM, 2000). High doses of vitamin E potentiate the antiplatelet effect of aspirin and other anticoagulant medications, such as coumadin, which can further the anticoagulant effect of these drugs (IOM, 2000; Wu & Croft, 2007).

Table 5-7 Vitamin E Food Sources

Vitamin E Source	Vitamin E Content, mg*
Sunflower seeds, dry roast, ¼ cup	8.35
Almonds, 1 oz (24)	7.33
Spinach, cooked, 1 cup	6.73
Canola oil, 1 tablespoon	2.39
Peanuts, 1 oz (28)	2.21

*Recommendation Reminder: RDA for adults—15 mg.
Source: Adapted from U.S. Department of Agriculture Nutrient Data Lab. Retrieved March 25, 2009, from http://www.nal.usda.gov/fnic/foodcomp

Research exists that supports the need to lower the UL for vitamin E because of negative outcomes at smaller intakes. A meta-analysis evaluating the findings of 19 trials found an increase in all-cause mortality with vitamin E supplementation of 400 international units/day or greater (Miller, Pastor-Barriuso, Riemersma, Appel, & Guallar, 2005). Reports have included an association between vitamin E supplements and increased risk of heart failure, ischemic events, and reduction in cardioprotective effects of statin drugs.

Wellness Concerns and Supplement Use

Supplements of vitamin E at varying high doses are widely available on the market. People may take vitamin E, choosing to believe it has cardioprotective or cancer-fighting powers. Some research supports a possible role for vitamin E in delaying the progression of already existing disorders, such as macular degeneration (Jager, Mieler, & Miller, 2008). Vitamin E supplementation to reduce the risk of Alzheimer's disease is less hopeful (Gray et al., 2008), but lack of consistent research findings does not stop some individuals from taking the supplement. When conducting a nursing assessment, the nurse should include an evaluation of dietary supplement intake and caution clients who are self-prescribing vitamins about the negative research outcomes at increased doses of vitamin E. Special attention should be paid to clients who are on aspirin and other anticoagulant treatment.

Vitamin K

Vitamin K plays an important role in health maintenance. New discoveries are underway that will expand the understanding of vitamin K function in humans.

Function

Vitamin K functions as a coenzyme in the synthesis of several proteins in the body. Some of these proteins are involved in the synthesis of blood-clotting factors, whereas others are important to bone health. Osteocalcin and matrix Gla protein are involved in bone metabolism, yet these proteins have reportedly been found in tissue outside the bone matrix, suggesting a possible undiscovered role for vitamin K (Van Winckel, DeBruyne, Van De Velde, & Van Biervliet, 2009).

Recommended Intake

The AI recommendation for vitamin K is 120 mcg/day for adult males and 90 mcg/day for adult females (IOM, 2001). During periods of low intake of vitamin K there may be preferential use of the vitamin for synthesis of blood-clotting factors at the expense of use in bone formation (Pearson, 2007). It is felt that the current AI for vitamin K may be too low to support optimal production of osteocalcin needed for bone formation, but no alternate recommendation currently exists (Pearson, 2007; Van Winckel et al., 2009).

Food Sources

Vitamin K is available in the diet from green leafy vegetables and some plant oils, such as soybean, cottonseed, canola, and

Table 5-8 Vitamin K Food Sources

Vitamin K Source	Vitamin K Content, mcg*
Kale, cooked, 1 cup	1,147
Collard greens, cooked, 1 cup	1,059
Spinach, cooked, 1 cup	1,027
Brussel sprouts, cooked, 1 cup	299
Broccoli, cooked, 1 cup	220

*Recommendation Reminder: AI for adult females—90 mcg, adult males—120 mcg.
Source: Adapted from U.S. Department of Agriculture Nutrient Data Lab. Retrieved March 25, 2009, from http://www.nal.usda.gov/fnic/foodcomp

olive oils. The form of vitamin K found in plants is called phylloquinone. The presence of fat in a food aids the absorption of vitamin K (Pearson, 2007). Vitamin K is also synthesized by bacteria in the large intestine. This form is called menaquinone. It is felt that the bacterial source of vitamin K alone is not sufficiently utilized by the body to support overall vitamin K requirements (IOM, 2001). Table 5-8 outlines sources of vitamin K in the diet.

Deficiency

Spontaneous cases of vitamin K-deficiency are unusual. In the neonate, vitamin K-deficiency bleeding is a rare life-threatening disorder. At birth infants have insufficient stores of vitamin K, and because of the sterility of the newborn's intestinal tract, adequate vitamin K has not been produced. It is a recommended practice for infants to receive an intramuscular injection of vitamin K at birth to prevent vitamin K deficiency bleeding (American Academy of Pediatrics, 2003). After feeding is initiated, infants receive vitamin K from breast milk or infant formula, in addition to the population of beneficial bacteria that develops in the intestine (American Academy of Pediatrics, 2003). Deficiency can occur related to disorders of fat absorption, such as biliary or pancreatic disease (IOM, 2001; Van Winckel et al., 2009). Suppression of menaquinone synthesis occurs with antibiotic treatment because the drugs alter gut flora and, therefore, the bacterial source of this form of the vitamin (IOM, 2001). Cystic fibrosis can lead to vitamin K deficiency because of chronic antibiotic use and both biliary and pancreatic insufficiency (Drury, Grey, Ferland, Gundberg, & Lands, 2008).

Deficiency results in alterations in vitamin K-dependent coagulation proteins, which leads to altered blood clotting, an elevated prothrombin time, and, ultimately, hemorrhaging (Van Winckel et al., 2009). Vitamin K is stored in the liver and turnover is rapid, resulting in quickly depleted stores in the absence of dietary intake (IOM, 2001). High intake of vitamin E can antagonize the anticoagulation effects of deficient vitamin K status (Booth et al., 2004).

Toxicity

No adverse effects have been reported with excess intake of vitamin K in healthy individuals not receiving anticoagulant therapy, and thus no UL exists for this vitamin (IOM, 2001).

Wellness Concerns and Supplement Use

Poor vitamin K intake and decreased circulating phylloquinones have been associated with increased risk of hip fracture (IOM, 2001; Pearson, 2007). It has been suggested that vitamin K plays a role in plasma calcium balance and bone health that is not yet fully understood (Pearson, 2007). The clinical significance of the relationship between bone health and plasma phylloquinones has yet to be established. The nurse should remain up to date on these research findings when counseling individuals on bone health and nutrition.

The nurse should be aware of the recommendation regarding vitamin K intake in clients prescribed the medication warfarin. Warfarin is prescribed for its anticoagulant effects in clients at risk for blood clot formation. This medication functions by interfering with vitamin K-related synthesis of clotting factors. Clients taking warfarin are advised to not vary the intake of vitamin K in the diet once a dose of warfarin has been established (National Institutes of Health [NIH], 2003). The nurse should advise clients of significant sources of vitamin K in the diet and the need to maintain an unvarying intake. When assessing intake of vitamin K, the nurse should include dietary supplements. Vitamin K present in dietary supplements, such as a multivitamin, is more bioavailable to humans than food sources and should not be overlooked (IOM, 2001). Bioavailability refers to how well a substance is absorbed and utilized by the body. Individuals on warfarin with low baseline intake of vitamin K are more likely to be sensitive to small changes in vitamin K intake, especially from supplements, than those with adequate intake (Johnson, 2005). A Client Education Checklist for this interaction is found in Chapter 25.

Water-Soluble Vitamins

Water-soluble vitamins include vitamin C and the B-complex vitamins, thiamin(B_1), riboflavin (B_2), niacin, pyridoxine (B_6), folate, the cobalamins (B_{12}), biotin, and pantothenic acid. As a rule, water-soluble vitamins are more easily destroyed by some handling and cooking processes than are fat-soluble vitamins. Many are cofactors of metabolism, and recommended intake is linked to overall energy needs. Additionally, water-soluble vitamins are stored in the body in lesser amounts than fat-soluble vitamins, which are stored in adipose. Together, these characteristics cause insufficient intake of water-soluble vitamins to lead more quickly to symptoms of deficiency than is seen with fat-soluble vitamins. Table 5-9 is an overview of water-soluble vitamins.

Vitamin C

Historical references to symptoms of vitamin C deficiency date back thousands of years. In the 1700s, a British Navy surgeon realized that these symptoms were prevented or cured with consumption of citrus fruit over the long months at sea; hence, the nickname "limeys" for the British Navy. It was not until the 1930s that the vitamin itself was isolated and named (Leger, 2008; Wang & Still, 2007).

Function

Vitamin C functions as an antioxidant and cofactor in the biosynthesis of many substances in the body. More specifically, vitamin C (IOM, 2000):

- Acts as an antioxidant scavenging free radicals, preventing oxidation in leukocytes, lung, and gastric mucosa
- Promotes the absorption of iron and may spare or regenerate vitamin E in the body
- Plays a role in the biosynthesis of collagen and connective tissue, important to the healing process
- Aids in synthesis of norepinephrine, epinephrine, carnitine, and the amino acid tyrosine

Recommended Intake

The RDA for vitamin C is 90 mg for adult males and 75 mg for adult females (IOM, 2000). The requirement for vitamin C in smokers is increased by 35 mg/day because of the oxidation stress of smoking on the body (IOM, 2000). The nurse should encourage increased intake of vitamin C by smokers, but underline that the extra intake of this antioxidant in no way negates the free-radical effects and disease risk from smoking. Individuals regularly exposed to passive or second-hand smoke have been reported to have low plasma levels of vitamin C similar to smokers, but the RDA does not include a recommendation for increased intake in this population (IOM, 2000).

Food Sources

Vitamin C is present in fruits and vegetables. Citrus fruits in particular, such as oranges, limes, kiwi, and grapefruit, are good sources of vitamin C. The nurse should encourage intake of at least five servings of fruits and vegetables per day as part of an overall healthy diet and note that this level of intake will contain more than adequate vitamin C. Table 5-10 outlines sources of vitamin C in the diet.

Deficiency

Scurvy is the name coined for vitamin C-deficiency symptoms. Fatigue is the early symptom of scurvy, which often goes unrecognized (Leger, 2008). The deficiency symptoms then progress to include deterioration in connective and elastic tissues (IOM, 2000). Pinpoint hemorrhages on the skin, called **petechiae,** and swollen, bleeding gums are well-noted symptoms of scurvy. Figure 5-4 ■ illustrates the effects of vitamin C deficiency on the gums, known as scorbutic gums. Wound healing can be compromised by poor vitamin C status at each stage in the healing process. Alterations in collagen synthesis cause capillary fragility, which contributes to the many symptoms of scurvy that, ultimately, can result in death from hemorrhaging (Wang & Still, 2007). Plasma levels of vitamin C can be checked to determine vitamin status. A level less than 0.1 mg/dL indicates a deficiency

Table 5-9 Water-Soluble Vitamins

Vitamin	Function	Adult DRI	Deficiency	Toxicity
Vitamin C	Antioxidant Collagen and connective tissue synthesis Promotes absorption of iron	RDA: 90 mg males, 75 mg females	Scurvy: Petechiae, bleeding gums, hemorrhage Poor wound healing	Diarrhea Abdominal cramping Nausea
Thiamin	Coenzyme in metabolism	RDA: 1.2 mg males, 1.1 mg females	Beri-beri: Fatigue, muscle weakness, neuropathy (dry beri-beri), edema (wet beri-beri) Wernicke-Korsakoff syndrome	No reports or adverse effects
Riboflavin	Coenzyme in metabolism Conversion of vitamin B_6 to active form	RDA: 1.3 mg males, 1.1 mg females	Ariboflavinosis: Magenta tongue, angular stomatitis, cheilosis	No reports of adverse effects
Niacin	Coenzyme, cofactor of metabolism	RDA: 16 mg NE males, 14 mg NE females	Pellagra: 4 Ds—diarrhea, dermatitis, depression, death Cheilosis Glossitis	Skin flushing Hepatotoxicity
Vitamin B_6	Coenzyme of metabolism Required for conversion of tryptophan to niacin	RDA: 1.3 mg	Seborrheic dermatitis Microcytic anemia Depression Convulsions	Peripheral neuropathy
Folate	Coenzyme of metabolism Cell division Needed for closure of neural tube in fetus	RDA: 400 mcg	Macrocytic anemia	Excessive doses can mask and potentiate vitamin B_{12} deficiency
Vitamin B_{12}	Coenzyme of metabolism Cell division Spinal column myelination	RDA: 2.4 mcg, supplement or fortified food for those over age 50 years	Macrocytic anemia Demyelination of spinal column Peripheral neuropathy Dementia	No reports of adverse effects
Biotin	Cofactor of metabolism	AI: 30 mcg	Alopecia Red scaly rash	No reports of adverse effects
Pantothenic Acid	Cofactor in synthesis of coenzyme A Fatty acid synthesis	AI: 5 mg	Irritability Restlessness Gastrointestinal complaints	No reports of adverse effects

Table 5-10 Vitamin C Food Sources

Vitamin C Source	Vitamin C Content, mg*
Pepper, red, raw, 1 each	283
Orange juice, 1 cup	124
Broccoli, cooked, 1 cup	101
Strawberries, raw, 1 cup	98
Orange, raw, 1 each	96
Grapefruit juice, 1 cup	94
Kiwi, 1 medium	71

CT? What advice would you give to a smoker about vitamin C in the diet?
*Recommendation Reminder: RDA for adult females –75 mg, adult males –90 mg.
Source: Adapted from U.S. Department of Agriculture Nutrient Data Lab. Retrieved March 25, 2009, from http://www.nal.usda.gov/fnic/foodcomp

(Wang & Still, 2007). Symptoms of vitamin C deficiency are outlined in Box 5-4.

Those at risk for vitamin C deficiency include individuals with poor intake of fruits and vegetables, and those who abuse alcohol or drugs (Leger, 2008). Smokers and those who receive dialysis treatment for renal failure have increased need for vitamin C, which, if unmet, predisposes them to deficiency (Wang & Still, 2007). Deficiency is rare in infants because both human milk and infant formulas contain adequate vitamin C (IOM, 2000). Vitamin C is a particularly labile vitamin and is easily destroyed by prolonged exposure to air or light and with some storage and cooking practices. Prolonged storage and cooking times destroy vitamin C as does boiling. Loss of vitamin C can ex-

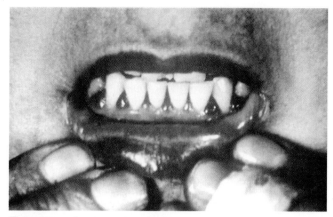

FIGURE 5-4 Scorbutic Gums.
Source: Centers for Disease Control and Prevention.

ceed 30% when food is reheated after 24 hours of cold storage (Galgano, Favati, Caruso, Pietrafesa, & Natella, 2007). In storage, losses approximate 40% of the vitamin over the course of a month (Galgano et al., 2007). When providing nutritional advice, the nurse should encourage short storage times for fruits and vegetables and preparation practices that minimize cooking time and exposure to water, such as steaming versus boiling vegetables. When reheating leftovers, vitamin C losses will be lessened by reheating small portions as needed rather than by whole batches repeatedly. Treatment for vitamin C deficiency can be accomplished quickly, with 1 gm/day given for up to 5 days followed by 300 to 500 mg/day for a week (Wang & Still, 2007). The nurse should collaborate with the client to determine easily accessible sources of vitamin C to include in the diet thereafter.

Toxicity

The UL for vitamin C intake is 2 gm, or 2000 mg, per day (IOM, 2000). Intake above this amount is associated with gastrointestinal side effects such as diarrhea, abdominal cramping, and nausea (IOM, 2000). In some individuals, especially

BOX 5-4	Symptoms of Vitamin C Deficiency

Early symptoms
Fatigue
Muscle weakness
Irritability

Later symptoms
Corkscrew-shaped hair
Petechiae—pinpoint hemorrhages on the skin
Scorbutic gums—swollen, bleeding gums
Poor wound healing
Hemorrhaging
Death

in those with existing renal disease or altered oxalate excretion, excess intake can increase risk of oxalate kidney stones (McGregor & Biesalski, 2006). Reports of dental enamel erosion and rebound scurvy following cessation of high-dose intake have been reported (IOM, 2000). Relative absorption of vitamin C is known to decrease with higher doses of intake; by-products of vitamin C appear in the urine above an intake of 100 mg (McGregor & Biesalski, 2006). It is felt that doses above 500 mg contribute little to vitamin C tissue storage. Intake above 200 mg contributes little to plasma levels of vitamin C (IOM, 2000). The nurse can advise those individuals who choose to take large doses of vitamin C of the doses associated with tissue saturation. Little research exists regarding any benefit to doses in excess of the UL.

Wellness Concerns and Supplement Use

The practice of taking vitamin C supplements to avoid the common cold is well known but not scientifically substantiated. It is agreed that intake of vitamin C above 200 mg can lessen the duration of an existing cold, but some argue that the effect is too small to be clinically significant (Hemila, Chalker, Treacy, & Douglas, 2007; IOM, 2000). When asked for advice on this practice, the nurse should not encourage chronic or excessive intake of vitamin C supplements, being mindful that there is little increased tissue levels at doses above 500 mg and that gastrointestinal side effects are dose related. Individuals prone to calcium oxalate kidney stones should be made aware that oxalate is a metabolite of vitamin C. Excess oxalate availability from vitamin C intake greater than 1,500 mg/ day can increase risk of this type of kidney stone in susceptible individuals (Borghi, Meschi, Maggiore, & Prati, 2006). Additionally, individuals taking supplements should be advised to stop intake 3 days before administration of a stool guaiac test, an assessment of blood in the feces, because higher intake can cause a false negative reading (Rabeneck, Zwaal, Goodman, & Zamkanei, 2008).

Thiamin

Thiamin was the first B vitamin to be identified and hence is often called vitamin B_1. Thiamin has been described as the "most urgently required of the B vitamins" because of the rapidness and seriousness of deficiency symptoms (Thomson, Cook, Touquet, & Henry, 2002).

Function

Thiamin functions as a coenzyme in the metabolism of carbohydrates and amino acids. The vitamin is involved in reactions that yield components of metabolism, which in turn enter the Kreb's cycle to generate energy. For this reason, the nurse should remember that any individual at risk for thiamin deficiency should receive thiamin supplementation when receiving intravenous glucose; failure to supplement thiamin while delivering glucose can cause rapid deterioration in thiamin status and serious side effects outlined here in the discussion on thiamin deficiency.

Recommended Intake

The RDA for thiamin in adults is 1.2 mg/day for males and 1.1 mg/day for females (IOM, 1998). The RDA is based on energy intake in these population groups. The DRI for infants is expressed as an AI based on the amount of thiamin found in human milk (IOM, 1998). The thiamin DRI for all age and gender groups is outlined in Appendix C.

Food Sources

Thiamin is available in a wide variety of foods. In the United States, the primary sources of thiamin are enriched bread, bread products, and ready-to-eat cereals; processed meats; and pork (IOM, 1998). Table 5-11 outlines thiamin content of selected foods in the diet.

Deficiency

Alcoholism is the most common cause of thiamin deficiency in developed countries (IOM, 1998). Of adults admitted to an emergency room for alcohol intoxication 15% are found to be thiamin deficient (Li, Jacob, Feng, & Kulkarni, 2008). Alcohol leads to poor thiamin status via several mechanisms; it decreases the absorption and liver storage of thiamin and increases its utilization, leading to compromised thiamin status in a population with already poor dietary intake (Agabio, 2005; Day, Bentham, Callaghan, Kuruvilla, & George, 2005). Thiamin absorption can decrease by almost 70% with chronic alcoholism (Thomson et al., 2002). Deficiency of thiamin can occur in less than 3 weeks because of the rapid turnover and low body storage of the vitamin (Kumar, 2007). Only 30 mg of thiamin is stored in the body, primarily in skeletal muscle with small amounts in the heart, liver, kidney, and nervous tissue (Wooley, 2008). Additional risk factors for thiamin deficiency include persistent vomiting, malabsorptive gastrointestinal diseases, and intestinal surgeries (Kumar, 2007; Thompson et al., 2008). Cultural food practices can lead to thiamine deficiency as outlined in Cultural Considerations: Cultural Food Practices and Thiamin.

Symptoms of thiamin deficiency begin with fatigue, muscle weakness, and neurological complaints such as numb-

Cultural Considerations

Cultural Food Practices and Thiamin

In parts of the world such as Southeast Asia, thiamin deficiency occurs where polished rice or raw fish are traditionally consumed (IOM, 1998). Polishing removes the hull of the grain where thiamin is contained. Raw fish contains an enzyme, thiaminase, which destroys the vitamin.

ness and tingling of the extremities (IOM, 1998). **Beri-beri** is the name given to thiamin deficiency, which is a Thai term translating to "I can't, I can't" because of the malaise and muscle complaints. Beri-beri can progress to more severe symptoms that include muscle wasting and worsened neurological complaints (dry beri-beri) or edema and cardiac failure (wet beri-beri). Wet beri-beri mimics the signs and symptoms of heart failure and can exacerbate these symptoms in those with existing heart failure (Wooley, 2008). Additionally, a condition known as **Wernicke-Korsakoff syndrome** can affect those with thiamin deficiency. Comprised of two disorders, Wernicke's encephalopathy and Korsakoff's psychosis, Wernicke-Korsakoff syndrome is a type of encephalopathy, or condition of the brain, where memory loss; disorientation; confabulation; altered gait **(ataxia);** and rapid, jerky eye movements **(nystagmus)** occur. The confused state, ataxia, and eye signs are considered the classic triad of symptoms of Wernicke's encephalopathy, but monitoring for only these three symptoms could lead to a missed diagnosis of thiamin deficiency (Thompson et al., 2008). Immediate thiamin supplementation is indicated when alcohol misuse is suspected or any symptoms of thiamin deficiency are present. Generally, the hospitalized individual is given high-dose intravenous thiamin for several days (Agabio, 2005; Day et al., 2005; Thomson et al., 2002). Left untreated (or undertreated), brain damage from cerebellar loss can become permanent in clients with Wernicke-Korsakoff syndrome (Thomson et al., 2002).

Toxicity

No UL recommendation exists for thiamin because of insufficient data on adverse effects (IOM, 1998). Absorption is diminished with increased oral doses of thiamin, and urinary excretion occurs with high plasma thiamin levels (IOM, 1998). There have been reports of anaphylactic reactions with high-dose parenteral thiamin, but these are rare (IOM, 1998; Thomson et al., 2002).

Wellness Concerns and Supplement Use

Clients who have undergone gastric bypass surgery for treatment of obesity have been reported to be at risk for thiamin deficiency, especially those with more extensive bypass or diversion surgery or when vomiting persists postoperatively (Bloomberg, Fleishman, Nalle, Herron, & Kini, 2005).

Table 5-11 Thiamin Food Sources	
Thiamin Source	**Thiamin Content, mg***
Barley, cooked, 1 cup	1.2
Cereal, fortified, ready-to-eat, 1 cup	Check label: can be 25–100% RDA
Rice, white, cooked, enriched, 1 cup	1.1
Pork loin, cooked, 3 oz	1.1
Dinner roll	0.4
Black beans, cooked 1 cup	0.4
Pasta, cooked, 1 cup	0.3

*Recommendation Reminder: RDA for adult females –1.1 mg, adult males –1.2 mg.
Source: Adapted from U.S. Department of Agriculture Nutrient Data Lab. Retrieved March 25, 2009, from http://www.nal.usda.gov/fnic/foodcomp

Peripheral neuropathy and Wernicke-Korsakoff syndrome has been described in this population (Bloomberg et al., 2005; Chang, Adams-Huet, & Provost, 2004; Koike et al., 2004). Vitamin supplementation is routine following gastric bypass and is outlined in Chapter 17.

The need for thiamin supplementation should be evaluated in the client with heart failure. Clients with advanced heart failure are already at risk for poor nutrition because of inadequate dietary intake due to fatigue, shortness of breath, and anorexia associated with the disease. Treatment of heart failure with medications called loop diuretics to manage fluid imbalance leads to increased urinary losses of thiamin, furthering the risk of thiamin deficiency (Wooley, 2008). This drug–nutrient interaction warrants attention in this population as a routine part of a nutrition assessment. Consumption of a multivitamin with the RDA of thiamin promotes adequate intake on a daily basis. Additional amounts can be given to those with poor intake or suspected of deficiency because risk of toxicity is low with an increased thiamin dose (Wooley, 2008).

Riboflavin

Riboflavin was identified subsequently to thiamin, earning it the name vitamin B_2. Like many B-complex vitamins, riboflavin is labile under certain conditions that destroy the vitamin. In particular, riboflavin is sensitive to light, which is why milk, an important source of riboflavin, is sold in opaque or waxed containers to block light.

Function

Riboflavin functions as a coenzyme in various reactions involving metabolism and energy production. Some of the reactions also are dependent on other B vitamins, such as niacin and thiamin (IOM, 1998). Additionally, riboflavin is involved in the conversion of vitamin B_6 to its active form.

Recommended Intake

The RDA for riboflavin in adults is 1.3 mg/day for males and 1.1 mg/day for females (IOM, 1998). Requirements are increased during pregnancy and lactation to support tissue synthesis and riboflavin losses in breast milk (IOM, 1998). Appendix C outlines the DRI for riboflavin.

Food Sources

Riboflavin is widely available in animal and plant foods. Dairy, meat, and dark-green leafy vegetables are important sources. In the United States breads and ready-to-eat cereals are enriched with riboflavin because of losses of the vitamin in processing. Table 5-12 outlines riboflavin content of foods in the diet.

Deficiency

Deficiency of riboflavin is called **ariboflavinosis.** A single deficiency of riboflavin is unusual; deficiency is generally accompanied by other nutrient deficiencies (McNulty & Scott, 2008). Those at risk for poor riboflavin status include individuals with little intake of dairy foods or meat. A single bowl

Table 5-12 Riboflavin Food Sources	
Riboflavin Source	**Riboflavin Content, mg***
Beef liver, cooked 3 oz	2.9
Cereal, fortified, ready-to-eat, 1 cup	Check label: can be 25–100% RDA
Milk, canned, evaporated, 1 cup	0.79
Wheat flour, white, enriched, 1 cup	0.62
Cornmeal, enriched, 1 cup	0.56
Yogurt, plain, 1 cup	0.53
Milk, skim, 1 cup	0.10

*Recommendation Reminder: RDA for adult females—1.1 mg, adult males—1.3 mg.
Source: Adapted from U.S. Department of Agriculture Nutrient Data Lab. Retrieved March 25, 2009, from http://www.nal.usda.gov/fnic/foodcomp

of enriched cereal with milk provides adequate riboflavin (Powers, 2003).

Symptoms of riboflavin deficiency include sore throat with edema of the pharyngeal and oral mucosa, a magenta-colored tongue with **glossitis** (atrophy of the taste buds), **angular stomatitis** (fissures at corners of mouth), cheilosis (swollen, fissured lips), and seborrheic dermatitis around the nasolabial folds (Friedlii & Saurat, 2004; IOM, 1998; McNulty & Scott, 2008). Figure 5-5 ■ illustrates these oral symptoms of riboflavin deficiency. Severe riboflavin deficiency impacts vitamin B_6 and niacin status because of the interrelationship of the respective metabolic pathways of these vitamins with riboflavin (IOM, 1998). Ariboflavinosis can contribute to anemia when iron status is already poor (Powers, 2003).

Toxicity

No UL for riboflavin exists because of insufficient evidence regarding adverse effects of high doses (IOM, 1998). Riboflavin is absorbed best in the presence of food, but a limited capacity exists for its absorption in the gastrointestinal tract; this factor may contribute to the lack of evidence regarding negative effects of high doses of riboflavin (IOM, 1998).

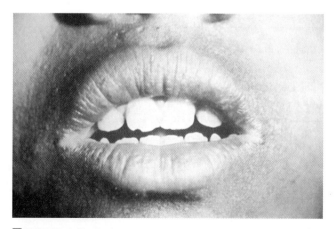

■ **FIGURE 5-5 Cheilosis.**
Source: Centers for Disease Control and Prevention.

Wellness Concerns and Supplement Use

The rarity of riboflavin deficiency coupled with the lack of reports of adverse effects from high doses of the vitamin leave little concern regarding general issues of wellness and riboflavin. Research on subclinical riboflavin deficiency and its relationship to other nutrient deficiencies as well as homocysteine and cardiac disease risk may provide new avenues of information on riboflavin in the future (Powers, 2003).

Niacin

Niacin was originally called the pellagra-preventing vitamin or vitamin B$_3$. Niacin has two forms: nicotinic acid and niacinamide. Additionally, the amino acid tryptophan can be converted to niacin by the body.

Function

Niacin acts as a coenzyme or cosubstrate in many biological reactions, including the metabolism of alcohol, proteins, fatty acids, lactate, and pyruvate and in the synthesis of steroids (IOM, 1998). High-dose supplemental niacin in the form of nicotinic acid is used as a pharmacological agent in the treatment of high blood lipid levels as discussed under Wellness Concerns and Supplement Use here.

Recommended Intake

The RDA for niacin is expressed as "niacin equivalents," taking into consideration the conversion of tryptophan content in foods to niacin. A 60-mg content of tryptophan yields 1 mg of niacin or 1 niacin equivalent (NE). The RDA for adults is 16 mg/day NE for males and 14 mg/day NE for females (IOM, 1998).

Food Sources

Important sources of niacin in the diet include "flesh foods," especially poultry and lean meats. Other high-protein foods, such as dairy foods, contain tryptophan that is converted to niacin. Whole grain breads, bread products, and ready-to-eat cereals also are important sources. Table 5-13 outlines niacin content of selected foods in the diet.

Table 5-13	Niacin Food Sources
Niacin Source	**Niacin Content, mg NE***
Beef liver, cooked, 3 oz	14.85
Chicken, light meat, cooked, 3 oz	11.23
Tuna fish salad, 1 cup	13.74
Pasta sauce, tomato, ready-to-serve	9.79
Rice, white, enriched, cooked, 1 cup	7.76
	7.38
Wheat flour, white, enriched, 1 cup	Check label: varies 25–100% RDA
Cereal, fortified, ready-to-eat, 1 cup	

*Recommendation Reminder: RDA for adult females—14 mg NE, adult males—16 mg NE.
Source: Adapted from U.S. Department of Agriculture Nutrient Data Lab. Retrieved March 25, 2009, from http://www.nal.usda.gov/fnic/foodcomp

Deficiency

Pellagra is the term used to denote niacin deficiency. Deficiency symptoms encompass the "4 Ds of pellagra": dermatitis, diarrhea, depression, and, ultimately, death. Pellagra (from the Italian *pelle* and *agra* for *skin* and *rough*, respectively) is so named because symptoms include a pigmented, symmetrical rash that is painful to the touch. The rash is present only where exposure to sunlight occurs and resembles a sunburn at first but changes to a cinnamon color with vesicles and bullae (Heygi, Schwartz, & Heygi, 2004). A necklace effect can occur in a broad band around the neck. Figure 5-6 ■ illustrates the dermatological effects of pellagra. Some say that "pellagra begins in the stomach" because gastrointestinal symptoms such as vomiting and diarrhea are common (Heygi et al., 2004). Cheilosis and glossitis similar to symptoms of other B vitamin deficiency also occur, making it difficult to differentiate a single deficiency. Symptoms can then progress to include neurological changes with depression, apathy, fatigue, and headache (IOM, 1998). Death can occur when niacin deficiency is left untreated for a number of years (Heygi et al., 2004).

Individuals at risk for poor niacin status are those with a poor overall diet lacking in protein as well as niacin. Populations that subsist on a corn-based diet as the primary grain are at risk because of the lack of the vitamin in this grain (Kumar, 2007). The conversion of tryptophan to niacin requires the B vitamins riboflavin and pyridoxine. Deficiency of these two vitamins can contribute to a secondary niacin deficiency as a result (Kumar, 2007). Alcoholism and metabolic disease involving altered tryptophan metabolism are risk factors for niacin deficiency (Heygi et al., 2004; IOM,

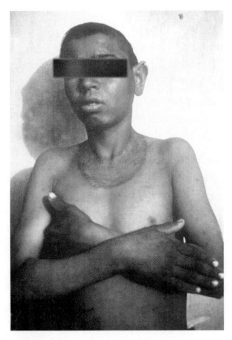

■ FIGURE 5-6 **Pellagra.**
Source: Centers for Disease Control and Prevention.

1998). Pellagra has been described in case reports of individuals with anorexia nervosa and following gastric bypass surgery (Ashourian & Mousdicas, 2006; Prousky, 2003).

Toxicity

The UL for niacin intake is 35 mg/day NE (IOM, 1998). No adverse effects have been reported for intake of naturally occurring niacin in foods, but supplements, fortified foods, and pharmacological agents containing niacin should be monitored. High intake of supplemental types of niacin can cause flushing of the skin because of a vasodilatory effect (IOM, 1998). This symptom is often encountered by individuals prescribed nicotinic acid as a treatment for hyperlipidemia and can be cause for some to discontinue this intervention (Davidson, 2008). High doses of nicotinic acid can lead to hepatotoxicity, which warrants monitoring of liver function when a pharmacological dose of niacin is prescribed as discussed later. The nurse should question clients about any self-prescribed treatment of high blood lipids because various forms of high-dose niacin are available over the counter.

Wellness Concerns and Supplement Use

Niacin is involved in fatty-acid metabolism and hence has been used to treat high blood cholesterol and triglycerides for a number of years. High-dose niacin in the nicotinic acid form is prescribed at doses in excess of 1 gm/day. The nurse should be aware of side effects and monitoring advice for the various types of niacin available. Flushing of the face, arms, and chest is a common complaint, especially in the beginning of niacin treatment and with the crystalline form (Davidson, 2008; IOM, 1998). Flushing includes redness and a burning or itching sense from dilation of small subcutaneous blood vessels. Long-acting or extended-release niacin can cause less flushing but carries a higher risk of hepatotoxicity and is more expensive than short-acting crystalline niacin (Davidson, 2008). The nurse should monitor clients for use of over-the-counter "no flush" niacin preparations because these have been found to contain no nicotinic acid, the active ingredient necessary to lower lipid levels (Davidson, 2008).

Special consideration for niacin supplementation should be given to clients with cirrhosis, dialysis treatment of renal disease, long-term isoniazid treatment for tuberculosis, or multiparous females because the RDA specifically does not meet the needs of these individuals (IOM, 1998). A registered dietitian can assess the proper supplementation dose for these individuals.

Vitamin B$_6$

Vitamin B$_6$ is comprised of pyridoxine and several related forms that are converted to pyridoxal phosphate in the body. Pyridoxal phosphate can be measured in plasma to determine vitamin B$_6$ status.

Function

Vitamin B$_6$ is a coenzyme for over 100 enzyme reactions in the metabolism of amino acids, glycogen, sphingolipids, neurotransmitters, and precursors to hemoglobin synthesis (IOM, 1998). Vitamin B$_6$ is required for the conversion of trytophan to niacin by the body.

Recommended Intake

The RDA for vitamin B$_6$ is 1.3 mg/day for males and females (IOM, 1998). In adults older than age 50 years, the requirement for vitamin B$_6$ increases slightly to maintain plasma levels of pyridoxal phosphate in a normal range (IOM, 1998). Specific age- and gender-related requirements for vitamin B$_6$ are listed in Appendix C.

Food Sources

Vitamin B$_6$ is well absorbed from food and supplements, even at high doses (IOM, 1998). Potatoes, bananas, and protein-containing foods such as poultry, pork, and beef are important sources of pyridoxine. Excessive heat can destroy pyridoxine in processing or cooking (Kumar, 2007). Table 5-14 outlines food sources of vitamin B$_6$.

Deficiency

Deficiency of vitamin B$_6$ leads to a seborrheic dermatitis similar to that of riboflavin deficiency (IOM, 1998). Vitamin B$_6$ deficiency can contribute to microcytic anemia where red blood cell size is diminished because of decreased hemoglobin. Reduced synthesis of neurotransmitters from poor vitamin B$_6$ status leads to convulsions, depression, and confusion (IOM, 1998; Kumar, 2007).

Single deficiency of vitamin B$_6$ is uncommon but can occur as a result of drug interactions with the nutrient. Isoniazid for tuberculosis and penicillamine, used in treatment of rheumatoid arthritis and lead poisoning, are two medications that compromise vitamin B$_6$ status by inhibiting formation of the active form of the vitamin. Individuals taking

Table 5-14   Vitamin B$_6$ Food Sources

Vitamin B$_6$ Source	Vitamin B$_6$ Content, mg*
Potato, baked, 1 whole medium	0.70
Banana, raw, 1 medium	0.68
Chickpeas, canned, ½ cup	0.57
Chicken breast, no bone, cooked, ½ breast	0.52
Cereal, fortified, ready-to-eat, 1 cup	Check label, varies 25–100% RDA
Roast beef, cooked, 3 oz	0.32
Sunflower seeds, roasted, 1 oz	0.23
Tuna, canned in water, 3 oz	0.18
Peanut butter, smooth, 2 tablespoons	0.15

*Recommendation Reminder: RDA for adults—1.3 mg.
Source: Adapted from U.S. Department of Agriculture Nutrient Data Lab. Retrieved March 25, 2009, from http://www.nal.usda.gov/fnic/foodcomp

such medications should be assessed for intake of the vitamin and any signs or symptoms of a deficiency to determine if a vitamin B_6 supplement is indicated.

Toxicity

The UL for vitamin B_6 is 100 mg/day. No adverse effects have been reported from high intake of vitamin B_6 from food sources, but large supplemental doses have been associated with development of peripheral neuropathy (IOM, 1998). Severe sensory neuropathy of the extremities occurs, exhibiting symptoms of a tingling sensation and, in some, inability to walk (Kumar, 2007). Symptoms abate with discontinued vitamin B_6 supplement use.

Wellness Concerns and Supplement Use

The nurse should be aware that supplemental vitamin B_6 is often recommended in the popular press for treatment of premenstrual syndrome (PMS) and carpal tunnel syndrome. There is little evidence that high-dose vitamin B_6 helps improve the symptoms of either condition, though there are some reports of improved symptoms of PMS at doses not exceeding the UL and increased pain tolerance with improved vitamin B_6 status in deficient clients with carpal tunnel syndrome ["Vitamin B-6 (Pyridoxine; pyridoxal 5'phosphate)," 2001; NIH, 2007b; Ryan-Harshman & Aldoori, 2007].

Folate

Folate exists in several forms depending on the source of the vitamin. The term *folate* generally denotes the vitamin as it is found naturally in foods, whereas folic acid is found in supplements and fortified foods. Folic acid is 50% more bioavailable for absorption by the body than is folate in foods (IOM, 1998; Johnson, 2007).

Function

Folate functions as a coenzyme in the metabolism of nucleic acids and amino acids (IOM, 1998). This involvement spans numerous reactions, including DNA synthesis and normal cell division, purine synthesis, and interconversion of several amino acids, such as homocysteine to methionine.

Folic acid plays a role in the prevention of neural tube defects, which are among the most common type of birth defects (American Academy of Pediatrics, 1999). Anencephaly, spina bifida, and encephalocele defects occur when the neural tube fails to close during fetal development within the first month of conception.

Recommended Intake

The RDA for folate is expressed as dietary folate equivalents to account for the difference in bioavailability of folate and folic acid (IOM, 1998). The RDA for adults is 400 mcg/day for males and females with more specific recommendations outlined for females of childbearing age, as outlined in Lifespan Box: Folic Acid for Women of Childbearing Age. Females of childbearing age are advised to consume 400 mcg/day of folic

Lifespan

Folic Acid for Women of Childbearing Age

Females of childbearing age are advised to consume 400 mcg/day of folic acid specifically from supplements or fortified foods in addition to folate in foods to decrease the risk of neural tube defect occurrence in a developing fetus. Because these birth defects occur in the very early stages of pregnancy when many females are unaware of the pregnancy, a blanket recommendation for all females of childbearing age is made. The RDA for pregnant females is 600 mcg/day (IOM, 1998).

acid specifically from supplements or fortified foods in addition to folate in foods to decrease the risk of neural tube defect occurrence in a developing fetus. The RDA for pregnant females is 600 mcg/day. Appendix C contains the DRI for folate for other age and gender groups.

Food Sources

Folate is present in green leafy vegetables, legumes (lentils, split peas, beans) and orange juice, among other sources. Beginning in 1998, wheat flour is enriched in the United States with 140 mcg folic acid per 100 gm flour, adding folic acid to the diet of the general population consuming any wheat flour-based product such as breads, cereals, pasta, and baked goods. This fortification was begun to target the improvement of folic acid intake by females of childbearing age to decrease the risk of neural tube defects. Fortification of flour has led to a 26% reduction in the incidence of neural tube defects in the United States (Centers for Disease Control and Prevention [CDC], 2004a). Table 5-15 and Practice Pearl: Folate outline sources of folate and folic acid in the diet.

Table 5-15 Folate Food Sources

Folate Source	Folate Content, mcg DFE*
Cereal, fortified, ready-to-eat, 1 cup	Check label, varies 25–100% RDA
Wheat flour, white, fortified, 1 cup	384
Lentils, cooked, 1 cup	358
Chickpeas, cooked, 1 cup	282
Spinach, cooked, 1 cup	263
Peas, green, cooked, 1 cup	148
Broccoli, cooked, 1 cup	140
Orange juice, 1 cup	74

C_T? What advice would you give to a female of childbearing age on how to obtain adequate folate and folic acid?

*Recommendation Reminder: RDA for adults—400 mcg.

Source: Adapted from U.S. Department of Agriculture Nutrient Data Lab. Retrieved March 25, 2009, from http://www.nal.usda.gov/fnic/foodcomp

PRACTICE PEARL

Folate

An easy way to remember foods that are rich in folate is to associate folate with *foliage,* green leaves. Green leafy vegetables are an excellent source of folate.

Folate is easily destroyed during food storage and cooking. The longer foods are heated or kept warm, the more substantial the losses of folate (McNulty & Scott, 2008). The nurse should encourage minimal cooking time of foods that are good sources of folate, such as green leafy vegetables.

Deficiency

The first sign of folate deficiency is a decreased folate content in plasma and then in red blood cells (IOM, 1998). Within weeks of deficiency, bone marrow changes lead to hypersegmented neutrophils and eventually increased red blood cell size (macrocytosis). Due to the long 120-day life of the red blood cell, these changes are not apparent in the early stages of deficiency. Gradually, macrocytic anemia occurs with decreased plasma hemoglobin and hematocrit values. Physical symptoms of anemia from folate deficiency are the same as those for other nutritional anemias: fatigue, difficulty concentrating, headache, shortness of breath on exertion, heart palpitations, and tachycardia (increased heart rate). Whenever deficiency of folate is suspected, vitamin B_{12} status should also be assessed because the two vitamins share metabolic pathways and hematological symptoms of deficiency. Provision of folate will correct the hematological changes of a vitamin B_{12} deficiency, dangerously masking and potentiating the vitamin B_{12} deficiency (IOM, 1998; Johnson, 2007).

Individuals at risk for folate deficiency include those with inadequate intake because of poor diet, such as alcoholics, individuals with restrictive eating patterns, or those with inadequate funds for food. Alcohol can worsen an already compromised folate status by both decreasing folate absorption and increasing its renal excretion (IOM, 1998). Folate deficiency associated with alcoholism can manifest symptoms in less than a few months (Kumar, 2007). Additionally, folate status can be compromised by liver disease because the liver stores 50% of the body's folate (IOM, 1998). Absorption of folate can be affected by gastric bypass surgery. The prevalence of folate deficiency has been reported to be up to 63% after such surgeries (Bloomberg et al., 2005).

A considerable amount of medications alter folate status by decreasing its absorption or exerting antifolate activity. Examples include some seizure medications, sulfasalazine used in treating inflammatory bowel disease, and methotrexate prescribed for psoriasis, among other conditions (IOM, 1998).

Survey data have revealed that 60% of U.S. females age 18 to 45 years report not meeting the recommended

400 mcg/day of folic acid (CDC, 2004b). Only 24% of those surveyed knew that folic acid can prevent neural tube defects. A mere 12% knew that folic acid should be taken during pregnancy. Although these females may not exhibit symptoms of folate deficiency, the nurse should routinely query females of childbearing age about folic acid intake and educate them on the importance of adequate intake.

Toxicity

The UL for folate is set at 1,000 mcg/day (1 mg) from fortified foods and supplements (IOM, 1998). The UL is exclusive of food folate. Folic acid supplements over 1,000 mcg are not available over the counter, but smaller doses that could be taken in multiples are readily sold. Individuals consuming a high proportion of fortified foods, such as breakfast cereal and bread products, can consume significant folic acid.

The UL of folate is established to avoid complications from the masking of a vitamin B_{12} deficiency with high-dose folic acid intake. Supplemental folic acid can potentiate the neurological damage of vitamin B_{12} deficiency and mask the deficiency by ameliorating the hematological changes (IOM, 1998; Johnson, 2007). These effects are serious and can be irreversible.

Wellness Concerns and Supplement Use

Elevated plasma homocysteine levels have been associated with an increased risk of cardiovascular disease in observational studies. Homocysteine is an amino acid that requires folate, vitamin B_{12}, and vitamin B_6 for its conversion to methionine. Supplemental folic acid along with vitamins B_{12} and B_6 have been reported to lower elevated homocysteine levels. However, clinical trials using the three vitamins to successfully lower homocysteine have not shown any effect on mortality or cardiovascular events in males and females at high risk for disease (Albert et al., 2008; Ebbing et al., 2008). In observational studies, elevated homocysteine levels have also been studied in relation to risk of Alzheimer's disease and other conditions. High-dose supplementation with vitamins B_6, B_{12}, and folic acid is not reported to slow cognitive decline in healthy individuals or those with impaired cognitive function (Aisen et al., 2008; Balk et al., 2007).

There is not conclusive evidence to warrant a change in the RDA for folate or folic acid supplementation to decrease the risk of vascular disease, cancers, or neurological disorders in individuals with adequate folate status (IOM, 1998). Folic acid supplementation to achieve the RDA for folate intake is advisable for females of childbearing age.

Vitamin B_{12}

Vitamin B_{12} refers to a group of compounds belonging to the cobalamin family. Absorption of vitamin B_{12} requires several factors for optimal bioavailability. An acid medium in the stomach is necessary to cleave the vitamin from protein to which it is bound in food. The vitamin then binds with an

R protein secreted by the stomach. Parietal cells in the stomach secrete intrinsic factor that in turn binds to vitamin B_{12} in the small intestine for absorption in the terminal ileum. About 50% of ingested vitamin B_{12} is absorbed under optimal conditions (IOM, 1998). Approximately 1% of high-dose crystalline B_{12} (not bound to protein) is passively absorbed in the small intestine, not requiring an acid stomach medium or

intrinsic factor (Carmel, 2008; IOM, 1998). Figure 5-7 ■ outlines vitamin B_{12} absorption.

Function

Vitamin B_{12} is a coenzyme in the metabolism of amino acids and reactions that produce nucleic acids, neurotransmitters, and the myelin sheaths of the central nervous system (IOM,

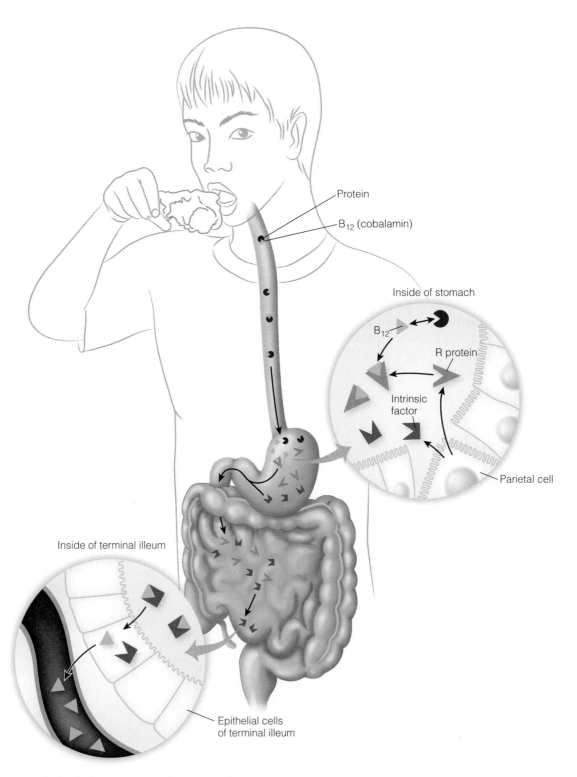

■ FIGURE 5-7 **Vitamin B_{12} Absorption and Deficiency Risk Factors.**

Lifespan

Vitamin B$_{12}$ Recommendations in the Older Adult

It is recommended that adults over age 50 years meet the vitamin B$_{12}$ requirement through fortified foods or a supplement because of the prevalence of malabsorption of the food-bound form of the vitamin in that population (IOM, 1998). **Atrophic gastritis** occurs in up to 30% of older adults, resulting in decreased production of both hydrochloric acid (achlorhydria) and intrinsic factor and impacting absorption of vitamin B$_{12}$ (IOM, 1998).

1998). Vitamin B$_{12}$ is required for cell division and normal neurological function.

Recommended Intake

The RDA for vitamin B$_{12}$ is 2.4 mcg/day in adults (IOM, 1998). Lifespan Box: Vitamin B$_{12}$ Recommendations in the Older Adult outlines specific recommendations for vitamin B$_{12}$ in the adult over age 50 years.

Food Sources

Vitamin B$_{12}$ is found in foods of animal origin and fortified foods, such as fortified breakfast cereals and some soy products. The microflora in the large intestine produce vitamin B$_{12}$, but it is excreted unabsorbed (IOM, 1998). Table 5-16 lists the vitamin B$_{12}$ content of selected foods.

Deficiency

Vitamin B$_{12}$ deficiency leads to hematological changes like those of folate deficiency. Added neurological symptoms differentiate deficiency of vitamin B$_{12}$ from that of folate. Increased mean red blood cell volume and anemia respond to treatment with vitamin B$_{12}$ or folate, but correction of neurological complications requires vitamin B$_{12}$ administration. Neurological symptoms of deficiency result from demyelina-

tion of axons and nerve tracts of the spinal column (Dali-Yousef & Andres, 2009). Resultant tingling and numbness of extremities, disorientation, visual disturbances, and dementia can ensue if the deficiency is left untreated. Neurological symptoms are reversible if vitamin B$_{12}$ treatment is given in a timely fashion but can be permanent. Neurological complications are evident in 75% to 90% of individuals with clinically observable vitamin B$_{12}$ deficiency. However, in 25% of clients with deficiency of vitamin B$_{12}$, neurological complications are the only manifestation of the deficiency (IOM, 1998).

Detection of vitamin B$_{12}$ status is measured via plasma cobalamin as well as methylmalonic acid and homocysteine, two intermediaries in vitamin B$_{12}$ metabolism. Elevated levels of each of the intermediaries can be indicative of deficiency, though both are also affected by factors unrelated to the vitamin. Methylmalonic acid can be elevated with renal disease whereas poor folate status can elevate homocysteine. Controversy exists as to the exact cutoff values for these when determining vitamin B$_{12}$ deficiency; it is suggested that more than one laboratory assay be used to diagnose vitamin B$_{12}$ deficiency to avoid the shortfalls of the individual tests (Carmel, 2008).

Individuals at risk for vitamin B$_{12}$ deficiency include those who have:

- Impaired intake
- Lack of adequate gastric acid or intrinsic factor production
- Malabsorptive conditions or bacterial overgrowth of the intestine

Food-cobalamin deficiency from inadequate gastric acid to cleave the protein-vitamin B$_{12}$ bond in food is the most common cause of poor vitamin B$_{12}$ status (Dali-Yousef & Andres, 2009). Older adults and individuals who use medications to buffer or diminish gastric acid production are at risk for food-cobalamin deficiency. Deficiency can progress more rapidly in individuals who lack intrinsic factor because vitamin B$_{12}$ contained in the enterohepatic recirculation of bile is not reabsorbed as it would be in those with adequate intrinsic factor (IOM, 1998). Breastfed children of mothers who consume no animal products are at risk for vitamin B$_{12}$ deficiency if the mother's diet is not supplemented with vitamin B$_{12}$. Maternal stores of vitamin B$_{12}$ do not cross the placenta. Instead vitamin B$_{12}$ available to the fetus and the breastfed infant rely on *current* maternal intake of the vitamin (Dror & Allen, 2008). Symptoms of deficiency are quick to appear in these children, and neurological damage can be permanent if not treated in a timely fashion (Dror & Allen, 2008; IOM, 1998). **Pernicious anemia** is an autoimmune disease associated with vitamin B$_{12}$ deficiency stemming from the destruction of the gastric mucosa and subsequent lack of intrinsic factor synthesis (Carmel, 2008). Figure 5-7 outlines the absorption of vitamin B$_{12}$ and deficiency risk factors.

Table 5-16	Vitamin B$_{12}$ Food Sources
Vitamin B$_{12}$ Source	**Vitamin B$_{12}$ Content, mcg***
Clams, cooked, 3 oz	28.0
Cereal, fortified, ready-to-eat, 1 cup	Check label, varies 25–100% RDA
Salmon, cooked, 3 oz	4.9
Beef, sirloin, lean, cooked, 3 oz	2.4
Yogurt, plain, 1 cup	1.4
Tuna, canned in water, 3 oz	1.4
Milk, skim, 1 cup	0.9
Pork, ham, roasted, 3 oz	0.6
Egg, boiled, 1 whole	0.6

CT? Where should an individual who consumes no animal products obtain dietary vitamin B$_{12}$?

*Recommendation Reminder: RDA for adults—2.4 mcg.

Source: Adapted from U.S. Department of Agriculture Nutrient Data Lab. Retrieved March 25, 2009, from http://www.nal.usda.gov/fnic/foodcomp

A dose of 1 to 2 mg of crystalline vitamin B_{12} is prescribed for vitamin B_{12} deficiency. Oral doses at this level are sufficiently absorbed by passive absorption, bypassing the need for intramuscular or parenteral administration of the vitamin in most individuals, especially those who are deficient because of decreased gastric acid production (Dali-Yousef & Andres, 2009). Some clinicians choose to administer monthly intramuscular vitamin B_{12} to ensure client adherence and prevent relapse of symptoms (Carmel, 2008).

Toxicity
No UL for vitamin B_{12} has been established because of a lack of reports on adverse effects with high doses (IOM, 1998). Fractional absorption decreases with increased intake, and this effect may contribute to low toxicity with increased consumption (IOM, 1998).

Wellness Concerns and Supplement Use
The DRI recommendations for vitamin B_{12} urge supplemental or food-fortified sources of the vitamin for those over age 50 years. Crystalline or free vitamin B_{12} in supplements or food does not require an acid stomach medium for absorption, which makes this form of a supplement ideal for the older adult and those who use medications to diminish gastric acid production. Synthetic vitamin B_{12} in a supplement or fortified foods is recommended for vegans because plant forms of the vitamin, though available on the market, are not bioavailable in humans.

When recommending supplements, the nurse should be aware that a nontraditional vitamin B_{12} form is required for individuals with Leber's optic atrophy, a genetic disorder from chronic cyanide poisoning. Cyanocobalamin is traditionally the form of the vitamin in supplements, but hydroxyocobalamin should instead be prescribed for its cyanide antagonistic effect (IOM, 1998).

Biotin
Biotin was discovered in 1927, but it was not recognized as a vitamin for another 40 years (IOM, 1998). Early research focused on the ability of biotin to counteract symptoms occurring in research animals after chronic intake of raw eggs. Avidin is a protein present in raw egg whites that binds biotin, preventing its absorption by the body (IOM, 1998). Cooking inactivates avidin.

Function
Biotin acts as a cofactor for enzymes in metabolic reactions involving gluconeogenesis, fatty acid metabolism, and catabolism of the amino acid leucine (IOM, 1998). It has been suggested that biotin may play a role in regulating transcription of proteins (Said, 2009).

Recommended Intake
Limited data exist on the adult requirement for biotin; thus the DRI is given as an AI rather than an RDA. The AI for biotin in adults is 30 mcg/day (IOM, 1998). Little research has been devoted to quantifying biotin distribution in the body or determining indices of biotin status in adults.

Food Sources
Information on biotin content of foods is limited. Traditional food composition tables do not contain information on biotin content of foods (IOM, 1998). Biotin is felt to be widely distributed in foods but can be protein bound in some foods, affecting its bioavailability (IOM, 1998; Said, 2009).

Biotin is synthesized by the microflora present in the gastrointestinal tract, though it is unknown whether this form contributes to biotin status in the body (IOM, 1998).

Deficiency
Biotin deficiency leads to loss of hair (alopecia) and hair color and a red scaly rash over the eyes, nose, and mouth. The dermatitis can resemble that of a zinc deficiency or candida infection. Central nervous system alterations can occur (IOM, 1998).

Individuals at risk for biotin deficiency are those who habitually consume raw egg whites or who have short-gut syndrome. A secondary deficiency occurs in the face of adequate intake of biotin because of an inborn error of metabolism lacking biotinadase, an enzyme required to cleave biotin from its food form (Hoffman, Simon, & Ficicioglu, 2005). Supplemental biotin can be given to compensate for this lack of biotinidase.

Toxicity
No UL exists for biotin because of insufficient data on which to base a recommendation (IOM, 1998). Doses as high as 200 mg orally have been used to correct or prevent deficiencies with no report of toxicity (IOM, 1998).

Pantothenic Acid
Although a vital component of metabolism, pantothenic acid is widely available and rarely deficient in the diet, thus seldom capturing the attention of health care providers.

Function
Pantothenic acid is involved in the synthesis of coenzyme A, an important cofactor of metabolism (IOM, 1998). The vitamin is also required for fatty acid synthesis.

Recommended Intake
The AI for pantothenic acid is 5 mg/day for adults (IOM, 1998). This estimate is derived primarily as a basis for replacing normal losses of the vitamin in urine.

Food Sources
Pantothenic acid is present in most foods, as denoted by its name "panto" or *all*. Protein-containing foods, such as meats, eggs, poultry, and dairy foods as well as plant foods are good sources of pantothenic acid.

Deficiency

Deficiency of pantothenic acid is rare and has been reported only in deliberate cases of semisynthetic diets devoid of the vitamin or by feeding of a vitamin antagonist (IOM, 1998). Symptoms of the deficiency range from irritability and restlessness to generalized gastrointestinal complaints, such as nausea, vomiting, and abdominal cramps (IOM, 1998).

Toxicity

Insufficient evidence exists to recommend a UL for pantothenic acid. No population subgroups have been identified as at risk for problems from excess pantothenic acid intake and there are no national estimates of intake of the vitamin from food or supplements (IOM, 1998).

Choosing a Vitamin Supplement

The nurse will often be asked for a recommendation on vitamin supplements. First, each person should be individually assessed to determine the indication of any need for a vitamin supplement. Overall diet, including fortified foods, should be considered. Medical conditions and treatments can limit dietary intake, warranting a vitamin supplement. However, the nurse should be wary of recommending a supplement to clients undergoing active treatment for cancer without first evaluating the effect that excess vitamins may have on the treatment. It should be kept in mind that some clients may already be taking supplements but have not volunteered this information, fearing disapproval. Hot Topic: Choosing a Vitamin Supplement outlines important factors to consider when giving vitamin supplement recommendations. If a supplement is deemed necessary, caution must be advised in the choice of a supplement that will meet but not exceed client needs. Additionally, the nurse should be aware that adult formulations are available in chewable and liquid forms.

hot Topic

Choosing a Vitamin Supplement

- Safety first. Vitamin supplements are not a substitute for medical treatment or an overall poor diet. Evaluate any possible interaction with medications.
- Do not chase headlines. Do not recommend changes in vitamin intake based on the results of a single study, observational studies, or quick-fix articles in the lay press.
- More is not better. Follow recommendations for intake based on the DRIs. Respect the Tolerable Upper Intake Limit guidelines.
- Expensive vitamins may not be worth the extra money. Buy supplements from respected companies, but those that cost more are not necessarily providing more benefit. Excessive doses of water-soluble vitamins are largely excreted.
- Usefulness of added vitamins in skin care products is uncertain. Little research has been devoted to investigate the absorption of vitamins from products that are applied to the skin.
- Natural is not synonymous with safe. The dose content of supplements is not restricted, leading some to believe that just because a product is natural, it poses no danger. Natural supplements can still interact with medications or lead to toxicity.

Source: Adapted from Food and Drug Administration, Office of Dietary Supplements, 2006.

NURSING CARE PLAN ## Client with Fatigue

CASE STUDY

Hilary is a 20-year-old-college student at a large university where she is a member of the gymnastics team. She has been a gymnast for many years and is thrilled to have achieved her dream of being a member of the team in a highly competitive environment. Lately, she has been feeling more fatigue than usual after daily practices. In addition, she carries 15 credits and tries to maintain a social life that includes a serious boyfriend. She has started to drink several cups of coffee a day to combat fatigue. Several months ago a friend told her that if she took a daily multivitamin tablet she would have more energy and not have to worry about what she ate. She was skeptical at the time but it seemed to work. However, now that the semester is underway she could feel the stress building and she is starting to doze in some of her classes. She thought someone in the Health Service could give her some advice to boost her energy. Figure 5-8 ■ outlines the nursing process for this case.

Applying the Nursing Process

ASSESSMENT

Hilary is pleasant in her interactions with the nurse and eager to talk about the gymnastics team. She is 5 feet 3 inches tall, weighs 98 pounds, and has a BMI of 18.3. Her weight had been stable since high school but decreased 2 pounds in the last 6 weeks. She has had numerous sprains and strains in the past but has no current injuries that trouble her. Her GPA is 3.4 and she says that she studies at least 4 hours every day, more on weekends when there are no competitions. She lives in a house with five other students. She describes herself as a vegetarian who is a "meat-avoider" who will drink milk or eat cheese. A typical day's intake is a granola bar on her way to class in the morning, salad with low-fat dressing for lunch, and spaghetti for dinner. She takes a multivitamin every day in the morning along with fruit juice if there is some available;

(continued)

Client with Fatigue *(continued)*

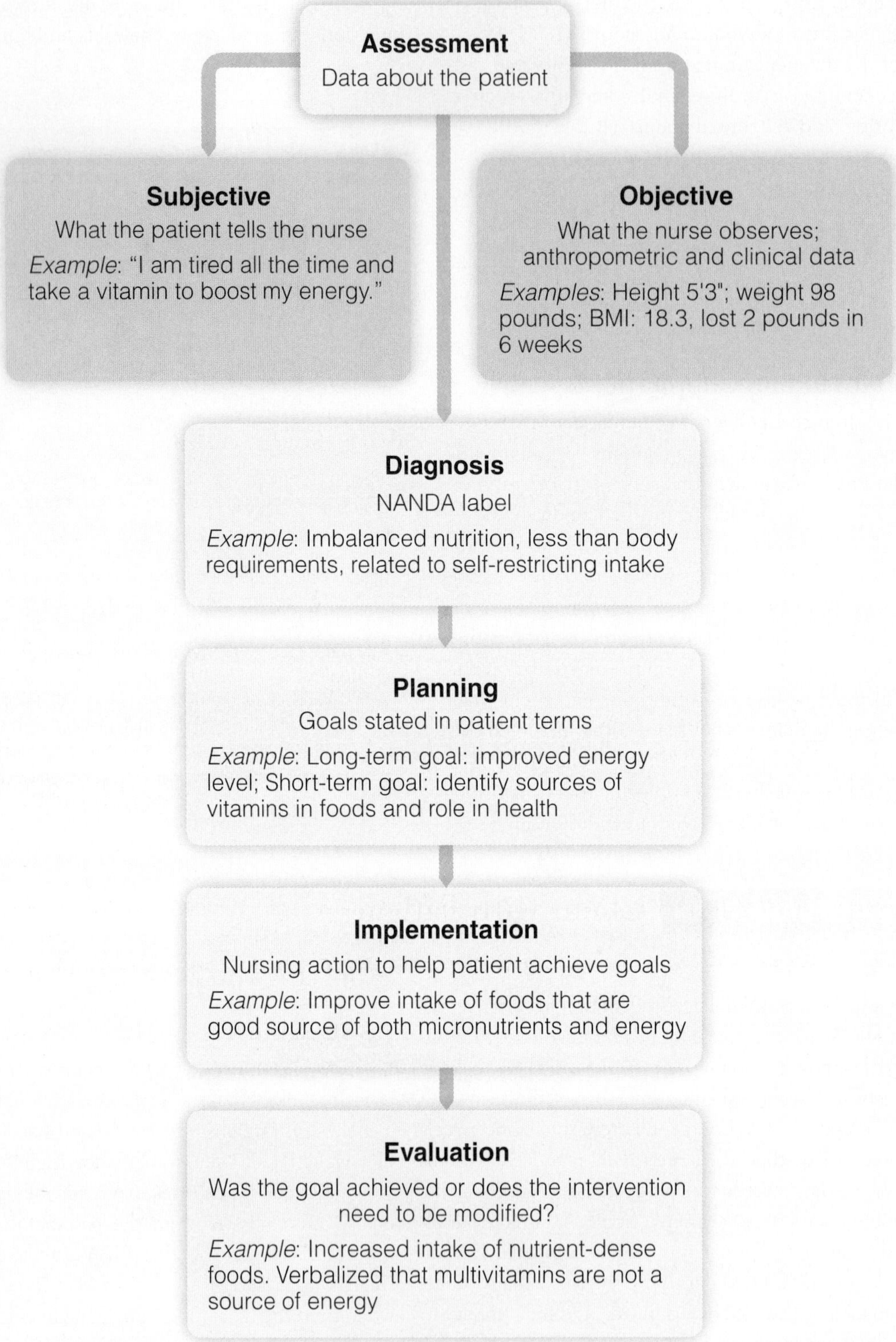

Assessment
Data about the patient

Subjective
What the patient tells the nurse
Example: "I am tired all the time and take a vitamin to boost my energy."

Objective
What the nurse observes; anthropometric and clinical data
Examples: Height 5'3"; weight 98 pounds; BMI: 18.3, lost 2 pounds in 6 weeks

Diagnosis
NANDA label
Example: Imbalanced nutrition, less than body requirements, related to self-restricting intake

Planning
Goals stated in patient terms
Example: Long-term goal: improved energy level; Short-term goal: identify sources of vitamins in foods and role in health

Implementation
Nursing action to help patient achieve goals
Example: Improve intake of foods that are good source of both micronutrients and energy

Evaluation
Was the goal achieved or does the intervention need to be modified?
Example: Increased intake of nutrient-dense foods. Verbalized that multivitamins are not a source of energy

■ FIGURE 5-8 **Nursing Care Plan Process: Client with Fatigue.**

Client with Fatigue *(continued)*

NURSING CARE PLAN

otherwise she drinks water or coffee. She describes herself as "tired all the time."

DIAGNOSES

Impaired nutrition, less than requirements, related to self-restricting intake

Knowledge deficit related to improper understanding of the role of supplementation in health maintenance

Disturbed sleep pattern related to lifestyle choices

Risk for activity intolerance related to inadequate diet

EXPECTED OUTCOMES

Verbalization of food choices that reflect knowledge of nutrient-dense foods that are acceptable on a vegetarian diet

Increased consumption of nutrient-dense foods

Development of a calendar that includes practice, classes, studying, eating, and sleeping

PLANNING

Obtain a 24-hour food and fluid recall

Discuss barriers that may affect food choices and meal preparation

Discuss schedule for practices, classes, and related activities

Teach about the consumption of vitamins from dietary sources and from supplements

Discuss the role of coffee and caffeinated beverages in providing true energy

Keep a food diary

EVALUATION

Hilary was relieved to know that some dietary changes could make a difference in energy level. Her food recall showed inadequate intake of all macro- and micronutrients. Her water intake was adequate but she also drank an average of 4 cups of coffee every morning. She had been reluctant to ask her parents for a larger allowance, but they readily increased it when she explained her plan to consume adequate nutrients and sufficient energy to maintain her weight by eating more balanced meals and snacks at her house. She eliminated coffee from her diet and said she now realized that fatigue was related to lack of sleep. Hilary began using a planner for recording her practice schedule and classes. She found that she could use time between classes and practices for study if she went to the library. Hilary found that if she planned most meals for the week she only needed to have a friend drive her to the store once weekly. Although she was still partial to fresh fruits and vegetables in a salad, she found that taking a sandwich of whole grain bread with cheese or hummus and vegetables made a good lunch choice. She continued to take a multivitamin but acknowledged that it was not for energy but to ensure that she had adequate vitamin intake.

Critical Thinking in the Nursing Process

1. **Hilary implied that her allowance was inadequate to purchase healthy food. What additional interventions by the nurse would have been appropriate if Hilary's parents had not increased her allowance?**

2. **Some vegetarians, like Hilary, merely avoid meat, poultry, and fish. Others also avoid dairy and eggs and products that contain them. How would the nurse modify teaching for a vegan who consumes no animal products?**

3. **What might be an appropriate way to explain why vitamins are not appropriate substitutes for food?**

CHAPTER SUMMARY

- Vitamin intake is necessary to maintain nutritional health.

- Vitamins function in the body as cofactors of metabolism, in growth and development, as antioxidants and hormones. Some are used as medications.

- Hypovitaminosis occurs because of decreased nutrient intake, altered absorption or metabolism, and with increased nutrient needs that are unmet.

- Hypervitaminosis generally occurs because of overuse of supplements and fortified foods.

- Vitamins are classified as either fat soluble or water soluble depending on their solubility in solutions. Vitamins A, D, E, and K are fat soluble, whereas vitamin C and B-complex vitamins are water soluble.

- The recommendations for vitamin intake are made as an RDA or an AI, depending on the amount of scientific evidence available. Some vitamins have UL recommendations when sufficient evidence exists to draw a conclusion.

- Poor vitamin health is a worldwide problem. The prevalence of vitamin A deficiency is high in underdeveloped countries. Poor vitamin D status is found in many developed countries. Intake of folic acid is a concern for all females of childbearing age. Older adults are at risk for inadequate vitamins D and B_{12} status. Alcohol intake affects the status of many of the B-complex vitamins, especially thiamin.

- The nurse must include an assessment of vitamin health in the nursing assessment. Information on intake of vitamin supplements and fortified foods should be included. It is essential that the nurse realize specific population groups at risk for poor vitamin status.

- The nurse should remain up to date about wellness issues and supplement use regarding vitamins and partner with the registered dietitian in relating accurate scientific recommendations on this subject to clients.

EXPLORE PEARSON **mynursingkit**™

MyNursingKit is your one stop for online chapter review materials and resources. Prepare for success with additional NCLEX®-style practice questions, interactive assignments and activities, web links, animations and videos, and more!

Register your access code from the front of your book at **www.mynursingkit.com.**

NCLEX® QUESTIONS

1. The mother of a newborn tells the nurse that she is concerned that her baby is not healthy because the baby got a "vitamin shot." How should the nurse respond?
   1. "Your baby is fine. You must have misunderstood what was said, but I will check and get back to you."
   2. "Vitamin K is given to all newborns to help their blood clot properly. Newborns do not yet have any vitamin K stores so a shot is given to them."
   3. "A vitamin shot is given to all newborns to get them off to a good nutritional start in life."
   4. "A vitamin C shot is given to help protect the newborn from infections. Your baby will be healthier because a shot was given."

2. The client asks the nurse why vitamin-enriched foods are a good choice. The nurse responds that:
   1. Vitamins are lost from foods during processing so enrichment adds them back to the food after processing.
   2. Extra vitamins are added to the processed foods to make them more nutritious.
   3. Additional vitamins are added so consumers do not need to eat as much of any given food to have the right amount of vitamins every day.
   4. Enriched foods are safer because vitamins that normally are not in foods are added during processing.

3. A toddler has been diagnosed with early-stage rickets. The nurse is counseling the mother and suggests increasing which of the following foods in the child's diet?
   1. Whole grain bread
   2. Apple juice
   3. Milk
   4. Green peas

4. A known alcoholic is admitted to the medical unit. What vitamin does the nurse expect will be part of the treatment plan?
   1. Thiamin
   2. Folic acid
   3. Vitamin D
   4. Vitamin C

5. The nurse determines that dietary teaching has been effective when a client who is planning pregnancy states which of the following food items has the highest folic acid content?
   1. Vanilla pudding
   2. Spinach salad
   3. Tuna salad
   4. Spaghetti with meatballs

REFERENCES

Agabio, R. (2005). Thiamin administration in alcohol-dependent patients. *Alcohol and Alcoholism, 40,* 155–156.

Aisen, P. S., Schneider, L. S., Sano, M., Diaz-Arrastia, R., van Dyck, C. H., Weiner, M. F., et al. (2008). High dose B vitamin supplementation and cognitive decline in Alzheimer disease. *Journal of the American Medical Association, 300,* 1774–1783.

Albert, C. M., Cook, N. R., Gaziano, J. M., Zaharris, E., MacFadyen, J., Danielson, E., et al. (2008). Effect of folic acid and B vitamins on risk of cardiovascular events and total mortality among women at high risk for cardiovascular disease. *Journal of the American Medical Association, 299,* 2027–2036.

Allen, L. H., & Haskell, M. (2002). Estimating the potential for vitamin A toxicity in women and young children. *Journal of Nutrition, 12,* 2907S–2919S.

American Academy of Pediatrics, Committee on Fetus and Newborn. (2003). Controversies concerning vitamin K and the newborn. *Pediatrics, 112,* 191–192.

American Academy of Pediatrics, Committee on Genetics. (1999). Folic acid for the prevention of neural tube defects. *Pediatrics, 104,* 325–327.

Ashourian, N., & Mousdicas, N. (2006). Images in clinical medicine: Pellagra-like dermatitis. *New England Journal of Medicine, 354,* 1614.

Balk, E. M., Raman, G., Tatsioni, A., Chung, M., Lau, J., & Rosenberg, I. (2007). Vitamin B-6, B-12, and folic acid supplementation and cognitive function. *Archives of Internal Medicine, 167,* 21–30.

Bloomberg, R. D., Fleishman, A., Nalle, J., Herron, D. M., & Kini, S. (2005). Nutritional deficiencies following bariatric surgery: What have we learned? *Obesity Surgery, 15,* 145–154.

Booth, S. L., Sacheck, J. M., Roubenoff, R., Dallal, G. E., Hamada, K., & Blumberg, J. B. (2004). Effect of vitamin E supplementation on vitamin K status in adults with normal coagulation status. *American Journal of Clinical Nutrition, 80,* 143–148.

Borghi, L., Meschi, T., Maggiore, U., & Prati, B. (2006). Dietary therapy in idiopathic nephrolithiasis. *Nutrition Reviews, 64,* 301–312.

Brown, S. J. (2006). The role of vitamin D in multiple sclerosis. *The Annals of Pharmacotherapy, 40*(6), 1158–1161.

Caire-Juvera, G., Ritenburgh, C., Wactawski-Wende, J., Snetselaar, L. G., & Chen, Z. (2009). Vitamin A and retinol intakes and the risk of fractures among participants of the Women's Health Initiative Observational Study. *American Journal of Clinical Nutrition, 89,* 1–8.

Cannell, J. J., & Hollis, B. W. (2008). Use of vitamin D in clinical practice. *Alternative Medicine Review, 13,* 6–20.

Carmel, R. (2008). How I treat cobalamin deficiency. *Blood, 112,* 2214–2221.

Cashman, K. D. (2007). Diet, nutrition, and bone health. *Journal of Nutrition, 137,* 2507S–2512S.

Cauley, J. A., LaCroix, A. Z., Wu, L., Horwitz, M., Danielson, M. E., & Bauer, D. C. (2008). Serum 25-hydroxyvitamin D concentrations and risk for hip fracture. *Annals of Internal Medicine, 149,* 242–250.

Centers for Disease Control and Prevention (CDC). (2004a). Spina bifida and anencephaly before and after folic acid mandate—United States 1995–1996 and 1999–2000. *Morbidity and Mortality Weekly Review, 53,* 362–365.

Centers for Disease Control and Prevention (CDC). (2004b). Use of vitamins containing folic acid among women of childbearing age—United States, 2004. *Morbidity and Mortality Weekly Review, 53,* 847–850.

Chang, C. G., Adams-Huet, B., & Provost, D. A. (2004). Acute post-gastric reduction surgery (APGARS) neuropathy. *Obesity Surgery, 14,* 182–189.

Cooney, R. V., Franke, A. A., Wilkens, L. R., & Kolonel, L. N. (2008). Elevated plasma gamma-tocopherol and decreased alpha-tocopherol in men are associated with inflammatory markers and decreased plasma 25-OH vitamin D. *Nutrition and Cancer, 60,* 21s–29s.

Dali-Yousef, N., & Andres, E. (2009). An update on cobalamin deficiency in adults. *Quarterly Journal of Medicine, 102,* 17–28.

Davidson, M. H. (2008). Niacin use and cutaneous flushing: Mechanisms and strategies for prevention. *American Journal of Cardiology, 101,* 14B–19B.

Davis, C. D. (2008). Vitamin D and cancer: Current dilemmas and future research. *American Journal of Clinical Nutrition, 88,* 565S–569S.

Dawson-Hughes, B. (2008). Serum 25-hydroxyvitamin D and functional outcomes in the elderly. *American Journal of Clinical Nutrition, 88,* 537S–540S.

Day, E., Bentham, P., Callaghan, R., Kuruvilla, T., & George, S. (2005). Thiamine for Wernicke-Korsakoff syndrome in people at risk from alcohol abuse (Review). *Cochrane Database of Systematic Reviews, 1,* CD004022 pub 2.

Debier, C. (2007). Vitamin E during pre- and postnatal periods. *Vitamins and Hormones, 76,* 357–373.

Dror, D. K., & Allen, L. H. (2008). Effect of vitamin B-12 deficiency on neurodevelopment in infants: Current knowledge and possible mechanisms. *Nutrition Reviews, 66,* 250–255.

Drury, D., Grey, V. L., Ferland, G., Gundberg, C., & Lands, L. C. (2008). Efficacy of high dose phylloquinone in correcting vitamin K deficiency in cystic fibrosis. *Journal of Cystic Fibrosis, 7,* 457–459.

Ebbing, M., Bleie, O., Ucland, P. M., Nordrehaug, J. E., Nilsen, D. W., Vollset, S. E., et al. (2008). Mortality and cardiovascular events in patients treated with homocysteine-lowering B vitamins after coronary angiography. *Journal of the American Medical Association, 300,* 795–804.

Eggermont, E. (2006). Recent advances in vitamin E metabolism and deficiency. *European Journal of Pediatrics, 165,* 429–434.

Food and Drug Administration, Office of Dietary Supplements. (2006). *What dietary supplements are you taking?* Retrieved December 12, 2008, from http://www.cfsan.fda.gov/~dms/ds-take.html

Friedlii, A., & Saurat, J. H. (2004). Images in clinical medicine: Oculo-orogenital syndrome—a deficiency of vitamins B_2 and B_6. *New England Journal of Medicine, 350,* 1130.

Galgano, F., Favati, F., Caruso, M., Pietrafesa, A., & Natella, S. (2007). The influence of processing and preservation on the retention of health-promoting compounds in broccoli. *Journal of Food Science, 72,* S130–S135.

Gaziano, J. M., Glynn, R. J., Christen, W. G., Kurth, T., Belanger, C., MacFayden, J., et al. (2009). Vitamins E and C in the prevention of prostate and total cancer in men. *Journal of the American Medical Association, 301,* 52–62.

Gray, S. L., Andersen, M. L., Crane, P. K., Breitner, J. C. S., McCormick, W., Bowen, J. D., et al. (2008). Antioxidant vitamin supplement use and risk of dementia or Alzheimer's disease in older adults. *Journal of the American Geriatric Society, 56,* 291–295.

Hathrock, J. N., Shao, A., Vieth, R., & Heaney, R. (2007). Risk assessment for vitamin D. *American Journal of Clinical Nutrition, 85,* 6–18.

Hemila, H., Chalker, E., Treacy, B., & Douglas, B. (2007). Vitamin C or preventing and treating the common cold. *Cochrane Database of Systematic Reviews, 3,* CD000980.

Heygi, J., Schwartz, R. A., & Heygi, V. (2004). Pellagra: Dermatitis, dementia and diarrhea. *International Journal of Dermatology, 43,* 1–5.

Hoffman, T. L., Simon, E. M., & Ficicioglu, C. (2005). Biotinidase deficiency: The importance of adequate follow-up for an inconclusive newborn screening result. *European Journal of Pediatrics, 164,* 298–301.

Holick, M. F. (2007). Vitamin D deficiency. *New England Journal of Medicine, 357,* 266–281.

REFERENCES   *(continued)*

Institute of Medicine (IOM), Food and Nutrition Board. (1998). *Dietary reference intakes for thiamin, riboflavin, niacin, vitamin B-6, folate, vitamin B-12, pantothenic acid, biotin and choline.* Washington, DC: National Academies Press.

Institute of Medicine (IOM), Food and Nutrition Board. (1999). *Dietary reference intakes for calcium, phosphorus, magnesium, vitamin D and fluoride.* Washington, DC: National Academies Press.

Institute of Medicine (IOM), Food and Nutrition Board. (2000). *Dietary reference intakes for vitamin C, vitamin E, selenium and carotenoids.* Washington, DC: National Academies Press.

Institute of Medicine (IOM), Food and Nutrition Board. (2001). *Dietary reference intakes for vitamin A, vitamin K, arsenic, boron, chromium, copper, iodine, iron, manganese, molybdenum, nickel, silicon, vanadium and zinc.* Washington, DC: National Academies Press.

Jager, R. D., Mieler, W. F., & Miller, J. W. (2008). Age-related macular degeneration. *New England Journal of Medicine, 358,* 2606–2617.

Johns Hopkins, Bloomberg School of Public Health. (2007). *Tables on the global burden of vitamin A deficiency among preschool children and women of reproductive age.* Retrieved December 10, 2008, from http://www.jhsph.edu/chn/globalVAD.html

Johnson, M. A. (2005). Influence of vitamin K on anticoagulant therapy depends on vitamin K status and the source and chemical forms of vitamin K. *Nutrition Reviews, 63,* 91–100.

Johnson, M. A. (2007). If high folic acid aggravates vitamin B-12 deficiency, what should be done about it? *Nutrition Reviews, 65,* 451–458.

Koike, H., Iilima, M., Mori, K., Hattori, N., Ito, H., Hirayama, M., et al. (2004). Postgastrectomy polyneuropathy with thiamine deficiency is identical to beriberi neuropathy. *Nutrition, 20,* 961–966.

Kumar, N. (2007). Nutritional neuropathies. *Neurologic Clinics, 25,* 209–255.

Leger, D. (2008). Scurvy: Reemergence of nutritional deficiencies. *Canadian Family Physician, 54,* 1403–1406.

Li, S., Jacob, J., Feng, J., & Kulkarni, M. (2008). Vitamin deficiencies in acutely intoxicated patients in the ED. *American Journal of Emergency Medicine, 26,* 792–795.

McGregor, G. P., & Biesalski, H. K. (2006). Rationale and impact of vitamin C in clinical nutrition. *Current Opinion in Clinical Nutrition and Metabolic Care, 9,* 697–703.

McNulty, H., & Scott, J. M. (2008). Intake of folate and related B-vitamins: Considerations and challenges in achieving optimal status. *British Journal of Nutrition, 99,* S48–S54.

Miller, E. R., Pastor-Barriuso, R., Riemersma, R. A., Appel, L. J., & Guallar, E. (2005). Meta-analysis: High dose vitamin E supplementation may increase all-cause mortality. *Annals of Internal Medicine, 142,* 37–46.

Moore, C., Murphy, M. M., Keast, D. R., & Holick, M. F. (2004). Vitamin D intake in the United States. *Journal of the American Dietetic Association, 104,* 980–983.

Munger, K. L., Levin, L. I., Hollis, B. W., Howard, N. S., & Ascherio, A. (2006). Serum 25-hydroxyvitamin D levels and risk of multiple sclerosis. *Journal of the American Medical Association, 296,* 2832–2838.

Munger, K. L., Zhang, S. M., O'Reilly, E., Hernan, M. A., Olek, M. J., Willett, W. C., & Ascherio, A. (2004). Vitamin D intake and incidence of multiple sclerosis. *Neurology, 62,* 60–65.

National Institutes of Health, Drug-Nutrient Interaction Task Force. (2003). *Important information for you when you are taking: Coumadin and vitamin K.* Retrieved July 12, 2005, from http://ods.od.nih.gov/factsheets/cc/coumadin1.pdf

National Institutes of Health, Office of Dietary Supplements. (2006). *Vitamin A and carotenoids.* Retrieved December 10, 2008, from http://ods.od.nih.gov/factsheets/vitamina.asp

National Institutes of Health, Office of Dietary Supplements. (2007a). *Dietary supplement fact sheet: vitamin E.* Retrieved December 10, 2008, from http://ods.od.nih.gov/factsheets/cc/vitd.html

National Institutes of Health, Office of Dietary Supplements. (2007b). *Dietary supplement fact sheet: vitamin B6.* Retrieved December 10, 2008, from http://ods.od.nih.gov/factsheets/vitaminb6.asp

National Institutes of Health, Office of Dietary Supplements. (2008). *Dietary supplement fact sheet: vitamin D.* Retrieved December 10, 2008, from http://ods.od.nih.gov/factsheets/cc/vitd.html

Pearson, D. A. (2007). Bone health and osteoporosis: The role of vitamin K and potential antagonism by anticoagulants. *Nutrition in Clinical Practice, 22,* 517–544.

Penniston, K. L., & Tanumihardjo, S. A. (2006). The acute and chronic toxic effects of vitamin A. *American Journal of Clinical Nutrition, 83,* 191–201.

Powers, H. J. (2003). Riboflavin (vitamin B-2) and health. *American Journal of Clinical Nutrition, 77,* 1352–1360.

Prousky, J. E. (2003). Pellagra may be a rare secondary complication of anorexia nervosa: A systematic review of the literature. *Alternative Medicine Review, 8,* 180–185.

Rabeneck, L., Zwaal, C., Goodman, J. H., & Zamkanei, M. (2008). Cancer Care Ontario guaiac fecal occult blood test laboratory standards: Evendentiary base and recommendations. *Clinical Biochemisty, 41,* 1289–1305.

Ryan-Harshman, M., & Aldoori, W. (2007). Carpal tunnel syndrome and vitamin B-6. *Canadian Family Physician, 53,* 1161–1162.

Said, H. M. (2009). Cell and molecular aspects of human intestinal biotin absorption. *Journal of Nutrition, 139,* 158–162.

Sesso, H. D., Buring, J. E., Christen, W. G., Kurth, T., Belanger, C., MacFayden, J., et al. (2008). Vitamins E and C in the prevention of cardiovascular disease in men. *Journal of the American Medical Association, 300,* 2123–2133.

Sheth, A., Khurana, R., & Khurana, V. (2008). Potential liver damage associated with over-the-counter vitamin supplements. *Journal of the American Dietetic Association, 108,* 1536–1537.

Thompson, A. D., Cook, C. H., Guerrini, I., Sheedy, D., Harper, C., & Marshall, J. E. (2008). Wernicke's encephalopathy: Plus ca change, plus c'est la meme chose. *Alcohol & Alcoholism, 43,* 180–186.

Thomson, A. D., Cook, C. C., Touquet, R., & Henry, J. A. (2002). The Royal College of Physicians report on alcohol: Guidelines for managing Wernicke's encephalopathy in the accident and emergency department. *Alcohol and Alcoholism, 37,* 513–521.

Van Winckel, M., DeBruyne, R., Van De Velde, S., & Van Biervliet, S. (2009). Vitamin K, an update for the paediatrician. *European Journal of Pediatrics, 168,* 127–134.

Vitamin B-6 (Pyridoxine; pyridoxal 5'phosphate) (Monograph). (2001). *Alternative Medicine Review, 6,* 87–92.

Wagner, C. L., Greer, F. R., & Section on Breastfeeding, Committee on Nutrition. (2008). Prevention of rickets and vitamin D deficiency in infants, children, and adolescents. *Pediatrics, 122,* 1142–1152.

Wang, A. H., & Still, C. (2007). Old world meets modern: A case report of scurvy. *Nutrition in Clinical Practice, 22,* 445–448.

Wooley, J. A. (2008). Characteristics of thiamin and its relevance to the management of heart failure. *Nutrition in Clinical Practice, 23,* 487–493.

Wooltorton, E. (2003). Too much of a good thing? Toxic effects of vitamin and mineral supplements. *Canadian Medical Association Journal, 169,* 47–48.

World Health Organization (WHO). (2008). *Micronutrient deficiencies: Vitamin A deficiency.* Retrieved December 10, 2008, from http://www.who.int/nutrition/topics/vad/en/

Wu, J. H., & Croft, K. D. (2007). Vitamin E metabolism. *Molecular Aspects of Medicines, 28,* 437–452.

Minerals 6

WHAT WILL YOU LEARN?

1. To examine the role of minerals in maintaining health.
2. To classify good dietary sources of major and trace minerals.
3. To analyze risk factors for poor mineral status, including interactions with foods and other nutrients.
4. To categorize signs and symptoms of mineral deficiency that can be found when conducting a nursing assessment.
5. To appraise the role of the nurse in identifying individuals at risk for altered health related to poor mineral status.

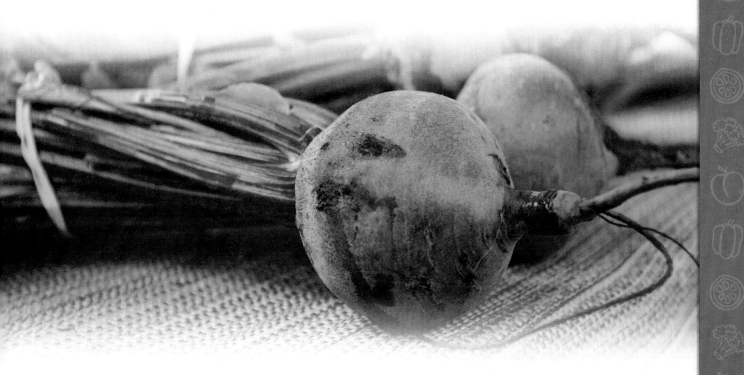

DID YOU KNOW?

▶ Consuming a calcium supplement at the same time as an iron supplement can decrease iron absorption.

▶ A mere teaspoon of table salt contains almost double the amount of sodium that is recommended in a day.

▶ Alcohol causes decreased absorption and increase urinary losses of zinc. Poor zinc status can impair sexual maturation.

▶ A symptom of poor potassium status is muscle cramping.

KEY TERMS

acrodermatitis enteropathica, *132*

bioavailability, *113*

fluorosis, *134*

goiter, *136*

koilonychia, *130*

osmolality, *124*

osteoporosis, *113*

pica, *130*

selenosis, *133*

tetany, *118*

Why Do We Need Minerals?

Minerals are inorganic elements that originate from rocks within the earth's crust. Minerals exist in a form that is electronically charged and therefore can gain or lose electrons. Unlike organic substances in the body, minerals do not break down during metabolism, though they can combine with other compounds or elements as they are incorporated into the body. For example, iron becomes part of hemoglobin in the red blood cell and zinc is incorporated into metabolic enzymes, but neither mineral is altered in such a way that it is no longer the same element or mineral. Like vitamins, minerals do not contain a source of energy for the body.

Minerals serve many general functions within the body: providing structure in the form of bones, teeth, and soft tissue; exerting osmotic pressure to maintain fluid balance; assisting in acid–base balance of fluids; serving as cofactors and coenzymes for metabolic and hormonal reactions; and playing a role in crucial nerve transmission and muscle contraction, including the heart. Minerals that are part of the structural components can be drawn on as a reserve when the mineral in needed for more urgent functions. For example, the calcium in bone serves as a depot for the tightly controlled amount of calcium present in the plasma. Table 6-1 outlines examples of mineral functions within the body.

What Affects Mineral Balance?

Mineral balance is affected by intake and excretion of minerals as well as by factors that interact or alter availability of the mineral. Poor mineral status can occur with insufficient intake to meet needs, mineral interactions, lowered mineral absorption, and increased mineral excretion, or any combination of these factors. Mineral balance is carefully orchestrated by the body, which is able to fine-tune absorption or excretion rates as needed. For example, if iron deficiency is present the percentage of iron absorbed in the intestine increases to improve iron status. The balance system does not entirely compensate for extreme situations of deficiency or toxicity. Mineral toxicity results when the body stores excessive mineral content because of increased intake, usually from supplements; altered metabolism; or environmental exposure, such as with mercury or lead.

Table 6-1 Examples of Mineral Functions

Mineral Function	Mineral Example	Role
Structure	Calcium, phosphorus, fluoride	Components of bones and teeth
Fluid balance	Sodium, potassium	Contribute to maintenance of fluid and plasma volume
Acid–base balance	Phosphorus	Assists in pH balance of blood and urine
Nerve cell transmission	Sodium, potassium Magnesium, calcium	Involved in active transport of substances across cell membranes Play role in neuromuscular activity
Muscle contraction	Calcium, magnesium, potassium	Involved in muscle contraction and relaxation, including the heart
Cofactor for enzymes and hormone activity	Iodine Zinc, selenium, copper	Component of thyroid hormones Enzyme cofactor

Mineral **bioavailability** refers to the absorbability of the mineral and is affected by the state of the mineral when it is in the intestine before absorption. Bioavailability affects mineral balance by influencing how well the mineral is absorbed. In humans, several naturally occurring substances in some foods render certain minerals less well absorbed than from other foods. For example, plant foods that contain phytates or oxalates as part of the plant fiber have reduced calcium and iron bioavailability because minerals bind to these two acid compounds and then are excreted. This net effect is most pronounced in the individual with poor baseline mineral status. Absorption of some minerals, such as iron, is diminished by lowered gastric acid content that can occur from aging, medical conditions, or medications. Other substances are known to improve mineral bioavailability, such as with the effect of vitamin C on certain types or iron.

Interactions among minerals and also between minerals and other substances can alter mineral balance. Minerals with similar ionic charge can compete with one another for absorption. Copper, zinc, iron, and calcium are frequently cited for the inverse relation that exists between them for intestinal absorption. This effect is most pronounced when mineral status is borderline and high amounts of one mineral are consumed. The individual with poor copper status can have worsened copper status if high-dose zinc supplements are taken, lowering the copper absorption rate. Likewise, zinc and calcium negatively affect iron absorption. Other examples of mineral interactions include the negative effect of caffeine on increased losses of calcium from urine and the positive effect of vitamin D and lactose on improved calcium absorption. Specific inhibitors and enhancers of mineral balance are outlined further within the discussions on specific minerals. Practice Pearl: Mineral Assessment offers some basic advice for the nurse to consider when beginning the evaluation of mineral status in a client.

PRACTICE PEARL

Mineral Assessment

To streamline the evaluation of risk factors for poor mineral health in a client, consider three questions:

1. *Is client intake of the mineral low?* Assessing why intake may be poor will allow meaningful advice to be offered to the client that is specific to needs.
2. *Are there increased mineral losses?* This can be from drug interactions, disease, or poor absorption.
3. *Is there an increased need for the mineral that is not being met?* Think about lifespan specific needs for growth and development especially.

Mineral Classification

There are 16 essential minerals needed in the diet for health. Essential refers to the fact that the body cannot make these nutrients and requires them from the diet. Essential minerals are classified as major minerals, which include electrolytes, and trace minerals. Major minerals are present in the body in amounts of 5 gm or more and require an intake of at least 100 mg/day. Trace minerals are present in amounts less than 5 gm and have recommended intakes of under 100 mg daily.

What Are the Major Minerals

Major minerals include calcium, phosphorus, magnesium, sulfur, sodium, potassium, and chloride. A summary of the function, food sources, and deficiency and toxicity symptoms of major minerals is outlined in Table 6-2.

Calcium

In recent years, the need for calcium in health and disease prevention has broadened to include more than just building strong bones and teeth. The role of calcium at the cell level, how it affects biological reactions in the body, and how it may lower risk of certain chronic diseases have all received attention by researchers.

Function

Calcium is an important part of the matrix that makes bone and teeth. Approximately 99% of the calcium in the body is in these structural components. A mere 1% is present in the plasma, body fluids, and tissues such as muscle. Although the majority of the body's calcium supports the structure of the body, the fraction present outside the bone is needed for crucial functions such as nerve impulse conduction and muscle contraction. Calcium in the bone serves as a storage depot of the mineral for this tightly controlled balancing act of plasma and fluid calcium. *Bone resorption* is the term used to describe the loss of bone, including calcium. Resorption of bone and calcium deposits in bone occurs continually over the lifespan, as discussed in Lifespan Box: Calcium.

Amenorrhea, or lack of menstruation, because of an eating disorder, a high level of physical activity, or any other cause also can lead to bone loss as seen in postmenopausal females related to a lowered estrogen environment in the body (National Institutes of Health [NIH], 2008a). Individuals who do not maintain adequate intake of calcium, poorly absorb calcium, or have increased calcium losses will have altered calcium balance and potentially diminished bone mass regardless of age. *Osteopenia* refers to diminished bone mass, whereas **osteoporosis** refers to a further reduction in bone mass with fragile, porous bones. These conditions are discussed in the upcoming text under Deficiency. Table 6-2

Table 6-2 Overview of Major Minerals

Major Mineral	Function	Food Sources	Deficiency Symptoms	Toxicity Symptoms
Calcium	• Structural component of bones and teeth • Nerve impulse conduction • Muscle contraction	Milk, yogurt, cheese, fish with edible bones, fortified soy products, fortified juices, green leafy vegetables	Osteopenia Osteoporosis	Risk of kidney stones in some High blood calcium → calcification of soft tissues
Phosphorus	• Structural component of bones • Synthesis of ATP, phospholipids • Acid–base balance	Protein-rich foods such as dairy, meats, poultry, legumes	Dietary deficiency rare Hypophosphatemia → anorexia, muscle weakness, confusion	Toxicity rare with normal kidney function Elevated blood phosphorus → calcification of tissues
Magnesium	• Coenzyme of metabolism • Maintenance of heart rhythm	Green leafy vegetables, whole grains, nuts	Low blood magnesium → neuromuscular excitability, cardiac arrhythmias, low blood potassium and calcium	Occurs with supplements only Diarrhea, mental status changes, muscle weakness, arrhythmias
Sulfate	• Component of some amino acids, bile • Synthesis of connective tissue, fibrinogen, estrogen	Drinking water, high-protein foods	Deficiency rare Growth stunting	Acute toxicity → osmotic diarrhea
Sodium	• Maintenance of plasma volume • Cell membrane potential and active transport of substances across cell membranes	Table salt, processed and convenience foods, smoked and pickled foods	Decreased extracellular fluid volume	Altered fluid volume and potential for increased blood pressure
Potassium	• Nerve cell transmission • Muscle contraction • Fluid balance	Fruits—banana, dried fruit, melon Vegetables—tuberous, root and green leafy (potato, sweet potato, carrot, spinach) Legumes Potassium chloride (KCl) salt substitute	Cardiac arrhythmia, muscle weakness, ↑ urinary calcium, glucose intolerance	Cardiac arrhythmia

Lifespan

Calcium

During periods of growth, such as childhood, bone deposition occurs at a greater rate than bone resorption. Peak bone mass is achieved by age 30 years, after which bone resorption and deposition balance out. This balance is upset when postmenopausal females and older males begin to lose more bone than is deposited. Estrogen has a positive effect on maintaining bone mass, and diminished estrogen production with menopause causes a dramatic loss of bone on the order of 3% to 5% of bone mass per year in the first 5 years after menopause (NIH, 2008a). Males experience an increase in bone resorption as well but do not present with symptoms of diminished bone density for 10 additional years compared to females (Tuck & Datta, 2007. In addition to increased bone loss with aging, absorption of calcium decreases compounding the effect. By age 65 years, calcium absorption is almost half that of adolescence (Straub, 2007).

outlines the functions of calcium in the body. Figure 6-1 ■ outlines the regulation of calcium in the body.

Recommended Intake

The dietary reference intake (DRI) for calcium is given as an adequate intake (AI) recommendation. In adults age 19 years to 50 years, the AI is 1,000 mg of calcium daily. Over age 50 years, the daily recommendation for males and females increases to 1,200 mg to offset increased bone resorption (Institute of Medicine [IOM],1997). During adolescence when bone deposition is increased, the AI is 1,300 mg/day. No increase in calcium requirement during pregnancy or lactation has been reported because of improved intestinal absorption of calcium during pregnancy and rapid replacement of bone loss from lactation during weaning (IOM, 1997). The nurse should stress the importance of adequate calcium intake in achieving peak bone mass in growing clients and minimizing bone loss in adult

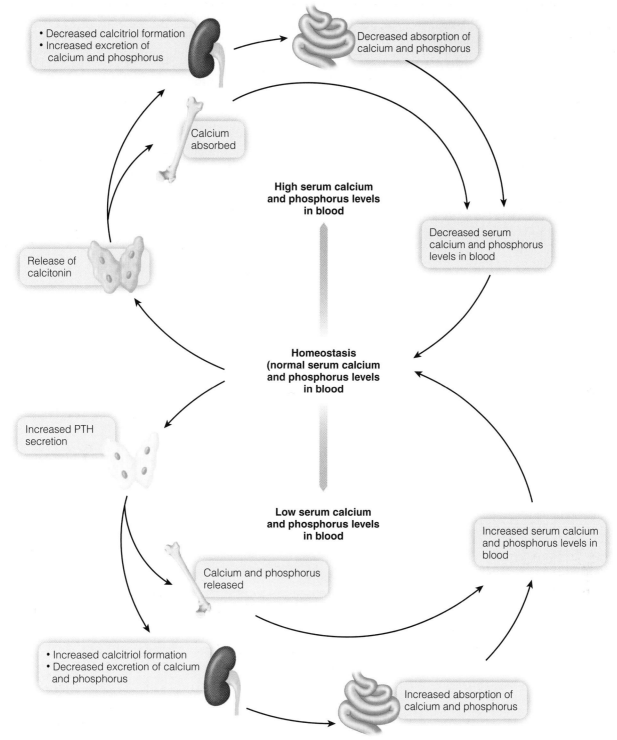

■ FIGURE 6-1 **Calcium Regulation in the Body.**

clients. The DRI recommendations, by definition, are intended for use with healthy individuals. Clients who have medical conditions or who are prescribed medications that affect calcium balance can have altered calcium requirements. Chapter 25 outlines medications that alter calcium balance. A registered dietitian should be consulted when working with these clients. The AI for calcium for all ages and genders is contained in Appendix C.

Sources

In the United States the major source of calcium in the diet is milk and other dairy foods (Cotton, Subar, Friday, & Cook, 2004). Other sources of calcium include some green leafy vegetables; fish with small bones, such as sardines and anchovies; and fortified products, such as calcium-fortified versions of juices, tofu, soy milk, and breakfast cereals. Some nuts, grains, and dried beans also contain some calcium.

Calcium bioavailability varies among foods. Oxalates and phytates present in plant fibers bind with calcium in foods, resulting in less availability of calcium for absorption. Soy and some green leafy vegetables, such as spinach and broccoli, contain these acids. As a result, calcium absorption from spinach is one-tenth of the absorption rate found with milk (IOM, 1997). Additionally, it has been reported that beverages fortified with calcium often have a precipitate form from the calcium unless the beverage container is shaken before consumption. Available calcium may not be adequately dissolved in the drink served (Heaney, Rafferty, & Bierman, 2005). Calcium absorption is improved in the presence of adequate vitamin D stores in the body. Without adequate vitamin D to enhance the active transport of calcium from the intestine, it is unlikely that adequate absorption of the mineral will occur (Heaney, 2008). The nurse should be aware of good sources of calcium in the diet and the effect that bioavailability has on calcium absorption. For example, one would need to consume 8 cups of cooked spinach to absorb the same amount of calcium found in 1 cup milk or 1.5 oz of cheddar cheese because of the low bioavailability of the calcium in the spinach (Weaver, Proulx, & Heaney, 1999). Table 6-3 outlines calcium food sources. The Client Education Checklist: Calcium offers advice that the nurse can give to improve intake.

Deficiency

Deficiency of calcium occurs because of chronically insufficient intake, altered absorption or metabolism, and increased losses of calcium. Insufficient intake of calcium results from a low intake of milk and dairy foods and restrictive eating

Table 6-3 Calcium Food Sources

Food	Calcium Content (mg)
Yogurt, plain, nonfat, 1 cup	488
Soy milk, calcium-fortified, 1 cup	368
Milk, skim, 1 cup	306
Milk, whole, 1 cup	276
Spinach, cooked, 1 cup	245
Chinese cabbage, cooked, 1 cup	158
Kale, cooked, 1 cup	94
Ice cream, vanilla, 1/2 cup	92

Source: USDA Nutrient Data Laboratory. Retrieved March 25, 2009, from http://www.nal.usda.gov/fnic/foodcomp/search

habits, including dieting. The average intake of calcium in the United States is inadequate at 892 mg/day, with females over age 70 years consuming even less (666 mg/day) (United States Department of Agriculture [USDA], 2005). Individuals may choose to not drink milk because of cost or taste preferences. Lactose intolerance can lead some individuals to eliminate dairy foods from the diet. A strict vegetarian lifestyle when no animal foods are consumed (vegan) will also contain no dairy products. Cultural Considerations Box: Calcium discusses these contributors to calcium intake. The nurse should assess the reason for low intake of calcium in an individual and make recommendations for good calcium sources that fit within the client's lifestyle.

CLIENT EDUCATION CHECKLIST   **Calcium**

1. Assess diet for sources of calcium. Include fortified foods and supplements.
2. Determine any reasons why calcium intake is low.
3. Assess diet for excess sodium, caffeine, or protein that will cause urinary calcium loss.
4. Educate the client on the role of calcium-containing foods in health.
   - Bone and teeth formation
   - Osteoporosis prevention
   - Alleviation of PMS symptoms
   - Blood pressure control
5. Customize advice based on causes of poor calcium intake. Suggestions follow each contributor to low-calcium intake.
   a) Lactose intolerance—Milk with lactase added, small amounts of aged cheese, yogurt with active cultures, calcium-fortified juice or soy products, fish with small bones (sardines, anchovies). (Also see Client Education Checklist 20-2: Lactose Intolerance.)
   b) Vegan diet—Calcium-set tofu, calcium-fortified soy or rice milk, calcium-fortified juice, kale, bok choy.

   c) Cost—Fortified breakfast cereals, lower cost cheeses, skim or low-fat milk. Green leafy vegetables, fortified soy milk and yogurt are more expensive sources of calcium.
   d) Dislike plain dairy foods—Add low-fat cheese to salads, pasta; make a smoothie with milk or yogurt and fresh or frozen fruit; cook with milk instead of water, making hot cereal, pancakes, or cocoa; make yogurt-based dips or salad dressing; make desserts with milk-like pudding, low-fat frozen yogurt, yogurt-fruit parfaits; fish with small bones; calcium sources listed under vegan advice.
   e) Knowledge deficit—Explain good sources of dietary calcium like milk, yogurt, cheese, kale, bok choy, and fortified juice, cereals, and soy products.

Calcium supplements for when food sources are not sufficient—Take in doses of 500 mg calcium or less; calcium carbonate is the least expensive form; vitamin D improves absorption; avoid oyster shell, bone meal, and dolomite preparations because of possible lead content; space intake away from timing of any iron supplements.

Cultural Considerations

Calcium

Consider cultural contributors to low-calcium intake. Tolerance to lactose in milk is found mainly in individuals of Northern European descent. Lactose intolerance is common in most other populations. Strict vegetarianism with no dairy intake may be followed because of religious beliefs. Clients following kosher law will not consume dairy when also consuming meat in a meal.

BOX 6-1	Foods Containing Phytates and Oxalates

Phytates

Whole grains
Legumes: beans, split peas, lentils
Nuts
Unleavened bread

Oxalates

Spinach	Beet greens
Rhubarb	Tea
Sweet potato	Chocolate
Nuts	Wheat bran

Calcium absorption or metabolism can be altered because of medical conditions or medications. Low production of gastric acid from age, gastric resection, or medications will lead to diminished calcium absorption. Poor vitamin D status decreases calcium absorption. Diseases that cause fat malabsorption can affect calcium, such as cystic fibrosis, inflammatory bowel disease, celiac disease, and short bowel syndrome. Medications such as steroids, some anticonvulsants, and tetracycline alter calcium absorption (NIH, 2008a; Straub, 2007). Alcohol may reduce calcium absorption, but this remains controversial, especially with moderate to low alcohol intake (NIH, 2008a; Straub, 2007). Carbonated sodas have been postulated as contributing to poor bone health because of the negative effects of the phosphorus content on calcium absorption (Tucker et al., 2006). It seems more likely that the negative association between soda intake and poor bone health is because of displacement of milk in the diet with soda and the caffeine in cola-type beverages, and not an effect of the phosphorus content (Heaney & Rafferty, 2001; Tucker et al., 2006). Additional dietary factors that affect calcium absorption include phytates and oxalates, which decrease calcium absorption from the food source itself, but not from other foods eaten at the same time (NIH, 2008a). Box 6-1 outlines foods containing phytates and oxalates.

Increased calcium excretion can contribute to poor calcium status. Long-term high caffeine intake has been associated with poor bone mineral density in older females, especially those with low-calcium intake (IOM, 1997; Straub, 2007). Caffeine fosters short-term urinary loss of calcium, but the small amount lost can be offset with the addition of a tablespoon of milk to the coffee or tea (NIH, 2008a). Likewise, a high-protein or high-sodium intake can lead to increased urinary calcium excretion, but the effects are minimal if calcium intake is adequate (IOM, 1997; NIH, 2008a). Table 6-4 outlines the effect of multiple factors on calcium balance, highlighting those that are risk factors for poor calcium status.

Seldom is a low blood level of calcium related to diet or poor calcium stores; rather hypocalcemia occurs from existing medical conditions or treatments (Moe, 2008). Examples include hypoparathyroid disease, pancreatitis, and certain cancers that cause increased calcium uptake into bone. Severe vitamin D deficiency can cause hypocalcemia (Moe, 2008). Hypocalcemia affects muscle contraction and nerve conduction and can result in cardiac arrhythmias, muscle

Table 6-4 Factors Affecting Calcium Balance

Balance Component	Effect	Cause of Imbalance
Calcium intake	Decreased	Weight loss/dieting Limited or no dairy intake: vegan diet, lactose intolerance, financial Limited intake of nondairy sources of calcium
Calcium absorption	Increased	Adequate vitamin D Presence of lactose in food
	Decreased	Fat malabsorption Oxalates and phytates Alkaline gastric pH: medications, aging, gastric resection Poor vitamin D status Medication interactions
Calcium excretion	Increased	Caffeine, high-protein intake, high-sodium intake

CT? Who might be following a high-protein diet? How should the nurse approach the issue of calcium balance in someone choosing to follow a high-protein diet?

MyNursingKit National Osteoporosis Foundation

cramps, and numbness in the extremities and around the mouth. **Tetany** is the term used to describe the physical symptoms of hypocalcemia. Trousseau's sign and Chvostek's sign are two clinical tests for hypocalcemia. The test for Trousseau's sign is performed by inflating a blood pressure cuff above the systolic pressure for 3 minutes and watching for a telltale hand spasm. Chvostek's sign is a facial muscle twitch that occurs when tapping over the facial nerve in front of the ear as shown in Figure 6-2 ■. Hypocalcemia is treated medically with intravenous or supplemental calcium (Moe, 2008).

Calcium deficiency manifests itself in the form of poor bone mineral density, and eventually osteopenia can go on to become osteoporosis. The large depot of calcium in the bones is used to maintain adequate calcium balance in the blood and other tissues. This calcium reservoir can be sacrificed over time when calcium intake or absorption are poor and fail to replete bone resorption. Decreased bone mineral density causes weakened architecture and fragility of the bones, which are risk factors for fractures (National Osteoporosis Foundation [NOF], 2008). Figure 6-3 ■ depicts this effect. Prevention and treatment of osteoporosis include an adequate intake of calcium and vitamin D as part of the medical approach, which may include medications and weight-bearing exercise (NOF, 2008). Vitamin D and calcium supplements that meet amounts for recommended intake have been shown to improve bone density in postmenopausal women but have no reported effect on risk of hip fracture (Jackson et al., 2006). Individuals who are unable to consume adequate dietary calcium may require calcium supplements, which are discussed under Wellness Concerns and Supplement Use here.

Toxicity

The tolerable upper intake level (UL) for calcium is 2,500 mg daily for those over 1 year of age (IOM, 1997). No UL has been established for infants under age 1 year because of insufficient research. As with most vitamins and minerals, the

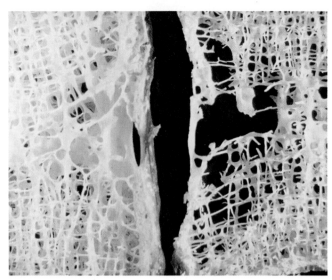

■ FIGURE 6-3 **Osteoporosis.**
Source: Michael Klein/Peter Arnold, Inc.

effects of excess calcium intake primarily occur from the use of dietary supplements, and not from naturally occurring dietary calcium sources. Excess intake of calcium can contribute to the development of calcium oxalate kidney stones in some individuals, though the evidence is weak for most healthy people (IOM, 1997). Alterations in fat absorption and excess oxalate consumption are associated with risk of kidney stone development in these individuals. Excessive calcium intake can cause hypercalcemia, which can lead to soft tissue deposits of calcium, renal damage, and, ultimately, death (IOM, 1997). Medical conditions, such as parathyroid disease and certain cancers, can also cause hypercalcemia. The nurse should conduct a careful diet history when a client presents with hypercalcemia to determine if excess intake of dietary calcium is a factor. Additionally, the nurse should screen those persons found to have high intake of calcium for risk of other mineral deficiencies. Calcium negatively interacts with iron, zinc, magnesium, and phosphorus absorption (IOM, 1997). High-dose intake of calcium can place vulnerable individuals with borderline mineral status at risk for deficiency. In particular, the nurse should warn clients with poor iron status to avoid taking calcium supplements with meals or with iron-containing supplements because the calcium will negatively affect the absorption of iron. If dual supplementation is indicated, the client with iron-deficiency should alter the timing to maximize absorption (Straub, 2007).

Wellness Concerns and Supplement Use

In addition to maintaining bone health, adequate calcium has been reported to play a role in blood pressure control and reduction of symptoms of premenstrual syndrome (PMS). Both observational studies and clinical trials have supported the consumption of adequate calcium from three dairy servings per day as part of an overall diet aimed at controlling blood pressure (Vollmer et al., 2001). The Dietary

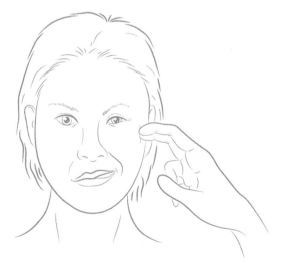

■ FIGURE 6-2 **Chvostek's Sign.**

Approaches to Stop Hypertension (DASH) diet includes plenty of fruits and vegetables, three servings of low-fat dairy, and is low in fat and sodium. It has been reported to lower blood pressure in both hypertensive and normotensive individuals (Vollmer et al., 2001). The DASH diet is outlined in Chapter 18. Adequate calcium has been reported to reduce symptoms of PMS in females. Calcium supplementation of 1,000 to 1,200 mg has been clinically shown to alleviate symptoms such as irritability and cramping (American Dietetic Association [ADA] & Dietitians of Canada, 2004; Thys-Jacobs, McMahon, & Bilezikian, 2007).

Research has linked adequate calcium intake with a reduction in colon cancer risk and improvement in weight management in some individuals, though results are far from conclusive. Some research supports the role of calcium in the diet or from supplementation in the reduction of nonmalignant tumors in the colon and risk of colon cancer (NIH, 2008a; Weingarten, Zalmanovici, & Yaphe, 2008). Further studies are needed before any conclusions or recommendations can be made. Although calcium from dairy foods has been postulated to play a role in weight management in overweight and obese adults, research results have been mixed, with the majority of studies finding no evidence to support a role of dairy or calcium in aiding weight loss (Lanou & Barnard, 2008; Zemel & Miller, 2004).

Calcium supplements and calcium-fortified foods are popular methods to increase dietary calcium intake. It is important that the nurse have accurate information about supplemental and fortified sources of calcium to relate to the client. Hot Topic Box: What Calcium Supplement Is Best? outlines information about choosing a calcium supplement. Some individuals choose to consume calcium-fortified foods that do not naturally contain calcium instead of taking a calcium supplement. Juices, soy products, breakfast cereals, and meal replacement bars are examples of foods that are available in a calcium-fortified version. The nutrition label will identify the amount of calcium in the product as a percentage of the AI of 1,000 mg. For example, a fortified juice with 30% of the recommended calcium for the day would have 300 mg of calcium in a serving. Clients should be advised to shake fortified beverage containers before pouring the drink to mix any calcium precipitate back into the solution (Heaney, Rafferty, Dowell, & Bierman, 2005). Bioavailability of calcium fortificants differ and research is ongoing to discover absorbability of these compounds that are added to foods.

Phosphorus

Phosphorus is found in both animal and plant tissues. Cells that have either a high content of ribonucleic acid (RNA) or nerve cells with a high myelin content have more phosphorus than other components of protoplasm (IOM, 1997). Outside these cells, phosphorus is found rather uniformly in plants and animals alike. In nature, phosphorus is combined

hot Topic

What Calcium Supplement Is Best?

Clients often ask for advice on what type of calcium is best. Calcium from food sources is the preferred source because these foods deliver other essential nutrients in addition to the calcium. Calcium in dairy foods is absorbed well because of the presence of vitamin D and lactose. For some individuals, calcium supplementation may be needed because of little or no intake of high-calcium foods because of dietary habits, beliefs, or tolerances. Several factors should be considered when considering calcium supplementation. Cost differs among the various types of supplements, and for a client on a budget, calcium carbonate provides the most inexpensive calcium source. For the client who has difficulty taking many pills, calcium carbonate provides more elemental calcium than other supplements of the same weight. Calcium carbonate is 40% elemental calcium, whereas calcium citrate is only 21% calcium by weight. Other forms of calcium compounds are available with varying calcium content as outlined in Figure 6-4 ■. Calcium carbonate and calcium citrate are absorbed almost equally well by most individuals, but the person with low gastric acidity or those on medications to lessen gastric acid would benefit from the citrate form. The nurse should advise clients against the use of "natural" calcium supplements derived from oyster shell or bone meal because these can contain lead. Coral calcium is marketed by manufacturers as a superior product but is no more than calcium carbonate. Clients should be instructed to consume 500 mg or less of a supplement at any time to optimize calcium absorption. For individuals using supplements to reach the full 1,000 mg AI, a divided dose is advisable, taking care to not take calcium with iron supplements or any medications with which there is an interaction, such as tetracycline, fluoroquinolone antibiotics, levothyroxine for thyroid disease, and the antiseizure medicine phenytoin.

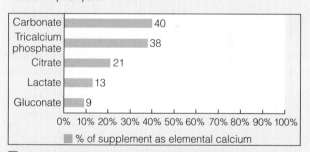

■ **FIGURE 6-4 Calcium Content of Supplements.**
Sources: Keller, Lanou, & Barnard, 2002; National Institutes of Health, Office of Dietary Supplements, 2008a; Straub, 2007.

with oxygen in the phosphate form. In the human body, the mineral exists as phosphate as well as a multitude of other phosphorus-containing compounds, such as phospholipids, nucleotides, and nucleic acids.

Function

The majority of phosphorus exists in bone, with only 10% to 15% of body stores occurring in soft tissue, plasma, and extracellular fluid (ECF) (IOM, 1997). Like calcium, the phosphorus present in bone is used as a structural component and a reservoir on which to draw for maintenance of crucial plasma and tissue levels. Phosphorus is a constituent of phospholipids present in cell walls and lipoproteins that act as carriers in the plasma. A tiny crucial fraction of the body's phosphorus plays an important role in maintaining pH control of blood and urine, providing substrate for synthesis of the high-energy adenosine triphosphate (ATP) and creatine phosphate, and catalyzing proteins involved in enzyme reactions. Table 6-2 outlines the functions of phosphorus. The body seeks to maintain a steady state between phosphorus absorption from the intestine and excretion in the urine while keeping a balance in the small ECF and plasma pool. In instances when phosphorus intake is high, healthy kidneys will filter out the excess into the urine. When intake is low, less phosphorus is excreted, and if necessary bone resorption of the mineral occurs. Phosphorus and calcium regulation are outlined in Figure 6-1.

Recommended Intake

The DRI for phosphorus exists as an RDA. In adults age 19 years and older, the RDA is 700 mg per day (IOM, 1997). Recommendations for phosphorus intake in other age groups are contained in Appendix C.

Sources

All plant and animal foods contain phosphorus. Foods that are protein rich tend to have more phosphorus content. Additionally, sodas and several food additives contain phosphorus for moisture retention, smoothness, and binding (IOM, 1997). Phosphorus is well absorbed in the intestine with the exception of plant foods containing phytates, where the phosphorus is a component of phytic acid and poorly absorbed. Table 6-5 outlines food sources of phosphorus.

Deficiency

A true dietary deficiency of phosphorus is rare because of the ubiquitous nature of the mineral in foods. However, decreased plasma phosphorus and altered phosphorus in extracellular fluid is more common. Low plasma phosphate is not indicative of overall poor phosphorus stores, but rather occurs because of altered absorption of phosphorus, intracellular shifts of phosphorus, or a change in phosphorus excretion.

Table 6-5   Phosphorus Food Sources

Food	Phosphorus Content (mg)
Chicken breast, cooked, 3½ oz	228
Chickpeas, canned, 1 cup	216
Roast beef, cooked, 3½ oz	212
Salmon, cooked, 3½ oz	200
Cheddar cheese, 1 oz	145
Ice cream, vanilla, ½ cup	76
Milk, skim, 1 cup	27

Source: USDA Nutrient Data Laboratory. Retrieved March 25, 2009, from http://www.nal.usda.gov/fnic/foodcomp/search

Aluminum-containing and calcium carbonate antacids and dietary supplements can alter phosphorus absorption. Pharmacological doses of calcium carbonate are needed for this effect to happen (IOM, 1997). Intracellular shifts of phosphorus occur with changes in cellular pH; following treatment for diabetic ketoacidosis; and with refeeding of clients who are malnourished, including those with prolonged postoperative starvation, anorexia nervosa and, alcohol abuse. As glucose enters cells, phosphorus shifts to provide substrate for ATP production and plasma phosphorus drops. This is called *refeeding syndrome* and is discussed in detail in Chapter 16. Phosphorus excretion can be altered in response to changes in plasma pH and from medications, such as diuretics and glucocorticoids, among other reasons.

Although hypophosphatemia seldom occurs from diet, the nurse should be aware of its risk factors and negative consequences. Hypophosphatemia can lead to anorexia, muscle weakness, confusion, alteration in blood clotting, and immune dysfunction. In severe cases, respiration and cardiac function can be affected by altered contractions of the diaphragm, decreased affinity of hemoglobin for oxygen, and cardiomyopathy (Moe, 2008). Generally, hypophosphatemia is treated with oral repletion under medical supervision (Moe, 2008).

Toxicity

The UL for phosphorus is 4,000 mg in adults (IOM, 1997). Symptoms from excess phosphorus in the diet are seldom seen in healthy individuals with healthy kidney function. Individuals with renal failure or vitamin D intoxication can develop hyperphosphatemia, or elevated plasma phosphate level, in response to excess dietary phosphorus intake (Moe, 2008). Hyperphosphatemia can alter hormonal balance of plasma calcium because of the related physiological balance between these two minerals. Additionally, metastatic calcification of nonskeletal tissues can occur if the mathematical product of serum calcium and serum phosphorus is greater than $72 \text{ mg}^2/\text{dL}^2$, resulting in deposition of a calcium-phosphorus compound in organs and other tissues (Friedman, 2005). The kidneys are particularly affected, which results in a downward spiral in kidney function that further complicates the hyperphosphatemia (Friedman, 2005). In those with chronic kidney disease and elevated plasma phosphorus, dietary phosphorus is not overly restricted because this can result in too little intake of protein (Shinaberger et al., 2008). Instead, phosphorus-binding medications are used to control hyperphosphatemia (Moe, 2008).

Wellness Concerns and Supplement Use

The balance between phosphorus, calcium, and vitamin D affects bone health. When intake of phosphorus is elevated and calcium and vitamin D decreased, poor bone health can result from improper mineralization. Although certain diseases can alter this delicate balance, such as chronic kidney disease because of limited activation of vitamin D in the kidney, dietary

EVIDENCE-BASED PRACTICE RESEARCH BOX

Does consuming large amounts of phosphorus from carbonated beverages increase the risk of bone fractures in children and adolescents?

Clinical Problem: American children and adolescents frequently consume large amounts of carbonated beverages, which have a high phosphorus content. Researchers are interested in what effect, if any, that has on bone health.

Research Findings: The consumption of carbonated beverages in the United States has increased steadily to the point that in 2005 over 28% of all nonalcoholic beverages consumed were carbonated soft drinks. Milk and bottled water were next at 10.9% and 10.7%, respectively (American Beverage Association, 2005). Bottled water is gaining in popularity and will likely surpass milk in the near future.

Exactly how much carbonated beverage consumption is by children and adolescents is unknown, but the quantity is believed to be significant as it replaces milk as the beverage of choice. Boys drink more beverages than girls and teens tend to drink more carbonated beverages than children (Forshee & Storey, 2003). Researchers have undertaken studies of children and adolescents to assess the effect that intake of carbonated beverages has on bone mineral density (BMD) in that age group.

An early study of 465 high school girls by Wyshak (2000) found an association (p = 0.002) between cola drinks and fractures in physically active adolescent girls. A similar association was not found with other types of carbonated beverages. A study of 1,335 adolescents in Northern Ireland found that consumption of cola and noncola carbonated beverages was inversely associated with heel BMD in girls but not boys (McGartland et al., 2003).

A total of 206 cases of upper limb fractures (hand, wrist, forearm, and upper arm) in children were matched with 206 control subjects. There was a weak association between cola consumption and fractures but no association with other carbonated beverages. The researchers believe that other factors, such as activity level, mediated the results (Ma & Jones, 2004).

Data from 1,125 men and 1,413 women in the Framingham Osteoporosis Study were reviewed with respect to carbonated beverage consumption. Interestingly, the researchers found significantly lower BMD in the hips of women who consumed cola beverages but not men. This association was not found with other carbonated beverages (Tucker et al., 2006).

Nursing Implications: There is a small but growing body of evidence that carbonated cola beverages may be associated with decreased BMD and, to a lesser extent, fractures. Nurses should continue to stress the importance of milk as a beverage of choice for children and adolescents to improve diet quality and prevent a decrease in BMD.

CRITICAL THINKING QUESTIONS:

1. How should the nurse respond to the parent who tells the nurse that the 10-year-old daughter will only drink lemonade or diet soda with meals?

2. A client asks the nurse about what age it is acceptable to give carbonated soft drinks to a child. What could the nurse share with the client?

---

alterations can also contribute. The Evidence-Based Practice Box: Colas and Bone Health discusses the question of whether phosphorus intake from sodas contributes to poor bone health.

Magnesium

The total body pool of magnesium exists primarily in bone and soft tissue. Approximately 50% to 60% of the body's magnesium is found in bone and of that, one-third is available as an exchange reservoir for maintaining plasma magnesium levels (IOM, 1997). Only 1% to 2% of the body's magnesium is found in the plasma, yet this fraction is often measured to determine overall magnesium status despite the fact that it has not been validated for this use (IOM, 1997; Moe, 2008). The kidney is the organ primarily responsible for maintaining magnesium homeostasis through excretion or reabsorption of magnesium as needed.

Function

Magnesium is involved in over 300 metabolic enzyme reactions in the body (IOM, 1997). The macronutrients, carbohydrate, protein, and fat, all require magnesium for some aspect of metabolism to generate energy. Glycogen breakdown, fat oxidation, protein synthesis, and ATP generation involve enzymes that have magnesium as a cofactor (IOM, 1997). Maintenance of normal heart rhythm requires adequate magnesium. Magnesium is essential in the regulation of sodium, potassium, and calcium homeostasis in intracellular and extracellular fluids. Excess or deficiency of magnesium can lead to detrimental alterations in these important minerals in the body.

Recommended Intake

The DRI for magnesium is given as an RDA. In males between ages 19 and 30 years, the RDA is 400 mg/day. This recommendation increases to 420 mg at age 31 years and beyond. Females require 310 mg/day from age 19 years to 30 years. After age 30, it is recommended that females consume 320 mg/day of magnesium (IOM, 1997). Magnesium intake should be slightly increased during pregnancy as outlined in Appendix C.

Sources

Green leafy vegetables, whole grains, seeds, and nuts are good sources of dietary magnesium. Animal products, such as poultry, fish, and milk products, also contain magnesium but in smaller amounts than in the plant foods. Drinking water contains varying amount of magnesium. Hard water, with high

Table 6-6 Magnesium Food Sources

Food	Magnesium Content (mg)
Halibut, cooked, 3½ oz	107
Almonds, dry roasted, 1 oz (22 nuts)	81
Lentils, cooked, 1 cup	71
Nuts, mixed, 1 oz	64
Peanut butter, 2 tbsp	49
Potato, baked with skin, medium	48
Yogurt, fruit, low fat, 1 cup	36

Source: USDA Nutrient Data Laboratory. Retrieved March 25, 2009, from http://www.nal.usda.gov/fnic/foodcomp/search

mineral content, generally contains more magnesium than soft-water sources (IOM, 1997). Processing of foods leads to magnesium loss; overall intake of magnesium is declining in the United States with the increased consumption of processed foods. Approximately 56% of Americans are not consuming adequate magnesium (USDA, 2005). The nurse should encourage intake of whole grains, fruits, and vegetables with minimal processing to maximize intake of magnesium. Table 6-6 outlines dietary sources of magnesium.

Deficiency

True deficiency of magnesium is rare because the bone maintains a large reservoir of the mineral. Plasma magnesium is used to assess for magnesium deficiency or toxicity even though it is not indicative of overall magnesium stores (Arnaud, 2008; Moe, 2008). Poor magnesium status in cellular fluids and plasma can lead to dangerous consequences even when total body magnesium remains within normal limits.

Reduced intake and renal and gastrointestinal losses of magnesium contribute to decreased available magnesium. Decreased intake results from poor-quality diet; a high intake of processed, rather than whole, foods; and overall diminished intake. Increased losses from the gastrointestinal tract occur with malabsorptive conditions, such as chronic diarrhea, Crohn's disease, and short bowel syndrome. Renal wasting of magnesium occurs because of glucose in the urine from uncontrolled diabetes and from medications (NIH, 2005). Alcohol, diuretics, and certain antibiotics and chemotherapeutic agents decrease magnesium retention by the kidneys, leading to increased excretion (Moe, 2008; NIH, 2005). The individual with a poor diet from increased alcohol intake is additionally at risk for poor magnesium status from the compounded effect of increased renal loss of the mineral.

Low levels of magnesium in the plasma cause neuromuscular hyperexcitability, which can lead to various cardiac arrhythmias and muscular contractions (IOM, 1997; Moe, 2008). Hypomagnesemia can cause concurrent hypokalemia, hypocalcemia, and increased intracellular calcium (Moe, 2008). The nurse should recall this association when caring for a client with arrhythmias or refractory hypokalemia be-

cause magnesium is not generally assessed in routine laboratory assays and can be a contributing cause with these conditions. Clients with cardiac disease who are on diuretic therapy can be at further risk for hypomagnesemia and, therefore, arrhythmias, because of the negative effect of low blood magnesium on intracellular potassium (IOM, 1997).

Toxicity

The UL for magnesium is for magnesium supplements only and does not include food sources of magnesium (IOM, 1997). Adverse effects of excess magnesium from the diet have not been reported in individuals with healthy kidney function. Healthy kidneys are able to rapidly respond to elevated plasma magnesium (Moe, 2008). The UL for magnesium supplements is greater than or equal to 350 mg/day (IOM, 1997).

Individuals at risk for magnesium toxicity include those with renal failure and those taking magnesium-containing medications. Laxatives such as magnesium sulfate and other magnesium salts are used for the effect of osmotic diarrhea; altered magnesium status can occur in those who use these laxatives without guidance and monitoring. Some antacids contain magnesium as well. Magnesium overdose from medications resulting in stroke-like symptoms has been reported (NIH, 2005). The nurse can read the label on these over-the-counter products to determine if magnesium is present.

Symptoms of magnesium toxicity include diarrhea, low blood pressure, and altered mental status. Other symptoms closely mimic those seen with magnesium deficiency such as arrhythmias, nausea, loss of appetite, and muscle weakness (Moe, 2008).

Wellness Concerns and Supplement Use

The nurse should warn clients with poor kidney function about taking supplemental magnesium or medications containing magnesium, unless specifically instructed otherwise. Magnesium supplementation may be indicated in certain individuals after careful assessment of need. Clients with arrhythmias or disorders where magnesium excretion is increased, such as alcoholism, can be evaluated for supplemental magnesium (IOM, 1997). Magnesium supplementation is one of the treatments of choice in hypertension of pregnancy (Leeman & Fontaine, 2008).

Magnesium may play a wellness role in prevention or management of hypertension and diabetes. Population studies have shown an association between adequate intake of magnesium and decreased risk of type 2 diabetes (Larsson & Wolk, 2007; NIH, 2005). It may be that glycosuria (glucose in the urine) is associated with magnesium losses, but there is also some evidence of altered magnesium absorption from the intestine in those at risk for diabetes (IOM, 1997). Additional clinical research is needed before a conclusion can be drawn. Analysis of current research makes it difficult to separate the effects of dietary magnesium from the other effects of a diet high in magnesium, which usually contains whole grains, fruits and vegetables, and minimal processed foods. For now the American Diabetes Association recommends magnesium supplements only for individuals with demonstrated hypomagnesemia (American Diabetes Association, 2008).

A diet with adequate magnesium has been associated with improved blood pressure regulation in population studies (IOM, 1997; NIH, 2005). No conclusion can be drawn that magnesium has an independent effect on lowering blood pressure because many diets studied were also high in potassium and low in sodium (NIH, 2005). Low intake of magnesium is associated with risk of metabolic syndrome, a condition associated with cardiovascular risk, in older adults (McKeown, Jacques, Zhang, Juan, & Sahyoun, 2008). The DASH diet, which is encouraged for treating hypertension, includes adequate magnesium.

Sulfate

Sulfur is abundant in the earth's crust and organic matter. The oxidation of sulfur yields sulfate, the most stable and abundant form of the mineral used by living organisms (Kormarnisky, Christopherson, & Basu, 2003). Some sulfate-containing compounds are crucial for health, whereas others threaten the environment. Industrial sources of sulfates, from burning of fossil fuels and by-products of mills, are producing increasing amounts of sulfur dioxide, which is an environmental pollutant partly responsible for acid rain (IOM, 2004).

Function

There are hundreds of sulfur-containing compounds in the body. The essential amino acids methionine and cysteine contain sulfur and, therefore, proteins in the body synthesized with these amino acids also contain the element. Bile salts and components of connective tissue, such as chondroitin sulfate are synthesized using the mineral (IOM, 2004). Heparin, fibrinogen, and estrogen are also synthesized from sulfate (Kormarnisky et al., 2003).

Recommended Intake

A separate recommendation for dietary sulfate does not exist, although the mineral is essential. Consuming the recommended protein intake should provide adequate sulfate with the ingestion of the amino acids methionine and cysteine (IOM, 2004). Drinking water and other foods will provide additional sulfate beyond the 2.8 gm per day of sulfate obtained from these protein sources (IOM, 2004).

Sources

Drinking water and many foods have a significant amount of sulfate. The amount of sulfate in drinking water varies with the source of the water; rural wells or sources near mines or industrial sites can have higher levels than some other sources (IOM, 2004). Water with high-sulfate levels will have an off-taste and strong odor, which is felt to self-regulate individuals from overconsumption (IOM, 2004). Plant foods grown in soil with high-sulfate content will contain more sulfate than those grown in poor soil. High-protein foods will contain sulfate because of the sulfur-containing amino acid content. Sulfates are also used as additives in medication and as browning agents and dough conditioners. Sulfites are another form of sulfur that is present in food. Sulfites occur naturally from fermentation in wine and are added as preservatives in other foods, such as dried fruit.

Deficiency

Deficiency of sulfate is rare in healthy humans consuming an adequate amount of protein. Growth stunting has been reported in experimentally induced sulfate deficiency (IOM, 2004).

Toxicity

There is a lack of sufficient data to establish a UL for sulfate (IOM, 2004). Reports have been published of osmotic diarrhea occurring as a result of drinking water with high-sulfate content. This is a particular concern in infants (IOM, 2004).

Wellness Concerns and Supplement Use

Deficiency of protein can negatively affect immune status. Cysteine and methionine, two sulfur-containing amino acids, are being investigated for potential roles in immune function and anti-inflammatory effects associated with disease. More research is needed into this area of nutrition and disease prevention (Grimble, 2006; Roth, 2007).

Electrolytes

Sodium, potassium, and chloride are major minerals in the body and are also called electrolytes. Electrolytes can exist in ionically charged forms, exerting an effect on fluid concentration, acid–base balance, nerve conduction, and membrane permeability in the body. Plasma levels of electrolytes are checked to determine the status of these minerals but do not always reflect intake because healthy kidneys can excrete excessive amounts to maintain the delicate balance needed in the plasma to effect crucial body processes.

Sodium and Chloride

Sodium and chloride are generally found together in the food supply as the compound sodium chloride, commonly referred to as salt. Balance of sodium and chloride in the body is maintained by hormones such as renin, angiotensin, and aldosterone, along with the sympathetic nervous system and intrarenal mechanisms. Under conditions of minimal sweat losses, the body seeks to keep a steady state between sodium intake and urinary losses. Sodium lost in sweat can vary according to ambient temperature, humidity, exertion level, and acclimatization by the individual. Intense exercise or toiling in extreme heat can lead to significant sodium losses through sweat as the body attempts to cool. The hormone systems and renal mechanisms respond to variations in blood volume affected by fluid and sodium loads in the body; the result is renal conservation or excretion of sodium to maintain proper plasma volume. Over time the body is able to adapt to very low intake of sodium with increased reabsorption of sodium by the renal tubules (IOM, 2004). This adaptation is markedly slowed with the aging process.

The taste preference for salt in foods is believed to be innate. Taste adaptation to a lower salt intake can take up to 8 to 12 weeks (Mattes, 1997).

Function

Almost 95% of the sodium in the body is found in the ECF compartment (IOM, 2004). Sodium is the principal cation in these fluids and, thus, along with chloride plays a central role in maintaining plasma volume by contributing to ECF **osmolality.** Osmolality refers to the concentration of charged particles in a solution. The body seeks to maintain a balance in osmolality and accomplishes this with fluid and electrolyte shifts. It is the relationship between plasma volume and sodium balance that is responsible for the effect of sodium intake on blood pressure, as discussed under Wellness Concerns and Supplement Use.

Sodium is also responsible for maintaining cell membrane potential and the active transport of substances across cell membranes (IOM, 2004). In addition to its role in fluid balance, chloride is a constituent of hydrochloric acid in the stomach.

Sodium added to the food supply functions as a preservative, extending the shelf life of products and controlling microbial growth (IOM, 2004). Sodium additives are also used to add texture or control leavening in baked goods.

Recommended Intake

The DRI for sodium and chloride exist as AI recommendations. Chloride recommendations are extrapolated from sodium recommendations to account for the molecular relationship between the two elements. Salt is 40% sodium and 60% chloride. The AI for sodium for adults age 19 to 50 years is 1.5 gm per day. The AI for chloride for the same age population is 2.3 gm per day, thereby achieving a recommendation of 3.8 gm of sodium chloride daily (IOM, 2004). For adults 50 to 70 years of age, the AI is 1.3 gm of sodium and 2.0 gm of chloride (IOM, 2004). Adults over age 70 years are advised to consume 1.2 gm of sodium and 1.8 gm of chloride (IOM, 2004). Although it has been reported that under maximal adaptation the body can maintain sodium balance with as little intake as 180 mg of sodium per day, the overall diet at this low a sodium intake is lacking in other important nutrients (IOM, 2004). The AI recommendation does not apply to individuals with a large volume of sodium and fluid loss through sweating, such as competitive athletes who are undergoing intense training or workers exposed to extreme heat and humidity (IOM, 2004).

Sources

Sodium is primarily found as sodium chloride in food. Only 12% of the sodium in food is naturally occurring, whereas almost 77% is added during food processing in many forms such as sodium chloride, monosodium glutamate, sodium ben-

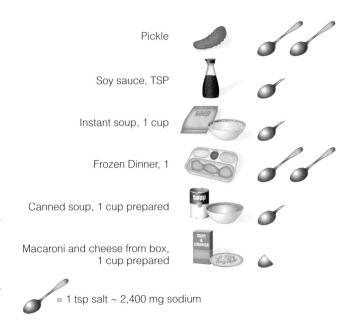

Pickle

Soy sauce, TSP

Instant soup, 1 cup

Frozen Dinner, 1

Canned soup, 1 cup prepared

Macaroni and cheese from box, 1 cup prepared

= 1 tsp salt ~ 2,400 mg sodium

■ FIGURE 6-5 **Sodium Content of Foods in Teaspoons.**

zoate, and sodium citrate (IOM, 2004). The remaining sodium in food is called discretionary sodium and is the result of salt added by the consumer during cooking or at the table. Approximately 20% of individuals add salt to food before tasting it (Mattes, 1997). One teaspoon of table salt contains 2.4 gm (or 2,400 mg) of sodium. A small fraction of intake of sodium chloride is from tap water (IOM, 2004). Figure 6-5 ■ compares the sodium content of foods to the amount of sodium in a teaspoon of salt.

The nurse should be aware that the primary contributor to sodium intake is from processed foods. Canned, smoked, pickled, and instant foods along with select condiments contain significant amounts of sodium. Luncheon meats, frozen entrees, instant soup, cheese, canned vegetables, and soy sauce are examples of high-sodium foods. Cultural Considerations Box: Sodium discusses the effects of cultural food habits on sodium intake.

Foods "closest to their original form" such as plain meats, fish, poultry, legumes, fruits, vegetables, milk, and

Cultural Considerations

Sodium

High-sodium foods are integral to the diets of many cultures. Kosher foods are processed with salt. In many forms of Chinese cooking, soy sauce, oyster sauce, black bean sauce, monosodium glutamate, and miso contribute high amounts of sodium. Teriyaki sauce is featured in Japanese foods. Mediterranean diets can have high-sodium cheese, like feta, and processed meats in an antipasto. Cheeses and refried beans are high-sodium contributors in a Mexican diet. Salted, smoked, and pickled fish are high in sodium and are foods found in many cultures.

Table 6-7	Sodium Content of Foods		
Over 1,500 mg/serving		**Greater than 250–500 mg serving**	
Large dill pickle		Pretzels, 1 oz	
Table salt, 1 tsp		American cheese, 1 slice	
Frozen meal		Olives, 10	
Ham, 3½ oz			
1,000–1,500 mg/serving		**100–250 mg/serving**	
Soup, canned, 1 cup prepared		Catsup, 1 tbsp	
Tomato sauce, canned, 1 cup		Worcestershire sauce, 1 tbsp	
Soy sauce, 1 tbsp		Mixed nuts, 1 oz	
		Anchovy, 1	
500–1,000 mg/serving		**Less than 100 mg/serving**	
Dehydrated soup, 1 cup prepared		Most fruits, vegetables, and plain grains	
Macaroni and cheese, prepared from box, 1 cup			
Cheese crackers, bite size, 1 cup			

Source: USDA Nutrient Data Laboratory. Retrieved March 25, 2009, from http://www.nal.usda.gov/fnic/foodcomp/search

grains generally contain little sodium. The nurse can remind clients that the more processed version of a food will have more sodium than the less processed version of the same food. Fresh foods have less sodium than the frozen counterpart. Generally, canned and dehydrated foods have more sodium than the frozen form, but labels should be checked. Table 6-7 outlines the sodium content of common foods.

Deficiency

In healthy people, a true deficiency of sodium is uncommon. Adaptation to low-sodium intake occurs but can be a challenge in the older adult with large fluid losses because of illness or surgery and a slowed adaptation process with age. The result can yield decreased plasma sodium and ECF volume. Increased losses of sodium in the urine can occur with uncontrolled diabetes because excess glucose in the urine leads to passive water and sodium loss (IOM, 2004). Excess sodium losses in sweat can occur with intense exercise, working in extreme heat, and with cystic fibrosis. Sodium losses because of excessive sweat loss should be replaced with an increased intake of salty foods. Lightly salting food or consuming salty snacks, such as pretzels, following intense exercise or manual work can supply needed sodium.

When sodium losses are excessive, low plasma sodium can occur. This condition is treated emergently because severe negative consequences, including coma and death, can occur from hyponatremia. Athletes who lose a large volume of sweat and fail to replace sodium when rehydrating can also develop hyponatremia. The risk and prevention of hyponatremia in athletes is discussed further in Chapter 11.

Toxicity

The UL is 2.3 gm for sodium and 3.6 gm for chloride per day (IOM, 2004). This recommendation is based on the progressive and continuous relationship between sodium intake and elevated blood pressure (IOM, 2004). Those with excessive sweat losses may have needs greater than the UL.

Sodium consumption in the United States is well above the UL recommendation. Over 85% of the population in the United States consumes more than the recommended sodium each day (USDA, 2005). Males age 12 years to 60 years have daily intakes greater than 4 gm of sodium, close to twice the UL. Females have high-sodium intake as well but slightly less than males because of overall lower energy intake. The nurse should advise clients with high-sodium intake of the relationship between sodium and blood pressure and offer suggestions for lowering intake of sodium as outlined in the Client Education Checklist: Sodium and in Chapter 18.

Wellness Concerns and Supplement Use

The major wellness concern relative to sodium is its relationship with blood pressure. Reduced sodium diets have been associated with improved blood pressure control in normotensive and hypertensive individuals (Bray et al., 2004). The response is greater in hypertensive than in normotensive individuals and further enhanced with intake of dietary potassium (Geleijnse, Kok, & Grobbee, 2003). Some individuals with high blood pressure have a heightened blood pressure response to sodium intake and are referred to as "salt sensitive." Salt-sensitive individuals, who include older adults, African Americans, and those with diabetes, renal failure, or hypertension, can benefit greatly from a reduction in sodium intake. The DASH diet, a low-fat diet with low sodium, high potassium and adequate dairy is recommended for prevention and treatment of hypertension.

Excess sodium intake fosters increased excretion of urinary calcium, which in turn can increase risk of calcium-based kidney stones (Worcester & Coe, 2008). Increased potassium intake may temper the effect of high-sodium intake on urinary calcium losses (Harrington, 2003; IOM, 2004).

Use of salt supplements is not recommended as a usual practice unless medically advised for those with chronic

MyNursingKit National Institutes for Health (NIH) Reduce Salt and Sodium in Your Diet

CLIENT EDUCATION CHECKLIST   Sodium

1. Assess diet for sources of sodium. Include salt added in cooking and at the table.
2. Determine any reasons why sodium intake is high.
3. Educate the client on the negative impact of a high-sodium intake on health.
   a) Blood pressure control
   b) Loss of calcium in urine—affects bone health and risk of kidney stone
4. Outline significant sources of sodium and offer alternatives.
   a) High-sodium food sources
   - Preserved, pickled, or smoked foods—cheese, pickles, olives, smoked meats, hot dogs, cold cuts, sausage, bacon, sauerkraut, canned meats, fish and vegetables, frozen entrees, prepared tomato products (canned or jarred tomato sauce, puree, tomatoes)
   - Convenience foods—dried or canned soup, mixes (gravies, rice, instant mashed potato, macaroni and cheese), instant hot cereal
   - Condiments—sauces (soy, teriyaki, oyster, steak, meat sauce, Worcestershire), catsup, salad dressing, marinades and tenderizers, MSG
   - Salty snacks—nuts, chips, pretzels
   b) Lower sodium alternatives
   - Fresh or frozen plain meats, fish, poultry
   - Fresh or frozen vegetables
   - Rice, potato, pasta cooked without salt
   - Fresh, frozen, or canned fruit or juice
   - Whole grain cereals and breads
   - Unsalted nuts, crackers, snack foods
   - Low-sodium version of salty condiments
   - Substitute herbs, spices, and citrus flavors for salt in cooking
   - Cover most holes in the salt shaker and gradually use less added salt
   - Taste food before deciding to add salt
   - If canned vegetables or beans must be used, rinse before use
5. Instruct on label reading—sodium content is listed on the nutrition label; 140 mg of sodium or less per serving is "low sodium;" check ingredient list for the words *salt* or *sodium*.

significant salt losses. Athletes and manual workers are advised to lightly salt food and to consume salty foods when sweat losses are high.

Potassium

Potassium is the major intracellular cation, but it is also found in ECFs, including plasma. The kidneys regulate potassium balance in the body by conserving or excreting potassium in the urine. Kidney disease and some medications can alter potassium balance by affecting urinary potassium.

Function

Although most of the body's potassium is present within cells, the small fraction in plasma and other ECFs is maintained within a narrow range that is delicately balanced to affect neural transmission and muscle contraction. Potassium is also involved in maintenance of fluid balance within the body. Potassium acts directly on the renal tubule to increase excretion of sodium in the urine.

Recommended Intake

The DRI for potassium pertains only to potassium from food and not from supplemental potassium sources. The recommendation is given as an AI. For all adults, the AI is 4.7 gm of potassium per day (IOM, 2004). Individuals with altered kidney function or those on specific medications may be advised to consume less potassium than the AI.

In both the United States and Canada, intake of potassium is well below the recommended level (IOM, 2004).

Mean intake of potassium for all age groups is 2.606 gm per day (USDA, 2005).

Sources

Potassium is plentiful in fruits, vegetables, legumes, and milk. In particular bananas, dried fruit, and melons are good fruit sources of potassium. Tuberous, root, and leafy green vegetables such as potato, sweet potato, carrots, and spinach are good vegetable sources of the mineral. Winter squashes and dried beans are additional sources. Table 6-8 outlines food sources of potassium.

Table 6-8   Potassium Food Sources

Food	Potassium Content (mg)
Baked potato with skin, medium	926
Spinach, cooked, 1 cup	839
Raisins, ½ cup	785
Lentils, cooked, 1 cup	731
Yogurt, fruit, low fat, 1 cup	490
Banana, medium	422
Honeydew melon, 1 cup	388
Orange, medium	232
Tomato juice, ½ cup	228
Whole wheat cereal flakes, 1 cup	132

Source: USDA Nutrient Data Laboratory. Retrieved March 25, 2009, from http://www.nal.usda.gov/fnic/foodcomp/search

Deficiency

A severe deficiency of potassium can lead to hypokalemia when plasma levels of the mineral are diminished below 3.5 mmol/L. The result can be cardiac arrhythmias, muscle weakness, increased calcium losses in the urine, and glucose intolerance. Reduced potassium levels alter the capacity of the pancreas to secrete insulin (IOM, 2004). At moderate levels of deficiency, hypokalemia may not be present, but risk of adverse effects such as elevated blood pressure, stroke, and kidney stones still exists (IOM, 2004). Using blood potassium level alone does not adequately assess potassium status, but it is the measure commonly employed.

Poor potassium status can occur from reduced intake, increased losses, or a combination of the two. Decreased potassium intake can occur with a poor quality diet with minimal fruits and vegetables or severe calorie restriction. Increased losses of potassium can occur in sweat with excessive exercise, in urine from use of certain diuretic medications, and from the gastrointestinal tract from diarrhea or laxative abuse. Potassium deficiency is commonly treated with potassium supplementation. The nurse should advise the client with a poor diet or chronic potassium losses about good dietary sources of potassium.

Toxicity

No UL for dietary potassium exists for healthy people with normal kidney function (IOM, 2004). Excess intake of potassium should be excreted by the kidney without negative effect. The nurse should not suggest an increased potassium intake for individuals with chronic kidney diseases, Addison's disease, or those on certain potassium-sparing medications used to treat hypertension before an evaluation of potassium status. Potassium toxicity has been reported in otherwise healthy persons who accidentally or intentionally ingested large quantities of potassium chloride supplements or potassium-containing salt substitutes (IOM, 2004).

Excess potassium in the blood leads to hyperkalemia. Elevated plasma potassium is a risk factor for life-threatening cardiac arrhythmias.

Wellness Concerns and Supplement Use

The nurse should encourage clients with normal kidney function to consume adequate amounts of potassium. In particular, increased intake of potassium can ameliorate the effects of high-sodium intake on blood pressure, especially in salt-sensitive hypertensive individuals, such as older adults and African Americans (IOM, 2004). Potassium supplements are not recommended as part of the dietary treatment of high blood pressure; instead a diet with ample fruits and vegetables and low-fat dairy to supply good sources of dietary potassium is recommended.

The nurse should be aware that some salt substitutes available on the market contain potassium as an alternative to sodium. The product label will list the ingredients to assist in the determination of the composition. For certain individuals, such as those on a potassium-wasting diuretic who require increased potassium intake, these salt substitutes may be appropriate. For others with compromised renal function, use of a potassium salt substitute could be dangerous. As part of a diet history, clients should be assessed for use of salt substitutes.

What Are Trace Minerals?

Trace minerals are iron, iodine, zinc, selenium, copper, fluoride, chromium, molybdenum, and manganese. These nutrients are classified as trace minerals because they are present in the body in amounts less than 5 gm and the daily requirement is less than 100 mg. A summary of functions, recommendations, and consequences of poor trace mineral status is outlined in Table 6-9. Other trace minerals exist in the body but are not considered essential in the diet. Boron, arsenic, nickel, silicon, and vanadium are examples of nonessential trace minerals with no established guidelines for recommended intake.

Iron

Knowledge and understanding about iron nutrition is essential for the nurse because iron deficiency is the most common nutritional deficiency worldwide (Clark, 2008). In the United States, infants, children, and females of childbearing age are particularly at risk for poor iron status.

Function

Iron is essential for oxygen transport throughout the body. Approximately two-thirds of the body's iron is part of the protein hemoglobin found in red blood cells. Hemoglobin carries oxygen from the lungs to the rest of the body. Iron is also present in myoglobin, an oxygen-carrying protein found in muscle, and cytochromes, where electron transport occurs within cells. Enzymes involved in oxidative metabolism and other biological reactions require iron. Iron that is being actively utilized is referred to as functional iron. In health, 25% of the body's iron is in the form of storage iron, as ferritin and hemosiderin, and transport iron, as transferrin (Centers for Disease Control and Prevention [CDC], 1998; IOM, 2001; Zimmerman & Hurrell, 2007). Transferrin transports absorbed iron via the plasma to the body's cells. Iron storage occurs primarily in the liver, spleen, and bone marrow when the body has adequate functional iron for its needs. Muscle and plasma also contain storage iron. The intestines regulate iron balance by altering absorption based on iron stores. When iron stores are low, relative iron absorption is increased compared to during normal or increased stores. The body is highly conservative in maintaining iron stores, and little iron is lost from baseline needs except during pregnancy or blood loss (IOM, 2001).

Table 6-9 Trace Mineral Overview

Trace Mineral	Function	Food Sources	Deficiency Symptoms	Toxicity Symptoms
Iron	Oxygen transport	Organ meats, animal flesh proteins, fortified grains, legumes, molasses, green leafy vegetables	Fatigue, rapid heart rate, developmental delays in children, pica, koilonychias, glossitis, cold intolerance, blue sclera	Hemochromatosis Organ damage
Zinc	Enzyme cofactor	Oysters, red meat, whole grains	Reduced appetite and taste acuity, stunted growth, hypogonadism in boys, diarrhea, poor wound healing	Impaired copper status, reduced immune response, decreased HDL cholesterol
Selenium	Antioxidant	Brazil nuts, beef, seafood, some plants	Rare. Hypothyroidism	Hair loss, garlicky breath, fatigue, intestinal complaints
Copper	Coenzyme, synthesis of connective tissue, collagen	Organ meats, seafood, nuts, grains	Anemia, bone demineralization	Vomiting, diarrhea, cirrhosis, liver failure
Fluoride	Mineralization of bones/teeth	Drinking water	Increased risk of dental caries	Fluorosis
Chromium	Cofactor in insulin activity	Red wine, animal flesh proteins	Rare. Impaired glucose tolerance	None reported
Iodine	Component of thyroid hormones	Seafood, iodized salt	Thyroid disease, goiter, congenital hypothyroidism	Thyroid disease
Manganese	Bone formation, metabolism	Legumes, grains, nuts	Slowed growth	Limited human data. Neurological symptoms
Molybdenum	Cofactor in metabolism	Legumes, grains, nuts	Neurological damage with inborn error of metabolism	Limited human data. Growth abnormalities in animals

Recommended Intake

The DRI for iron is given as an RDA for all population groups except infants, where an AI recommendation is made because of insufficient data. Iron needs change over the lifespan because of differences in needs to support growth and because of menstrual blood losses in the female of childbearing age. Lifespan Box: Iron discusses these effects. The RDA for males

Lifespan

Iron

Iron needs vary throughout the lifespan. During times of growth and development, such as infancy, young childhood, and adolescence, iron needs are increased. Infants require a source of iron from fortified cereal or formula by age 6 months, when stores acquired in utero are diminished. Adolescents require increased iron to support increased lean body mass and corresponding blood supply. During pregnancy, iron needs increase to support increased maternal blood volume, placenta, and the needs of the fetus. Females of childbearing age have increased iron needs to compensate for iron loss with menstruation. Relative iron requirements are decreased in healthy adult males and postmenopausal females because of little iron loss and lack of growth.

CT? How should the nurse factor in these recommendations considering the iron needs of a pregnant teen who is still growing?

age 19 years and older is 8 mg of iron per day (IOM, 2001). Females of childbearing age are advised to consume 15 mg of iron from age 14 to 18 years and then 18 mg of iron daily until age 50 years (IOM, 2001). During pregnancy, iron absorption efficiency is increased and 27 mg of iron per day is recommended (IOM, 2001). The CDC and the ADA recommend that pregnant females take a 30-mg iron supplement to ensure that they meet this increased iron requirement, whereas other authorities advise an individualized approach to iron supplementation (American College of Obstetricians and Gynecologists [ACOG], 2008; ADA, 2008; CDC, 1998; NIH, 2007). Infants born to mothers with iron deficiency anemia are at risk for low birth weight and preterm delivery. Healthy, full-term babies should have sufficient fetal iron stores to last until age 4 to 6 months (IOM, 2001). Iron needs during pregnancy are discussed in detail in Chapter 13. Recommendations for iron intake for all groups are outlined in Appendix C.

Sources

Iron is present in food in two forms: heme and nonheme iron. Heme iron is derived from animal foods, which have a hemoglobin source, such as red meat, poultry, and fish. Nonheme iron is found in plant foods, fortified and enriched foods, iron supplements, and animal foods. Heme iron is better absorbed than nonheme iron by two- to threefold, yet nonheme iron sources comprise the primary dietary source of iron (CDC 1998; IOM, 2001). Gastric pH and bioavailability of iron impacts the ability of the body to absorb the iron from the gastrointestinal tract. Nonheme iron can have enhanced absorption with a normal acidic gastric pH, or if consumed with a vitamin C source, which helps render the iron into a more absorbable form. An alkaline gastric environment because of a medical condition or medications that diminish gastric acid will reduce iron absorbability because the iron is not converted to the more readily absorbed form that requires an acid medium. Absorption of nonheme iron can be inhibited by a number of substances in foods, such as polyphenols in tea that decrease iron absorption significantly when consumed within an hour of an iron source (Nelson & Poulter, 2004). One cup of tea decreases iron absorption by almost 50% in healthy adults and by more than 60% in iron deficient individuals (Thankachan, Walczyk, Muthayya, Kurpad, & Hurrell, 2008). Other enhancers and inhibitors of iron bioavailability are listed in Box 6-2.

Heme sources of iron include meat, poultry, and fish. Nonheme sources of iron include dried beans, peas and lentils, leafy green vegetables, dried fruit, fortified and enriched grains, and molasses. Children under the age of 1 year should consume an iron-fortified cereal or iron-fortified infant formula by age 6 months to obtain the recommended iron (Kazal, 2002). Cow's milk is a poor source of iron and can cause iron losses through occult bleeding in the intestinal

Table 6-10	Iron Food Sources	
Heme Iron	**Nonheme Iron**
Clams	Fortified cereals
Oysters	Lentils
Chicken and beef liver	Spinach
Beef	Tofu
Tuna	Dried fruit
Pork	Beans (kidney, chickpea, black)
Poultry, dark meat	Enriched breads
	Blackstrap molasses

tract when given to children under age 1 year; hence it is not recommended for this age population (CDC, 1998). The nurse should be aware that, in particular, females of childbearing age have been reported to consume insufficient iron with only a mean intake of 13.1 mg daily (USDA, 2005). The nurse should routinely include an assessment of iron nutrition when assessing clients with increased iron needs. Advice should be offered, outlining good sources of iron in the diet when indicated. Table 6-10 outlines heme and nonheme iron foods.

Deficiency

Iron deficiency can occur because of poor diet, poor iron bioavailability or absorption, and increased iron losses. Poor intake of iron can occur from limited intake of nutrient-dense foods, restrictive eating habits, or lack of knowledge about iron sources. During periods of rapid growth with increased iron needs, inadequate intake magnifies the risk of iron deficiency. Iron bioavailability becomes a factor when iron status is poor or intake is exclusively comprised of nonheme iron sources, such as with a vegetarian diet. Iron availability from a plant-based diet is 10% compared with up to 35% from heme sources of iron found in animal foods (Zimmerman & Hurrell, 2007). A vegetarian individual, therefore, must be mindful of consuming good sources of iron and enhancing iron absorption with foods containing vitamin C whenever possible. Altered iron absorption because of limited gastric acid production or alkalinizing medication use can place an individual at risk for iron deficiency. Gastric bypass surgery also diminishes iron absorption (Clark, 2008). Lastly, increased iron losses are a risk factor for poor iron status. Blood loss from surgery, gastrointestinal bleeding, or heavy menstruation can upset iron balance and lead to a deficiency. Box 6-2 outlines risk factors for iron deficiency.

Symptoms of iron deficiency arise from the decreased efficiency of the body to deliver oxygen via hemoglobin to cells. Fatigue, diminished work performance, and increased heart rate can occur. In children, slowed cognitive and social development is seen and is significant because some poor functioning can persist despite treatment. The school nurse may note problems with social inattentiveness, decreased school

---

BOX 6-2	**Factors Affecting Iron Balance**

Decreased iron intake:
- Poor-quality diet
- Inappropriate use of cow's milk in children under age 1 year

Decreased iron absorption:
- Reduced iron bioavailability—phytates, polyphenols (tea, coffee, red wine), high-calcium intake, soy protein
- Alkaline gastric pH—gastric resection, medications (antacids and other ulcer or gastritis medications), aging
- Hookworm
- Malabsorptive disease

Increased iron losses:
- Surgery
- Menstruation
- Gastrointestinal or genitourinary losses of blood

Increased iron needs:
- Growth
- Pregnancy

■ Which factors should the nurse consider for each stage in the lifespan?

performance, and diminished motor activity in children with iron deficiency (Zimmerman & Hurrell, 2007). Additional symptoms can include an inability to maintain body temperature (with a complaint of always feeling cold), blue sclera, and glossitis. **Koilonychia,** or upward curved and ridged fingernails, can be found. **Pica** can be present in some individuals with iron deficiency. This craving and ingesting nonfood items has been reported in pregnant females with iron deficiency, but it is uncertain whether this consumption habit leads to iron deficiency or is a result of it. The nurse should screen pregnant females for consumption of nonfood items, such as ice, freezer frost, laundry starch, clay, and burnt match tips because ingestion of all of these has been reported with pica. Consumption of clay, dirt, or small stones is of particular concern because of possible contamination. It is important to discuss pica practices in a nonjudgmental way because some individuals may be embarrassed about this practice and not divulge it if feeling judged. In some cultures, pica is more common than in others, as outlined in Cultural Considerations Box: Pica. Pica is discussed in more detail in Chapter 13.

Laboratory tests to assess for iron deficiency can differentiate between low-iron stores and poor functional iron status. Iron deficiency occurs along a continuum and is often slow occurring unless acute blood loss is experienced. Iron deficiency and iron deficiency anemia are not interchangeable terms. Iron deficiency occurs in the early stage of mineral deficiency when iron intake and stores are insufficient, but no hematological changes have occurred in red blood cell morphology. When functional iron is limited, hemoglobin synthesis is compromised and iron deficiency anemia develops. Iron deficiency anemia alters red blood cell parameters, causing a smaller red blood cell, called microcytosis, and leads to a more severe magnitude of deficiency symptoms. Table 6-11 outlines laboratory tests used to assess for iron status in the adult.

Treatment for iron deficiency anemia generally involves iron supplementation as outlined in Wellness Concerns and Supplement Use. Hemoglobin values may begin to rise incrementally after several weeks of treatment, whereas reple-

Cultural Considerations

Pica

Pica is practiced around the world and has been for centuries with records of this practice found in ancient civilizations. The exact reason that pica occurs is not understood. In some cultures, the eating of nonfood substances is considered abnormal, whereas in others it is commonplace and may be especially linked to beliefs about fertility, childbirth, treatment of pregnancy symptoms, or femininity. In the United States pica is practiced more commonly among African American or Mexican American females than among whites. Those living in rural areas or have a family history of pica are also more likely to engage in pica. In some cultures, consuming clay is felt to help treat diarrhea. Baked clay is available for purchase in some ethnic food markets. Others consume starches to quell nausea from morning sickness and as a source of kcalories when food is scarce.

In pregnant females, an assessment of pica practices should occur with each prenatal visit, especially in females with anemia. A nonjudgmental approach is essential. Embarrassment is felt by many in association with practicing pica and perception of a judging attitude by the nurse could cause some individuals to withhold information about pica. Cultural reasons for pica should be explored so that they can be understood when formulating any needed intervention. Not all pica associated with iron deficiency disappears when the deficiency is treated. The client should be educated about any health concerns related to pica, such as the contamination of soil with lead or protozoa.

Sources: Corbett, Ryan, & Weinrich, 2003; Mills, 2007; Stokes, 2006.

tion of iron stores can take up to 6 months (Clark, 2008). Client Education Checklist: Iron outlines advice that the nurse can give about improving iron intake.

Toxicity

The UL for iron is 45 mg per day in healthy adults (IOM, 2001). This recommendation does not apply to individuals with iron deficiency because they may require additional intake under medical supervision. Symptoms of toxicity initially

Table 6-11 Laboratory Assessment of Iron Status in Adults

Laboratory	Iron Deficiency Value	Iron Compartment **
Hemoglobin	Less than 13 gm/dL males, less than 12 gm/dL females	Functional
Hematocrit	Less than 39.9% males, less than 35.7% females	Functional
Mean corpuscular volume	Less than 80 fL	Functional
Erythrocyte protoporphyrin	Greater than 70 mcg/dL erythrocyte or greater than 30 mcg/dL whole blood	Functional
Ferritin	Less than 15 mcg/ L	Storage
Total Iron-Binding Capacity (TIBC)	Greater than 400 mcg/dL	Storage
Transferrin saturation	Less than 16%	Storage

** Early detection of iron deficiency can be made by checking storage iron indices. Functional iron decreases later in the deficiency state.
Source: Centers for Disease Control and Prevention (CDC), 1998; Institute of Medicine (IOM), Food and Nutrition Board, 2001.

MyNursingKit National Digestive Diseases Information Clearinghouse: Hemochromatosis

CLIENT EDUCATION CHECKLIST — Iron

1. Assess the client's diet for iron intake. Include fortified foods and supplements.
2. Assess diet for inhibitors to iron absorption such as coffee, tea, calcium supplements.
3. Educate about the role of iron in health such as transporting oxygen to cells, importance during growth and development/pregnancy.
4. Customize advice given.
   a) Low intake
      • Heme iron sources—meat and poultry (especially organ meats), fish
      • Nonheme iron sources—legumes (beans, split peas, lentils), dried fruit, fortified grain products, blackstrap molasses, leafy greens
   b) Altered absorption
      • Avoid coffee and tea within 1 hour of iron intake.
   • Avoid calcium supplements at the same time as iron source.
   • Add vitamin C source to meals with iron such as fruits, vegetables, juice.
   • Cook acid foods with cast iron to contribute added iron.
5. Lifespan note:
   Babies require iron supplementation by age 4–6 months in formula, drops, or fortified cereal.
   Children under age 1 year should not drink cow or goat milk.
   Children consuming more than 24 oz milk/day often do so at the expense of iron intake.
   Pregnant females require 30 mg/day of iron and may require a supplement to achieve this intake.

include nausea and diarrhea. Excess storage of iron follows, with liver, kidney, and heart damage as a result (IOM, 2001). The severity of symptoms and damage is in proportion to the amount of excess iron that was ingested. Individuals with preexisting liver disease are more susceptible to adverse effects of excess iron intake (IOM, 2001).

Wellness Concerns and Supplement Use

Excess iron can be fatal to children. An accidental iron overdose is the most common cause of poisoning death among children in the United States (IOM, 2001). The nurse should advise clients taking iron supplements to keep the pill container tightly closed and away from a child's reach.

Hemochromatosis is a genetic disorder that causes increased iron storage. Organ damage can result from excess iron storage. Clients with hemochromatosis should not take iron supplements because this can accelerate the damage (NIH, 2007).

Individuals with iron deficiency anemia and those who are unable to consume adequate dietary iron may be advised to take iron supplements. Iron salts in the ferrous form are better absorbed than in the ferric form (NIH, 2007). Ferrous fumarate, gluconate, and sulfate are commonly the prescribed forms of iron supplements. The nurse should advise clients to read the supplement label for dosage of elemental iron when purchasing an over-the-counter iron supplement because this value varies depending on the formulation. Ferrous fumarate has a higher percentage of elemental iron at a given weight than do ferrous sulfate or gluconate (NIH, 2007). The potential for gastrointestinal side effects increases with increasing doses. Additionally, because the amount of iron absorbed decreases with increasing doses, it is advised that clients with iron deficiency anemia take iron supplements in divided doses. Box 6-3 outlines suggestions that the nurse can give for improving tolerance and absorbability of iron supplements.

Zinc

Zinc is responsible for a variety of functions because of its association with many enzymes in the body. Newer roles for zinc are being researched, but no consensus on a valid clinical measure of zinc status exists, making conclusions difficult to draw.

Function

Over 100 different enzymes in the body rely on zinc as a cofactor or coenzyme for catalytic reactions, enzyme structure, and regulation. Alcohol dehydrogenase and alkaline

BOX 6-3 — Nursing Interventions with Iron Supplementation

• Advise client of side effects of supplements: black stool, possible abdominal discomfort, nausea, diarrhea, or constipation.
• Divide supplement doses to two or three times a day to minimize side effects and improve absorption.
• Iron can be taken with a meal if side effects are present.
• Choose form of supplement to fit individual need. Fumarate form provides more elemental iron in a smaller-weight pill than sulfate or gluconate forms.
• Optimize iron absorption: Cook with cast iron pans, include vitamin C source with meals or supplement. Avoid tea or coffee 1 hour before or after supplement timing.
• Avoid mineral interactions: Separate timing of calcium supplements from iron supplements. "Calcium with your toothbrush and iron with a meal" is an easy way to help clients taking both types of supplements to remember this.
• Postmenopausal females and males should not take iron supplements unless prescribed.

phosphatase are two examples of zinc-related enzymes. Zinc is involved in DNA expression, cell growth, and differentiation. Zinc plays an important role in immune response via the development of T-lymphocytes, a component of the white blood cell for fighting infection (IOM, 2001; Ruz, 2006).

Zinc homeostasis is in part regulated by the gastrointestinal tract. Absorption of both dietary and endogenous sources of zinc occurs in the small intestine. Endogenous zinc is secreted into the intestinal tract in pancreatic enzymes, bile, and intestinal cell sloughing. This endogenous zinc secretion is conserved by reabsorption in the small intestine. Malabsorptive disorders, including chronic diarrhea, can reduce the conservation of endogenous zinc, upsetting zinc balance in the body. Small amounts of zinc are also lost daily in the urine, sweat, and with other body fluids (IOM, 2001).

Recommended Intake

The DRI for zinc is given as an RDA. The recommendation for adult females is 8 mg of zinc daily, whereas 11 mg daily is recommended for adult males (IOM, 2001). A small increase in zinc intake is recommended during pregnancy and lactation as outlined in Appendix C. Vegetarians may require up to 50% more zinc in the diet than nonvegetarians because of the limited bioavailability of zinc from many plant-based foods like whole grains, soy, and other beans (IOM, 2001). Despite the potential for reduced zinc absorption in this population, no separate recommendation for zinc intake exists for vegetarians.

Sources

Zinc is present in many foods. Oysters contain the highest zinc per serving compared with other foods (NIH, 2008b). Red meats, other seafood, wheat germ, wheat bran, and fortified breakfast cereals are sources of zinc. Zinc is better absorbed in the presence of protein. Zinc from animal protein sources is better absorbed than that from plant protein sources. Phytates present in whole grains and legumes, like soy and other beans, complex with zinc, rendering it poorly absorbed.

Deficiency

Poor zinc status can occur because of insufficient zinc intake or absorption, increased zinc losses, or a combination of the two. A rare inborn error of metabolism exists that alters zinc metabolism and leads to zinc deficiency if left untreated. Overt zinc deficiency is uncommon in the United States but is seen in developing nations where diet quality and medical conditions place individuals at risk (IOM, 2001). Decreased intake is the most common cause of zinc deficiency (Roberts, Martin-Clavijo, Winston, Dharmagunawardena, & Gach, 2007). Poor diet from food insecurity or limited intake can lead to marginal zinc status that is easily worsened with other precipitating factors. Diminished absorption of zinc can result from a high-fiber, or high-phytate diet. In developing countries where there is a high reliance on cereals in the diet, zinc is poorly absorbed because of this effect (Prasad, 2008). Interactions with other minerals, particularly iron, can lessen zinc absorption. Mineral interactions become clinically significant in the individual with existing marginal zinc status who then takes dietary supplements of the interacting mineral (IOM, 2001). Alcohol decreases zinc absorption and increases its excretion in the urine. It is estimated that 30% to 50% of chronic alcoholics have poor zinc status (IOM, 2001; Olivares, Pizarro, & Ruz, 2007). Malabsorptive conditions, such as inflammatory bowel disease, fat malabsorption, and short bowel syndrome, can lead to decreased zinc absorption and increased fecal losses of zinc. Chronic diarrhea puts an individual at risk for zinc deficiency because of losses of zinc from small bowel fluids; this zinc is normally reabsorbed. The nurse should consult with a registered dietitian when caring for a client with a chronic or large volume of small bowel fluid loss from diarrhea or an ostomy in order to get advice on zinc replacement therapy.

Symptoms of zinc deficiency vary with the magnitude of the deficit. Mild deficiency states can foster reduced growth velocity in children. Reduced appetite and diminished taste acuity can occur and has been reported as a contributing cause of these changes that can occur with aging (Stewart-Knox et al., 2005). Response to zinc supplementation is often used to judge whether a mild zinc deficiency exists because no reliable biochemical measurement exists to easily test zinc status in the clinical setting (IOM, 2001; Lowe, 2005; Roberts et al., 2007).

More severe zinc deficiency leads to additional symptoms. Growth retardation in children, alopecia, diarrhea, delayed sexual maturation with hypogonadism in boys, poor wound healing, and eye and skin lesions can be found (IOM, 2001; Fischer Walker, & Black, 2004). Skin changes initially include a scaly rash that becomes a bullous, pustular dermatitis, primarily at friction sites (Prasad, 2008; Roberts et al., 2007). The nurse should suspect zinc deficiency in a client with protein malnutrition in conjunction with undiagnosed skin changes (Roberts et al., 2007). Development of diarrhea because of the deficiency and its effect on decreased resistance to infection can lead to increased zinc losses, a vicious cycle that is difficult to correct with diet alone (Fischer Walker & Black, 2004). The term **acrodermatitis enteropathica** has been used to describe a congenital zinc deficiency caused by a recessive gene. Infants with this condition present with a scaly rash, alopecia, and failure to thrive (Roberts et al., 2007). Treatment is supplemental zinc in amounts equivalent to 2 mg/kg of body weight. Symptoms should diminish within 5 days (Roberts et al., 2007).

Plasma zinc is often used to estimate zinc status, but this is an insensitive measure of total body zinc. Deficiency symptoms have been reported while plasma zinc has remained within normal limits (IOM, 2001; Lowe, 2005).

Toxicity

The UL for zinc is 40 mg per day for all adults (IOM, 2001). Above this level of intake, absorption of copper can be compromised because the two minerals share some absorptive mechanisms (IOM, 2001). This effect is significant when copper status is marginal or excess zinc intake is chronic. Other symptoms of excess zinc include diminished immune response and lowered high-density lipoprotein (HDL cholesterol) (IOM, 2001). Gastrointestinal distress is a symptom of acute zinc toxicity, with vomiting occurring from single doses over 200 mg (IOM, 2001).

The UL recommendation for zinc does not apply to those with deficiency or those being treated for Wilson's disease, a disorder of copper metabolism. Increased zinc is prescribed to clients with Wilson's disease to deliberately decrease copper absorption and avoid excess copper storage (IOM, 2001).

Wellness Concerns and Supplement Use

Zinc has received attention for a possible role in treating the common cold. Laboratory experiments have shown decreased replication of several rhinoviruses that cause a cold when zinc is present in vitro. Results in humans have yielded mixed results using zinc lozenges, nasal gels, and sprays. Varying zinc preparations and cold virus strains contribute to the lack of consistent results; further research is needed before the nurse can draw conclusions about this treatment (Caruso, Prober, & Gwaltney, 2007; IOM, 2001).

When advising individuals in need of zinc supplementation, the nurse should warn that zinc supplements interact with iron and copper supplements and the antibiotics tetracycline and fluroquinolones. Separation of these medications by a 2-hour time span should be advised (MedlinePlus Health Information, 2008). Additionally, high-dose zinc supplements are associated with gastric bleeding, a factor that may become significant in those taking chronic supplements, such as for macular degeneration (MedlinePlus Health Information, 2008).

Selenium

Selenium is an antioxidant that works in concert with the antioxidant vitamin E. Soil content of selenium varies worldwide and leads to a wide range of selenium content in crops and animals fed local crops. Some areas of the United States, like Nebraska and the Dakotas, have high-selenium soil content and many of the coastal areas of the country have lower levels. China is known for its low-selenium soil content and resultant low-selenium status of its population (NIH, 2004).

Function

Selenium is bound with proteins as enzymes involved in prevention of oxidative damage to cells. This function of selenium has generated much investigation into a possible role for selenium in cancer prevention. Selenium also plays a role in maintenance of thyroid and immune function.

Recommended Intake

The RDA for selenium is 55 mcg for all adults (IOM, 2000). There is insufficient data to establish an RDA for selenium in infants, and an AI recommendation is instead extrapolated, as outlined in Appendix C.

Sources

Plants grown in soil with high-selenium content contain higher selenium than plants grown in selenium-poor soil. Beef, poultry, and seafood also contain selenium. Brazil nuts contain high-selenium content. In the United States, the mean selenium intake far exceeds the RDA for all ages (USDA, 2005).

Deficiency

Deficiency of selenium is unusual but has been reported in areas where soil content of the mineral is poor, such as China (Boosalis, 2008). Because of the role of selenium in thyroid health, a hypothyroid effect can result from selenium deficiency. Lack of adequate selenium may potentiate the negative effect of iodine deficiency on the thyroid (NIH, 2004). Selenium deficiency can make some individuals more prone to several rare diseases, such as Kashan's disease, Kashin-Beck disease, and a form of congenital hypothyroidism (Boosalis, 2008).

Toxicity

The UL for selenium is 400 mcg per day (IOM, 2000). Toxicity is rare and usually a result of industrial overexposure (NIH, 2004). Symptoms are labeled as **selenosis** and include hair loss, garlicky breath, fatigue, irritability, gastrointestinal complaints, and nerve damage (Boosalis, 2008; See, Lavercombe, Dillon, & Ginsberg, 2006). Death can result from liver necrosis, cerebral and pulmonary edema, and cardiac arrest (See et al., 2006).

Wellness Concerns and Supplement Use

Observational studies have associated a low blood selenium level with increased risk of certain types of cancers (Boosalis, 2008). Clinical studies thus far are inconclusive but are ongoing. A large-scale trial of selenium supplementation with vitamin E and prostate cancer risk will be completed in 2013 (Lippman et al., 2005). Accidental acute selenium poisoning and death has been reported in a male who took excessive selenium, hoping to lessen risk of prostate cancer based on reading unsubstantiated Internet-based information on the subject (See et al., 2006). The nurse should await the outcome of long-standing trials before considering the recommendation of selenium supplementation.

Copper

Knowledge about copper requirements is evolving. Only with the most recent DRI recommendations was an RDA established for dietary copper. Research on copper covers a wide range of health topics from bone health to heart disease.

MyNursingKit National Digestive Diseases Information Clearinghouse: Wilson's Disease

Function

Copper is a constituent of many catalytic enzymes involved in antioxidant reactions and metabolism (IOM, 2001). Copper is needed for the binding of iron to the transport protein transferrin and is important in collagen and connective tissue synthesis. Wound healing requires adequate copper because copper is an essential component of an enzyme used in the synthesis of collagen and elastin (Higdon, 2007).

Recommended Intake

The RDA for copper is 900 mcg per day for adolescents and all adults (IOM, 2001). Appendix C outlines copper recommendations for other populations.

Sources

Copper is widespread in the diet. Organ meats, such as liver, seafood, and nuts are good sources of copper. Grain products also contain copper and, unlike selenium, are unaffected by the copper in the soil in which it is grown (IOM, 2001). Fruits and vegetables generally are low in copper content. The mean intake of copper in the United States by adults exceeds the RDA (USDA, 2005).

Deficiency

Copper deficiency contributes to anemia and bone demineralization (IOM, 2001). Deficiency of this mineral alone is rare, but it is seen in conjunction with other nutritional problems, like overall malnutrition, excess zinc supplementation, or an exclusive diet of cow's milk in infants (Higdon, 2007; IOM, 2001). Menke's syndrome is a rare genetic defect of copper absorption, metabolism, and excretion that leads to copper deficiency with abnormal connective tissue, heart, and bone development in infants. A common symptom for copper deficiency is a microcytic anemia that is not responding to iron treatment (Higdon, 2007).

Toxicity

The UL for copper is 10,000 mcg or 10 mg per day (IOM, 2001). Copper toxicity is rare unless a result of Wilson's disease, an inborn error of copper metabolism that results in excess copper storage. Vomiting and diarrhea can occur with acute high intake of copper. Chronically high-copper intake or Wilson's disease leads to increased copper storage in the liver, brain, and eye (Brewer, 2008). The result, if left untreated, can be cirrhosis and liver failure. Wilson's disease is treated with anticopper medications, which include zinc because of the interaction between these two minerals (Brewer, 2008).

Fluoride

The requirement for fluoride exists across the lifespan despite earlier beliefs that it was necessary only for proper tooth formation. Approximately 99% of the body's fluoride is found in calcified tissue, such bone and teeth (IOM, 1997).

Function

Fluoride has a high affinity for calcium and thus aids in mineralization of bone and teeth (IOM, 1997). It can assist in the

Lifespan

Fluoride

Fluoride provided to children up to age 8 years to 12 years improves the mineralization of dental enamel in pre-eruptive teeth; later in life fluoride continues to provide benefit through topical inhibition of bacterial action in dental plaque (ADA, 2005; IOM, 1997; Morin, 2006). The overall effect is a reduction in risk of dental caries.

stimulation of new bone formation and lifelong resistance to dental caries (ADA, 2005; IOM, 1997). Lifespan Box: Fluoride outlines the role of fluoride in the mineralization of teeth.

Recommended Intake

The DRI for fluoride is given as an AI recommendation of 2 mg per day for adult females and 3 mg for adult males (IOM, 1997). Community water fortification with fluoride is recommended at a rate of 1 ppm (IOM, 1997).

Sources

The primary source of fluoride intake is drinking water and the beverages made with it (IOM, 1997). Small amounts of fluoride are found in most other foods. Dental products such as rinses, gels, and foams also supply fluoride. Fluoride is well absorbed from most sources unless it is consumed along with calcium, which decreases absorption by 10% to 25% (IOM, 1997).

Deficiency

Inadequate fluoride intake has been shown to increase the risk of dental caries compared with risk in those who consume adequate fluoride. With cross-transportation of beverages and foods among areas of varying drinking water fluoride, the prevalence of low intake of fluoride is less than in the past (IOM, 1997).

Toxicity

The UL for fluoride intake is 10 mg per day (IOM, 1997). Excess exposure to fluoride in children under age 12 years can lead to dental enamel **fluorosis** of permanent teeth (ADA, 2005). Enamel develops opaque horizontal striations in the early stages of fluorosis. With prolonged high intake, teeth become stained and pitted, though not at risk for increased caries (ADA, 2005). High-fluoride intake after all teeth have emerged is not considered a risk for fluorosis.

Skeletal fluorosis can develop with long-term overexposure to fluoride. Calcification of ligaments and vertebra can result (IOM, 1997).

Wellness Concerns and Supplement Use

Routine fluoride supplementation for children is not recommended as it has been in the past. Supplemental fluoride in community drinking water at recommended levels results in adequate fluoride intake for most individuals. The CDC recommends fluoride supplementation only for children living in areas without fluoridated water if they are considered at high risk for caries (CDC, 2001). The nurse should advise clients using well water for drinking to have it tested for fluoride content before considering fluoride supplements (ADA, 2005). Exclusive use of bottled or filtered water may not provide adequate fluoride and overall intake should be assessed under these circumstances (Morin, 2006). Additionally, children under age 6 years should be supervised while brushing teeth and warned against chronic swallowing of fluoridated toothpaste, which can lead to enamel fluorosis. Only a pea-size amount of toothpaste should be given to young children while brushing teeth (ADA, 2005).

Chromium

Chromium naturally exists in foods in small amounts in its trivalent form (Cr 3+). This form of the mineral should not be confused with the hexavalent form (Cr 6+), a known toxin found in industrial pollution.

Function

Chromium acts as a cofactor in the action of insulin in the body, maintaining blood glucose homeostasis. It is not fully understood how chromium acts in this regard. Chromium also seems to function in the metabolism of proteins and fats, but this too is poorly understood (NIH, 2005b).

Recommended Intake

The DRI recommendation for chromium is made as an AI recommendation. In adult males up to age 50 years, 35 mcg per day is recommended, whereas females of the same age are advised to consume 25 mcg daily (IOM, 2001). It is recommended that adults over age 50 years decrease intake of chromium by 5 mcg per day from the baseline recommendation. This is a minute amount and too difficult to track for most any individual.

Sources

No database exists with information on chromium content of foods. Chromium can be gained or lost during food processing and is poorly absorbed from the diet (IOM, 2001). Meats, poultry, and fish contain approximately 1 to 2 mcg per serving, whereas diary foods are a poor source of chromium (IOM, 2001). Red wine and some beers are high in chromium.

Deficiency

Chromium deficiency is reported to cause glucose intolerance (Balk, Tatsioni, Lichtenstein, Lau, & Pittas, 2007). It is difficult to measure chromium status because no biochemical marker is known that represents body stores (Drake, 2007a). Some researchers use toenail chromium content, but this is not universally utilized nor is it routinely available in the clinical setting.

Toxicity

No UL recommendation exists for chromium (IOM, 2001). A potential for toxicity has been outlined for individuals with preexisting renal or liver failure who take chromium supplementation (Drake, 2007a; IOM, 2001). These individuals should limit intake of supplemental chromium.

Wellness Concerns and Supplement Use

Research into the use of chromium supplementation in the population with diabetes to improve glucose tolerance has received considerable attention. Results have been variable and inconsistent (Drake, 2007a). The American Diabetes Association does not recommend chromium supplementation for persons with diabetes unless chromium deficiency is known (American Diabetes Association, 2008). Likewise, research into possible benefits to improve blood lipid profiles with chromium supplementation have been inconclusive (Balk et al., 2007). More research is needed to provide the clinician with better assessment measurements of chromium status and improved information on chromium content of foods before future clinical trials on chromium supplementation can yield meaningful results.

Chromium picolinate is a supplemental form of chromium that is better absorbed than other types of chromium supplements. It is marketed to athletes and those wishing to lose weight, but the evidence of any benefit is lacking.

Chromium supplements can interfere with the effectiveness of certain medications, such as beta blockers, niacin in the form of nicotinic acid used to treat high blood lipids, and nonsteroidal anti-inflammatory drugs (NIH, 2005b). Additionally, medications that alter gastric pH, such as antacids and proton-pump inhibitors, impair chromium absorption or increase its excretion (NIH, 2005b). The nurse should carefully evaluate medication and dietary supplement use to assess for these interactions.

Iodine

Poor iodine status was more common in the United States in the past when iodine in some soil and availability of seafood were limited to large parts of the population. It remains a problem in some parts of Europe, Africa, and Asia.

Function

Iodine comprises the majority of the weight of two thyroid hormones, thyroxine (T_4) and triiodothyronine (T_3) (IOM, 2001). These two hormones are responsible for regulation of temperature, metabolic rate, and enzyme action in the body.

Recommended Intake

The RDA for iodine is 150 mcg per day for adults (IOM, 2001). The median intake of iodine in the United States exceeds this recommendation (IOM, 2001).

Sources

Iodine content of food varies depending on the soil where plants are grown or the feed given to animals. Seafood is a good source of dietary iodine. In the United States table salt is available fortified with iodine because the mineral is lost in the normal processing of sea salt.

Deficiency

Iodine deficiency is a common cause of preventable brain damage (Drake, 2007b). Insufficient iodine alters the production of

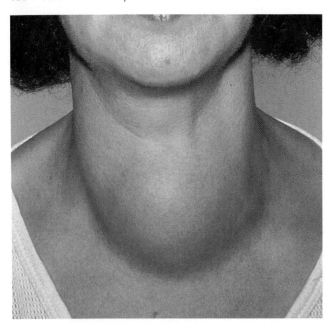

■ FIGURE 6-6 **Goiter.**
Source: Custom Medical Stock Photo, Inc.

thyroid hormones, leading to lethargy and weight gain. Iodine deficiency during pregnancy results in congenital hypothyroidism in the fetus, a condition characterized by mental retardation, and short stature (Drake, 2007b; IOM, 2001). Prolonged iodine deficiency causes the thyroid gland to become enlarged as it compensates for lack of iodine. An enlarged thyroid gland is called **goiter.** Figure 6-6 ■ illustrates the physical finding of goiter in an individual with iodine deficiency. Once treated with iodine, goiter may resolve or it can remain (IOM, 2001).

Toxicity
The UL for iodine is 1,100 mcg (or 1.1 mg) per day (IOM, 2001). Iodine toxicity is rare but can occur in those with thyroid autoimmune disease (Drake, 2007b; IOM, 2001). Goiter develops with iodine toxicity as it does for iodine deficiency, and thyroid-stimulating hormone (TSH) becomes elevated with resultant hypothyroid function (IOM, 2001).

Wellness Concerns and Supplement Use
Certain medications and foods contain significant iodine. The nurse should be aware that the medication amiodarone, used in cardiac arrhythmia management, contrast dye, food coloring, and water purification tablets are examples (IOM, 2001). Individuals with thyroid autoimmune disease may have sensitivity to increased iodine intake from these sources, whereas other individuals will experience no adverse effects.

Manganese and Molybdenum
Manganese is involved in the formation of bone and a constituent in the metabolism of carbohydrate, protein, and fat. The DRI for manganese is an AI of 2.3 mg per day for males and 1.8 mg per day for females (IOM, 2001). Manganese is poorly absorbed from food. Deficiency of manganese is not clearly associated with a low manganese diet. Symptoms of deficiency include impaired growth, reproductive function, and glucose tolerance and a low blood cholesterol (IOM, 2001). The UL for manganese is 11.0 mg per day for adults. Because manganese is excreted in bile, risk of toxicity is greatest in conditions that result in decreased excretion of bile, such as in neonates and with liver disease (IOM, 2001). Occupational exposure to manganese dust and disorders of bile secretion have been reported to lead to symptoms that mimic Parkinson's disease (IOM, 2001). An elevated blood manganese level is found with toxicity.

Molybdenum is a cofactor in the catabolism of sulfur-containing amino acids, purines, and pyridines (IOM, 2001). The RDA for molybdenum is 45 mcg per day for adults (IOM, 2001). Mean intake in the United States for adults exceeds this recommendation; thus a deficiency state is unusual except in cases of an inborn error of metabolism that results in neurological damage (IOM, 2001). Molybdenum is found in legumes, grains, and nuts and little is known of its bioavailability. The UL is 2 mg per day for adults (IOM, 2001). Little data are available on toxicity in humans, though impaired growth and skeletal abnormalities have been reported in animals (IOM, 2001).

Nonessential Trace Minerals
Arsenic, boron, nickel, silicon, and vanadium are trace minerals found in the body for which no recommendations exist for daily intake. No clear metabolic role has been established in humans, nor are there known consequences of deficiency.

Arsenic has a suggested role in metabolism and gene expression. It is found in dairy foods, meat, poultry, and fish. No UL has been established for organic arsenic found in foods. Inorganic arsenic is a known human poison at doses over 1 mg/kg/day (IOM, 2001). Case reports of arsenic toxicity from dietary kelp supplements have been noted because of contamination (Amster, Tiwary, & Schenker, 2007). Symptoms of toxicity include gastrointestinal symptoms, anemia, and toxicity to the liver (IOM, 2001). Chronic toxicity at lower doses can cause a change in skin pigmentation and neurological and gangrene-like symptoms (IOM, 2001). The nurse should look for skin changes associated with chronic toxicity, such as eczema, alopecia, altered skin pigmentation, and brittle nails with white lines (Amster et al., 2007).

Boron has been the topic of much research, yet no clear role has been established for the mineral. Abnormal bone mineralization has been reported in animals with boron deficiency, suggesting a role in bone health (IOM, 2001). Boron is found in fruits, tuberous vegetables, and legumes. The UL for boron is 20 mg per day. Symptoms of excess boron include skin flushing, convulsions, and depression and reduced fertility in animals (IOM, 2001).

Nickel is felt to be a cofactor in the function of several enzymes. It is found in grains and legumes. No adverse effects have been reported for nickel from naturally occurring food sources (IOM, 2001). Adverse effects have been reported for soluble nickel salts and in individuals with oral nickel sensitivity (IOM, 2001). The UL is 1 mg per day (IOM, 2001). Gastrointestinal symptoms and shortness of breath can occur with excess intake. Nickel sensitivity causes contact dermatitis-like symptoms.

Silicon seems to play a role in the formation of collagen and bone (IOM, 2001). No adverse effects have been reported with high levels of silicon intake from food or water.

Vanadium seems to mimic insulin and is involved in cell proliferation and division (IOM, 2001). It is poorly absorbed from foods and present in varied sources such as mushrooms, shellfish, beer, wine, black pepper, and dill (IOM, 2001). The UL for vanadium is 1.8 mg per day for adults (IOM, 2001). Insufficient data exist to establish a UL for other populations. Toxicity from food sources is highly unlikely. Excess intake can cause mild gastrointestinal effects, renal toxicity, and anemia. Green tongue and fatigue have also been reported (IOM, 2001).

NURSING CARE PLAN   Iron and a Vegan Diet in Children

CASE STUDY

Laura and Matt have been vegans since adolescence. Now in their late 20s, they are determined that they will raise their 3-year-old daughter, Emily, as a vegan. Laura has recently returned to work as a bank teller and Emily is enrolled in day care. Laura packs a lunch for Emily every morning and puts it in a lunch box that Emily picked out. Emily has always been a "picky" eater and now her lunch is coming back home with little having been eaten. Emily has been even fussier at meals, refusing to eat what is prepared and begging for "good" cookies for a snack. Laura and Matt have met with the day care staff and learned that Emily refuses to eat most of her own lunch and frequently asks the other children to share with her. She plays well with the other children but gets to be a pest at mealtime, so other children will often give her an extra cookie or sweet. They also make fun of the "funny food" that Emily brings. The staff suggests they find a few things Emily likes to eat and send those for her lunch. It is time for a regular checkup so Laura and Matt decide to ask the nurse for suggestions about maintaining their dietary decisions and how to meet the needs for a good diet for Emily.

Applying the Nursing Process

ASSESSMENT

Emily weighs 27 pounds, is 36 inches tall (BMI: 14.6), and her weight-for-stature percentile is 5. She sits quietly on her mother's lap and is holding a stuffed bear as she watches her parents and the nurse. She is well groomed and has bright eyes and smooth skin. She responds to the nurse with a soft voice and says she has to eat "icky" food at school. She says she has a friend named Charley at her school and likes to chase him. Her hemoglobin is 7.9 g/dL and her hematocrit is 27%. Laura and Matt are articulate and explain that they want what is best for Emily but that a vegan diet is something they practice for moral reasons. They also state that they are frustrated with a day care provider who does not seem to uphold their dietary wishes.

DIAGNOSES

Imbalanced nutrition: Less than body requirements related to diminished oral intake, including overall calories and iron

Deficient knowledge related to lack of information about adequate dietary needs for a toddler

Readiness for enhanced knowledge related to questions about supplying adequate dietary nutrients

Potential for impaired parenting related to frustrations dealing with toddler eating habits

EXPECTED OUTCOMES

Emily will gain 1 pound in 2 months

Parents will confer with a dietitian about increasing the variety and acceptability of vegan foods for a toddler, including good sources of dietary iron and vitamin C to enhance iron absorption

Parents will continue to interact with day care staff to develop plans for supporting the family dietary wishes

Parents will acquire information about toddler growth and development patterns and eating habits via a parenting class or reading

PLANNING

Keep a food diary for Emily

List foods frequently included in Emily's lunch

Identify parenting classes at a local social service agency

Supply a list of books about parenting toddlers

Refer to a dietitian who will work closely with the family to plan menus that will meet their needs

Develop a plan for meeting with day care staff and sharing information about vegan diets

EVALUATION

Emily has gained half a pound in 2 months. The parents met weekly for a total of four visits with a dietitian who was supportive of their dietary habits. The dietitian elaborated on the information that Matt and Laura learned in a parenting book about toddler eating habits and "food

(continued)

Iron and a Vegan Diet in Children *(continued)*

NURSING CARE PLAN

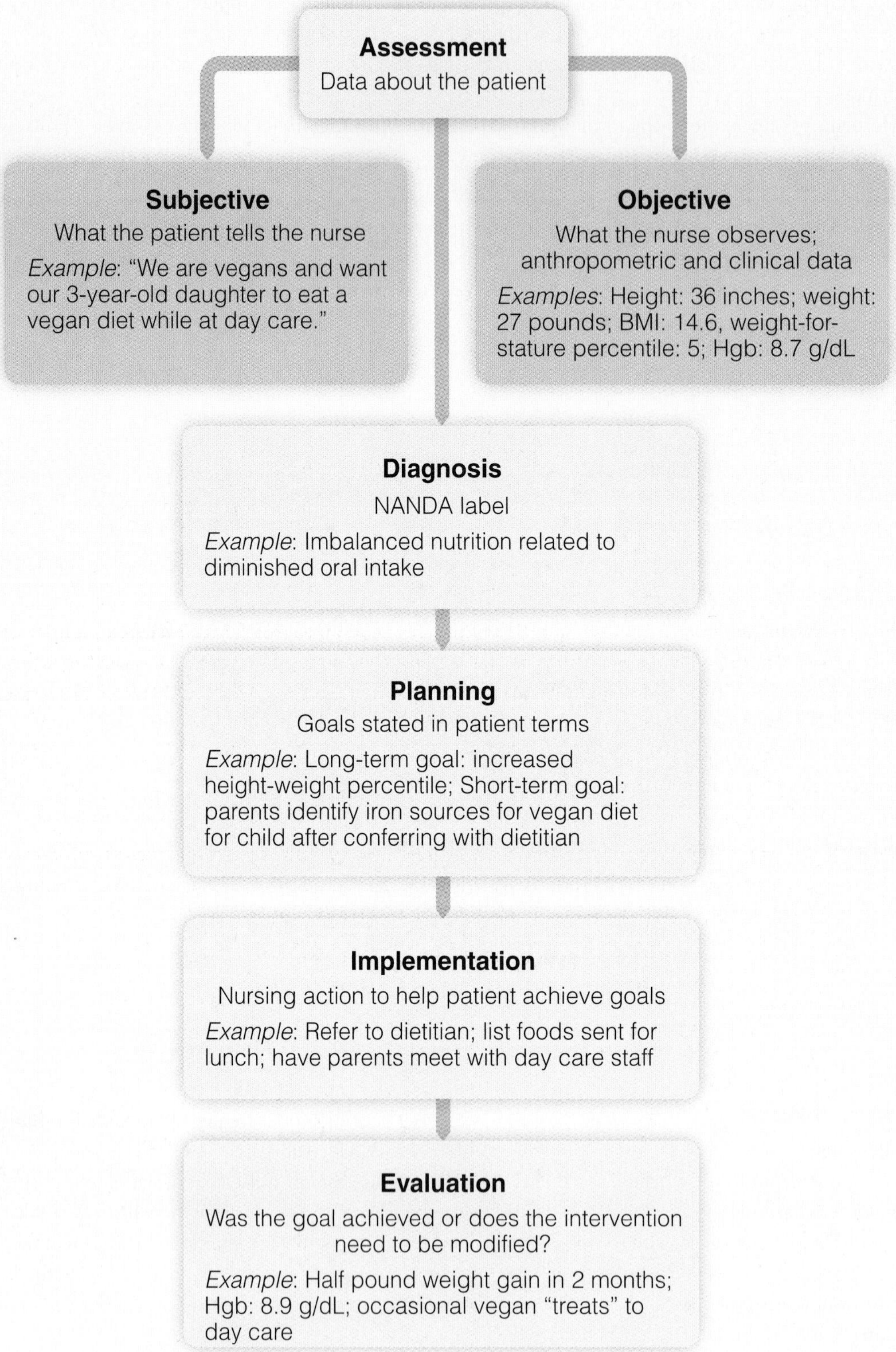

Assessment
Data about the patient

Subjective
What the patient tells the nurse

Example: "We are vegans and want our 3-year-old daughter to eat a vegan diet while at day care."

Objective
What the nurse observes; anthropometric and clinical data

Examples: Height: 36 inches; weight: 27 pounds; BMI: 14.6, weight-for-stature percentile: 5; Hgb: 8.7 g/dL

Diagnosis
NANDA label

Example: Imbalanced nutrition related to diminished oral intake

Planning
Goals stated in patient terms

Example: Long-term goal: increased height-weight percentile; Short-term goal: parents identify iron sources for vegan diet for child after conferring with dietitian

Implementation
Nursing action to help patient achieve goals

Example: Refer to dietitian; list foods sent for lunch; have parents meet with day care staff

Evaluation
Was the goal achieved or does the intervention need to be modified?

Example: Half pound weight gain in 2 months; Hgb: 8.9 g/dL; occasional vegan "treats" to day care

■ FIGURE 6-7 **Nursing Care Plan Process: Iron and a Vegan Diet in Children.**

Iron and a Vegan Diet in Children *(continued)*

NURSING CARE PLAN

jags." They met with the day care staff and discussed the importance of their dietary needs. Laura prepared treats for Emily to take to day care to share with the other children. They decided to send small quantities of simple foods in Emily's lunch that looked appealing. They stated that they were no longer as worried about Emily's food preferences because they understand that toddlers can be fussy eaters and will outgrow that if the parents continue to serve appropriate foods. Emily's hemoglobin is now 8.9 g/dL and it will be monitored every 2 months. Figure 6-7 ■ outlines the nursing process for this case.

Critical Thinking in the Nursing Process

1. Hemoglobin is the iron-carrying factor in the blood. What are some iron-rich foods that the nurse can suggest to vegan families?

2. What signs and symptoms of iron deficiency in children should the nurse share with parents who are vegans?

CHAPTER SUMMARY

- Minerals serve many general functions within the body, providing structure in the form of bones, teeth, and soft tissue; exerting osmotic pressure to maintain fluid balance; assisting in acid–base balance of fluids; serving as cofactors and coenzymes for metabolic and hormonal reactions; and playing a role in crucial nerve transmission and muscle contraction, including the heart.

- Minerals that are part of structural components can be drawn on as a reserve when the mineral is needed for more urgent functions.

- Poor mineral status can occur with insufficient intake to meet needs, mineral interactions, lowered mineral bioavailability, and increased mineral excretion, or any combination of these factors.

- Exceeding the RDA for mineral intake can lead to excessive mineral storage and negative health effects. Clients

are advised to not exceed the recommended levels of mineral intake unless specifically directed by a primary health care provider.

- Mineral balance in the blood is carefully orchestrated. In healthy individuals, the body is able to fine-tune absorption or excretion rates as needed to maintain blood levels of minerals.

- Some chronic diseases and conditions are associated with mineral status. Osteoporosis is linked with poor calcium status. Blood pressure control can be improved with a diet that is low in sodium and contains good sources of potassium from food. Premenstrual syndrome symptoms improve with adequate intake of calcium.

PEARSON

EXPLORE **mynursingkit**™

MyNursingKit is your one stop for online chapter review materials and resources. Prepare for success with additional NCLEX®-style practice questions, interactive assignments and activities, web links, animations and videos, and more!

Register your access code from the front of your book at
www.mynursingkit.com.

NCLEX® QUESTIONS

1. The nurse determines that teaching has been effective when a client who needs to be on a sodium-restricted diet states that which of the following foods should be avoided?
   1. Whole milk
   2. Sirloin steak
   3. Salami
   4. Poached egg

2. The nurse is discussing the importance of fluoride in dental health of children with a client. The nurse would want to be sure to state which of the following?
   1. Fluoride should be taken with calcium to ensure strong teeth.
   2. Minute amounts of fluoride are added to most public water supplies to prevent dental caries.
   3. Children who have adequate fluoride will not need to worry about dental caries as an adult.
   4. Fluoride supplements will prevent dental problems.

3. The nurse determines that a client has an adequate understanding of potassium restrictions when the client makes the following selection from a lunch menu.
   1. Fruit salad with blueberries, strawberries, and cantaloupe
   2. Baked potato with broccoli and melted cheese
   3. Cottage cheese on a pear half
   4. Vanilla milk shake

4. A client has started taking a daily iron supplement. The nurse suggests that the client take the supplement with which of the following foods to increase the absorption of the iron?
   1. Leafy green vegetables
   2. Milk
   3. Whole wheat bread
   4. Orange juice

5. A middle-age female client tells the nurse that she feels an increasing desire to consume ice chips, now amounting to at least 6 cups a day. The nurse will want to assess the client for which of the following conditions?
   1. Sodium deficiency
   2. Dehydration
   3. Iron deficiency
   4. Potassium excess

REFERENCES

American Beverage Association. (2005). *What America drinks: Our favorite beverages.* Retrieved March 31, 2007, from http://www.ameribev.org/all-about-beverage-products-manufacturing-marketing-consumption/what-america-drinks/index.aspx

American College of Obstetricians and Gynecologists (ACOG). (2008). Anemia in pregnancy. *Obstetrics and Gynecology, 112,* 201–207.

American Diabetes Association. (2008). Nutrition recommendations and interventions for diabetes. *Diabetes Care, 31,* S61–S78.

American Dietetic Association (ADA). (2005). Position of the American Dietetic Association: The impact of fluoride on health. *Journal of the American Dietetic Association, 105,* 1620–1628.

American Dietetic Association (ADA). (2008). Position of the American Dietetic Association: Nutrition and lifestyle for a healthy pregnancy outcome. *Journal of the American Dietetic Association, 108,* 553–561.

American Dietetic Association (ADA) and Dietitians of Canada. (2004). Position of the American Dietetic Association and

Dietitians of Canada: Nutrition and women's health. *Journal of the American Dietetic Association, 104,* 984–1001.

Amster, E., Tiwary, A., & Schenker, M. B. (2007). Case report: Potential arsenic toxicosis secondary to herbal kelp supplement. *Environmental Health Perspectives, 115,* 606–608.

Arnaud, M. J. (2008). Update on the assessment of magnesium status. *British Journal of Nutrition, 99,* S24–S36.

Balk, E. M., Tatsioni, A., Lichtenstein, A. H., Lau, J., & Pittas, A. G. (2007). Effect of chromium supplementation on glucose metabolism and lipids. *Diabetes Care, 30,* 2154–2163.

Boosalis, M. G. (2008). The role of selenium in chronic disease. *Nutrition in Clinical Practice, 23,* 152–160.

Bray, G. A., Vollmer, W. M., Sacks, F. M., Obarzanek, E., Svetkey, L. P., Appel, L. J. et al. (2004). A further subgroup analysis of the effects of the DASH diet and three dietary sodium levels on blood pressure: Results of the DASH-Sodium Trial. *American Journal of Cardiology, 94,* 222–227.

Brewer, G. J. (2008). The risks of free copper in the body and the development of useful anti-copper drugs. *Current Opinion in Clinical Nutrition and Metabolic Care, 11,* 727–732.

Caruso, T. J., Prober, C. G., & Gwaltney J. M. (2007). Treatment of naturally acquired common colds with zinc: A structured review. *Clinical Infectious Disease, 45,* 569–574.

Centers for Disease Control and Prevention (CDC). (1998). Recommendations to prevent and control iron deficiency in the United States. *Morbidity and Mortality Weekly Report, 47,* 1–36.

Centers for Disease Control and Prevention (CDC). (2001). Recommendations for using fluoride to prevent and control dental caries in the United States. *Morbidity and Mortality Weekly Report Recommendation Report, 50,* 1–42.

Clark, S. F. (2008). Iron deficiency anemia. *Nutrition in Clinical Practice, 23,* 128–141.

Corbett, R. W., Ryan, C., & Weinrich, S. P. (2003). Pica in pregnancy: Does it affect outcomes? *American Journal of Maternal Child Nursing, 28,* 183–189.

REFERENCES   *(continued)*

Cotton, P. A., Subar, A. F., Friday, J. E., & Cook, A. (2004). Dietary sources of nutrients among US adults, 1994 to 1996. *Journal of the American Dietetic Association, 104,* 921–930.

Drake, W. (2007a). *Chromium.* Retrieved December 23, 2008, from http://lpi.oregonstate.edu/infocenter/minerals/chromium/

Drake, W. (2007b). *Iodine.* Retrieved December 23, 2008, from http://lpi.oregonstate.edu/infocenter/minerals/iodine/

Fischer Walker, C., & Black, R. E. (2004). Zinc and the risk for infectious disease. *Annual Review of Nutrition, 24,* 255–275.

Forshee, R. A., & Storey, M. L. (2003). Total beverage consumption and beverages choices among children and adolescents. *International Journal of Food Sciences & Nutrition, 54*(4), 297–307.

Friedman, E. A. (2005). Consequences and management of hyperphosphatemia in patients with renal insufficiency. *Kidney International, 67,* S1–S7.

Geleijnse, J. M., Kok, F. J., & Grobbee, D. E. (2003). Blood pressure response to changes in sodium and potassium intake: A metaregression analysis of randomised trials. *Journal of Human Hypertension, 17,* 471–480.

Grimble. R. F. (2006). The effects of sulfur amino acid intake on immune function in humans. *Journal of Nutrition, 136,* 1660S–1665S.

Harrington, M. (2003). High salt intake appears to increase bone resorption in postmenopausal women, but high potassium intake ameliorates this adverse effect. *Nutrition Reviews, 61,* 179–183.

Heaney, R. P. (2008). Vitamin D and calcium interactions: Functional outcomes. *American Journal of Clinical Nutrition, 88,* 541S–544S.

Heaney, R. P., & Rafferty, K. (2001). Carbonated beverages and urinary calcium excretion. *American Journal of Clinical Nutrition, 74,* 343–347.

Heaney, R. P., Rafferty, K., & Bierman, J. (2005). Not all calcium-fortified beverages are equal. *Nutrition Today, 40,* 39–44.

Heaney, R. P., Rafferty, K., Dowell, S., & Bierman, J. (2005). Calcium fortification systems differ in bioavailability. *Journal of the American Dietetic Association, 105,* 807–809.

Higdon, J. (2007). *Copper.* Retrieved December 23, 2008, from http://lpi.oregonstate.edu/infocenter/minerals/copper/

Institute of Medicine (IOM), Food and Nutrition Board. (1997). Dietary reference intakes for calcium, phosphorus, magnesium, vitamin D and fluoride. Washington, DC: National Academies Press.

Institute of Medicine (IOM). Food and Nutrition Board (2000). *Dietary reference intakes for vitamin C, vitamin E, selenium, and carotenoids.* Washington, DC: National Academies Press.

Institute of Medicine (IOM), Food and Nutrition Board. (2001). Dietary reference intakes for vitamin A, vitamin K, arsenic, boron, chromium, copper, iodine, iron, manganese, molybdenum, nickel, silicon, vanadium and zinc. Washington, DC: National Academies Press.

Institute of Medicine (IOM), Food and Nutrition Board. (2004). *Dietary reference intakes for water, potassium, sodium, chloride, and sulfate.* Washington, DC: National Academies Press.

Jackson, R. D., LaCroix, A. Z., Gass, M., Wallace, R. B., Robbins, J., Lewis, C. E., et al. (2006). Calcium plus vitamin D supplementation and the risk of fractures. *New England Journal of Medicine, 354,* 669–683.

Kazal, L. A. (2002). Prevention of iron deficiency anemia in infants and toddlers. *American Family Physician, 66,* 1217–1224.

Keller, J. I., Lanou, A. J., & Barnard, N. D. (2002). The consumer cost of calcium form food and supplements. *Journal of the American Dietetic Association, 102,* 1669–1671.

Kormarnisky, L. A., Christopherson, R. J., & Basu, T. K. (2003). Sulfur: Its clinical and toxicologic aspects. *Nutrition, 19,* 54–61.

Lanou, A. J., & Barnard, N. D. (2008). Dairy and weight loss hypothesis: An evaluation of the clinical trials. *Nutrition Reviews, 66,* 272–279.

Larsson, X., & Wolk, X. (2007). Magnesium intake and risk of type 2 diabetes: A meta-analysis. *Journal of Internal Medicine, 262,* 208–214.

Leeman, L., & Fontaine, P. (2008). Hypertensive disorders of pregnancy. *American Family Physician, 78,* 93–100.

Lippman, S. M., Goodman, P. J., Klein, E. A., Parnes, H. L., Thompson, I. M., Kristal, A. R., et al. (2005). Designing the selenium and vitamin E cancer prevention trial SELECT. *Journal of the National Cancer Institute, 97,* 94–100.

Lowe, N. M. (2005). In search of a reliable marker of zinc status—are we nearly there yet? *Nutrition, 21,* 883–884.

Ma, D., & Jones, G. (2004). Soft drink and mild consumption, physical activity, bone mass, and upper limb fractures in children: A population-based case-control study. *Calcified Tissue International, 75*(4), 286–291.

Mattes, R. D. (1997). The taste for salt in humans. *American Journal of Clinical Nutrition, 65,* 692S–697S.

McGartland, C., Robson, P. J., Murray, L., Cran, G., Savage, M. J., Watkins, D., et al. (2003). Carbonated soft drink consumption and bone mineral density in adolescence: The Northern Ireland Young Hearts project. *Journal of Bone and Mineral Research, 18*(9), 1563–1569.

McKeown, N. M., Jacques, P. F. Zhang, X., Juan, W., & Sahyoun, N. R. (2008). Dietary magnesium intake is related to metabolic syndrome in older Americans. *European Journal of Nutrition, 47,* 210–216.

MedlinePlus Health Information. (2008). *Medline Plus herbs and supplements: Zinc.* Retrieved December 20, 2008, from http://www.nlm.nih.gov/medlineplus/druginfo/natural/client-zinc.html

Mills, M. E. (2007). Craving more than food: The implications of pica in pregnancy. *Nursing for Women's Health, 11,* 266–273.

Moe, S. M. (2008). Disorders involving calcium, phosphorus, and magnesium. *Primary Care: Clinics in Office Practice, 35,* 215–237.

Morin, K. (2006). Fluoride: Action and use. *Maternal Child Nursing, 31,* 127.

National Institutes of Health, National Institute on Aging. (2008). *Postmenopausal health concerns.* Retrieved March 25, 2009, from http://www.nia.nih.gov/NR/rdonlyres/638AB293-EC0D-4F02-9947-F9F851612595/9533/04_bone.jpg

National Institutes of Health, Office of Dietary Supplements. (2004). *Selenium.* Retrieved December 20, 2008, from http://ods.od.nih.gov/factsheets/selenium.asp

National Institutes of Health, Office of Dietary Supplements. (2005). *Magnesium.* Retrieved December 20, 2008, from http://ods.od.nih.gov/factsheets/magnesium.asp

National Institutes of Health (NIH), Office of Dietary Supplements. (2005b). *Chromium.* Retrieved June 15, 2009, from http://ods.od.nih.gov/factsheets/chromium.asp

National Institutes of Health, Office of Dietary Supplements. (2007). *Iron.* Retrieved December 20, 2008, from http://ods.od.nih.gov/factsheets/iron.asp

National Institutes of Health, Office of Dietary Supplements. (2008a). *Calcium.* Retrieved December 20, 2008 from http://ods.od.nih.gov/factsheets/calcium.asp

National Institutes of Health, Office of Dietary Supplements. (2008b). *Zinc.* Retrieved December 20, 2008, from http://dietary-supplements.info.nih.gov/FactSheets/Zinc.asp

National Osteoporosis Foundation. (2008). *Clinician's guide to the prevention and treatment of osteoporosis.* Retrieved December 19, 2008, from http://nof.org/professionals/NOF_Clinicians_Guide.pdf

Nelson, M., & Poulter, J. (2004). Impact of tea drinking on iron status in the U.K.: A review. *Journal of Human Nutrition and Dietetics, 17,* 43–54.

REFERENCES *(continued)*

Olivares, M., Pizarro, M. T., & Ruz, M. (2007). New insights about iron bioavailability inhibition by zinc. *Nutrition, 23,* 292–295.

Prasad, A. S. (2008). Zinc in human health: Effect of zinc on immune cells. *Molecular Medicine, 14,* 353–357.

Roberts, C. M. L., Martin-Clavijo, A., Winston, A. P., Dharmagunawardena, B., & Gach, J. E. (2007). Malnutrition and rash: Think zinc. *Clinical Dermatology, 32,* 654–657.

Roth, E. (2007). Immune and cell modulation by amino acids. *Clinical Nutrition, 26,* 535–544.

Ruz, M. (2006). Zinc supplementation and growth. *Current Opinion in Clinical Nutrition and Metabolic Care, 9,* 757–762.

See, K. A., Lavercombe, P. S., Dillon, J., & Ginsberg, R. (2006). Accidental death from acute selenium poisoning. *Medical Journal of Australia, 185,* 388–389.

Shinaberger, C. S., Greenland, S., Kopple, J. D., Van Wyck, D., Mehrotra, R., Kovesdy, C. P., et al. (2008). Is controlling phosphorus by decreasing dietary protein intake beneficial or harmful in persons with chronic kidney disease? *Amercian Journal of Clinical Nutrition, 88,* 1511–1518.

Stewart-Knox, B. J., Simpson, E. E. A., Parr, H., Rae, G., Polito, A., Intorre, F., et al. (2005). Zinc status and taste acuity in older Europeans: The ZENITH study. *European Journal of Clinical Nutrition, 59,* S31–S36.

Stokes, T. (2006). The earth-eaters. *Nature, 444,* 543–544.

Straub, D. A. (2007). Calcium supplementation in clinical practice: A review of forms, doses, and indications. *Nutrition in Clinical Practice, 22,* 286–296.

Thankachan, P., Walczyk, T., Muthayya, S., Kurpad, A. V., & Hurrell, R. F. (2008). Iron absorption in young Indian women: The interaction of iron status with the influence of tea and ascorbic acid. *American Journal of Clinical Nutrition, 87,* 881–886.

Thys-Jacobs, S., McMahon, D., & Bilezikian, J. P. (2007). Cyclical changes in calcium metabolism across the menstrual cycle in women with premenstrual dysphoric disorder. *Journal of Clinical Endocrinology and Metabolism, 92,* 2952–2959.

Tuck, S. P., & Datta, H. K. (2007). Osteoporosis in the aging male: Treatment options. *Clinical Interventions in Aging, 2,* 521–536.

Tucker, K. L., Morita, K., Qiano, N., Hannan, M. T., Cupples, L. A., & Kiel, D. P. (2006). Colas, but not other carbonated beverages, are associated with low bone mineral density in older women: The Framingham Osteoporosis Study. *American Journal of Clinical Nutrition, 84*(4), 936–942.

United States Department of Agriculture (USDA). (2005). *What we eat in America, NHANES, 2001–2002: Usual nutrient intakes from food compared with DRIs.* Retrieved December 19, 2008, from http://www.ars.usda.gov/SP2UserFiles/Place/12355000/pdf/usualintaketables2001-02.pdf

Vollmer, W. M., Sacks, F. M., Ard, J., Appel, L., Bray, G. A., Simons-Morton, D. G., et al. (2001). Effects of diet and sodium intake on blood pressure: Subgroup analysis of the DASH sodium trial. *Annals of Internal Medicine, 135,* 1019–1028.

Weaver, C. M., Proulx, W. R., & Heaney, R. (1999). Choices for achieving adequate dietary calcium with a vegetarian diet. *American Journal of Clinical Nutrition, 70,* 543S–548S.

Weingarten, X., Zalmanovici, X., & Yaphe, X. (2008). Dietary calcium supplementation for preventing colorectal cancer and adenomatous polyps. *Cochrane Database Systematic Review, 23,* CD 003548.

Worcester, E. M., & Coe, F. L. (2008). Nephrolithiasis. *Primary Care: Clinics in Office Practice, 35,* 369–391.

Wyshak, G. (2000). Teenaged girls, carbonated beverage consumption, and bone fractures. *Archives of Pediatrics & Adolescent Medicine, 154*(6), 610–613.

Zemel, M. B., & Miller, S. L. (2004). Dietary calcium and dairy modulation of adiposity and obesity risk. *Nutrition Reviews, 62,* 125–131.

Zimmerman, M. B., & Hurrell, R. F. (2007). Nutritional iron deficiency. *Lancet, 370,* 511–520.

Fluid 7

WHAT WILL YOU LEARN?

1. To examine the role of water in maintaining health.
2. To relate sources of water, caffeine, and alcohol in the diet.
3. To illustrate methods of assessing fluid requirements.
4. To translate the current consensus regarding the role of caffeine and alcohol in overall health.
5. To summarize signs and symptoms of altered fluid status that can be found when conducting a nursing assessment.
6. To evaluate the role of the nurse in identifying individuals at risk for altered health related to poor fluid status or excessive intake of caffeine or alcohol.

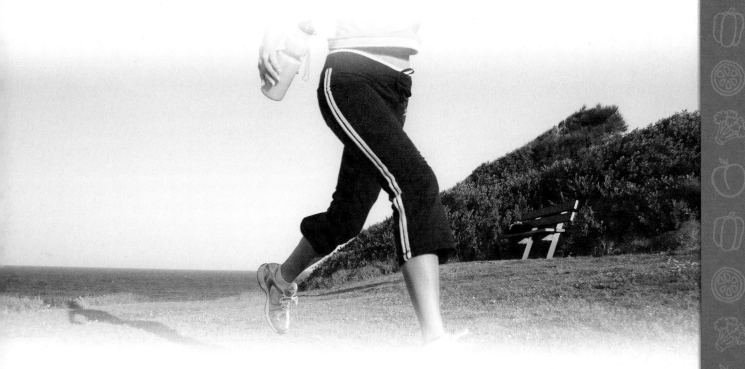

DID YOU KNOW?

▶ You can weigh yourself immediately before and after exercise to determine the amount of water lost from sweat during exercise.

▶ Caffeinated and alcoholic beverages both lead to short-term water loss but can be counted toward overall daily water needs.

▶ Light beer has almost the same alcohol content as regular beer.

▶ Moderate alcohol intake is associated with increased "good" cholesterol, or HDL, but is also considered a risk factor for breast cancer.

▶ Caffeine intake causes increase loss of calcium in the urine. The amount of calcium lost from moderate intake of coffee can be offset with intake of just 1 cup of milk in the day.

KEY TERMS

dehydration, *144*

euhydration, *144*

hyperhydration, *144*

hypohydration, *144*

insensible water loss, *144*

osmolality, *145*

sensible water loss, *144*

solutes, *145*

solvent, *144*

Water

Water is the largest single constituent of the human body (Institute of Medicine [IOM], 2004). The average adult is approximately 60% water, whereas children and individuals with ample muscle have a higher percentage of total body water. Most older adults have diminished total body water because of the loss of muscle with aging; the water content of muscle is higher than that of fat (IOM, 2004; Sawka et al., 2007).

Function of Water

Water is the **solvent,** or medium, in which biochemical reactions in the body take place. It also acts as a solvent for the transportation and elimination of substances in the body. Nutrients are transported in a water medium. Blood, lymph, and gastrointestinal secretions are other water-based modes of transporting substances in the body. By-products of metabolism and waste products are eliminated via water in urine and feces.

The regulation of body temperature is dependent on water. Water is able to absorb the heat produced from metabolism and physical activity and dissipate it to maintain an even core body temperature. Sweating allows water to transport heat to the surface of the skin where it is lost with conduction and evaporation to cool the body. This water loss is called **insensible water loss** because it is difficult to measure. Other sources of insensible water loss include respiratory and fecal water losses. Water loss that is measurable is called **sensible water loss** and includes water lost in urine.

Other functions of water include provision of structure and shape to cells; lubrication and protection of joints, spinal column, and the eyes; and acting as a constituent of mucous membrane tissue. Box 7-1 outlines the functions of water in the body. Figure 7-1 ■ depicts the distribution of water in the body.

BOX 7-1	Functions of Water in the Body

Solvent for biochemical reactions

Transport nutrients and other substances

Remove waste products

Regulation of core body temperature

Lubricant for joints, eyes, mucous membranes

Shock-absorbent protection for spinal cord, eyes, fetus

Structure for cells, skin integrity

Constituent of gastrointestinal secretions for digestion, absorption, and excretion

Maintenance of vascular volume

Water Balance in the Body

Water balance refers to the difference between total water gain and total water losses in the body (IOM, 2004). Water balance is delicately maintained within 0.2% of body weight over the course of an entire day in healthy individuals (IOM, 2004). Short-term water imbalances occur as a result of excess gains or losses of fluid, but in healthy individuals the body's neurological and hormonal balancing mechanisms should correct these over time. Water is gained by the body through dietary intake and as an end product of metabolism of carbohydrates, proteins, and fats. Water is lost through urine, the gastrointestinal tract, skin, and respiration. Unless water is consumed through food or beverages, water balance will become negative because daily losses exceed the water gained from just the end product of metabolism. The state of being in water balance is referred to as **euhydration. Hyperhydration** results when there is an excess of water while **hypohydration** refers to a water deficit. **Dehydration** and hypohydration are often used interchangeably, but the term *dehydration* can include loss of solutes along with water.

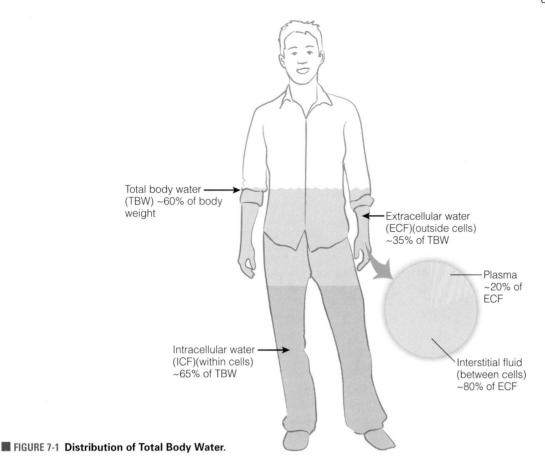

Total body water (TBW) ~60% of body weight

Extracellular water (ECF)(outside cells) ~35% of TBW

Plasma ~20% of ECF

Intracellular water (ICF)(within cells) ~65% of TBW

Interstitial fluid (between cells) ~80% of ECF

■ FIGURE 7-1 **Distribution of Total Body Water.**

Water moves across membranes within the body in an attempt to equalize the concentration of **solutes** between intracellular fluid (ICF) and extracellular fluid (ECF) compartments. Solutes are particles dissolved in a solution (or solvent); in the body solvents include plasma, interstitial fluid, and ICFs. Solutes include electrolytes and protein particles such as sodium, potassium, chloride, magnesium, and plasma proteins. Although the amounts and types of solutes differ between ICF and ECF, the net concentration is the same in both fluid compartments. The measure of the solute concentration is referred to as **osmolality.** Osmolality is measured as the milliosmoles of solute particles in a kilogram of solvent (mOsm/kg). A loss or gain of water or solutes from the body, such as with excessive sweating or conversely excessive water drinking, can cause a change in the osmolality of the plasma or ICF that then signals the body to initiate its fluid-balancing mechanisms. A proportionate loss of both water and solutes will not lead to a change in osmolality and the body relies on a secondary fluid-balancing mechanism when this change occurs.

At the cellular level, changes in osmolality are initially met with a shift in water to equalize osmolality on both sides of a cell membrane. Normal osmolality of the body is 280 to 290 mOsm/kg (IOM, 2004). Excess loss of extracellular water signals osmoreceptors in the brain and vascular and gastrointestinal systems that detect alterations in osmolality, leading to a secretion of vasopressin from the hypothalamus and pituitary glands. Vasopressin acts on the kidney to increase water reabsorption from the renal tubules. When both water and solutes are lost from ECF, the renin-angiotensin-aldosterone system is activated to retain sodium and water by the kidneys. Conversely, the body reacts to any gain in water by increasing water excretion by the kidney. A toxic level of excess water gain is discussed under Wellness Concerns.

The kidneys are the primary route by which the body regulates retention or excretion of water imbalances. Osmoreceptors play an additional role by modulating thirst, signaling drinking behavior when osmolality is elevated. Corrections to fluid imbalance via the thirst mechanisms occur more slowly than with renal mechanisms. Thirst does not lead to a short-term correction of fluid deficits; it assists in volume repletion over 24 hours and may not be initiated until plasma volume has become depleted by up to 2% of body

BOX 7-2	Risk Factors for Alterations in Fluid Balance in Older Adults

Physiological

↓ baseline of total body water with loss of muscle mass

↓ sensitivity to vasopressin (renal tubule response to reabsorb water blunted)

↓ ability to concentrate urine (higher urine volume needed to excrete solutes)

↓ sensitivity to thirst

Medical

Alteration in cognition because of disease or medications

Swallowing difficulties can cause poor intake of food and fluids

Medications—diuretics, medications with thirst-altering side effects

Gastrointestinal losses—vomiting, gastric suction, diarrhea

Urinary losses—diuretic use, polydipsia with poorly controlled diabetes

Exudative wounds or decubiti

Insensitive fluid losses with extreme heat, humidity, fever, ↑ respiratory rate

Social

Dependency on others can limit access to fluids when thirsty

Toileting difficulties, incontinence, or diuretic prescription can foster deliberate decreased fluid intake to limit frequency of urination in those with limited mobility, vision problems, pain, or other health issues

---

weight (Armstrong, 2005; IOM, 2004). Aging blunts both the renal and thirst responses to alterations in fluid balance, placing the older adult at increased risk of dehydration. Medical and social risk factors further contribute to risk. Box 7-2 outlines risk factors for altered fluid balance in the older adult.

Hydration Assessment

An assessment of hydration is important when considering fluid requirement recommendations for an individual. General fluid recommendations exist for healthy population groups but do not include specific recommendations for individuals with increased fluid needs. The nurse should utilize available tools for assessing hydration status when making fluid intake recommendations for athletes or those involved in heavy labor, especially when environmental conditions foster excess water losses with perspiration. Further discussion on fluid needs in these populations is contained in this chapter.

No gold standard exists for assessing hydration status. Available tools vary in specificity and sophistication. In the research setting, labeled water using tracer methodology is accurate with 1% to 2% in measuring total body water but is impractical and costly in the clinical setting (Armstrong, 2007; IOM, 2004). Plasma parameters are often used in the clinical setting and have varying specificity. Elevated levels of these blood values can indicate loss of water, leading to hemoconcentration. Serum osmolality is the most widely used blood measurement for determining hydration status (Armstrong, 2005). Blood hematocrit and urea nitrogen can be assessed, but if used alone could give an inaccurate assessment because of confounding by such factors as anemia or kidney disease. An elevated serum sodium level can signal loss of water from ECF. Mild hypohydration does not always lead to hemoconcentration; assessing urinary parameters of

hydration is recommended as an adjunct to hematological indices because no single parameter can accurately be used to assess hydration status (Armstrong, 2007). It should be noted that up to one-third of individuals with altered hydration status have no evident changes in laboratory measurements (Vivanti, Harvey, Ash, & Battistutta, 2008).

Urinary indices of hydration can be measured more easily than hematological indices in most settings, making them a practical alternative to hydration assessment when specificity is not needed (Armstrong, 2005). Urine osmolality and urine specific gravity correlate with one another and become elevated with dehydration and lowered with hyperhydration. Urine specific gravity of 1.030 or more is indicative of dehydration, whereas a value below 1.012 can signal excess water intake (Armstrong, 2005). Normal kidney function is needed for this assessment to be useful (Thomas et al., 2008).

A simple observation of urine volume and color is an educational tool for the nurse to share with individuals trying to manage hydration status, such as competitive athletes, where a crude measure of hydration can be used to gauge hydration practices. Urine volume of less than 30 mL/hour can signal dehydration because healthy, hydrated individuals have a urine output of approximately 100 mL/hour (IOM, 2004). High urine output should result when excessive fluid intake occurs in individuals with healthy renal function. A relationship exists between urine color and hydration status that can be part of an assessment for overhydration or underhydration. Pale yellow or straw-colored urine is felt to indicate euhydration, whereas darker-colored urine can reflect hypohydration (Armstrong, 2007). The nurse should educate the healthy client that taking vitamins or some medications alters urine color, negating the usefulness of this tool in such cases. Clients with bilirubin or blood in the urine from medical conditions should not rely on this tool to assess hydration.

Short-term changes in body weight can be used to assess for hydration, especially dehydration. Metabolic loss of body weight does not occur at as rapid a rate as does weight loss from water loss; thus weight lost in a matter of hours is because of water loss. Water has a density of 1 mL/kg; any net change in volume of total body water is reflected by an equal change in body weight. The nurse can teach an athlete, those doing physical labor, or those exposed to extreme environmental conditions to use short-term changes in body weight to estimate insensible water loss that, in turn, warrants repletion. The individual must first measure body weight after voiding for a baseline value and then remeasure weight after voiding following the physical activity. Each pound of weight loss warrants replacement with 1 pound of water, which has a volume of 16 ounces. Fluid replacement in the athlete is discussed further in Chapter 10.

Scales exist to quantify thirst as a tool in determining hydration. Although thirst can indicate dehydration, it is not a sensitive indicator by which to gauge fluid status. Thirst aids in repletion of water deficits over the course of 24 hours, not in the short-term (IOM, 2004). In people, drinking even a small amount brings relief of a dry mouth sensation and thus satisfies the sensation of thirst before there is correction of any fluid deficit (Bourque, 2008). Immersion in water blunts the feedback mechanisms for thirst and suppresses drinking (Sagawa et al., 1992); the nurse should advise competitive swimmers of this significant alteration when discussing hydration. The thirst mechanism in humans is also influenced by gastric distention from drinking and the palatability of liquid consumed, which includes its temperature, flavor, color, and odor (Bourque, 2008; IOM, 2004; Sawka et al., 2007). The effect of gastric distention in terminating drinking is altered in the older adult, resulting in less fluid intake following dehydration compared with younger adults (Farrell et al., 2008). Thus, replacement of water based on feedback mechanisms is gradual; short-term assessment of thirst may not reflect hydration accurately. Client Education Checklist: Hydration Monitoring outlines educational pointers that the nurse can offer to individuals who need to closely monitor hydration status because of physical exertion or exposure to extreme heat.

Physical findings can be assessed in conjunction with other methods for assessing hydration. The nurse can inspect mucous membranes, skin turgor, and vital signs as outlined in Table 7-1. Although it is common to test skin turgor for dehydration by lightly pinching a small skinfold to test for a lasting skinfold when the pinch is released, called "tenting," this finding is not a reliable measure of hydration in the older adult because of subcutaneous tissue loss and changes in skin elasticity associated with aging (Thomas et al., 2008). An overview of hydration assessment parameters is presented in Table 7-1.

Recommended Intake

The recommendation for daily water intake includes water from beverages and water contained in foods. A recommendation for total water intake is given as an adequate intake (AI) guideline with the goal of preventing dehydration (IOM, 2004). Although advice exists regarding water intake for chronic disease prevention, such as that outlined in Wellness Concerns in this chapter, the dietary reference intake (DRI) for water is given only for maintenance of hydration in a well population (IOM, 2004).

The AI for total water in adults age 19 years and older is 3.7 L/day for males and 2.7 L/day for females (IOM, 2004). Males are advised to consume 3.0 L/day of water from beverages, whereas females are urged to consume 2.2 L/day (IOM, 2004). Older adults have diminished total body water and blunted thirst and fluid balance homeostasis, yet the recommendations for this age group remains the same as in younger adults to ensure that intake is not limited (IOM, 2004). Water needs with pregnancy and lactation are increased to support maternal intracellular and extracellular water gains during pregnancy and production of breast milk during lactation.

CLIENT EDUCATION CHECKLIST 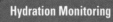 **Hydration Monitoring**

Clients who are exercise in extreme environmental conditions or those who perform physical labor should be educated to monitor hydration status. The nurse can teach the following:

• Develop a personalized fluid replacement prescription. After voiding determine body weight before and after physical activity. Any acute weight difference is from water loss. Each pound of weight loss requires a replacement of 16 oz of water. Once replacement volume is learned, replace water loss before and during physical activity. Recalculate fluid replacement needs when environmental conditions change, such as with intense heat or humidity.

• Monitor urine volume and color as indicators of hydration. Urine should be pale, straw color. Darker urine or decreased volume can indicate a water deficit. Urine color can be affected by vitamin intake, medications, and blood or bilirubin in the urine.

• Do not rely on thirst alone to gauge fluid intake. Thirst is quenched short term by simply moistening the mouth. Swimmers can have blunted thirst because of the effects of water immersion on thirst perception.

• Monitor for signs of dehydration, such as dry mucous membranes (mouth, long tongue furrows, dry axillae, sunken eyes), lethargy, lightheadedness, confusion.

• The general recommendation for fluid intake from beverages is 2.2 L/day for females and 3.0 L/day for males. Fluid needs are increased in those with increased insensible losses because of sweating and excessive gastrointestinal, urinary, or respiratory losses. Insensible respiratory water loss is increased with dry hot or cold air.

Table 7-1 Hydration Assessment*

	Euhydration	Dehydration	Overhydration
Hematological Indices	• Plasma osmolality 290 mOsm • Normal plasma sodium, BUN, creatinine, hematocrit	• Plasma osmolality greater than 290 mOsm • ↑ Plasma sodium, BUN, creatinine, hematocrit	• Plasma osmolality less than 290 mOsm • ↓ Plasma sodium, BUN, creatinine, hematocrit
Urinary Indices	• Urine color pale, straw • Urine volume approximates fluid intake	• Urine color darkened • ↓ Urine output	• Urine color clear • ↑ Urine output
Physical Findings	• Moist mucous membranes • Good skin turgor • Stable body weight	• Dry mucous membranes (long tongue furrows, dry mouth, dry axillae, sunken eyes) • Dry skin with "tenting" or lasting skinfold • Acute weight loss • Lightheadedness, altered cognition, muscle weakness, ↑ core temperature, ↑ heart rate, ↓ blood pressure	• Moist mucous membranes • Edema possible with toxic water ingestion • Acute weight gain • Altered cognition, muscle weakness, lung congestion

*Each parameter used in hydration assessment can be altered because of disease or conditions unrelated to hydration. The nurse is reminded to use multiple tools to assess hydration.

Infants and children need slightly less daily water because of smaller body mass. These needs are outlined in Appendix C.

No tolerable upper intake level (UL) for water is set for healthy individuals. The kidneys should be able to maintain water balance and excrete excess ingested water under normal conditions (IOM, 2004). Acute water toxicity has been reported and is discussed under Hyperhydration.

Sources

When developing recommendations for total water intake, it was observed that most individuals consume approximately 20% of water needs from food, whereas the remaining 80% comes from beverages (IOM, 2004). Bottled water has become a popular way to maintain hydration and meet fluid requirements, though its superiority to other forms of water varies, as outlined in Hot Topic Box: Bottled Water. All bev-

type of water must be on the label. Bottled water from a public water system is listed as *drinking water* on the label.
- Groundwater from a well, spring, or underground aquifer, such as with many municipal sources, can be used to produce bottled water.
- Disinfectant antimicrobial agents can be added to bottled water. Check with the bottler to determine what is being used when there is a concern.
- Fluoride may be added to bottled water and must be listed on the label.

What is not defined in the bottled water regulations?
- Catchy titles that infer pristine quality like *natural, pure, mountain, glacier* or *alpine*.
- Bottled waters with more than fluoride or disinfectants added (e.g., flavored bottled water). These are regulated as another type of beverage.

What are some of the municipal tap-water regulations?
- Municipal drinking water is regulated by the Environmental Protection Agency (EPA).
- Local water suppliers test water for quality. Consumers can inquire about contaminants detected, disinfectant practices, and obtain a copy of these reports.

What about people with compromised immune systems?
- Individuals with compromised immune systems, such as with AIDS or cancer treatment, may need to take special precautions when consuming water.
- Boiling water or using some filtration devices may avoid some waterborne bacteria.
- Bottled water from protected wells and spring water are safer bets than bottled water from untreated municipal sources.
- Both local water authorities and water bottlers can provide information on the safety and disinfectant practices of their product.

Unless there are known safety risks associated with municipal water, the choice to consume bottled water rests simply on personal preference.

Source: Adapted from Environmental Protection Agency (EPA), 2005.

hot Topic

Bottled Water

Bottled water consumption is on the rise and is expected to soon become the second-leading beverage choice in the United States. Some consumers purchase bottled water under the assumption that it is of superior quality to municipal tap water. When offering advice on hydration, the nurse should point out that both municipal and bottled waters are regulated by the federal government. Some popular bottled waters even come from municipal water sources.

What is regulated with bottled water?
- Bottled water is regulated by the Food and Drug Administration (FDA) as a food.
- Artesian, ground, mineral, sparkling bottled, and spring waters all have specific definitions in the food code. The

Table 7-2   Water Content of Foods

Food	Water Volume (mL)
Liquids	
Beer, 12 oz	327
Coffee, 8 oz	236
Milk, skim, 8 oz	223
Soup, chicken noodle, 8 oz	222
Tea, 8 oz	236
Fruits	
Apple, whole, medium	118
Melon, average, small ⅛	92
Orange, medium	114
Strawberries, ½ cup sliced	75
Vegetables	
Celery, 1 stalk	38
Green beans, raw, 1 cup	99
Lettuce, iceberg, 1 cup	53
Potato, baked with skin, medium	130

Source: United States Department of Agriculture, Nutrient Data Laboratory. Retrieved March 27, 2009, from http://www.nal.usda.gov/fnic/foodcomp/search

erages are considered toward water needs, including alcohol and caffeinated beverages that previously had been excluded from recommendations because of their short-term diuretic effects (IOM, 2004). Limited and inconclusive data suggest that high doses of caffeine (over 180 mg) can contribute to increased urine volume, but the effect is transient and not felt to warrant special fluid recommendations regarding caffeinated beverages (IOM, 2004; Tunnicliffe, Erdman, Reimer, Lun, & Shearer, 2008). Alcohol acts as a short-term diuretic but is also reported to have an antidiuretic effect 6 to 12 hours after ingestion (IOM, 2004).

Foods with high moisture content contribute to total water intake. In particular, most fruits and vegetables contain a significant weight percentage of water content. Table 7-2 outlines the water content of select foods.

Metabolic production of water provides a source of fluid to the body but is insufficient to maintain water balance. Carbohydrates, proteins, and fats yield carbon dioxide and water as an end product of metabolism. Carbohydrates yield 15 gm of water/100 kilocalories, whereas protein and fat yield slightly less (IOM, 2004). The result is less than 500 mL/day in most individuals.

Hypohydration/Dehydration

Underhydration can occur with insufficient intake, increased water losses, or a combination of the two factors. Older adults can become at increased risk of dehydration when presented with physical stressors, such as illness, because of lower total body water and blunted response to poor hydration (Sawka et al., 2007). Almost 8% of hospitalized older adults are diag-

nosed with dehydration, which in turn is a risk factor for morbidity and mortality (Thomas et al., 2008). Fluid status in the older adult is discussed further in Chapter 15. Intake of total water can diminish in the individual with swallowing difficulties; altered cognition, such as Alzheimer's disease; or blunted water homeostasis because of age or disease. Dependency on others is a risk factor for diminished fluid intake. Often, clients with poor appetite and decreased intake overall also have decreased intake of total water. Older adults trying to manage toileting difficulties may deliberately restrict fluid intake. Athletes participating in weight-class sports, such as wrestling and crew, may deliberately restrict fluid intake to foster dehydration in order to "make weight" for competition; such a practice is dangerous and has resulted in death (Centers for Disease Control and Prevention [CDC], 1998; Sawka et al., 2007).

Increased losses of water negatively affect water balance. Gastrointestinal, perspiration, respiratory, and urinary losses can become extreme under certain conditions and warrant monitoring when hydration is a concern. Normal gastrointestinal water loss from feces is less than 200 mL/day (IOM, 2004). Excess fluid loss occurs with diarrhea and gastric suction used in the treatment of some intestinal disorders. Laxative abuse can present a hydration challenge with ongoing fluid loss. Vomiting causes fluid losses and often results in decreased fluid intake as well. The gastrointestinal tract produces over 3 L/day of fluid that is normally reabsorbed; gastrointestinal illnesses can lead to loss of this fluid with vomiting, diarrhea, or malabsorption.

Respiratory water loss is insensible but can become significant with environmental stressors. High altitude and dry air conditions, in both heat and cold, each lead to increased respiratory water loss. Such losses become more crucial in the individual with increased ventilatory volume because of exercise or respiratory conditions. Athletes exercising during cold, dry conditions will likely not perceive the increased water loss and need to be reminded to follow hydration guidelines outlined in Chapter 10.

Insensible loss of water through the skin occurs with diffusion of less than 500 mL/day. More significant water loss occurs with sweat, which is the body's cooling mechanism when heat is generated from physical activity or fever. Evaporation of sweat from the skin surface leads to the dissipation of heat. Humid climate conditions do not allow sweat evaporation compared with drier conditions; the result is that more sweat is produced in humid weather as the body tries to cool. Heavy clothing that traps body heat and lessens evaporation fosters increased sweat losses. Daily sweat lost in hot climates can exceed 3 liters (IOM, 2004). Physical exertion, especially in heat and humidity, will lead to significant water loss that can be individually assessed by monitoring body weight. For example, athletes and military personnel exercising in extreme heat or with two-a-day sessions can have greatly increased insensible fluid losses, especially when such conditions occur in sequential days and a fluid deficit accumulates (Sawka et al., 2007). Draining wounds and burns contribute to increased skin losses of water. Nutrition care for individuals with wounds and burns is discussed in Chapter 22.

Urinary losses of water are generally in proportion to water intake in the healthy individual. Disproportionate water loss can contribute to dehydration. Conditions such as uncontrolled diabetes lead to increased urine production to excrete glucose present in the urine. Diuretic use can lead to water imbalance when not carefully monitored. Box 7-3 outlines risk factors for dehydration.

Symptoms of dehydration occur along a continuum. Mild hypohydration may not yield changes in hematological values, yet still can cause physical symptoms. A water deficit as little as 1% to 2% of body weight can impair cognitive function and physical performance (Armstrong, 2005; Sawka et al., 2007; Thomas et al., 2008). Persistent subclinical dehydration is associated with hallucinations and delusion in older adults (Thomas et al., 2008). Long-term memory, attention, and arithmetic efficiency are impaired with dehydration of over 2% of body weight (IOM, 2004). Aerobic power and physical work capacity are likewise diminished with the worst effects seen in children (IOM, 2004). It is possible that some of the cognitive and physical performance effects of dehydration reported during exercise are also related to the heat and physical stress of the exercise itself (Grandjean & Grandjean, 2007). Alterations in cardiovascular, central nervous system, and body heat regulation are cited as contributors to the negative effects. It is an interaction of all these factors, including an increased body core temperature, which degrades physical performance with dehydration (Sawka et al., 2007). Core temperature regulation

is reported to be offset with as little as 1% of body weight loss of water (IOM, 2004). Dehydration can worsen the effects of exposure to extreme heat by lessening evaporative heat loss with diminished sweat production. Wound healing is impaired by dehydration (Thomas et al., 2008). Poor fluid status affects delivery of blood flow, oxygen, and nutrients to the wound site to facilitate healing.

Symptoms of further dehydration include more severe cardiovascular, neurological, and laboratory abnormalities. Symptoms will vary depending on the amount of fluid deficit and whether or not electrolytes have been lost along with water. Progressive dehydration is increasingly detrimental to cardiovascular function and regulation of body temperature (Murray, 2007). Ultimately, death can result from untreated severe dehydration. Table 7-1 outlines symptoms of dehydration. The nurse should be aware that dehydration symptoms can be overlooked or mistaken as symptoms of other disorders, especially in the older adult who may inch slowly into dehydration with a corresponding slow decline in cognition that should not be considered a normal part of aging. Keen assessment skills and careful monitoring of fluid intake and output (I & Os) are central to prevention and treatment of dehydration. The nurse should first assess the reason for dehydration in order to formulate appropriate interventions to prevent recurrence of dehydration. For example, those who exercise in extreme environmental conditions can be advised to drink to a schedule and monitor body weight for daily changes that signal dehydration. The institutionalized older adult with cognitive changes may benefit from frequent cueing to drink, brightly colored cups or straws, and access to preferred beverages to improve intake. Reliance on thirst alone to prevent dehydration may not always be appropriate, as outlined in the Evidence-Based Practice Box: Is Thirst an Adequate Measure of Hydration Status? Treatment of individuals losing more than 10% of body weight as water must rely on medical intervention rather than simply on nutritional repletion (IOM, 2004).

Hyperhydration/Water Toxicity

Under normal circumstances, excess intake of water can be excreted by healthy kidneys, which is why no UL for water has been established. The healthy kidney can excrete a maximum of 0.7 L to 1 L/hour of urine (IOM, 2004). Nevertheless, acute intake of large volumes of water can lead to water toxicity, a dangerous imbalance of water within the ECF compartment, resulting in diluted plasma and lowered concentration of serum sodium. Low serum sodium, or hyponatremia, can be life threatening when it leads to an increase in ICF as the body attempts to balance water and electrolyte concentrations between compartments. The result can be edema of the brain and lungs.

Water toxicity can occur with endurance athletes who attempt to maintain hydration but do not replace lost electrolytes sufficiently along with the lost water. Psychogenic

---

BOX 7-3	Risk Factors for Dehydration

Decreased water intake:

- Anorexia
- Nausea and vomiting
- Dependency on others
- Altered cognition
- Swallowing difficulty
- Blunted thirst because of aging or medications

Increased water losses:

- Gastrointestinal—gastric suction, vomiting, diarrhea, laxative abuse
- Respiratory—dry air conditions, high altitude, ↑ respiratory rate
- Skin—wounds, burns, physical activity in extreme heat or humidity, fever
- Urinary—diuretic use, polydipsia

Is thirst an adequate measure of hydration status?

Clinical Problem: Thirst is a driving force in fluid consumption in healthy individuals. When individuals satisfy thirst with fluid consumption, is the individual likely to be adequately hydrated?

Research Findings: Thirst is regulated by a complicated set of physiological processes that may be stimulated by febrile illness, increased activity, or sweating because of increased ambient temperature (McKinley, Denton, Oldfield, De Oliveira, & Mathai, 2006; McKinley et al., 2004; Parsons and Coffman, 2007).

Studies conducted with healthy adults and exercise-induced dehydration found that thirst increased early in the activity but then reached a plateau beyond which thirst decreased (Maresh et al., 2004; Shirreffs, Merson, Fraser, & Archer, 2004). In other studies, forced dehydration demonstrated decreased saliva production (Walsh et al., 2004), decreased body mass (Maresh et al., 2004; Maughan, Shirreffs, & Leiper, 2007; Szinnai, Schachinger, Arnaud, Linder, & Keller, 2005; Walsh et al., 2004;), and increased

tiredness with decreased alertness (Szinnai et al., 2005; Shirreffs et al., 2004). When subjects were rehydrated by *ad lib* consumption with fluids of choice, physiological parameters returned to normal.

However, children and the elderly have different thirst sensation and body-cooling mechanisms than adults. In addition, younger children have significantly greater body water than adults. Children and independently living adults may consume adequate fluid (D'Anci, Constant, & Rosenberg, 2006; Kenney & Chiu, 2001; Mentes, 2006;), but those dependent on caregivers may become dehydrated because of inability to respond to thirst by self-regulated hydration.

Nursing Implications: Adults respond to thirst and dehydration by consumption of fluids. The elderly and children may not respond to the same cues of thirst as healthy adults; therefore, nurses need to be vigilant to signs of dehydration in those groups and take appropriate action to hydrate them.

CRITICAL THINKING QUESTION:

1. How would the nurse respond to the elderly client who states that fatigue is an increasing problem in the summer, even after short periods of working in the garden?

---

polydipsia is a phenomenon seen in some individuals with psychiatric illness, especially schizophrenia. This disorder results in chronically excessive fluid intake unless regulation of drinking behavior is enforced. It is poorly understood why polydipsia occurs in this population (IOM, 2004). SIADH, or syndrome of inappropriate antidiuretic hormone, is a disorder that results in low plasma sodium levels that are normally associated with water toxicity. However, total body water is generally normal with this condition. Treatment includes a combination of medications and a fluid restriction to lower total body water, which will increase the concentration of sodium in the plasma (Gross, 2008). Treatment of water intoxication with hyponatremia requires medical attention and is not handled with dietary manipulation.

Wellness Concerns

Adequate intake of water is important in the prevention and treatment of certain medical conditions. Low urine volume is a risk factor for the development of a recurrent kidney stone. Sufficient intake of fluids is associated with a reduced recurrence rate of kidney stones because it helps to prevent urinary supersaturation that causes kidney stones to crystallize (Manz, 2007). The nurse should advise clients with a history of kidney stones to consume enough fluid to promote at least 2 L/day of urine output; generally this recommendation amounts to an intake of almost 3 L/day of beverages but varies depending on individual insensible losses (Krieg,

2005). A higher urine volume lessens the relative concentration of solutes, such as calcium, that produce stones in the bladder, lowering the chance of a stone precipitating in the solution. Kidney stones are discussed further in Chapter 21.

Common advice is often given to increase fluid intake to treat constipation. Little evidence exists in the medical literature to support this advice unless the individual is poorly hydrated (Manz, 2007). Increasing fluid intake beyond recommended levels has not been shown to treat constipation in well-hydrated individuals (Leung, 2007).

Bladder and colon cancer risk have been linked with low intake of fluid, but evidence is inconsistent and not sufficient to warrant advice to increase intake above recommended levels (IOM, 2004; Manz, 2007).

The risk of developing blood clots, called thromboembolisms, fatal cardiac disease, and stroke is reported to increase with dehydration. The effect is believed to be related to increased blood coagulation affected by plasma volume (Manz, 2007). Individuals at risk for development of thromboembolism, including those traveling long distance and sitting for an extended time, are advised to stay well hydrated.

Caffeine

Caffeine is the most widely used central nervous stimulant in the world (IOM, 2001; Shapiro, 2008). It exerts both pharmacological and physiological effects on the heart, lungs, kidneys, and smooth muscle with stimulation of the central

MyNursingKit Caffeine, Medline Plus

nervous system through the release of hormones such as nor-epinephrine, dopamine, and serotonin. The effect is also mediated through caffeine's inhibition of specific enzymes. In addition to the intended nervous system stimulation, the end result can be cardiac stimulation, antiasthmatic action, and short-term diuresis.

The effects of caffeine vary among individuals because of half-life differences, genetics, and personal tolerance. Peak caffeine levels reach the bloodstream within 30 to 120 minutes, and the half-life of caffeine ranges from 3 to 6 hours in adults (Mort & Kruse, 2007). Half-life is prolonged during pregnancy, especially in the third trimester, or with use of oral contraceptives; it is shortened with smoking (Care Study Group, 2008; IOM, 2001). Improved tolerance to caffeine occurs after several days of regular ingestion. The cardiostimulatory effect on heart rate and blood pressure is lessened in as little as 3 days, but the tolerance effects begin to diminish when caffeine intake ceases for as little as 1 day (Greenberg, Boozer, & Geliebter, 2006).

Sources of Caffeine

As much as 87% of the U.S. population consumes caffeine, with adults and male teens consuming the most (Frary, Johnson, & Wang, 2005). Caffeine is found in coffee, tea, soft drinks, energy drinks, chocolate, and medications. In the United States, 71% of ingested caffeine is from coffee, with soft drinks placing second at 16% (Frary et al., 2005). The amount of children consuming caffeine-containing beverages is higher among children in the United States versus Canada (56% vs. 36%, respectively) (Knight, Knight, & Mitchell, 2006). Table 7-3 outlines the caffeine content of select beverages, foods, and medications.

Wellness Concerns

The initial wellness concern with caffeine intake is the avoidance of high intake and toxic side effects. In a review of poison center reports related to dietary supplements, almost half were because of caffeine-containing substances (Haller et al., 2008). Excessive caffeine intake can result in irritability, agitation, nervousness, and insomnia. This effect is a concern in children and adolescents because of behavioral effects and sleep disturbances (IOM, 2001; Orbeta, Overpeck, Ramcharran, Kogan, & Ledsky, 2006). Caffeine toxicity can lead to vomiting, seizures, and tachyarrythmias, where heart rate is both elevated and of an abnormal rhythm. An acute lethal dose of caffeine is considered to be 10 gm or higher or a blood caffeine level of over 80 mcg/gm (Holmgren, Norden-Pettersson, & Ahlner, 2004). Excessive intake is defined in excess of 400 to 500 mg daily. Factors affecting individual caffeine tolerance can alter the level at which intake produces acute negative side effects.

Table 7-3	Caffeine Content of Foods, Beverages, and Medications	
Product	**Caffeine Content (mg)**
Chocolate	
• Chocolate bar, average, 1 oz	15
• Chocolate milk, 8 oz	8
• Fudge, 1oz	11
• Hot cocoa, 8 oz	5
Coffee, 8 oz*	
• Brewed, home drip	135
• Brewed, specialty coffee shop	250
• Espresso, 2 oz	70
• Ice cream, coffee, average	58
• Latte	35
Medications, over-the-counter, 1 tablet, average	
• Analgesics	30–65
• Cold remedies	30
• Stimulants (caffeine tablets)	100
Soft drinks, 12 oz**	
• Cola	35–45
• Energy drinks	50–100
• Root beer	0–25
Tea, 8 oz*	
• Brewed	7–35
• Green	30
• Iced	20–35

*Caffeine content of coffee and tea varies with brand, brewing method, and steeping time.
**Soft drink labels should be checked for added caffeine on the ingredient list.
Sources: American Beverage Organization, 2009; Harland, 2000; United States Department of Agriculture, Nutrient Data Laboratory. Retrieved March 27, 2009, from http://www.nal.usda.gov/fnic/foodcomp/search

The safety of moderate caffeine intake on long-term health is a topic of constant debate in the media and in medical research. Conclusions on the subject are difficult because of various methodological challenges with caffeine research. Personal caffeine tolerance can lead to no caffeine effects in one individual and a pronounced effect in another. Genetic differences in caffeine metabolism play a role in health risk from caffeine in some individuals, especially as it relates to cardiovascular disease or poor pregnancy outcomes (Cornelius & El-Sohemy, 2007; Grosso & Bracken, 2005; Tunnicliffe et al., 2008). Research focusing on population studies using questionnaires is employed in many studies and relies on accurate recall of intake, including portion sizes. In addition, caffeine in coffee and tea is affected by brand, brewing method, and steeping time. Cultural Considerations Box: Coffee Brewing Method and Health discusses the effect of brewing methods on health. Table 7-4 summarizes the effects of caffeine on wellness issues across the lifespan.

Table 7-4 Wellness Concerns with Caffeine Intake

Caffeine Concern	Caffeine Conclusion
Benign breast disease	No longer considered to have a causal relationship with fibrocystic benign breast disease. Some report improved symptoms with reduced intake.
Bone health	Caffeine causes urinary calcium losses that can be offset with as little intake as 1 cup/day of milk.
Cardiac • High cholesterol • Myocardial infarction (MI) • Arrhythmia • Hypertension	Boiled coffee with no filter use ↑ cholesterol. Risk of MI in some felt to be related to genetically slow caffeine metabolism. More research needed. Moderate intake not associated as independent risk factor for arrhythmia in healthy individuals. Acute rise in blood pressure with intake; may lessen with tolerance. More pronounced in those with existing high blood pressure or high anxiety level.
Diabetes	Long-term coffee intake may substantially ↓ risk of type 2 diabetes.
Gastrointestinal • Gastroesophageal reflux/gastritis • Gallstones	• Coffee and caffeine ↑ gastric acid production and ↓ lower esophageal sphincter pressure, leading to symptoms. • Coffee intake associated with ↓ risk of symptomatic gallstone development.
Hydration	Short-term causes ↑ urine output but with no long-term risk for dehydration.
Medication interactions	Caffeine ↑ effect of stimulatory drugs and counters the effect of sedative/antianxiety medications.
Parkinson's disease	Intake associated with ↓ risk of Parkinson's.
Pregnancy and lactation	Recommendation is to not exceed intake of 300 mg/day because of potential risk of spontaneous abortion and low birth weight babies with higher intake, especially in smokers. Effects on delayed conception inconclusive. In nursing infants, note that half-life of caffeine is longer in infants.
Psychological disorders • Anxiety • Stress	• Can worsen anxiety or panic attacks in those with existing anxiety. • Can heighten sensation of stress in those without habitual intake.
Sports performance	Caffeine may enhance aerobic sport performance via ↑ fatty acid availability. Chapter 11 outlines guidelines.

CT? The nurse should consider cultural practices in coffee preparation because boiled coffee with no filter use is associated with elevated blood cholesterol. What cultures traditionally boil coffee? What can the nurse suggest to an individual who boils coffee and has elevated cholesterol?

Sources: Adapted from Care Study Group, 2008; Cornelius & El-Sohemy, 2007; Institute of Medicine (IOM), Food and Nutrition Board, 2001; Sawka et al., 2007; Shaffer, 2006; van Dam, 2008.

Cultural Considerations

Coffee Brewing Method and Health

Coffee brewing methods differ among cultures. Brewing coffee using a paper or metal mesh filter is commonplace. Boiling coffee with no filter is practiced in some traditional cultures, such as those in Scandinavia, Turkey, and Greece. Use of a French press to make coffee is also considered a form of boiled coffee. Naturally occurring substances called diterpenoid alcohols that are present in the coffee bean end up in the brewed coffee when it is boiled and no filter is used. These compounds are reported to contribute to elevated blood cholesterol levels.

Source: Campos & Baylin, 2007; Cornelius & El-Sohemy, 2007; van Dam, 2008.

Alcohol

Alcohol is considered a drug because of its stimulant and depressant effects on the body. Unlike other drugs, alcohol also provides a source of energy, with approximately 7 calories/gm. Alcohol is absorbed in the stomach and small intestine before reaching the liver where it is degraded by the alcohol dehydrogenase (ADH) enzyme. Women produce less ADH than do men and thus have a lowered capacity to handle any increased metabolism because of excessive alcohol intake. When the amount of ingested alcohol exceeds the ability of the body to degrade it, excess alcohol remains in the plasma and crosses the blood-brain barrier, exerting its effects on the central nervous system. This effect is more pronounced in females because of lower body water than males, increasing the relative concentration of alcohol in the blood (National Institute on Alcohol Abuse and Alcoholism [NIAAA], 2000a).

Alcohol ingested by a pregnant female acts as a direct toxin on the developing fetal brain and can lead to permanent neuronal damage. Alcohol passes from the mother's blood and into that of the fetus, where it is more slowly metabolized than in an adult, exerting its damaging effects for a longer amount of time. Although all organs are affected, detrimental effects on the brain are most noted (Mengel, Searight, & Cook, 2006). Additionally, alcohol constricts blood vessels, limiting blood flow to the placenta and fetus (U.S. Department of Health and Human Services, 2007). Alcohol intake at any time in pregnancy can lead to fetal alcohol spectrum disorder, a condition that causes a range of physical defects and mental and behavioral disabilities. A safe threshold of alcohol intake is not known. Consuming one or more drinks per day or binge drinking places the fetus at highest risk (United States Surgeon General, 2005). Permanent brain damage, central nervous system defects, facial anomalies, learning disabilities, and problems with language, social skills, and impulse control are lifelong impairments that are part of this disorder (Mengel et al., 2006).

Peak plasma alcohol levels are reached within 30 to 45 minutes following consumption of a single alcoholic beverage. When more than a single drink is consumed over a short period, peak plasma alcohol levels are achieved in a similar time frame but at a higher peak, and the length of time that the blood alcohol level remains elevated is prolonged (NIAAA, 2000a). The metabolization of alcohol by the liver produces metabolic end products that include excess hydrogen molecules capable of disturbing the body's normal redox state. The result can be acidosis, elevated ketones, triglycerides in the plasma, development of fatty liver, and decreased gluconeogenesis. The nurse should be aware that impairment in gluconeogenesis leads to hypoglycemia. This consequence is of increased clinical significance when alcohol is consumed in a fasting state, especially by those who have diabetes mellitus and are taking hypoglycemic medications. Alcohol consumed on an empty stomach is absorbed more rapidly than when food is present (NIAAA, 2000a).

Nutritional antidotes to the negative side effects of alcohol, including hangover, are receiving popular attention despite the ineffectiveness of these practices. Research on these products is reviewed in Hot Topic Box: Nutritional Antidotes to Alcohol.

Alcohol has direct negative effects on the absorption and metabolism of nutrients in the diet. Absorption is inhibited by the effects of alcohol on the gastric mucosa and pancreas. In turn, nutrients that are absorbed have altered transportation, storage, and excretion because of alcohol. In addition to these secondary effects of alcohol on nutrition, excessive alcohol intake contributes to primary malnutrition when adequate intake of food is replaced with alcohol. Table 7-5 outlines the effects of alcohol on nutrition status.

hot TOPIC

Nutritional Antidotes to Alcohol

Nutrition products are marketed on the Internet and elsewhere as antidotes to the short-term effects of alcohol intoxication. Altered motor coordination and visual-spatial skills, lightheadedness, headache, and nausea can follow excessive alcohol intake as part of an alcoholic hangover. There is little research to substantiate the effectiveness of these antidotes. The research that does exist has the following conclusions:

- Energy drinks containing sugars, caffeine, and taurine, an amino acid, marketed as alcohol mixers and used in an attempt to ward off a hangover have been investigated for any benefit. Although the drinker's perception of alcohol on motor coordination may be improved, objective measures of visual-motor skills show no change from consuming alcohol alone (Ferreira, deMello, Pompeia, & deSouza-Formagioni, 2006). Guidelines in Europe and Canada warn against mixing energy drinks with alcohol and suggest daily limits on intake to curtail caffeine intake (Reissig, Strain, & Griffiths, 2009). No such labels or regulations exist in the United States.

- Multiple nutritional supplements, such as various plant abstracts marketed as alcohol antidotes, were found to have no compelling evidence of benefit in the prevention or treatment of an alcoholic hangover (Pittler, Verster, & Ernst, 2005).

CT? What safety concerns should the nurse have regarding use of energy drinks with alcohol intake? What advice should the nurse offer regarding use of nutritional supplements as antidotes to alcohol intoxication?

Sources of Alcohol

Alcohol is found in wine, beer, and distilled spirits or hard liquor, such as vodka, whiskey, rum, and gin. A single serving of alcohol contains 13 to 14 gm of ethanol and is considered to be one 12 oz beer, 1.5 oz of 80-proof hard liquor, or 5 oz of

Table 7-5	Effects of Alcohol on Nutrition
Alcohol Effect	**Affected Nutrient**
Primary malnutrition	Excessive alcohol intake replaces food intake
Decreased nutrient absorption	Thiamin Folate Vitamin B_{12} Fat and fat-soluble vitamins A, D, E, K
Decreased nutrient storage	Folate Riboflavin Vitamin B_6
Increased urinary nutrient losses	Folate Magnesium Zinc

Sources: Adapted from Lieber, 2000; National Institute on Alcohol Abuse and Alcoholism (NIAAA), 2000b; Stickel, Hoehn, Schuppan, & Seitz, 2003.

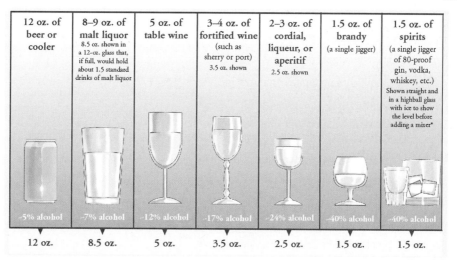

FIGURE 7-2 What Is a Standard Drink?

Source: National Institutes of Health, National Institute on Alcohol Abuse and Alcoholism, 2005.

wine (United States Department of Agriculture [USDA], 2005). Figure 7-2 ■ illustrates serving sizes of standard drinks for various beverages. The nurse should educate those who drink light beer about the alcohol content as outlined in Practice Pearl: Light Alcoholic Beverages.

Current recommendations on alcohol intake in adults advise that women and small men limit intake to one drink per day. Moderation is considered two drinks per day in other men (USDA, 2005). Children, pregnant or lactating females, individuals with medical conditions or who are taking medications that interact with alcohol, and those who cannot limit alcohol intake are advised to avoid alcohol intake completely. Many screening tools exist to assess alcohol intake and whether or not alcohol abuse exists. On-line versions of screening tools can be part of a nursing assessment. The MyNursingKit link is one example of such a tool.

The nurse should remind clients who choose to drink alcoholic beverages to consider both the caloric content of the beverage as well as any mixes used to prepare the drink. Table 7-6 outlines the alcohol and calorie content of alcoholic beverages.

Wellness Concerns

Alcohol is considered a double-edged sword. Moderate intake of alcohol by a healthy adult can have some health ben-

efits, while at the same time health risks exist associated with alcohol intake. Moderate intake of alcohol can advantageously increase HDL or "good" cholesterol (Ashen & Blumenthal, 2005; Ellison et al., 2004; O'Keefe, Bybee & Lavie, 2007). This effect is achieved with any type of alcohol, though much attention focuses on intake of red wine for its additional antiplatelet effect that can alter blood clotting. The effect of alcohol on risk of cardiovascular disease is discussed further in Chapter 18.

Table 7-6   Alcohol and Calorie Content of Beverages

Beverage	Alcohol (gm)	Calories
Beer, 12 oz		
• Light	11	103
• Regular	14	153
Distilled spirits, 80-proof, 1.5 oz Gin, rum, vodka, whiskey	14	97
Wine, 5 oz		
• Red	16	125
• White	15	122
Wine, sweet, 3 oz	13.5	142
Cocktails		
• Daiquiri, 4 oz	28	225
• Martini, 4 oz	38	274
• Piña colada, 4 oz	12	219
Drink mixes, 8 oz		
• Cola	0	91
• Cranberry juice cocktail	0	137
• Orange juice	0	112
• Tonic water	0	83

Source: United States Department of Agriculture, Nutrient Data Laboratory. Retrieved March 27, 2009, from http://www.nal.usda.gov/fnic/foodcomp/search

PRACTICE PEARL

Light Alcoholic Beverages

Although the calorie content can differ between light and regular types of beer, the alcohol content is not drastically different between the two beverages. When educating clients about the recommendations for moderate alcohol intake, consuming light beer does not afford a higher serving allowance.

Table 7-7   Wellness Concerns with Alcohol Intake

Condition	Research
Cancer • Breast • Gastrointestinal	↑ risk with moderate consumption. ↑ risk of oral, liver, colon.
Heart disease • Hypertension • Atherosclerosis • Atrial fibrillation	↑ blood pressure with ↑ intake. ↑ HDL cholesterol with moderate intake. Red wine may have additional benefit related to antiplatelet effect. ↑ risk with excessive intake.
Digestive disease • Ulcer • Pancreatitis • Liver disease	↑ risk with ↑ intake. ↑ risk with ↑ intake. ↑ risk with ↑ intake.
Gout	↑ risk with ↑ intake.
Hydration	↑ urinary output with intake can delay rehydration.
Medication interactions	Alcohol potentiates or inhibits the effect of many medications. See Chapter 25.

CT? What overall advice should the nurse give when asked about alcohol intake and disease risk?

Sources: Adapted from Choi, Atkinson, Karlson, Willett, & Curhan, 2004; Djousse et al., 2004; Franke, Teyssen, & Singer, 2005; National Heart, Lung, and Blood Institute (NHLBI), 2004; Sawka et al., 2007; United States Department of Agriculture (USDA), 2005.

The benefits of alcohol intake on heart disease risk can be offset by the association of alcohol intake on breast cancer risk even at a moderate intake level. There appears to be a dose-related risk between alcohol intake and breast cancer risk in females; even one drink a day increases risk by 10% compared with females who are nondrinkers (USDA, 2005). The mechanism for this increased risk is not fully understood, but it may be related to alterations in folate metabolism and interactions between alcohol and existing risk factors for breast cancer, such as family history, including genetics (Boffetta & Hashibe, 2006). The nurse should advise women who are on hormone replacement therapy or have a family history of breast cancer of the clinical significance of alcohol intake on breast cancer risk in those populations (USDA, 2005).

The effects of alcohol on pancreatic, liver, and gastrointestinal health are reviewed in Chapter 20. Other wellness concerns, including the effects of alcohol on blood pressure and risk of other cancers, are outlined in Table 7-7. Lifespan Box: Alcoholic Avoidance Advice outlines particular wellness concerns for the pregnant or lactating female and children because of the negative effects of alcohol on brain development and function. Discussion of fetal alcohol spectrum disorders is outlined in Chapter 13.

Lifespan

Alcohol Avoidance Advice

Avoidance of alcohol is recommended for children and pregnant and lactating females. The nurse should recommend abstinence from alcohol for the following reasons:

• Alcohol intake during pregnancy is associated with lifelong neurocognitive deficits, behavior problems, and malformation in offspring called fetal alcohol spectrum disorders. No safe level of alcohol intake has been determined that avoids these consequences.

• Breast milk alcohol level mirrors that of the mother's blood and can negatively affect the infant. Alcohol does not have a positive influence on milk production.

• Alcohol intake is associated with risk of trauma, the most prevalent cause of death in children and adolescents. Elevated blood alcohol levels result more quickly in the young than in adults because of smaller body size. Children who begin drinking by age 15 years are four times as likely to abuse alcohol as adults than children who do not drink before age 21 years. Psychosocial development can be impaired. Disease risks from alcohol intake reflect that of adults.

Sources: Adapted from American Academy of Pediatrics, Committee on Substance Abuse, 2001; Centers for Disease Control and Prevention (CDC), 2005; United States Department of Agriculture (USDA), 2005.

NURSING CARE PLAN   Nutrition and Dehydration

CASE STUDY

Mr. McGillicudy is a 78-year-old widower who lives in an assisted-living facility. He no longer drives much so he enjoys the companionship of the residents and the occasional group excursions to local events. He is increasingly troubled by arthritis in his hips and knees but otherwise has no chronic medical conditions. Since the medication for his arthritis was changed about a month ago, he has experienced frequent bouts of diarrhea. Now he reports to the nurse at the clinic that the diarrhea seems to be "letting up a bit," but that he feels tired. He used to go to the dining area for meals, but the coffee just does not "taste right" and he does not like the skim milk they give him instead. He admits to drinking less later in the day because frequent trips to the bathroom cause knee pain. He says his appetite is fine but that he feels sluggish. He does not believe he has lost any weight recently. He asks the nurse what can be done to return things to the way they were a few months ago.

Applying the Nursing Process

ASSESSMENT

Weight: 163 pounds Height: 5 feet 9 inches BMI: 24
Mucous membranes pink and dry
Skin warm and dry
T 98.1 P 80 R 14 BP 152/84

DIAGNOSES

Deficient fluid volume related to voluntary restriction of intake and diarrhea
Mobility impaired related to joint degeneration
Chronic pain related to joint degeneration

EXPECTED OUTCOMES

Adequate hydration and moist mucous membranes
Increased socialization with residents at mealtimes
Diminished pain in hips and knees

INTERVENTIONS

Determine fluid preferences
Have fluid of choice available at meals
Diet recall to determine if food choices may be causing diarrhea
Refer to physician to determine if change in medication or dosage is indicated
Weigh monthly to monitor for weight loss
Suggest moderate exercise to prevent additional decrease in mobility
Teach importance of maintaining regular fluid intake, even if not thirsty

EVALUATION

Two months later, Mr. McGillicudy reports that he is feeling better. His physician decreased the dose of his arthritis medication and increased his pain medication. He feels that the combination is having the desired effect because he has less frequent diarrhea. He has joined an exercise class that meets twice a week at the residence and feels more "limber." As a result, he does not feel the need to restrict fluid intake later in the day to avoid bathroom trips. His daughter brought him small bottles of the fruit punch he likes, so he sometimes takes one to the dining center to have with his meal. He maintains he is too old to change what he likes so still refuses milk if the coffee is not up to his standards. Figure 7-3 ■ outlines the nursing process for this case study.

Critical Thinking in the Nursing Process

1. **Why is the nurse particularly concerned about the hydration status of elderly clients?**
2. **What fluids can the nurse recommend to the elderly to maintain adequate hydration?**

(continued)

Nutrition and Dehydration *(continued)*

Assessment

Data about the patient

Subjective

What the patient tells the nurse

Example: "I've been having more diarrhea since my medications were changed. Coffee doesn't taste right and I don't like skim milk."

Objective

What the nurse observes; anthropometric and clinical data

Examples: Height: 5 feet 9 inches; weight: 163 pounds; BMI: 24, dry mucous membranes

Diagnosis

NANDA label

Example: Deficient fluid intake related to voluntary restriction and diarrhea

Planning

Goals stated in patient terms

Example: Long-term goal: sustained intake of at least 2,000 mL of fluid daily; Short-term goal: mucous membranes are moist

Implementation

Nursing action to help patient achieve goals

Example: allow fluid of choice at meals; encourage drinking water between meals or with snacks

Evaluation

Was the goal achieved or does the intervention need to be modified?

Example: drinks bottled fruit punch for meals and snacks

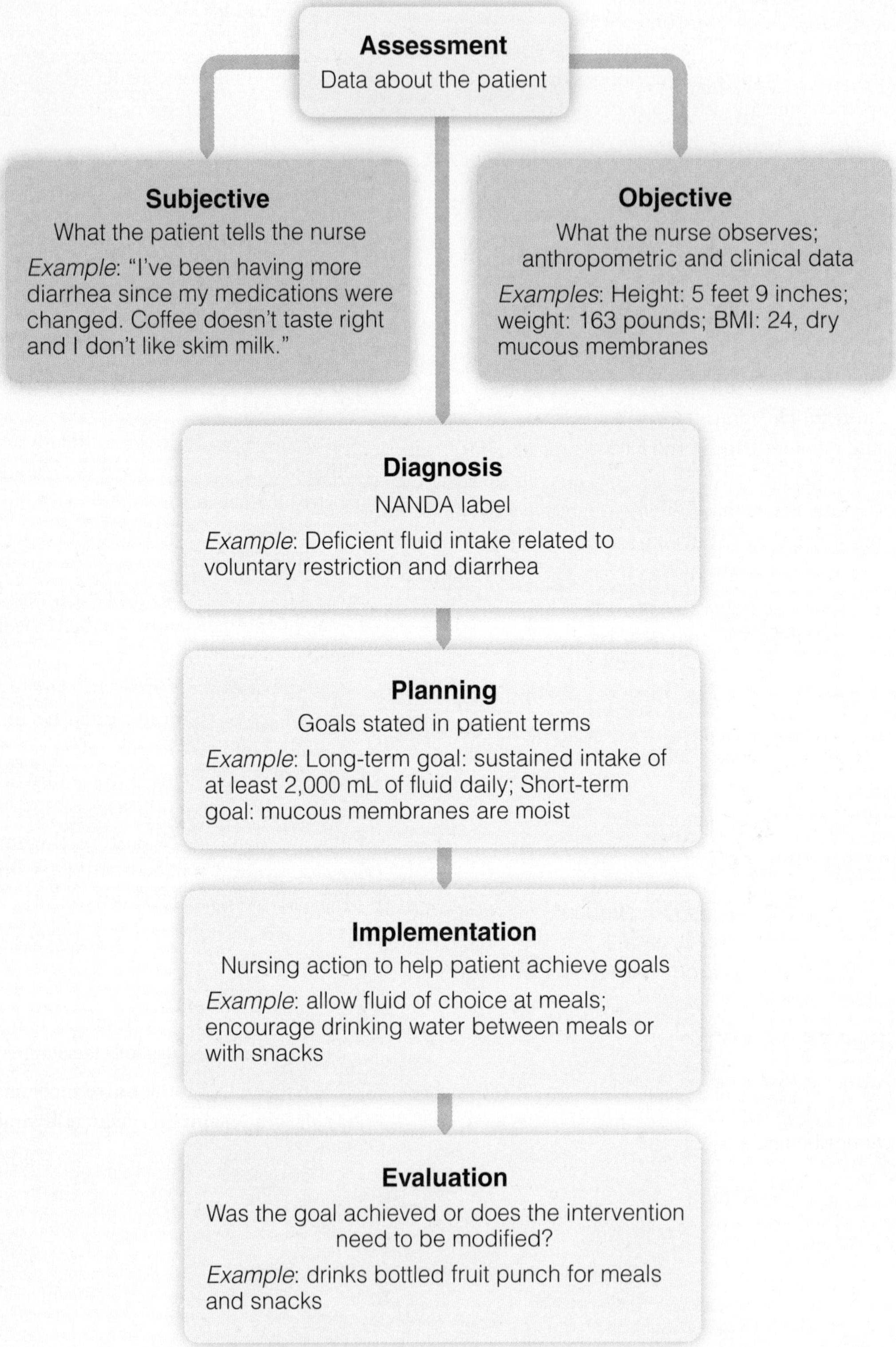

■ FIGURE 7-3 **Nursing Care Plan Process: Nutrition and Dehydration.**

CHAPTER SUMMARY

- Water comprises 60% of total body weight and is essential as a medium for metabolic reactions, body temperature maintenance, joint lubrication, transport and excretion of substances in the body, and maintenance of vascular volume and skin integrity.

- Water balance is a delicate process that is controlled by many neurological and hormonal factors.

- There is no one measurement for assessing hydration status. It is best to use multiple tools, such as laboratory measurements and physical examination.

- Recommendations for water intake can be met with both fluids and foods.

- There are health risks to both dehydration and water toxicity that require medical attention.

- The effects of caffeine on health vary and may differ among individuals.

- Alcohol is considered a drug with both stimulant and depressive effects.

- There are positive health effects associated with a moderate intake of alcohol. Increased intake does not confer additional health benefits, but rather is associated with health risks.

EXPLORE PEARSON **mynursingkit™**

MyNursingKit is your one stop for online chapter review materials and resources. Prepare for success with additional NCLEX®-style practice questions, interactive assignments and activities, web links, animations and videos, and more!

Register your access code from the front of your book at
www.mynursingkit.com.

NCLEX® QUESTIONS

1. A 24-year-old office worker tells the nurse about hearing that drinking alcohol will help prevent heart disease. How should the nurse respond to this statement?
   1. "What specific kind of alcohol are you talking about?"
   2. "Alcohol may be beneficial if used in moderate amounts."
   3. "The risk of alcoholism is too great to recommend consumption of alcohol to prevent heart disease."
   4. "Alcohol consumption is a risk factor in many disease processes so it should be avoided."

2. What assessment data is the nurse certain will be present in a client who is known to be dehydrated?
   1. Pale skin
   2. Dry skin
   3. Diminished muscle tone
   4. Dry mouth

3. The nurse is caring for each of the following clients. Which one will require increased fluid intake?
   1. A middle-age client receiving antibiotics for an upper respiratory condition
   2. An elderly client with intermittent diarrhea
   3. A middle-age client with severe heart failure
   4. An elderly client receiving diuretics

4. How should the nurse respond to the middle-age client who reported hearing that coffee is "bad" because it causes dehydration?
   1. "Coffee is bad because it contains caffeine, which raises the heart rate, and that may be a problem as people age."
   2. "That is not true. Coffee contains beneficial substances like antioxidants."
   3. "That is only true about caffeinated coffee, not decaffeinated coffee."
   4. "Coffee acts as a mild diuretic but does not cause dehydration because it is almost all water."

5. A client reports to the nurse that the urine seems to be very yellow and has a mild odor. Which of the following is the most appropriate response by the nurse?
   1. "This is a normal variation and is of no concern."
   2. "This indicates that the urine is very concentrated and you should try to increase consumption of water."

3. "Tell me all of the medications you are currently taking; they may be affecting the urine."
4. "Call your health care provider immediately and share your concern."

REFERENCES

American Academy of Pediatrics, Committee on Substance Abuse. (2001). Alcohol use and abuse: A pediatric concern. *Pediatrics, 108,* 185–189.

American Beverage Organization. (2009). *Caffeine.* Retrieved January 17, 2009, from http://www.ameribev.org/swf/ingredients.swf?_default=1

Armstrong, L. E. (2005). Hydration assessment techniques. *Nutrition Reviews, 63,* S40–S54.

Armstrong, L. E. (2007). Assessing hydration status: The elusive gold standard. *Journal of the American College of Nutrition, 26,* 575S–584S.

Ashen, M. D., & Blumenthal, R. S. (2005). Low HDL cholesterol levels. *New England Journal of Medicine, 353,* 1252–1260.

Boffetta, P., & Hashibe, M. (2006). Alcohol and cancer. *The Lancet, Oncology, 7,* 149–156.

Bourque, C. W. (2008). Central mechanisms of osmosensation and systemic osmoregulation. *Nature Reviews. Neuroscience, 9,* 519–531.

Campos, H., & Baylin, A. (2007). Coffee consumption and risk of type 2 diabetes and heart disease. *Nutrition Reviews, 65,* 173–179.

Care Study Group. (2008). Maternal caffeine intake during pregnancy and risk of fetal growth restriction: A large prospective observational study. *British Medical Journal, 337,* a2332.

Centers for Disease Control and Prevention (CDC). (1998). Hyperthermia and dehydration-related deaths associated with intentional rapid weight loss in three collegiate wrestlers. *Morbidity and Mortality Weekly Report, 47,* 105–108.

Centers for Disease Control and Prevention (CDC). (2005). Surgeon General's advisory on alcohol use in pregnancy. Retrieved January 17, 2009, from http://www.cdc.gov/mmwr/preview/mmwrhtml/mm5409a6.htm

Choi, H. K., Atkinson, K., Karlson, E. W., Willett, W., & Curhan, G. (2004). Alcohol intake and risk of incident gout in men: A prospective study. *Lancet, 363,* 1277–1281.

Cornelius, M. C., & El-Sohemy, A. (2007). Coffee, caffeine, and coronary heart disease. *Current Opinion in Clinical Nutrition and Metabolic Care, 10,* 745–751.

D'Anci, K. E., Constant, F., & Rosenberg, I. H. (2006). Hydration and cognitive function in children. *Nutrition Reviews, 64*(10), 457–464.

Djousse, L., Levy, D., Benjamin, E. J., Blease, S. J., Larson, M. G., Massaro, J. M., et al. (2004). Long-term alcohol consumption and the risk of atrial fibrillation in the Framingham Heart Study. *American Journal of Cardiology, 93,* 710–713.

Ellison, R. C., Zhang, Y., Quershi, M. M., Knox, S., Arnett, D. K., & Province, M. A. (2004). Lifestyle determinants of high-density lipoprotein cholesterol: The National Heart, Lung, and Blood Institute Family Heart Study. *American Heart Journal, 147,* 529–535.

Environmental Protection Agency (EPA). (2005). *Water health series: Bottled water basics.* Retrieved January 17, 2009, from http://www.epa.gov/safewater/faq/pdfs/fs_healthseries_bottlewater.pdf

Farrell, M. J., Zamirripa, F., Shade, R., McKinley, M., Phillips, P. A., & Fox, P. T. (2008). Effect of aging on regional cerebral blood flow responses associated with osmotic thirst and its satiation by water drinking: A PET study. *Proceedings of the National Academy of Sciences, 105,* 382–387.

Ferreira, S. E., deMello, M. T., Pompeia, S., & deSouza-Formagioni, M. L. (2006). Effects of energy drink ingestion on alcohol intoxication. *Alcoholism, Clinical and Experimental Research, 30,* 598–605.

Franke, A., Teyssen, S., & Singer, M. V. (2005). Alcohol-related diseases of the esophagus and stomach. *Digestive Diseases, 23,* 204–213.

Frary, C. D., Johnson, R. K., & Wang, M. Q. (2005). Food sources of intakes of caffeine in the diets of persons in the United States. *Journal of the American Dietetic Association, 105,* 110–113.

Grandjean, A. C., & Grandjean, N. R.(2007). Dehydration and cognitive performance. *Journal of the American College of Nutrition, 26,* 549S–554S.

Greenberg, J. A., Boozer, C. N., & Geliebter, A. (2006). Coffee, diabetes, and weight control. *American Journal of Clinical Nutrition, 84,* 682–693.

Gross, P. (2008). Treatment of hyponatremia. *Internal Medicine, 47,* 885–891.

Grosso, L. M., & Bracken, M. B. (2005). Caffeine metabolism, genetics, and perinatal outcomes: A review of exposure assessment considerations during pregnancy. *Annals of Epidemiology, 15,* 460–466.

Haller, C., Kearney, T., Bent, S., Ko, R., Benowitz, N., & Olson, K. (2008). Dietary supplement adverse events: Report of a one-year poison center surveillance project. *Journal of Medical Toxicology, 4,* 84–92.

Harland, B. (2000). Caffeine and nutrition. *Nutrition, 16,* 522–526.

Holmgren, P., Norden-Pettersson, L., & Ahlner, J. (2004). Caffeine fatalities—four case reports. *Forensic Science International, 139,* 71–73.

Institute of Medicine (IOM), Food and Nutrition Board. (2001). *Caffeine for the sustainment of mental task performance: Formulations for military operations.* Washington, DC: National Academies Press.

Institute of Medicine (IOM), Food and Nutrition Board. (2004). *Dietary reference intakes for water, potassium, sodium, chloride and sulfate.* Washington, DC: National Academies Press.

Kenney, W. L., & Chiu, P. (2001). Influence of age on thirst and fluid intake. *Medicine and Science in Sports and Exercise, 33*(9), 1524–1532.

Knight, C. A., Knight, I., & Mitchell, D. C. (2006). Beverage caffeine intakes in young children in Canada and the U.S. *Canadian Journal of Dietetic Practice & Research, 67,* 96–99.

Krieg, C. (2005). The role of diet in the prevention of common kidney stones. *Urologic Nursing, 25,* 451–456.

Leung, F. W. (2007). Etiologic factors of chronic constipation—review of the scientific evidence. *Digestive Disease Science, 52,* 313–316.

Lieber, C. S. (2000). Alcohol: Its metabolism and interaction with nutrients. *Annual Review of Nutrition, 20,* 395–430.

Manz, F. (2007), Hydration and disease. *Journal of the American College of Nutrition, 26,* 535S–541S.

Maresh, C. M., Gabaree-Boulant, C. L., Armstrong, L. E., Judelson, D. A., Hoffman, J. R., Castellani, J. W., et al. (2004). Effect

REFERENCES   *(continued)*

of hydration status on thirst, drinking, and related hormonal responses during low-intensity exercise in the heat. *Journal of Applied Physiology, 97,* 39–44.

Maughan, R. J., Shirreffs, S. M., & Leiper, J. B. (2007). Errors in the estimation of hydration status from changes in body mass. *Journal of Sports Sciences, 25,* 797–804.

McKinley, M. J., Cairns, M. J., Denton, D. A., Egan, G., Mathai, M. L., Uschakov, A., et al. (2004). Physiological and pathophysiological influences on thirst. *Physiology and Behavior, 81,* 795–803.

McKinley, M. J., Denton, D. A., Oldfield, B. J., De Oliveira, L. B., & Mathai, M. L. (2006). Water intake and the neural correlates of the consciousness of thirst. *Seminars in Nephrology, 26,* 249–257.

Mengel, M. B., Searight, R., & Cook, K. (2006). Preventing alcohol-exposed pregnancies. *Journal of the American Board of Family Medicine, 19,* 494–505.

Mentes, J. (2006). Oral hydration in older adults. *American Journal of Nursing, 106,* 40–49.

Mort, J. R., & Kruse, H. R. (2007). Timing of blood pressure measurement related to caffeine consumption. *Annals of Pharmacotherapy, 42,* 105–110.

Murray, B. (2007). Hydration and physical performance. *Journal of the American College of Nutrition, 26,* 542S–548S.

National Heart, Lung, and Blood Institute (NHLBI). (2004). *Seventh report of the Joint National Committee on the Prevention, Detection, Evaluation and Treatment of High Blood Pressure.* Accessed April 20, 2006, from www.nhlbi.nih.gov/guidelines/hypertension/jnc7full.pdf

National Institute on Alcohol Abuse and Alcoholism (NIAAA). (2000a). Alcohol metabolism. *Alcohol Alert, 35,* PH371. Retrieved January 17, 2009, from http://pubs.niaaa.nih.gov/publications/aa35.htm

National Institute on Alcohol Abuse and Alcoholism (NIAAA). (2000b). Alcohol and nutrition. *Alcohol Alert, 22,* PH346. Retrieved January 17, 2009, from http://pubs.niaaa.nih.gov/publications/aa22.htm

National Institutes of Health, National Institute on Alcohol Abuse and Alcoholism. (2005). *Helping patients who drink too much.* Retrieved March 27, 2009, from http://pubs.niaaa.nih.gov/publications/Practitioner/CliniciansGuide2005/guide.pdf

O'Keefe, J. H., Bybee, K. A., & Lavie, C. J. (2007). Alcohol and cardiovascular disease. *Journal of the American College of Cardiology, 50,* 1009–1014.

Orbeta, R. L., Overpeck, M. D., Ramcharran, D., Kogan, M. D., & Ledsky, R. (2006). High caffeine intake in adolescents: Associations with difficulty sleeping and feeling tired in the morning. *Journal of Adolescent Health, 38,* 451–453.

Parsons, K. K., & Coffman, T. M. (2007). The renin-angiotensin system: It's all in your head. *Journal of Clinical Investigation, 117,* 873–876.

Pittler, M. H., Verster, J. C., & Ernst, E. (2005). Interventions for preventing or treating alcohol hangover: Systematic review of randomised controlled trials. *British Medical Journal, 331,* 1515–1518.

Reissig, C. J., Strain, E. C., & Griffiths, R. R. (2009). Caffeinated energy drinks—A growing problem. *Drug & Alcohol Dependence, 1,* 1–10.

Sagawa, S., Miki, K., Tajima, F., Choi, J. K., Keil, L. C., Shiraki, K., et al. (1992). Effect of dehydration n thirst and drinking during immersion in men. *Journal of Applied Physiology, 72,* 128–134.

Sawka, M. N., Burke, L. M., Eichner, E. R., Maughan, R.J., Montain, S. J., & Stachenfeld, N. S. (2007). American College of Sports Medicine position stand: Exercise and fluid replacement. *Medicine, Science, Sports, & Exercise, 39,* 377–390.

Shaffer, E. A. (2006). Gallstone disease: Epidemiology of gallbladder stone disease. *Best Practice & Research: Clinical Gastroenterology, 20,* 981–996.

Shapiro, R. E. (2008). Caffeine and headaches. *Current Pain and Headache Reports, 12,* 311–315.

Shirreffs, S. M., Merson, S. J., Fraser, S. M., & Archer, D. T. (2004). The effects of fluid restriction on hydration status and subjective feelings in man. *British Journal of Nutrition, 91,* 951–958.

Stickel, F., Hoehn, B., Schuppan, D., & Seitz, H. K. (2003). Nutrition therapy in alcoholic liver disease. *Alimentary Pharmacology and Therapeutics, 18,* 357–373.

Szinnai, G., Schachinger, H., Arnaud, M. J., Linder, L., & Keller, U. (2005). Effect of water deprivation on cognitive-motor performance in healthy men and women. *American Journal of Physiology. Regulatory, Integrative, Comparative Physiology, 289,* 275–280.

Thomas, D. R., Cote, R., Lawhorne, L., Levenson, S. A., Rubenstein, L. Z., Smith, D. A. et al. (2008). Understanding clinical dehydration and its treatment. *Journal of the American Medical Directors Association, 9,* 292–301.

Tunnicliffe, J. M., Erdman, K. A., Reimer, R. A., Lun, V., & Shearer, J. (2008). Consumption of dietary caffeine and coffee in physically active populations: Physiological interactions. *Applied Physiology, Nutrition & Metabolism, 33,* 1301–1310.

United States Department of Agriculture (USDA). (2005). *Dietary guidelines for Americans.* Retrieved January 17, 2009, from http://www.healthierus.gov/dietaryguidelines

United States Department of Health and Human Services, Substance Abuse and Mental Health Services Administration. (2007). *Effects of alcohol on a fetus.* Retrieved January 17, 2009, from http://www.fasdcenter.samhsa.gov/documents/wynk_effects_fetus.pdf

United States Surgeon General. (2005). *U.S. Surgeon General releases advisory on alcohol use in pregnancy.* Retrieved January 17, 2009, from http://www.surgeongeneral.gov/pressreleases/sg02222005.html

van Dam, R. M. (2008). Coffee consumption and risk of type 2 diabetes, cardiovascular diseases, and cancer. *Applied Physiology, Nutrition & Metabolism, 33,* 1269–1283.

Vivanti, A., Harvey, K., Ash, S., & Battistutta, D. (2008). Clinical assessment of dehydration in older people admitted to hospital: What are the strongest indicators? *Archives of Gerontology and Geriatrics, 47,* 340–355.

Walsh, N. P., Laing, S. J., Oliver, S. J., Montague, J. C., Walters, R., & Bilzon, J. L. (2004). Saliva parameters as potential indices of hydration status during acute dehydration. *Medicine and Science in Sports and Exercise, 36,* 1535–1542.

8 Energy Balance

WHAT WILL YOU LEARN?

1. To define energy and categorize how it is supplied by the diet.
2. To summarize the components of energy expenditure.
3. To examine energy balance and factors that contribute to altered energy balance.
4. To formulate nursing interventions that target improving energy balance for weight loss or weight gain.

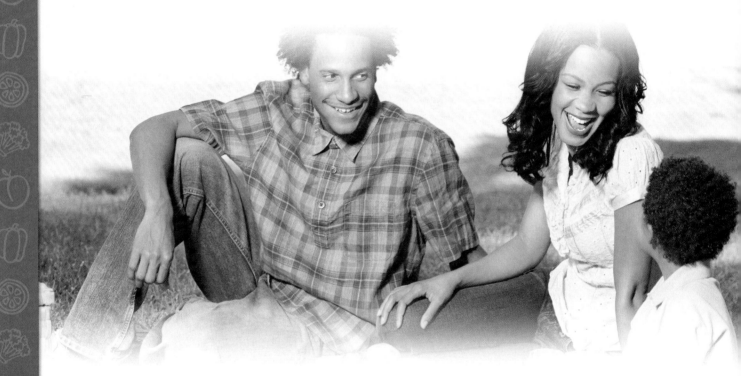

DID YOU KNOW?

▶ A calorie is really a kilocalorie and contains 1,000 calories.

▶ Alcohol contains almost twice the amount of kilocalories per gram compared with carbohydrate or protein.

▶ Recommended levels of moderate physical activity can be accumulated during the day to reach the same energy expenditure compared with the same amount of moderate activity done in one time span.

▶ Metabolic rate can be indirectly measured by measuring oxygen consumption and carbon dioxide production.

▶ To gain or lose a pound of body fat, energy balance must be altered by approximately 3,500 kilocalories.

KEY TERMS

bomb calorimeter, *163*

energy balance, *163*

energy expenditure, *163*

indirect calorimetry, *168*

kilocalories, *163*

kilojoule, *163*

nonexercise activity thermogenesis (NEAT), *167*

thermic effect of food, *166*

What Is Energy and Energy Balance?

Energy is a term used to describe available usable power, whether it is in chemical, mechanical, electrical, or other form. Fossil fuel used to power an engine and solar radiation used to generate electricity are forms of energy. In the human body, available energy is derived from the stored chemical energy in the foods we eat to allow us to power our bodies and produce heat to maintain body temperature.

Energy balance is the relationship between energy intake and energy used by the body to perform physical functions, such as respiration or digestion, as well as physical activity. The term **energy expenditure** is used to describe all the energy used by the body.

The chemical form of energy in foods is measured in units called **kilocalories,** or kcalories (kcals). One calorie is the amount of energy it takes to raise the temperature of 1 gm of water by 1°C, whereas a kilocalorie denotes the energy needed to do the same but with 1,000 gm (or 1 kg) of water. Although most people refer to the energy in food simply as *calories,* the correct term is actually *kilo*calories because it contains 1,000 times more energy than a calorie.

The basis for measuring the kilocalories in foods is a device called the **bomb calorimeter.** Food is burned inside the calorimeter surrounded by a chamber of water that is insulated on the outside. The heat energy derived from the combustion of the food's chemical energy will increase the temperature of the water in the calorimeter and can thus be measured. Figure 8-1 ■ depicts a bomb calorimeter. Likewise, the amount of energy expended by the body can be measured by the heat that is produced using similar science where a person is immersed in water and temperature is monitored under laboratory conditions. These methods of measuring kilocalories in food and those expended by the body are used in the laboratory setting but not in general practice. More practical methods are discussed later in the chapter.

Kilojoule is another term used around the world to measure energy. A kilojoule is a term from physics meaning the amount of energy or force needed to move 1 kg with an acceleration of 1 meter per second. More simply, 1 kilojoule is equivalent to 0.239 kilocalories.

Energy Intake

The body derives energy from the metabolism of carbohydrate, protein, fat, and alcohol that are contained in foods and beverages. Carbohydrate and protein each yield 4 kilocalories/gm. Alcohol contains 7 kilocalories/gm, whereas fat has 9. The end products of metabolism are carbon dioxide, water, and energy in the form of adenosine triphosphate, or ATP. Figure 8-2 ■ depicts the interrelationship of the metabolism of the macronutrients carbohydrate, protein, and fat and the resulting formation of the body's source of energy for physical functioning, ATP. Alcohol metabolism yields some by-products that enter this

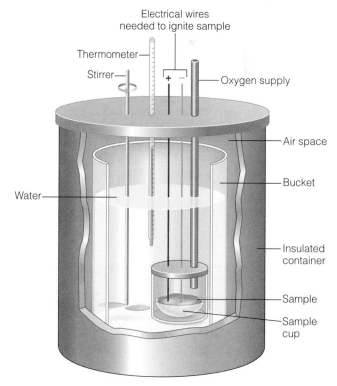

■ **FIGURE 8-1 Bomb Calorimeter.**

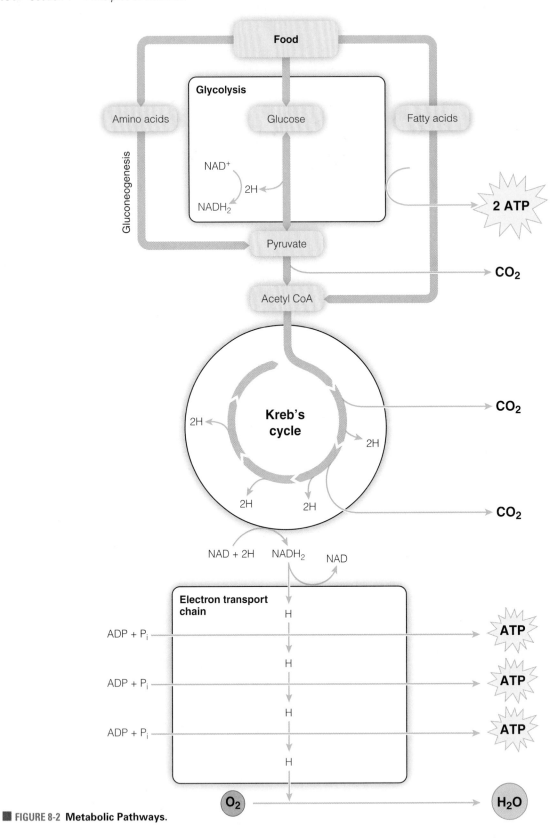

■ FIGURE 8-2 **Metabolic Pathways.**

same general metabolic cycle, but the remainder takes another pathway that yields production of long-chain fatty acids.

How Is Energy Intake Measured?

It is impractical for all foods to be burned in a bomb calorimeter to determine the energy content. Instead, simple calculations are done based on basic knowledge about food content. Scientific databases exist that contain analyses of the nutritional content of foods based on laboratory study and food manufacturer information. The United States Department of Agriculture's well-known Nutrient Data Laboratory is an example and is available online and in book form. Additionally, many commercially available computer software programs exist that use such databases and are available for a fee online or for downloading to a computer or similar device. An individual can record all dietary intake for a day or series of days. Information on the energy intake or a single food can be calculated using these available resources or a manufacturer label, combining any items used in a recipe to arrive at a total. When only amounts of carbohydrate, protein, fat, and alcohol are known, calculations can be easily done to determine kcalorie content. Box 8-1 outlines an example of how this is done.

Energy Expenditure

The total amount of energy used by the body over the course of a day is comprised of several components that result in each person having a unique energy requirement based on these variables. Energy expenditure can be measured indirectly or calculated using various equations.

What Affects Energy Expenditure?

Total energy expenditure, often abbreviated TEE, is the sum of all energy-requiring processes in the body as well as any physical activity.

Basal Metabolism

Basal metabolism refers to the energy required for the vital functions of the body at complete rest. This component of total energy expenditure is also referred to as basal metabolic rate (BMR). This component of energy expenditure encompasses the energy required to sustain metabolic activity in cells and tissues and maintain respiration, circulation, and the function of the brain and other organs (Institute of Medicine [IOM], 2002). The production of heat to maintain core body temperature requires energy that is also part of these basic energy needs. Additionally, any energy required for synthesizing new tissue, as occurs in growth and development, is included as part of basal metabolism. When BMR is expressed as kcalories expended over 24 hours, it is called the basal energy expenditure, or BEE. A related term, *resting energy expenditure* (REE), differs from BEE in that it includes the energy used to rest quietly and awake following a meal. REE is also expressed as kcalories/24 hours.

The BMR of individuals varies depending on body size, and more specifically on fat-free body mass. Fat-free mass includes muscle and other tissue, such as organs, which are more metabolically active than fat tissue. The brain, heart, and liver are the most metabolically active tissues in the body (IOM, 2002). These tissues require more energy to function than does an equal weight of fat tissue. Individuals with higher body weight or greater fat-free mass have higher basal metabolic needs than lower weight or less muscular individuals of otherwise similar size. Gender differences in energy expenditure may be largely due to larger skeletal muscle mass and organ size rather than any gender-specific differences in tissue metabolism (IOM, 2002). It is a subject of debate whether BEE automatically declines with age or is more closely related to loss of muscle mass, which could be overcome with resistance training. Traditional belief is that, despite a stable body weight, metabolic rate declines by 1% to 2% per decade of adulthood with a greater decline beginning in the fifth decade (IOM, 2002). Common lore is that metabolism declines following menopause in women and later in men. The Evidence-Based Practice Box: Menopause and Weight Gain addresses the issue of basal metabolic changes with aging.

BOX 8-1	Calculating Kilocalories

The amount of kcalories in a food can be determined whenever the amount of protein, fat, carbohydrate, and alcohol are known. This is based on the knowledge that:

- Carbohydrate has 4 kcals/gm
- Protein has 4 kcals/gm
- Fat has 9 kcals/gm
- Alcohol has 7 kcals/gm

Example: Emma is a collegiate field hockey player and wants to know whether she is meeting her target kcalorie intake of 2,500 kcals but only collected information on carbohydrate, protein, and fat intake from the food labels that she had in her apartment. On 1 day, she consumed 75 gm of protein, 30 gm of fat, and 350 gm of carbohydrate.

75 gm protein × 4 kcal/gm = 300 kcals
30 gm fat × 9 kcal/gm = 270 kcals
350 gm carbohydrate × 4 kcal/gm = 1,400 kcals
Total 1,970 kcals

- What feedback could the nurse give to Emma about her kcalorie intake? If Emma suggested including a cereal bar that had no fat, 10 gm of protein, and 30 gm of carbohydrate in a serving before practice, how many kcalories would this add to her intake?

EVIDENCE-BASED PRACTICE RESEARCH BOX

Menopause and Weight Gain

Clinical Problem: Menopausal women frequently report weight gain, expanded waistlines, and increased abdominal fat. Is this an inevitable consequence of menopause?

Research Findings: Menopause is precipitated by hormonal changes, primarily a decrease in estrogen and progesterone production by the ovaries. Following menopause, women are more prone to develop cardiovascular disease and metabolic syndrome. There is increased deposition of abdominal fat that seems to be related to decreased circulating estrogen (Koskova, Petrasek, Vondra, & Skibova, 2007; Toth, Tchernof, Sites, & Poehlman, 2000). Further, administration of estrogen seems to ameliorate that effect (D'Eon, Rogers, Stancheva, & Greenberg, 2008; Jensen et al., 2003; Mattsson & Olsson, 2007). Concurrent with menopause, aging results in decreased BMR, REE, and TEE when skeletal muscle mass diminishes (Day, Gozansky, Van Pelt, Schwartz, & Kohrt, 2005; Roberts & Dallal, 2005).

Given the menopausal changes that occur independent of BMI upon entering menopause, researchers have studied interventions that ameliorate the effects of menopause on weight gain and body composition changes. Longitudinal studies of large cohorts of racially and ethnically diverse women have demonstrated that regular physical activity (walking or participating in a "10,000 steps" program) is associated with a lower BMI, less body fat, and better serum lipid profile. There were small, but statistically insignificant, changes in waist and hip circumference, leading researchers to conclude that regular physical activity can prevent or attenuate weight gain and increases in BMI (Brown, Williams, Ford, Ball, & Dobson, 2005; Evans & Racette, 2006; Krumm, Dessieux, Andrews, & Thompson, 2006; Sternfeld, Bhat, Wang, Sharp, & Quesenberry, Jr., 2005; Sternfeld et al., 2004; Thompson, Rakow, & Perdue, 2004).

Nursing Implications: There is convincing evidence that weight gain, increased waist circumference, and elevated lipid levels are not inevitable with menopause. Lifestyle interventions through management of dietary intake and physical activity should be encouraged as women approach and proceed through menopause.

CRITICAL THINKING QUESTION

1. How should the nurse respond to the 50-year-old woman who says she is resigned to gaining weight and getting flabby as she goes through menopause?

Regulation of body temperature utilizes differing amounts of energy depending on body size. Infants and children have relatively greater loss of heat through the skin surface because of the higher body surface area-to-weight ratio in a smaller body (Donahoo, Levine, & Melanson, 2004). This results in increased energy expenditure to maintain body temperature when that calculation is expressed in relation to body weight. Maintenance of core body temperature occurs within a very narrow range of temperature for healthy individuals. When this thermoregulation is challenged, there can be an alteration in energy used for heat production. Fever causes elevated energy expenditure as the body responds to this condition with increased heart rate and respiration as well as heat production. A long-held clinical nutrition practice is to adjust energy expenditure calculations by a 7% increase for every 1°F elevation in body temperature above normal. Although this may not result in significantly elevated metabolic needs in a mildly ill individual, it has been demonstrated to be of clinical significance in the already critically ill client who has elevated metabolic needs because of illness (Frankenfield, Smith, Cooney, Blosser, & Sarson, 1997). Extreme ambient temperatures may also alter energy expenditure. Temperatures low enough to cause shivering as a way to produce heat will result in increased energy expenditure to support the mechanical work of increased muscle activity associated with shivering (IOM, 2002). Shivering associated with the chills from a fever will compound the increased energy expenditure of the elevated body temperature alone (Holtzclaw, 2004). Very high ambient temperatures may temporarily increase energy expenditure when performing physical tasks, but this effect is quickly lessened as the individual becomes acclimatized to the environmental conditions (IOM, 2002). Under normal temperature ranges, the body is able to maintain core temperature with little change in energy expenditure.

Growth and development are variables that affect basal energy needs. Infancy, childhood, adolescence, and pregnancy are times when synthesis of new tissue requires additional energy over that of baseline needs. Additionally, increased energy is required during lactation in order to produce breast milk. Lifespan Box: Energy Expenditure during Growth and Development outlines further how growth and development affect BEE.

Thermic Effect of Food

The digestion, metabolism, and storage of nutrients require energy. This metabolic cost is referred to as the **thermic effect of food.** In the past, the term *specific dynamic action* was used to describe this effect, but its use is waning. On average, the energy expenditure from the thermic effect of food is approximately 10% of the energy value of the food itself (IOM, 2002). This majority of this increase in expenditure occurs within a few hours of a meal before returning to baseline (Compher, Frankenfield, Keim, & Roth-Yousey, 2006). Protein has the highest thermic effect at 20% to 30% of the energy value of the food consumed because of the energy required to metabolize

MyNursingKit NAT Energy Calculator

Lifespan

Energy Expenditure during Growth

Growth refers to increasing height and weight as well as changes in body composition and organ systems. Energy needs are elevated during growth for tissue synthesis and energy deposits.

Infancy: Energy requirements for growth when expressed per kilogram of body weight are highest during the first month of life when 35% of energy needs are for growth. Infants double birth weight by age 6 months and triple it at age 1 year.

Childhood: Energy requirements for growth drop to 3% of total energy requirements through childhood.

Adolescence: Energy requirements for growth and development increase during puberty to about 4% of total needs. Increased muscle, adipose, an expanded cardiovascular system, and increased bone mass are among the new tissues requiring energy for synthesis.

Pregnancy: Energy requirements increase during pregnancy to support the needs for fetal growth and development as well as the synthesis of new maternal tissue, such as breast tissue and adipose.

Lactation: Energy requirements during lactation are increased to support the synthesis of breast milk. Breast milk contains 0.67 kcalorie/gm of milk, amounting to a daily energy cost of approximately 500 kcalories.

Source: IOM, 2002.

amino acids, synthesize proteins, and metabolize urea and glucose from proteins. Alcohol has a thermic effect ranging up to 13%, higher than that of carbohydrate at 5% to 10%. In alcoholics, the thermic effect of alcohol can be elevated even further because of a change in the pathway of alcohol metabolism when excessive quantities are chronically consumed (Compher et al., 2006; Lieber, 1991). The thermic effect of fat is less than 5% of the energy contained in the food. Overall, the thermic effect of food influences TEE in a minor way.

Physical Activity

In addition to the energy required for the inner functions of the body, energy is required to perform physical work of any kind. Whether it is a nonstrenuous activity such as sitting or extreme physical work, such as chopping wood or running a triathlon, there is a metabolic cost to performing the physical work. Some use the term *activity thermogenesis* to describe the energy used (and heat production) from physical activity. Whichever term is preferred, the physical activity component of energy expenditure can be further subdivided to include actual exercise and nonexercise activities, also called **nonexercise activity thermogenesis (NEAT).** NEAT includes any activity that involves some muscle contraction and encompasses activities of daily living, including talking and sitting. Fidgeting is considered a component of NEAT and may contribute to the increased TEE observed between the lean "couch potato" and their heavier "couch potato" coun-

terpart (Levine et al., 2005). Some researchers report that the energy expended from fidgeting and other spontaneous forms of physical activity can total hundreds of kcalories in a day or more (Levine, 2007; Ravussin, 2005).

The energy expenditure associated with each of these physical activity components varies widely, depending on the intensity and duration of the activity. Intensity refers to how strenuous the activity is, which in turn is related to oxygen consumption during the activity. The more intense the activity, the higher the energy expenditure is per minute. Likewise, the longer the duration of the activity, the higher the overall energy expenditure is for that activity. The energy expended from physical activity is usually expressed as a ratio or percentage of BEE, referred to as physical activity level, or PAL. PALs are categorized as sedentary, low active, active, and very active by the IOM. More commonly, the terms *sedentary, moderate, and vigorous activity* are used to describe activity level. Based on laboratory measurements of energy expenditure during physical activity, data are available that make it possible to calculate the energy (kcalories) used per minute of a given activity for various body weights. An example of this is included in Table 8-1 and is also available from a multitude of Internet-based and computer software programs. Any given activity expends more energy per minute in a heavier person compared with someone lighter because of a basic rule of physics regarding moving mass over a distance. It takes more energy to move a heavier mass than it does a lighter mass.

How Is Energy Expenditure Measured?

Energy expenditure can be measured directly under experimental conditions that resemble a creation of a bomb calorimeter for humans where heat transfer into a small body of water or thermally sealed metabolic chamber is carefully measured under controlled conditions. This is not practical

Table 8-1 Physical Activity Level		
Activity Level	**Kcalories/min 125 pounds**	**Kcalories/min 160 pounds**
Sedentary		
• Cooking	2.7	3.5
• Light housework	2.3	3.0
• Sitting	1.2	1.5
Moderate		
• Gardening, yard work	5.0	6.7
• Golf, walking w/clubs	4.6	6.2
• Mowing lawn, power mower	3.5	4.8
• Walking, 4 mph	4.5	6.1
Vigorous		
• Jogging, 5 mph	9.3	12.4
• Skating, roller or ice	5.9	7.9
• Skiing, downhill	5.7	7.6
• Swimming, 55 yd/min	7.8	10.3
• Tennis	6.0	7.9

in most conditions and not a method often employed except in some research settings. Instead, **indirect calorimetry** is used to measure energy expenditure using several types of technology.

Indirect calorimetry measures energy expenditure using the knowledge that carbon dioxide, water, and heat are products of metabolism in proportion to the amount of oxygen consumed. Indirect calorimetry calculates energy expenditure by measuring these two respiratory gases and comparing oxygen consumption with carbon dioxide production. Respiratory gases are analyzed in a metabolic chamber or by using a canopy hood system, a portable metabolic cart that uses a mask or mouthpiece, or with handheld devices.

The nurse working in the critical care setting should be familiar with the use of indirect calorimetry because it is felt to be more accurate than simply using predictive equations described here, provided that correct technique is used (Compher et al., 2006). Additionally, the use of handheld devices is becoming commonplace in wellness locations that offer fitness and nutrition assessment services, such as gyms and sports centers. It is essential that proper technique be used or measurement error will occur. An individual should be in the resting state and have avoided any substances, such as caffeine, that affect metabolic rate. Box 8-2 describes some practice guidelines for measuring energy expenditure with indirect calorimetry.

A doubly labeled water technique is now being used in the research setting to more accurately measure energy expenditure than by gas exchange methods. The turnover of labeled isotopes of water is monitored after many days to assess their disappearance from urine. A comparison between the two isotopes allows an estimate of carbon dioxide production without all the cumbersome measurements associated with indirect calorimetry (Heymsfield, Harp, Rowell, Nguyen, & Pietrobelli, 2006). The source of carbon dioxide produced during metabolism is from oxygen consumption, which in turn is related to the water produced during metabolism. Such technology was used to develop the latest recommendations for energy intake across many age groups in the general population (IOM, 2002).

When indirect calorimetry is not an available option, predictive equations are used to estimate energy expenditure. Harris-Benedict, Mifflin–St. Jeor, and many other equations have been developed to estimate energy needs based on height, weight, gender, and age. Box 8-3 outlines the more commonly used equations.

Despite the widespread use, such equations are prone to a higher margin of error compared with actual measured expenditure because they have been derived on a set population, often with small sample size, and yet are generalized for use with the general population. Some equations were developed using healthy, normal weight individuals yet are used

---

| BOX 8-2 | Indirect Calorimetry Guidelines |

Energy expenditure measured using indirect calorimetry must be done under controlled conditions to minimize factors known to alter metabolic rate. The following influences should be monitored before measuring energy expenditure:

Activity level:

Rest: Client should rest 10–20 minutes before beginning measurement and be in a comfortable sitting or reclining position.

Prior physical activity: Vigorous activity should be avoided 14 hours prior to measurement. Moderate activity should be avoided 2 hours prior.

Intake:

Fasting: A minimum fast of 5 hours should be observed to avoid the thermic effect of food.

Alcohol: No alcohol should be had during the fast.

Caffeine: No caffeine should be had during the fast.

Dietary supplements: No stimulant-type dietary supplements, such as bitter orange or synephrine, should be taken 4 hours before measurement.

Nicotine:

No nicotine should be used for 2 hours before the measurement.

Note: Handheld devices may not be used to measure energy expenditure in individuals who are on a respirator. Some medications, such as sedatives, and fever alter metabolic rate. Repeat measurements should be done when these effects are present or end.

- What effect would smoking or a weight-loss pill with bitter orange have on the measurement of energy expenditure with indirect calorimetry?

Sources: Branson & Johanninian, 2004; Compher et al., 2006; Haugen, Chan, & Li, 2007.

---

with the critically ill or obese, leading to estimation errors. For example, the Harris-Benedict equation estimates energy expenditure within 10% of measured expenditure in approximately 64% of obese individuals but results in error 36% of the time. Thirty percent of these errors are overestimates of energy needs (American Dietetic Association Evidence Analysis Library, 2008). Mifflin–St Jeor accurately estimates energy needs in the same population 80% of the time and is the preferred equation for use in predicting the metabolic needs of nonobese and obese individuals (Frankenfield et al., 2005). It is a practice of some clinicians to alter these equations by using ideal or adjusted body weight when estimating the energy needs of the obese population. This practice leads to unacceptable errors in estimation and is not supported as a best practice (American Dietetic Association, 2008; Frankenfield et al., 2005; Ireton-Jones, 2005). No well-accepted equation exists that is specific to the older adult and

BOX 8-3	**Predictive Equations for Estimating Energy Expenditure (kcalories)**

Harris-Benedict
- Males = 66.45 + 13.75 × wt + 5 × ht − 6.75 × age
- Females = 655.09 + 9.56 × wt + 1.84 × ht − 4.67 × age

Mifflin–St Jeor
- Males = 9.99 × wt + 6.25 × ht − 4.92 × age + 5
- Females = 9.99 × wt + 6.25 × ht − 4.92 × age − 161

World Health Organization
- Males, age 18–30 years = 15.3 × wt + 679
- Females, age 18–30 years = 14.7 × wt + 496

Age: in years, wt = weight in kg, ht = height in meters.

- Some practitioners use the rough estimate of 1 kcal/kg/hour to estimate basal metabolic needs. How do the results compare to these equations if you use yourself as an example? What factors are omitted with this type of estimate?

Sources: Food & Agriculture Organization/World Health Organization/United Nations University, 1985; Harris & Benedict, 1919; Mifflin et al., 1990.

research is limited regarding the accuracy of standard equations when used with this population.

Energy Balance

Energy balance is the relationship between energy intake and energy expenditure as depicted in Figure 8-3 ■. A balance occurs when intake approximates expenditure. Unlike vitamin or mineral balance where alterations may not be readily apparent, imbalances in energy can be monitored through body weight (IOM, 2002). For most healthy adults, energy balance fosters weight maintenance because there is neither an excess nor a deficit of kcalories to support gain or loss of body mass. In children, energy balance should foster normal growth and development. Negative energy balance results when there is insufficient energy available to support the needs of the body and weight loss occurs. Negative energy balance occurs because of insufficient intake, increased expenditure, or a combination of the two. Positive energy balance occurs when energy intake exceeds energy expenditure because of increased intake, decreased expenditure, or a combination of the two. Parents or caregivers might express concern to the nurse about a child's energy balance. Practice

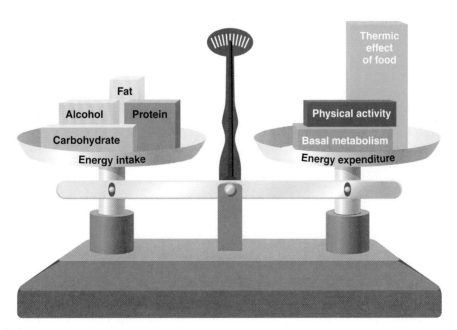

■ FIGURE 8-3 **Energy Balance.**

PRACTICE PEARL

Energy Balance in Children

Parents or caregivers may express concern about whether a child is eating sufficiently. The nurse can assure them that normal growth and development is a positive indicator that the child's energy needs are being met. Children who do not receive sufficient energy intake can develop a slowed growth rate, also called growth faltering.

Pearl: Energy Balance in Children offers a quick way to assess a child's energy balance.

In theory, energy balance is a simple equation that compares intake and expenditure. In reality, many more components influence this balance directly or indirectly. Some individuals are able to maintain body weight within a small range despite fluctuations in energy balance, whereas for others such fluctuations result in weight change. Biology, including genetics and hormones, and a host of other factors can influence appetite, satiety, and metabolism in ways that make the energy balance equation less simple than it appears. Hot Topic Box: Is Energy Balance Only About Intake and Expenditure? discusses some of these influences and how they may affect energy balance.

hot Topic

Is Energy Balance Only About Intake and Expenditure?

Energy balance seems to be just a math equation: Energy Intake = Energy Expenditure. Although basic energy balance does constitute these components, there are many influences that affect the equation, especially why or how much energy intake occurs. These are just a few examples that are under current investigation:

Hormonal influences—There are many hormones that affect appetite and modulate satiation, the feeling of fullness and satisfaction that terminates eating and delays onset of the next meal or snack. A host of peptides, protein-based substances, are responsible for the cascade of response to hunger and satiety that involves the gastrointestinal tract and feedback to the brain. Ghrelin is one that is synthesized in the stomach and small intestine and stimulates appetite. Research has focused on why some individuals have high baseline ghrelin levels while others have low. Weight loss is found to increase ghrelin. Leptin is another peptide and is produced by adipose tissue in proportion to fat stores, acting on the brain to decrease feeding. Individuals have varying levels of leptin and some respond differently following food intake. Additional peptides are being investigated for both short- and long-acting influences on appetite and feeding. Exercise has been reported to alter some peptides and not others, leading to a short-term reduction in appetite soon after moderate exercise. More research is needed before firm conclusions can

be made regarding the hormonal influence on energy intake in general.

Food types—Much focus has been given to the type of foods provided or consumed and the effect on energy intake. From a food behavior standpoint, it has been shown that simply providing larger portions of foods leads to increased intake at the given meal and overall; individuals do not seem to compensate for the increased portion at later meals. This has been reported for both restaurant and family meals as well as in food packaging.

Liquid forms of intake is another topic of much debate. Most liquids elicit little satiation yet can deliver significant kcalories to the diet, which largely go uncompensated. Clear beverages, such as soda, some juices, sports drinks, alcohol, and flavored teas or coffees, do not cause lasting fullness yet can be significant sources of kcalories in the diet. In both school-age children and adults, caloric beverages intake has risen over the last 30 years and now provides up to 20% of all kcalories. Large-portioned beverages that are frequently offered in restaurants as a value option are popular despite the caloric price tag.

The effect of protein-containing foods is another area of research on satiation and energy balance. Protein is believed to have a greater effect on satiation than an equal kcalorie serving of carbohydrate or fat and, therefore, may contribute to less energy intake. The metabolism of protein also has a higher thermic effect on energy expenditure than does carbohydrate or fat. More research is needed to determine at what level of overall protein intake this potential benefit is seen and what negative consequences are associated with elevated protein intake before advice can be offered to the general population.

CT? The nurse should include assessment of liquid intake when assessing overall dietary intake. What advice can the nurse offer to the client who has gained unwanted weight regarding liquid intake?

Sources: Cummings & Overduin, 2007; Mattes, 2006; Paddon-Jones et al., 2008; Storey, Forshee, & Anderson, 2006.

Recommendations for Energy Intake and Expenditure

The subject of energy balance is widespread in both the popular press and medical literature because of the burgeoning obesity epidemic in North America. Consider that two-thirds of Americans are overweight or obese and that over half of all waking hours are spent doing sedentary activities (Centers for Disease Control and Prevention [CDC], 2008; Matthews et al., 2008). Over 60% of adults never participate in any type of vigorous physical activity (Plies & Lethbridge-Cejku, 2007). Among older adults, approximately 30% do not engage in any leisure-time physical activity (Kruger, Ham, & Sanker, 2008) despite reports that those who are active have lower mortality rates in healthy older adulthood than healthy but inactive peers (Manini et al., 2008). Over 65% of school-age children do not meet weekly recommended levels of physical activity yet over 35% watch 3 or more hours of television daily (Eaton et al., 2008). Considering the energy consumption side of the energy balance equation, it is reported that the increasing propensity to serve larger food portions, whether in a restaurant or through food packaging, leads to an increased intake and overall increased energy consumption by both children and adults (Diliberti, Bordi, Conklin, Roe, & Rolls, 2004; Fisher & Kral, 2008). It is with the public health issue of obesity in mind that national recommendations are made regarding energy balance with the goal of preventing obesity while providing adequate energy for nutritional health.

The IOM delineates estimated energy requirements (EER) for adults and children across the lifespan with the goal of meeting energy needs for important body functions, growth and development, physical activity, and good health. These are recommendations that are made for population groups as a whole; individual differences will occur because of unique physical needs and physical activity levels. A regis-

tered dietitian is able to assess these differences for individuals and recommend specific advice when there is a question about energy balance. Recommendations do not encompass advice for managing energy imbalances leading to weight gain or weight loss, which are discussed in Chapter 17. In addition, the IOM makes specific recommendations regarding physical activity as part of its overall approach to energy balance. *The Dietary Guidelines for Americans* is another national scientific body of advice that outlines energy and physical activity recommendations. Table 8-2 outlines both of these national recommendations along with the Surgeon General's advice on physical activity.

Wellness Concerns

Wellness concerns regarding energy balance include the effects of both negative and positive energy balance. Before the nurse can address appropriate interventions for energy imbalance, the cause of the imbalance must be discerned using

---

Table 8-2   Energy and Physical Activity Recommendations*

Estimated Energy Requirements (EER) (kcalories)

Children: 0–36 mos = Total energy expenditure + energy deposition
- 0–3 mos = (89 × wt − 100) + 175
- 4–6 mos = (89 × wt − 100) + 56
- 7–12 mos = (89 × wt − 100) + 22
- 13–36 mos = (89 × wt − 100) + 20
- 3–8 yrs, female = 135.3 − (30.8 × age) + PA × (10 × wt + 934 × ht) + 20
- 3–8 yrs, male = 88.5 − (61.9 × age) + PA × (26.7 × wt + 903 × ht) + 20
- 9–18 yrs, female = 135.3 − (30.8 × age) + PA × (10 × wt + 934 × ht) + 25
- 9–18 yrs, male = 88.5 − (61.9 × age) + PA × (26.7 × wt + 903 × ht) + 25

Adults:
- Females = 354 − (6.91 × age) + PA × (9.36 × wt + 726 × ht)
- Males = 662 − (9.53 × age) + PA × (15.91 × wt + 539 × ht)

Pregnancy:
Prepregnancy EER + increased energy expended with pregnancy + energy deposition
- 1st trimester = EER + 0 + 0
- 2nd trimester = EER + 160 + 180
- 3rd trimester = EER + 272 + 180

Lactation:
Lactation EER = prepregnancy EER + milk energy – loss of energy stores
- 1st 6 mos = EER + 500 − 170
- After 6 mos = EER + 400 − 0

Age: in years, wt: weight in kg, ht: height in meters.
PA: physical activity factor of 1, 1.16, 1.31, or 1.56 based on sedentary, light active, active, or very active overall activity, respectively.

Physical Activity Recommendations

Children:
- At least 60 minutes of moderate physical activity on most days.
- Minimize sedentary behavior by limiting television watching and video viewing to 2 hours or less per day.

Adults:
- At least 30 minutes of moderate activity on most days.
- Many adults may require up to 60 minutes of moderate activity most days to prevent weight gain.
Physical activity can be initiated slowly and increased over time to meet recommendations.
Activities can be split into increments and combined to meet total time recommendation.
More activity can be incorporated into everyday life activities.

---

*Energy needs for each lifespan stage are discussed further in the respective chapters on pregnancy, lactation, children, and adults.
Sources: AAP, 2003; IOM, 2002; Surgeon General, 2007; USDA & Department of Health and Human Services, 2005.

the team approach. In addition to any medical reasons for altered energy balance, a thorough assessment of energy intake and expenditure should be done. Nutrition assessment is discussed in detail in Chapter 12.

Positive Energy Balance: Weight Gain

Positive energy balance can occur because of any combination of excessive energy consumption compared to needs or from too little physical activity. An excess energy balance of 3,500 kcalories can lead to a gain of 1 pound of body fat. This can occur over weeks, months, or more. When weight gain increases risk of other diseases or conditions such as diabetes mellitus or hypertension, nutrition intervention is indicated. Nursing interventions for positive energy balance should target the aspects of energy consumption or expenditure that contribute to the imbalance. Portion size, caloric density of food choices, and frequency of intake are possible targets. Caloric density refers to the amount of kcalories in a given weight or portion of food. For example, a 12-ounce soda has 150 kcalories, whereas an equal portion of water has zero. The soda is more calorically dense. Similarly, toast with butter has more calories than toast with jelly. Foods that contribute high-caloric value but have little or no nutritional value are said to be sources of "empty calories." The nurse can explore with a client what foods contribute significant kcalories or empty calories and solutions to modifying intake of these. The nurse can brainstorm with the client ways to create a 3,500 kcalorie deficit over weeks or months by adjusting energy intake or expenditure. For example, a 100 kcalorie deficit/day over 35 days will yield a 3,500 kcalorie negative energy balance. Client Education Checklist: Altering Energy Balance presents a preliminary approach to this issue. Chapter 17 discusses this in detail.

The nurse should also address physical activity level and assist the client in improving opportunities to be more physically active when appropriate. Barriers to physical activity should be assessed in order to collaboratively brainstorm solutions to them. Almost 25% of school-age children do not participate in moderate to vigorous physical activity for 60 minutes on even 1 day of the week (Eaton et al., 2008). For children, unsafe neighborhoods or inability to walk or bicycle to school can be a barrier to adequate physical activity. The nurse can suggest safe indoor activities, such as dancing or an exercise video. Cultural Considerations Box: Ethnicity

---

CLIENT EDUCATION CHECKLIST	Altering Energy Balance
Intervention	**Example**
Assess reason for energy imbalance.	Assess energy intake and expenditure.
Explain energy imbalance and provide examples that pertain to the individual.	Energy balance is the relationship between energy intake and energy expenditure. Energy is derived from carbohydrates, protein, fats, and alcohol in the diet. Weight gain occurs when energy intake exceeds energy expenditure. Weight loss occurs when energy intake is less than energy expenditure. An imbalance of 3,500 kcalories will alter weight by 1 pound.
Brainstorm with the client solutions to the energy imbalance issue.	Examples of contributors to energy imbalance include: Portion size of food: Serving more food will result in larger portion consumption. Energy content of foods: Consuming foods high in fat or sugar can result in more energy consumption in a given portion compared with lower fat and sugar foods. Clients should read food labels to learn the calorie content of food portions. Food form: Liquid foods generally are less filling and can result in increased intake without notice.
Refer clients with complicated energy imbalance (large weight gain, unplanned weight loss, or growth failure) to a registered dietitian.	A full team approach is necessary when energy imbalance threatens overall health.

Cultural Considerations

Ethnicity and Physical Activity

In both observational and survey research, it has been noted that physical inactivity is higher among certain ethnic populations than in others. This has been reported in both children and adults. In school-age children, the prevalence of no participation in 60 minutes or more of physical activity on any day is highest among black (32%) and Hispanic (27.1%) students compared with white students (22.4%) (Eaton et al., 2008). Additionally, in the same report black students had a higher prevalence (62.7%) of watching 3 or more hours of television per weekday than Hispanic (43%) or white (27.2%) students. Immigrant school-age children in all race/ethnic groups are less physically active than native children in the United States (Singh, Yu, Siahpush, & Kogan, 2008). Hispanic adults are reported to engage in less leisure-time physical activity than black or white adults (Ahmed et al., 2005). Within each racial or ethnic group, inactivity is increased among those of lower socioeconomic status, minimizing the evidence for an association between race/ethnic group and inactivity when adjusting for this factor (Marshall et al., 2007). Social class, not occupational physical activity, affected the relationship between race/ethnic group and leisure-time physical activity.

and Physical Activity discusses the effect of ethnic background on the amount of leisure-time and overall physical activity. Although some point to ethnic background as an influence on overall physical activity, such associations disappear when socioeconomic status is considered. Populations that are of lower socioeconomic status have lower physical activity levels than those of higher status (Marshall et al., 2007). Educating all individuals about the benefits of physical activity and healthy weight should be part of nursing interventions targeting wellness.

Negative Energy Balance: Weight Loss

Negative energy balance can occur because of any combination of insufficient energy consumption or excess physical activity compared to energy intake. When weight loss increases health risks associated with poor nutrition or slowed growth occurs in children, nutrition intervention is indicated. Nursing interventions for negative energy balance should target the aspects of energy consumption or expenditure that contribute to the imbalance. Again, a team approach is necessary to evaluate any medical contributors to

negative energy balance, such as undiagnosed diabetes mellitus, gastrointestinal disease, medication side effects, or an eating disorder. Children may experience growth faltering or failure because of negative energy balance and fail to gain expected weight or stature as a result. A pediatric health care team that is expert in this field should be consulted, as outlined in Chapter 14. As part of a nutritional assessment, the amount, quantity, type, and timing of foods consumed is needed. For example, children may fail to take in adequate energy at a meal if allowed to drink large quantities of fluid at the beginning of a meal or to snack on empty calorie foods too close to mealtime. An older adult who has experienced unplanned weight loss might be found to have a good appetite but trouble chewing because of poorly fitting dentures. Chapter 15 discusses negative energy balance in the older adult in detail.

The nurse should also include an assessment of physical activity levels when considering negative energy balance. Exercise type, intensity, frequency, and duration should be evaluated to determine if this aspect is contributing to negative energy balance. Chapter 11 discusses this in more detail. In some cases when energy intake cannot be modified sufficiently to accommodate a level of physical activity, exercise amount must be curtailed at least temporarily until balance can be achieved. Such is the case in treatment of some eating disorders as outlined in the chapter on weight management.

Energy Balance in Critical Illness

During some illnesses, injuries, or conditions, the body responds to the physiological stress of the situation by elevating energy expenditure through a metabolic response that involves a cascade of hormones and other substances. Burns, fractures, trauma, and surgery are examples of situations that result in this hypermetabolic response by the body. When such conditions occur, typical predictive equations to estimate energy expenditure should not routinely be used because these were formulated for a healthy population and do not consider critical illness. Instead, indirect calorimetry is the preferred method to determine energy expenditure in order to formulate nutrition interventions (Frankenfield et al., 2007; Stucky, Moncure, Hise, Gossage, & Northrop, 2008). When indirect calorimetry is not available, a modified approach to estimating energy requirements is needed, as outlined in Chapter 22. The nurse is a crucial member of the health care team managing the nutritional needs of the critically ill.

NURSING CARE PLAN | Client in an Automobile Accident

CASE STUDY

Ann Marie, age 28 years, was involved in a serious automobile accident on her way to work as respiratory therapist. She sustained fractures in both legs, a ruptured spleen, as well as numerous cuts and bruises. Extensive surgery was required to set the fractures and to remove her spleen. Her hospital stay was extended when she developed an infection at the surgical site in her left leg. She has lots of friends and family who visit regularly, but she frequently expresses frustration at her immobility and the slow course of recovery. Previous to this, she described herself as having excellent health and enjoying roller blading for exercise. In addition, she worries about how she will manage in her apartment, when she can return to work, and the expense of a prolonged hospital stay. She eats little from her hospital tray and says her stomach is upset from the antibiotics and pain medications she takes. Today she has refused physical therapy and asks to be left alone.

Applying the Nursing Process

ASSESSMENT

Height: 5 feet 6 inches Weight: 128 pounds (prior to injury) BMI: 21

Current weight: 116 BMI: 18.9

T101.2 BP 104/62 P 92 R 18

Dressing changes to open wound on left leg every 8 hours

Intravenous (IV) antibiotics every 8 hours; oral pain medication every 4 hours PRN

DIAGNOSES

Nutrition, Imbalanced: less than body requirements related to elevated temperature and wound infection evidenced by 12-pound weight loss

Skin Integrity, Impaired related to injuries from accident evidenced by surgical incisions

Pain, acute related to injuries from accident and surgery evidenced by requests for pain medication

EXPECTED OUTCOMES

Temperature returns to normal

Wound begins healing

Weight returns to normal within 2 weeks of hospital discharge

Pain is managed with nonnarcotic medication

INTERVENTIONS

Consult with dietitian about protein and calorie needs to promote healing and weight regain

Find out food preferences

Monitor wound for signs of healing

Pain medication as needed

EVALUATION

The dietitian recommended a high-calorie, high-protein diet to promote healing. A daily multivitamin was prescribed. Ann Marie did not care for hospital food and asked to have family and friends bring favorite foods from home. Her leg is healing slowly but will not be fully healed by discharge, so Ann Marie will be referred to a wound clinic for follow-up treatment. She will need to continue the recommended diet after discharge. The nursing process for this case study is outlined in Figure 8-4 ■.

Critical Thinking in the Nursing Process

1. When a hospitalized client is on a special diet and does not like the foods that are part of that diet or states that the food does not taste good, what are some strategies that the nurse can use to ensure that the integrity of the diet is maintained?

Client in an Automobile Accident *(continued)*

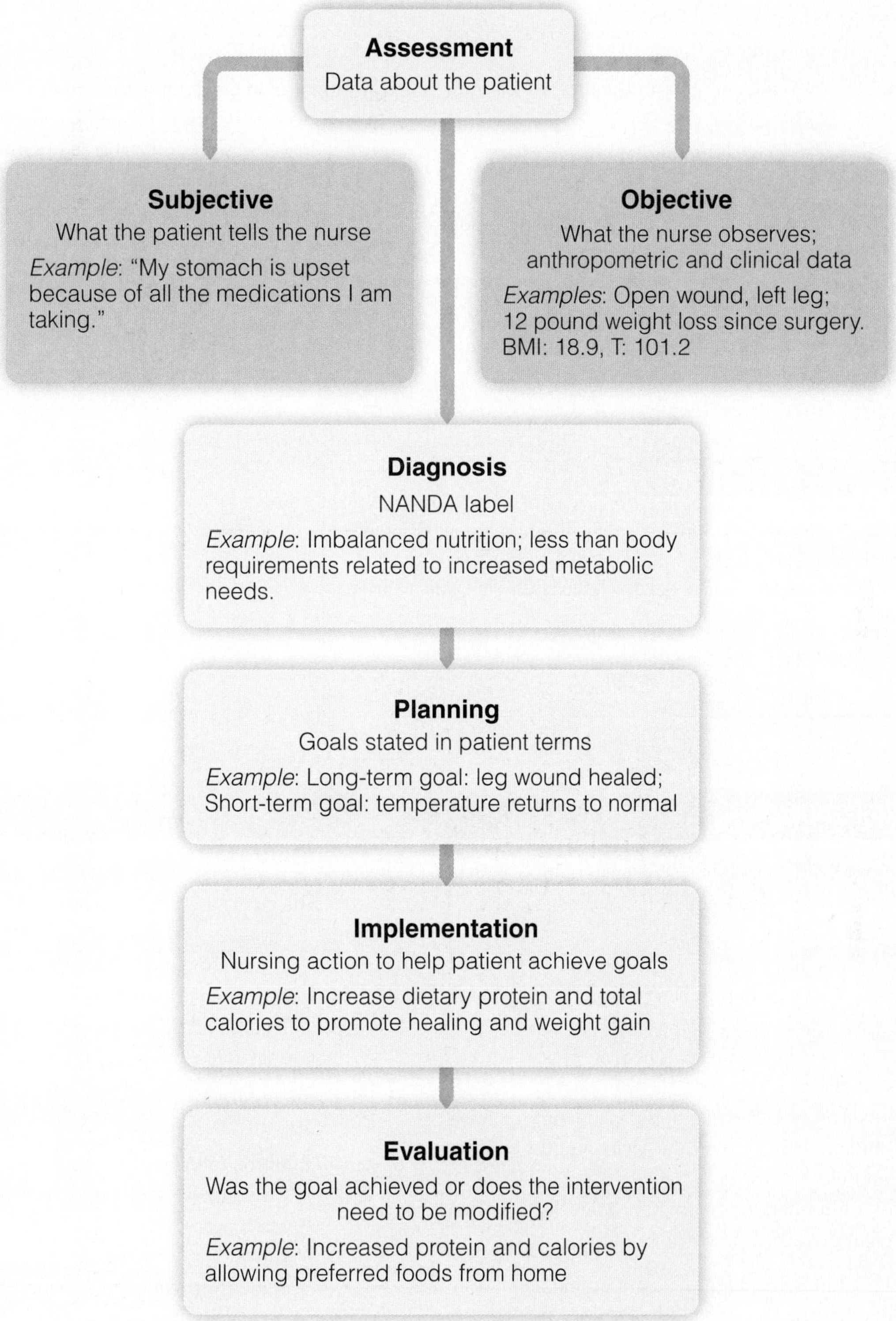

Assessment
Data about the patient

Subjective
What the patient tells the nurse

Example: "My stomach is upset because of all the medications I am taking."

Objective
What the nurse observes; anthropometric and clinical data

Examples: Open wound, left leg; 12 pound weight loss since surgery. BMI: 18.9, T: 101.2

Diagnosis
NANDA label

Example: Imbalanced nutrition; less than body requirements related to increased metabolic needs.

Planning
Goals stated in patient terms

Example: Long-term goal: leg wound healed; Short-term goal: temperature returns to normal

Implementation
Nursing action to help patient achieve goals

Example: Increase dietary protein and total calories to promote healing and weight gain

Evaluation
Was the goal achieved or does the intervention need to be modified?

Example: Increased protein and calories by allowing preferred foods from home

FIGURE 8-4 Nursing Care Plan Process: Patient in an Automobile Accident.

CHAPTER SUMMARY

- Energy balance is the relationship between energy consumption and expenditure.

- Energy in humans is measured in units called kilocalories or kilojoules.

- Carbohydrates, fats, protein, and alcohol are sources of energy in the diet.

- Energy expenditure is comprised of basal metabolic needs, thermic effect of food, and physical activity.

- Basal metabolic needs describe the energy needed for vital functions of the body, including organ function, nerve conduction, growth, and maintenance of cells and tissues.

These needs are closely associated with the amount of fat-free mass in the body.

- National guidelines exist that advise energy intake and physical activity levels for age-based population groups. Individual needs may differ based on unique basal metabolism and physical activity levels.

- Energy imbalances occur when energy consumption and expenditure are not equal and can ultimately lead to a change in body weight.

- The nurse is part of the health care team that evaluates the causes of energy imbalance and formulates interventions to address them.

EXPLORE PEARSON mynursingkit™

MyNursingKit is your one stop for online chapter review materials and resources. Prepare for success with additional NCLEX®-style practice questions, interactive assignments and activities, web links, animations and videos, and more!

Register your access code from the front of your book at
www.mynursingkit.com.

NCLEX® QUESTIONS

1. A client tells the nurse that "slow metabolism" is the reason for being overweight. What is the best response from the nurse?
   1. "Everyone has the same metabolic rate so we need to explore some of the other reasons you might be having a problem with your weight."
   2. "Let's see what we can do to increase your metabolic rate."
   3. "A person's metabolic rate is dependent on many things, including physical activity and the amount of muscle."
   4. "Your information is correct; people who are overweight do have a slower metabolism."

2. The school nurse explains to a class of middle school students that the energy contained in a specific amount of a food is measured in:
   1. Grams
   2. Ounces
   3. Kilowatts
   4. Calories

3. A client has read technical information about the thermic dynamic action of foods and wonders how to apply it. Which of the following foods will the nurse tell the client uses the most energy for the body to metabolize?
   1. Beef steak, 6 ounces
   2. Beer, 12 ounces
   3. Celery, 2 stalks
   4. Orange juice, 8 ounces

4. Children who spend 3 or more hours a day watching television and using a computer will likely have which of the following?
   1. Impaired glucose tolerance
   2. A positive energy balance
   3. Diminished caloric intake
   4. A higher resting energy expenditure

5. A client wants to lose 10 pounds in the next 10 weeks. By how many calories per day will the client need to reduce intake or increase expenditure to lose that amount of weight?
   1. 350 kcalories
   2. 500 kcalories
   3. 750 kcalories
   4. 1,000 kcalories

REFERENCES

Ahmed, N. U., Smith, G. L., Flores, A. M., Pamies, R. J., Mason, H. R., Woods, K. F., et al. (2005). Racial/ethnic disparity and predictors of leisure-time activity among U.S. men. *Ethnicity & Disease, 15*, 40–52.

American Academy of Pediatrics (AAP). (2003). Policy statement: Prevention of pediatric overweight and obesity. *Pediatrics, 112*, 424–430.

American Dietetic Association Evidence Analysis Library. (2008). *Nutrition assessment*. Retrieved August 14, 2008, from http://www.adaevidencelibrary.com/topic.cfm?cat=1151

Branson, R. D., & Johanninian, J. A. (2004). Measurement of energy expenditure. *Nutrition in Clinical Practice, 19*, 622–636.

Brown, W. J., Williams, L., Ford, J. H., Ball, K., & Dobson, A. J. (2005). Identifying the energy gap: Magnitude and determinants of 5-year weight gain in midage women. *Obesity Research, 13*, 1431–1441.

Centers for Disease Control and Prevention (CDC), National Center for Health Statistics. (2008). *Fast Stats A–Z: Overweight*. Retrieved September 8, 2008, from http://www.cdc.gov/nchs/fastats/overwt.htm

Compher, C., Frankenfield, D., Keim, N., & Roth-Yousey, L., for the Evidence Analysis Working Group. (2006). Best practices methods to apply to measurement of resting metabolic rate in adults: A systematic review. *Journal of the American Dietetic Association, 106*, 881–903.

Cummings, D. E., & Overduin, J. (2007). Gastrointestinal regulation of food intake. *The Journal of Clinical Investigation, 117*, 13–23.

Day, D. S., Gozansky, W. S., Van Pelt, R. E., Schwartz, R. S., & Kohrt, W. M. (2005). Sex hormone suppression reduces resting energy expenditure and {beta}-adrenergic support of resting energy expenditure. *The Journal of Clinical Endocrinology and Metabolism, 90*, 3312–3317.

D'Eon, T., Rogers, N., Stancheva, Z., & Greenberg, A. (2008). Estradiol and the estradiol metabolite, 2-hydroxyestradiol, activate amp-activated protein kinase in c2c12 myotubes. *Obesity, 18*, 1284–1288.

Diliberti, N., Bordi, P. L., Conklin, M. T., Roe, L. S., & Rolls, B. J. (2004). Increased portion size leads to increased energy intake in a restaurant meal. *Obesity Research, 12*, 562–568.

Donahoo, W. T., Levine, J. A., & Melanson, E. L. (2004). Variability in energy expenditure and its components. *Current Opinion in Clinical Nutrition and Metabolic Care, 7*, 599–605.

Eaton, D. K., Kann, L., Kinchen, S., Shanklin, S., Ross, J., Hawkins, J., et al. (2008). Youth risk behavior surveillance—United States, 2007. *Morbidity and Mortality Weekly Review, 57*, 1–131.

Evans, E. M., & Racette, S. B. (2006). Menopause and risk for obesity: How important is physical activity? *Journal of Women's Health, 15*, 211–213.

Fisher, J. O., & Kral, T. V. (2008). Super-size me: Portion size effects on young children's eating. *Physiology of Behavior, 94*, 39–47.

Food & Agriculture Organization/World Health Organization/United Nations University. (1985). *Energy and protein requirements. Report of a joint FAO/WHO/UNU expert consultation*. WHO Technical Report Series 724. Geneva: World Health Organization.

Frankenfield, D., Hise, M., Malone, A., Russell, M., Gradwell, E., Compher, C., et al. (2007). Prediction of resting metabolic rate in critically ill adult patients: Results of a systematic review of the evidence. *Journal of the American Dietetic Association, 107*, 1552–1561.

Frankenfield, D., Roth-Yousey, L., Compher, C., for the Evidence Analysis Working Group. (2005). Comparison of predictive equations for resting and metabolic rate in healthy nonobese and obese adults: A systematic review. *Journal of the American Dietetic Association, 105*, 775–789.

Frankenfield, D. C., Smith, J. S., Cooney, R. N., Blosser, S. A., & Sarson, G. Y. (1997). Relative association of fever and injury with hypermetabolism in critically ill patients. *Injury, 9/10*, 617–621.

Harris, J. A., & Benedict, F. G. (1919). *A biometric study of baseline metabolism in man*. Publication 279. Washington, DC: Carnegie Institute.

Haugen, H. A., Chan, L., & Li, F. (2007). Indirect calorimetry: A practical guide for clinicians. *Nutrition in Clinical Practice, 22*, 377–388.

Heymsfield, S. B., Harp, J. B., Rowell, P. N., Nguyen, A. M., & Pietrobelli, A. (2006). How much may I eat? Calorie estimates based upon energy expenditure prediction equations. *Obesity Reviews, 7*, 361–370.

Holtzclaw, B. J. (2004). Shivering in acutely ill vulnerable populations. *AACN Clinical Issues, 15*, 267–279.

Institute of Medicine (IOM). (2002). *Dietary reference intakes for energy, carbohydrate, fat, fatty acids, cholesterol, protein, and amino acids*. Washington, DC: The National Academies Press.

Ireton-Jones, C. (2005). Adjusted body weight, con: Why adjust body weight in energy expenditure calculations? *Nutrition in Clinical Practice, 4*, 468–473.

Jensen, L. B., Vestergaard, P., Hermann, A. P., Gram, J., Eiken, P., Abrahamsen, B., et al. (2003). Hormone replacement therapy dissociates fat mass and bone mass, and tends to reduce weight gain in early postmenopausal women: A randomized controlled 5-year trial of the Danish Osteoporosis Prevention Study. *Journal of Bone Mineral Research, 18*, 333–342.

Koskova, I., Petrasek, R., Vondra, K., & Skibova, J. (2007). Weight, body composition and fat distribution changes of Czech women in the different reproductive phases: A longitudinal study. *Prague Medical Report, 108*(3), 226–242.

Kruger, J., Ham, S. A., & Sanker, S. (2008). Physical inactivity during leisure time among older adults—behavioral risk factor surveillance system, 2005. *Journal of Aging and Physical Activity, 16*, 280–291.

Krumm, E. M., Dessieux, O. L., Andrews, P., & Thompson, L. (2006). The relationship between daily steps and body compositin in postmenopausal women. *Journal of Women's Health, 15*, 202–210.

Levine, J. A. (2007). Nonexercise activity thermogenesis—liberating the life-force. *Journal of Internal Medicine, 262*, 273–287.

Levine, J. A., Lanningham-Foster, L. M., McCrady, S. K., Krizan, A. C., Olson, L. R., Kane, P. H., et al. (2005). Interindividual variation in posture allocation: Possible role in human obesity. *Science, 307*, 584–586.

Lieber, C. S. (1991). Perspectives: Do alcohol calories count? *American Journal of Clinical Nutrition, 54*, 976–982.

Manini, T. M., Everhart, J. E., Patel, K. V., Shoeller, D. A., Colbert, L. H., Visser, M., et al. (2008). Daily activity energy expenditure and mortality among older adults. *Journal of the American Medical Association, 296*, 171–179.

Marshall, S. J., Jones, D. A., Ainsworth, B. E., Reis, J. P., Levy, S. S., & Macera, C. A. (2007). Race/ethnicity, social class, and leisure-time physical inactivity. *Medicine, Science, Sports & Exercise, 39*, 44–51.

Mattes, R. D. (2006). Fluid energy—where's the problem? *Journal of the American Dietetic Association, 106*, 1956–1961.

Matthews, C. E., Chen, K. Y., Freedson, P. S., Buchowski, M. S., Beech, B. M., Pate, R. R., et al. (2008). Amount of time spent in sedentary behaviors in the United States, 2003–2004. *American Journal of Epidemiology, 167*, 875–881.

Mattsson, C., & Olsson, T. (2007). Estrogens and glucocorticoid hormones in adipose tissue metabolism. *Current Medicinal Chemistry, 14*, 2918–2924.

Mifflin, M. D., St. Jeor, S. T., Hill, L. A., Scott, B. J., Daugherty, S. A., & Koch, Y. O. (1990). A new predictive equation for resting energy expenditure in healthy individuals. *American Journal of Clinical Nutrition, 5*, 1241–1247.

Paddon-Jones, D., Westman, E., Mattes, R. D., Wolfe, R. R., Astrup, A., &

REFERENCES *(continued)*

Westerterp-Plantenga, M. (2008). Protein, weight management, and satiety. *American Journal of Clinical Nutrition, 87S*, 1558S–1561S.

Plies, J. R., & Lethbridge-Cejku, M. (2007). Summary health statistics for U.S. adults: National Health Interview Study, 2006. *Vital Health Statistics, 235*, 1–153.

Ravussin, E. (2005). A NEAT way to control weight. *Science, 307*, 530–531.

Roberts, S. B., & Dallal, G. E. (2005). Energy requirements and aging. *Public Health Nutrition, 8*, 1028–1036.

Singh, G. K., Yu, S. M., Siahpush, M., & Kogan, M. D. (2008). High levels of physical inactivity and sedentary behavior among U.S. immigrant children and adolescents. *Archives of Pediatric and Adolescent Medicine, 162*, 756–763.

Sternfeld, B., Bhat, A. K., Wang, H., Sharp, T., & Quesenberry, C. P., Jr. (2005). Menopause, physical activity, and body composition/fat distribution in midlife women. *Medicine and Science in Sports and Exercise, 37*, 1195–1202.

Sternfeld, B., Wang, H., Quesenberry, C. P., Jr, Abrams, B., Everson-Rose, S. A., Greendale, G. A., et al. (2004). Physical activity and changes in weight and waist circumference in midlife women: Findings from the Study of Women's Health Across the Nation. *American Journal of Epidemiology, 160*, 912–922.

Storey, M. L., Forshee, R. A., & Anderson, P. A. (2006). Beverage consumption in the U.S. population. *Journal of the American Dietetic Association, 106*, 1992–2000.

Stucky, C. H., Moncure, M., Hise, M., Gossage, C., & Northrop, D. (2008). How accurate are resting energy expenditure prediction equations in obese trauma and burn patients? *Journal of Parenteral and Enteral Nutrition, 32*, 420–426.

Surgeon General. (2007). *Overweight and obesity: What you can do*. Retrieved September 8, 2008, from http://www.surgeongeneral.gov/topics/obesity/calltoaction/fact_whatcanyoudo.html

Thompson, D. L., Rakow, J., & Perdue, S. M. (2004). Relationship between accumulated walking and body composition in middle-aged women. *Medicine and Science in Sports and Exercise, 36*, 911–914.

Toth, M. J., Tchernof, A., Sites, C. K., & Poehlman, E. T. (2000). Menopause-related changes in body fat distribution. *Annals of the New York Academy of Sciences, 904*, 502–506.

United States Department of Agriculture (USDA) & Department of Health and Human Services. (2005). *Dietary Guidelines for American* (6th ed.). Washington, DC: U.S. Government Printing Office.

Section 2

Community Nutrition and Health Promotion

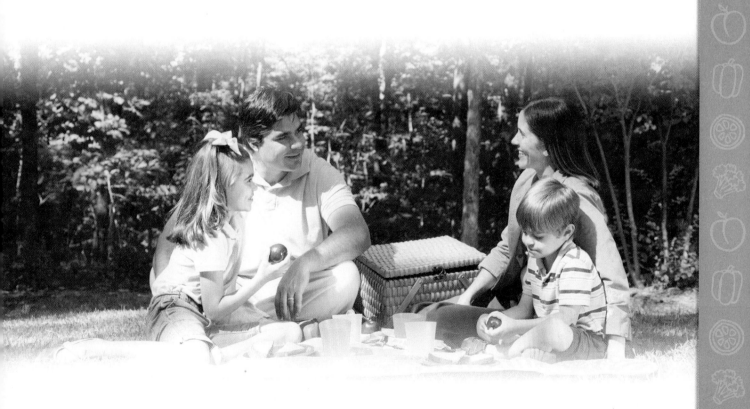

Susan Prion

Nutrition Recommendations and Standards 9

WHAT WILL YOU LEARN?

1. To describe dietary reference intakes and how they are used by health care professionals.
2. To define the basic diet planning principles of balance, moderation, variety, adequacy, nutritional density, and enjoyment.
3. To summarize the overall dietary recommendations contained in the *Dietary Guidelines for Americans*.
4. To compare and contrast the dietary recommendations for disease prevention given by national health organizations.
5. To interpret how to read a food label and decipher nutrient content claims.
6. To formulate nursing interventions that target nutrition misinformation.

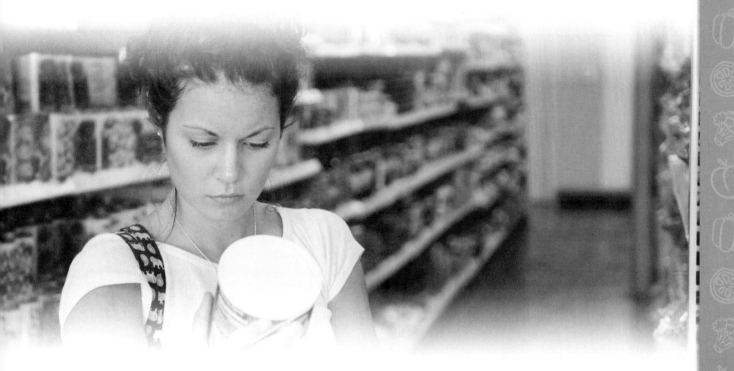

DID YOU KNOW?

▶ Dietary reference intakes (DRIs) are only meant for healthy people and should not be used for those who have malnutrition or illness.

▶ MyPyramid has guidelines so consumers can budget discretionary calories to moderate intake of fats, added sugars, and alcohol.

▶ Food labels are not permitted to claim that the product can treat or cure a disease.

▶ Many consumers are confused by the information included on food labels.

▶ No government preapproval is required to substantiate food or dietary supplement labels or advertising with health-related claims.

KEY TERMS

acceptable macronutrient distribution range (AMDR), *184*

adequate intake (AI), *183*

daily value, *192*

estimated average requirements (EAR), *183*

estimated energy requirement (EER), *184*

health claim, *194*

nutrient content claims, *193*

nutrient dense, *185*

recommended daily allowance (RDA), *183*

structure-function claims, *194*

tolerable upper intake levels (UL), *183*

What Is a Healthy Diet?

A healthy diet should provide adequate calories and all of the essential nutrients to avoid nutritional deficiencies, but not so much that nutrient excesses develop leading to chronic problems such as cardiovascular disease, diabetes, and cancer. Compared with the past when nutritional deficiencies were common, nutrient deficiencies are now rare in the United States except among vulnerable populations, such as the elderly, substance abusers, the poor, malnourished children, and some hospitalized clients. Yet nutrient excesses, especially of simple carbohydrates in the form of added sugar, saturated fat, cholesterol, and calories, increase each year. Poor diet choices were linked with 4 of the top 10 causes of death in America in 2005 that are listed in Box 9-1 (Centers for Disease Control and Prevention [CDC], 2008). Diet is implicated in the development and progression of heart disease, cancer, stroke, and diabetes. Fortunately, as understanding of the role of diet in the disease process has increased, the death rates for cardiac disease, cancer, strokes, and accidents have decreased (Jemal, 2005).

Most Americans admit that they would like to make healthier food choices and lose "a few pounds." Yet even as the prevalence of overweight and obesity has increased, fewer American consumers perceive themselves as overweight or obese (Johnson-Taylor, Fisher, Hubbard, Starke-Reed, & Eggers, 2008). The ethnic variation in self-reported weight and

height as studied by the Third National Health and Nutrition Examination Survey shows even greater discrepancies between actual body mass index values and respondents' perceptions of overweight and obesity (Gillum & Sempos, 2005). Studies show that these same consumers do not understand nutritional labeling, are confused about macro- and micronutrients, and lack the information and confidence to implement healthier diet and fitness habits (Rothman et al., 2006; Tufts University Health and Nutrition Letter, 2006). Personal preferences, habits and values related to food, cultural traditions, food availability, convenience, cost, emotional state, body image, and perceived nutritional and health benefits are additional influences on consumer diet and food choices.

Nurses have a unique opportunity to help these consumers become healthier. By asking routine dietary screening questions at regular intervals, modeling healthy behaviors, and serving as community resources, nurses can have significant influence on the health and wellness of American consumers (McCullough et al., 2002).

Nutritional Recommendations and Standards

Nutritional recommendations and standards have been developed by government and private health organizations to provide advice to the public about the amounts of energy

BOX 9-1	The 10 Leading Causes of Death in the United States in 2005 in Descending Order

1. Heart disease
2. Cancer
3. Stroke
4. Chronic obstructive pulmonary disease
5. Accidents

6. Diabetes
7. Pneumonia/flu
8. Alzheimer's disease
9. Kidney disease
10. Blood infections

Source: Centers for Disease Control and Prevention, 2008.

(measured as kilocalories), macro- and micronutrients, essential and nonessential dietary elements, and physical activity that promote health and wellness. Many of these recommendations and standards are the result of research studies conducted by health professionals and nutrition experts. Nutritional recommendations and standards are necessary because consumers and health care professionals need clear, evidence-based guidelines for dietary intakes. Some recommendations are given that are nutrient specific, such as the DRIs. Others base advice on recommendations for overall diet, such as those offered by health organizations targeting disease prevention.

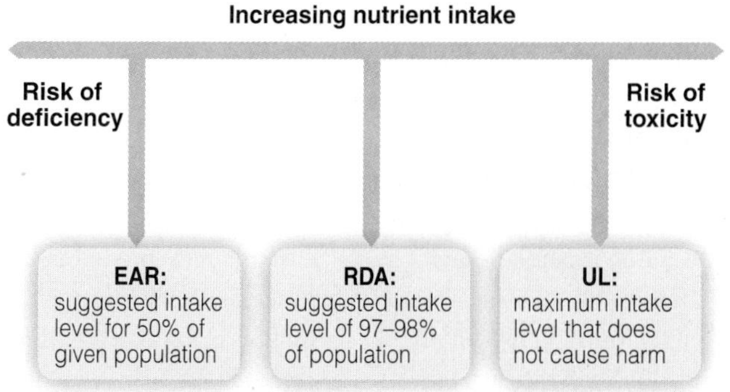

What Are Dietary Reference Intakes?

The DRIs, developed by researchers in the United States and Canada, present recommendations for optimal nutrient intake levels. Before the development of DRIs, the recommended dietary allowances (RDAs) in the United States and the recommended nutrient intakes (RNIs) in Canada were used as the guidelines for recommended levels of nutrient intake. The purpose of these guidelines was to prevent consumers from diseases caused by inadequate and nutritionally deficient diets. As a growing amount of research highlighted the interactions of chronic diseases and diet, it became clear that nutrient excesses were also of great concern, and that new recommendations were needed that defined intake levels for both the prevention of nutrient deficiencies and avoidance of nutritional excess. The DRIs are intended for use with healthy individuals. The recommendations are not intended for use with individuals who are malnourished or have a medical condition.

In 1997, the older RDA/RNI guidelines were replaced by the DRIs. The initial guidelines described optimal dietary intake for five important nutrients: calcium, phosphorus, magnesium, vitamin D, and fluoride. Additional reports since have proposed intake guidelines for vitamins, minerals, macronutrients, cholesterol, fiber, electrolytes, and fluids. In 2005, a report was issued by the Food and Nutrition Information Center of the U.S. Department of Agriculture detailing the DRI guidelines for bioactive compounds such as phytoestrogens and other phytochemicals. Finally, a report was issued describing the role of lifestyle choices, specifically alcohol abuse and smoking, on health and disease.

DRI values are determined by the Food and Nutrition Board of the National Academy of Sciences, at the request of the U.S. Department of Agriculture. Unfortunately, many consumers are not familiar with the DRI recommendations, and even health professionals can be overwhelmed by the extremely technical nature of the DRI reports. DRI values are defined for nutrients, not foods, so it can be difficult for consumers to apply DRIs to health food choices.

DRIs have been established for a variety of nutrients, including vitamins, minerals, macronutrients, cholesterol, fiber, electrolytes, and fluids. There is also a DRI report specifically

FIGURE 9-1 DRIs along Continuum of Intake.

for older Americans, aged 51 years and above. The DRI recommendations involved four different values: estimated average requirements (EAR), RDA, adequate intake (AI), and tolerable upper intake levels (UL). Figure 9-1 ■ depicts the relationship of the various components of the DRI.

Estimated average requirements (EAR) is the average daily nutrient intake value that is estimated to meet the requirements of 50% or more of healthy individuals in a life stage and gender group (Institute of Medicine [IOM], 2000). The EAR is based on sophisticated physiological research and is used to assess minimum dietary adequacy. It forms the basis of the RDA.

Recommended daily allowance (RDA) is the average daily amount of a given nutrient that is sufficient to meet the nutrient requirement of 97% to 98% of healthy individuals in a particular life stage and gender group (IOM, 2000). The RDA is the nutrient goal recommended for individuals. For example, research evidence on folate is sufficient to establish an RDA for that vitamin.

Adequate intake (AI) is the *recommended* nutrient intake by a group of healthy people when the RDA cannot be determined, usually because of insufficient research evidence (IOM, 2000). Adequate intake is an estimation that appears to be adequate for most people and is believed to meet or exceed the needs of those individuals. The recommendation is derived from observation of intake level in well-nourished individuals or from available limited data. Often, AI recommendations for children are derived from those made for adults. Examples of nutrients with AI recommendations include calcium and vitamin D.

Tolerable upper intake levels (UL) is the highest average daily intake level of a nutrient that is likely to present little or no risk to most individuals in a given life stage and gender group (IOM, 2000). This form of recommendation grew out of the increasing use of dietary supplements and fortified foods that result in increased intake of some nutrients. A UL exists for some nutrients, but not all. For example, B-vitamins folate and niacin have a UL recommendation, whereas B_{12} does not. The nurse should caution clients to not misinterpret the UL as an endorsement of high levels of nutrient intake.

In addition to recommendations for adequate or optimal nutrient levels, the DRI system also defined two additional values related to energy. The **acceptable macronutrient distribution range (AMDR)** and the **estimated energy requirement (EER)** make recommendations about dietary intake needed to meet average daily energy needs.

EER is the dietary energy intake level predicted to achieve and maintain energy balance in healthy, normal weight individuals of a given age, height and weight, gender and physical activity level (IOM, 2002). The EER recommendation is consistent with good health and maintenance of ideal weight goals. EER is the energy equivalent to the EAR values made for micronutrients. Weight gain or loss can occur when an individual respectively exceeds or falls short of the recommended EER.

AMDR is defined as the suggested intake range for a given macronutrient (carbohydrate, protein, or fat) that is sufficient for essential nutrients but not associated with an increased risk of chronic disease (IOM, 2002). AMDR values are reported as percentages of daily calories consumed. Daily intake above or below this recommended percentage can increase or decrease the risk of chronic disease development, respectively. According to the DRIs (IOM, 2002), acceptable macronutrient distribution ranges for adults are as follows:

Carbohydrate	45% to 65% of total daily calories consumed
Protein	10% to 35% of total daily calories consumed
Fat	20% to 35% of total daily calories consumed
Linoleic acid	5% to 10% of total daily calories consumed
Alpha-linolenic acid	0.6% to 1.2% of total daily calories consumed

How to Use the DRIs

There are several important points to remember when using nutrient and energy recommendations for nutritional counseling. The DRI values can be confusing to health care professionals and consumers because they define the suggested intake levels of specific nutrients rather than actual food items. The translation from specific nutrient intake to healthy food choices can be difficult, even for the most well-intentioned and informed person. But compliance with these recommendations depends on a functional understanding of nutrients and the ability to apply these standards to healthy food choices (Barr, Murphy, & Poos, 2002). Specific strategies for healthy eating are discussed later in this chapter.

The DRI values are explicitly written for healthy persons. They are further detailed by age and gender, and some require accommodation for activity levels. The DRI values

are intended to prevent the risk of chronic disease development as a result of nutritional causes. They are not intended to serve as references for clients who have special nutrient needs because of illness or disease.

DRI values serve as an evidence-based starting point for nutritional interventions. They define neither minimum nor maximum recommended levels, but offer a range of suggested intake values. A healthy balance and variety of dietary intake is assumed with the DRI values, which describe an average intake recommendation rather than specifying absolute values for each nutrient.

Finally, it is crucial to recognize that the DRI values are intended as general guidelines for a population group rather than an individual. Their purpose is to suggest general nutrient intake ranges rather than to serve as a specific guideline for daily dietary planning and food selection.

Is it possible to individualize these nutrient recommendations? With careful planning and adherence to the intention of the DRI ranges, it is quite possible to individualize these evidence-based recommendations for daily use.

Five variables must be accommodated in order to successfully translate population suggestions into actual food choices for a client. These include age; body size; daily energy expenditure; any relevant medical conditions; and dietary habits including culture, religion, and personal preferences. Integrating these unique and personal characteristics with the DRI ranges allows the health care professional to suggest food choices that will have the greatest chance of acceptance by the client. National recommendations that are based on the total diet instead of those that are nutrient specific are easier tools to use when educating consumers.

Diet-Based Nutrition Recommendations

One of the first questions many consumers ask is, "What is a healthy diet?" The media constantly provides updates on the latest medical and nutritional research, often confusing even the most informed consumer with contradictory results and advice. The specifics of a healthy diet may be modified by new research, but the basic foundational principles remain the same: balance, moderation, variety, adequacy, nutrient density, and enjoyment.

A *balanced* diet is one that contains a sufficient quantity of each type of food. Balance means consuming all of the essential macronutrients and micronutrients in the recommended quantity through a combination of different food types. For example, calcium is abundant in dairy products. Meat, fish, and poultry are rich in iron but calcium poor. A balanced diet would contain adequate amounts of both dairy and meat products, in addition to grains, vegetables, and fruits, which contribute other essential nutrients.

Moderation refers to the practice of regularly eating foods low in saturated fat, cholesterol, and added sugars and infrequently splurging on foods that are high in these nutrients.

Foods high in fat and sugar are delicious to eat but high in calories and, habitually, high intake increases the risk of developing chronic conditions such as obesity, cardiovascular disease, and diabetes. Moderation usually is associated with a balanced diet and adequate levels of nutrients. Moderation is also positively associated with weight management.

A *varied* diet contains food from each of the food groups each day. By alternating food choices within each food group, the consumer increases adequate consumption of vital nutrients and decreases potential exposure to food contaminants. For example, cantaloupe is a good source of vitamin A, whereas bananas are a good source of potassium. If one eats only melon, then nutrient adequacy will be difficult to achieve without a variety of other fruits and vegetables.

Adequacy means that the diet provides sufficient amounts of all micro- and macronutrients for the nutritional needs of a healthy person. An underlying principle of many dietary guidelines is that balance and variety in the diet will lead to nutrient adequacy.

A food is **nutrient dense** if it contains a significant amount of nutrients for the least amount of calories. Another way to think about nutrient density it to consider the nutrient contributions contained in a single serving of a food. For example, a serving of fat-free milk (1 cup) offers about 300 mg of calcium in 85 kcalories. One banana contributes only 7 mg of calcium but offers 450 mg of potassium in about 70 kcalories. The cup of milk is nutritionally dense for calcium (6.7 mg/kcal) and the banana is nutritionally dense for potassium (6.43 mg/kcal). Obviously, a balanced consumption of both fat-free milk and bananas will lead to adequate daily intake for both of these important micronutrients. Conversely, a high-calorie food, such as candy, soda, or French fries, is not considered nutrient dense despite the high caloric content because of the lack of significant nutrients.

Last, but definitely not least, is the principle of *enjoyment*. If you do not like it or do not enjoy eating it, you probably will not include it in your diet choices. It is important to recognize that not everyone enjoys every food. But if there are healthy and nutrient-dense foods that are not included in a consumer's diet, it is important to replace the nutritional contributions of that food with another similar food. For example, kiwi fruit is an excellent source of vitamin C. Some consumers do not like the taste of kiwi or other citrus fruit, but they can substitute another good source of vitamin C, such as green leafy vegetables.

There are a wealth of dietary guidelines and resources that are available to assist consumers in making healthy food choices. Such guidelines incorporate the evidence of nutrient-specific research combined with that concerning diet and health to offer advice that guides overall dietary choices rather than for a specific nutrient, food, or meal.

Dietary Guidelines for Americans

The *Dietary Guidelines for Americans* is published every 5 years by a partnership of the U.S. Department of Health and Human Services and the U.S. Department of Agriculture (USDA). The primary goal of the dietary guidelines is to provide evidence-based nutritional advice to consumers based on a synthesis of the latest scientific research. The recommendations are intentionally presented as suggestions for food choice patterns and total diet planning rather than emphasizing specific foods or set numerical intake levels. Following these guidelines can assist consumer and health care professionals in making healthy food choices that fulfill the specific nutrient values defined by the DRIs.

The dietary guidelines emphasize a balance of exercise and healthy diet choices, including fruits, vegetables, whole grains, and fat-free or low-fat milk and milk products, lean meats, poultry, fish, beans, eggs, and nuts and foods that are low in saturated fats, trans fats, cholesterol, salt (sodium), and added sugars. Consumer resources provide suggestions about how to choose healthy snacks and healthier options when dining out, ensure more variety between and among food groups, optimize intake of nutrient-dense foods, read nutrition labels, follow food safety tips, and limit alcohol intake. The dietary guidelines are summarized in Box 9-2. Combining the guidelines with MyPyramid provides a consumer-friendly tool for the nurse to use when educating individuals about healthy eating patterns.

BOX 9-2	**U.S. Dietary Guidelines**

ADEQUATE NUTRIENTS WITHIN CALORIE NEEDS
Key Recommendations

- Consume a variety of nutrient-dense foods and beverages within and among the basic food groups while choosing foods that limit the intake of saturated and trans fats, cholesterol, added sugars, salt, and alcohol.
- Meet recommended intakes within energy needs by adopting a balanced eating pattern, such as the USDA Food Guide or the DASH Eating Plan.

WEIGHT MANAGEMENT
Key Recommendations

- To maintain body weight in a healthy range, balance calories from foods and beverages with calories expended.
- To prevent gradual weight gain over time, make small decreases in food and beverage calories and increase physical activity.

(continued)

BOX 9-2	**U.S. Dietary Guidelines** *(continued)*

PHYSICAL ACTIVITY
Key Recommendations

- Engage in regular physical activity and reduce sedentary activities to promote health, psychological well-being, and a healthy body weight.
- To reduce the risk of chronic disease in adulthood: Engage in at least 30 minutes of moderate-intensity physical activity, above usual activity, at work or home on most days of the week.
- For most people, greater health benefits can be obtained by engaging in physical activity of more vigorous intensity or longer duration.
- To help manage body weight and prevent gradual, unhealthy body weight gain in adulthood: Engage in approximately 60 minutes of moderate- to vigorous-intensity activity on most days of the week while not exceeding caloric intake requirements.
- To sustain weight loss in adulthood: Participate in at least 60 to 90 minutes of daily moderate-intensity physical activity while not exceeding caloric intake requirements. Some people may need to consult with a health care provider before participating in this level of activity.
- Achieve physical fitness by including cardiovascular conditioning, stretching exercises for flexibility, and resistance exercises or calisthenics for muscle strength and endurance.

FOOD GROUPS TO ENCOURAGE
Key Recommendations

- Consume a sufficient amount of fruits and vegetables while staying within energy needs. Two cups of fruit and 2½ cups of vegetables per day are recommended for a reference 2,000-calorie intake, with higher or lower amounts depending on the calorie level.
- Choose a variety of fruits and vegetables each day. In particular, select from all five vegetable subgroups (dark green, orange, legumes, starchy vegetables, and other vegetables) several times a week.
- Consume 3 or more ounce-equivalents of whole-grain products per day, with the rest of the recommended grains coming from enriched or whole-grain products. In general, at least half the grains should come from whole grains.
- Consume 3 cups per day of fat-free or low-fat milk or equivalent milk products.

FATS
Key Recommendations

- Consume less than 10 percent of calories from saturated fatty acids and less than 300 mg/day of cholesterol, and keep trans-fatty acid consumption as low as possible.
- Keep total fat intake between 20 to 35 percent of calories, with most fats coming from sources of polyunsaturated and monounsaturated fatty acids, such as fish, nuts, and vegetable oils.
- When selecting and preparing meat, poultry, dry beans, and milk or milk products, make choices that are lean, low-fat, or fat-free.

- Limit intake of fats and oils high in saturated and/or trans-fatty acids, and choose products low in such fats and oils.

CARBOHYDRATES
Key Recommendations

- Choose fiber-rich fruits, vegetables, and whole grains often.
- Choose and prepare foods and beverages with little added sugars or caloric sweeteners, such as amounts suggested by the USDA Food Guide and the DASH Eating Plan.
- Reduce the incidence of dental caries by practicing good oral hygiene and consuming sugar- and starch-containing foods and beverages less frequently.

SODIUM AND POTASSIUM
Key Recommendations

- Consume less than 2,300 mg (approximately 1 tsp of salt) of sodium per day.
- Choose and prepare foods with little salt. At the same time, consume potassium-rich foods, such as fruits and vegetables.

ALCOHOLIC BEVERAGES
Key Recommendations

- Those who choose to drink alcoholic beverages should do so sensibly and in moderation—defined as the consumption of up to one drink per day for women and up to two drinks per day for men.
- Alcoholic beverages should not be consumed by some individuals, including those who cannot restrict their alcohol intake, women of childbearing age who may become pregnant, pregnant and lactating women, children and adolescents, individuals taking medications that can interact with alcohol, and those with specific medical conditions.
- Alcoholic beverages should be avoided by individuals engaging in activities that require attention, skill, or coordination, such as driving or operating machinery.

FOOD SAFETY
Key Recommendations

To avoid microbial foodborne illness:

- Clean hands, food contact surfaces, and fruits and vegetables. Meat and poultry should not be washed or rinsed.
- Separate raw, cooked, and ready-to-eat foods while shopping, preparing, or storing foods.
- Cook foods to a safe temperature to kill microorganisms.
- Chill (refrigerate) perishable food promptly and defrost foods properly.
- Avoid raw (unpasteurized) milk or any products made from unpasteurized milk, raw or partially cooked eggs or foods containing raw eggs, raw or undercooked meat and poultry, unpasteurized juices, and raw sprouts.

Source: U.S. Department of Health and Human Services, 2005.

MyPyramid

MyPyramid is an interactive consumer resource based on the *Dietary Guidelines for Americans*. It translates the dietary guidelines into a total diet plan that limits dietary components often consumed in excess and encourages consumption of health components often deficient in American diets. MyPyramid features an extensive educational component, including Web-based interactive and print-based resources for consumers. The Pyramid's Education Framework identified what changes most Americans need to make for healthier living choices, how to make these changes, and why these changes are important to health. These recommendations include the following:

- Increased intake of vitamins, minerals, dietary fiber, and other essential nutrients that are often deficient in typical American diets
- Lowered intake of saturated fats, trans fats, and cholesterol
- Increased intake of fruits, vegetables, and whole gains

- Caloric intake balanced with energy and fitness needs to prevent weight gain or maintain a healthy weight

The MyPyramid recommendations can be organized by four general themes: variety, proportionality, moderation, and activity, which are all denoted in the pictorial of the pyramid in Figure 9-2 ■. *Variety* means eating from all food groups and subgroups frequently. The vertical stripes in the pyramid represent all the food groups. *Proportionality* refers to eating more of some healthy foods such as whole grains, fruits, and vegetables and less of other foods high in sugar, saturated or trans fat, cholesterol, and alcohol. The thickness of the pyramid stripes in Figure 9-2 indicates the proportionality of the food groups in relation to one another. *Moderation* means eating healthy quantities of food low in saturated or trans fat, sugar, cholesterol, salt, and alcohol. The pyramid offers advice about moderating discretionary calories from fats, added sugars, and alcohol to remain within guidelines for both disease prevention and weight management.

Anatomy of MyPyramid

One size doesn't fit all

USDA's new MyPyramid symbolizes a personalized approach to healthy eating and physical activity. The symbol has been designed to be simple. It has been developed to remind consumers to make healthy food choices and to be active every day. The different parts of the symbol are described below.

Activity
Activity is represented by the steps and the person climbing them, as a reminder of the importance of daily physical activity.

Moderation
Moderation is represented by the narrowing of each food group from bottom to top. The wider base stands for foods with little or no solid fats or added sugars. These should be selected more often. The narrower top area stands for foods containing more added sugars and solid fats. The more active you are, the more of these foods you can fit into your diet.

Personalization
Personalization is shown by the person on the steps, the slogan, and the URL. Find the kinds and amounts of food to eat each day at MyPyramid.gov.

Proportionality
Proportionality is shown by the different widths of the food group bands. The widths suggest how much food a person should choose from each group. The widths are just a general guide, not exact proportions. Check the website for how much is right for you.

Variety
Variety is symbolized by the 6 color bands representing the 5 food groups of the Pyramid and oils. This illustrates that foods from all groups are needed each day for good health.

Gradual Improvement
Gradual improvement is encouraged by the slogan. It suggests that individuals can benefit from taking small steps to improve their diet and lifestyle each day.

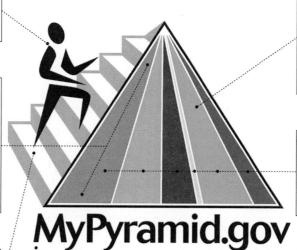

USDA U.S. Department of Agriculture Center for Nutrition Policy and Promotion April 2005 CNPP-16

USDA is an equal opportunity provider and employer.

| GRAINS | VEGETABLES | FRUITS | OILS | MILK | MEAT & BEANS |

■ **FIGURE 9-2 MyPyramid.**
Source: United States Department of Agriculture, MyPyramid.gov.

MyNursingKit The British Nutrition Society Eatwell Plate

Moderate amounts of *activity* are recommended on a daily basis. Stairs running up the side of the pyramid denote the need for exercise.

The nurse can use the many tools contained within MyPyramid when educating clients about a healthy diet. Specifically, individuals can obtain personal and specific advice about energy intake and servings in each food group needed to meet nutritional needs. Tutorials exist online to further explain each food group. Box 9-3 outlines examples of the advice given for various levels of daily calorie need.

Critics of the 2005 *Dietary Guidelines for Americans* and the MyPyramid recommendations complain that these continue to recommend too much refined starch, do not differentiate between protein sources by their fat content, and advocate extra calories through unnecessary dairy products to ensure adequate calcium intake (Mitka, 2005). Many of the resources are available only online, limiting their accessibility to consumers with computer and Internet access. Despite these concerns, the MyPyramid tool is felt to align with other national recommendations that target reducing the risk of chronic disease (Krebs-Smith & Kris-Etherton, 2007). MyPyramid emphasizes moderation in intake of fat and saturated fat, sodium, and added sugars and encourages intake of fiber through fruits, vegetables, and whole grains similar to guidelines published by private groups such as the American Heart Association, American Diabetes Association, and American Institute for Cancer Research.

MyPyramid can also be used for children in the form of MyPyramid for kids. Similar resources are available for the nurse to use when educating children but with age-appropriate messages and recommendations. Use of this tool for children is supported by the American Dietetic Association (ADA), the nation's professional organization of registered dietitians (ADA, 2008). Figure 9-3 ■ depicts the pyramid used for children.

Pyramids and Guidelines from around the World

Nutrition researchers at the Harvard School of Public Health created the Healthy Eating Pyramid in response to the deficits they had identified in the *Dietary Guidelines for Americans* and the subsequent MyPyramid. The Healthy Eating Pyramid, depicted in Figure 9-4 ■, uses the current research-based evidence about the relationships between dietary choices and disease to recommend significant changes in the American diet. The authors of the Healthy Living Pyramid believe that the modest changes in diet and fitness proposed may reduce the risk of premature cardiac disease, type 2 diabetes mellitus, and colon cancer by 70% to 90% (Willett, 2001).

The base of the Healthy Eating Pyramid is daily exercise and weight control. This is considered the "foundation" of healthy living because of the multiple benefits of daily fitness and careful balancing of caloric intake and output. Emphasis is placed on daily intakes of whole grains, plant oils, and vegetables. Daily calcium and multivitamin, multimineral supplements are recommended. Americans are cautioned to limit their intake of red meat, butter, white rice, white bread, potatoes, pasta, and sweets. Each of these dietary modifications increases the amount of nutrient-dense foods that a person consumes and decreases the amount of saturated fat, simple carbohydrates, cholesterol, and excess sugar that have been positively associated with obesity, cardiac disease, and diabetes mellitus.

BOX 9-3	MyPyramid Food Intake Patterns

Listed are the suggested amounts of food to consume from the basic food groups, subgroups, and oils to meet recommended nutrient intakes at 12 different calorie levels. Nutrient and energy contributions from each group are calculated according to the nutrient-dense forms of foods in each group (e.g., lean meats and fat-free milk). The table also shows the discretionary calorie allowance that can be accommodated within each calorie level, in addition to the suggested amounts of nutrient-dense forms of foods in each group.

Daily Amount of Food from Each Group

Calorie Level	1,000	1,200	1,400	1,600	1,800	2,000	2,200	2,400	2,600	2,800	3,000	3,200
Fruits	1 cup	1 cup	1.5 cups	1.5 cups	1.5 cups	2 cups	2 cups	2 cups	2 cups	2.5 cups	2.5 cups	2.5 cups
Vegetables	1 cup	1.5 cups	1.5 cups	2 cups	2.5 cups	2.5 cups	3 cups	3 cups	3.5 cups	3.5 cups	4 cups	4 cups
Grains	3 oz-eq	4 oz-eq	5 oz-eq	5 oz-eq	6 oz-eq	6 oz-eq	7 oz-eq	8 oz-eq	9 oz-eq	10 oz-eq	10 oz-eq	10 oz-eq
Meat and Beans	2 oz-eq	3 oz-eq	4 oz-eq	5 oz-eq	5 oz-eq	5.5 oz-eq	6 oz-eq	6.5 oz-eq	6.5 oz-eq	7 oz-eq	7 oz-eq	7 oz-eq
Milk	2 cups	2 cups	2 cups	3 cups	3 cups	3 cups	3 cups	3 cups	3 cups	3 cups	3 cups	3 cups
Oils	3 tsp	4 tsp	4 tsp	5 tsp	5 tsp	6 tsp	6 tsp	7 tsp	8 tsp	8 tsp	10 tsp	11 tsp
Discretionary calorie allowance	165	171	171	132	195	267	290	362	410	426	512	648

Source: Retrieved March 30, 2009, from http://www.mypyramid.gov/downloads/MyPyramid_Food_Intake_Patterns.pdf

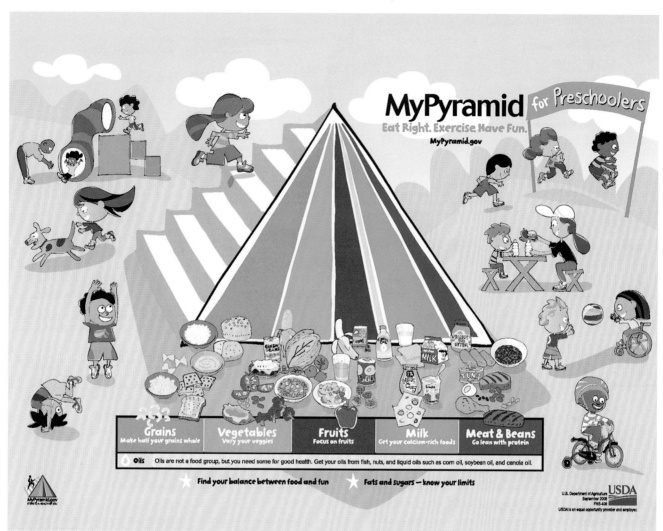

■ FIGURE 9-3 **MyPyramid for Children.**

Source: United States Department of Agriculture, MyPyramid.gov

Many other countries have pyramids, or other pictorial shapes, that depict dietary guidelines. The nurse may consider becoming familiar with the guidelines given for a client's native country in order to incorporate advice or specific foods into health education. Cultural Considerations Box: Nutrition Recommendations around the World outlines examples of guidelines offered by other countries.

Cultural Considerations

Nutrition Recommendations around the World

The Healthy Living Pyramid and MyPyramid are all excellent diet-planning references. But many countries offer healthy living advice using a variety of formats. Japan organizes the dietary advice from the Ministry of Health, Labor and Welfare and the Ministry of Agriculture, Forestry and Fisheries into a "spinning top" format, with grain dishes at the large end of the top and fruits and milk products at the

pointed end that "spins." The picture is different, but the serving recommendations are very similar to the old USDA Food Guide Pyramid that has been replaced by MyPyramid.

The British Nutrition Society advocates the "eatwell plate," a guide to both type of foods and amounts. The round "plate" lists show visually (rather than by percentages) the amount of fruits and vegetables, bread and starches, meat, milk, and dairy products that should be included in a healthy diet.

Canada offers a food guide that is similar in format to MyPyramid. It organizes the food groups into "bands" of different types of foods and also includes serving size suggestions.

Another useful resource is the on-line availability of various healthy guides developed specifically for different cultures. Some of the resources are offered in English but include foods that are familiar to the specific cultural group. Others are printed in the client's native language and include familiar foods. They can be viewed at the USDA Food and Nutrition Information Center's Web site.

MyNursingKit Japanese Food Guide Spinning Top   MyNursingKit Eating Well with Canada's Food Guide   MyNursingKit USDA Ethnic/Cultural Food Pyramid

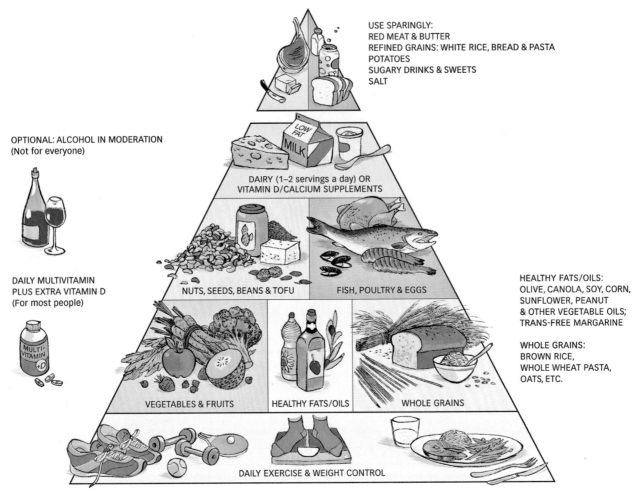

USE SPARINGLY:
RED MEAT & BUTTER
REFINED GRAINS: WHITE RICE, BREAD & PASTA
POTATOES
SUGARY DRINKS & SWEETS
SALT

OPTIONAL: ALCOHOL IN MODERATION
(Not for everyone)

DAIRY (1–2 servings a day) OR
VITAMIN D/CALCIUM SUPPLEMENTS

DAILY MULTIVITAMIN
PLUS EXTRA VITAMIN D
(For most people)

HEALTHY FATS/OILS:
OLIVE, CANOLA, SOY, CORN,
SUNFLOWER, PEANUT
& OTHER VEGETABLE OILS;
TRANS-FREE MARGARINE

WHOLE GRAINS:
BROWN RICE,
WHOLE WHEAT PASTA,
OATS, ETC.

NUTS, SEEDS, BEANS & TOFU

FISH, POULTRY & EGGS

VEGETABLES & FRUITS

HEALTHY FATS/OILS

WHOLE GRAINS

DAILY EXERCISE & WEIGHT CONTROL

■ **FIGURE 9-4 Healthy Eating Pyramid.**

Source: Copyright © 2008. For more information about The Healthy Eating Pyramid, please see The Nutrition Source, Department of Nutrition, Harvard School of Public Health, http://www.thenutritionsource.org, and *Eat, Drink, and Be Healthy,* by Walter C. Willett, M.D. and Patrick J. Skerrett (2005), Free Press/Simon & Schuster Inc.

Fruit and Veggies—More Matters Program

The 5- to 9-a-day program has now become the "Fruit and Veggies—More Matters" program. Cosponsored by the CDC, the American Cancer Society, and the U.S. Department of Health and Human Services, this diet-planning program is intended to increase the consumption of fruits and vegetables by American consumers. The program's Web site offers a wide variety of consumer-friendly information in both English and Spanish. Content includes the benefits of fruit and vegetable consumption, a guide to serving size for fruits and vegetables, recipes, and helpful tips for increasing fruit and vegetable intake for all ages. The site describes fruits and vegetables as nutrient-dense foods to assist in weight loss, provide vital nutrients, and prevent acute and chronic illness.

Fruit and Veggies—More Matters is the product of the National Fruit and Vegetable Program. This program is a result of the change in fruit and vegetable recommendations included in the *Dietary Guidelines for Americans*. Previous dietary guidelines like the Food Pyramid recommended a range of 5 to 9 servings of fruits and vegetables a day. The new guidelines recommend 2 to 6 1/2 cups of fruits and vegetables a day or the equivalent of 4 to 13 servings. Through consumer research, experts realized that describing a cup as a serving size is a more understandable tool for helping consumers visualize the amount of fruits and vegetables to be consumed each day. Client Education Checklist: Increasing Fruit and Vegetable Intake outlines advice that the nurse can offer when educating clients about increasing intake of fruits and vegetables.

The New American Plate

The New American Plate was created by the American Institute for Cancer Research in the hopes of decreasing dietary risk factors that lead to cancer. The emphasis is on a predominately plant-based diet to reduce the risk of cancer. Whole grains, fruits, vegetables, and other plant-based foods

MyNursingKit The American Institute for Cancer Research Guidelines for Cancer Prevention

CLIENT EDUCATION CHECKLIST	Increasing Fruit and Vegetable Intake
Intervention	**Example**
Explain the role of fruits and vegetables in a balanced diet.	Fruits and vegetables provide vitamins, minerals, fiber, and phytochemicals (plant chemicals) believed to be beneficial in overall health and reduction of disease risk.
Outline dietary recommendations for intake.	At least 2 cups of fruits and vegetables are recommended. Some guidelines suggest daily intake of 8 servings or more.
Describe serving sizes.	*Dietary Guidelines for Americans* describes servings in cups. Other guidelines consider a serving to be the following: 1 piece of fruit 1 cup chopped fruit ½ cup 100% fruit juice ¼ cup dried fruit 1 cup raw vegetable ½ cup cooked vegetable or vegetable juice
Encourage choice of fruits and vegetables high in fiber.	Choose fruit and vegetables that are less processed—an unpeeled apple vs. apple juice is an example. Consume edible skins and seeds.
Modify existing intake to meet recommendations.	Replace low-fiber processed fruits and vegetables with less processed forms. Add fruits and vegetables to existing dishes. Example: add peas to macaroni and cheese; have vegetable pizza; add fruit to a smoothie drink, yogurt, or cereal; add vegetables to plain casseroles; add spinach or dark greens to a sandwich. Try new fruits and vegetables to add to those already in the diet. Adding one per month makes it an easy idea.
Address existing barriers to adequate intake.	*Cost:* Purchase only seasonal fruits and vegetables or frozen. If canned are used, rinse before using. *Dental problems:* Cut or mash, use riper or softer forms that require less chewing (melon, banana, whipped squash, tomato sauce). *Taste:* Experiment with different types and recipes. *Convenience:* Frozen fruits and vegetables retain more nutrition than canned and are convenient for when fresh produce is not available. Dried fruit is also an option.

contain a variety of cancer-protective ingredients and can also help limit excess caloric intake. The recommended healthy eating strategies are as follows (American Institute for Cancer Research, 2007):

Strategies for Cancer Prevention:
1. Eat mostly plant-based foods, which are low in energy density.
2. Be physically active.
3. Maintain a healthy weight (via steps 1 and 2, as well as reducing portion size).

Strategies for Weight Loss:
1. Eat a greater proportion of plant-based foods, which are low in energy density.
2. Be physically active.
3. Reduce your portion size.

Food Labels

One of the most effective ways to make healthy food choices is to read the labels on foods. Legally required on all packaged foods except for a few foods without significant nutritional value, such as coffee, tea, and spices, food labels offer a wealth of information for the informed consumer. Yet consumers remain confused about the terminology and unsure about the validity of the nutrient content, structure-function, and health claims included on food labels. In addition, there is some evidence that food advertising is intentionally targeted at ethnic and cultural groups at higher risk for obesity and chronic disease conditions related to unhealthy and uninformed food choices (Henderson & Kelly, 2005). In addition, the majority of Saturday morning food advertisements on children's programming are for products that are high in fat, sugar, and sodium or low in nutrients (Batada, Dock Seitz, Wootan, & Story, 2008). Such marketing makes it all the more important for consumers to learn how to read food labels and bypass the advertising hype meant to catch the eye. There are three parts of the food label that the nurse can emphasize with the client: the ingredient list, the nutrition facts panel, and use of any nutritional claims.

MyNursingKit The National Health, Lung, and Blood Institute Food Label Activity

Ingredient List

By law, the ingredient list must include all ingredients in the food source in descending order by weight. So for most foods, the ingredient listed first is the largest contributor to the food's caloric and nutrient value. A can of fruit that lists in order of weight "sugar, water, fruit" will not offer the consumer a lot of nutrient density for the caloric count compared with one that lists fruit as the first ingredient. A juice-based drink that lists "sugar, water, coloring, flavoring" before actual fruit products will also not add much nutritional value to a diet. Real juice, and not a juice drink, would have fruit listed as the first ingredient.

Beginning in 2004, ingredient lists must also contain a separate subsection that lists any common food allergens contained in the product (Food and Drug Administration [FDA], 2004a). The allergens must be listed in common language so that consumers can clearly understand what the product contains. For example, if an ingredient list contains casein, a protein found in milk, the allergen subsection would list a warning that the product contains milk, making it much clearer to those with milk allergy, than using technical jargon or complicated ingredient names. The law requires that eight major food allergens be highlighted if present: milk, egg, fish, crustacean shellfish, tree nuts, peanuts, wheat, and soy (FDA, 2004a). Figure 9-5 ■ depicts an ingredient list with food allergen information.

Nutrition Facts Panel

The nutrition facts panel must follow a standard format that is shown in Figure 9-6 ■. It allows the consumer to see information on serving size, calories, and key nutrients in the product. A daily values section allows comparison with the nutrition recommendations for a 2,000 kcal diet.

> **Ingredients**: Enriched flour (**wheat** flour, malted barley, niacin, reduced iron, thiamin mononitrate, riboflavin, folic acid), sugar, partially hydrogenated soybean oil, and/or cottonseed oil, high fructose corn syrup, whey (**milk**), **eggs**, vanilla, natural and artificial flavoring) salt, leavening (sodium acid pyrophosphate, monocalcium phosphate), lecithiin (**soy**), mono-and diglycerides (emulsifier)

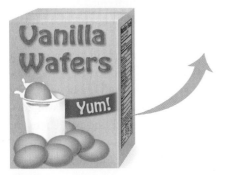

■ **FIGURE 9-5 Ingredient List.**

The nurse can teach a client to read the nutrition facts panel by following the steps in Figure 9-6. Serving size should be looked at first because it refers to the amount of the food source that constitutes one serving. Checking other parts of the label without knowing serving size can lead to inaccurate assumptions about the nutrient content of the food. The FDA has established standardized serving sizes for many foods and requires all producers of those foods to use the mandated serving size. Serving sizes can be listed in either metric (e.g., millimeters, milligrams, and grams) or U.S. customary units (e.g., cups, ounces, tablespoons, and teaspoons). Serving size can be confusing; potato chips marketed as "big grab" size, implying a single serving, actually contain 2 or more servings and twice the expected caloric count. Checking the serving size instead of just reading the marketing on the package would let the consumer know the actual number of servings contained in the product. To further confuse matters, some food labels list serving sizes that do not correlate with the USDA Food Guide suggestions (Herring, Britten, Davis, & Tuepker, 2002). The USDA records a serving of rice as ½ cup, yet many products list a serving as 1 cup. A research study completed by Basiotis, Lino, and Dinkins in 2002 found that individuals' perceptions of their consumption of food groups differed greatly from actual consumption, especially for serving size, and probably based on a misunderstanding of what constitutes a serving size.

The middle section of the panel contains information on key nutrients associated with health. In addition to calorie information, total, saturated, and trans fat content are listed along with sodium. The nurse can teach the client that it is recommended that intake of these nutrients be moderated in the diet. Information on fiber, vitamins A and C, calcium, and iron should be emphasized so that consumers can choose products that contribute to an adequate intake of these micronutrients.

Nutritional facts on a food label are required to present nutrient information in both quantities (milliequivalents, milligrams, or grams) and as a percentage of a standard known as **daily value.** The daily value for a macro- or micronutrient is the amount that is recommended for health, based on ongoing research. The FDA established the daily values system for use on food labels to allow consumers to compare the amount contained in the food source with the amount of that nutrient suggested for daily intake. This allows the consumer to know if the product is high or low in a nutrient and how it may fit in with overall intake.

Daily values for food labels have been established for these nutrients: fat, saturated fat, cholesterol, total carbohydrate, fiber, protein, sodium, potassium, vitamin C, vitamin A, calcium, and iron. These daily values are calculated on a 2,000-calorie diet, but most labels also list the daily values for a 2,500-calorie diet. Individuals who consume a 2,000-calorie diet can calculate their nutrient intake by adding the percentages from each of their food choices during the day. Consumers can also easily determine if a po-

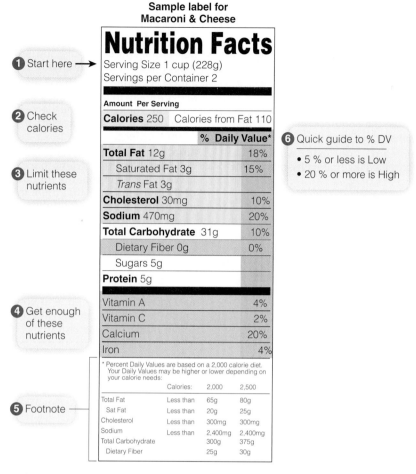

FIGURE 9-6 How to Read a Food Label.

tential food is nutritionally dense for an individual nutrient. If Food A contains 50% of the daily value for iron, then one serving would be a good source of that micronutrient. If Food B contained only 5% of the daily value for iron, it would not compare favorable to Food A as a significant source of iron. A daily value of 20% or more of a nutrient is considered high, whereas a daily value of 5% or less is low (FDA, 2004b).

Nutritional Claims

One of the most confusing areas of consumer nutritional education is a claim about the health benefits of individual nutrients. Often, the discrepancy between the legal or regulatory definition of "low fat" or "reduced sodium" and the consumer perception of those same terms can be significant. Label claims can be made in three areas: nutrient content, structure-function associations, and health. The following is a description of common nutritional claims and the actual definitions.

Nutrient Content Claims

The following terms often appear in bold, colorful letters in advertisements and on the packaging of common food items.

The FDA-approved definitions of these terms are often not what the consumer might expect. It is very important to understand exactly what these terms mean legally so informed food choices can be made to support a healthy diet. These terms were originally specified in the 1990 Nutrition Labeling and Education Act (NLEA, 1990).

Nutrient content claims describe the level of a nutrient in the product, using terms such as *free, high,* and *low,* or they compare the level of a nutrient in a food to that of another food, using terms such as *more, reduced,* and *lite.* The "comparison food" in the definitions refers to a reference food, usually the original food source to which the nutrient content has been compared. For example, a hot dog that claims to have "reduced fat" is in reference to a traditional hot dog. Unfortunately, "reduced fat" does not mean that the hot dog is actually *low* in fat, just that it has at least 25% less fat than the reference hot dog. So a hot dog with 12 grams of saturated fat per serving can be labeled "reduced fat" if the comparison food (traditional hot dog) has 16 grams of saturated fat. It is not surprising that consumers are confused by nutrient content claims. The FDA definitions for nutrient claims are listed in Box 9-4.

BOX 9-4	Label Nutrient Claims: Definitions

"Low" means an amount that would allow frequent consumption of a food without exceeding the daily value of the nutrient. Labels may also list this as "few" or "low source of."

"Reduced" refers to at least 25% less of a given nutrient or calories than the comparison food. This characteristic is also listed as "less" and "fewer."

"Free" is also listed as "zero," "no," and "without." It means that a food provides insignificant amounts of a nutrient.

"Light" is often charmingly misspelled as "lite." Both terms refer to a food that has one-third (1/3) fewer calories, or 50% or less of the fat or sodium than the comparison food. It is also used when referring to a characteristic of the food, such as "light in color" or "light in texture."

If a food is a **"good source,"** it provides between 10% and 19% of the daily value for that nutrient per serving. Note that this is less than 20% of the recommended daily intake of the nutrient, so additional sources of the nutrient are necessary to meet the body's requirements.

If a food is **"high"** or **"rich in"** a specified nutrient, by law it means that it provides at least 20% or more of the daily value of that nutrient. Foods that meet this requirement are also labeled an **"excellent source"** of the nutrient.

"More" means that there is at least 10% more of the daily value of the nutrient than the comparison food. It does not mean that the food is a significant source of the nutrient, only that there is more of the nutrient in this food than in the reference sample.

A **"lean"** food is one that contains less than 10 grams of fat, 4.5 grams of saturated fat and trans fat combined, and no more than 95 mg of cholesterol either per serving or per 100 grams of meat, poultry, and seafood. If a food is labeled **"extra lean,"** it contains only 5 grams of fat, 2 grams of saturated fat and trans fat combined, and not more than 95 mg of cholesterol either per serving or per 100 grams of meat, poultry, and seafood.

■ An overweight client with high blood pressure reports switching to "light" potato chips to "help with the diet." What should the nurse say about this change?

Source: FDA, 2003a.

After reviewing the NLEA regulations for nutritional content claims, it is easy to understand why consumers become confused and potentially misled by the statements made in advertisements and on the packaging of food sources. Nurses have an important responsibility to help these clients become more informed about reading nutritional labels and comparing this information with packaging claims.

Structure-Function Claims

Structure-function claims describe a food or dietary supplement in regard to a normal structure or function in the body or general well-being (FDA, 2003a). For example, a label may tout the need for calcium for bone health. Structure-function claims may not refer to a specific disease or symptoms. Food marketers can claim that a food item will "stop aging," "improve memory," or "support healthy joints" but cannot say that the food will "cure arthritis." No premarket approval is required for structure-function claims, nor is there a requirement to submit evidence to the FDA regarding the claim. Labels with structure-function claims must not be misleading to the consumer and must have a disclaimer that states that the product "is not intended to diagnose, treat, cure or prevent any disease" (FDA 2003a). The onus to police misleading claims or those that infer that a disease can be treated is the burden of the FDA once the product is already on the market. The sheer volume of products on the market and the limited personnel to police products makes this a slow process that results in products being sold that do not meet regulations.

Health Claims

A **health claim** is a statement about the hypothesized or proven relationship between a nutrient or ingredient in a food or dietary supplement and a known disease or health-related condition (FDA, 2003a). Health claims fall into three categories, all of which require scientific review by the FDA: authorized health claims, claims based on authoritative statements, and qualified health claims. Authorized health claims are allowed under the 1990 NLEA law and include statements about scientifically well-established links between diet and disease. Examples include calcium and osteoporosis and sodium and hypertension. Authoritative statements are only those from government scientific organizations or the National Academy of Sciences. An example is the positive effects of a high-potassium diet on lowering blood pressure, an authoritative statement based on recommendations from the National Heart, Lung, and Blood Institute. Qualified health claims are those for which there is emerging evidence of a health benefit, but the level of evidence is not sufficient for the FDA to issue an authoritative statement. Manufacturers must petition the FDA for consideration of a qualified health claim

MyNursingKit Federal Trade Commission Guidance Documents: Diet, Health, and Fitness

BOX 9-5 Grading of Label Health Claims

A **grade A health claim** means that the level of confidence in the validity of the statement is high, and there is significant scientific research to support this assertion. Grade A claims do not require any disclaimers on the food label.

A **grade B health claim** has a moderate level of confidence in the validity of the statement. The FDA requires that the following disclaimer be included on the food label: "[Health claim]: Although there is scientific evidence supporting the claim, the evidence is not conclusive."

A **grade C health claim** has a less than moderate level of confidence in its validity, often due to inconclusive or insufficient research. The FDA requires food labels to include this statement: "Some scientific evidence suggests [Health Claim]. However, the FDA has determined that this evidence is limited and not conclusive."

A **grade D health claim** has very low confidence of validity, with little or no research supporting it. The FDA requires the following disclaimer on the food label: "Very limited and preliminary scientific research suggests [Health Claim]. FDA concludes that there is little scientific evidence supporting this claim."

Source: FDA, 2003b.

and undergo a review process. An example of a qualified health claim is the beneficial effect of omega-3 fatty acids on reduced risk of heart disease. Qualified health claims must include a disclaimer that denotes the level of confidence that exists for the available evidence. The FDA recognizes four levels of health claims in descending order of confidence: Grade A, B, C, and D claims (FDA, 2003b). Box 9-5 outlines the health care grading definitions.

The FDA attempts to alert consumers to the relative merits of various health claims for nutrients and food components through statements on the food label. However, criticism exists that the majority of consumers cannot differentiate between the grade levels of evidence or the types of nutrition claims found on labels (Hasler, 2008). A nonjudgmental discussion between the nurse and a client can help underline the true definition of a label claim made for a product that the client is purchasing and its health implications. Often clients are surprised to learn that structure-function claims are about well-being and are not to imply that a condition can be treated with use of the product. For example, a product touting that it "helps memory" may be taken by a client who believes that it will prevent or treat dementia. Only medications are allowed to make claims about disease treatment after careful government scrutiny, a process that does not exist for foods or dietary supplements. Unfortunately, many consumers have turned to the Internet for information about foods and health, and the health claims

made on Web sites and by devotees of specific approaches to prevention and disease treatment often make unsubstantiated claims without intervention from any regulatory agency. The Food Label and Package Survey (FLAPS) is an FDA study of food labels for processed and packaged food to ensure that the food industry is following current governmental policy about nutritional labeling and food safety (LeGault et al., 2004).

Nutritional Misinformation

Nutrition misinformation occurs for a number of reasons, including lack of understanding, a misinterpretation of nutritional research or facts, susceptibility to inaccurate claims reported by friends or the media, or a deliberate attempt by an unscrupulous promotion of a food or product for financial gain (ADA, 2006). The wide availability of health information in the media and on the Internet, coupled with confusion about the validity of advertising and label claims, can further blur the line between fact and fiction. Whatever the reason for the nutritional misinformation, nurses have an opportunity and an obligation to help the consumer become more informed and practical about their food choices. A nonjudgmental, objective, and respectful approach is useful to change consumer awareness and knowledge of nutritional misinformation.

Nurses must be nonjudgmental in order to elicit truthful information from the client about their food choices and the reasons for those choices. Nutrition misinformation can lead to harmful effects, especially if it causes an interaction or delay in medical treatment. Such effects need to be communicated to the client. If a client reports a harmless food belief that is not supported by research, the nurse must decide whether addressing the practice will alienate the client to future dietary teaching. Some nutrition misinformation results in economic consequences when costly products are purchased that have no therapeutic effect. An example includes the many bogus weight loss products that are marketed as miracle cures for overweight. Figure 9-7 ■ depicts the Federal Trade Commission's (FTC) mock advertisement for an unproven weight loss product with the corrected information also featured. The FTC is responsible for overseeing the advertising aspects of nutritional claims.

Objectivity and sensitivity are important when responding to client reports of nutritional misinformation. Many health claims for specific foods are deeply engrained in culture, religion, or lifestyle habits. Detaching the client from a long-standing food practice requires professional tact, interpersonal skill, and current knowledge. It is important to not overreact when addressing nutrition misinformation because the client can lose perspective and believe that either everything causes harm or conversely that the practitioner is an alarmist and nothing really is dangerous (ADA, 2006).

It is also important that the message from different health care professionals be consistent. Because nutritional

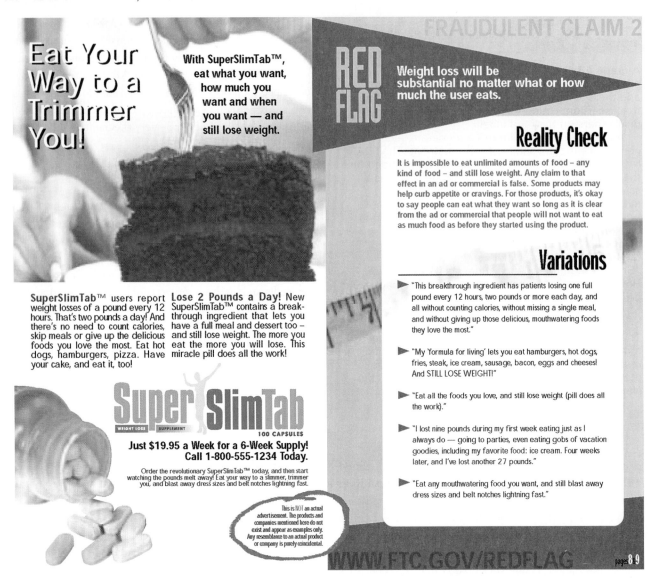

■ FIGURE 9-7 **Mock Nutrition Advertising.**

Source: Federal Trade Commission (2003). Red flag bogus weight loss claims. Retrieved November 9, 2009, from http://www.ftc.gov/bcp/edu/pubs/business/adv/bus60.pdf

information can be complicated, it is imperative that the client receives a similar message from all of the members of the health care team. Other team members who are not current or complete in the nutritional information they communicate to the client can unwittingly sabotage effective health teaching. A consistent message that the nurse can offer is that there is no such thing as good foods or bad foods, but there are good diets and bad diets. No one nutrient, food, or product should be emphasized as superior to another. Rather, it is overall dietary intake that matters. Hot Topic Box: When Nutrition Advertising Is Too Good to Be True discusses nutrition misinformation and some examples that the nurse can use when discussing this topic with clients.

hot TOPic

When Nutrition Advertising Is Too Good to Be True

It probably will not surprise you that false health claims for nutritional products costs unwary consumers billions of dollars a year. Unfortunately, if it sounds too good to be true, it probably is. But people who suffer from acute or chronic illness, especially those that are life-threatening, are especially vulnerable to unvalidated structure-function claims. What are the most popular treatments? Those that promise to "cure" cancer, HIV/AIDS, and arthritis. The Federal Trade Commission (FTC) estimates that consumers spend $2 billion each year on arthritis cures alone. In addition to delaying or interacting with proven health treatments, these treatments often carry safety risks for people because of contaminated compounds or medically active ingredients.

The FTC oversees advertising of food and dietary supplements to make sure that all types of advertising— print, television, or other types—is not misleading to the consumer or that food- and nutrition-related products are not advertised in a way that infers that they have drug-like properties that can treat medical conditions. Unfortunately, the process to screen and react to misleading advertisements happens after products are already on the market and is time-consuming. Following are some examples of bogus health claims for nutrition products on which the FTC has taken action.

- A Florida-based company had to pay almost $400,000 in settlement charges for marketing deceptive, unsubstantiated claims that its dietary supplement made kids taller. The product promised clinical proof that children and young adults would grow an additional 2 to 3 inches in 6 months and have an overall gain in height of up to 35% if used regularly. The settlement charges were to reimburse all the consumers who had purchased the product.
- A $1 million settlement was paid by a manufacturer of two products that had unsubstantiated label claims. Part of the settlement went to consumers who had purchased a dietary supplement that promised to improve mood and concentration in adults and children. Structure-function claims were used to tout that the product improved the ability to "focus." The second supplement contained an amino acid and herb combination that promised to improve male sexual performance.
- Several natural foods and dietary supplement companies have been implicated for claiming that their products treat attention-deficit hyperactivity disorder and improve scholastic performance in children who have trouble focusing on school work. Such claims imply that the products treat a condition and are not allowed as a label claim.
- Several manufacturers of zinc supplements have advertised that the products treat or prevent the common cold, a medical condition. The FTC has taken action that such unsubstantiated claims be removed from the advertising of these products. In order for the zinc products to make a claim about cold relief, they would have to undergo the review process in place for medications.

The nurse should note the significant settlement charges for some of these misleading claims and advertisements and realize that the amounts awarded are proportionate to the sales. Although some of the label claims outlined may seem far-fetched, a great number of consumers have purchased these products. The FTC seeks to protect consumers from health fraud, including that which arises from misleading nutrition claims. The nurse can use the on-line resources available from the FTC to remain up to date about bogus nutrition claims found in the marketplace.

Additionally, the adage "if it sounds too good to be true, it is" should be applied to nutrition-related advertising. The FTC offers these ideas to spot false claims:

- Be skeptical. If it sounds too good to be true, it is.
- Be cautious of products that offer a quick cure-all for a variety of conditions, such as pain, cancer, heart problems.
- Avoid nutrition products or dietary supplements that promise to cure or treat a disease.
- Think twice when words like "scientific breakthrough" and "miracle" are used or if there is an ancient or secret ingredient.
- Watch out for impressive medical jargon that really has no scientific meaning. An example is a product claiming to reset the "hunger stimulation point."
- Use of testimonials and anecdotes as evidence should not be confused with scientific evidence.
- Economic warning signs of a product include promises of money-back guarantees (which most consumers are too embarrassed to seek) and the implication that there is a limited supply of the product warranting quick payment.

Chapter 25 discusses labeling and marketing of these products in more detail.

Source: Federal Trade Commission, 2008.

NURSING CARE PLAN The Language of Nutrition

CASE STUDY

Nichelle, age 27, an administrative assistant in the school district main office, comes to the clinic because she has had some recent problems controlling her asthma. After reviewing her current medications, Nichelle tells the nurse that she would like to do a "little something" about her diet. She explains that she knows she is not really overweight, but she gets so confused by all she hears on television or reads on the computer that she does not really know where to start to make some improvements. She asks how she can figure out where to find "the truth" about what she should eat or avoid. She said she does not want to become "some kind of health food nut"; she just wants to do the right thing given her modest budget.

Applying the Nursing Process

ASSESSMENT

Height: 5 feet 6 inches Weight: 143 pounds BMI: 23.2 BP 124/76 P 78 R 18

(continued)

The Language of Nutrition *(continued)*

NURSING CARE PLAN

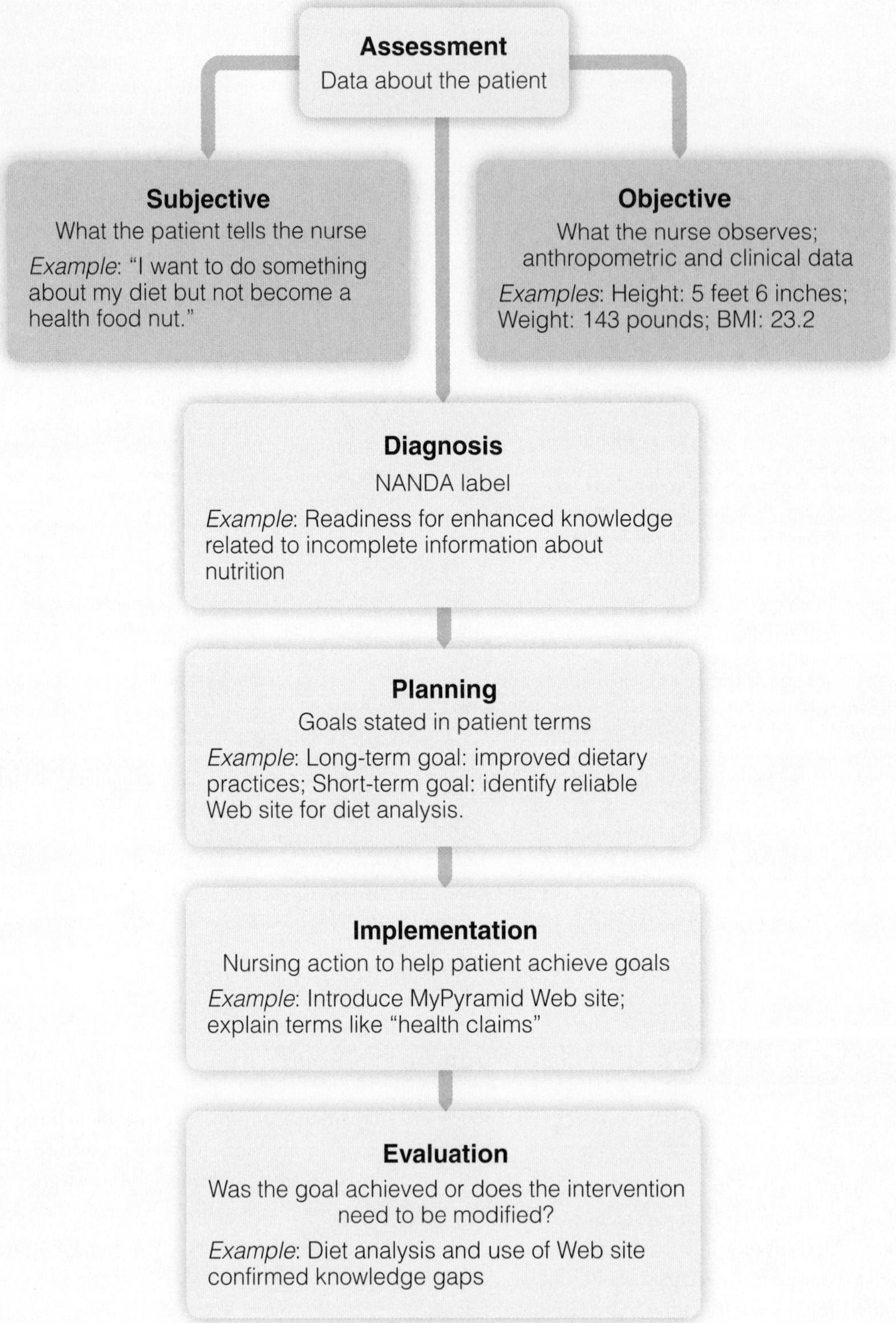

Assessment
Data about the patient

Subjective
What the patient tells the nurse

Example: "I want to do something about my diet but not become a health food nut."

Objective
What the nurse observes; anthropometric and clinical data

Examples: Height: 5 feet 6 inches; Weight: 143 pounds; BMI: 23.2

Diagnosis
NANDA label

Example: Readiness for enhanced knowledge related to incomplete information about nutrition

Planning
Goals stated in patient terms

Example: Long-term goal: improved dietary practices; Short-term goal: identify reliable Web site for diet analysis.

Implementation
Nursing action to help patient achieve goals

Example: Introduce MyPyramid Web site; explain terms like "health claims"

Evaluation
Was the goal achieved or does the intervention need to be modified?

Example: Diet analysis and use of Web site confirmed knowledge gaps

■ FIGURE 9-8 **Nursing Care Plan Process: The Language of Nutrition.**

The Language of Nutrition *(continued)*

DIAGNOSIS

Readiness for enhanced knowledge related to incomplete information evidenced by questions about improving diet

EXPECTED OUTCOMES

Identify new sources for enhancing knowledge

Ask relevant questions about the quality of new knowledge and evidence for the information

Incorporate new information in dietary practices

INTERVENTIONS

Clarify current sources of information that Nichelle uses

Use the interactive MyPyramid Web site for a diet assessment

Explain relevant terms like "DRI" or "health claims"

Share sources of trusted dietary information

Answer questions and clarify misconceptions about nutrients and diets

EVALUATION

Nichelle expressed gratitude for being directed to helpful Web sites because that is how she gets most of her current information. She keeps reading about studies that claim that particular foods are good in certain quantities or should be avoided, but now finds it easier to use the *Dietary Guidelines for Americans* or the MyPyramid Web site for reliable information. She said that she thought she had a pretty good idea all along what she should be doing, but it was nice to skip over some of the claims she reads on the Internet and go to more trusted sites. Figure 9-8 ■ outlines the nursing process for this case.

Critical Thinking in the Nursing Process

1. **How should the nurse respond to the client who says that it is hard to know what to believe when there are so many sources of information about nutrition and that there are so many abbreviations like DRI or UL or RDA?**

CHAPTER SUMMARY

- Nutrient deficiencies are rare in the United States, but nutrient excesses, especially of simple carbohydrates, saturated fat, cholesterol, and calories, increase each year.

- Studies show that consumers do not understand nutritional labeling, are confused about macro- and micronutrients, and lack the information and confidence to implement healthier diet and fitness habits.

- Nutritional recommendations and standards have been developed by government and private groups to provide advice to consumers to describe the amounts of energy (measured as calories), macro- and micronutrients, essential and nonessential dietary elements, and physical activity that promote health and wellness.

- Dietary reference intakes (DRIs) are recommendations and standards for optimal nutrient intake levels for calcium, phosphorus, magnesium, vitamin D, fluoride, vitamins, minerals, macronutrients, cholesterol, fiber, electrolytes, and fluids.

- The DRI recommendations involved four different values: estimated average requirements (EAR), recommended daily allowance (RDA), adequate intake (AI), and tolerable upper intake levels (UL).

- The DRI system also defined two values related to energy. The acceptable macronutrient distribution range (AMDR) and the estimated energy requirement (EER) make recommendations about dietary intake needed to meet average daily energy needs.

- The DRI recommendations can be individualized by considering the client's age; body size; daily energy expenditure; any relevant medical conditions; and dietary habits, including culture, religion, and personal preferences.

- Healthy diet principles for all consumers include balance, moderation, variety, adequacy, nutrient density, and enjoyment.

- A variety of diet-planning guides are available to help consumers to make healthy food choices. The *Dietary Guidelines for Americans*, Healthy Living Pyramid, New American Plate, MyPyramid, Fruit and Veggies—More Matters, and exchange lists are all examples of easy-to-use approaches that are available for American consumers.

- Food labels are an excellent source of information about the nutritional content of a food product. Daily value is the amount of micronutrient or macronutrient that is recommended for health based on ongoing research.

Daily values for food labels have been established for fat, saturated fat, cholesterol, total carbohydrate, fiber, protein, sodium, potassium, vitamin C, vitamin A, calcium, and iron. These daily values are calculated on a 2,000-calorie diet, but most labels also list the daily values for a 2,500-calorie diet.

- The U.S. Food and Drug Administration regulates the nutrient content, health, and structure-function claims that manufacturers and producers can place on food labels.

- Registered nurses are optimally suited to help consumers develop this skill and to reinforce their healthy food choices for protection and prevention of chronic conditions such as cardiovascular disease, diabetes, and cancer.

EXPLORE **mynursingkit** PEARSON

MyNursingKit is your one stop for online chapter review materials and resources. Prepare for success with additional NCLEX®-style practice questions, interactive assignments and activities, web links, animations and videos, and more!

Register your access code from the front of your book at
www.mynursingkit.com.

NCLEX® QUESTIONS

1. A young mother asks the clinic nurse about DRIs and why they are important. How should the nurse respond?
   1. "They are guidelines for how many calories your child should consume."
   2. "They are the standards by which health care providers determine obesity."
   3. "They provide guidance about recommended intake of nutrients, including vitamins and minerals."
   4. "They are used by dietitians to calculate calories and plan diets to treat diseases."

2. The nurse who is teaching a client about food product labels points out that a package of cookies that is labeled "low fat" contains cookies that have:
   1. Very little fat per serving
   2. Half the fat calories of traditional cookies
   3. No saturated fat
   4. Fewer calories than traditional cookies

3. The nurse explains the concept of nutrient density to a client as:
   1. The nutrient being widely available in a variety of foods

2. The practice of consuming foods from each food group every day
3. Foods that contain a significant amount of specific nutrients for the least amount of calories
4. Those foods that are at the base of MyPyramid

4. The nurse uses the example of "milk builds strong bones" to explain the concept of:
   1. A nutrient content fact
   2. A structure-function claim
   3. A health claim
   4. An exaggerated health claim

5. A client expresses a desire to have a healthier diet. What could the nurse suggest as a first step?
   1. Read the dietary reference intakes (DRIs).
   2. Do a diet analysis using the MyPyramid Web site.
   3. Read current nutritional pamphlets from a health food section at the grocery store.
   4. Check the United States Department of Agriculture (USDA) Web site.

REFERENCES

American Dietetic Association (ADA). (2006). Position of the American Dietetic Association: Food and nutrition misinformation. *Journal of the American Dietetic Association, 106,* 601–607.

American Dietetic Association (ADA). (2008). Position of the American Dietetic Association: Nutrition guidance for healthy children ages 2 to 11 years. *Journal of the American Dietetic Association, 108,* 1038–1047.

American Institute for Cancer Research. (2007). *Food, nutrition, physical activity, and cancer prevention: A global perspective.* Retrieved June 24, 2009, from http://www.dietandcancerreport.org/downloads/summary/english.pdf

Barr, S. I., Murphy, S. P., & Poos, M. I. (2002). Interpreting and using the Dietary References Intakes in dietary assessment of individuals and groups. *Journal of the American Dietetic Association, 102* (6), 780–788.

Basiotis, P. P., Lino, M., & Dinkins, J. M. (2002). Consumption of food group servings: People's perceptions vs. reality. *Family Economics and Nutrition Review, 14* (1), 67–70.

Batada, A., Dock Seitz, M., Wootan, M. G., & Story, M. (2008). Nine out of ten food advertisements shown during Saturday morning children's programming are for foods high in fat, sodium, added sugar, or low in nutrients. *Journal of the American Dietetic Association, 108,* 673–678.

Centers for Disease Control (CDC) and Prevention, National Center for Health Statistics. (2008). *Deaths/mortalities.* Retrieved October 30, 2008, from http://www.cdc.gov/nchs/fastats/deaths.htm

Federal Trade Commission. (2008). *Miracle health claims: Add a dose of skepticism.* Retrieved October 30, 2008, from http://www.ftc.gov/bcp/edu/pubs/consumer/health/hea07.shtm

Food & Drug Administration (FDA). (2003a). *Claims that can be made for conventional foods and dietary supplements.* Retrieved October 30, 2008, from http://www.cfsan.fda.gov/~dms/hclaims.html

Food & Drug Administration (FDA). (2003b). *Interim procedures for qualified health claims in the labeling of conventional human food and human dietary supplements.* Retrieved October 30, 2008, from http://www.cfsan.fda.gov/~dms/hclmgui3.html

Food & Drug Administration (FDA). (2004a). Food Allergen Labeling and Consumer Protection Act of 2004. Title II of Public Law 108-282. Retrieved October 30, 2008, from http://www.fda.gov/Food/LabelingNutrition/FoodAllergensLabeling/GuidanceComplianceRegulatoryInformation/ucm106187.htm

Food & Drug Administration (FDA). (2004b). *How to understand and use the nutrition facts label.* Retrieved October 30, 2008, from http://www.cfsan.fda.gov/~dms/foodlab.html

Food & Drug Administration (FDA). (2008).*A food labeling guide.* Retrieved April 25, 2008, from http://www.cfsan.fda.gov/~dms/2lg-toc.html

Gillum, R. F., & Sempos, C. T. (2005). Ethnic variation in validity of classification of overweight and obesity using self-reported weight and height in American women and men: the Third National Health and Nutrition Examination Survey. *Nutrition Journal, 4.* Retrieved April 21, 2008, from: http://www.nutritionj.com/content/4/1/27

Hasler, C. M. (2008). Health claims in the United States: An aid to the public or a source of confusion? *Journal of Nutrition, 138,* 1216S–1220S.

Henderson, V. R., & Kelly, G. (2005). Food advertising in the age of obesity: Content analysis of food advertising on general market and African American television. *Journal of Nutrition Education Behavior, 37,* 191–196.

Herring, D., Britten, P., Davis, C., & Tuepker, K. (2002). Serving sizes in the Food Guide Pyramid and on the nutrition facts label: What's different and why? *Family Economics and Nutrition Review, 14* (1), 71–73.

Institute of Medicine (IOM). (2000). *Dietary reference intakes: Applications in dietary assessment.* Washington, DC: The National Academies Press.

Institute of Medicine (IOM). (2002). *Dietary reference intakes for energy, carbohydrate, fat, fatty acids, cholesterol, protein, and amino acids.* Washington, DC: The National Academies Press.

Jemal, A. (2005). Trends in the leading causes of death in the United States, 1970–2002. *Journal of the American Medical Association, 294,* 1255–1259.

Johnson-Taylor, W. L., Fisher, R. A., Hubbard, V. S., Starke-Reed, P., & Eggers, P. S. (2008). The change in weight perception of weight status among the overweight: Comparison of NHANES III (1988–1994) and 1999–2004 NHANES. *The International Journal of Behavioral Nutrition and Physical Activity, 5* (9). Retrieved April 15, 2008, from http://www.ijbnpa.org/content/5/1/9

Krebs-Smith, S. M., & Kris-Etherton, P. (2007). How does MyPyramid compare to other population-based recommendations for controlling disease? *Journal of the American Dietetic Association, 107,* 830–837.

LeGault, L., Brandt, M. B., McCabe, N., Adler, C., Brown, A., & Brecher, S. (2004). 2000–2001 Food label and package survey: An update on prevalence of nutrition labeling and claims on processed, packaged foods. *Journal of the American Dietetic Association, 104* (6), 952–958.

Making the most of nutrition facts labels. (2006). *Tufts University Health & Nutrition Letter, 24* (10), 4–5.

McCullough, M. L., Feskanich, D., Stampfer, M. J., Giovannucci, E. L., Rimm, E. B., Hu, F. B., et al. (2002). Diet quality and major chronic disease risk in men and women: Moving toward improved dietary guidance. *American Journal of Clinical Nutrition, 76,* 1261–1271.

Mitka, M. (2005). Government unveils new pyramid: Critics say nutrition tool is flawed. *Journal of the American Medical Association, 293,* 2581–2582.

Nutrition Labeling Education Act (NLEA). (1990). Pub. L. No. 101-535. Washington, DC.

Rothman, R. L., Housam, R., Weiss, H., Davis, D., Gregory, R., Gebretsadik, T., et al. (2006). Patient understanding of food labels: the role of literacy and numeracy. *American Journal of Preventive Medicine, 31* (5), 391–398.

U.S. Department of Health and Human Services. (2005). *Dietary Guidelines for Americans.* Retrieved October 30, 2008, from http://www.health.gov/dietaryguidelines/dga2005/document/pdf/ExecutiveSummary.pdf

Willett, W. C. (2001). *Eat, drink and be healthy: The Harvard Medical School guide to healthy eating.* New York: Simon & Schuster.

10

Susan Prion

Community Nutrition

WHAT WILL YOU LEARN?

1. To examine the powerful influence of community on individual health behaviors.
2. To evaluate the relationship between healthy living behaviors and decreased risk of chronic diseases.
3. To categorize how America's food safety is regulated and monitored.
4. To differentiate between food intolerances and food allergies and summarize nutrition care for each.
5. To relate common causes of foodborne illness and formulate nursing interventions to prevent it.
6. To provide sensitive and competent nutritional care to clients from diverse cultural, ethnic, and religious groups.

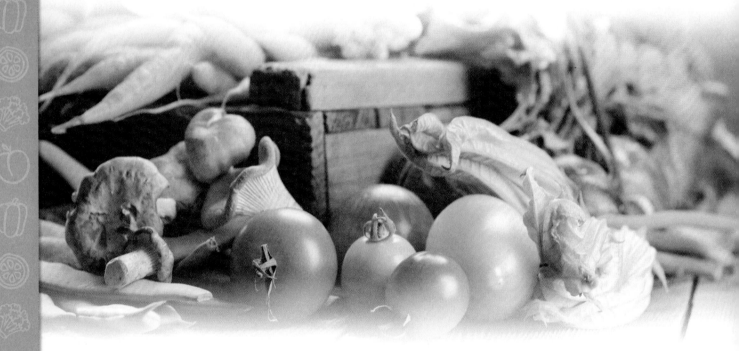

DID YOU KNOW?

▶ Four of the top 10 causes of death in the United States are related to diet.

▶ The Centers for Disease Control and Prevention (CDC) reports that at least 76 million Americans will experience a foodborne illness this year and that 5,000 people will die because of it.

▶ Environmental contamination of food and water sources is causing an increased number of acute and chronic health problems.

▶ Cultural, ethnic, and religious influences determine what most of us eat on a daily basis.

KEY TERMS

What Is a Community?

Communities are very important in health care. Communities are defined in a variety of ways depending on the context but generally refer to a collection of people with like characteristics. The World Health Organization (WHO) defines a **community** as "a collective body of individuals identified by geography, common interests, concerns, characteristics or values" (WHO, 1974). A community can also be conceptualized as a self-selecting gathering of people who have creativity and capacity for solving shared problems (McKnight, 2002). A study of community members' definitions of "community" revealed that the respondents defined a community as "a group of people with diverse characteristics who are linked by social ties, share common perspectives, and engage in joint action in geographical locations or settings" (MacQueen, et al., 2001, p. 1935). These researchers argued that the diverse nature of communities necessitates "the need for multiple models of collaboration for public health research and programs" (MacQueen, et al. 2001, p. 1935). Nurses must recognize that communities are composed of members with shared values and common goals, and that those members have a common system of communication and helping patterns that promote both individual and collective goodwill. Working in partnership with community members is essential to successful **health prevention** and **health promotion** activities.

Communities may be formed around similar interests (e.g., a hobby), similar needs (e.g., breastfeeding mothers), common experiences (e.g., caregivers of spouses with dementia), religion, culture, ethnicity, gender, and a host of other characteristics and conditions that people may share. The important thing to recognize is that the existence of a community and the interactions among and between community members offer powerful opportunities for nurses to influence the health and wellness choices of those people. In health promotion at the community level, changes occur at multiple levels usually beginning with individuals and ultimately encompassing the entire community (Shuster & Goeppinger, 2004).

Why Are Community Nutrition and Health Promotion Important?

If intact communities provide ready opportunities for influencing health behaviors, what types of information and assistance can nurses attempt to offer? Minkler and Wallerstein (2002) propose that community health promotion models are based on four assumptions:

1. Individual behaviors are shaped and influenced significantly by community values and norms.
2. Communities can change individual actions by promoting desirable behaviors and environments that encourage those individual changes.
3. Participation of community leaders is essential for change to occur.
4. Community members must be part of the planned changes, giving them a sense of responsibility about the outcomes.

For nurses, that means developing respect for existing community values, identifying positive strategies for community change, and working in partnership with community leaders and members to enact healthy living changes. Control of community-based health promotion activities must always be with the community members.

In order to understand the possibilities for community health promotion, it is necessary to review the types and levels of health promotion and prevention activities. Health promotion can be defined as "the science and art of helping people change their lifestyle to move toward a state of optimum health" (O'Donnell, 1987, p. 4). Kreuter and Devore

(1980) defined health promotion as "the process of advocating health in order to enhance the probability that personal (individual, family and community), private (professional and business), and public (federal, state and local government) support of positive health practices will become a societal norm" (p. 26). Health promotion can be contrasted with health prevention, which can be strictly defined as aversion to future disease development (Edelman & Mandle, 2002). Leavell and Clark (1965) defined prevention more broadly to include all of the actions one could take to limit the progression of a disease. Included in their definition was the concept of health promotion.

Levels of Health Prevention

Health care professionals categorize health prevention and promotion activities into three general levels: primary, secondary, and tertiary as listed in Figure 10-1 ■ (Leavell & Clark, 1965). *Primary* prevention activities are those that can prevent a health condition from developing. They include health promotion and specific protection activities.

Primary prevention

Health promotion activities such as
- Health education
- Healthy nutrition choices appropriate for developmental level
- Genetic screening
- Regular physical exams
- Provision of satisfactory housing and working conditions

Secondary prevention

Early diagnosis and treatment
- Screening surveys for physical and mental illnesses
- Specific examinations to identify disease processes, prevent communicable disease spread, prevent complications, decrease potential for disability

Tertiary prevention

Restoration and rehabilitation
- Agency and community resources to optimize remaining capacities and overall client wellness
- Integration of client into workforce as fully as possible

■ FIGURE 10-1 **Levels of Health Promotion with Definitions and Examples.**
Source: Adapted from Leavell & Clark, 1965.

Examples of primary health prevention activities include nutrition education for school-age children and fluoride added to municipal water supplies. Primary health prevention is most often delivered in a community-based model, because that is the most effective method for reaching the greatest number of people with the information. *Secondary* health prevention activities are those aimed at early detection of potential health conditions. Examples of secondary health promotion include cholesterol testing, blood pressure screening, and routine electrocardiograms (ECGs). Secondary health prevention strategies are individually based but are often publicized through a community-based model because of the importance of community influence on the individual community member. *Tertiary* health prevention activities are targeted at management and prevention of progression of existing clinical conditions. Examples of tertiary health prevention activities include diet modification interventions for clients with cardiac disease and smoking cessation support for clients with chronic pulmonary disease. Tertiary health prevention activities are the most individualized of all health prevention approaches, yet they would be unnecessary if adequate primary and secondary health prevention strategies were effective. The most productive and potentially influential health prevention and promotion activities for nurses are community based.

Community-based health prevention and promotion strategies are the most effective but are often difficult to deliver and manage. The constant interaction between community members and the community can be an important asset in nurses' attempts to encourage healthy living actions. There are also other influences that can enhance or distract from individual motivation and compliance with healthy living behaviors.

Peers can have great influence over individual community members, especially at specific developmental life stages. For example, adolescents and the elderly can be greatly influenced in their diet and fitness choices by their peers. Peers can also exert positive influence to promote healthy living behaviors, especially if personal improvements can be readily observed. The use of celebrity spokespersons in advertising for weight-loss programs is predicated on the observable, quantifiable weight loss that viewers can recognize for themselves. Similarly, significant health improvements such as weight loss, cessation of smoking, and decreased reliance on hypertension or antiglycemic medications can be powerful positive peer influences to impact positive lifestyle changes among community members. This is especially true if the community members share similar health care concerns.

Just as peers can influence healthy lifestyle choices, the community can promote or prevent those choices (Pender, Murdaugh, & Parsons, 2006). The content of the workshops offered at the local community center, the emphasis placed on healthy choices by community leaders, and the resources avail-

EVIDENCE-BASED PRACTICE RESEARCH BOX

Is there an association between food insecurity and obesity?

Clinical Problem: Food insecurity is widespread in the United States and throughout the world. Obesity is an increasing problem in developed countries among all age groups. Is the presence of food insecurity associated with the increased obesity among all age groups?

Research Findings: A broad definition of food insecurity comes from the Life Sciences Research Office: "the availability of nutritionally adequate and safe foods or the ability to acquire acceptable foods in socially acceptable ways is limited or uncertain" (Anderson, 1990). This definition has been adapted and used in numerous studies since then. A meta-analysis by Dinour, Bergen, and Ming-Chen (2007) reviewed 14 studies for findings about the relationship of food insecurity and obesity. They determined that studies that used children and adolescents as the populations had inconsistent findings about the presence of obesity when food insecurity existed; in some, there was significant obesity and in others there was not. However, in adults and especially women, food insecurity was correlated to obesity. The researchers developed several hypotheses to explain these findings; a novel hypothesis being that food stamp recipients experienced food insecurity because the aid did not span the entire month, forcing recipients to rely on energy-dense (i.e., high calorie and inexpensive) but not nutrient-dense food. This was seen as particularly true of mothers who may have "sacrificed" meeting their nutrient needs in favor of their children receiving adequate nutrition.

A study of rural childbearing women suggested that obesity led to food insecurity, but that women who were obese and food insecure had a significantly greater weight gain during and following pregnancy (Olson & Strawderman, 2008). Another study of very low-income food-insecure families concluded that maternal stressors were more closely associated with obesity in their children than the food insecurity (Gunderson, Lohman, Garasky, Stewart, & Eisenmann, 2008). A recent study found that among adults who were food insecure, those consuming fast food, and participation in government food programs and receipt of food stamps had a significantly higher BMI. They also found that adults who receive food stamps for more than 6 consecutive months had a lower BMI than those who had participated for less than 6 months, leading researchers to suggest that long-term use of food stamps may help alleviate the concern of not knowing when food would be available again (Webb, Schiff, Currivan, & Villamor, 2008).

Nursing Implications: The nurse must avoid concluding that low-income individuals who are overweight or obese are overeating and do not need assistance with access to nutrition programs or food stamps.

CRITICAL THINKING QUESTION:

1. How should the nurse respond to the client who says that the family's food stamps run out before the end of the month so they have to eat processed foods such as instant ramen noodles and packaged macaroni and cheese?

---

able to community members can significantly determine the overall success of health prevention and promotion activities.

In preparing for health promotion teaching activities, professional nurses should always conduct an individual needs assessment and also try to obtain information about the nutritional, fitness, and health concerns of the community. Much of the information collected by local, state, and national public health agencies is readily available online. By recognizing peer and community influences, the possibilities for successful health behavioral change can be increased. The Evidence-Based Practice Box: Is There an Association between Food Insecurity and Obesity? is an example of how an individual assessment is important before beginning health promotion education.

Nutrition in Health Promotion

A healthy diet and lifestyle prevents a myriad of health problems. Eating the proper amount of carbohydrates, fats, protein, vitamins, minerals, and fluids decreases the risk of chronic diseases such as cardiac disease, cancer, diabetes, and hypertension. Nutrient deficiencies are rare in the United States except among vulnerable populations such as the el-

derly, substance abusers, the poor, malnourished children, and some hospitalized clients. Yet nutrient excesses, especially of simple carbohydrates, saturated fat, cholesterol, and calories, increase each year. Poor diet choices are linked with 4 of the top 10 causes of death in America. Diet is implicated in the development and progression of heart disease, cancer, stroke, and diabetes. Fortunately, as understanding of the role of diet in the disease process has increased, the death rates for cardiac disease, cancer, and strokes have decreased (Centers for Disease Control and Prevention, 2009; Jemal, 2005).

Smoking and physical inactivity are also associated with poor diet choices. In fact, smoking, diet, inactivity, and alcohol intake are factors that contribute to almost 40% of deaths in the United States (Mokdad, Marks, Stroup, & Gergerding, 2004). Risk factors can be defined as any condition or activity associated with an increased disease frequency but not proven to be causal. Leading risk factors for chronic diseases include obesity, cigarette smoking, hypertension, elevated serum cholesterol, physical inactivity, and a diet high in saturated fats and low in vegetables, fruits, and whole grains (CDC, 2004). It is important to note that the likelihood of developing a chronic disease will increase with the number of risk factors present. In other words, risk factors together and dramatically increase the probability of a disease developing. Conversely, the fewer risk factors present, the less likely that a chronic disease will develop. Presence or absence of chronic disease is also associated with quality of life for that person. Helping clients to make healthy life choices based on evidence should be the goal of professional nursing nutritional practice.

Guidelines and Resources for Nutrition and Health Promotion

Consumers are bombarded with information about nutrition and health promotion on a daily basis. Many of the advertisements and information sources are credible and legitimate, but others prey on Americans' desire for healthier lives with a minimum of effort. The advent of the Internet has opened up millions of resources to consumers with availability to computers. Some of the Web sites that are credible and provide reliable information to consumers are listed in the media links for this chapter. These on-line resources contain many useful tools available to assist consumers in changing their diet and exercise habits. Many of these resources are provided free of charge by government agencies and professional organizations. There are also many fee-based Web sites that promise individualized support, nutritional and exercise planning, and healthy living information. In addition to the nutrition recommendations outlined in Chapter 9 that include *Dietary Guidelines for Americans* and various nutrition pyramids, the nurse can direct a client seeking additional information on improving nutritional health to these on-line resources, many of which are interactive and offer personalized advice. Examples include the American Heart Association and the National Heart, Lung, and Blood Institutes, which outline the role of nutrition in reducing risk of hypertension and other cardiovascular diseases.

Healthy People 2010

Healthy People 2010 is a national public health initiative under the control of the Department of Health and Human Services. The program identifies national health priorities and provides guidelines for policies for health promotion and prevention activities. The nurse working in the area of public health can use these guidelines that include some nutrition-focused objectives when formulating nursing interventions in the community. A new *Healthy People* initiative is distributed at the start of each decade and sets goals for improving the nation's health for the next 10 years. *Healthy People 2010* (United States Department of Health and Human Services, 2000) uses leading indicators to measure the nation's overall health during the 10-year period. Leading indicators include:

- Physical Activity
- Overweight and Obesity

- Tobacco Use
- Substance Abuse
- Responsible Sexual Behavior
- Mental Health
- Injury and Violence
- Environmental Quality
- Immunization
- Access to Health Care

The overall goal of *Healthy People 2010* is "improving the quality of life and eliminating disparity in health among racial and ethnic groups" (United States Department of Health and Human Services, 2000). Obviously, many of the goals focus on healthy nutritional practices, and the relationship between diet and obesity is emphasized in many of the goals. Box 10-1 outlines the nutrition-focused goals.

Healthier US and Steps to Healthier US are community-based companion programs to translate the *Healthy People 2010* goals into individual and community activities. The "pillars" of Healthier US are four broad strategies: physical fitness, nutrition, prevention, and make healthy choices. Steps to Healthier US provides support to evidence-based community programs and interventions with the goal of reducing the incidence of chronic diseases and related risk behaviors.

Healthy Eating Index

The healthy eating index (HEI) was created by the Department of Agriculture's Center for Nutrition Policy and Promotion to measure the conformance of American diets to the current healthy eating recommendations and federal dietary guidelines. It was originally created in 1995 and revised to reflect the current *Dietary Guidelines for Americans*. The scoring sheet uses components of the original MyPyramid and the *Dietary Guidelines for Americans* to determine how closely respondents were following recommended guidelines. A score of 100 means complete compliance with these guidelines and a score of 0 means the respondent completely ignored the dietary recommendations. The total score is comprised of evaluating the amount and type of intake in each food group. For example, the intake of fruit vs. fruit juice and total vegetables vs. dark green and orange vegetables are evaluated. The HEI is pictured in Table 10-1.

Evaluation of the data found that men who scored highest on the **healthy eating index,** most closely approximating the United States Department of Agriculture's (USDA) guidelines, reduced their overall risk of developing cancer, cardiac, or other types of chronic diseases by 11% over the 8 to 12 years of follow-up when compared with men who scored lower on the HEI. On the other hand, women who scored highest on the HEI were only 3% less likely to develop a chronic disease than other women who did not follow federal guidelines as closely (McCullough et al., 2002).

| BOX 10-1 | **Nutrition and Overweight Objectives from *Healthy People 2010*** |

19-1. Increase the proportion of adults who are at a healthy weight.

19-2. Reduce the proportion of adults who are obese.

19-3. Reduce the proportion of children and adolescents who are overweight or obese.

19-4. Reduce growth retardation among low-income children under age 5 years.

19-5. Increase the proportion of persons aged 2 years and older who consume at least two daily servings of fruit.

19-6. Increase the proportion of persons aged 2 years and older who consume at least three daily servings of vegetables, with at least one-third being dark green or orange vegetables.

19-7. Increase the proportion of persons aged 2 years and older who consume at least six daily servings of grain products, with at least three being whole grains.

19-8. Increase the proportion of persons aged 2 years and older who consume less than 10 percent of calories from saturated fat.

19-9. Increase the proportion of persons aged 2 years and older who consume no more than 30 percent of calories from total fat.

19-10. Increase the proportion of persons aged 2 years and older who consume 2,400 mg or less of sodium daily.

19-11. Increase the proportion of persons aged 2 years and older who meet dietary recommendations for calcium.

19-12. Reduce iron deficiency among young children and females of childbearing age.

19-13. Reduce anemia among low-income pregnant females in their third trimester.

19-14. (Developmental) Reduce iron deficiency among pregnant females.

19-15. (Developmental) Increase the proportion of children and adolescents aged 6 to 19 years whose intake of meals and snacks at school contributes to good overall dietary quality.

19-16. Increase the proportion of worksites that offer nutrition or weight management classes or counseling.

19-17. Increase the proportion of physician office visits made by patients with a diagnosis of cardiovascular disease, diabetes, or hyperlipidemia that include counseling or education related to diet and nutrition.

19-18. Increase food security among U.S. households and in so doing reduce hunger.

Source: United States Department of Health and Human Services, 2001.

The **alternate healthy eating index** was also created by researchers at the Harvard School of Public Health to measure compliance with the principles emphasized in the Healthy Living Pyramid. Approximately 100,000 female nurses and male health care professionals taking part in another long-term study completed both the HEI and the alternative HEI. The scoring process for the alternative HEI was similar to the HEI, but the results were significantly different. Men who scored highest on the alternative HEI were 20% less likely to develop a chronic disease than their counterparts who had lower scores. Women who scored highest on the alternative HEI were 30% less likely to develop a chronic disease than their female peers who did not follow the Health Eating Pyramid guidelines (McCullough et al., 2002).

Food Intolerances and Allergies

Many people experience gas, abdominal bloating, constipation, or diarrhea after eating certain foods. Most experts term those symptoms "food intolerance" because there is not an immune response initiated by the food source. Lactose intolerance is an example. Food intolerances do not involve the immune system and are not life threatening, yet individuals may inappropriately label a food intolerance as a food allergy; this is not accurate.

Food allergy is a type of **food hypersensitivity** reaction triggered by antigens in the food source. A true food allergy triggers an immune response, often a type 1 hypersensitivity reaction, caused by release of immunoglobulin E (IgE) and degranulation of mast cells, releasing histamine. Symptoms of histamine release as a response to an allergen range from gastrointestinal symptoms, itching, and hives to life-threatening bronchial constriction and anaphylaxis. Anaphylaxis occurs when histamine causes complete obstruction of the respiratory bronchi, resulting in hypoxia, organ failure, and death if not treated promptly. The nurse should be aware that symptoms of food allergy in children can manifest as food aversions or altered behavior related to certain foods as the child tries to avoid a food that has caused some physical symptoms (Lack, 2008).

Adults and children have different stimuli for food allergies. Food allergies are prevalent in less than 3% of the adult population, whereas in children the prevalence is closer to 8% (Lack, 2008). For adults, the most common allergens are shrimp, lobster, crab, and other shellfish; fish; peanuts; tree nuts such as walnuts and other nuts; and eggs. For children, cow's milk, peanuts, eggs, and tree nuts are the primary allergens (Lack, 2008). Other common allergens include soy and wheat. Egg and milk allergies are more commonly outgrown by age 5 years, whereas peanut and tree nut allergies are less likely to resolve (Lack, 2008; Lee & Burks, 2006).

Table 10-1   Healthy Eating Index—2005 Components and Standards for Scoring[1]

Component	Maximum Points	Standard for Maximum Score	Standards for Minimum Score of Zero
Total Fruit (includes 100% juice)	5	≥0.8 cup equiv. per 1,000 kcal	No Fruit
Whole Fruit (not juice)	5	≥0.4 cup equiv. per 1,000 kcal	No Whole Fruit
Total Vegetables	5	≥1.1 cup equiv. per 1,000 kcal	No Vegetables
Dark Green and Orange Vegetables and Legumes[2]	5	≥0.4 cup equiv. per 1,000 kcal	No Dark Green or Orange Vegetables or Legumes
Total Grains	5	≥3.0 oz equiv. per 1,000 kcal	No Grains
Whole Grains	5	≥1.5 oz equiv. per 1,000 kcal	No Whole Grains
Milk[3]	10	≥1.3 cup equiv. per 1,000 kcal	No Milk
Meat and Beans	10	≥2.5 oz equiv. per 1,000 kcal	No Meat or Beans
Oils[4]	10	≥12 grams per 1,000 kcal	No Oil
Saturated Fat	10	≤7% of energy[5]	≥15% of energy
Sodium	10	≤0.7 gram per 1,000 kcal[5]	≥2.0 grams per 1,000 kcal
Calories from Solid Fats, Alcoholic Beverages, and Added Sugars (SoFAAS)	20	≤20% of energy	≥50% of energy

[1]Intakes between the minimum and maximum levels are scored proportionately, except for Saturated Fat and Sodium (see note 5).
[2]Legumes counted as vegetables only after Meat and Beans standard is met.
[3]Includes all milk products, such as fluid milk, yogurt, and cheese, and soy beverages.
[4]Includes nonhydrogenated vegetable oils and oils in fish, nuts, and seeds.
[5]Saturated Fat and Sodium get a score of 8 for the intake levels that reflect the 2005 Dietary Guidelines, <10% of calories from saturated fat and 1.1 grams of sodium/1,000 kcal, respectively.
Source: Center for Nutrition Policy and Promotion, 2008.

Nurses and parents need to be aware of the spectrum of food allergies from moderate gastrointestinal involvement to life-threatening anaphylaxis. Before a treatment plan can be initiated, the food or foods causing the allergic reaction must be identified. Typically, the health care provider would ask the child or parent to keep a food diary, detailing every food product ingested and the amount. By correlating when allergic symptoms occur with the food diary, the offending food may be identified. An oral food challenge under a physician's supervision may be scheduled because it is considered the gold standard for diagnosing food allergy. The client is given a very small amount of the suspected food and monitored for an allergic reaction. Skin prick tests and blood assessment of food-specific IgE antibody levels can also be used (AAAAI Work Group, 2003; Niggemann & Beyer, 2005). Leading professional allergy organizations do not consider use of tests such as cytotoxic testing, provocation-neutralization, and kinesiology as valid diagnostic tools for allergy (Bernstein et al., 2008). Despite mainstream criticism of these alternative testing methods, they remain available to the susceptible consumer looking for answers to solve the reason for physical symptoms and who may end up with false diagnoses and unnecessary dietary restrictions because of the invalid and unreliable tests (Senna, Passalacqua, Lombardi, & Antonicelli,

2004; Wuthrich, 2005). It is essential, especially in growing children, that correct diagnoses be made using recommended testing methods and that unnecessary restrictions be avoided that could jeopardize nutritional health, growth, and development. Case reports exist of children who have followed restrictive diets that eliminate foods erroneously thought to cause food allergy symptoms and where malnutrition has resulted (Noimark & Cox, 2008).

Treatment for a food allergy is straightforward: avoiding the offending food in any form. Evidence that food allergies can be prevented by various measures is lacking (Heine & Tang, 2008). Care must be taken to avoid cross-contamination with the offending food allergen. For example, using a cutting board or knife to cut a peanut butter sandwich and then using the same surface or utensil to prepare food for an individual with peanut allergies will cross-contaminate the allergic person's food with peanut butter. Cross-contamination in restaurants as well as the home is a risk that must be avoided. The client and his or her parents must be vigilant in checking for the ingredient on food labels and in medications. Sometimes, the food has another name and the label must be checked to make sure it is not present. For example, casein and whey are components of milk and would need to be avoided by those with milk allergy. Current federal law requires that ingredient labeling list the top eight food allergens in plain language so that they can be easily recognized on the food label. This includes the allergens milk, egg, fish, shellfish, tree nuts, peanuts, wheat, and soy. Drug excipients, the fillers and other inactive ingredients in medications, can be a source of food allergens and also be a problem for those with food intolerances. Lactose is a common excipient in up to 20% of prescription medications (NIDDK, 2003). The nurse should collaborate with the pharmacist to assist the food allergic client with determining the excipients in any over-the-counter or prescription medications. Chapter 24 discusses drug excipients and food allergy and intolerance in more detail.

Emergency medicine may be prescribed in case the client accidentally ingests the offending food and suffers an allergic reaction. An injectable form of epinephrine is the medication used in emergency situations when risk of an allergic reaction is high.

Pediatric and school nurses can help children and parents develop strategies to avoid the offending food and to safely handle any accidental ingestion. The school nurse can be involved in developing an individualized plan of care for students while at school as well as strategies for field trips, classroom food activities, food sharing, and student and staff education (Weiss, Munoz-Furlong, Furlong, & Arbit, 2004). The Food Allergy and Anaphylaxis Network has Web-based forms for developing plans for children at schools and camps. Friends and caregivers may need to be taught how to administer emergency medicines if the client becomes incapacitated by the allergic reaction. An on-line tutorial for administration of epinephrine is available for teaching. Individuals, especially children, with multiple or complicated food allergies should be referred to a registered dietitian experienced in treatment of food allergies to ensure that nutritional needs are being met while dietary restrictions are followed. The nurse can encourage parents of a child with food allergies to join local allergy support groups as an additional resource.

Food Safety

The safety of food is an important issue for all Americans. Many government and nongovernmental agencies work tirelessly to ensure that consumers have access to food that is safe from **foodborne illnesses, environmental contaminants,** naturally occurring toxins, **pesticides,** and other potentially harmful substances. The food safety chain involves farmers and ranchers who grow the food, shippers who deliver food to stores or manufacturers, manufacturers who process food, and grocers who store and supply the finished food products to the public.

Who Is in Charge of Food Safety?

There are four governmental agencies charged with monitoring **food safety** in the United States: the Food and Drug

Administration (FDA), the USDA, the CDC, and the Environmental Protection Agency (EPA). Each agency has unique functions and also provides overlapping levels of protection to the American public.

The Food and Drug Administration

The FDA is part of the Department of Health and Human Services. Its professed goal is protection of the American consumer. The FDA is the scientific regulatory agency responsible for monitoring the safety and purity of all dietary supplements; monitoring any foods that are processed and distributed interstate (except meat, poultry, and eggs, which are controlled by the USDA); inspecting plants distributed as food; inspecting all imported foods; and establishing the federal standards for both composition of foods and their labeling. The FDA also regulates all cosmetics, drugs, biologics, medical devices, and radiological products.

The Center for Food Safety and Applied Nutrition (CFSAN) is one of six centers within the FDA. CFSAN is charged with "promoting and protecting the public's health by ensuring that the nation's food supply is safe, sanitary, wholesome, and honestly labeled, and that cosmetic products are safe and properly labeled." CFSAN also works with international organizations such as the WHO and foreign governments to assist in their understanding of U.S. requirements and to help standardize international food regulations.

United States Department of Agriculture

The USDA is responsible specifically for the safety, quality, and wholesomeness of meat, poultry, and eggs produced in the United States. It is also charged with conducting nutrition research and helping the public to better understand nutrition and health. The USDA is responsible for MyPyramid and offers a wealth of consumer-oriented resources such as Nutrition.gov, What's in the Foods You Eat Search Tool, a meat and poultry hotline, food preservation and home canning information, and on-line links to child nutrition programs. The agency also offers a current on-line listing of all recalled products and on-line resources to assist consumers in reading nutrition labels.

Centers for Disease Control and Prevention

The CDC is a branch of the Department of Health and Human Services that is responsible for many functions, including monitoring foodborne diseases. The CDC has four overarching health protection goals: healthy people in every stage of life; healthy people in healthy places; people prepared for emerging health threats; and healthy people in a healthy world. The CDC also manages the Office of Minority Health and Health Disparities (OMHD) and the Office of Women's Health. The CDC publishes the *Morbidity and Mortality Weekly Report*, providing current information about infectious disease outbreaks and food safety issues that may cause

MyNursingKit Food Allergy and Anaphylaxis Network

MyNursingKit Epinephrine Administration

public concern. The CDC offers many resources for consumers, including an on-line body mass index (BMI) calculator, a search engine for healthy fruit and vegetable recipes, and podcasts on a wide variety of health-related subjects.

The Environmental Protection Agency

The EPA is the government agency charged with protecting human health and the environment. Specifically, the EPA regulates pesticide use with foods and establishes water quality and safety standards. The EPA enforces the Clean Water and Clean Air Acts and is also responsible for hazardous waste cleanup and dealing with oil spills and other environmental disasters. Finally, the EPA oversees efforts to eradicate lead, mercury, asbestos, and mold from public and private spaces.

Why Should We Be Concerned about Food Safety?

The media is full of news about food-related illnesses. Issues of food safety related to foodborne illness and food contamination are of concern. The Partnership for Food Safety, a joint project of representatives from food industry associations, professional societies in food science, nutrition and health consumer groups, the USDA, the EPA, the Department of Health and Human Services, the CDC, and the FDA, estimates that foodborne illnesses are the leading food safety concern because episodes of food poisoning are the most common manifestation of food-related illnesses. The CDC reports that some 76 million American experience some manifestation of foodborne illness each year, including approximately 5,000 people who die because of it (CDC, 2006). The severity of foodborne illness is determined by the vulnerability of the host: Immunosuppressed and immunocompromised clients, the very old and the very young, pregnant women, and those with poor nutritional status are at much greater risk than those with functioning immune systems and adequate nutrition.

Foodborne Illness

Foodborne illnesses are commonly called "food poisoning." Yet there are actually two distinct types of foodborne illness: foodborne infection, caused by a pathogen carried on or in the food source, and food intoxication, caused by a toxin contained by the food source. Symptoms can include nausea, vomiting, abdominal cramps, diarrhea, and, sometimes, fever. One of the most common foodborne infections is caused by *Salmonella*, a bacterium contaminating undercooked poultry and unpasteurized milk. Raw animal products, such as meat, poultry, fish, milk, and eggs are more common sources of foodborne illness. Raw fruits and vegetables are also of concern (CDC, 2005). Table 10-2 outlines common foodborne infections. The most common cause of food intoxication is the toxin released by *Staphylococcus aureus*. *Clostridium botulinum* produces a deadly toxin in anaerobic conditions such as home-canned foods. Both types of

foodborne illness, infection and intoxication, are extremely unpleasant for the victim and may cause serious damage or death if not treated immediately.

Industry and Marketplace Food Safety

As food distribution becomes more of a global phenomenon, the importance of monitoring the safety of worldwide food production, distribution, and preparation becomes even more important.

The Hazard Analysis Critical Control Points (HAACP) system is a systematic approach to the identification, evaluation, and control of food safety hazards. It is administered by the FDA, USDA, and the Center for Food Safety and Nutrition and is "designed for use in all segments of the food industry from growing, harvesting, processing, manufacturing, distributing, and merchandising to preparing food for consumption" (FDA and USDA, 2008). This system has been adopted by most governments, trade associations, and food industry professionals globally. The HAACP standards outlined in Box 10-2 attempt to assure consumers that our food is free from any predictable hazards, including contamination by infectious agents or other types of potentially dangerous substances like lead, mercury, or environmental pesticides.

Consumer Awareness

Of course, one of the most powerful preventive strategies against food hazards is consumer awareness and adequate consumer information. When shopping for foods, consumers can make sure to purchase items before the "sell by" date. Careful inspection of perishable items to ensure intactness of seals and packaging, rejection of canned goods that are damaged or bulging, and attention to basic food safety guidelines when handling and preparing foods are all important consumer actions. Being alert to announcements about food contamination, toxins, and food recalls can help protect consumers and their family from foodborne illnesses.

When eating outside the home, consumers can check on the cleanliness of restaurants, and inquire with local public health officials when the cleanliness of an establishment is in question. Although state and local regulations govern restaurant operations, consumers can also prevent foodborne illnesses when dining outside the home by:

- Washing hands before meals and after coughing, sneezing, or using the bathroom
- Demanding that hot foods be served hot and cold foods be served cold
- Limiting use of shared condiments and other foods stored at room temperature
- Not frequenting restaurants if there is a concern about the cleanliness of the facilities and the safe preparation of food
- Refrigerating "doggy bags" within 2 hours of the meal or toss them in the garbage

Table 10-2 Common Foodborne Illnesses

Foodborne Organism	Most Frequent Food Sources	Prevention Methods
Campylobacter	Raw and undercooked poultry meat, unpasteurized milk, contaminated drinking water	Cook foods thoroughly to recommended temperature; choose only pasteurized milk and milk products; do not drink questionable water; always follow safe food-handling methods.
Cyclospora cayetanensis	Contaminated swimming and drinking water, contaminated raw produce, unpasteurized juices	Wash all raw vegetables and fruits before peeling and eating; use only pasteurized milk and milk products; do not swallow water while swimming; do not drink questionable water.
Escherichia coli	Undercooked ground beef, unpasteurized milk and juices, raw fruits and vegetables, contaminated water, person-to-person contact	Cook foods thoroughly to recommended temperature; choose only pasteurized milk and milk products; do not drink questionable water; always follow safe food-handling methods; wash all raw vegetables and fruits before peeling and eating.
Norwalk virus	Raw foods and salads, person-to-person contact	Always follow safe food-handling methods.
Giardia intestinalis	Contaminated water, uncooked foods	Always follow safe food-handling methods; avoid raw fruits and vegetables if parasites are suspected; dispose of raw sewage safely.
Hepatitis	Undercooked or raw shellfish	Cook foods thoroughly to recommended temperature; avoid sushi if infection is suspected.
Listeria monocytogenes	Unpasteurized milk and cheese, processed meats, and hot dogs	Cook foods thoroughly to recommended temperature, refrigerate food promptly, choose only pasteurized milk and milk products; always follow safe food-handling methods.
Salmonella	Raw or undercooked eggs, meats, raw milk and milk products, shrimp, coconut, chocolate, and yeast	Cook foods thoroughly to recommended temperature; refrigerate food promptly; choose only pasteurized milk and milk products; always follow safe food-handling methods.
Shigella	Raw foods, salads, sandwiches, contaminated water, person-to-person contact	Cook foods thoroughly to recommended temperature; refrigerate food promptly; always follow safe food-handling methods.
Vibrio vulnificus	Raw or undercooked seafood and contaminated water	Cook foods thoroughly to recommended temperature; always follow safe food-handling methods.

BOX 10-2 HAACP Principles

- Analyze hazards. Potential hazards associated with a food and measures to control those hazards are identified. The hazard could be biological, such as a microbe; chemical, such as a toxin; or physical, such as ground glass or metal fragments.
- Identify critical control points. These are points in a food's production—from its raw state through processing and shipping to consumption by the consumer—at which the potential hazard can be controlled or eliminated. Examples are cooking, cooling, packaging, and metal detection.
- Establish preventive measures with critical limits for each control point. For a cooked food, for example, this might include setting the minimum cooking temperature and time required to ensure the elimination of any harmful microbes.
- Establish procedures to monitor the critical control points. Such procedures might include determining how and by whom cooking time and temperature should be monitored.
- Establish corrective actions to be taken when monitoring shows that a critical limit has not been met—for example, reprocessing or disposing of food if the minimum cooking temperature is not met.
- Establish procedures to verify that the system is working properly—for example, testing time-and-temperature recording devices to verify that a cooking unit is working properly.
- Establish effective recordkeeping to document the HAACP system. This would include records of hazards and their control methods, the monitoring of safety requirements and action taken to correct potential problems. Each of these principles must be backed by sound scientific knowledge: for example, published microbiological studies on time-and-temperature factors for controlling foodborne pathogens.

Source: Adapted from Food and Drug Administration, 2001.

MyNursingKit Fight Bac

Home and Kitchen Safety

Foodborne illness is also a cause of concern in home kitchens. The government's Fight Bac Web site lists four actions that can prevent most foodborne illnesses in the home (Partnership for Food Safety Education, 2006).

1. *Clean:* Wash hands often and keep all food preparation areas clean. Wash any items used in food preparation with hot soapy water.
2. *Separate:* Avoid cross-contamination. Pathogens on the surface of food, especially raw meat, eggs, and poultry, can recontaminate other cooked foods, especially if the food preparation items were not cleaned between preparations.
3. *Cook:* Keep hot foods hot. Cook foods until they reach the temperature at which internal microbes are successfully killed, and maintain the temperature until the food is served to prevent bacterial growth. See Table 10-3 for recommended safe temperatures for meat and eggs.
4. *Chill:* Keep cold foods cold. Any perishable food should be promptly refrigerated and not left at room temperature. Frozen foods should be defrosted properly to prevent microbial growth.

Dietary Guidelines for Americans includes recommendations for home food safety, including the following (USDA, 2005):

- Clean hands, food contact surfaces, and fruits and vegetables. Meat and poultry should not be washed or rinsed.

- Separate raw, cooked, and ready-to-eat foods while shopping, preparing, or storing foods.
- Cook foods to a safe temperature to kill microorganisms, as listed in Table 10-3.
- Chill (refrigerate) perishable food promptly and defrost foods properly.
- Avoid raw (unpasteurized) milk or any products made from unpasteurized milk, raw or partially cooked eggs or foods containing raw eggs, raw or undercooked meat and poultry, unpasteurized juices, and raw sprouts.

Special care should be taken by specific populations, such as pregnant women, the elderly, young children, and those who are immunocompromised.

- Do not eat or drink raw (unpasteurized) milk or any products made from unpasteurized milk, raw or partially cooked eggs or foods containing raw eggs, raw or undercooked meat and poultry, raw or undercooked fish or shellfish, unpasteurized juices, and raw sprouts.
- Only eat certain deli meats and frankfurters that have been reheated to steaming hot.

Food safety is an important concern for most Americans. The regulatory monitoring of governmental agencies, informed consumers, and basic home food safety guidelines outlined in Box 10-3 can decrease the risk of foodborne illness and increase quality of life for those especially susceptible to its effects. Nurses are an instrumental part of this education, especially because 80% of food safety problems arise from lack of education or awareness (American Dietetic Association [ADA], 2003). The nurse can use Client Education Checklist: Preventing Foodborne Illness when educating clients on reducing risk of foodborne illness. Practice Pearl: Food Safety Myths lists some common food safety myths that the nurse may encounter when providing food safety education. Chapter 23 discusses the issue of foodborne illness in clients with cancer or human immunodeficiency virus (HIV) in more detail.

Table 10-3	Internal Temperatures for Meats and Eggs
Temperature	**Food**
0 degrees (Fahrenheit)	Freezer temperature
40 degrees	Refrigerator temperature
40–140 degrees	DANGER ZONE: Don't keep any food at this temperature for > 2 hours or > 1 hour if air temperature is more than 90 degrees
140 degrees	Holding temperature for most hot foods
145 degrees	Internal temperature for medium-rare steaks, roast, veal and lamb
160 degrees	Internal temperature for medium-well meats, eggs and egg dishes, pork and ground meats
165 degrees	Internal temperature for stuffing, poultry, reheating leftovers
170 degrees	Internal temperature for well-done meats

Source: Adapted from United States Department of Agriculture (USDA), Food Safety and Inspection Service, 2006.

BOX 10-3	Consumer Food Safety Suggestions

1. Wash your hands often and thoroughly.
2. Keep a clean kitchen.
3. Avoid cross-contamination.
4. Keep hot foods hot.
5. Keep cold foods cold.
6. Don't reuse disposable containers.
7. If you don't know, throw it out.
8. Don't buy products with broken seals or damaged packaging.
9. Always follow the label instructions for storing and preparing foods.

CLIENT EDUCATION CHECKLIST	Preventing Foodborne Illness
Intervention	**Example**
Assess knowledge about foodborne illness.	Review how food is purchased, stored, prepared, served, and consumed by the client. Note refrigeration and other food storage practices. Ask about cooking methods and temperatures.
Explain major areas of food handling where foodborne illness risk exists and appropriate practices to prevent illness.	1. Cleanliness: Good personal hygiene when working with food and food products such as proper and frequent hand washing, appropriate dress, covering any open wounds, and staying away from food preparation when sick. Use clean work surfaces and utensils. Keep refrigerator clean, discarding out-of-date food. Rinse fruits and vegetables and scrub those with tough skins. 2. Cross-contamination: Avoid cross-contamination of one food by another from unsanitized cutting boards, kitchen utensils, dirty towels and sponges, unwashed hands, and contact with pets. Avoid contact between raw meats, fish, eggs, and poultry with uncooked produce while shopping and in the refrigerator. 3. Temperature: Time and temperature principles such as using a food thermometer to cook foods to proper temperatures and keeping hot foods hot and cold foods cold during holding periods. Do not leave food at temperatures between 40°F and 140°F for 4 hours or longer. Thaw frozen foods in the refrigerator, not at room temperature.

PRACTICE PEARL

Food Safety Myths

Many clients hold inaccurate beliefs about food and food safety. The following are the most popular food myths and a short explanation of why it is not true.

1. *If it tastes O.K., it's safe to eat.*

   Fact: Your senses can't tell you if the food is contaminated or unsafe to eat. An estimated 75 million Americans experience a foodborne illness each year.

2. *"Food poisoning" occurs immediately and goes away quickly.*

   Fact: It can be weeks before a foodborne illness is detected in your system. Foodborne illnesses can be very serious and sometimes fatal.

3. *GI distress (nausea, vomiting, and diarrhea) is the most serious consequence of foodborne illness.*

   Fact: Central nervous system damage, paralysis, and death are potential consequences of a foodborne illness.

4. *If no one else got sick, then the food is probably fine.*

   Fact: Young children, pregnant and nursing women, the elderly, and anyone with immunosuppression are much more at risk for a foodborne illness than someone with a healthy immune system.

5. *I can protect a food that is unrefrigerated by covering it. If a food has been unrefrigerated for more than 2 hours, I can make it safe by making it really hot or freezing the food.*

   Fact: Foods should be properly stored within 2 hours of preparation, regardless of type of food or ingredients. A lid will not protect against bacterial contamination, and many bacteria are not destroyed by temperature changes.

Environmental Contaminants

One untoward effect of our increasingly industrialized world is growing concern about the contamination of foods by environmental toxins. Industrial wastes and processes pollute the land and water, and those contaminants are absorbed by plants and animals. When humans consume those food sources, the environmental pollutants are subsequently absorbed by our bodies. Unfortunately, environmental contaminants have the potential to cause acute and chronic disease and to decrease quality of life by their presence.

The food chain is the interrelated system of dependence of bigger organisms on smaller organisms as a food source. For example, little fish eat plants and plankton, big fish eat little fish, and humans eat fish. Any contaminant that is absorbed by bottom-dwelling plants or plankton is ultimately integrated into the person who eats the fish. This effect of the food chain is depicted in Figure 10-2 ■. Environmental contaminants are especially dangerous because they persist over time. Many contaminants are inorganic substances that do not break down. Mercury and pesticides are both examples of persistent environmental toxins that can bioaccumulate in people.

Mercury Contamination

Mercury is a metal that is heavier than water. That means that mercury that is dumped into water will sink to the bottom of that reservoir. When mercury is exposed to water, it turns into methylmercury. Methylmercury (CH_3Hg^+) is a potentially fatal neurotoxin that is the most common form of mercury to bioaccumulate in humans. Methylmercury can

MyNursingKit EPA Mercury Information

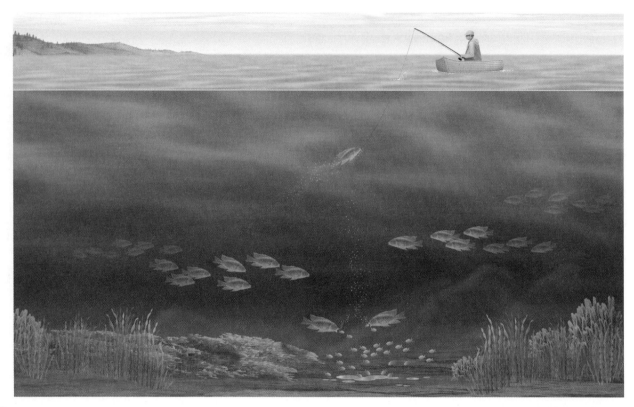

■ FIGURE 10-2 **Food Chain Contaminants.**

also cause permanent damage to the brain and kidneys and has been suggested to cause cancer. Effects on brain functioning may result in irritability, shyness, tremors, changes in vision or hearing, and memory problems. Methylmercury poisoning is especially harmful to developing fetuses and young children.

Plants and plankton that have been exposed to mercury are eaten by bottom-dwelling fish, mollusks, and crustaceans. In turn, those animals are eaten by larger fish that eventually make their way into the human food system. As the mercury is passed from animal to animal, it becomes more concentrated. The more fish and seafood a person consumes, the greater the bioaccumulation of mercury and the greater the potential health risk.

The EPA has set a limit of 2 parts of mercury per billion parts of drinking water (2 ppb) (EPA, 2006). The FDA has set a maximum permissible level of 1 part of methylmercury in a million parts of seafood (1 ppm) (FDA, 2009).

The best way to protect against methylmercury contamination is to be aware of and strictly follow any local or regional alerts about mercury contamination in fish and seafood. Lifespan Box: Mercury and Seafood outlines the advice that the EPA and FDA offer for those most at risk for mercury contamination. The United States Geological Services (2009) has developed a National Fish Mercury Model that can predict the mercury content of certain species of fish at different times of the year and in different geographical locations. The EPA offers on-line resources

Lifespan

Mercury and Seafood

Mercury ingestion can be a serious issue for people at different times in the lifespan. Methylmercury can cause nervous system disorders in adults and can cause permanent neurological damage in growing infants and children.

General dietary principles include the following for women who may become pregnant, pregnant women, nursing mothers, and young children to avoid some types of fish and eat fish and shellfish that are lower in mercury.

1. Do not eat shark, swordfish, king mackerel, or tilefish because they contain high levels of mercury.
2. Eat up to 12 ounces (2 average meals) a week of a variety of fish and shellfish that are lower in mercury.
   - A commonly eaten fish, albacore ("white") tuna has more mercury than canned light tuna. So, when choosing your two meals of fish and shellfish, you may eat up to 6 ounces (one average meal) of albacore tuna per week.
3. Check local advisories about the safety of fish caught by family and friends in your local lakes, rivers, and coastal areas. If no advice is available, eat up to 6 ounces (one average meal) per week of fish you catch from local waters, but don't consume any other fish during that week.

Follow these same recommendations when feeding fish and shellfish to a young child, but serve age-appropriate smaller portions.

Source: Adapted from Environmental Protection Agency (EPA), 2004.

about mercury in local waters and educational brochures in English, Cambodian, Chinese, Hmong, Portuguese, Korean, and Vietnamese.

Pesticides

Pesticides are also known as fungicides, herbicides, and rodenticides. They are powerful chemical compounds that can kill insects, animals, and other pests that can cause harm or disease. Unfortunately, pesticides also can kill or harm pets, nonharmful animals, and humans. Laboratory studies have linked pesticides to cancers, nerve damage, and birth defects (ADA, 2003). Biological pesticides that use naturally occurring substances for pest eradication are considered safer than other types of synthetic pesticides, but all can cause harm if they infiltrate the human food chain. Children are particularly vulnerable to the effects of pesticides because of immature organs and low body weight in relation to the amount of food and beverages consumed compared with adults (ADA, 2003). The EPA ranks pesticides as highly toxic, moderately toxic, slightly toxic, and relatively toxic.

In 2004, the United Nations signed a treaty banning 12 of the most dangerous pesticides, known as persistent organic pollutants (POPs), including aldrin, chlordane, DDT, dieldrin, endrin, heptachlor, mirex, toxaphene, polychlorinated biphenols (PCBs), hexachlorobenzene, dioxins, and furans. As the press release for the treaty signing noted: "Every human carries traces of POPs, which circulate globally through a process known as the 'grasshopper effect.' POPs released in one part of the world can, through a repeated process of evaporation and deposit, be transported through the atmosphere to regions far away from the original source. Though not soluble in water, they are readily absorbed in fatty tissue, where concentrations can become magnified by up to 70,000 times the background levels. Fish, predatory birds, mammals and humans high up the food chain absorb the greatest concentrations. When they travel, POPs go with them" (United Nations News Center, 2004).

Water Contamination

Water may be the source of life, but it can also transmit many harmful pathogens. *Cryptosporidium* and *Cyclospora*, often associated with contaminated fruits and vegetables, are actually carried through the water system. Water can also contain heavy metals and environmental toxins, including pesticides.

Drinking water comes from one of two sources: surface water and groundwater. Surface water includes lakes, streams, reservoirs, and, sometimes, the ocean. Groundwater is found in underground reservoirs that are less readily contaminated than surface sources of water. Groundwater is more difficult to access for drinking water, which is why most municipal water supplies come from surface water. Surface water can become contaminated more easily than groundwater, but it is amenable to a variety of "purification" strategies. Groundwater that becomes contaminated by environmental toxins is permanently altered.

Water can be treated, or purified, by three general strategies. Most municipal water systems use a disinfectant to kill bacteria, and add chlorine and fluoride to prevent common public health problems. When traveling to areas where sanitation is poor and available water is unsafe to drink, the CDC recommends buying bottled water, boiling water, or using chemical disinfection, which can improve water safety. Using untreated water to make other beverages or ice should be avoided (CDC, 2007). Home water treatment systems use some type of carbon filter or reverse osmosis process to filter bacteria, heavy metals, and organic contaminants. Bottled water, which is increasingly popular in the United States, is often disinfected with ozone and has been distilled or deionized to remove undesirable compounds and pathogens. Consumers may purchase bottled water with the belief that it is superior to tap water. However, at least 25% of bottled water sold in the United States originates from a municipal water source and, therefore, is essentially tap water (Natural Resources Defense Council [NRDC], 2008). Additionally, it should be noted that many bottled waters contain little to no fluoride, whereas many municipal sources are fluoridated as a public health initiative to prevent dental caries (Napier & Kodner, 2008). The nurse should assess the use of bottled water for mixing infant formula or by children to ensure that adequate fluoride is obtained in the diet. Bottled water may be cleaner than tap water known to contain contaminants, but otherwise the choice to use bottled water is based on personal preference. Environmental groups point to the staggering recycling problems created by millions of plastic bottles entering the waste stream as a result of this consumption trend.

Naturally Occurring Contaminants

These substances may be naturally occurring, but they are still potentially harmful. Mother Nature has given some of her children sophisticated and dangerous toxins to combat predators.

Poisonous mushrooms are the most familiar example of naturally occurring toxicants. The American Association of Poison Control Centers (Bronstein et al., 2008) reports that more than 7,000 cases of acute mushroom poisoning are reported to poison control centers each year. Of the 5,000 types of mushrooms in the United States, only about 100 are capable of causing serious harm and death. Children under 6 years of age are most likely to become ill or die because of mushroom ingestion. There is currently no antidote to the serious hepatic and renal damage caused by poisonous mushrooms, so consumers are cautioned to be extremely careful and purchase mushrooms only from a knowledgeable source.

Cabbages, Brussels sprouts, cauliflower, broccoli, and other brassica family vegetables contain small amounts of substances known as **goitrogens,** which are capable of hypertrophying and decreasing the function of the thyroid gland. Large quantities of goitrogens can cause acute hypothyroidism in normothyroid clients and can exacerbate decreased thyroid function in hypothyroid clients.

Cyanogens are inactive compounds that can be activated by certain plant enzymes into poisonous cyanide. Lima beans and fruit seed such as apricot pits are the most familiar examples of cyanogen-containing foods.

Solanine is a natural poison found in potatoes. Solanine is a powerful narcotic when consumed in large amounts. It is found in the green layer of potatoes that have been exposed to light, extreme cold, or heat. It should be sliced off the potato because cooking does not inactivate the poison.

Can Contaminants Be Limited in the Diet?

Fear of ingested toxins, food and water contamination are enhanced by concerns about global warming and environmental health. The environmental cost of shipping peaches from South America to the Northeastern United States in January is high when measured in carbon dioxide production and energy use. It is estimated that the United States imports almost as much food as it exports, and that recent changes are related to increased imports of fruits and vegetables (ADA, 2007). Most experts recommend a general strategy of "think globally and eat locally." The more technical term for that philosophy, *sustainable agriculture*, is that which conserves resources and is environmentally sound while also being commercially competitive (USDA, 1999). Part of the initiatives to support sustainable agriculture is the motivation to lessen the impact of food systems on the environment, such as reducing energy use and pollution. This includes reduction of ecological concerns stemming from use of pesticides and the contamination of water. All of these factors, in turn, have an impact on human health. Sustainable agriculture promotes the use of foods grown for the local or regional market. Foods grown within a 100-mile radius of home are more likely to reflect the best produce available during that season, and consumers are more aware of potential food safety issues when dealing with locally grown items. Such food is also minimally processed, thus preserving nutrients with little need for food additives (ADA, 2007).

The Slow Food USA movement "envisions a future food system that is based on the principles of high quality and taste, environmental sustainability, and social justice—in essence, a food system that is good, clean and fair" (Slow Food USA, 2008). They encourage a variety of activities (defending biodiversity, reviving American food traditions, taste education, and garden to table projects) as a proactive response to environmentally damaging food practices. Hot Topic Box: Slow Foods discusses this aspect of changing how we eat.

One of the most effective strategies for limiting pesticide exposure is to choose organic or foods that have minimal pesticide exposure. Small family-owned farms may be more likely to limit pesticide use than large commercial farm operations. Sustainable agriculture practices limit use of pesticides, hor-

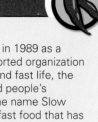

Slow Foods

The Slow Food movement started in Italy in 1989 as a nonprofit, ecogastronomic member-supported organization that was started to counteract fast food and fast life, the disappearance of local food traditions, and people's dwindling interest in the food they eat. The name Slow Food is meant as a direct contrast to the fast food that has become common in the diets of many individuals. The movement also considers how our food choices affect the rest of the world. Many of America's most famous chefs and "foodies" like Michael Pollan and Alice Waters are supporters of the movement. Critics say that it is elitist, and following its principles will raise the cost of food because it discourages cheaper alternative methods of growing or preparing food and seeks to eliminate large industrial food production to the benefit of small, local producers.

What exactly is "Slow Food"? Slow Food is more than what one eats or how quickly one eats it. It refers to a fundamental paradigm shift in how one views the relationship between food, health, and the environment. As noted on their website, Slow Food is "going beyond the passive role of a consumer and taking interest in those that produce our food, how they produce it and the problems they face in doing so. In actively supporting food producers, we become part of the production process."

The Slow Food Foundation for Biodiversity, an related organization to Slow Food USA, is concerned that industrial farming, poor animal husbandry techniques, and an increased dependence on a limited number of fruit and vegetable varieties is leading to a dramatic loss in the world's biodiversity. The mission of this organization is to organize and fund projects that defend our world's heritage of agricultural biodiversity and gastronomic traditions while respecting local cultural identities, the earth's resources, sustainable animal husbandry, and the health of individual consumers.

The philosophy behind support of Slow Food is one which supports the idea of enjoying and appreciating foods while also being mindful of the social and environmental consequences of food choices.

Sources: Pietrykowski, 2004; Slow Food International, http://www.slowfood.com; Slow Food USA, http://www.slowfoodusa.org/index.html

mones, and nontherapeutic antibiotics in foods (ADA, 2007). In addition to eating local foods, consumers can decrease pesticide residue by washing all fresh produce in warm, soapy water. Discarding the outer leaves of vegetables and peeling waxed fruits and vegetables can decrease pesticide exposure. Eating a wide variety of fruits and vegetables can limit specific exposure to specific pesticides that are used only for a single type of plant. If it is not evident from the food label or packaging, always ask the grocer or store clerk whether the food was exposed to pesticides. The FDA requirements for labeling food as organic are outlined in Box 10-4.

Exposure to pesticides increases with foods higher on the food chain. Pesticides that bioaccumulate in fat cells and foods such as eggs, milk, meat, and cheese can increase human exposure to these substances (ADA, 2007). Organically

BOX 10-4	**Organic Food Claims**

Foods that make organic claims can only do so under the Organic Foods Production Act that assures the consumer that the production and processing practice for the food has been certified to meet standards laid out by the law. The nurse can help consumers understand label claims regarding organic food:

100% organic: all ingredients must meet standard for being organically produced and processed. The USDA organic seal may be used on the label with this claim.

Organic: at least 95% of ingredients must be organically produced. Remaining ingredients can only be from an approved list of agricultural products. The USDA organic seal may be used on the label with this claim.

Made with organic ingredients: at least 70% of ingredients meet organic standard. Up to three ingredients that are organic can be listed in the title of the food. For example, a label could say pie made with organic apples and wheat, but not organic apple pie. The USDA organic seal cannot be used on these products.

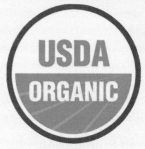

Source: United States Department of Agriculture.

- Some consumers confuse the word *natural* with *organic*. The definition of natural is that no artificial ingredients are in the product; it is not synonymous with organic. What should the nurse say to the clients who say they need not worry about what is in their foods because they buy all natural products?

Source: United States Department of Agriculture, Agricultural Marketing Service, 2008.

grown foods usually have far less pesticide exposure than nonorganically grown foods, but their health benefits have yet to be proven in long-term research. For example, it is known that children who consume a conventional, nonorganic diet have blood levels of pesticide metabolites that far exceed those of their peers who consume at least a 75% organic diet. However, despite evidence that some pesticides cause neurological damage in laboratory animals, such a correlation has not been definitively drawn in children (Kligler, 2007). It is also known that organic produce has higher levels of some nutrients, such as vitamin C and beneficial phytochemicals such as phenols, than conventionally grown produce (Edlich et al., 2007). There are many who subscribe to the Precautionary Principle regarding pesticide use. This principle supports the use of caution when there is sufficient suspicion of harm instead of waiting for more definitive evidence before action is taken. Deliberately taking reasonable measures to reduce pesticide exposure now seems a wise alternative to waiting for more proof, all the while continuing existing exposure to these chemicals.

Cultural Influences on Dietary Practices

Culture refers to the way of life of a community at a given time. It is a value and belief system that is learned from other community members, and it determines what is "normal" for that community. A very important source of cultural information is the family. Culture is often grouped together with race, ethnicity, and geographic region. Race is a biological term used to distinguish a group of people with distinct physical characteristics. For example, skin color, hair texture, dominant eye color, and facial features are all characteristics of race. A racial group is a community of the same race that share common cultural values and features (Queralt, 1996). An ethnic group refers to a community of people that share customs, socialization, and cultural patterns (Giddens, 1996). A minority group can refer to a group of people who have not received their share of wealth, power, or social status (Persell, 1990).

Food Practices

When describing the significance of culture to diet and food habits, one must appreciate that culture encompasses a wide variety of eating practices. Culture defines its own foodway; that is, the rules and expectations about many aspects of food habits that are important to that culture. Culture determines what is edible, the role of food in the diet, how food is prepared, the use of foods for celebration and other functions, how food is eaten, meal-related rituals, and the number and timing of meals.

What Is Edible?

Culture defines what is edible and what is not edible. In most cultures, good sources of nutrients that are necessary to meet daily needs are included as food sources. Yet there are interesting cultural variants. In the United States, we do not eat insects or snakes as protein. In other cultures, these foods are important contributors to daily protein intake. When traveling, one sometimes enjoys a strange food without knowing its origin. Once the source is known, cultural rules may change perceptions and dictate that it is inedible or unpleasant.

Nurses need to understand that different cultures accept or reject food sources that may be familiar to American tastes. Sensitivity to other cultural norms about what is defined as food is very important in order to deliver optimum care to clients.

Important Food Roles

Different foods have different roles in each culture. Core foods are essential to cultural food habits and offer a good source of calories or protein, or both. Common core foods include grains and starchy vegetables. Secondary foods are accessory tastes that often provide the identifiable cultural or ethnic characteristics. Secondary foods include types of vegetables, nuts, and meats that are not always available but are eaten as often as possible. Occasional foods are usually served only at special events like celebrations or funerals and are not readily available year-round.

Food Preparation

The decision to serve a food cooked or raw, or some variation in between, is certainly a cultural distinction. Traditional food preparation methods, including seasonings, are highly characteristic of a culture. Of course, food preparation is rooted in food availability. If fresh fruit is available all the time, preparation of that food probably involves simply chopping or eating out of hand.

Use of Foods

The use of foods for celebration, mourning, and emotional comfort is deeply rooted in one's culture. Certain foods carry great symbolism, such as the association of eggs with fertility in many cultures. Culture determines the distinction between snack and meal foods, masculine and feminine foods, food rewards and punishments, demonstration of religious compliance, and how foods may be used to signify life events.

Every culture uses food in its celebratory activities. Special foods can be reserved for specific events, such as cake for birthdays and weddings and champagne for happy celebrations. Potato salad and hot dogs are emblematic of the Fourth of July national holiday in the United States, and most cultures have very well-defined food habits around important religious holidays like Christmas, Thanksgiving, Davali, Ramadan, and Passover.

Comfort foods serve as a vital link to our past. Different foods become comfort foods for different cultures. When we are emotionally or physically stressed, ill, or need to relax, we often turn to familiar and well-loved comfort foods. Unfortunately, some of our comfort foods can be high in sugar, saturated fat, or salt.

Number and Timing of Meals

Most cultures eat at least once a day. Many eat five or six times per day, including snacks and "tea breaks." Culture determines when meals are eaten. In hot climates, the evening meal may begin as late as 9 or 10 P.M. to allow the heat of the day to pass. During the winter, when darkness falls early, some cultures eat as early as 5 P.M. to take advantage of the daylight. In caring for clients from different cultures, the nurse can assess the expected mealtimes and try to schedule inpatient meals to better conform to those times. Many hospitals now allow clients to order their meals for delivery at preferred times.

How Food Is Eaten

Utensils to eat food vary worldwide. In some cultures, bread is used as the primary food implement. In many Asian cultures, chopsticks are used to eat. In some African cultures, it is considered disrespectful to your fellow diners if you do not use your hands to eat out of the shared food bowl.

Culture also dictates eating etiquette. Most American children are instructed to chew with their mouths closed, to refrain from talking while chewing, to chew quietly, and to keep elbows off the dining table. In other cultures, loud chewing and smacking sounds are a compliment to the host or hostess and silence while eating indicates displeasure with the food.

Despite what our parents taught us, it is often more culturally acceptable to respect the customs of our dining companions and "when in Rome, do as the Romans do."

Health Beliefs about Food and Dietary Habits

Food serves many vital functions in different cultures. Certain foods can promote wellness, cure disease, or rebalance important body systems. Sometimes these cultural beliefs are confirmed by scientific evidence discovered much later, and sometimes there is no apparent validity to those beliefs. It is still very important to respect and honor cultural beliefs about the health benefits of certain foods, unless there is evidence that the food could be damaging to the client.

Meal-Related Habits

In many cultures, meals do not begin until the entire family is present. In others, it is desirable to have a guest at the table so that the meal will be especially blessed. Sometimes, the men in the family are served first and the women do not eat until the men have left the dining area. Whatever the cultural practice, nurses need to understand that meal-related habits are deeply ingrained and difficult to change. Some basic understanding about culture meal habits can help provide culturally respectful care to the client and his or her family.

Beliefs about Relationship between Body Size and Health

Despite American beliefs about the relationship between weight and healthiness, many cultures have different values. For some cultures, large body sizes and a BMI greater than 25 implies wealth and health. For others, excessive body weight signifies a lack of self-discipline and is considered quite offensive. Before applying cultural values on a large person, nurses need to gather information about the beliefs for body size and health in that culture.

Acculturation and Assimilation of Dietary Practices

Acculturation and assimilation of dietary practices are important processes that nurses need to recognize as they provide care to diverse individuals and communities. **Acculturation** occurs when people move into a new community and begin to adopt the beliefs, values, attitudes, and practices of that community. It occurs whenever a person transitions to a new community, regardless of whether there is a geographical change. Individuals who become acculturated to their new community are more likely to try new foods that are important to the community or symbolize a desirable attribute (like wealth or sophistication) to community members. For example, immigrants may be unfamiliar with "American" foods like hamburgers or fries but seek out those foods because they serve as a visible connection with the new culture. Foods emphasized by the new community may be substituted for more traditional foods, sometimes with negative health consequences. Newcomers may have eaten a traditional diet high in fruits and vegetables with minimal animal-based proteins but adopt a more meat-based, caloric-intense diet when acculturating to American dietary practices. It may also be difficult to purchase traditional foods because they are unavailable or prohibitively expensive. Children may be especially prone to reject the traditional foods of their parents because they are heavily influenced by their peers and want to appear as "American" as possible. Hopefully, school-based nutritional education provides children with information on the health risks associated with unhealthy dietary choices, whether traditional or American foods.

Assessing Acculturation

When nurses plan care for clients from different cultures, a basic understanding of cultural practices is essential. Important questions to ask include the following:

- What culture does the client identify with?
- How long has the client lived in the United States?
- What traditional foods does the client eat? How often (daily, weekly, occasionally)?
- Has the client deleted or substituted for any traditional foods?
- What are the client's food preferences, both traditional and "new"? What are the client's favorite foods from both cultures?
- What are the client's beliefs about the relationship between health and diet? Body size and health?
- Who is responsible for food preparation in the client's family?
- Who is the "learner" if teaching is needed? In other words, are there others who should be included in dietary teaching sessions?
- Does the client wish to become acculturated or is the client trying to balance traditional and new cultural identities?
- What questions does the client have about diet, nutrition, and health?

Guidelines for Respecting Cultural Dietary Practices

Dignity and respect are two characteristics of every professional nurse and client interaction. When providing nutritional counseling for clients of diverse cultural groups, there are several important guidelines to follow.

Be Familiar with and Respect Traditional Dietary Practices

A basic understanding of traditional dietary practices for that client is essential. It is permissible for the nurse to ask questions of the client and elicit this information, but the practices should be treated with respect and not judged by the nurse's individual dietary standards.

Be Knowledgeable about Common Diet-Influenced Health Problems in the Client's Culture

Familiarity with common health problems in clients' cultural, ethnic, or religious group can be useful in prioritizing health teaching. For example, the incidence of cardiovascular disease is higher in Pacific Islanders, so a discussion of strategies to decrease saturated fat and cholesterol intake might be included in each teaching session with these clients.

Be Aware of Possible Dietary Acculturation Practices

Completing an acculturation assessment is necessary to better understand the client's current dietary habits and to help determine his or her diet and health goals. If the client has replaced traditional plant-based foods with unhealthy fat-laden fast foods, this information provides an important basis for education about healthy eating.

Another useful source of information for clients is a Web site of nutrition facts for the 10 most popular fast-food restaurants. Because they are inexpensive, ubiquitous, and uniquely American, many immigrants eat a large proportion of their calories at fast-food establishments, especially breakfast and lunch. The Fast Food Nutrition Fact Explorer provides information about the foods sold at Arby's, Blimpie, Burger King, Domino's, Hardee's, KFC, Papa John's, Pizza Hut, Wendy's, Subway, McDonald's, and Taco Bell. The site is easy to use and allows consumers to search their favorite foods by fat calories, total calories, percentage of calories from fat, total fat, saturated fat, cholesterol, sodium, carbohydrates, fiber, and protein. It is offered only in English.

Promote Healthy Food Choices

There are many opportunities for nurses to learn more about cultural practices, and any interaction with a client from a different culture is an opportunity to advance one's understanding and respect for diverse food practices. The Nutrition Education for New Americans Project at the

MyNursingKit *"Fast Food Nutrition Fact Explorer"*

MyNursingKit Nutrition Education for New Americans University of Georgia

MyNursingKit The Southeastern Michigan Dietetics Association

University of Georgia is an excellent reference for specific nutritional and diabetes-related handouts. Nutritional resources are available in 35 languages other than English, and bilingual diabetes handouts are available in 29 languages. The Southeastern Michigan Dietetics Association offers a variety of downloadable food pyramids organized by culture, ethnicity, and religion. There is a wealth of on-line information available to assist nurses in providing culturally relevant dietary information. Many of those resources are available in English and in the selected language, and most of the recommendations include traditional foods familiar to the client.

Culturally Sensitive Nutritional Counseling

If diet teaching is required, it must be sensitive and responsive to cultural characteristics. The following guidelines are useful:

- Assess language fluency and literacy levels of the client and his or her family. It may be necessary to enlist others to assist with dietary teaching. Family members may not be appropriate, skilled enough in the language, or the content to adequately substitute for a trained health care interpreter.
- Use respectful and appropriate body language. Different cultures have different norms for nonverbal communication actions, and it is disrespectful to ignore those behavioral rules.
- Choose resources that are relevant and appropriate for the client. Many Web sites offer nutritional information in the client's preferred language and use foods that are traditional and well known.

Communities exert great influence on health behaviors. When providing care to an individual, the professional nurse must recognize the potential impact of the client's intersecting communities. Culturally sensitive and competent care can ease the stress of an illness and communicate acceptance. Knowledge of health habits and common cultural expectations can help provide exemplary and individualized care to the individual, the family, and the community.

NURSING CARE PLAN Safe Food Handling

CASE STUDY

Alice, 31 years old, comes to the clinic with concerns about intermittent bouts of diarrhea over the last 3 months. She is a single parent who lives with her 8- and 11-year-old daughters in a mobile home park. Her work as a receptionist in a small real estate firm provides a modest income but no health insurance. She makes it clear that she wants as little diagnostic testing as possible because she does not know how she will pay for it. Upon further questioning, she reveals that the diarrhea is accompanied by abdominal discomfort and maybe a low fever, but it always resolves after a few days. She says that her children sometimes have it at the same time as she does, but other times they do not have it. They have all missed occasional days of school and work. When the nurse asks about food preparation and storage, Alice says she tries to be careful but their mobile home is cramped for the three of them and that space is at a premium. She describes the refrigerator as "old and tiny" and she is not sure it keeps things very cold. When she knows she will be using a food soon, she frequently leaves it on the counter or in the sink, rather than trying to find a place for it in the refrigerator. For instance, she often packs leftovers for lunches the night before and leaves them in insulated lunch bags on the table for everyone to grab as they go out the door. She says that she does her best to keep the home tidy and clean but that space is so tight it is hard to make a difference.

Applying the Nursing Process

ASSESSMENT

Height: 5 feet 4 inches; Weight: 128 pounds; BMI: 22
T 98.7 P 80 R 16 BP 126/72
Skin warm and dry
Moist mucous membranes
Active bowel sounds

DIAGNOSES

Diarrhea related to possible bacterial contamination from unsafe food storage evidenced by intermittent loose, watery stools
Knowledge, deficient related to lack of information about safe food storage practices evidenced by disclosure of current food storage practices

EXPECTED OUTCOMES

Bowel elimination pattern will return to normal
Alice will discuss causative factors and preventive practices

INTERVENTION

Stool specimen to identify causative organism(s)
Discuss importance of fluid intake during diarrhea episodes
Discuss safe food preparation and storage guidelines
Stress importance of hand washing during food preparation and after using the bathroom

Safe Food Handling (continued)

NURSING CARE PLAN

Assessment
Data about the patient

Subjective
What the patient tells the nurse
Example: "My children and I are having bouts of intermittent diarrhea. Leftovers left out of the refrigerator overnight."

Objective
What the nurse observes; anthropometric and clinical data
Examples: Height: 5 feet 4 inches; Weight: 128 pounds; BMI: 22, active bowel sounds

Diagnosis
NANDA label
Example: Diarrhea realted to unsafe food handling and storage practices

Planning
Goals stated in patient terms
Example: Long-term goal: safe food storage and preparation practices implemented; Short-term goal: normal bowel elimination pattern

Implementation
Nursing action to help patient achieve goals
Example: Explain safe food handling practices, including hand washing

Evaluation
Was the goal achieved or does the intervention need to be modified?
Example: No further diarrhea; leftovers refrigerated within 30 minutes

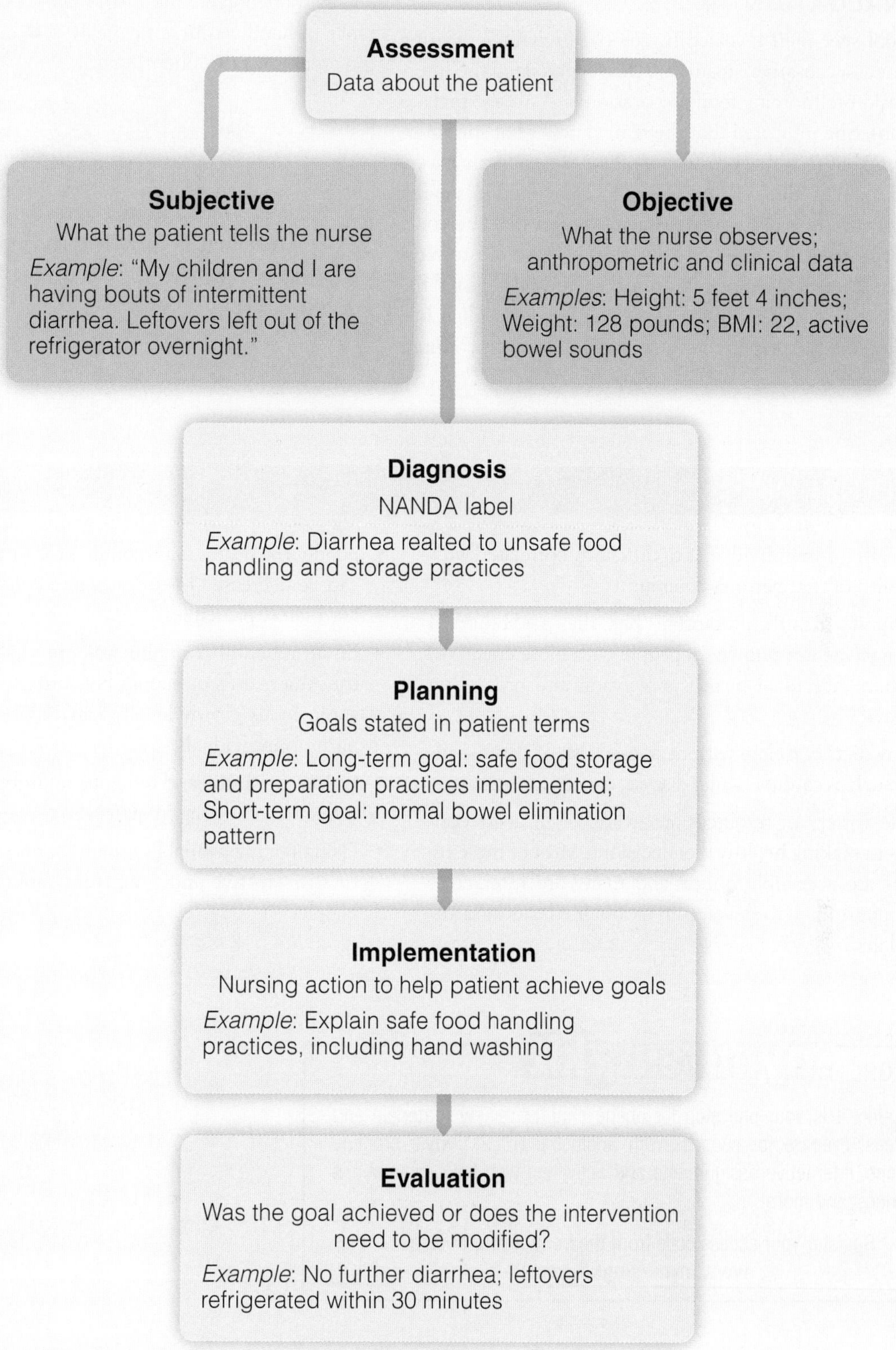

■ FIGURE 10-3 **Nursing Care Plan Process: Safe Food Handling.**

(continued)

Safe Food Handling *(continued)*

NURSING CARE PLAN

EVALUATION

Stool specimen revealed *E. coli* overgrowth, indicating that as a causative organism. Alice appreciated the information reinforcing food preparation and storage precautions. She indicated that she really knew what should be done, but that maybe she was taking shortcuts that were not helpful. She said she was purchasing food in smaller quantities so she would not have leftovers that she could not store safely. She had talked to the landlord to have the refrigerator temperature checked; he had adjusted the temperature after finding it was set too low. Alice had completely scrubbed the bathroom and kitchen counters and reminded everyone in the family about the importance of hand washing. Figure 10-3 ■ outlines the nursing process for this client.

Critical Thinking in the Nursing Process

1. **What are some specific suggestions about safe food handling, preparation, and storage that the nurse could make to a client who may have a foodborne infection?**

CHAPTER SUMMARY

- The health of an individual is significantly correlated with the health of that person's community.

- Community health promotion has the possibility of reaching a greater number of people with more effectiveness than individual health prevention and promotion efforts.

- Healthy diets correlate with decreased risk of chronic illnesses such as cardiovascular disease, cancer, and diabetes.

- A wide variety of resources are available to assist consumers in making healthy diet decisions. Most of these resources are accessible online and many are interactive with opportunity to develop individualized diet and fitness plans.

- Foodborne illness is a common problem for Americans but can be decreased by industry and consumer awareness of food safety principles.

- Environmental contaminants are a growing problem for the American food supply, but strategies such as eating organic foods grown locally can reduce the potential for harm to individuals.

- Cultural, ethnic, and religious traditions exert significant influence on dietary practices.

- Using readily available resources, nurses can provide culturally sensitive and competent care to diverse groups of people.

EXPLORE PEARSON **mynursingkit™**

MyNursingKit is your one stop for online chapter review materials and resources. Prepare for success with additional NCLEX®-style practice questions, interactive assignments and activities, web links, animations and videos, and more!

Register your access code from the front of your book at
www.mynursingkit.com.

NCLEX® QUESTIONS

1. The nurse who is interested in primary prevention will participate in which of the following activities?
   1. Teaching the spouse of a client with renal disease about a low-sodium diet
   2. Recommending multivitamin supplements to parents of school-age children
   3. Teaching high school students examples of low-fat snacks
   4. Suggesting foods to a middle-age client who is struggling with chronic constipation

2. A client tells the nurse that he knows he is experiencing food poisoning. What is the first thing the nurse should ask the client?
   1. What did you eat?
   2. When did you last eat something?
   3. What are your symptoms?
   4. Who else in your family is sick?

3. A mother tells the nurse at the clinic that she frequently adds a raw egg to her 5-year-old daughter's milkshakes because she is such a picky eater and this adds more nutrition to the one food she readily consumes. How should the nurse respond?
   1. "I am glad you are adding a good source of protein to the milkshakes."
   2. "Raw eggs contain *Salmonella*, a kind of bacteria, so they should never be added to foods that will not be cooked."
   3. "Raw eggs are hard to digest so they should be added to milkshakes no more than once per week."
   4. "Raw eggs frequently induce vomiting so do not use them in foods that a child enjoys."

4. The nurse knows that a client who consumes unpasteurized milk is at a greater risk for:
   1. Food allergy
   2. Foodborne intoxication
   3. Cancer
   4. Foodborne infection

5. When a client tells the nurse that every time someone in the family develops a fever the sick person gets served chicken soup, the nurse recognizes that this is an example of:
   1. A commonly accepted way to treat a fever
   2. A comfort food used to treat illness
   3. Assimilation of dietary practices
   4. Acculturation

REFERENCES

American Academy of Allergy, Asthma, & Immunology (AAAAI) Work Group. (2003). *Current approach to the diagnosis and management of adverse reactions to food.* Retrieved November 7, 2008, from http://www.aaaai.org/members/academy_statements/practice_papers/adverse_reactions_to_foods.pdf

American Dietetic Association (ADA). (2003). Position of the American Dietetic Association: Food and water safety. *Journal of the American Dietetic Association, 103,* 1203–1218.

American Dietetic Association (ADA). (2007). *Healthy land, healthy people: Building a better understanding of sustainable food systems for food and nutrition professionals.* Retrieved November 3, 2008, from http://www.eatright.org/ada/files/Sustainable_Primer.pdf

Anderson, S. A. (1990). Core indicators of nutritional state for difficult-to-sample populations. *Journal of Nutrition, 120,* 1559–1560.

Bernstein, I. L., Li, J. T., Bernstein, D. I., Hamilton, R., Spector, S., Tan, R., et al. (2008). Allergy diagnostic testing: An updated practice parameter. *Annals of Allergy, Asthma, and Immunology, 100,* S1–S148.

Bronstein, A. C., Spyker, D. A., Cantilena, L. R., Green, J. L., Rumack, B. H., & Heard, S. E. (2008). 2007 annual report of the American Association of Poison Control Centers' National Poison Data Systems: 25th annual report. *Clinical Toxicology, 46,* 927–1057.

Center for Nutrition Policy and Promotion. (2008, June). *Healthy eating index—2005.* Alexandria, VA: Author. Retrieved March 30, 2009, from http://www.cnpp.usda.gov/Publications/HEI/healthyeatingindex2005factsheet.pdf

Centers for Disease Control and Prevention (CDC). (2004). *The burden of chronic diseases and their risk factors: National and state perspectives 2004.* Atlanta, GA: U.S. Department of Health and Human Services. Retrieved June 24, 2009, from http://www.cdc.gov/nccdphp/burdenbook2004

Centers for Disease Control and Prevention (CDC). (2005). *Foodborne illness.* Retrieved November 7, 2008, from http://www.cdc.gov/ncidod/dbmd/diseaseinfo/foodborneinfections_g.htm#

Centers for Disease Control and Prevention (CDC). (2006). Preliminary FoodNet data

on the incidence of infection with pathogens transmitted commonly through food—10 states, 2006. *Morbidity and Mortality Weekly Report, 56*(14), 336–339.

Centers for Disease Control and Prevention (CDC). (2007). *Water treatment methods.* Retrieved March 16, 2009, from http://wwwnc.cdc.gov/travel/content/water-treatment.aspx

Centers for Disease Control and Prevention (CDC). (2009). *Deaths: Final data for 2006.* Retrieved June 24, 2009, from http://www.cdc.gov/nchs/fastats/lcod.htm

Dinour, L. M., Bergen, D., & Ming-Chen, Y. (2007). The food insecurity-obesity paradox: A review of the literature and the role food stamps may play. *Journal of the American Dietetic Association, 107,* 1952–1961.

Edelman, C. L., & Mandle, C. L. (2002). *Health promotion throughout the lifespan* (5th ed.). St. Louis, MO: Mosby.

Edlich, R. F., Drake, D. B., Rodeheaver, G. T., Kelley, A., Greene, J. A., Gubler, K. D., et al. (2007). Revolutionary advances in organic food. *Internal and Emergency Medicine, 2,* 182–187.

REFERENCES *(continued)*

Environmental Protection Agency (EPA). (2004). *What you need to know about mercury in fish and shellfish.* Retrieved November 7, 2008, from http://www.epa.gov/waterscience/fish/advice/index.html

Environmental Protection Agency (EPA). (2006). *EPA ground water and drinking water. Consumer fact sheet: Mercury.* Retrieved November 7, 2008, from http://www.epa.gov/ogwdw/dwh/c-ioc/mercury.html

Food and Drug Administration (FDA). (2001). *HAACP: A state-of-the-art approach to food safety.* Retrieved March 16, 2009, from http://www.cfsan.fda.gov/~lrd/bghaccp.html

Food and Drug Administration (FDA). (2009). *Action levels, tolerances, and guidance levels for poisonous or deleterious substances in seafood.* Retrieved November 7, 2009, from http://www.fda.gov/Food/FoodSafety/Product-SpecificInformation/Seafood/FederalStatePrograms/NationalShellfishSanitationProgram/ucm053987.htm

Giddens, A. (1996). *Introduction to sociology* (2nd ed.). New York: W. W. Norton.

Gunderson, C., Lohman, B. J., Garasky, S., Stewart, S., & Eisenmann, J. (2008). Food security, maternal stressors, and overweight among low-income US children: Results from the National Health and Nutrition Examination Survey (1999–2002). *Pediatrics, 122*(3), 529–540.

Heine, R. G., & Tang, L. K. (2008). Dietary approaches to the prevention of food allergy. *Current Opinion in Clinical Nutrition and Metabolic Care, 11,* 320–328.

Jemal, A. (2005). Trends in the leading causes of death in the United States, 1970–2002. *Journal of the American Medical Association, 294,* 1255–1259.

Kligler, B. (2007). Ask the experts. *Explore, 3,* 640.

Kreuter, M., & Devore, R. (1980). Update: Reinforcing the case for health promotion. *Family and Community Health, 10,* 106.

Lack, G. (2008). Food allergy. *New England Journal of Medicine, 359,* 1252–1260.

Leavell, H., & Clark, A. E. (1965). *Prevention medicine for doctors in the community.* New York: McGraw-Hill.

Lee, L. A., & Burks, W. A. (2006). Food allergies: Prevalence, molecular characterization, and treatment/prevention strategies. *Annual Review of Nutrition, 26,* 539–565.

MacQueen, K. M., McLellan, E., Metzger, D. S., Kegeles, S., Strauss, R. P., Scotti, R., et al. (2001). What is community? An evidence-based decision for participatory public health. *American Journal of Public Health, 91*(12), 1929–1938.

McCullough, M. L., Feskanich, D., Stampfer, M. J., Giovannucci, E. L., Rimm, E. B., Hu, F. B., et al. (2002). Diet quality and major chronic disease risk in men and women: moving toward improved dietary guidance. *American Journal of Clinical Nutrition, 76*(6), 1261–71.

McKnight, J. L. (2002). Two tools for well-being: health systems. In M. Minkler (Ed.), *Community organizing and community building for health* (pp. 20–29). New Brunswick, NJ: Rutgers University Press.

Minkler, M., & Wallerstein, N. B. (2002). Improving health through community organization and community building. In K. Glanz, B. K. Rimer, & F. M. Lewis (Eds.), *Health behavior and health education theory, research and practice* (3rd ed., pp. 279–311). San Francisco: Jossey-Bass.

Mokdad, A. H., Marks, J. S., Stroup, D. F., & Gergerding, J. L. (2004). Actual causes of death in the United States, 2000. *Journal of the American Medical Association, 291*(10), 1238–1245.

Napier, G. L., & Kodner, C. M. (2008). Health risks and benefits of bottled water. *Primary Care Clinics in Office Practice, 35,* 789–802.

National Institutes of Health (NIH), National Institute of Diabetes and Digestive and Kidney Diseases (NIDDK). (2003). *Lactose intolerance.* Retrieved November 7, 2008, from http://www.digestive.niddk.nih.gov/ddiseases/pubs/lactoseintolerance/index.htm

Natural Resources Defense Council (NRDC). (2008). *Bottled water.* Retrieved November 7, 2008, from http://www.nrdc.org/water/drinking/qbw.asp

Niggemann, B., & Beyer, K. (2005). Diagnostic pitfalls in food allergy in children. *Allergy, 60,* 104–107.

Noimark, L., & Cox, H. E. (2008). Nutritional problems related to food allergy in children. *Pediatric Allergy Immunology, 19,* 188–195.

O'Donnell, M. (1987). Definition of health promotion. *American Journal of Health Promotion, 1*(1), 4.

Olson, C. M., & Strawderman, M. S. (2008). The relationship between food insecurity and obesity in rural childbearing women. *Journal of Rural Health, 24*(1), 60–66.

Partnership for Food Safety Education. (2006). *Fight Bac.* Retrieved November 7, 2008, from http://www.fightbac.org

Pender, N. J., Murdaugh, C. L., & Parsons, M. A. (2006). *Health promotion in nursing practice.* Upper Saddle River, NJ: Pearson Prentice Hall.

Persell, C. H. (1990). *Understanding society* (3rd ed.). New York: Harper Collins College.

Pietrykowski, B. (2004). You are what you eat: The social economy of the Slow Food movement. *Review of Social Economy, 3,* 307–321.

Queralt, M. (1996). *The social environment and human behavior.* Boston: Allyn and Bacon.

Senna, G., Passalacqua, G., Lombardi, C., & Antonicelli, L. (2004). Position paper: Controversial and unproven diagnostic procedures for food allergy. *European Annals of Allergy and Clinical Immunology, 36,* 139–145.

Shuster, G. F., & Goeppinger, J. (2004). Community as client: Using the nursing process to promote health. In M. Stanhope & J. Lancaster (Eds.), *Community and public health nursing* (pp. 306–329). St. Louis, MO: Mosby.

Slow Food USA. (2008). *Mission statement.* Retrieved February 22, 2008, from http://www.slowfoodusa.org/index.html

United Nations News Center. (2004). *UN-backed treaty banning most dangerous pesticides to come into force in May.* Retrieved February 22, 2008, from http://www.un.org/apps/news/story.asp?NewsID=9808&Cr=Pollutants&Cr1=

United States Department of Agriculture (USDA). (1999). *Sustainable agriculture: Definitions and terms.* Retrieved October 28, 2008, from http://desearch.nal.usda.gov/cgi-bin/dexpldcgi?qry1861764957;2

United States Department of Agriculture (USDA), Agricultural Marketing Service. (2008). *National Organic Program: Organic labeling and marketing information.* Retrieved November 7, 2008, from http://www.ams.usda.gov/AMSv1.0/getfile?dDocName=STELDEV3004446

United States Department of Agriculture (USDA), Food Safety and Inspection Service. (2006). *Is it done yet? Internal temperatures for cooking meats and eggs.* Retrieved March 16, 2009, from http://www.fsis.usda.gov/Is_It_Done_Yet/Brochure_Text/index.asp

United States Department of Health and Human Services. (2000). *Healthy People 2010: Understanding and improving health.* Washington, DC: U.S. Government Printing Office.

United States Department of Health and Human Services. (2001). *Healthy People 2010: Nutrition and overweight.* Retrieved March 16, 2009, from http://www.healthypeople.gov/Publications/

United States Department of Health and Human Services. (2005). *Dietary Guidelines for Americans.* Retrieved February 22, 2008, from http://www.health.gov/dietaryguidelines/default.htm

United States Geological Services. (2009). *Nation fish mercury model.* Retrieved June 24, 2009, from http://toxics.usgs.gov/highlights/mercury_model.html

Webb, A. L., Schiff, A., Currivan, D., & Villamor, E. (2008). Food Stamp Program participation but not food insecurity is associated with higher adult BMI in Massachusetts residents living in low-income neighbourhoods. *Public Health Nutrition, 11*(12), 1248–1255.

Weiss, C., Munoz-Furlong, A., Furlong, T. J., & Arbit, J. (2004). Impact of food allergies on school nursing practice. *The Journal of School Nursing, 20,* 268–274.

World Health Organization (WHO). (1974). *Community health nursing: Report of a WHO expert committee.* Technical Report Series No. 558. Geneva: Author.

Wuthrich, B. (2005). Unproven techniques in allergy diagnosis. *Journal of Investigative Allergology and Clinical Immunology, 15,* 86–90.

Nutrition in Sports 11

WHAT WILL YOU LEARN?

1. To differentiate the roles of carbohydrate, protein, and fat in the diet of the athlete.
2. To formulate nursing interventions to promote adequate intake of calories, protein, and carbohydrate by physically active clients.
3. To relate the effect of mineral nutrition on athletic performance.
4. To develop hydration strategies for athletes of all levels and ages.
5. To apply guidelines for nutrition in exercise to individuals in unique stages of the lifespan.
6. To evaluate the role of dietary supplements marketed for sports performance.

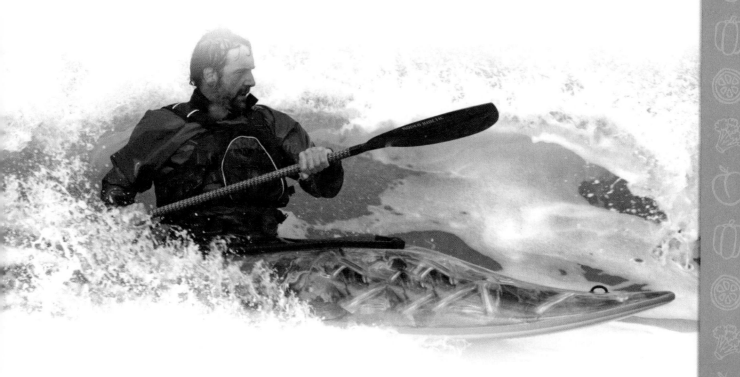

DID YOU KNOW?

▶ Carbohydrates are the preferred source of fuel for exercising muscle.

▶ Consuming enough protein but not enough kcalories will result in protein being sacrificed for use as fuel instead of as a building block.

▶ Exercising to work up a "good sweat" that results in immediate postexercise weight loss is only a loss of water. Dehydration of as little as 1% to 2% of body weight has a negative effect on sports performance and health.

▶ Lack of menses in a nonpregnant female results in loss of bone, which can predispose an athlete to stress fractures.

▶ No sports nutrition supplement will compensate for a poor diet.

MyNursingKit Gatorade Sports Science Institute

KEY TERMS

aerobic, *226*

amenorrhea, *228*

anaerobic, *226*

energy availability, *228*

ergogenic aids, *238*

female athlete triad, *228*

glycemic index, *228*

hyponatremia, *235*

Why Is Sports Nutrition Important?

Optimal nutrition has a positive effect on exercise performance for every level of athlete. Both competitive and recreational athletes benefit from a nutrition strategy that provides the right fuel and fluids to sustain exercise training and recovery. The popularity of sports nutrition products, supplements, and advice from the lay public presents a challenge to the athlete who is trying to improve overall fitness without jeopardizing health. Often, athletes obtain sports nutrition information from unreliable sources or hold erroneous beliefs about nutrition and fitness. The nurse can serve as a resource for reliable advice on choosing foods, fluids, and supplements to optimize sports performance and training recovery.

What Fuels Exercise?

The primary sources of energy during exercise are derived from carbohydrates and fats. Metabolism of these nutrients yields adenosine triphosphate (ATP) that in turn is broken down to yield the energy needed for muscle contraction. Glucose and fatty acids derived from carbohydrate and fat sources are present in the blood and muscle as energy substrates. Glucose is used to generate an immediate energy source for contracting muscle fibers or is stored as glycogen in muscle and the liver for later conversion back to glucose. Exercise that is strenuous with a short "all out" burst of energy is referred to as **anaerobic** in nature because it requires no oxygen during metabolism. Anaerobic exercise, such as weight lifting or sprinting, relies on glucose as the sole energy source. The body is capable of generating energy with anaerobic metabolism for up to 2 minutes. After that time frame, either fatigue sets in or metabolism is shifted to a pathway using oxygen. **Aerobic** exercise requires oxygen for metabolism and utilizes a mix of both glucose and fat sources for fuel. Fat utilization cannot yield energy immediately when physical activity begins. Examples of aerobic activities include jogging and swimming laps. Protein sources provide some energy during prolonged endurance events, such as a marathon, but should not be a primary source of fuel except under such extreme metabolic conditions. Instead, dietary protein serves as a building block for muscle recovery and enhancement.

Overall, the mix of fuel required to fuel any activity depends on two factors: the intensity and duration of the activity. High-intensity, short-duration activities, which are strenuous and require bursts of energy, require a greater proportion of glucose to fuel the activity than less strenuous activities. Longer-duration activities, such as distance running, are fueled by a mix of glucose and fats. Many activities are a combination of intensities and duration and thus switch back and forth between fuel mixes. Soccer and other field sports are examples with a combination of running and sprinting. When asked for sports nutrition recommendations, the nurse should first point out the importance of a diet containing sufficient calories. The mix of fuels utilized for anaerobic-type or aerobic-type exercises is almost irrelevant if the athlete is not consuming adequate fuel to support physical activity. The nurse can also stress that adequate carbohydrate as a source of glucose is essential for both types of exercise. On-line resources are available with nutrition education materials to assist those working with athletes.

Energy Recommendations

Physical activity requires varying amounts of energy depending on how strenuous the activity is and its duration. Achieving energy balance in the healthy weight athlete is crucial to both providing adequate fuel to support physical activity and for health maintenance. Estimates of the energy needed for physical activity are outlined in Table 11-1. The nurse can assist a client in determining the fuel needs of an activity using these estimates. Overall energy needs are determined by adding the specific energy requirements of activity to the other components of the resting metabolic rate as outlined in Chapter 8. Internet tools designed for this purpose are an additional resource.

Some physically active people want to alter body composition through weight gain or loss. The nurse should help the active person explore the rationale for any weight change goal, emphasizing the concept that weight or body fat alone do not determine performance ability. Genetic predisposi-

MyNursingKit Nutrition Analysis Tool Energy Calculator

Table 11-1 Estimating Energy Requirements of Exercise

Expended Calories/Hour*	Activity
1,000+	Running 9 mph or faster
750–1,000	Jumping rope Rowing, competitive Running 7 mph Skiing cross-country 5 mph or faster
500–750	Basketball, vigorous Biking greater than 10 mph Football Hockey, field and ice Jogging 5 mph Martial arts Rock/mountain climbing Skiing downhill Soccer Swimming, breast stroke, butterfly, or crawl Wrestling
350–500	Aerobics Skating Tennis Walking 4.5 mph Weight lifting, vigorous effort
200–350	Baseball Biking less than 10 mph Dancing Golf, carrying clubs Hiking Weight lifting, light effort Walking 3.5 mph

*Estimates are based on a body weight of 70 kg (154 lb). Athletes with a greater weight will expend more calories per hour and those who are lighter will expend less.

tion, age, gender, training, rest, and overall diet play important roles in body composition and exercise performance. In both the competitive and recreational athlete, the emphasis should be on healthful dietary choices from a variety of foods and avoidance of too low an energy intake to sustain physical activity when trying to reduce body weight (American Dietetic Association [ADA], Dietitians of Canada [DC], & American College of Sports Medicine [ACSM], 2009).

The goal of weight change or altered body composition in the competitive athlete should be evaluated by the health care team and, if indicated, occur during the off-season and under the close supervision of an expert in the sports nutrition field to ensure that body fat does not drop too low or that muscle is not sacrificed to meet fuel needs, compromising power, strength, endurance, and health. Registered dietitians (RDs) with the additional C.S.S.D. credential are board cer-

tified in sports dietetics and are considered the nutrition experts in this field. Hot Topic: Making Weight outlines important points for the nurse to consider when working with athletes who are in weight-class sports, such as wrestling or rowing, and utilizing unsafe methods to reach a desired weight. School nurses and those working in collegiate health, sports medicine, and pediatric and adolescent health should be aware of these practices.

hot Topic

Making Weight

Weight-class sports group competitors by weight-range categories. Wrestling, rowing, and the martial arts are examples of weight-class sports. Rapid weight loss to quickly meet weight criteria before competition is employed by some athletes in these sports, often on a regular basis during the sport season. Techniques used for quick weight loss include calorie deprivation with excessive exercise, fasting, or eating and purging; and promotion of dehydration with use of diuretics and laxatives, sauna, rubber or plastic suits, or a steam room. Some athletes perform combinations of these activities, such as drinking no fluids while exercising in a steam room wearing a rubber suit. The athlete may intend to be only temporarily dehydrated for the weigh-in, thinking that there is time to rehydrate before competition. However, adequate rehydration takes many hours and, therefore, the athlete enters competition in a dangerous, dehydrated state. The death of three collegiate wrestlers who had employed dehydrating practices to make weight has prompted a change in weight guidelines for that sport at the high school and collegiate levels, resulting in strict weigh-in and weight-loss guidelines that have demonstrated beneficial outcomes (Centers for Disease Control and Prevention [CDC], 1998; NCAA, 2009; National Federation of State High School Associations [NFHS], 2006; Oppliger, Utter, Scott, Dick, & Klossner, 2006). Other weight-class sports have yet to make stricter guidelines.

Measures to discourage the use of dangerous weight loss practices include the following:

Weigh-in practices:
- Check urine specific gravity to detect dehydration. Athlete not allowed to compete with value greater than 1.020–1.025 (NCAA, 2009; NFHS, 2006).
- Weigh-ins should be timed no greater than 1–2 hours before competition. Athletes may not compete below lowest certified weight class for the individual.

General weight guidelines:
- Establish minimal body fat guidelines for athletes and utilize when determining appropriate weight class (e.g., males not less than 7% of body fat) (NCAA, 2009).
- Limit amount of weight that can be lost in a week (e.g., high school and collegiate wrestlers may not lose greater than 1.5% of body weight/week) (NCAA, 2009; NFHS, 2006).
- Educate about healthy weight and athletic performance.
- Educate about safe and healthy ways to achieve and maintain healthy body weight. Refer athletes needing to gain or lose weight to a registered dietitian (AAP, 2005).
- Educate about healthy hydration practices and the negative effects of dehydration. Use of impermeable suits, rubber shirts, and the like is prohibited (NCAA, 2009).

Female athletes are at particular risk for poor energy balance. The emphasis on leanness in many sports, along with the Western cultural emphasis on thinness, causes some athletes to consume suboptimal calories or overexercise to achieve a lower body weight. Some athletes simply do not realize the high-energy demands of training and fail to consume sufficient calories. When energy expenditure exceeds energy intake, the result is called low **energy availability.** This energy deficit, whether inadvertent or intentional, results in diminished reproductive hormone production and secretion and irregular or absent menstruation, called **amenorrhea** (Nattiv et al., 2007). Bone loss, which can manifest as a stress fracture in an athlete, occurs because of the endocrine disturbance, and it is much like the reduced bone mineral density that is found in postmenopausal females. Risk of a stress fracture is increased at least twofold in the athlete with amenorrhea compared with those with normal menstrual function (Nattiv et al., 2007). Growth and regulation of body temperature are additional physiological effects affected by low-energy availability. Together, the consequences of low-energy availability, reduced bone mineral density, and amenorrhea are referred to as the **female athlete triad.** The symptoms of the triad occur along a continuum and proceed to an eating disorder and osteoporosis in some athletes in addition to the amenorrhea. Practice Pearl: The Female Athlete Triad describes symptoms of the female athlete triad.

Female athletes should be screened for all components of the female athlete triad at preparticipation physical exams or annual physicals (Nattiv et al., 2007). On-line resources are available for the health professional including screening forms for the triad. Treatment of the female athlete triad should focus on improving energy availability with any combination of increased intake or decreased physical activity. When disordered eating is a contributor, the athlete should be referred to a mental health professional. Participation in specific sports that emphasize thinness, such as gymnastics, ballet, or figure skating, places the athlete at increased risk of developing an eating disorder (Nattiv et al., 2007). The competitive nature of sports and pressure from a coach or parent to lose weight further escalate risk.

As part of preventive education, the focus should be on food as a needed source of fuel for both training and recovery. Emphasis should be given to preservation of bone health through proper diet and sufficient energy intake to maintain hormone function (Nattiv et al., 2007).

Carbohydrate Recommendations

Adequate carbohydrate intake is essential to fuel exercise and to restore glycogen levels before the next exercise session. Physically active individuals who train more than once in a day or on successive days especially must pay close attention to carbohydrate intake to avoid diminished glycogen stores and poor performance. Athletes need to learn to match carbohydrate intake to the demands of the individual sport. High-intensity and long-duration sports cannot rely on fat in the diet or adipose stores to supply sufficient ATP rapidly enough for the needs of the athlete (Coleman, 2006). Recommendations for carbohydrate intake are given in relation to body weight instead of as a percentage of total energy intake. Use of the calorie percentage approach should be avoided because it is not user friendly and can short-change carbohydrate in smaller- to medium-weight athletes and overestimate intake in large athletes (ADA, DC, & ACSM, 2009; Coleman, 2006). Daily carbohydrate recommendations include:

- 6 to 10 gm of carbohydrate per kilogram of body weight (ADA, DC, & ACSM, 2009) are needed.
- Higher amounts may be needed by endurance athletes who train many hours per day.
- Lower amounts may be needed by the recreational athlete who exercises an hour or less per day.
- A sports nutrition specialist can educate athletes how to adjust carbohydrate intake according to training level.

Often an athlete will ask about the recommended type of carbohydrate when making food choices. Some believe that one type of carbohydrate is better than another because of how quickly or slowly it elevates blood sugar levels. Research outcome varies on the usefulness of categorizing individual foods this way, a method that is referred to as the **glycemic index.** Foods are ranked as having a low, moderate, or high glycemic index based on the blood sugar response to ingesting a 50 gm of carbohydrate portion of the single food compared with the response seen with the same amount of carbohydrate from either glucose or white bread. A lower glycemic index food will raise blood sugar less over an equal amount of time than a higher glycemic index food. Some athletes try to ingest low- or moderate-glycemic foods before exercise, believing that

PRACTICE PEARL

The Female Athlete Triad

The American College of Sports Medicine warns that when a female athlete presents with any one component of the female athlete triad, she should be screened for the presence of the other two components.

- Some athletes view amenorrhea as an acceptable sign of a high training level and thus may not report it.
- Stress fracture injury is a red flag for potential bone loss occurrence.
- Insufficient caloric intake can lead to an "energy drain" or low-energy availability that alters reproductive hormone secretion and may or may not result in weight loss, depending on the extent of the deficit.

Source: Adapted from Bonci et al., 2008; Loucks, 2007; Nattiv et al., 2007; NCAA, n.d.

high-glycemic foods cause a quick elevation of blood glucose and rapid drop from the insulin response that should be avoided during exercise. This school of thought reserves high-glycemic foods for after exercise when restoring glycogen levels is a priority. Although most high-fiber complex carbohydrates tend to have a lower glycemic index than simple sugars, it is difficult to make generalizations about the glycemic index of foods. Preparation techniques and combining foods together change the glycemic index by altering the digestion and absorption rate of the carbohydrate. Glycemic index tables are long and cumbersome, but they are used by some highly motivated athletes seeking to fine-tune the diet. Client Education Checklist: Carbohydrate Recommendations contains some examples of glycemic index values.

Timing of carbohydrate intake before, during, and after exercise affects the availability of glucose to the exercising muscle. During exercise, the body relies on existing glycogen stores to maintain blood glucose level and to fuel muscle

CLIENT EDUCATION CHECKLIST	Carbohydrate Recommendations
Intervention	**Example**
Review the importance of carbohydrate as a fuel source for athletic training.	• Carbohydrate provides the body with substrate for glucose synthesis. • Glucose is utilized to fuel activity that is short-burst and maximal effort (anaerobic). • Glucose and fat are used to fuel activity that lasts longer than several minutes and is less than maximal effort (aerobic). • Glycogen is the storage form of glucose and becomes diminished during exercise. • Glycogen stores should be restored after exercise as part of recovery and preparation for the next exercise session.
Calculate overall carbohydrate needs based on level of training.	• 5–7 gm/kg for exercise less than 1 hour/day or general training • 7–10 gm/kg for intense exercise 1–4 hours/day or endurance training • 11–12 gm/kg for intense exercise greater than 4 hours/day or ultraendurance training
Educate client on dietary sources of carbohydrate.	• Carbohydrate is found in plant-based foods (grains, fruits, legumes, vegetables), some dairy foods, and treats. • Animal proteins (meat, poultry, fish, cheese), fats, and oils are not carbohydrate sources **10–15 gm carbohydrate** Bread, 1 slice Candy, hard, 3 pc or lollipop, ½ oz Green peas, ½ cup, cooked Marshmallow, 20 mini Melon, 1 cup Milk, 1 cup Raisins, mini box, ½ oz Yogurt, plain, 1 cup Waffle, toaster, 1 **15–20 gm carbohydrate** Beans, lentils, ½ cup cooked Fruit, fresh, less than 3″ diameter Oatmeal, 1 cup Pita bread, small, 4″ diameter Pretzels, 1 oz Soy nuts, 4 TBSP Sports drink, 8 oz Waffle, toaster **20–25 gm carbohydrate** Carbohydrate gel, 1 packet Cereal, cold, 1 cup avg (check label, varies) Pasta, ½ cup Potato, baked, med or mashed, ½ cup Rice, ½ cup Roll, hamburger or hotdog Tortilla, flour, 12″

(continued)

CLIENT EDUCATION CHECKLIST	✓	Carbohydrate Recommendations *(continued)*

Intervention	Example
	25–30 gm carbohydrate Banana, 7″ Candy, soft sugar gummy type, 1 oz Chocolate milk, low fat, 1 cup English muffin, 1 std Fruit juice, avg, 1 cup Grapes, 1 cup Pancake, from mix, 6″ diameter Pudding, avg, 1 cup Soup, noodle, avg, 12 oz
	30+ gm carbohydrate Applesauce, 1 cup Apricots, figs, dried, 5 Bagel, large Raisins, ⅓ cup Yogurt, frozen, 1 cup Yogurt, fruit flavored, 1 cup
Discuss the potential for varying glycemic index of carbohydrate on performance.	• Glycemic index refers to the glucose response from foods consumed alone compared to a standard. • Combining foods or altering preparation alters the glycemic index of the food. • Low- to moderate-glycemic index foods elevate blood glucose less dramatically compared with high-glycemic foods and may be useful before exercise. • High-glycemic foods consumed after exercise may replenish glycogen stores more quickly than lower glycemic foods. **Low-glycemic foods** • Chickpeas and hummus, kidney beans, lentils • Dried apricots • Fruit with edible skin (apples, peach, pear) • Peanuts, cashews • Whole grain cereal, high fiber cereal • Yogurt, fat-free or sugar-free **Moderate-glycemic foods** • Green peas • Ice cream • Juice, apple, orange, pineapple • Milk, cow and soy • Oranges • Pasta, plain • Rice, converted **High-glycemic foods** • Bagels • Bananas • Bread, wheat, pita • Carbohydrate gels • Cereal, cold (varies with sugar content and grain) • Corn • Doughnuts • Honey • Pretzels • Raisins • Rice, long-grain • Soda • Sports drinks • Sugar candy—jelly beans, candy corn, gummy candy, etc.
Strategize timing of carbohydrate intake with client.	• Begin exercise following guidelines for carbohydrate intake (see Box 11-1). • Consume 30–60 gm of carbohydrate/hour during exercise. • Follow recommendations for postexercise carbohydrate depending on level of training (see Box 11-1). • Carbohydrate can be solid or liquid, depending on tolerance. • Practice intake of varying carbohydrate sources during training to learn tolerance to form and glycemic index of carbohydrate.

contraction. The nurse should emphasize the importance of meeting overall carbohydrate needs throughout the day to both fuel exercise and maintain glycogen stores. Additional recommendations about timing include:

Before exercise: Carbohydrate-containing foods or liquids consumed within hours of exercise serve to "top off" a source of glucose when exercise time exceeds an hour.

During prolonged exercise: 30 to 60 gm of carbohydrate/ hour should be consumed in a tolerated solid or liquid form in order to sustain blood glucose levels (ADA, DC, & ACSM, 2009). Some athletes can tolerate solid foods before or during exercise and others find sports drinks or carbohydrate gels necessary.

After exercise: Glycogen repletion is an essential part of recovery nutrition. Carbohydrates should be consumed within one-half hour of exercise and at 2-hour intervals up to 6 hours following exercise for maximal glycogen repletion (ADA, DC, & ACSM, 2009). This advice is important for the athlete who trains daily, twice a day, or is involved in tournament play over the course of 1 or more days but is not significant for the athlete with 1 or more days between intense exercise sessions.

The nurse should stress the importance of practicing nutritional strategies during the training process so tolerance to timing and types of food can be learned before competition. Client Education Checklist: Carbohydrate Recommendations can assist the athlete needing overall carbohydrate guidance. Box 11-1 outlines strategies for carbohydrate timing.

Protein Recommendations

Increased intake of protein is needed by the very active athlete to support both increases in lean muscle mass and post-exercise repair of microdamage to muscle fibers (ADA, DC, & ACSM, 2009). Additionally, increased protein is required for endurance athletes because small amounts of protein are used as fuel during prolonged physical activity (Institute of Medicine [IOM], 2002). Most sports nutrition professionals recommend a daily protein intake of 1.2 to 1.4 gm/kg for the endurance athlete and 1.2 to 1.7 gm/kg for strength training (ADA, DC, & ACSM, 2009). Despite this practice, the recommended dietary allowance (RDA) for protein does not differ for the athlete compared with a sedentary individual at 0.8 gm/kg, citing improved efficiency of protein metabolism in the very active population (IOM, 2002). Vegetarian athletes who follow a high-fiber diet may require close attention

---

BOX 11-1	**Carbohydrate Timing**

Before exercise

- Approximately 1 gm of carbohydrate/kg of body weight/hour prior to exercise is recommended. This amount translates to 1 gm of carbohydrate/kg if timing is 1 hour before exercise, 2 gm/kg if 2 hours before exercise, up to 4 gm/kg for intake 4 hours before exercise.
- Individual tolerance to the amount, type, and timing of carbohydrate varies. The athlete should choose familiar foods that digest easily to avoid gastrointestinal distress.
- Either solid foods or liquids can be chosen depending on tolerance.
- Athletes should use training time to assess any personal response to varying glycemic index of foods ingested before exercise.

During exercise

- Performance with exercise lasting greater than 1 hour or stop-and-go or anaerobic sports benefits from carbohydrate consumption during exercise to sustain blood glucose levels and endurance.
- Approximately 30–60 gm carbohydrate/hour recommended if exercise exceeds 1 hour.
- Consumption of carbohydrate during exercise is underscored in athletes who have not consumed a preexercise meal or have insufficient intake overall.
- Solid foods or liquids can be chosen depending on tolerance. Liquids assist with dual goal of maintaining hydration.

- Consumption of low glycemic index foods *during* exercise is of little value unless exercise is quite prolonged.

After exercise less than 90 minutes or with 1–2 days between intense workouts

- Glycogen repletion will be accomplished during the 24 hours after exercise and intake does not need to fit into a strict time table.
- Athletes should be encouraged to meet overall nutritional needs over the course of a day, being mindful of total carbohydrate recommendations.

After strenuous exercise greater than 90 minutes or with close timing of workouts

- Glycogen repletion is best accomplished with ingestion of immediate sources of carbohydrate rather than delaying intake greater than 2 hours.
- Consumption of 1.5 gm carbohydrate/kg immediately and 2 hours later is recommended.
- Any type of carbohydrate can be chosen because intolerance issues lessen after exercise. Moderate-to high-glycemic index carbohydrates are recommended for glycogen recovery when intense exercising will recur in less than 24 hours.
- Some athletes complain of no hunger after strenuous exercise yet can be encouraged to consume high-carbohydrate drinks, or even candies, to meet needs.

Sources: Adapted from ADA, DC, & ACSM, 2009; Coleman, 2006; Jeukendrup, 2007; Kersick et al., 2008.

to protein intake as outlined in Cultural Considerations Box: Vegetarian Diets and the Athlete.

When advising an athlete about protein needs for training, the nurse should stress that first adequate calorie intake is required for protein in the diet to be used for muscle-building or recovery. Without adequate energy intake, dietary protein intake will be sacrificed for fuel instead (Rodriguez, Vislocky, & Gaine, 2007). Conversely, in the presence of adequate calorie and protein intake, excess protein serves as a source of excess calories. The nurse should assess the types of protein choices that an athlete is making. Consuming protein following strength training can enhance muscle repair and synthesis (ADA, DC, & ACSM, 2009). Milk, whey, and casein, all dairy proteins, or soy proteins are cited as beneficial following resistance exercise (Tang & Phillips, 2009). Assessment of the types of protein consumed should also be reviewed to avoid excessive intake of saturated fats that are found in many animal proteins. The role of saturated fat in the risk of cardiovascular disease is discussed in Chapter 18.

Protein supplements are not needed for muscle building because adequate nutrition can be found in the diet and most athletes already consume more than the recommended amounts (ADA, DC, & ACSM, 2009; Tipton & Witard, 2007). Box 11-2 shows an example comparing the protein content of powder supplements and foods. Collegiate ath-

Cultural Considerations

Protein and the Vegetarian Athlete

Athletes may follow a vegetarian diet for a number of reasons, including religious beliefs such as Hinduism and Seventh Day Adventism. As with any dietary pattern, the individual's food preferences will dictate whether a vegetarian diet provides adequate nutrition for the athlete. Diets that are high in fiber from numerous plant-based foods can be also high volume and, therefore, filling, making it a challenge to consume sufficient calories to meet the demands of physical activity. Protein needs can be met with consumption of a variety of plant proteins, such as lentils, dried beans, nuts, seeds, and grains, but may fall short if personal preference or time factors limit intake. Athletes who travel may face particular meal-planning challenges. When assessing the adequacy of dietary protein in the vegetarian athlete, the nurse should first assess for adequacy of calorie intake, including any weight loss coinciding with an increase in physical activity. Protein sources and amounts should then be evaluated as outlined in Chapter 3. Daily protein needs for vegetarian athletes are 1.3 gm to 1.8 gm/kg body weight to account for intake of plant proteins that are less well digested. The vegetarian athlete can benefit from the same type of nutrition education as other athletes faced with the challenge of high-energy demands. Provided that adequate energy and a variety of vegetarian protein sources are consumed, a well-planned vegetarian diet can meet the nutritional demands of the athlete.

Sources: ADA, DC, & ACSM, 2009; Larson-Meyer, 2006; Tipton & Witard, 2007.

BOX 11-2	Protein Comparison: Supplements vs. Foods

Where can you find 20 gm of protein?

Canned tuna, 3 oz		Protein powder, 1–2 scoops
OR		OR
Chicken breast, 3 oz	**vs.**	Amino acid pills (many because only few milligrams/pill)
OR		

1 cup milk, 1 tbsp peanut butter, 2 slices toast

STOP
- Consuming whole foods provides a less expensive source of protein than from supplements. What other benefits to whole foods could the nurse reinforce with the athlete?

Source: U.S. Department of Agriculture Nutrient Data Lab. Retrieved March 25, 2009, from http://www.nal.usda.gov/fnic/foodcomp and manufacturer's labels

letes are warned against the use of protein supplements, which are a banned substance by the National Collegiate Athletic Association (NCAA) (NCAA, 2008). Box 11-3 outlines an example of suggested protein intake in a strength-trained athlete seeking to increase muscle mass.

Fat Recommendations

Fat is an important energy source, a vehicle for the absorption and delivery of fat-soluble vitamins to cells, central to regulation of core temperature and organ protection, and a substrate for synthesis of substances such as steroid hormones and vitamin D. The recommendation for fat intake of 20% to 35% of total calorie intake is based on the amount needed to provide essential fats while also reducing the effects of chronic disease associated with high-fat intake (IOM, 2002). The recommendation for fat intake does not differ between athletes and nonathletes.

Aerobic conditioning improves the efficiency of fat oxidation in endurance athletes. The result is that over time and with training, the proportion of fat used as energy during exercise increases while the proportion of carbohydrates decreases, sparing glycogen stores and prolonging time to exhaustion in this population (ADA, DC, & ACSM, 2009). For this reason, some athletes experiment with a fat-loading diet under the mistaken belief that endurance performance will be enhanced, which has not been shown to be true (Burke & Kiens, 2006). The nurse should discourage the practice of fat loading because it can worsen performance by jeopardizing needed glycogen stores owing to inadequate carbohydrate intake.

Some athletes overly restrict fat intake in an attempt to decrease body fat. This practice is popular among body builders. The result can be insufficient fat intake to support growth and development in the young athlete, deficiency of essential fats, and diminished production of reproductive hormones in males and females (Jonnalagadda, 2006). Lack of sufficient testos-

BOX 11-3   Protein Needs in the Athlete

Protein needs range from 0.8 gm/kg of body weight/day up to 1.7 gm/kg/day depending on an athlete's level of training. The following example outlines how protein needs can be met for Paul, a 70 kg (154 lb) wrestler trying to build muscle in the off-season with a regimen of strength training and intake of the upper limit of the protein recommendation.

- Protein calculation for strength training: 1.7 gm/kg × 70 kg/day = 119 gm of protein/day
- Sample protein intake (grams of protein in parenthesis):

Breakfast (23)

1 cup cereal (2)
1 cup milk, soy or cow's (8)
2 slices toast (5) with 1 tbsp peanut butter (8)

Lunch (38)

1 cup bean soup (10)
Sandwich w/ 2 slices of bread (5) and 2 oz cheese (15)
1 cup milk, soy or cow's (8)

Dinner (24)

2 soy vegetarian meatballs (11) on 1 cup pasta (7)
1 slice Italian bread (2)
½ cup cooked green peas (4)

Snacks (41)

1 cup yogurt (12)
3″ Bagel (6) with 2 tbsp hummus (8)
½ cup almonds (15)

Total protein: 126 gm

- How should the nurse respond to Paul when he asks about the need for a protein supplement to quicken muscle building? This meal plan may not contain adequate calories for an active adult. How will insufficient calorie intake affect Paul's muscle-building goal?

Source: Food values from the U.S. Department of Agriculture Nutrient Data Lab. Retrieved March 25, 2009, from http://www.nal.usda.gov/fnic/foodcomp

terone production has a negative effect on the maintenance of skeletal muscle, an outcome that is counterproductive to any athlete's efforts (Lambert, Frank & Evans, 2004).

Vitamins and Minerals

Vitamins and minerals have an essential role in the metabolic reactions that occur with physical activity and recovery from exercise. Metabolism of carbohydrate, protein, and fat relies on micronutrients for energy production. The transfer of oxygen to cells and the repair and building of tissue, such as bone and muscle, also require vitamins and minerals. The athlete needs to attend to both energy and micronutrient intake when optimizing diet and performance.

Whether the vitamin and mineral needs of an athlete are greater than that of an inactive individual is the subject of great debate and much research. Requirements for B-complex vitamins are increased proportionate to increased requirements for overall energy and can be met through a high-energy diet (ADA, DC, & ACSM, 2009). Antioxidant vitamins A, C, and E are marketed to athletes as an antidote to the stress incurred by muscles during exercise, but little evidence exists to support such claims (ADA, DC, & ACSM, 2009).

General nutrient supplementation is not recommended in the athlete unless intake is limited (Volpe, 2007). Low intakes of calcium and iron are reported in some athletes, especially females, with a resultant negative impact on exercise performance (ADA, DC, & ACSM, 2009). Restrictive eating and avoidance of certain foods, such as red meats or dairy foods, contributes to poor iron and calcium intake. Lengthy indoor training limits sun exposure, a vitamin D source, which in turn affects calcium absorption. The nurse should assess the vitamin D intake of athletes involved in indoor sports such as competitive skating or gymnastics and make recommendations for improvement when indicated. Calcium and vitamin D nutrition are discussed in detail in Chapters 5 and 6. Poor calcium status increases the risk of bone loss and stress fractures, especially in the athlete with existing menstrual dysfunction (Nattiv et al., 2007). Poor intake of iron is magnified when iron losses are increased. Up to 60% of female athletes have some level of iron depletion (Volpe, 2007). Iron deficiency directly affects sports performance because of impaired oxygen delivery to cells that in turn affects muscle function and work capacity (ADA, DC, & ACSM, 2009). Box 11-4 outlines considerations for the nurse when assessing iron status in the athlete.

Hydration: Fluid and Electrolytes

Physically active people need more fluid on a daily basis because of increased fluid losses (IOM, 2004). Activity that produces high fluid losses via sweating also causes loss of sodium and small amounts of potassium, iron, and calcium (ADA, DC, & ACSM, 2009). Some athletes can lose sodium in excess of 1 gm/L of sweat (Sawka et al., 2007). The nurse should emphasize the importance of balanced hydration on overall performance and health. Hydration with adequate fluid and electrolytes is essential for temperature regulation, maintenance of circulating blood volume, and tissue perfusion. Exercising muscles produce heat that needs to be dissipated to maintain core body temperature. Heat dissipation occurs through radiation and evaporation. Radiation brings heat to the surface of the skin where it can dissipate into the environment when ambient temperature is less than body temperature. Evaporation cools the body when sweat vaporizes into the environment, dissipating the heat along with it. The increase in fluid loss that occurs because of exercise drives the increased need for fluid. The focal point of adequate hydration in the

BOX 11-4	Iron and the Athlete

Risk factors for iron deficiency include poor intake, iron losses, or a combination of the two. The consequences of iron deficiency negatively affect sports performance. The nurse should consider all aspects of poor iron status when providing intervention to the athlete.

Iron intake or absorption diminishes because of

- Restrictive eating to maintain a given body weight or to lose weight
- Avoidance of good sources of iron, such as red meat and poultry
- Reliance on insufficient amounts of plant sources of iron, such as legumes, fortified grains, and dried fruit
- Inhibition of absorption with simultaneous intake of calcium supplements, coffee, tea, red wine, or high fiber

Iron losses increase with

- Menstrual loss
- Increased sweat loss
- Gastrointestinal bleeding with intense jarring activities (e.g., distance running)

- Red blood cell rupture with foot-strike activities (e.g., running)
- Loss of myoglobin in urine from muscle damage

Performance consequences of iron deficiency

- Decreased delivery of oxygen to tissues
- Decreased aerobic capacity
- Decreased endurance
- Altered thermoregulation

Nutrition advice

- Optimize intake of adequate amounts of animal and plant sources of iron (see Chapter 6).
- Optimize absorption of iron with simultaneous intake of vitamin C sources.
- Separate intake of iron sources by at least 1 hour from intake of calcium supplements, coffee, tea, red wine, and excessive fiber.
- Avoid iron supplementation unless medically indicated. Supplementation will not improve performance in those with adequate iron status and runs the risk of excess iron storage (hemochromatosis).

---

athlete is to begin any exercise in a hydrated state and replace fluid and electrolytes lost during exercise.

When fluid needs are not met, dehydration can occur. Increased sweating and insensible respiratory loss of fluid contribute significantly to risk of dehydration in the athlete. The nurse should be aware that exercising in certain environmental conditions alters fluid losses. High ambient temperature or humidity lessens the ability of the body to radiate or evaporate heat. As a result, sweat rate increases in an attempt to cool the body. Some athletes can lose up-

ward of 1.8 liters of sweat/hour under extreme heat and humid conditions (Sawka et al., 2007). Exercising in dry or cold air increases respiratory losses of fluid, which can go unnoticed by the athlete. Winter sport clothing that traps heat can increase fluid losses because sweat rate increases when there is a lack of evaporation to cool the body. Some athletes consume less fluid before winter exercise to avoid the inconvenience of using the bathroom when wearing heavy gear. Box 11-5 outlines risks, signs, and symptoms of dehydration.

BOX 11-5	Dehydration in the Athlete

Risk factors for dehydration

Increased fluid loss

- High ambient temperature
- High humidity
- Cold or dry air
- High altitude
- Heavy clothing or equipment
- Deliberately curtailing sweat evaporation—sauna, rubber shirt, plastic suit

Decreased fluid intake

- Deliberately restrict because of inconvenient bathroom access (winter gear, outdoor activity, not wanting to stop during endurance event)
- Deliberately restrict to lose weight for weight-class sport
- High altitude—poor appetite

- Difficulty carrying beverage—endurance events, cold weather
- No access to fluids
- Altered thirst with age

Symptoms of dehydration

Chills along with head/neck heat flush sensation

Dark urine

Dizziness

Fatigue

Headache

Irritability

Muscle cramping

Nausea

Thirst

Vomiting

Dehydration has many negative consequences for an athlete. Fluid loss of as little as 1% of body weight impairs heat dissipation and increases heart rate because of diminished plasma volume (von Duvillard, Braun, Markofski, Beneke, & Leithauser, 2004). Loss of 2% or more of body weight affects speed, reaction time, cognitive performance, and muscle coordination. Larger fluid losses put an athlete at risk for heat illness, including heat stroke (ADA, DC, & ACSM, 2009; Sawka et al., 2007).

Some athletes, especially those in weight-class sports such as rowing or wrestling, deliberately dehydrate themselves prior to an event in order to "make weight" for a precompetition weigh-in. This dangerous practice has been associated with a fatal outcome in athletes because of dehydration.

When excess water is consumed or when fluid and sodium intake does not sufficiently match sodium content of sweat loss, hyponatremia can develop. **Hyponatremia,** a blood sodium less than 135 mEq/L, leads to fluid shifts in the body in an attempt to overcome unequal electrolyte concentrations across cell membranes. Initial symptoms include bloating, headache, and swollen fingers. Pulmonary and cerebral edema occurs in severe cases and can lead to death. Novice endurance athletes, those who run slowly, sweat less, or are overvigilant about hydration are at risk for hyponatremia (Sawka et al., 2007). Drinking to maintain and not gain body weight during an event and eating a salty diet are recommended for avoidance of hyponatremia (Sawka et al., 2007). Client Education Checklist: Fluid and Sodium Recommendations further outlines recommendations for avoiding hyponatremia.

Muscle cramps that are associated with exercise can result from improper hydration and insufficient sodium and potassium replacement of sweat losses. Consuming a liberally salted diet rich in fresh fruits, vegetables, and whole grains should be adequate for most athletes. Those with high sweat rates may require an addition of up to 1/4 tsp of salt to 500 mL of sports beverages consumed surrounding exercise to compensate for sodium lost (Armstrong et al., 2007).

Fluid and Electrolyte Recommendations

No blanket recommendation for fluid or electrolyte intake exists for all exercising individuals. Instead daily fluid recommendations are based on calculations that customize fluid advice based on fluid losses during exercise. Replacement of sodium lost in sweat is less precise because of difficulty in determining exact loss. General sodium replacement guidelines are outlined in Client Education Checklist: Fluid and Sodium Recommendations. The nurse can assist the athlete in determining exercise-related fluid needs using the calculations outlined in Box 11-6.

Additional recommendations exist to guide the athlete in maintaining hydration before, during, and after exercise as outlined in Box 11-7. It is important to realize that the rate

of gastric emptying during exercise affects fluid absorption. Gastric emptying is maximized when gastric volume of fluid is kept between 500 and 1,000 mL. This fact underscores the need to drink to a schedule during prolonged exercise. High-carbohydrate concentrations (greater than 8%) slow gastric emptying, which is why sugary beverages are not recommended during exercise (ADA, DC, & ACSM, 2009). Dehydration diminishes gastric emptying, placing the athlete at risk for further dehydration. Athletes need to practice drinking to a schedule during training to avoid competition-day fluid imbalance. Using thirst alone to guide drinking is not considered a reliable tool. Assessment of fluid status and an outline of general fluid requirements for adults are discussed in detail in Chapter 7.

Who Needs a Sports Drink?

Sports drinks with catchy names and fluorescent colors are marketed to the general population as an everyday beverage. The nurse should be aware that not all exercising individuals need sports drinks. Sports beverages with a carbohydrate intake of 6% to 8% can be recommended to the athlete who exercises continually for longer than 1 hour (Sawka et al., 2007). The nurse can also recommend a sports beverage to athletes engaged in high-intensity stop-and-go sports that benefit from ready glucose to support anaerobic metabolism. Examples include strength training and field sports like soccer, lacrosse, or field hockey, in which athletes are constantly moving and at times sprinting. Beverages with a carbohydrate content above or below that range are not recommended during exercise because of negative effects that slow gastric emptying. The nurse can help the client apply this beverage guideline by teaching them to look for a drink with 14 to 19 gm of carbohydrate in an 8 oz portion. Diluting sports beverages for consumption during exercise is not advised. Diluting beverages intended for use during exercise will not provide a beneficial amount of carbohydrate replacement and can slow gastric emptying compared with the recommended concentration. High concentrations of carbohydrate in a beverage ingested during exercise slow gastric emptying and cause gastric distress in some. Athletes who have difficulty consuming adequate carbohydrate from food can benefit from high-carbohydrate beverages following exercise when gastric emptying is less of a concern and glycogen and fluid replacement are a priority. The nurse should advise other physically active people that a sports drink is simply providing calories without additional nutritional benefit.

Do Alcohol and Caffeine Affect Performance?

Some athletes use caffeine in an attempt to improve performance. Caffeine stimulates the central nervous system, acting as a potential ergogenic aid by altering alertness and

CLIENT EDUCATION CHECKLIST	Fluid and Sodium Recommendations

Intervention	Example
Review the importance of adequate fluid and sodium for sports performance.	Adequate hydration is needed for: • Core temperature regulation through evaporation of sweat • Preservation of plasma volume to deliver oxygen to exercising muscle • A medium for metabolic processes Adequate sodium is needed for: • Maintenance of fluid concentration in cells • Nerve conduction and muscle contraction
Teach the client to assess hydration status.	• Use urine color as indication of hydration with a goal of straw color urine. • Calculate fluid losses during exercise by measuring dry body weight before and after exercise. • Thirst is not a sensitive indicator of hydration status.
Teach the client to monitor for signs of altered fluid or sodium status.	Signs and symptoms of dehydration: • Irritability • Headache • Weakness • Muscle cramping • Dark urine • Thirst • Chills with head or neck heat flush • Nausea and vomiting Signs and symptoms of hyponatremia: • Swollen fingers, feet, or legs • Rapid weight gain and bloating • Confusion • Dizziness • Headache • Muscle cramping • Nausea • Wheezy breathing • Seizure
Calculate fluid needs.	• Weigh after voiding before and after exercise. • Replace weight loss with 1–1.5 oz of fluid for each 1 oz lost during exercise (for every 1 lb lost replace with 16–24 oz fluid). • Recalculate needs with changes in climate (heat, humidity, altitude).
Strategize with client how to "drink to a schedule."	• Begin exercise hydrated. • Distribute fluid requirements evenly over the duration of the exercise using calculated fluid needs. • 1 oz fluid = one adult-size "gulp." • Plan ahead for fluid availability. • Practice drinking recommended amounts during training and not just on competition date.

Educate the client about recommended beverage choices during exercise.	• Water alone suffices for exercise of less than 1 hour.
	• Sports beverages are beneficial for greater than 1 hour or stop-and-go sports with maximal effort.
	• Carbonated fluids linked with gastric discomfort during exercise.
	• Gastric emptying promoted by:
	  1. Cool beverages
	  2. Carbohydrate concentration of 4–8%
	  3. Topping off gastric fluid volume to keep it in the 600-ml range

Strategize with the client on how to consume recommended sodium.	Choose sports beverage with 300–700 mg/L of sodium. Following exercise of long duration, high sweat volume, high humidity or heat: • Add salt to foods to offset sodium lost in sweat. • Consume salty foods such as salted snacks, convenience soup, pickles, cheese, commercial vegetable juices.

BOX 11-6	Fluid Calculations for Athletes

Exercise-related fluid recommendations are determined based on fluid losses during exercise. A post-void weight is recorded just before and after exercise. Weight lost during exercise is from fluid and warrants replacement at a rate of 100–150% of loss. The following outlines the necessary calculations:

1. Obtain "dry" weight (after voiding) immediately before exercise.
2. Obtain "dry" weight (after voiding without wet clothing) immediately following exercise.
3. Calculate weight lost during exercise.
4. Match replacement fluid at a rate of 1–1.5 oz per 1 oz of weight lost (1 lb = 16 oz weight lost = 16 oz fluid weight lost).
5. Try to consume increased fluid during next exercise session to better approximate losses. Make a drinking schedule to spread the needed volume over time. Recalculate fluid needs with changes in climate (humidity, altitude, temperature).

Example: Michael is training in the winter for a warm-weather marathon in spring and experiencing symptoms of dehydration after his longer runs.

1. Dry weight before long run: 200 lb
2. Dry weight after long run: 197 lb
3. Weight lost during long run: 3 lb (48 oz)
4. Fluid required to match losses: 48 oz $\times$ 1–1.5 oz fluid/oz weight lost = 48–72 oz fluid (6–9 cups)
5. The nurse advises Michael that he needs 48–72 oz of fluid to replace his sweat losses and that he should make a drinking schedule for his next long run to ensure that he consumes this additional fluid during exercise with the goal of maintaining hydration. An option is to aim for 48 oz (1-1/2 quarts) over a 2-hour run at a rate of 6 oz every 15 minutes. Michael is also advised to recalculate his sweat losses when he begins training in hotter and humid weather.

- When offering these recommendations, it is important to be sure that Michael begins his run hydrated. What easy way can Michael use to assess his own hydration?

BOX 11-7	Fluid Recommendations for Athletes

Fluid before exercise:

Start exercise already well hydrated.

- Hydrate well over the day before training.
- Drink 400–600 mL (up to 20 oz) of fluid 2–3 hours before exercise.
- Make sure urine color is light and not dark.

Fluid during exercise:

Top off fluid at regular intervals to promote ongoing gastric emptying and hydration.

- Drink 150–350 mL (6–12 oz) fluid every 15–20 minutes during exercise. Plan ahead and carry fluid or know where fluid is readily available during exercise.
- One adult-sized "gulp" is 1 oz of fluid.
- Choose water if exercise is less than 1 hour in duration or a drink with 4–8% carbohydrate content for longer durations. Avoid high-carbohydrate concentrations because they slow gastric emptying.

- Fluids containing sodium in a concentration of 0.5–0.7 gm/L replace sodium loss from sweat and promote thirst.
- Do not drink enough to cause weight gain during exercise.
- Practice drinking to a schedule during training before competition occurs.
- Do not rely on thirst as an indicator of hydration during exercise.

Fluid after exercise:

Calculate personal fluid deficit as outlined in Box 11-6.

- Consume sufficient fluid to match or slightly exceed fluid losses.
- If weight gain occurs during exercise, drink less fluid during the next session.
- Include sodium in fluid or consume salty foods to replace sodium lost in sweat.

Sources: Adapted from ADA, DC, & ACSM, 2009; American Medical Athletic Association (AMAA), 2005; NATA, 2000; Sawka et al., 2007.

neurocognitive performance (Deldicque & Francaux, 2008). **Ergogenic aids** are substances that increase work performance. It is also theorized that caffeine in high amounts beneficially increases fat oxidation, therefore sparing glycogen in endurance training (ADA, DC, & ACSM, 2009). Caffeine doses in the range of 5 to 6 mg/kg of body weight are amounts used by athletes seeking this effect. This level of intake amounts to 500 to 600 mg of caffeine intake by the 100 kg (220 lb) athlete. Caffeine pills or high-caffeine beverages are used by athletes to achieve this intake. Potential side effects result from the stimulatory effects of the drug. Insomnia, irritability, rapid heart rate, anxiety, and fluid loss have been documented, all with the potential to negatively affect athletic performance (Tunnicliffe, Erdman, Reimer, Lun, & Shearer, 2008). High-caffeine use is limited by the NCAA because of the stimulant effects. Athletes are tested for excessive use and cannot exceed 15 mcg/L of urine (Keisler & Armsey, 2006). When asked about the use of caffeine in sports, the nurse should point out that the negative side effects could outweigh any benefit to the athlete. Athletes who choose to use caffeine for ergogenic purposes should be advised to avoid trying this tactic for the first time on the day of competition and that there is no demonstrated benefit to intake higher than 5 to 6 mg/kg of body weight. This research is discussed in the Evidence-Based Practice Box: What is the evidence of caffeine extending endurance in athletes?

Alcohol negatively affects sports performance for a variety of reasons, both direct and indirect. Alcohol acts directly as a central nervous system depressant and is directly linked to the rate of injuries in sporting events (El-Sayed, Ali, & El-Sayed, 2005). Indirectly, alcohol in the diet has been shown to replace needed carbohydrate, impeding recovery from intense exercise. Alcohol has also been reported to decrease glucose uptake by exercising muscle and potentially impede glycogen repletion after exercise (El-Sayed et al., 2005). Rapid rehydration efforts following exercise can be hampered by alcohol because of its transient diuretic effect (IOM, 2004; Sawka et el., 2007).

Nutrition Considerations for Younger and Older Athletes

Adequate nutrition is crucial in the young athlete who must meet needs for growth and development as well as training. Overall calories, iron, and calcium intake remain

---

EVIDENCE-BASED PRACTICE RESEARCH BOX

What is the evidence for caffeine extending endurance in athletes?

Clinical Problem: Caffeine is a widely available stimulant, but questions exist among athletes about its value in endurance sports.

Research Findings: Caffeine is a generally mild stimulant that causes physiological and psychological changes in the body. It is considered the most commonly ingested drug in the world and has gained wide acceptance as an ergogenic aid (Paluska, 2003), being widely available in drinks, gels, and diet aids. Questions linger about its efficacy in various types of endurance versus short-burst activities.

One study analyzed the effect of caffeine ingestion on performance during lab-simulated 100-km cycling time trials. Eight highly trained cyclists were given either a placebo or 6 mg/kg of caffeinated drinks. In three separate events, there was no significant difference in endurance between the groups, although the subjects who received the caffeinated drinks had a higher heart rate (Hunter, St. Clair-Gibson, Collins, Lambert, & Noakes, 2002).

A recent study of ironman triathletes found that caffeinated products were used by 89% of the athletes prior to or during the competition. A self-report survey of the athletes indicated they used coffee, energy drinks, gels, and tablets as the source of caffeine. Blood analysis of 50 athletes after the event showed plasma concentrations of 3 mg/kg or more (Desbrow & Leveritt, 2006). However, the researchers did not correlate the presence of caffeine to fin-

ish time, limiting the usefulness of the data for athletes contemplating using caffeine for improving endurance.

Recent studies in simulated settings with highly trained cyclists examined the effects of caffeine on power output (Doherty, Smith, Hughes, & Davison, 2004) and performance time (Wiles, Coleman, Tegerdine, & Swaine, 2006). Subjects who ingested 5 mg/kg of caffeine were compared with subjects who received placebos. In both groups the high-intensity, short-burst power output, speed, and performance time were significantly higher in the test subjects than the control groups.

Nursing Implications: Health care providers should be aware that caffeine is widely believed to be an inexpensive means to gain an edge in competition or to enhance one's personal performance. Studies of highly trained athletes provide support for its ability to increase performance, enhance endurance, and reduce fatigue only for short-duration and high-intensity exercise without risk of dehydration. Athletes who compete in sports under the auspices of the NCAA should be aware of guidelines for the use of substances containing caffeine.

CRITICAL THINKING QUESTIONS:

1. How should the nurse respond to the high school athlete who really wants to improve endurance and time in a 400-meter freestyle event?

2. What response would the nurse give to the middle-age female who jogs 5–7 miles 4 days a week and wants to know if the caffeinated sports drinks will help improve her time for the run she has entered in 2 weeks?

concerns, as with the adult athlete. Insufficient intake of energy and nutrients can delay the onset of puberty, increase risk of injury, slow recovery, and impair bone mineral density (Petrie, Stover, & Horswill, 2004). Female athletes and athletes participating in weight-class sports are particularly vulnerable to this effect when utilizing energy restriction to make weight. The nurse can assist the young athlete with optimizing intake by exploring any reasons for insufficient intake and strategizing ideas for improvement. A hectic pace and lack of time can contribute to poor intake if planning ahead for the day's food is left to chance. The nurse can make suggestions for well-balanced snacks and meals for the child or adolescent who spends most waking hours in school or at athletic practice. Juices, fruit, iron-fortified cereals, trail mix with dried fruit, yogurt, cheese sticks, crackers, and peanut butter are examples of snack options.

The nurse should also be mindful of hydration status in the exercising child or adolescent. Children may be at greater risk of dehydration during exercise than adults, especially in high heat or humidity, because of the following:

- Greater body surface area relative to body mass that results in greater heat gain or loss
- Higher relative heat production from exercise
- Decreased sweating capacity that results in less heat dissipation
  (American Academy of Pediatrics [AAP], 2000; Rowland, 2008)

In addition to limiting exercise time and intensity during extreme conditions, the AAP recommends enforced intake of water or a sports-type beverage every 20 minutes during exercise even if a child does not feel thirsty (AAP, 2000).

Athletic older individuals have the same nutritional needs as the younger adult athlete who is training at the same intensity and volume (Tarnopolsky, 2008). Conversely, older athletes who are beginning a training program or have lessened training volume require less energy than younger counterparts because of potential age-associated loss of muscle mass, which results in lower metabolic rate (Campbell & Geik, 2004). The nurse can assist the older client in assessing dietary adequacy by monitoring body weight and overall nutrient intake. Hydration needs in the older athlete are the same as the younger athlete (Tarnopolsky, 2008). However, age-associated changes in fluid balance mechanics can predispose the older athlete to dehydration. Altered thirst and changes in hormonal feedback mechanisms and kidney function can impede adequate hydration if left to thirst alone (Campbell & Geik, 2004). The nurse can advise the older athlete to drink to a schedule during training after determining fluid needs as outlined in Box 11-6.

What Sports Supplements Work and Which Are Safe?

Competitive athletes strive to improve performance and some consider the use of dietary supplements as a route to achieving that goal. Although such supplements have been popular with adult athletes for decades, use by young athletes is becoming increasingly popular (Calfee & Fadale, 2006). Purported performance-enhancing supplements make up a multimillion-dollar industry that capitalizes on athletes' quest to excel. The most common reasons cited for taking supplements includes maintenance of strength, avoidance of illness or injury, and improved endurance (Petroczi et al., 2008).

The Food and Drug Administration (FDA) regulates dietary supplements, including vitamins, minerals, botanicals, and sports supplements, as foods despite the fact that many have medicinal-like effects. Product labels for dietary supplements are permitted to make claims about the effect of the product on any bodily function or structure, so long as no claims are made regarding disease prevention or cure. Thus, supplements targeted at the athlete are permitted to make claims about athletic or physical performance, but not about treating an injury or condition. First and foremost, the nurse should advise the athlete that such supplements do not undergo any premarket approval process by the FDA, nor is there mandated product testing required assuring that the claims made are valid. Issues such as impurities, contamination, lack of active ingredients, and doping with pharmaceutical products have been reported in dietary supplements as outlined in Chapter 25. The result for a competitive athlete could be inadvertent intake of a banned substance and disqualification from competition. Before considering any dietary supplement use, the nurse can help the athlete scrutinize the product as outlined in Box 11-8.

Popular supplements used by athletes generally are marketed to increase energy, build muscle, or decrease body fat. Long-term research is lacking on most supplements and many clinical studies are carried out with only a small number of participants, making generalization to all athletes difficult. Little to no research exists on the effects of these supplements on young athletes, which should not be mistaken for an indication of product safety. Table 11-2 outlines examples of popular dietary supplements used by athletes and nursing recommendations. Further information on dietary supplements is outlined in Chapter 25.

Carbohydrate gels and energy bars are marketed to athletes and nonathletes as dietary supplements, snacks, and meal replacements. The advent of new products is never ending and driven by the financial success of this industry. Hot Topic: Carbohydrate Gels and Energy Bars discusses these products and nursing recommendations.

BOX 11-8	Evaluating Sports Supplements

Large-scale clinical research on sports supplements is scarce, which makes it difficult to offer evidence-based advice to clients who ask about use of sports supplements. The nurse should teach the client to consider the following points when contemplating supplement use:

What is the evidence?

- *Are there any clinical, published studies done on the product? If so, what was the study population?*
- *Is the "evidence" only in the form of anecdotal comments?*
- *Does the product advertisement tout a "new breakthrough," secret or ancient formula, or miracle, no-work solution?*

Good evidence is derived from larger studies on diverse populations. Research on six elite cyclists using a supplement for a week does not constitute research that the nurse should apply to a college-age wrestler looking to take a supplement for months on end! Research on adults cannot be generalized to children and pregnant or lactating females. Beware of marketing strategies like anecdotes and catchy scientific-sounding words parading as evidence.

What is the marketing claim?

- *Are the claims reasonable or too good to be true?*
- *Is the term "natural" touted to hint that the product is safe?*

Claims that are too good to be true generally are just that! Any supplement promising a quick-fix, no-work solution is suspect of this type of claim. Improvements in sports performance happen with training, rest, and good nutrition. The term "natural" on any supplement carries no promise of safety or efficacy. Arsenic is "natural" but also a poison! Prohormone supplements are "natural" precursors to steroids but do not improve performance and have negative side effects.

Who is manufacturing and promoting the product?

- *Is the product being promoted by a celebrity?*
- *Is the manufacturer a well-known company or a small unknown?*

As a rule, larger and well-known companies, especially those that also manufacture medications, have a reputation to uphold and have the funds to conduct research and quality assurance control compared with a fly-by-night manufacturer. Clients can check the Food and Drug Administration and the Federal Trade Commission Web sites for any negative information on a manufacturer. Celebrity endorsement of any supplement does not constitute the effectiveness or safety of any product. Products with a USP code (*United States Pharmacopoeia*) have been voluntarily tested to ensure potency and purity, but this code should not be interpreted to also mean that the product is safe or lives up to its claims; it just means that what the manufacturer says is in the product actually is!

What are the short-term effects of use?

- *Is the supplement banned by a sports governing body?*
- *Are there side effects to the product?*
- *Will the supplement interact with medications?*

Little is known about the side effects of most supplements. Even less is known about the effects on children and pregnant or lactating females. The potential for interaction with both over-the-counter and prescription medications should be investigated before use. The nurse should assess the use of any dietary supplements before surgery in any client because some supplements negatively affect blood clotting and anesthesia. Competitive athletes at the college, professional, or elite level need to be familiar with which supplements are banned by sports governing bodies and adhere to policy. The banning or limiting of any supplement should be a red flag to all athletes.

What are the long-term effects of use?

- *Is there any information on long-term use?*
- *Are there any long-term side effects?*

Often what research that does exist on a supplement is of a short duration and long-term effects are not known. For that reason, it is not recommended that children and pregnant or lactating females use dietary supplements other than recommended vitamins and minerals. Lack of negative reports on a supplement does not imply that the product is indeed safe; it can simply mean that there has been no research.

Would improving diet quality yield the same effect promised for supplement use?

- *Is the client looking to build muscle or have more energy?*
- *Does a diet history reveal that there is room for nutritional improvements?*

Building muscle and having more energy are common goals of an athlete. Adequate calories, carbohydrate, and protein in the diet are essential to accomplish these goals. Consuming expensive supplements does not compensate for a poor diet.

Table 11-2 Dietary Supplements Used by Athletes

Dietary Supplement	Marketing Claim	Nursing Recommendation
Ergogenic		
Bee pollen	↑ Energy and stamina	No scientific evidence to support use. Caution avoidance in clients with bee sting allergy.
Branched chain amino acids—isoleucine, leucine, valine	Exercise-induced fatigue	Research inconclusive on whether these amino acids affect central nervous system perception of fatigue. Supplements not shown to delay fatigue.
Ginseng and Siberian ginseng	↑ Energy and stamina	No scientific evidence to support use. Caution clients about potential alteration in blood clotting.
Stimulants • Caffeine • Ephedra • Guarana • Synephrine (bitter orange, citrus aurantium)	Improved performance by stimulating muscle fibers and central nervous system	All products in this category are limited or banned by many sport governing organizations. Controlled caffeine dose can improve performance but risk of central nervous system stimulation negatively affecting performance exists. Ephedra associated with dizziness, risk of stroke, heart attack, and death and thus removed from the market. Replaced by synephrine in products, which may have similar profile. Guarana has two times the caffeine of coffee.
Muscle Building		
Creatine	Provides energy substrate for muscle-building activity	Naturally found in diet from meat and poultry. Used by contracting muscle as energy substrate during anaerobic activity, allowing maximal effort that in turn could build muscle. No benefit found in aerobic activity. Athletes regularly consuming food with creatine sources may find no added benefit to supplementation. Side effects include bloating and intramuscular water weight gain, dehydration, muscle cramping, gastrointestinal complaints. No information on long-term effects. Not recommended in athletes less than 18 years.
Amino acids	Provide building blocks of protein for muscle development or recovery	No more effective than food proteins, which already contain amino acids. Glutamine, a nonessential amino acid in healthy people, researched with mixed results for its effect on immunity and carbohydrate sparing.
Prohormones (steroid precursors) • "Andro" (Androstenedione) • Dehydroepiandrosterone (DHEA)	Metabolic precursors to testosterone for "natural" elevation of testosterone and muscle building	Androstenedione now considered a controlled substance, requiring a prescription. DHEA formerly required a prescription. No scientific evidence of ↑ athletic performance. Negative side effects of ↓ HDL cholesterol and ↑ estradiol (estrogen precursor).
β-hydroxy β-methylbutyrate (HMB)	↓ Muscle breakdown from exercise	Metabolite of leucine, an amino acid. Mixed results from clinical studies. No long-term safety data available.
Fat Cutting		
Stimulants	"Fat burner"	See Ergogenics. No evidence that stimulants alone burn fat. Caffeine potentiates the effects of ephedra.
Chromium	Improves carbohydrate metabolism	Essential mineral found in beef, poultry, eggs, whole grains. No evidence to support its use for fat loss. Excessive intake can lead to excess stores.

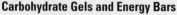

hot Topic

Carbohydrate Gels and Energy Bars

Carbohydrate gels and energy bars are increasing in popularity among athletes, driving up the variety of products in these categories as large and small companies try for a market share in this profitable line of business. In particular, energy bars are widely marketed to both athletes and the general public as a snack or meal replacement. What place do these products have in the diet, if any?

Energy bars are:

- Calorie sources—"energy" on a food label denotes the presence of calories, not the ability of the product to give you instant "energy."
- Available with varying amounts of calories, carbohydrate, protein, and fat. Some are low carbohydrate. Some are the nutritional equivalent of a candy bar.
- Convenient, portable snacks when carrying whole foods is not feasible.
- A before-competition carbohydrate for the athlete who cannot tolerate whole foods close to the event time.
- Carbohydrate sources for the athlete competing in endurance events, such as a triathlon, or multievents, such as track and field or gymnastics, when whole foods are difficult to carry or may not be tolerated well.
- Postexercise sources of carbohydrate for the athlete needing to replace glycogen.
- Overused. Whole foods can be substituted in many cases where energy bars are used. A mini-bagel or juice and crackers are substitutes for standard bars.
- Expensive sources of nutrition compared with whole foods.

Energy bars are not:

- Recommended if they are low in carbohydrate. Low-carbohydrate versions defeat the purpose of supplying a convenient source of this needed nutrient.
- Needed by people who do not expend many calories with physical activity.

- Everyday snacks or meal replacement foods.
- A substitute for whole foods or a balanced diet.

The nurse can help a client evaluate the usefulness of energy bars in the overall diet, while discouraging the habitual replacement of whole foods by these products.

Carbohydrate gels are:

- A concentrated source of carbohydrate in semisolid form, usually containing 25 gm of carbohydrate per portion.
- Made with different types of carbohydrate, such as maltodextrin and fructose. More recently, honey and certain brands of jelly beans are being marketed to compete with gels.
- Used by athletes as a portable carbohydrate source during all day or endurance events, such as a marathon.
- A quick source of needed carbohydrate to replenish glycogen after exercise in the athlete who has no tolerance for food or is not hungry after grueling exercise.
- Best used during an event only after practicing use during training. Some individuals do not tolerate this concentrated source of carbohydrate or are adverse to the texture.
- Expensive compared to other carbohydrate sources.
- A personal preference rather than a product that offers a competitive edge compared with other quick carbohydrate sources.

Carbohydrate gels are not:

- A substitute for sports beverages containing carbohydrate because most lack electrolytes and fluid replacement is still needed. Athletes using carbohydrate gels must be conscientious about hydration along with carbohydrate needs.
- Superior to other carbohydrate sources such as sports beverages, honey, or candy marketed to athletes.

The nurse can help the athlete evaluate whether a carbohydrate gel would be an effective source of carbohydrate in the training regimen while ensuring that hydration needs are not overlooked.

NURSING CARE PLAN   Inadequate Carbohydrate Intake for Exercise

CASE STUDY

Peter, 43, is a self-described "weekend warrior." He works as an accountant for a large company. He typically works 8- to 10-hour days, skipping breakfast and eating just a sandwich from home at his desk for lunch. When he gets home, he helps his wife prepare dinner and has been reducing his intake of potato and other starches to try to lose a few pounds. In nice weather, he and his wife take a quick walk to talk over the events of the day and to have a little quiet time. Peter reports that on weekends he makes up for all he could not do during the week; he goes to the gym to lift weights and uses the treadmill both days, he plays at least one round of golf, and he takes care of the house repairs and yard work. Lately he has noticed that he cannot keep up the pace on the treadmill or do the usual number of reps with the weights and that he is worn out by the time the yard work is done. He has come to the clinic for a check and specifically wants to know if there are any natural supplements he could take to increase his strength and stamina.

Applying the Nursing Process

ASSESSMENT

Peter is 5 feet 10 inches (178 cm) tall and weighs 180 pounds (82 kg) with a BMI of 26. Vital signs are T 98.9, P 78, R 18; BP 128/88. He is pleasant and states that he has no health concerns beyond not having the stamina he used to have. He admits to "not having the greatest diet" but states that he always takes his lunch to work and the family rarely eats out. He says he has to get more energy soon or he is afraid he will turn into a "couch potato" like his overweight father. Lately, he has reduced his intake of carbohydrates based on a neighbor's advice about how to lose weight.

DIAGNOSES

Deficient knowledge related to questions about use of supplements and avoiding carbohydrates

Readiness for enhanced nutrition

Anxiety related to concern about consequences of not exercising

EXPECTED OUTCOMES

Peter will develop a plan for energy expenditure realistic for age and nutrient intake

Identify facts and myths about both carbohydrates and supplements that are marketed to enhance strength

Develop a plan for nutrient intake that uses the principles of the U.S. Dietary Guidelines and MyPyramid

INTERVENTIONS

Do a 24-hour food recall

Review lab data for iron deficiency

Suggest options for spreading exercise and activity throughout the week to maximize the benefits of those activities

Develop an individualized MyPyramid plan that is acceptable to Peter and his family and that contains adequate carbohydrate sources

Discuss the role of supplements in enhancing physical fitness

EVALUATION

After 6 weeks Peter reports feeling more rested and increased stamina. The family has agreed to eat dinner later one evening a week so Peter can go the gym for an hour. The children have enjoyed using the computer to see how foods that the family eats affect the pyramid and they have begun to plan weekly grocery lists. Peter tries to take a 15-minute walk at lunch with a colleague and finds he enjoys the socialization and has more energy to tackle work. He has improved his carbohydrate intake with cereal and milk for breakfast and fruit along with his lunch. At dinner, he has a baked potato or a serving of rice or pasta. He sometimes buys skim milk from the vending machine, but otherwise he drinks water. Peter was surprised to find that he lost 2 pounds by increasing his activity during the week and eating more balanced intake. He reviewed the educational information and prices for supplements and decided that he would concentrate on eating more balanced meals and getting more regular exercise to improve strength and endurance instead of considering supplements. His hemoglobin was 15.1 so no interventions were indicated. Figure 11-1 ■ outlines the nursing process for this case.

Critical Thinking in the Nursing Process

1. **How can the nurse incorporate MyPyramid as part of diet teaching with clients and families?**

(continued)

Inadequate Carbohydrate Intake for Exercise *(continued)*

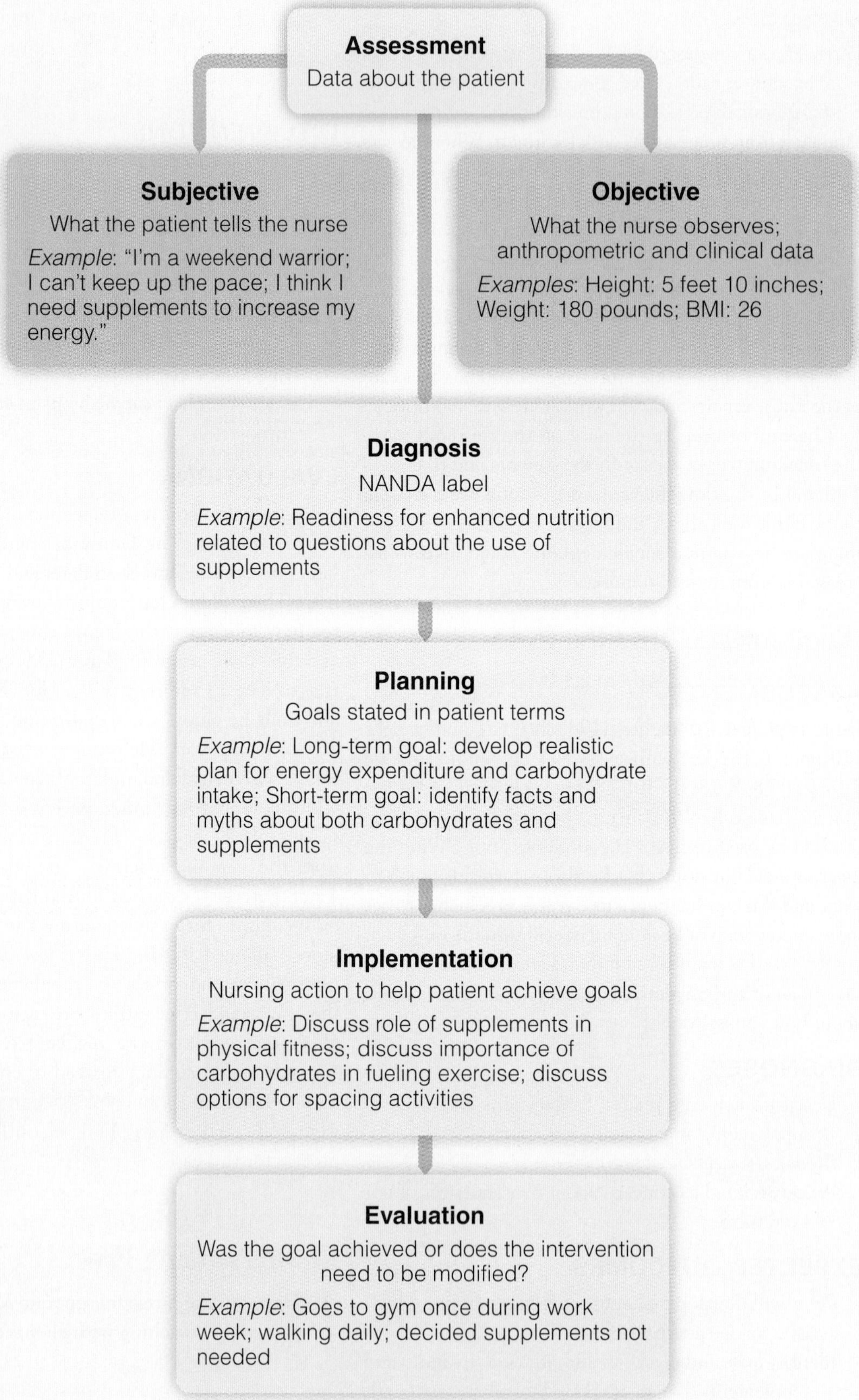

Assessment
Data about the patient

Subjective
What the patient tells the nurse

Example: "I'm a weekend warrior; I can't keep up the pace; I think I need supplements to increase my energy."

Objective
What the nurse observes; anthropometric and clinical data

Examples: Height: 5 feet 10 inches; Weight: 180 pounds; BMI: 26

Diagnosis
NANDA label

Example: Readiness for enhanced nutrition related to questions about the use of supplements

Planning
Goals stated in patient terms

Example: Long-term goal: develop realistic plan for energy expenditure and carbohydrate intake; Short-term goal: identify facts and myths about both carbohydrates and supplements

Implementation
Nursing action to help patient achieve goals

Example: Discuss role of supplements in physical fitness; discuss importance of carbohydrates in fueling exercise; discuss options for spacing activities

Evaluation
Was the goal achieved or does the intervention need to be modified?

Example: Goes to gym once during work week; walking daily; decided supplements not needed

■ FIGURE 11-1 **Nursing Care Plan Process: Inadequate Carbohydrate Intake for Exercise.**

CHAPTER SUMMARY

- Nutrition plays a central role in training and recovery from athletic activity.

- Carbohydrate is a preferred fuel source for anaerobic and aerobic activity. The nurse can educate the client about types and timing of carbohydrate ingestion for training.

- Intake of sufficient calories is a priority when fueling exercise, repleting glycogen stores after exercise and building muscle.

- Female athletes who fail to meet fuel requirements are at risk for development of the female athlete triad of disordered eating, amenorrhea, and osteoporosis.

- Athletes competing in weight-class sports should receive nutrition education on healthy weight management.

- Muscle building requires additional protein in the diet along with adequate calorie intake.

- Vitamin and mineral requirements for exercise can be met through the diet. Iron and calcium intake can be low in female athletes and those in weight-class sports.

- Hydration with adequate fluid and sodium intake is essential for sport performance and overall health. The nurse should strategize with the client on how to stay well hydrated.

- The nurse should assess nutrition and hydration practices of physically active children and older adults to ensure that needs are met.

- Dietary supplements marketed to the athlete are popular, but many lack scientific evidence on safety or efficacy.

EXPLORE **PEARSON mynursingkit**™

MyNursingKit is your one stop for online chapter review materials and resources. Prepare for success with additional NCLEX®-style practice questions, interactive assignments and activities, web links, animations and videos, and more!

Register your access code from the front of your book at
www.mynursingkit.com.

NCLEX® QUESTIONS

1. The nurse has been working with an adolescent soccer player who wants to use foods with a high-glycemic index after matches during weekend tournaments. The nurse knows teaching has been successful when which of the following foods is selected by the young person?
   1. Milk
   2. Plain bagel
   3. Dried apples
   4. Guacamole

2. A 150-pound (70 kg) athlete beginning a strict training program told the nurse that protein consumption of 105 grams/day was part of the regimen. The nurse should respond that:
   1. It would be more appropriate to decrease carbohydrate consumption.
   2. The addition of creatine supplements will enable the protein to be metabolized more efficiently.
   3. This amount of protein should be sufficient to meet training needs.
   4. It is more important to minimize fat consumption.

3. The nurse is teaching a group of adolescents about diet and exercise. A member of the swim team asks the nurse if creatine is safe for high school athletes who want to build up muscles. The nurse should respond that:
   1. Creatine is not recommended for teenage athletes.
   2. Creatine should only be taken with a physician's supervision.
   3. It has no proven benefits so it should be avoided.
   4. The side effects are not well tolerated by teens.

4. Which of the following statements given by a 17-year-old gymnast would the nurse feel warrants further investigation?
   1. She always drinks a full bottle of water during meets.
   2. She takes an occasional vitamin and mineral supplement.
   3. She has not had a menstrual period in 2 months.
   4. She is tired after practice.

5. An athlete asks the nurse about following a high-carbohydrate diet. The nurse should explain that such diets are:
   1. Beneficial for the athlete who engages in prolonged continuous exercise on a regular basis
   2. Beneficial only if the carbohydrates are composed of simple sugars
   3. Necessary before any planned exercise
   4. Useful only for highly trained athletes

REFERENCES

American Academy of Pediatrics (AAP), Committee on Sports Medicine and Fitness. (2000). Climactic heat stress and the exercising child and adolescent. *Pediatrics, 106,* 158–159.

American Academy of Pediatrics (AAP), Committee on Sports Medicine and Fitness. (2005). Promotion of healthy weight-control practices in athletes. *Pediatrics, 116,* 1557–1564.

American Dietetic Association (ADA), Dietitians of Canada (DC), and American College of Sports Medicine (ACSM). (2009). Position of the American Dietetic Association, Dietitians of Canada, and the American College or Sports Medicine: Nutrition and athletic performance. *Journal of the American Dietetic Association, 109,* 509–527.

American Medical Athletic Association. (2005). *The right way to hydrate for marathons.* Retrieved March 23, 2009, from http://www.aamasports.med.org

Armstrong, L. E., Casa, D. J., Millard-Stafford, M., Moran, D. S., Pyne, S. W., & Roberts, W. O. (2007). American College of Sports Medicine position stand: Exertional heat illness during training and competition. *Medicine & Science in Sports and Exercise, 39,* 556–572.

Bonci, C. M., Bonci, L. J., Granger, L. R., Johnson, C. L., Malina, R. M., Milne, L. W., et al. (2008). National Association of Athletic Trainers position: Preventing, detecting, and managing disordered eating in athletes. *Journal of Athletic Training, 43,* 80–108.

Burke, L. M., & Kiens, B. (2006). "Fat adaptation" for athletic performance—the nail in the coffin? *Journal of Applied Physiology, 100,* 7–8.

Calfee, R., & Fadale, P. (2006). Popular ergogenic drugs and supplements in young athletes. *Pediatrics, 117,* e577–e589.

Campbell, W. W., & Geik, R. A. (2004). Nutritional considerations for the older athlete. *Nutrition, 20,* 603–608.

Centers for Disease Control and Prevention (CDC). (1998). Hyperthermia and dehydration-related deaths associated with intentional rapid weight loss in three collegiate wrestlers. *Morbidity and Mortality Weekly Review, 47,* 105–108.

Coleman, E. (2006). Carbohydrate and exercise. In M. Dunford (Ed.), *Sports nutrition: A practice manual for professionals* (4th ed.). Chicago: American Dietetic Association.

Deldicque, L., & Francaux, M. (2008). Functional food for exercise: Fact or foe? *Current Opinion in Clinical Nutrition and Metabolic Care, 11,* 774–781.

Desbrow, B., & Leveritt, M. (2006). Awareness and use of caffeine by athletes competing at the 2005 Ironman Triathlon World Championships. *International Journal of Sport Nutrition and Exercise Metabolism, 16,* 545–558.

Doherty, M., Smith, P., Hughes, M., & Davison, R. (2004). Caffeine lowers perceptual response and increases power output during high-intensity cycling. *Journal of Sports Sciences, 22,* 637–643.

El-Sayed, M. S., Ali, N., & El-Sayed, A. Z. (2005). Interaction between alcohol and exercise: Physiological and hematological implications. *Sports Medicine, 35,* 257–269.

Hunter, A. M., St. Clair-Gibson, A., Collins, M., Lambert, M., & Noakes, T. D. (2002). Caffeine ingestion does not alter performance during a 100-km cycling time-trial performance. *International Journal of Sport Nutrition and Exercise Metabolism, 12,* 438–452.

Institute of Medicine (IOM), Food and Nutrition Board. (2002). *Dietary reference intakes for energy, carbohydrate, fiber, fat, fatty acids, cholesterol, protein and amino acids (macronutrients).* Washington, DC: National Academies Press.

Institute of Medicine (IOM), Food and Nutrition Board. (2004). *Dietary reference intakes for water, potassium, sodium, chloride, and sulfate.* Washington, DC: National Academies Press.

Jeukendrup, A. (2007). *Carbohydrate supplementation during exercise: Does it help? How much is too much?* Retrieved March 23, 2009, from http://www.gssiweb.com/Article_Detail.aspx?articleid=757

Jonnalagadda, S. S. (2006). Dietary fat and exercise. In M. Dunford (Ed.), *Sports nutrition: A practice manual for professionals* (4th ed.). Chicago: American Dietetic Association.

Keisler, B. D., & Armsey, T. D. (2006). Caffeine as an ergogenic aid. *Current Sports Medicine Reports, 5,* 215–219.

Kersick, C., Harvey, T., Stout, J., Campbell, B., Wilborn, C., Kreider, R., et al. (2008). International Society of Sports Nutrition position stand: Nutrient timing. *Journal of the International Society of Sports Nutrition, 5,* 17.

Lambert, C. P., Frank, L. L., & Evans, W. J. (2004). Macronutrient considerations for the sport of bodybuilding. *Sports Medicine, 34,* 317–327.

Larson-Meyer, D. E. (2006). Vegetarian athletes. In M. Dunford (Ed.), *Sports nutrition: A practice manual for professionals* (4th ed.). Chicago: American Dietetic Association.

Loucks, A. B. (2007). Energy availability and fertility. *Current Opinion in Endocrinology, Diabetes & Obesity, 14,* 470–474.

National Athletic Trainers' Association (NATA). (2000). Position statement: Fluid replacement for athletes. *Journal of Athletic Training, 35,* 212–224.

National Collegiate Athletic Association (NCAA). (2008). *NCAA sports medicine handbook 2008–2009.* Retrieved March 23, 2009, from http://www.ncaa.org/wps/ncaa?ContentID=1446

National Collegiate Athletic Association (NCAA). (n.d.). *Coaches' handbook: Managing the female athlete triad.* Retrieved March 23, 2009, from http://www.ncaa.org/wps/ncaa?ContentID=1123

National Collegiate Athletic Association (NCAA). (2009). *NCAA 2010–2011 wrestling rules and interpretations.* Retrieved November 9, 2009, from http://www.ncaapublications.com/Uploads/PDF/Wrestling_Rules_2009f2010fab-a10b-4d72-b0c6-c77067ebe273.pdf

National Federation of State High School Associations (NFHS). (2006). *2006–2007 Wrestling rules changes.* Retrieved October 5, 2006, from http://www.oiasports.com/files/content/sports/wrestling/WrestlingRuleChanges2006.pdf

Nattiv, A., Loucks, A. B., Manore, M. M., Sanborn, C. F., Sundgot-Borgen, J., & Warren, M. (2007). American College of Sports Medicine position stand: The female athlete triad. *Medicine & Science in Sports and Exercise, 39,* 1867–1882.

Oppliger, R. A., Utter, A. C., Scott, J. R., Dick, R. W., & Klossner, D. (2006). NCAA rule changes improve weight loss among national championship wrestlers. *Medicine and Science in Sports and Exercise, 38,* 963–970.

Paluska, S. A. (2003). Caffeine and exercise. *Current Sports Medicine Reports, 2,* 213–219.

Petrie, H. J., Stover, E. A., & Horswill, C. A. (2004). Nutritional concerns for the child and adolescent competitor. *Nutrition, 20,* 620–631.

REFERENCES *(continued)*

Petroczi, A., Naughton, D., Pearce, G., Bailey, R., Bloodworth, A., & McNamee, M. (2008). Nutritional supplement use by elite young U.K. athletes: Fallacies of advice regarding intake. *Journal of the International Society of Sports Nutrition, 5,* 22.

Rodriguez, N. R., Vislocky, L. M., & Gaine, P. C. (2007). Dietary protein, endurance exercise, and human skeletal-muscle protein turnover. *Current Opinion in Clinical Nutrition and Metabolic Care, 10,* 40–45.

Rowland, T. (2008). Thermoregulation during exercise in the heat in children: Old concepts revisited. *Journal of Applied Physiology, 105,* 718–724.

Sawka, M. N., Burke, L., Eichner, E. R., Maughan, R. J., Montain, S. J., & Stachenfeld, N. S. (2007). American College of Sports Medicine position stand: Exercise and fluid replacement. *Medicine & Science in Sports and Exercise, 39,* 377–390.

Tang, J. E., & Phillips, S. M. (2009). Maximizing muscle protein anabolism: The role of protein quality. *Current Opinion in Clinical Nutrition and Metabolic Care, 12,* 66–71.

Tarnopolsky, M. (2008). Nutritional considerations in the aging athlete. *Clinical Journal of Sports Medicine, 18,* 531–538.

Tipton, K. D., & Witard, O. C. (2007). Protein requirements and recommendations for athletes: Relevance of ivory tower arguments for practical recommendations. *Clinics in Sports Medicine, 26,* 17–36.

Tunnicliffe, J. M., Erdman, K. A., Reimer, R. A., Lun, V., & Shearer, J. (2008). Consumption of dietary caffeine and coffee in physically active populations: Physiological interactions. *Applied Physiology, Nutrition & Metabolism, 33,* 1301–1310.

Volpe, S. L. (2007). Micronutrient requirements for athletes. *Clinics in Sports Medicine, 26,* 119–130.

von Duvillard, S. P., Braun, W. A., Markofski, M., Beneke, R., & Leithauser, R. (2004). Fluids and hydration in prolonged endurance performance. *Nutrition, 20,* 651–656.

Wiles, J. D., Coleman, D., Tegerdine, M., & Swaine, I. L. (2006). The effects of caffeine ingestion on performance time, speed and power during a laboratory-based 1 km cycling time-trial. *Journal of Sports Sciences, 24,* 1165–1171.

Section 3

Nutrition in the Life Cycle

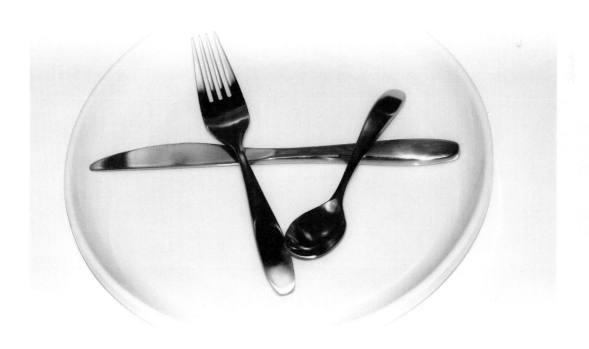

Nutritional Assessment 12

WHAT WILL YOU LEARN?

1. To summarize risk factors that affect nutritional health.
2. To differentiate between nutritional screening and nutritional assessment.
3. To categorize the major components of a nutritional assessment.
4. To relate the components of a nutrition history and techniques for gathering nutrition history data.
5. To distinguish the anthropometric measurements and physical findings that comprise the physical assessment portion of the nutritional assessment.
6. To illustrate appropriate laboratory data for use in an assessment.
7. To differentiate between normal and abnormal findings in a nutritional assessment.
8. To strategize how to incorporate a nutritional assessment into the nursing process.

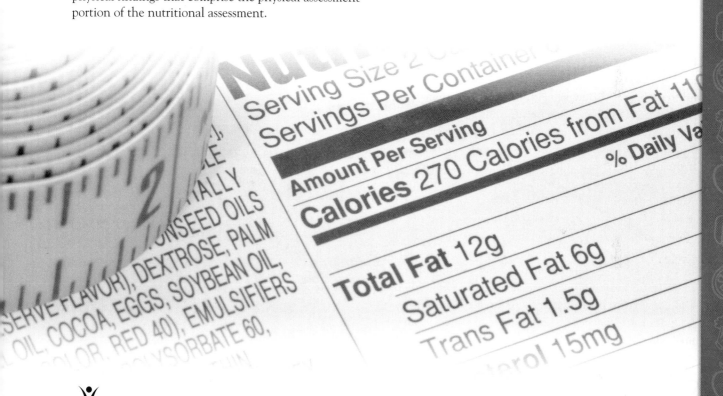

DID YOU KNOW?

▶ A very muscular person can seem overweight when assessed using only the body mass index (BMI).

▶ Alternative methods exist to measure height when a client cannot stand freely to be measured. Measuring arm span is an example.

▶ Standing scales that also measure body fat use bioelectrical impedance analysis to send an electrical current from one foot through the leg and lower body to the opposite leg and foot.

▶ Storage levels of most nutrients cannot be measured easily with routine laboratory assays.

▶ Hair is affected by poor nutrition. Balding, sparse hair, and changes in hair texture can be a physical finding of protein-calorie malnutrition.

KEY TERMS

anabolism, *269*

anergy, *268*

anthropometric measurements, *256*

Bitot's spots, *266*

catabolism, *269*

diet recall, *253*

flag sign, *266*

food frequency questionnaire, *255*

immunocompetence, *268*

infantometer, *258*

nutritional screening, *253*

overnutrition, *252*

somatic protein, *262*

undernutrition, *252*

visceral proteins, *265*

xerophthalmia, *266*

Nutritional Health

Across the lifespan, nutritional health affects overall health. An assessment of nutritional health should be included in the nursing process. Nutritional deficiencies affect the growth and development of infants and young children. The nutritional health of a pregnant female affects the health of the fetus. In the adult and older adult, nutritional deficiencies can contribute to the development of chronic disease, such as osteoporosis or anemias. **Undernutrition,** also called *malnutrition,* is a term used to describe compromised nutritional status that results from insufficient intake or low body stores of one or more nutrients. Most often this term is synonymous with protein-calorie malnutrition. Protein-calorie malnutrition is associated with poor wound healing; loss of muscle mass; functional decline; altered immune status; and in children, growth faltering (Norman, Pichard, Lochs, & Pirlich, 2008). **Overnutrition** is a term used to describe poor nutritional health that results from intake or stores of nutrients that exceeds recommended amounts. Obesity, hypercholesterolemia, and toxic levels of stored vitamins from oversupplementation are examples of overnutrition. Both undernutrition and overnutrition are associated with negative health consequences. Overnutrition and undernutrition are not mutually exclusive conditions. For example, an individual who abuses alcohol can be deficient in thiamine yet be overweight. An obese child who consumes excessive fat but no fruits and vegetables can have both overnutrition and undernutrition. The presence of risk factors for overnutrition or undernutrition should become apparent during the assessment process. The nurse should be aware of the risk factors for poor nutritional health before beginning the nutritional screening or assessment process. Table 12-1 outlines risk factors for undernutrition and overnutrition.

Table 12-1	Risk Factors for Poor Nutritional Health

Undernutrition

Medical:
- Chronic disease, acute illness, injury, or wounds
- Disease symptoms, including pain
- Treatment side effects such as nausea, anorexia
- Polypharmacy
- Drug–nutrient interactions
- Gastrointestinal complaints, malabsorption
- Chewing or swallowing difficulties
- Poor dental health—loose or missing teeth, caries, poorly fitting dentures
- Alcohol and drug abuse
- Depression

Altered functional status:
- Cognitive changes
- Inability to self-feed
- Visual impairment
- Poor muscle strength
- Diminished ability to perform activities of daily living or instrumental activities of daily living such as shopping and food preparation.

Diet:
- Poor quality intake
- Poor quantity intake— poor appetite, missed meals, restrictive eating (e.g., dieting, faddism, limited intake because of cultural or religious beliefs, disordered eating)

Socioeconomic:
- Food insecurity—limited access to food because of finances or living situation
- Sadness, bereavement, social isolation
- Limited knowledge or skills about food and health

Overnutrition

Excessive intake of one or more nutrients such as calories, saturated fats, vitamins, or minerals

Excessive intake of dietary supplements

Alcohol abuse

Sedentary activity level

Limited knowledge or skills about food and health

CT? What are some circumstances where both undernutrition and overnutrition exist in the same individual?

Nutrition Screening and Assessment

Either a **nutritional screening** or a nutritional assessment should be included in the nursing process. A nutritional screening is less comprehensive than an assessment and is done to identify the presence of risk factors for poor nutritional health. This abbreviated evaluation process is not intended to diagnose nutritional problems, but rather serves as a basic initial step toward identifying individuals requiring further assessment. Nutritional screening is a cost-effective way of determining the need for a full nutritional assessment (American Dietetic Association [ADA], 1994). Generally, a nutrition screening is brief and noninvasive, containing just a few questions or parameters to be checked. Examples include weight, weight history, and ability to take oral nutrition. In all health care settings, a nutrition screening is required within the first 24 hours of a client's admission (Charney, 2008). Most often, the nurse is responsible for this initial screening as part of the nursing assessment (Charney, 2008; Chima, Dietz-Seher, & Kushner-Benson, 2008).

A nutritional assessment serves as the foundation on which nutritional intervention goals are based. Generally a comprehensive nutritional assessment is the responsibility of a registered dietitian (RD) in most health care facilities. The nurse can also complete a nutritional assessment and in some settings is the primary clinician gathering and evaluating nutritional data. The nurse is ideally situated to facilitate early intervention for clients with compromised nutritional health.

A complete nutritional assessment is comprised of three major components:

- Nutrition history
- Physical assessment
- Laboratory measurements

No single assessment component or any one parameter provides the necessary scope of information needed for a complete assessment. Findings obtained during the physical assessment or from a single laboratory value are affected by factors other than nutrition, such as disease, the environment, or medications. The nurse should gather as much data as possible when conducting a nutritional assessment. Relying on limited data, or worse, a single parameter, can lead to inaccurate or missed nutritional diagnoses. Poor nutritional health occurs along a continuum. The nurse should be aware of any alteration in assessment parameters, even if findings remain within established normal limits. Always, sharp clinical judgment is a necessary adjunct to the available data when completing an assessment.

Nutrition History

The nutrition history portion of the nutritional assessment contains one or more components. Each of these components is subjective in nature, relying on self-reporting by the client. When time permits, the nurse should use more than one component to provide an information cross-check.

Diet Recall

A **diet recall** is also called a 24-hour recall because it involves the client's recollection of everything consumed in a set 24-hour time span. The client should be prompted to recall in sequence all the food, liquids, and dietary supplements consumed at all meals and snacks throughout the day. The nurse should make note of the time and location of intake, portion sizes, food preparation methods, use of fortified versions of foods, and types and doses of dietary supplements. Hot Topic Box: Why Ask about Dietary Supplements? outlines the importance of including information about dietary supplements in an assessment.

hot Topic

Why Ask about Dietary Supplements?

Vitamins, minerals, weight loss and sports nutrition products, herbs, and other plant products are all regulated by the federal government as foods, yet many of these substances act like medications, interfere with medications, or have other health effects. Many consumers assume that dietary supplements have been tested for safety when, in fact, no premarket safety testing is required. Drug-supplement interactions, alterations in platelet activity, and product contamination are among the concerns with dietary supplements.

The use of dietary supplements by people of all ages is on the rise in the United States, while the reporting of this use to health care providers is poor. Estimates range as high as 75% of adults in the United States use dietary supplements at least intermittently when vitamins and minerals are included in the definition. Up to 20% of adults in the United States and Canada reported using nonvitamin/nonmineral types of supplements over a 12-month period (Kelly et al., 2005; Singh & Levine, 2006). Use of nonvitamin/nonmineral supplements by adults over age 65 years doubled between the years 1998 and 2002 (Kelly et al., 2005). Over half of all older adults who take prescription drugs also take at least one dietary supplement (Qato et al., 2008). The nurse should be aware that the prevalence of dietary supplement use is higher among children with a chronic disease or condition compared with healthy peers. Over 60% of chronically ill children use dietary supplements with almost one-third of those using a supplement that was not recommended by a health care provider (Ball, Kertesz, & Moyer-Mileur, 2005). Further, in 80% of the cases of supplement use, no communication occurred with the health care provider about the supplement, a dismal statistic that has been approximated by other studies in children and adults (Ball et al., 2005; Gardiner, Buettner, Davis, Phillips, & Kemper, 2008).

Given the increasing prevalence of dietary supplement use combined with the possibility of drug interactions and health consequences, the nurse should routinely ask clients, parents, or caregivers specifically about supplement use. It is a common practice to encourage new clients to bring all prescribed and over-the-counter medications to a first health care visit; the nurse should also encourage the client to include dietary supplements in that initial assessment. Dietary supplements are discussed further in Chapter 25.

BOX 12-1	Sample Portion Estimates for Use in a Nutrition History

It is not always practical to have food models or other portion facsimiles available in a health care or community setting. The following verbal analogies can be helpful when estimating intake.

1 cup dry weight (not volume) measure = small, clenched woman's fist

2 tbsp = a single golf ball

4 tbsp = 4 thumb's tips, from knuckle to fingertip

1 oz cubed cheese = small-sized wooden match box or 2 dominoes

3 oz cooked animal protein = deck of cards

Piece of fruit, small potato, or dinner roll = computer mouse

Small pancake, tortilla = compact disc

Proper estimation of portion sizes is needed to accurately judge intake. Visual portion comparisons help a client estimate intake by providing a point of reference. Photographs and life-size food models can be helpful, especially if age- and culturally appropriate foods are depicted. Large-size portion models are available to represent customarily consumed portions because large portions tend to be underreported (Harnack, Steffen, Arnett, Gao, & Luepker, 2004). Portion analogies to common items like a deck of cards can universally be adapted to the recall process in any setting. Box 12-1 contains portion analogies for use in estimating intake. Clients responding to questions with statements such as "it depends" or "probably" should be asked further questions to clarify answers. Using visuals for portion estimates can be helpful for clarification.

Open-ended, nonjudgmental questions should be used during the interview. Open-ended questions allow the individual to answer with more than a simple *yes* or *no* and provide important details about intake. Nonjudgmental questions are essential to establish rapport with the client and to obtain valid and reliable information. Hinting at a correct answer, such as asking "what did you have for lunch?" when the person may have skipped lunch, or appearing to judge a client can lead to fabricated answers and other misreporting. Table 12-2 illustrates positive and negative examples of questions for a diet recall. The nurse should be aware that body language, word choice, and tone of voice can contribute to the client's responses (Livingstone & Black, 2003). An individual may overreport or underreport intake in order to avoid judgment or to gain approval by the nurse (Kristal, Andrilla, Koepsell, Diehr, & Cheadle 1998). Intake of alcohol tends to be underreported (Nevitt & Lundak, 2005; Walker & Cosden, 2007). Those who are obese or have a low socioeconomic or educational level are more likely to underreport overall intake than others (Scagliusi et al., 2008). Additionally, clients on a therapeutic diet may underreport foods that are restricted by the diet prescription (Foster & Leonard, 2004). Intake of fruits and vegetables tends to be overreported because of perceived social approval with such answers (Miller, Abdel-Maksoud, Crane, Marcus, & Byers, 2008). Conducting the diet recall in a nonjudgmental fashion helps establish an interview climate that fosters full answers by the client.

Table 12-2 Sample Diet Recall Questions

Question	Do Ask	Do Not Say
Beginning the recall	"When was the first time you had something to eat or drink (name the day)?"	"What did you have for breakfast?"
Clarifying meal or snack content	The nurse listens as the client lists what was consumed, gently prompting the client to remember by asking "Was there anything else with that?"	"So that was breakfast" when perhaps the client had more to eat at the meal but was slow or forgetful at reporting it.
Sequence of intake	"And then when was the next time you had something to eat or drink?"	"What did you have for lunch?" or "Did you have lunch?"
Food portions	"What portion of ice cream did you have compared to this container?" (Show picture, food model, or use Box 12-1 examples.)	"You said you had a cup of coffee?" The nurse then records the portion as 8 oz without clarifying the portion with the client.
Food preparation methods	"Who prepared the chicken? Can you tell me about how it was prepared?"	"Was that chicken baked or fried?"
Supplement use	"Dietary supplements include vitamins, minerals, herbs, and sports and weight loss products. Have you ever bought or taken any of these? Are you currently taking any dietary supplements? What was your reason for wanting a supplement? For how long have you been taking this? What is the dose? Where did you get the supplement?"	"Do you take any supplements?"

Because the diet recall provides only a snapshot view of intake, it cannot be exclusively used to generalize usual intake. The nurse can conduct a recall for several sample days to better assess intake. Asking for an example of a work and nonwork day would be an example. Food intake and habits can vary in an inconsistent manner that is not apparent in a diet recall. Significant alterations in intake occur occasionally and will be missed by a diet recall. For example, intake of alcohol or dietary supplements may not occur regularly, but each has significant effect on nutritional health. Table 12-3 outlines the strengths and weaknesses of the diet recall and other components of the nutrition history.

Food Frequency Questionnaire

A **food frequency questionnaire** is used to assess usual intake of a variety of foods or food groups over time. Specific foods or general food groups are listed on the questionnaire and frequency of intake by the day, week, month, or longer is recorded by the nurse or the client. Food frequency questionnaires will not provide information regarding the distribution or pattern of intake unless the nurse asks specifically about this intake when administering the tool. Food preparation methods generally are not included, making this tool less detailed than the diet recall. Informational gaps from a diet recall can be filled when a food frequency questionnaire is conducted in combination with the recall. For example, an individual may report no dairy intake during a 24-hour recall, but the nurse may learn from the food frequency questionnaire that a gallon of milk is consumed per week. Formal food frequency tools exist that are often derived from epidemiological research. When using an existing formal questionnaire, care should be taken to choose a tool that is population spe-

cific. Long questionnaires can be a time burden to the client and the nurse. Brief questionnaires are quicker and can be administered verbally as part of the history. Table 12-4 illustrates a nutrition history form used in the college health setting with a food frequency questionnaire that is administered verbally.

Food Record

A food record is a diary of recorded intake that is filled out by the client in an ongoing fashion. Intake is reported for several days or more to estimate usual intake. Food records run the same risks of misreporting as the diet recall. The nurse should use a food record as an assessment tool in a limited fashion to avoid overburdening the client, which can cause the client to resort to retrospective recording of intake that will affect reliability of the information.

Focused Interview

Combining the diet recall and food frequency questionnaire with a focused interview provides a comprehensive view of intake. The diet recall process serves as the foundation of the interview, providing a base from which to ask further questions than is possible with the recall or questionnaire alone. Interview questions cover both present and past nutritional habits. For example, when assessing an overweight client, the nurse can inquire about weight history, past dieting attempts and successes, supplement use, sources of dieting information, and social support. When assessing a pregnant female, information regarding preconception nutritional health would be important historical data to include. Box 12-2 outlines nutrition history data to gather during the focused interview. Data specific to concerns across the lifespan are included in Lifespan Box: Lifespan Considerations with a Nutrition History.

Table 12-3   Nutrition History Tools: Strengths and Weaknesses

Component	Strengths	Weaknesses
Diet Recall	Quick and easy	Relies on memory Subject to misreporting and reporting bias Portion size estimates difficult Not representative of overall intake since a snapshot in time
Food Frequency Questionnaire	Short versions are quick and easy Can be used with diet recall to fill information gaps	Relies on memory Needs to be population specific with familiar foods Does not represent eating patterns or food distribution
Food Record	May estimate usual intake over time Does not rely on memory	Cumbersome to maintain May erroneously be filled out retrospectively Subject to misreporting Some clients alter intake because of record Requires writing skills Portions size estimates may be difficult
Focused Interview	In-depth review of intake, habits, and beliefs Allows more time to establish rapport with client	Time consuming Misreporting possible

Table 12-4 Nutrition History Form

NUTRITION EVALUATION

NAME: _____ DATE: _____
SCHOOL ADDRESS/CLASS: _____ PHONE: _____
AGE: _____
HOME ADDRESS: _____ REFERRED BY: _____
SIGNED CONSENT/DATE: _____

HEIGHT	WEIGHT	RECENT WT CHANGE	MAX/MIN WEIGHTS	WEIGHT HISTORY
BODY COMPOSITION MEASUREMENTS	BODY FAT %	EXERCISE	EXERCISE FREQ/DURATION	OTHER ACTIVITIES
MEDICAL HISTORY	MEDICATION: RX,OTC	VITAMINS/MINERALS	HERBS	OTHER SUPPLE-MENTS
PREVIOUS DIETS	FOOD ALLERGIES/ INTOLERANCES	DORM REFRIG/COOKING LIVING WITH?	RESTRICTIVE? BINGE? PURGE? LAXATIVES? OTHER?	CLIENT'S SELF-REPORTED NUTRITION GOAL

Diet History:
M-F

Diet History:
Weekends

Food Frequency (note per week, day, month, or other)

Fruit: fresh other		Dairy:		Fluids: note type, include caffeine, water	
juice		Starches/grains:		Alcohol:	
Vegetables:		note type		Sugar/Sweets:	
green or orange		Animal Protein:		Fats: note type	
other		Plant Protein:		Supplements:	List above

Physical Assessment

The physical assessment component of the nutritional assessment includes both **anthropometric measurements** and a head-to-toe review of systems. Anthropometric measurements are any scientific measurement of the body, such as weight, height, and body fat. The nurse should routinely incorporate the nutritional aspects of a physical assessment into the nursing process. Not all physical assessment parameters can be practically evaluated in all health care situations. Some parameters are only population specific. A complete nutritional assessment should include as many assessment parameters as is feasible because no single physical parameter is specifically predictive of nutrition status.

Anthropometric Measurements

Assessment of body measurements ideally includes both current and historical values. The nurse should measure current weight and height and avoid simply asking the client for these values. The client or caregiver can be asked about weight history, but this information should be corroborated with documentation in medical records where available. Omitting this portion of the assessment or simply relying on client-supplied values can lead to overlooked nutrition risk or poor reference values if nutrition health declines and historical comparison is needed.

Height

Accurate measurement of height is essential in both children and adults. In adults, accurate height is needed to properly assess weight status. Inaccurate height can lead to mistaken

BOX 12-2	**Comprehensive Nutrition History Data**

Food

- All meals and snacks: frequency, number, missed meals
- All liquids: volume, type including water, alcohol, caffeinated and sugary beverages
- Portion sizes
- Use of fortified foods
- Location of meals and snacks; e.g., restaurant, home, school, vending machine, car
- Food preparation methods
- Grocery habits
- Food allergies and intolerances
- Food idiosyncrasies, foods avoided, or aversions
- Therapeutic diet prescription

Beliefs and Practices

- Cultural and religious influences on diet
- Faddism—trendy beliefs and practices
- Lifestyle food choices; e.g., vegetarianism, organic, extremely low fat
- Pica—eating of nonfood substances like clay, ice, laundry starch
- Knowledge, skills relative to food and health
- Source of food and health knowledge

Medical/Physical

- Medical history, including symptoms, treatment
- Gastrointestinal complaints and remedies
- Substance abuse
- Appetite
- Chewing and swallowing ability
- Functional capacity, including strength, sensory evaluation, and activities of daily living
- Physical activity level including type, frequency, and duration of activity

Supplement and Medication Use

- Vitamin and mineral use, including dose
- Use of herbal products, including dose and source
- Use of other dietary supplements such as weight loss or sports nutrition products
- Over-the-counter medications
- Prescribed medications
- Folk or home remedies; e.g., baking soda as an antacid, cider vinegar for general health

Socioeconomic Factors

- Education and literacy level
- Social environment and support; e.g., isolated, preparing food for others or only self
- Food security—access to food and sufficient funds for food

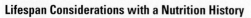

Lifespan

Lifespan Considerations with a Nutrition History

In addition to the standard data included in a nutrition history in Box 12-2, the nurse should consider the following when assessing specific populations:

Infants
- Breastfed vs. bottle fed

Breastfed infant:
Number and lengths of feedings
Number of wet diapers
If mother is vegan, assess mother for synthetic source of vitamin B$_{12}$ intake

Bottle-fed infant:
Type and volume of feeding
- Iron source by age 4–6 months with concomitant vitamin C source to improve absorption
- Intake of solids: note age at introduction, appropriateness to developmental stage, types and amount, intolerances, food allergies
- Medical conditions that affect diet: therapeutic diet, medication side effects, feeding difficulties, nutrient–drug interactions
- Food beliefs and practices of caregiver

- Inappropriate food practices: early introduction of solids, cereal added to bottle, putting to bed with bottle, nonprescribed dietary supplements, cow's milk before age 1 year

Children and Adolescents
- Meal and snack pattern, including number and frequency of meals, missed meals or meals on the run
- Self-prescribed restrictive food habits or diets
- Body satisfaction in older children and adolescents
- Activity level

Adults
- Meal and snack pattern, including number and frequency of meals, missed meals, or meals on the run
- Self-prescribed restrictive food habits or diets
- Adequacy of calcium, iron, and folic acid intake in females of childbearing age
- Nutrition health promotion beliefs and practices
- Activity level

Pregnant/Lactating Female
- Folic acid, calcium, vitamin D, and iron intake
- Caffeine and alcohol intake
- Fluid intake

(continued)

MyNursingKit CDC Growth Charts Training
MyNursingKit U.S. Department of Health and Human Services (USDHHS) Growth Charts

Lifespan (continued)

- Mercury exposure from consuming fish
- Food aversions or cravings
- Cultural beliefs related to food during pregnancy and lactation
- Prescribed and self-prescribed dietary supplement use
- Dietary treatments of pregnancy-associated symptoms (e.g., heartburn, constipation, nausea)

Older Adults

- Therapeutic diet use
- Food intolerances
- Alcohol intake
- Meal pattern and setting (assess for dining alone or missed meals)
- Alterations in sense of taste, smell, vision, or hearing that affect intake
- Functional capacity to prepare and eat food, self-feed
- Food insecurity
- Drug-nutrient interactions

Each lifespan chapter in this text provides further detail on assessing the nutritional health of individuals across each stage of the lifespan.

conclusions about overweight, underweight, or normal weight status. Height is monitored over time in children to assess growth. The nurse should compare the child's measured height to standard references. These references are classified by population percentiles, allowing the nurse to estimate how the child's anthropometric measurements compare to a large population of age and gender-matched peers. The best use of percentile classifications is in the monitoring of a child over time, being alert to any changes in the child's percentile channel. Percentile charts from the Centers for Disease Control and Prevention (CDC), developed for children 20 years of age and under, are available in Appendix A. On-line training tools for using growth charts are available from the CDC.

Height is ideally measured in children and adults using a standing measure. Alternative measurements are indicated when the individual cannot stand freely without assistance or has altered posture because of kyphosis from osteoporosis or other conditions. Proper technique for obtaining a standing height is contained in Figure 12-1 ■. Reliance on self-reported heights can overestimate true height as discussed in the Evidence-Based Practice Box: Are self-reported height and weight accurate enough for screening purposes with overweight individuals? If self-reported height must be used, the nurse should document its use in the medical record.

Recumbent length is an alternative to standing height and is used in the measurement of young children or individuals who cannot stand freely, such as frail older adults or individuals who must stay in bed. The client must be able to lie flat for an accurate measurement. An **infantometer** is a formal tabletop device developed for recumbent length measurements in infants and young children. The child is placed on

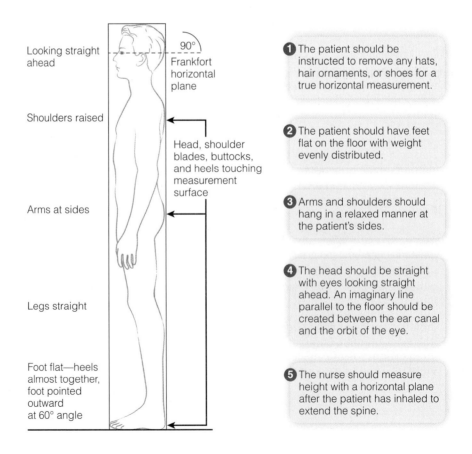

Looking straight ahead

Shoulders raised

Arms at sides

Legs straight

Foot flat—heels almost together, foot pointed outward at 60° angle

90°
Frankfort horizontal plane

Head, shoulder blades, buttocks, and heels touching measurement surface

❶ The patient should be instructed to remove any hats, hair ornaments, or shoes for a true horizontal measurement.

❷ The patient should have feet flat on the floor with weight evenly distributed.

❸ Arms and shoulders should hang in a relaxed manner at the patient's sides.

❹ The head should be straight with eyes looking straight ahead. An imaginary line parallel to the floor should be created between the ear canal and the orbit of the eye.

❺ The nurse should measure height with a horizontal plane after the patient has inhaled to extend the spine.

■ **FIGURE 12-1 Measurement of Standing Height.**

EVIDENCE-BASED PRACTICE RESEARCH BOX

Are self-reported height and weight accurate enough for screening purposes with overweight individuals?

Clinical Problem: Many people prefer not to get weighed when visiting a health care provider. This preference is particularly true for overweight and obese individuals. If an accurate body mass index (BMI) could be calculated from self-reported height and weight, the usefulness of screening programs could be increased.

Research Findings: Numerous studies have been conducted using children, adolescents, and adults to determine the accuracy of self-reported height and weight and, therefore, the accuracy of BMI. Because BMI is useful in classifying individuals as underweight, normal, overweight, or obese, knowledge of BMI can be used for determining individuals at risk for disease.

Studies of older schoolchildren and adolescents in several countries have shown that males and females are usually inaccurate in self-reporting height and weight. Most often, weight was underreported by both boys and girls and height was overreported. Girls underreported weight to a greater degree than boys, and boys overreported height to a greater degree than girls. Youth who were overweight consistently underreported weight to a greater extent than those who had normal weight. Interestingly, those who were underweight tended to overreport weight (Brener, McManus, Galuska, Lowry, & Wechsler, 2003; Goodman, Hinden, & Khandelwal, 2000; Hauck, White, Cao, Woolf, & Strauss, 1995; Jacobson & DeBock, 2001; Jansen, van de Looij-Jansen, Ferreira, de Wilde, & Brug, 2006; Morrissey, Whetstone, Cummings, & Owen, 2006; Tokmakidis, Christodoulos, & Mantzouranis, 2007; Tsigilis, 2006; Wang, Patterson, & Hills, 2002). When the BMI was calculated using self-report data and compared with measured height and weight, the data were less clear. The bias of self-report resulted in BMI values that ranged from 0.5 to 2.6 units higher in measured versus self-report data (Brener et al., 2003; Morrissey et al., 2006). The percentage of misclassification of overweight (BMI greater than 25) or obesity (BMI greater than 30) by self-report ranged from 4% to 31% (Goodman et al., 2001; Hauck et al., 1995; Morrissey et al., 2006; Tokmakidis et al., 2007; Wang et al., 2002).

One study of adolescents added an additional variable, body weight perception, in which students were asked if they perceived themselves as underweight, normal weight, or overweight. In the sample of 2,032 youth, 34.8% perceived themselves as underweight, 42.9% saw themselves as about right, and 22.3% perceived themselves as overweight. On the basis of BMI calculated from measured height and weight, only 1.5% of students were classified as underweight, whereas 51.2% were normal weight and 47.4% were overweight (Brener, Eaton, Lowry, & McManus, 2004).

Similar data exist for adults; women tend to understate weight and men tend to overstate height. Self-reported data also led to misclassification of BMI, especially in those who were already overweight or obese (Brunner-Huber, 2007; Engstrom, Paterson, Doherty, Trabulsi, & Speer, 2003; Kuczmarski, Kuczmarski, & Najjar, 2001; Nawaz, Chan, Abdulrahmann, Larson, & Katz, 2001; Nyholm et al., 2007; Rossouw, Senekal, & Stander, 2001; Spencer, Appleby, Davey, & Key, 2002; Taylor et al., 2006). There were no significant differences for African Americans or Hispanics compared to individuals of European descent (Avila-Funes, Gutierrez-Robledo, & Ponce De Leon Rosales, 2004; Brunner-Huber, 2007; Gillum & Sempos, 2005).

Nursing Implications: The current evidence is clear that individuals across the lifespan do not accurately report height and weight. Although the reasons for self-report inaccuracies were not explored, it is clear that discrepancies exist. Because the BMI is calculated to identify individuals at risk for disease and self-reported height and weight lead to inaccurate calculation of BMI, actual measurement should be performed by nurses to gather clinically accurate data.

CRITICAL THINKING QUESTIONS:

1. When a client who is on a weight reduction program asks why it is necessary to come to the clinic for a weight check, how should the nurse respond?

2. A community organization is planning to use a telephone survey to determine the prevalence of overweight and obesity in an area. How might the nurse respond when asked to volunteer time for such an effort?

---

the table in a supine position with head and feet flat against the fixed headboard and sliding footboard. The child's arms should be at the side, eyes looking straight ahead, and knees straightened. The nurse may find it easier to perform an accurate measurement on a frightened child when a parent or caregiver assists by soothing the child and gently holding the head in position. Figure 12-2 ■ shows an example of an infantometer.

Recumbent length measurement of older individuals is done at the bedside. The individual must lie flat in the same supine position as is used with the infantometer, with soles of the feet perpendicular to the bed. Any straightedge object, such as a book, is placed flat against the feet and then head

to mark those positions lightly with a pencil on the bed linens. The client should not move until both positions are marked. A measuring tape is used to measure the distance between the marks. Recumbent length overestimates height by up to 2% because of spinal compression that occurs with standing (American Medical Directors Association, 2001). The use of a recumbent rather than standing measurement should be documented when recording height.

Individuals who cannot stand freely nor lie flat for recumbent measurements require indirect measurements of height. Direct measurements are preferred because indirect measurements are less accurate (Luft, Beghetto, Castro, &

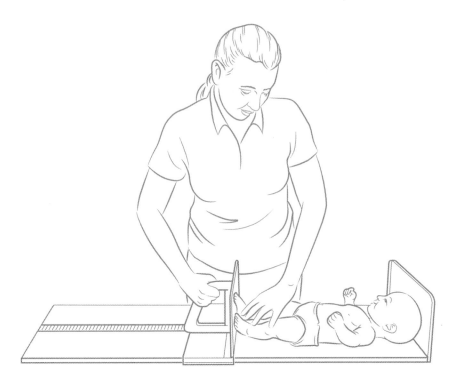

■ **FIGURE 12-2 Infantometer.**

deMello, 2008).The nurse should choose the best indirect measurement suitable to a client's situation.

- *Knee height* measurements are used with clients who have the flexibility to keep one foot bent at a 90-degree angle to the leg but who cannot stand freely. A sliding knee-height caliper is used to measure the distance between the bottom of the foot and the knee. Using the measurements, age and gender-specific predictive equation estimates height.
- *Armspan and demi-armspan* indirectly measure height in individuals who can fully and comfortably extend one or both arms in a straight line out to the side at shoulder level. The armspan measurement is made from right-hand fingertips to left-hand fingertips using a flexible tape. Demi-armspan is calculated by doubling the distance from either hand fingertips to the sternal notch. Predictive equations for demi-armspan are also used, including the following equation recommended by the World Health Organization (WHO 1999, chap. 9, p. 37):

$$\text{Height (m)} = [0.73 \times < 2 \times \text{demi-armspan (m)}>] + 0.43$$

Weight and Weight History

Documentation of current weight is a vital component of a nutritional assessment and should be standard practice. Additionally, the use of body weight to determine medication and anesthesia dosing underscores the need for accurate measurement (Jensen et al., 2003). The client should be weighed with a minimum of clothing, no shoes, and after voiding. Any deviation from this standard, such as the presence of a leg brace or heavier clothing, should be noted when the weight is recorded. The nurse should also note and quantify the presence of any edema when recording body weight. Assessment of clients with renal failure and receiving dialysis treatment should be done using a dry weight that is obtained following a dialysis session. Clients with an eating disorder should be assessed for any hidden objects intended to weight the scale. Pockets and underwear can be used to conceal heavy items. In such clients, the nurse would be prudent to cross-check urine specific gravity to assess for the dilutional effect of excessive liquid intake deliberately consumed just beforehand to increase the weight measurement temporarily. Waiting until the end of the data gathering and interview to obtain first the urine and then a weight is wise with these clients.

A variety of scales exist for measuring weight. Standing beam scales are used for individuals who can stand freely without grasping the scale, wall, cane, or other object to maintain balance. These types of scale have the advantage of movable weights and a balance to maintain accuracy with regular calibration. It is advisable to balance, or zero, the scale at the start of each clinical day (United States Department of Health and Human Services [USDHHS], n.d.). Other types of scales without balances, such as those intended for minimal home use, should be regularly cross-checked with a balanced scale if used in a clinical setting. Clients who cannot stand without assistance should be weighed in a chair scale. Bed scales are used to weigh the client who must remain in bed. Figure 12-3 ■ depicts use of a bed scale.

Additional weight calculations are needed when recording the weight of clients with missing limbs. It is difficult to accurately assess weight status or make later weight comparisons without adjusting for missing limbs. Calculations are done referencing the weight contributions of all limbs. Figure 12-4 ■ outlines the reference values used

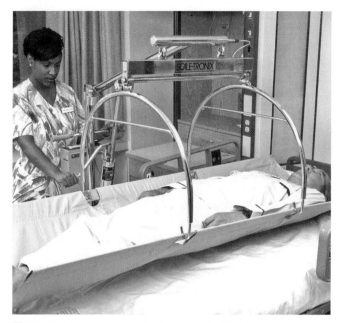

■ **FIGURE 12-3 Using a Bed Scale to Obtain Weight.**

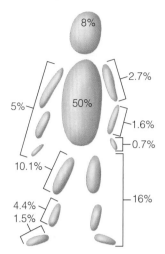

■ **FIGURE 12-4 Limb Weight Contributions.**
Source: Osterkamp, 1995.

are required for calculation of BMI using the following formula: BMI = weight (kg)/height^2 (m). The National Heart, Lung and Blood Institute (NHLBI) and the WHO have established parameters to categorize normal weight,

in calculating adjustments in weight. Table 12-5 outlines weight calculation examples for an individual with an amputated limb.

The nurse should obtain a weight history during the nutritional assessment. This information can be gathered during the focused interview and corroborated with any documentation in the medical record. Weight history is important in the assessment of children and the pregnant female especially but is also needed to assess for unplanned weight loss or weight gain patterns in adults and older adults. An unplanned weight loss of 5% of body weight or more in 1 month or 10% or more in 6 months is considered significant. Box 12-3 outlines a calculation of weight change.

Body Mass Index

Body mass index (BMI) is used to assess weight status in both children and adults. Accurate height and weight

BOX 12-3	Weight Change Calculations

Weight change calculations are done by using present weight, prior weight, and weight loss amount. Unplanned weight loss of greater than 5% in 1 month or greater than10% in 6 months is considered significant.

1. Subtract current weight from prior weight to calculate weight loss.
2. Divide weight loss amount by prior weight to calculate weight loss percentage.

Example A client seen in home care weighs 130 lb and the medical record reports a weight of 145 lb on admission to the hospital 2 months ago.

1. 145 lb prior weight − 130 lb current weight = 15 lb weight loss
2. 15 lb weight loss ÷ 145 lb prior weight = 0.10 or 10% weight loss

Table 12-5	Sample Body Weight Calculations with Missing Limb

A client is being assessed by the nurse in a rehabilitation hospital 10 days after a below-the-knee amputation (BKA). His preoperative weight was 81 kg. He was not weighed postoperatively and currently weighs 75 kg.

1. Determine weight contribution of missing limb.	BKA = 1.5% (foot)+ 4.4% (leg) = 5.9% body weight
2. Calculate estimated weight of missing limb.	75 kg × 0.059 = 4.425 kg
3. Add estimated weight of limb to current body weight for adjusted weight estimate.	75 kg + 4.425 kg = 79.425 kg
4. Use adjusted weight to calculate BMI.	The nurse can record height and assess weight status using 79.425 kg to calculate BMI from Figure 12-4.
5. Use current adjusted weight to compare weight history prior to loss of limb.	The nurse can compare 79.425 kg to the documented preoperative weight of 81 kg. The client has lost almost 2 kg in addition to the weight of the amputated limb.

Table 12-6 Body Mass Index (BMI) Classifications for Adults

BMI	Classification
Less than 16	Severe malnutrition
16–16.99	Moderate malnutrition
17–18.49	Mild malnutrition
18.5–24.9	Normal
25–29.9	Overweight
30–34.9	Obese class 1
35–39.9	Obese class 2
Greater than or equal to 40	Obese class 3

CT? What is the drawback to relying only on BMI to assess weight?

Sources: Adapted from NHLBI Obesity Education Initiative Expert Panel, 1998; Willett, Dietz, & Colditz, 1999; World Health Organization (WHO), 1999 (Table 13, p. 38).

overweight, obesity, and underweight in adults based on BMI. These classifications are illustrated in Table 12-6. Quick reference tables and nomograms are available to make the BMI calculations easier. If self-reported height or weight is used, BMI could be miscalculated because of underreporting of weight and overreporting of height.

The CDC has growth charts for children 2 to 20 years of age that outline BMI by percentile, and these are contained in Appendix A. In children over age 2 years, risk of overweight and overweight are defined as BMI-for-age of greater than the 85th percentile and 95th percentile, respectively (CDC, 2009). Underweight is defined as less than the 5th percentile. These parameters should be used as screening criteria for assessing weight status, but not as a diagnostic criterion (Cunningham, 2004). A child should be monitored for any change in percentile channel compared with prior measurements.

Use of BMI exclusively to determine weight status has limitations. Because the BMI equation factors in only height and weight, its use assumes that all persons of any given weight also have identical body composition. This assumption is false and limits use of BMI as a physical assessment parameter. Physically fit individuals with little body fat can be misclassified as overweight because of the contribution of ample muscle. Other individuals can have a normal weight status using BMI but have excess body fat and little muscle mass. Older adults typically lose muscle with age but can also gain fat, maintaining a steady weight; BMI masks this change in body composition. Racial and ethnic differences in body composition exist, but no population-specific BMI classifications are yet in existence (Lear, Humphries, Kohli, & Birmingham, 2007; Wen et al., 2009).

Waist Circumference

Excess adipose specifically situated along the waistline is considered an independent risk factor for type 2 diabetes, elevated

PRACTICE PEARL

Measuring Waist Circumference
Place the client in front of a mirror when measuring waist circumference. Stand behind the client to locate the lateral border of the ileum by palpating the right hip. Place a mark at that location. Use the mirror to make sure that the measurement tape is kept horizontal to the floor. Hold the measuring tape taut but not tight (CDC, 2000).

blood lipids, hypertension, and cardiovascular disease in adults (NHLBI, n.d.; Zhang, Rexrode, van Dam, Li, & Hu, 2008). Inclusion of a waist circumference measurement in a nutritional assessment is recommended in the adult, especially when cardiovascular risk factors are present. The NHLBI advises that a waist circumference greater than 102 cm (40 in) in adult males and greater than 88 cm (35 in) in adult females is an indicator of cardiovascular risk (NHLBI, 1998). These cut points are for BMIs within the range of 25 to 34.9 only. Waist circumference in individuals with a BMI *greater than* 35 loses its predictive power of estimating health risk (NHLBI, n.d.).

The nurse should measure the waist circumference using a spring-loaded measuring tape to ensure even tension with each measurement. Establishment of a bony landmark to guide the measurement is best, though there is some disagreement as to the best landmark to use (CDC, 2000). The CDC recommends use of the lateral border of the ileum (CDC, 2000). Measurement should be done directly over the skin and not over clothing. Avoid measuring waist circumference using the umbilicus as a reference point because its position can be altered with obesity. Practice Pearl: Measuring Weight Circumference is used to perform a reliable waist circumference.

Waist circumference measurements are not a valid nutrition assessment tool for all adults. Pregnant females and clients with increased abdominal girth from medical conditions, such as ascites, edema, or an abdominal mass should not have waist circumference measured as part of a nutrition assessment. Additionally, not all increases in body fat are reflected by changes in waist circumference, limiting its use (Lean & Han, 2002). Waist circumference will not give an accurate assessment of abdominal adiposity in clients with pendulous abdominal fat when gravity causes the excess fat to no longer remain along the waistline.

Body Composition

Measurement of weight, waist circumference, or BMI does not give the nurse specific information about body composition. Muscle mass, also called skeletal protein, **somatic protein,** or lean body mass, cannot directly be determined by these simple measurements. Body fat, bone mass, total body water, and other components of body composition are not determined easily, yet are important. Measurement of body composition is done indirectly using varying techniques with different levels of reliability and sophistication. Simple analysis techniques, like skinfold measures, assess only lean body mass and body fat, whereas more sophisticated technology can differentiate among the lean components to calculate protein, bone mass, and water. Because of variability in accuracy between different methods, it is recommended that serial monitoring of body composition be assessed using the same method each time (Hetzler, Kimura, Haines, Labotz, & Smith, 2006).

Skinfold Measurements   Skinfold measurements are performed using a caliper on up to eight sites on the body. Measurements are then used to estimate subcutaneous body fat. The most common site for skinfold measurement is the tricep skinfold. Other sites include specific points on the chest, abdomen, medial calf, upper thigh, and subscapular, supraailiac, and midaxillary sites. Professional grade calipers should be used. Plastic calipers are available but quickly become unreliable with use. The nurse should become practiced at doing skinfold measurements before reliably performing them on clients because specific technique is essential. Subsequent skinfold measurements on an individual should be repeated by the same clinician. When different clinicians perform an assessment on the same client, there is individual variability in measurements that will affect reliability and the ability to detect changes (Woodrow, 2009). On-line tutorials exist that demonstrate skinfold and other anthropometric measurements. Box 12-4 and Figure 12-5 ■ illustrate the tricep skinfold technique.

The best use of skinfold measurement results is in the monitoring of a client over time. Prior measurements serve as

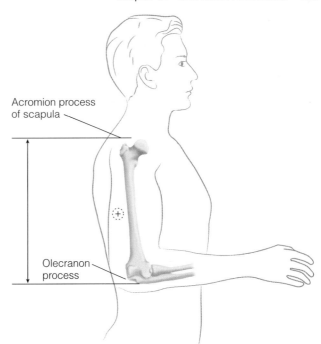

FIGURE 12-5 Site of Tricep Skinfold Measurement.

a self-reference against which client progress can be compared. The nurse should keep in mind that small and short-term changes are difficult to detect using skinfold measurements.

In addition to using serial skinfold measurements as a self-reference, measurements can be compared against reference values. Reference values exist for specific population groups and are age and gender specific. The nurse can compare the client's skinfold measurements with the reference value for the same measurement in a similar gender and age population group. These references are generally presented as percentiles. Age, fitness level, race, and gender each affect body composition and require specific reference values. Specific references for all groups do not exist, limiting the use of existing references. Older adults have loss of skin elasticity and changes in total body water, muscle mass, and fat distribution because of age; this change requires skinfold reference values that are unique to this population (Institute of Medicine [IOM], 2000; Kuczmarski, Kuczmarski, & Najjar, 2000; Woodrow, 2009). Lean muscle mass, fat distribution, and total body water are affected by disease states, such as renal failure or human immunodeficiency virus (HIV) infection (Aghdassi, Arendt, Salit, & Allard, 2007; DeLegge & Drake, 2007). Specific reference values should be used for these populations as well. More research is needed to develop additional reference values to represent the existing diverse population.

Circumference Measurements   Calf and midarm circumferences can be included in a body composition analysis. Measurements are done at the site of maximum calf width and the midpoint between the olecranon process and the acromium process, respectively. A spring-loaded measuring

---

BOX 12-4	Tricep Skinfold Technique

1. Instruct the individual to flex the right arm at a 90-degree angle for ease in finding the bony landmarks.
2. Measure length of the arm from the posterior edge of the acromium process to the olecranon process.
3. Establish and mark on the back of the arm the midpoint of that distance.
4. Instruct the individual to allow the arm to hang freely once marked.
5. Just above the marked site, grasp both the subcutaneous fat and skinfold layer between the thumb and forefinger, creating a fold parallel to the arm. Avoid grasping the underlying muscle by carefully pulling skinfold away from body.
6. Place the skinfold caliper perpendicular to the skinfold.
7. Grasp the skinfold with the caliper jaws while maintaining skinfold grasp with the other hand. Let go of the caliper's lever and read the measurement to the nearest 0.1 mm within few seconds.
8. Repeat the measurement at least once and average the results.

Source: Adapted from CDC, 2000 (Section 3.3.1.9 Skinfolds, pp. 3–34).

MyNursingKit National Center for Health Statistics: Skinfold and Anthropometric Measurements

Lifespan

Anthropometric Measurements across the Lifespan

Anthropometric measurements are an important part of a nutritional assessment, but lose their reliability when used incorrectly. Measurements intended for use in the adult, such as waist circumference, have no merit when used to assess nutritional health in a child. Likewise, head circumference should be used only up to age 3 years. Age and gender-specific body composition references are needed when using skinfold calipers or more advanced technology such as bioelectrical impedance analysis (BIA). Body composition changes across the lifespan; using references that are intended for a young adult to instead assess an older adult who has altered skin elasticity and loss of muscle will yield incorrect results.

tape is used. Measurement values are felt to reflect the relationship between body volume and body mass (Wagner & Heyward, 1999). Predictive equations based on the midarm circumference and tricep skinfold are used to estimate body fat and fat-free mass while correcting for the underlying bone.

Head circumference is measured in children up to age 3 years. This measurement is not part of an assessment of body composition, but rather an indirect measurement of nutritional health, growth, and development. Lifespan Box: Anthropometric Measurement across the Lifespan discusses the topic of anthropometric measurements and age.

Technology and Body Composition   Several noninvasive tools exist that measure body composition. Some require a laboratory setting and expensive equipment, whereas others are portable. Bioelectrical impedance analysis (BIA) is based on the principles of electroconduction. Electricity is conducted more easily through tissues with a high water and electrolyte content, such as muscle and body fluids, than through fat tissue. The original version of a BIA device used electrodes and a nonconductive table surface to measure conduction from foot to hand. There is less error associated with BIA than with skinfold measurements (Aghdassi et al., 2007). Newer handheld and standing versions are available that only measure conduction through the arm or leg segments. Hand-to-hand and leg-to-leg devices are not as accurate as traditional devices (Buchholz, Bartok, & Schoeller, 2004). The nurse working in sports medicine or wellness is likely to encounter these devices. Bathroom scales that measure body fat use this technology. Overhydration, including edema; dehydration; or altered skin temperature can cause measurement errors with BIA (DeLegge & Drake, 2007). The use of BIA is not recommended in individuals with a pacemaker because of the associated small electrical current (Lee & Gallagher, 2008).

Near-infrared interactance devices predict body fat by passing infrared light through tissue and measuring light reflection. The bicep is a common site used in this measurement. These devices are convenient handheld tools but have

a greater standard error than BIA or skinfold measurements, especially in the overweight person (DeLegge & Drake, 2007). These devices are often used in the wellness setting, such as at health fairs. The nurse should use population-specific predictive equations based on gender, fitness level, height, and weight.

Other methods for measuring body composition include underwater weighing, dual x-ray absorptiometry (DEXA), and plethysmography. These methods are more commonly utilized in the research rather than clinical setting because of high cost. Underwater weighing measures water displacement when the individual is completely submerged beneath the water. Predictive equations calculate body composition based on known densities of fat and fat-free tissue. DEXA is capable of measuring all components of body composition, including bone and total body water, unlike most other methods and uses x-ray technology. Plethysmography measures the body's composition via air displacement in a chamber called a BOD POD. Figure 12-6 ■ illustrates plethysmography being used on a client.

Body Fat Standards   Reference values for body composition are used to compare an individual to existing data gathered for a similar specific population. For example, reference values for body fat exist for various types of athletes as outlined in Chapter 11. Standards differ from references and should not be confused. A standard is a value that is believed to be a health target and is not the same as a population norm or reference value. Reference values for weight using BMI would reflect the distribution or underweight, normal weight, and overweight individuals in a population; this distribution differs from the recommended standard of "healthy" BMI of 20 to 24.9. Standards for total body fat specifically do not currently exist, but rather a range is recommended. The nurse should be careful not to

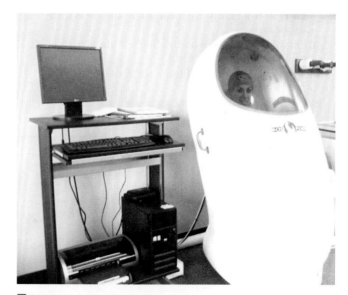

■ **FIGURE 12-6 Air Plethysmography.**

recommend a specific body fat target to an individual. Individual differences in essential fat and the known measurement error associated with predicting body composition make too specific a recommendation unreliable. In adults, a total body fat of 12% to 20% in males and 20% to 30% in females is recommended, but more population-specific research is yet to be published (Gallagher et al., 2000).

Physical Findings

When conducting the physical assessment of any individual, the nurse should be aware of any physical findings that impact nutritional status or indicate altered nutritional health. A head-to-toe assessment and review of systems yields important information. Findings such as poor dental health, swallowing difficulties, gastrointestinal complaints, limited strength, and alterations in cognition or vision problems negatively affect intake. Medical conditions and treatment can lead to nutritional challenges. Any functional or physical findings that impact nutrition status or are suggestive of an existing nutrition problem should be documented.

Physical changes related to altered nutritional health do not occur acutely. Any physical findings that are present indicate a nutritional issue that has been occurring for weeks, months, or longer. Deficiency of a fat-soluble vitamin is slow to manifest itself physically because of the storage of these vitamins in adipose tissue and the liver. Deficiency of water-soluble nutrients is more likely to occur sooner than fat-soluble nutrients because of limited body pools of these nutrients. Initially, deficiencies occur subclinically and are difficult to detect upon physical examination. Many of the physical findings that occur with poor nutritional health can also occur because of medical conditions or environmental effects. For example, hair texture and amount is affected with protein-calorie malnutrition, medications, and harsh hair treatments. Therefore, the nurse should combine the physical assessment with other nutritional parameters for a broader assessment. Use of the examination alone will not provide complete data for an accurate assessment. Table 12-7 outlines a review of physical findings and the possible nutritional implications. Further information about vitamin and mineral deficiencies is contained in Chapters 5 and 6.

Laboratory Assessment

No one laboratory measurement can uniquely assess nutritional status. The nurse should consider confounding medical conditions and laboratory value limitations when completing this portion of the nutritional assessment.

Plasma Proteins

Plasma proteins are synthesized in the liver and are often called **visceral proteins** along with the proteins found in organs. Albumin, prealbumin, and transferrin are plasma proteins that are commonly used as part of a nutritional assessment. Each of these proteins has a different half-life, or time span over which half the body pool breaks down. The nurse should recall that the shorter the half-life of the protein, the more current the reflection of visceral protein status. Additionally, these proteins are acute-phase reactant proteins that provide substrate to the body for reacting to the physiological stresses of infection or inflammation, such as with trauma, burns, or sepsis. As a result, during infection or inflammatory responses, these plasma proteins decrease unrelated to nutritional status.

Albumin is a routine laboratory value commonly used in a nutritional assessment. Normal plasma albumin is 3.5 gm/L to 5 gm/L. It has a long half-life (14 days to 21 days) and a large body pool, which detracts from its sensitivity as a marker of current nutritional status despite its wide use. Decreased plasma levels can be indicative of altered nutrition status as outlined in Table 12-8. It has been suggested that a slightly higher threshold of 3.8 gm/L be used to mark low normal albumin in the assessment of older adults because of the risk of undernutrition in that population (IOM, 2000). Albumin less than 3.5 mg/dL is associated with increased risk of morbidity and mortality in the older adult following discharge from the hospital (Carriere et al., 2008; Sullivan, Roberson, & Bopp, 2005). The nurse should be aware that any condition leading to dehydration or fluid overload will result in hemoconcentration or dilution, respectively, and a false measurement of albumin status. Additionally, disease states such as liver disease or nephrotic syndrome can lead to decreased albumin unrelated to nutritional status. Because of the many confounding variables affecting albumin, there are many who believe it is more an indicator of morbidity and mortality risk than an exclusive indicator of current nutrition status in adults and children (DeLegge & Drake, 2007; Horowitz & Tai, 2007; Horwich, Kalantar-Zadeh, MacLellan, & Fonarow, 2008).

Prealbumin is also called thyroxine-binding prealbumin or transthyretin. Normal plasma prealbumin is 150 mg/L to 350 mg/L. Similar alterations occur during inflammation or infection but to a lesser extent than seen with albumin. Prealbumin is felt to be a better nutrition screening tool, reflecting a more current picture of visceral protein status than albumin in part because of its shorter half-life of 2 to 3 days (Robinson et al., 2003). Like albumin, low prealbumin is associated with increased risk of morbidity and mortality in the older adult (Carriere et al., 2008).

Transferrin has a role in iron binding and transport in the body. Normal transferrin is above 200 mg/dL. The half-life of transferrin is 8 to 10 days, reflecting a more current picture of nutrition status than with albumin but less current than prealbumin. Transferrin levels are altered during physiological stress because of its role as an acute phase reactant protein, limiting its use as a true indicator of nutrition status under such conditions. Transferrin values derived in the laboratory from total iron-binding capacity value will be affected by low iron states.

Table 12-7 Overview of Nutritional Findings during Physical Assessment

System or Body Part	Clinical Finding	Examples	Potential Nutrient Deficiency
Hair	Dull, sparse, easily pluckable, brittle, **flag sign** (band of hair without pigment)	*Source:* Centers for Disease Control and Prevention (CDC)	Protein
	Alopecia		Protein, biotin, zinc
Eyes	Night blindness, blindness, foamy spots (**Bitot's spots**), dry and hard mucosa (**xerophthalmia**)	*Source:* Centers for Disease Control and Prevention (CDC)	Vitamin A
	Pale conjunctiva		Iron
Mouth	Cracks at corners of lips (angular stomatitis), inflamed lips (cheilosis)	*Source:* Centers for Disease Control and Prevention (CDC)	Riboflavin, niacin, pyridoxine
	Smooth, magenta or beefy red tongue (glossitis)	*Source:* Centers for Disease Control and Prevention (CDC)	Riboflavin, niacin, pyridoxine

Table 12-7 Overview of Nutritional Findings during Physical Assessment *(continued)*

System or Body Part	Clinical Finding	Examples	Potential Nutrient Deficiency
	Diminished taste buds (atrophic papillae)		Iron
	Complaint of diminished taste		Zinc
	Delayed eruption of teeth in children		Vitamin D
	Development of caries in infant or young child		Check if child is being put to bed with bottle (baby bottle tooth decay)
	Mottled enamel		Overexposure to fluoride
	Spongy, bleeding gums	*Source:* Centers for Disease Control and Prevention (CDC)	Vitamin C
Head and Neck	Facial pallor		Iron
	Moon face		Protein
	Increased thyroid size		Iodine
	Increased parotid size		Protein and calories, assess for bulimia
Skeleton/Trunk	Ascites		Protein
	Growth stunting		Protein and calories, zinc
	Rickets (bowed legs), widened epiphyses, narrow chest, rachitic rosary (beading on ribs)	*Source:* Centers for Disease Control and Prevention (CDC)	Vitamin D
	Muscle and fat wasting		Protein, calories
Limbs	Muscle and fat wasting		Protein, calories
	Edema of lower limbs	*Source:* Centers for Disease Control and Prevention (CDC)	Protein

(continued)

Table 12-7 Overview of Nutritional Findings during Physical Assessment *(continued)*

System or Body Part	Clinical Finding	Examples	Potential Nutrient Deficiency
Nails	Koilonychia (spoon-shaped nails), ridges in nails		Iron
Skin	Bruising		Vitamins C and K
	Pinpoint hemorrhages (petechiae)		Vitamin C
	Dry scaly skin		Vitamin A, essential fatty acids
	Follicular hyperkeratosis (goosebump flesh)		Vitamins A and C
	Poor wound healing		Protein, calories, vitamin C, zinc
	Symmetrical rash on sun-exposed areas only	*Source:* Centers for Disease Control and Prevention (CDC)	Niacin
Genitalia	Hypogonadism		Zinc
Nervous system	Hyporeflexia, confabulation, neuropathy		Thiamine
	Neuropathy, confusion, ataxia		Vitamin B$_{12}$
	Tetany		Calcium, magnesium
Cardiac	Tachycardia		Iron, folic acid, vitamin B$_{12}$
	Arrhythmia		Magnesium, potassium

Source: CDC, Public Health Image Library. (1970). Retrieved March 20, 2009, from http://phil.cdc.gov/phil/home.asp

Immunocompetence

An assessment of a client's immune status, or **immunocompetence,** can be included in a nutritional assessment. Undernutrition is associated with a decline in immune function, which can be reflected in laboratory assessments of the immune system. Many disease states and medications, such as HIV, autoimmune diseases, and chemotherapy also impact immune status, limiting the use of these parameters as nutritional indicators in these clients.

Total lymphocyte count (TLC) and delayed skin hypersensitivity testing are used to assess immunocompetence. Decreased TLC can indicate poor immunocompetence and potential malnutrition as outlined in Table 12-8. TLC is calculated using the white blood cell (WBC) count and lymphocyte percentage using the formula:

$$TLC = WBC \times \% \text{ lymphocytes}$$

Delayed skin hypersensitivity testing detects delayed or absent immune response to common antigens, such as streptococcus. An altered response can indicate poor immunocompetence, undernutrition, or simply lack of exposure to the antigen. Testing is done by administering intradermal injections of a panel of antigens while monitoring the injection sites for signs of hypersensitivity, such as induration and erythema, occurring within 48 hours. A positive reaction with induration of at least 0.5 cm is indicative of a good immune status. No response to the antigens despite known exposure is called **anergy** and indicates poor immune status.

Nitrogen Balance Assessment

A nitrogen balance assessment estimates the adequacy of dietary intake and is used in the monitoring of the nutrition status of an individual. A client is in nitrogen balance when nitrogen intake from protein equals nitrogen output by the

Table 12-8 Common Laboratory Measurements Used in Nutritional Assessment

Laboratory	Normal Value	Mild Malnutrition	Moderate Malnutrition	Severe Malnutrition	Half-life (days)	Nonnutritional Causes of Altered
Albumin	3.5–5 gm/L	2.8–3.4 gm/L	2.1–2.7 gm/L	Less than 2.1 gm/L	14–20	Inflammation, infection, liver disease, renal losses
Transferrin	200–400 mg/L	180–200 mg/L	160–180 mg/L	Less than 160 mg/L	8–10	Inflammation, infection, iron deficiency, liver disease, renal losses
Prealbumin	150–350 mg/L	110–150 mg/L	50–109 mg/L	Less than 50 mg/L	2–3	Inflammation, infection, liver disease, renal losses
Total lymphocyte count (TLC)	2,000–3,500 cells/ m³	1,200–1,500 cells/m³	800–1,200 cells/m³	Less than 800 cells/m³	N/A	Immune suppressive disease or treatment

Sources: Adapted from Beck & Rosenthal, 2002; Fuhrman, Charney, & Mueller, 2004; Omran & Morley, 2000; Shenkin, Cederblad, Ellia, & Isaksson, 1996.

body. Nitrogen output is measured with a 24-hour urine urea nitrogen; insensible nitrogen losses from hair, feces, and skin are accounted for in the nitrogen balance equation. Negative nitrogen balance arises when protein intake is low or nitrogen losses are high, or both. Negative nitrogen balance can occur with poor quantity or quality intake or **catabolism,** the breakdown of stored proteins by the body. **Anabolism,** or synthesis of tissue, requires a positive nitro-gen balance. Box 12-5 outlines the nitrogen balance equation and a sample calculation that a nutrition support nurse or dietitian uses.

Laboratory Measures of Nutrient Status

Laboratory values of select nutrients can be included in a nutrition assessment where available. Indices that screen for nutritional anemias should be included in a nutritional

---

BOX 12-5	Nitrogen Balance Calculations

Nitrogen balance studies can be used to estimate whether a client is receiving adequate nutrition. A client is said to be "in nitrogen balance" when nitrogen intake from protein and nitrogen output are equal. Negative nitrogen balance occurs when intake is too low or losses are too great and this leads to catabolism. Positive nitrogen balance occurs when intake exceeds losses, and tissue synthesis, or anabolism, is possible. Calculations will not be pertinent in clients with abnormal urine output, such as in renal failure.

Nitrogen balance = nitrogen in (from protein) – nitrogen losses (from urine and insensible loss)

Nitrogen in = calculation of 24-hour protein intake (gm) / 6.25 gm nitrogen per gram of protein

Nitrogen out = 24-hour urine urea nitrogen collection (UUN) + 4 gm nitrogen insensible loss

Example:

The nutrition support nurse suggests a nitrogen balance study for a client transitioning from a feeding tube to oral intake. The 24-hour intake from diet, liquids, and feeding formula is recorded by the nursing staff. A 24-hour urine collection is sent to the laboratory. The client is estimated to have consumed 120 gm protein. The 24-hour UUN reveals 10 gm nitrogen.

Nitrogen in = 120 gm protein / 6.25 gm nitrogen per gram protein = 19.2 gm nitrogen

Nitrogen out = 10 gm UUN + 4 gm insensible loss = 14 gm nitrogen

Nitrogen balance = 19.2 gm nitrogen in – 14 gm nitrogen out = positive nitrogen balance of 5.2 gm

 ▪ What level of protein intake would put this client in negative nitrogen balance?

assessment. Hemoglobin, hematocrit, red blood cell volume, and measures of folic acid and vitamin B_{12} status provide the nurse with useful information to include in the assessment.

Low serum cholesterol, defined as less than 160 mg/dL, is associated with frailty and risk of mortality in the older adult but debated by others as to its clinical use as a nutrition parameter (Okamura et al., 2008; Spada et al., 2007). Currently, the use of cholesterol-lowering medications limits the use of low serum cholesterol in many individuals as an independent indicator of undernutrition.

Plasma levels of many nutrients are not valid measures of nutrient status. For example, serum calcium accounts for only a small fraction of total body calcium and is not directly related to calcium intake. Although serum calcium is included in routine laboratory assays, it is evaluated for medical purposes and not as a routine part of a nutritional assessment. For other nutrients, measurement of the nutrients' total body pool cannot be measured via the plasma, but blood levels do reflect overall stores. Plasma vitamin C levels are an example (Mosdol, Erens, & Brunner, 2008). Measurement of plasma and tissue levels of most nutrients is generally reserved for research and is not a routine nutrition assessment practice. Use of hair analysis to assess nutrient status is a controversial topic and is outlined in Hot Topic Box: Hair Analysis of Mineral Status.

Laboratory Measurements Associated with Overnutrition

Hypercholesterolemia, defined as a serum cholesterol greater than 200 mg/dL, is associated with risk of cardiovascular disease and overnutrition. Elevated fasting triglyceride levels are also considered a cardiac risk factor. Increased fasting glucose and hemoglobin A1C levels are associated with glucose intolerance and diabetes and should be noted. Medical nutrition therapy for hyperlipidemia and diabetes are discussed in detail in the respective chapters dedicated to those diagnoses.

Oversupplementation with some dietary supplements affects platelet function and clotting time, especially in the client taking medications that also alter blood clotting. Vitamin E, ginkgo biloba, feverfew, and ginseng are examples. Alterations in clotting time should be noted in an assessment and the client should be questioned about supplement use. Chapters 24 and 25 outline the effects of dietary supplements on platelet function and discuss interactions between supplements and medications.

Cultural Considerations

Cultural competency is an important factor in providing effective health care. During the nutritional assessment, the nurse should be mindful of the influence that culture has on food and nutrition habits and also on the conduct of the assessment itself. During the focused interview, the nurse should ask specific questions about the influence of culture

hot Topic

Hair Analysis of Mineral Status

Laboratory Hair Analysis: Fact, Fiction, or Fraud?
Laboratory analysis of hair is used in forensic medicine to detect mineral or heavy metal contamination. The deaths of both President Andrew Jackson and Napoleon Bonaparte have been attributed by some to poisoning, supported by present-day analysis of hair strands indicating that they suffered from lead exposure and arsenic and cyanide poisoning, respectively (Deppisch, Centeno, Gemmel, & Torres, 1999; Kintz, Ginet, Marques, & Cirimele, 2007). Mercury poisoning can also be detected through hair analysis, though levels are not considered as accurate as those from blood or urine assays (Ng, Chan, Soo, & Lee, 2007). Many companies exist that will provide hair analysis and some sell vitamin and mineral supplements based on the laboratory findings. Almost $10 million is spent yearly on hair analysis in the United States (Seidel, Kreutzer, Smith, McNeel, & Gilliss, 2001). Should the use of laboratory hair analysis be a part of a comprehensive nutritional assessment?

The nurse should warn any individual considering hair analysis that ongoing evidence does not support its use as a part of a nutritional assessment (Barrett, 2001; Seidel et al., 2001; Steindel & Howanitz, 2001). A correlation between dietary intake of minerals and the amount found in hair is lacking (Gonzalez-Munoz, Pena, & Meseguer, 2008). Uniform standards for hair mineral content are not established. Environmental factors and hair treatment choices affect the analysis. Little research has been conducted about the relationship between mineral content of the hair and overall mineral status (Seidel et al., 2001). The American Medical Association (AMA) opposes the use of hair analysis in determining the need for medical therapy and believes the potential for health care fraud exists with this practice (AMA, 2004).

on food beliefs and practices. The nurse should not make assumptions about how an individual belonging to any cultural or religious population adheres to generalized beliefs. Food and health beliefs vary within and among ethnic groups and the nurse should inquire about how an individual interprets and practices these beliefs. Acculturation can influence nutrition practices of individuals who have immigrated to a new country and adopted some or many new food habits. Cultural Considerations Box: Cultural Considerations with a Nutrition Assessment outlines key points for the nurse to consider during the nutrition assessment.

Cultural and religious beliefs can influence the physical assessment portion of the nutritional assessment. Beliefs that discourage touch by members of the opposite gender or the removal of certain garments present obstacles to the gathering of anthropometric measurements and the physical examination. The nurse should ask the client or a translator about the presence of these issues and explain the physical assessment process before attempting to begin this portion of the nutritional assessment. In some cases, the nurse may

Cultural Considerations

Cultural Considerations with a Nutrition Assessment

Culture can influence food and health beliefs and practices. The nurse should take into consideration any of these influences when gathering data for a nutritional assessment.

Assess for:

- Core foods in the diet.
- Food preparation methods and types of ingredients used, such as type of fat for frying.
- Dietary laws observed such as kosher, vegetarian, or vegan practices or avoidance of other specific foods.
- Use of fasting as part of religious observation. Assess frequency and duration of fast.
- Foods consumed as part of traditional celebrations or religious observations.
- Foods believed to have health or curative powers (such as consuming "hot" foods to balance "cold" health conditions, yin and yang foods, or foods felt to assist with childbirth).
- Use of dietary supplements, including herbs and other plant products.
- Influence of family on reinforcing cultural practices.
- Changes in diet because of acculturation; note healthful and unhealthful changes like addition of fats, processed foods, extra sugar, and elimination of traditional healthy foods.

need to seek assistance from another nurse of the same gender as the client; in other cases, certain portions of the assessment may need to be modified to accommodate the client's beliefs. The nurse should engage in decision making with the client about how to proceed when these issues are present.

Nutrition Screening and Assessment Tools

Incorporation of a nutrition screening or assessment tool into the nursing process can streamline the identification of nutritionally at-risk individuals. Screening tools are not meant to diagnose malnutrition or overnutrition, but rather serve to identify factors associated with nutritional problems and deserving of further assessment. Screening tools generally can be performed by most members of a health care team in a variety of settings (ADA, 1994). In contrast, assessment tools are used to determine nutritional status. Many screening and assessment tools exist and new tools are constantly being developed. No consensus exists on the most reliable parameters to measure in a nutritional assessment or on an absolute definition of malnutrition; this contributes to the ongoing quest for the most effective tool. When choosing to use a screening or assessment tool, the nurse should choose one that is population specific and has research supporting it as both reliable and valid for its intended use. Screening tools mistakenly

used instead for nutritional assessment or assessment tools used in an unintended population can lead to missed diagnoses and delayed nutrition intervention.

Malnutrition Universal Screening Tool (MUST)

The Malnutrition Universal Screening Tool (MUST) is a nutrition screening tool for use in adults. This instrument is supported by evidence-based research that validates its use (Anthony, 2008). Only three parameters are part of this quick screen: BMI, weight history, and the effect of disease on ability to take oral nutrition. Clients at risk of malnutrition are either monitored or referred to a dietitian, depending on level of risk. An on-line version of the tool is available that contains instructions and scoring.

MyPyramid

MyPyramid, the food guide pyramid that is based on the *Dietary Guidelines for Americans*, was not developed as a nutritional screening or assessment tool, but it can easily be used to provide a quick assessment of intake using a food record or diet recall. The nurse can compare an individual's intake to the quantity and distribution of food groups recommended within MyPyramid for a general assessment of the reported diet. MyPyramid can be used as a quick point of reference by the nurse conducting an estimate of dietary intake in adults and children.

In health care settings with access to the Internet, an interactive tool utilizing MyPyramid can be used by the nurse and as a teaching tool for the client seeking to improve intake.

Tools for Use in Older Adults

Older adults are at a disproportionate risk of malnutrition compared with other age groups. The aging process and medical conditions and treatments are among the reasons this disparity exists. Chapter 15 discusses undernutrition in the older adult in detail. Screening and assessment tools have been developed in an effort to address the incidence of undernutrition in this population.

Nutrition Screening Initiative

The Nutrition Screening Initiative (NSI) consists of three tools aimed at improving the routine nutrition screening and assessment of older adults in the community (NSI). This broad-based public health strategy was developed by the American Academy of Physicians, the American Dietetic Association, and the National Council on Aging. One of the three tools is a checklist using the mnemonic DETERMINE and is intended for exclusive use as a screening tool. Nine risk factors for undernutrition are surveyed in the checklist: **D**isease, **E**ating poorly, **T**ooth loss/mouth pain, **E**conomic hardship, **R**educed social contact, **M**ultiple medications,

MyNursingKit DETERMINE Tool

MyNursingKit Mini Nutrition Assessment (MNA)

BOX 12-6	Minimum Data Set Nutrition Parameters

Section G 1h Eating:
Assess how the resident eats and drinks (regardless of skill). Include source of nutrients from feeding tube, parenteral nutrition. Note if feeding assistance is required or not.

Section K: Oral/Nutritional Status

K1.	ORAL PROBLEMS	Chewing problem		a.
		Swallowing problem		b.
		NONE OF ABOVE		d.
K2.	HEIGHT AND WEIGHT	*Record (a.) height in inches and (b.) weight in pounds. Base weight on most recent measure in last 30 days; measure weight consistently in accord with standard facility practice—e.g., in a.m. after voiding, before meal, with shoes off, and in nightclothes*		
		a. HT (in.)	b. WT (lb.)	
K3.	WEIGHT CHANGE	a. Weight loss—5% or more in last 30 days, or 10% or more in last 180 days 0. No 1. Yes		
		b. Weight gain—5% or more in last 30 days, or 10% or more in last 180 days 0. No 1. Yes		
K5.	NUTRITIONAL APPROACHES	*(Check all that apply in last 7 days)*		
		Parenteral/IV	a.	On a planned weight change program	h.
		Feeding tube	b.	*NONE OF ABOVE*	i.
K6.	PARENTERAL OR ENTERAL INTAKE	*(Skip to Secton M if neither 5a or 5b is checked)* a. Code the proportion of total calories the resident received through parenteral or tube feedings in the last 7 days 0. None 3. 51% to 75% 1. 1% to 25% 4. 76% to 100% 2. 26% to 50%		
		b. Code the average fluid intake per day by IV or tube in last 7 days 0. None 3. 1001 to1500 cc/day 1. 1 to 500 cc/day 4. 1501 to 2000 cc/day 2. 501 to 1000 cc/day 5. 2001 or more cc/day		

Source: Centers for Medicare and Medicaid Services (CMS), 2000 (Chapter 3 MDS Sections G & K).

Involuntary weight loss/gain, **N**eeds assistance with self-care, **E**lder years above age 80 years. The *Determine Your Nutritional Health Checklist* can be filled out by the older adult or by those interacting with older adults in the community, such as at a congregate meal site. The checklist should not be used in the in-patient setting because it is not validated for that use (Sahyoun, Jacques, Dallal, & Russell, 1997). Individuals with high scores are encouraged to seek nutritional health advice.

Minimum Data Set

The Minimum Data Set (MDS) is used in all Medicare-certified health care institutions as a component of the Resident Assessment Instrument (Centers for Medicare and Medicaid Services [CMS], 2000). Nutritional parameters are included in the MDS and must be assessed on a regular basis as mandated. Additionally, any nutritional status change in a client warrants a full reassessment and response by the health care team (IOM, 2000). Box 12-6 outlines the MDS criteria pertaining to nutritional status.

Mini Nutrition Assessment

The Mini Nutrition Assessment (MNA) is an assessment tool validated for use with the older adult (Guigoz, 2006). The nurse working with older adults in a variety of health care and community settings can use the MNA as a routine and quick assessment tool to evaluate nutritional status. Anthropometric measurements and general physical and nutritional assessment questions comprise the tool. A Web-based version of the tool is available in many languages for use in settings with easy Internet access, such as an office, a clinic, or home care.

| NURSING CARE PLAN | Nutrition Assessment for Weight Management |

CASE STUDY

Louis is a 55-year-old married man who has dropped by the clinic's yearly health fair to find out about weight loss planning. His only daughter is getting married in 8 months and his wife has been asking him about losing some weight before the big event. He works as a laborer at a meat packing plant and has health insurance. He states that he is entitled to one checkup a year but he has not taken advantage of that for several years because he is in good health and does not want "to raise the cost of health care" any more than necessary. He says he is 5'10" tall and weighs about 220 pounds, "give or take a couple." His weight has been stable in recent years, but he admits he rarely steps on a scale and acknowledges that he might be "a bit overweight." He says he needs to eat "a lot" to keep up his energy for work and because he simply likes to eat almost anything. Activities outside work hours include only sedentary pastimes such as watching television or playing cards. He asks for some kind of diet plan so he can lose about 40 pounds before the wedding.

Applying the Nursing Process

ASSESSMENT

BMI based on stated data: 31.6
Measured height: 5 feet 9.5 inches Measured weight:
   235 pounds Measured BMI: 34.3
BP 152/86 P 78 R18
Waist measurement: 54 inches

DIAGNOSES

Imbalanced nutrition: more than body requirements related to greater caloric intake versus expenditure
Readiness for enhanced nutrition related to request for a diet plan

EXPECTED OUTCOMES

Weight loss of 1 pound per week; approximately 30 pounds by the time of the wedding
Verbalization of meal plans for weight reduction
Participation in daily physical activity

INTERVENTIONS

More complete nutrition history with 24-hour food recall and weight and dieting history
Keep a food and activity diary for 1 week
Preliminary reduction of dietary intake by 500 calories per day with referral to a dietitian for more detailed dietary advice
Obtain laboratory values to assess general health and risk for overnutrition
Increase physical activity following medical clearance; begin by reducing time watching television and sitting at home

EVALUATION

Louis answers the phone call from the nurse 2 months later. He has decided not to follow through on the visit to the dietitian and states that he "knows what he has to do" to lose weight based on the information from the nurse. Besides, he says it is a waste of good money to return to the clinic for checkups when he can just call in his weight. He says he has lost a "few" pounds. The nurse explains that it important to have accurate measurements to track health status and that laboratory work and a thorough nutrition history is part of the assessment plan. Louis says he will do the best he can and get back to the nurse with any questions or problems. Figure 12-7 ■ outlines the nursing process for this case.

Critical Thinking in the Nursing Process

1. **How can the nurse respond to the client who states that he knows his height and weight because he weighs himself weekly and therefore does not need to get weighed at the clinic?**

2. **What are the minimum data that the nurse should gather as part of a health screening?**

(continued)

NURSING CARE PLAN

Nutrition Assessment for Weight Management *(continued)*

Assessment
Data about the patient

Subjective
What the patient tells the nurse
Example: I am a bit overweight and need to lose 40 pounds for my daughter's wedding in 8 months.

Objective
What the nurse observes; anthropometric and clinical data
Examples: Height: 5 feet, 9 inches; Weight: 235 pounds; BMI: 34.3; Waist 54 inches; BP: 152/86; Cholesterol: 262

Diagnosis
NANDA label
Example: Imbalanced nutrition: more than body requirements related to caloric intake exceeding caloric expenditure

Planning
Goals stated in patient terms
Example: Long-term goal: 40-pound weight loss in 8 months; Short-term goal: lose 1-2 pounds per week; participate in daily physical activity of choice

Implementation
Nursing action to help patient achieve goals
Example: Refer to dietitian; reduce intake by 500 kcal per day

Evaluation
Was the goal achieved or does the intervention need to be modified?
Example: Declined referral to dietitian; has lost "a few" pounds; not interested in follow-up

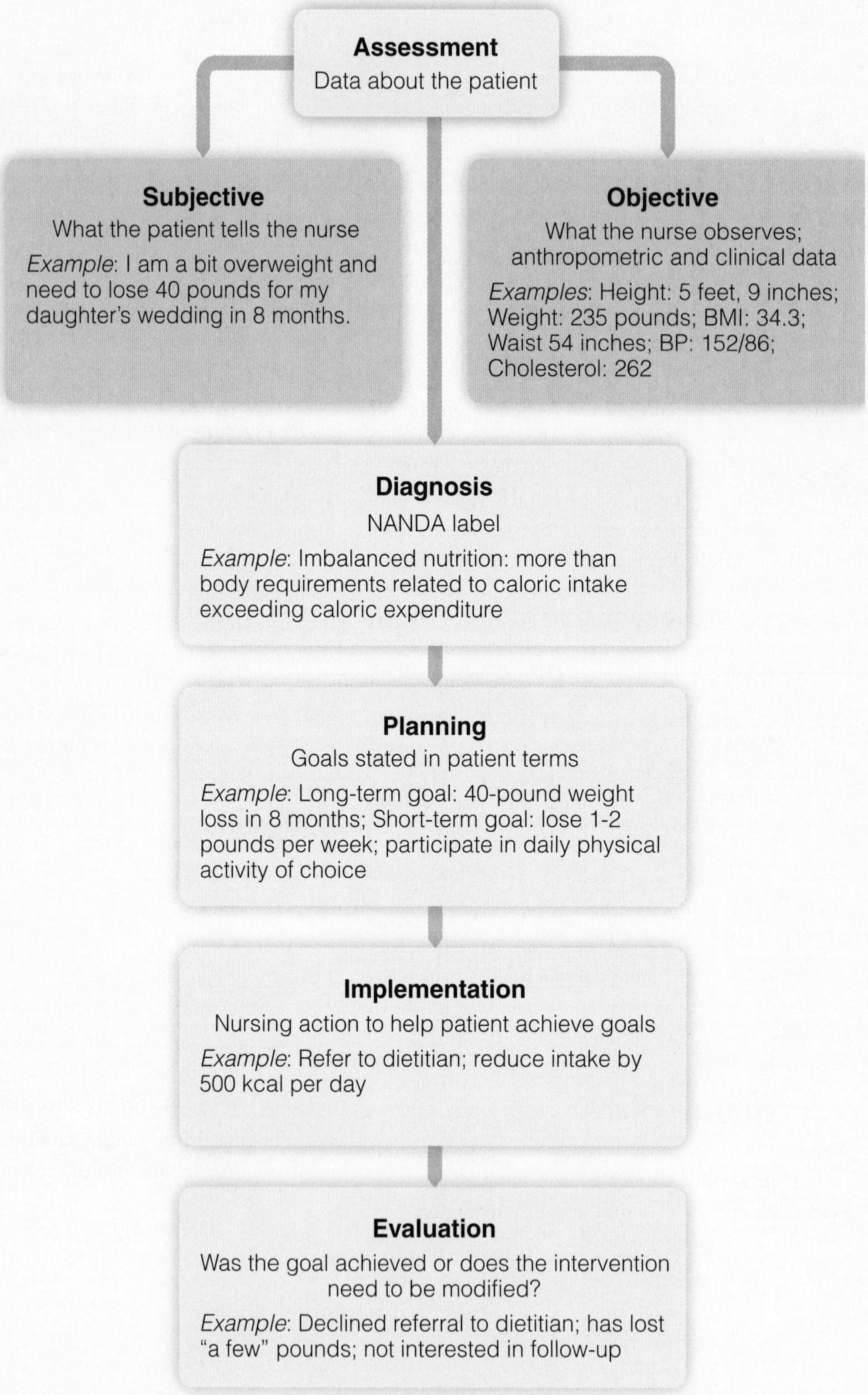

■ FIGURE 12-7 **Nursing Care Plan Process: Nutrition Assessment for Weight Management.**

CHAPTER SUMMARY

- A nutrition assessment is an important component of a nursing assessment.

- Components of a nutrition assessment include a nutrition history, a physical assessment, and evaluation of laboratory values.

- No single component used in an assessment uniquely reflects nutritional health. The nurse is urged to use more than one component when conducting an assessment.

- A nutrition history includes a diet recall, food frequency questionnaire, food record, and the focused interview.

- Physical assessment of nutrition status includes both anthropometric measurements, such as weight, height, and body composition measures and a head-to-toe review of systems.

- Most laboratory values used to assess nutritional status are affected by other conditions such as medical conditions or treatment. The nurse should consider factors that will confound laboratory results.

- Validated tools exist that the nurse can use to streamline nutrition screening or assessment. Attention must be given to choose a tool that is appropriate for its intended use.

PEARSON

EXPLORE **mynursingkit**™

MyNursingKit is your one stop for online chapter review materials and resources. Prepare for success with additional NCLEX®-style practice questions, interactive assignments and activities, web links, animations and videos, and more!

Register your access code from the front of your book at www.mynursingkit.com.

NCLEX® QUESTIONS

1. When using a nomogram to determine a client's body mass index (BMI), the nurse should be aware that:
   1. It is the most accurate assessment of weight in relation to height that is available.
   2. It may represent a muscular athlete as overweight.
   3. It does not factor in the metabolic rate of the individual.
   4. It is useful to determine if an individual is pear shape or apple shape.

2. When analyzing data from a nutritional assessment of a middle-age female client, which of the following would suggest to the nurse that the client is underweight?
   1. Waist measurement of 25 inches
   2. Hematocrit of 39
   3. BMI of 19
   4. Presence of fine wrinkles on the face

3. During a routine screening, the nurse determines that a middle-age male client has a BMI of 33. An appropriate nursing diagnosis for this client would be:
   1. Risk for obesity, related to above-normal BMI
   2. Imbalanced nutrition, related to excessive caloric intake
   3. Risk for altered metabolism, related to advancing age
   4. Imbalanced nutrition, related to deficient knowledge

4. An elderly client who comes to the clinic and has difficulty standing reports a height of 5 feet 8 inches and weight of 150 pounds. The nurse should:
   1. Record the values as "height and weight reported by the client"
   2. Assist the client to stand on the scale so an accurate measure of height and weight can be obtained
   3. Use a bed scale for weight and take a supine measurement of height
   4. Use a chair scale for weight and a knee height measurement for height

5. While evaluating a client for malnutrition, the nurse wants to gather which of the following data?
   1. Fasting blood glucose
   2. Albumin
   3. Serum cholesterol
   4. Serum triglyceride

REFERENCES

Aghdassi, E., Arendt, B., Salit, I. E., & Allard, J. P. (2007). Estimation of body fat mass using dual-energy x-ray absorptiometry, bioelectrical impedance analysis, and anthropometry in HIV-positive male subjects receiving highly active retroviral therapy. *Journal of Parenteral and Enteral Nutrition, 31*, 135–141.

American Dietetic Association, Council on Practice Quality Management Team. (1994). Identifying patient at risk: ADA's definitions for nutrition screening and nutrition assessment. *Journal of the American Dietetic Association, 94*, 838– 839.

American Medical Association (AMA). (2004). *Policy H-175.955 Hair analysis—a potential for medical abuse*. Retrieved March 20, 2009, from http:www.ama-assn.org

American Medical Directors Association (2001). *Altered nutritional status: Clinical practice guideline*. Washington, DC: Author.

Anthony, P. S. (2008). Nutrition screening tools for hospitalized patients. *Nutrition in Clinical Practice, 23*, 373–382.

Avila-Funes, J. A., Gutierrez-Robledo, L. M., & Ponce De Leon Rosales, S. (2004). Validity of height and weight self-report in Mexican adults: Results from the national health and aging study. *The Journal of Nutrition, Health & Aging, 8*, 355–361.

Ball, S. D., Kertesz, D., & Moyer-Mileur, L. J. (2005). Dietary supplement use is prevalent among children with chronic illness. *Journal of the American Dietetic Association,105*, 78–84.

Barrett, S. (2001). *Commercial hair analysis: A cardinal sign of quackery*. Retrieved March 21, 2009, from http://www.quackwatch.org/01QuackeryRelatedTopics/hair.html

Beck, F. K., & Rosenthal, T. C. (2002). Prealbumin: A marker for nutritional evaluation. *American Family Physician, 65*, 1575–1578.

Brener, N. D., Eaton, D. K., Lowry, R., & McManus, T. (2004). The association between weight perception and BMI among high school students. *Obesity Research, 12*, 1866–1874.

Brener, N. D., McManus, T., Galuska, D. A., Lowry, R., & Wechsler, H. (2003). Reliability and validity of self-reported height and weight among high school students. *Journal of Adolescent Health, 32*, 281–287.

Brunner-Huber, L. R. (2007). Validity of self-reported height and weight in women of reproductive age. *Maternal and Child Health Journal, 11*, 137–144.

Buchholz, A. C., Bartok, C., & Schoeller, D. A. (2004). The validity of bioelectrical impedance models in clinical populations. *Nutrition in Clinical Practice, 19*, 433–446.

Carriere, I., Dupuy, A. M., Lacroux, A., Cristol, J. P., Delcourt, C., & Pathologies oculaires liees a l'age study group. (2008). Biomarkers of inflammation and malnutrition associated with early death in healthy elderly people. *Journal of the American Geriatric Society, 56*, 840–846.

Centers for Disease Control and Prevention (CDC), National Center for Health Statistics. (2000). *Anthropometry procedures manual*. Retrieved March 21, 2009, from http://www.cdc.gov/nchs/data/nhanes/nhanes_01_02/body_measures_year_3.pdf

Centers for Disease Control and Prevention (CDC). (2009). *Defining childhood overweight and obesity*. Retrieved March 21, 2009, from http://www.cdc.gov/obesity/childhood/defining.html

Centers for Medicare and Medicaid Services (CMS). (2000). *Minimum data set (version 2.0)*. Retrieved March 21, 2009, from http:/www.cms.hhs.gov/medicaid/mds20/mds0900b.pdf

Charney, P. (2008). Nutrition screening vs. nutrition assessment: How do they differ? *Nutrition in Clinical Practice, 23*, 366–372.

Chima, C. S., Dietz-Seher, C., & Kushner-Benson, S. (2008). Nutrition risk screening in acute care: A survey of practice. *Nutrition in Clinical Practice, 23*, 417–423.

Cunningham, E. (2004). Is body mass index for children and adolescents assessed differently than for adults? *Journal of the American Dietetic Association, 104*, 694.

DeLegge, M. H., & Drake, L. M. (2007). Nutritional assessment. *Gastroenterology Clinics of North America, 36*, 1–22.

Deppisch, L. M., Centeno, J. A., Gemmel, D. J., & Torres, L. (1999). Andrew Jackson's exposure to mercury and lead: Poisoned president? *Journal of the American Medical Association, 282*, 569–571.

Engstrom, J. L., Paterson, S. A., Doherty, A., Trabulsi, M., & Speer, K. L. (2003). Accuracy of self-reported height and weight in women: An integrative review of the literature. *Journal of Midwifery and Women's Health, 48*, 338–345.

Foster, B. J., & Leonard, M. B. (2004). Measuring nutritional status in children with chronic kidney disease. *American Journal of Clinical Nutrition, 80*, 801–814.

Fuhrman, M. P., Charney, P., & Mueller, C. M. (2004). Hepatic proteins and nutrition assessment. *Journal of the American Dietetic Association, 104*, 1258–1264.

Gallagher, D., Heymsfield, S. B., Heo, M., Jebb, S. A., Murgatroyd, P., & Sakamoto, Y. (2000). Healthy percentage body fat ranges: An approach for developing guidelines based on body mass index. *American Journal of Clinical Nutrition, 72*, 694–701.

Gardiner, P., Buettner, C., Davis, R. B., Phillips, R. S., & Kemper, K. J. (2008). Factors and common conditions associated with adolescent dietary supplement use: An analysis of the National Health and Nutrition Exam Survey (NHANES). *BMC Complementary and Alternative Medicine, 31*, 9.

Gillum, R. F., & Sempos, C. T. (2005). Ethnic variations in validity of classification of overweight and obesity using self-reported weight and height in American women and men: The Third National Health and Nutrition Examination Survey. *Nutrition Journal, 4*, 27.

Gonzalez-Munoz, M. J., Pena, A., & Meseguer, I. (2008). Monitoring heavy metal contents in food and hair sample of young Spanish subjects. *Food & Chemical Toxicology, 46*, 3048–3052.

Goodman, E., Hinden, B. R., & Khandelwal, S. (2000). Accuracy of teen and parental reports of obesity and body mass index. *Pediatrics, 106*, 52–58.

Guigoz, Y. (2006). The Mini Nutrition Assessment (MNA) review of the literature—what does it tell us? *Journal of Nutrition, Health & Aging, 10*, 466–485.

Harnack, L., Steffen, L., Arnett, D. K., Gao, S., & Luepker, R. V. (2004). Accuracy of estimation of large food portions. *Journal of the American Dietetic Association, 104*, 804–806.

Hauck, F. R., White, L., Cao, G., Woolf, N., & Strauss, K. (1995). Inaccuracy of self-reported weights and heights among American Indian adolescents. *Annals of Epidemiology, 5*(5), 386–392.

Hetzler, R. K., Kimura, I. F., Haines, K., Labotz, M., & Smith, J. (2006). A comparison of bioelectrical impedance and skinfold measurements in determining minimum wrestling weights in high school wrestlers. *Journal of Athletic Training, 41*, 46–51.

Horowitz, I. N., & Tai, K. (2007). Hypoalbuminemia in critically ill children. *Archives of Pediatric and Adolescent Medicine, 161*, 1048–1052.

Horwich, T. B., Kalantar-Zadeh, K., MacLellan, R. W., & Fonarow, G. C. (2008). Albumin levels predict survival in patients with systolic heart failure. *American Heart Journal, 155*, 883–889.

Institute of Medicine (IOM). (2000). *The role of nutrition in maintaining health in the nation's elderly: Evaluating coverage of nutrition services for the Medicare population*. Washington DC: National Academies Press.

Jacobson, B. H., & DeBock, D. H. (2001). Comparison of body mass index by self-reported versus measured height and weight. *Perceptual and Motor Skills, 92*, 128–132.

Jansen, W., van de Looij-Jansen, P. M., Ferreira, I., de Wilde, E. J., & Brug, J. (2006). Differences in measured and self-reported height and weight in Dutch adolescents. *Annals of Nutrition & Metabolism, 50*, 339–346.

REFERENCES   *(continued)*

Jensen, G. L., Friedmann, J. M., Henry, D. K., Skipper, A., Beiler, E., Porter, C., et al. (2003). Noncompliance with body weight measurement in tertiary care teaching hospitals. *Journal of Parenteral and Enteral Nutrition, 27*, 89–90.

Kelly, J. P., Kaufman, D. W., Kelley, K., Rosenberg, L., Anderson, T. E., & Mitchell, A. A. (2005). Recent trends in use of herbal and other natural products. *Archives of Internal Medicine, 165*, 281–286.

Kintz, P., Ginet, M., Marques, N., & Cirimele, V. (2007). Arsenic speciation of two specimens of Napoleon's hair. *Forensic Science International, 170*, 204–206.

Kristal, A. R., Andrilla, H. A., Koepsell, T. D., Diehr, P. H., & Cheadle, A. (1998). Dietary assessment instruments are susceptible to intervention-associated response set bias. *Journal of the American Dietetic Association, 98*, 40–43.

Kuczmarski, M. F., Kuczmarski, R. J., & Najjar, M. (2000). Descriptive anthropometric reference data for older Americans. *Journal of the American Dietetic Association, 100*, 59–66.

Kuczmarski, M. F., Kuczmarski, R. J., & Najjar, M. (2001). Effects of age on validity of self-reported height, weight and body mass index: Findings from the Third National Health and Nutrition Examination Survey 1988–1994. *Journal of the American Dietetic Association, 101*, 28–34.

Lean, M. J., & Han, T. S. (2002). Waist worries. *American Journal of Clinical Nutrition, 76*, 699–700.

Lear, S. A., Humphries, K. H., Kohli, S., & Birmingham, C. L. (2007). The use of BMI and waist circumference as surrogates of body fat differs by ethnicity. *Obesity, 15*, 2817–2824.

Lee, S. Y., & Gallagher, D. (2008). Assessment methods in human body composition. *Current Opinion in Clinical Nutrition and Metabolic Care, 11*, 566–572.

Livingstone, M. B., & Black, A. E. (2003). Markers of the validity of reported energy intake. *Journal of Nutrition, 133*, 895S–920S.

Luft, V. C., Beghetto, M. G., Castro, S. M., & deMello, E. D. (2008). Validation of a new method developed to measure the height of adult patients in bed. *Nutrition in Clinical Practice, 23*, 424–428.

Miller, T. M., Abdel-Maksoud, M. F., Crane, L. A., Marcus, A. C., & Byers, T. E. (2008). Effects of social approval bias on self-reported fruit and vegetable consumption: A randomized controlled study. *Nutrition Journal, 27*, 18.

Morrissey, S. L., Whetstone, L. M., Cummings, D. M., & Owen, L. J. (2006). Comparison of self-reported and measured height and weight in eighth grade students. *Journal of School Health, 76*, 512–515.

Mosdol, A., Erens, B., & Brunner, E. J. (2008). Estimated prevalence and predictors of vitamin C deficiency within U.K.'s low-income population. *Journal of Public Health, 30*, 456–460.

National Heart, Lung, and Blood Institute (NHLBI). (n.d). *Guidelines on overweight and obesity: Electronic textbook.* Retrieved March 17, 2009, from http://www.nhlbi.nih.gov/guidelines/obesity/e_txtbk/index.htm

National Heart, Lung, and Blood Institutes (NHLBI), Obesity Education Initiative Expert Panel (1998). *Clinical guidelines on the identification, evaluation and treatment of overweight and obesity in adults: The evidence report.* Retrieved March 21, 2009, from http://www.nhlbi.nih.gov/guidelines/obesity/ob_gdlns.pdf

Nawaz, H., Chan, W., Abdulrahmann, M., Larson, D., & Katz, D. L. (2001). Self-reported weight and height: Implications for obesity research. *American Journal of Preventative Medicine, 20*, 294–298.

Nevitt, J. R., & Lundak, J. (2005). Accuracy of self-reports of alcohol offenders in a rural midwestern county. *Psychology Reports, 96*, 511–514.

Ng, D. K., Chan, C. H., Soo, M. T., & Lee, R. S. (2007). Low-level chronic mercury exposure in children and adolescents: Meta-analysis. *Pediatrics International, 49*, 80–87.

Norman, K., Pichard, C., Lochs, H., & Pirlich, M. (2008). Prognostic impact of disease-related malnutrition. *Clinical Nutrition, 27*, 5–15.

Nyholm, M., Gullberg, B., Merlo, J., Lundqvist-Persson, C., Rastam, L., & Lindblad, U. (2007). The validity of obesity based on self-reported weight and height: Implications for population studies. *Obesity (Silver Spring), 15*, 198–208.

Okamura, T., Hayakawa, T., Hozawa, A., Kadowaki, T., Murakami, Y., Kita, Y., et al. (2008). Lower levels of serum albumin and total cholesterol associated with decline in activities of daily living and excess mortality in a 12-year cohort study of elderly Japanese. *Journal of the American Geriatric Society, 56*, 529–535.

Omran, M. L., & Morley, J. E. (2000). Assessment of protein-energy malnutrition in older persons, part II: Laboratory evaluation. *Nutrition, 16*, 131–140.

Osterkamp, L. K. (1995). Current perspective on assessment of human body proportions of relevance to amputees. *Journal of the American Dietetic Association, 95*, 215–218.

Qato, D. M., Alexander, G. D., Conti, R. M., Johnson, M., Schumm, P., & Lindau, S. T. (2008). Use of prescription and over-the-counter medications and dietary supplements among older adults in the United States. *Journal of the American Medical Association, 300*, 2867–2878.

Robinson, M. K., Trujillo, E. B., Mogensen, K. M., Rounds, J., McManus, K., & Jacobs, O. (2003). Improving nutritional screening of hospitalized patients: The role of prealbumin. *Journal of Parenteral and Enteral Nutrition, 27*, 389–395.

Rossouw, K., Senekal, M., & Stander, I. (2001). The accuracy of self-reported weight by overweight and obese women in an outpatient setting. *Public Health Nutrition, 4*, 19–26.

Sahyoun, N. R., Jacques, P. F., Dallal, G. E., & Russell, R. M. (1997). Nutrition Screening Initiative checklist may be a better awareness/educational tool than a screening one. *Journal of the American Dietetic Association, 97*, 760–764.

Scagliusi, F. B., Ferriolli, E., Pfrimer, K., Laureano, C., Sanita Cunha, C., Gualano, B., et al. (2008). Underreporting of energy intake in Brazilian women varies according to dietary assessment: A cross-sectional study using doubly labeled water. *Journal of the American Dietetic Association, 108*, 2031–2040.

Seidel, S., Kreutzer, R., Smith, D., McNeel, S., & Gilliss, D. (2001). Assessment of commercial laboratories performing hair analysis. *Journal of the American Medical Association, 285*, 67–72.

Shenkin, A., Cederblad, G., Ellia, M., & Isaksson, B. (1996). Laboratory assessment of protein energy status. *Clinica Chimica Acta, 253*, S5–S59.

Singh, S. R., & Levine, M. A. (2006). Natural health product use in Canada: Analysis of the National Population Health Survey. *Canadian Journal of Clinical Pharmacology, 13*, e240–e250.

Spada, R. S., Toscano, G., Cosentino, F. I., Iero, I., Lanuzza, B., Tripodi, M., et al. (2007). Low total cholesterol predicts mortality in the nondemented oldest old. *Archives of Gerontology & Geriatrics, 44*, 381–384.

Spencer, E. A., Appleby, P. N., Davey, G. K., & Key, T. J. (2002). Validity of self-reported height and weight in 4808 EPIC-Oxford participants. *Public Health Nutrition, 5*, 561–565.

Steindel, S. J., & Howanitz, P. J. (2001). The uncertainties of hair analysis for trace metals. *Journal of the American Medical Association, 285*, 83–85.

Sullivan, D. H., Roberson, P. K., & Bopp, M. M. (2005). Hypoalbuminemia 3 months after hospital discharge: Significance for long-term survival. *Journal of the American Geriatric Society, 53*, 1222–1226.

Taylor, A. W., Dal Grande, E., Gill, T. K., Chittleborough, C. R., Wilson, D. H., Adams, RJ., et al. (2006). How valid are self-reported height and weight? A comparison between CATI self-report and clinic measurements using a large cohort study. *Australia and New Zealand Journal of Public Health, 30*, 238–246.

REFERENCES *(continued)*

Tokmakidis, S. P., Christodoulos, A. D., & Mantzouranis, N. I. (2007). Validity of self-reported anthropometric values used to assess body mass index and estimate obesity in Greek school children. *Journal of Adolescent Health, 40*, 305–310.

Tsigilis, N. (2006). Can secondary school students' self-reported measures of height and weight be trusted? An effect size approach. *European Journal of Public Health, 16*(5), 532–535.

United States Department of Health and Human Services (USDHHS), Maternal Child Health Bureau. (n.d.). *Accurately weighing and measuring infants, children and adolescents: Equipment.* Retrieved March 21, 2009, from http://depts.washington.edu/growth/index.htm

Wagner, D. R. & Heyward, V.H. (1999). Techniques of body composition assessment:

A review of laboratory and field methods. *Research Quarterly for Exercise and Sport, 70,* 135–149.

Walker, S., & Cosden, M. (2007). Reliability of college student self-reported drinking behavior. *Journal of Substance Abuse Treatment, 33,* 405–409.

Wang, Z., Patterson, C. M., & Hills, A. P., (2002). A comparison of self-reported and measured height, weight and BMI in Australian adolescents. *Australia and New Zealand Journal of Public Health, 26,* 473–478.

Wen, C. P., David Cheng, T. Y., Tsai, S. P., Chan, H. T., Hsu, H. L., Hsu, C. C., et al. (2009). Are Asians at greater mortality risk for being overweight than Caucasians? Redefining obesity for Asians. *Public Health Nutrition, 12,* 497–506.

Willett, W. C., Dietz, W. K., & Colditz, G. A. (1999). Guidelines for healthy weight. *New England Journal of Medicine, 341,* 427–434.

Woodrow, G. (2009). Body composition analysis techniques in the aged adult: Indications and limitations. *Current Opinion in Clinical Nutrition and Metabolic Care, 12,* 8–14.

World Health Organization (WHO). (1999). *Management of malnutrition: A manual for physicians and other senior healthcare workers.* Retrieved February 28, 2005, from http://www.who.int/nutrition/publications/severemalnutrition/en/manage_severe_malnutrition_eng.pdf

Zhang, C., Rexrode, K. M., van Dam, R. M., Li, T. Y., & Hu, F. B. (2008). Abdominal obesity and the risk of all-cause, cardiovascular, and cancer mortality: Sixteen years of follow-up on U.S. women. *Circulation, 117,* 1658–1667.

Pregnancy and Lactation 13

WHAT WILL YOU LEARN?

1. To relate the importance of preconception nutrition to factors associated with healthy pregnancy outcomes.

2. To examine the macro- and micronutrients required during pregnancy and lactation.

3. To translate appropriate nutrition interventions for medical conditions that affect both diet and pregnancy outcome.

4. To compare the nutritional recommendations for pregnant females who have unique needs, such as adolescents or vegetarians, with general nutrition recommendations.

5. To formulate nursing interventions for improving nutritional intake during pregnancy and lactation.

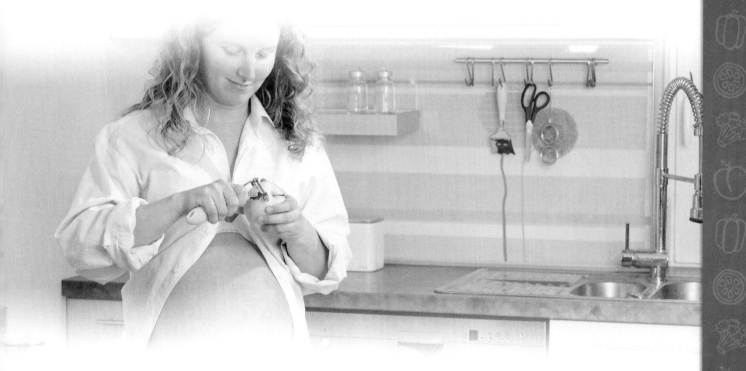

DID YOU KNOW?

▶ Neural tube defects develop in the first weeks of pregnancy when many females are unaware of the pregnancy.

▶ Unusual cravings for nonfood items, such as dirt, during pregnancy can be related to iron deficiency.

▶ Alcohol is absorbed into the fetal bloodstream and metabolized at a slower rate than that of the mother, leading to many detrimental effects on the infant.

▶ Pregnant and lactating females should restrict intake of high mercury seafood because of negative effects on fetal and infant brain development.

279

KEY TERMS

Pregnancy

The gift and the responsibility of bearing and nurturing a new human being are incredible. Although people may be excited by the prospect of bringing a new person into the world, they can also be overwhelmed. Thus, during pregnancy, the support of a health care professional can truly be a lifeline. The nurse is ideally situated to provide the knowledgeable guidance and reassurance that is profoundly needed by prospective parents.

The dietary and lifestyle habits of a woman prior to pregnancy can have substantial effects on the health and wellness of her child. Unfortunately, many females of childbearing years are not actively engaged in healthy lifestyle practices commensurate with optimal pregnancy outcome, and many do not receive appropriate preventive health care that targets reproduction. This lack of preparation is not surprising, given that approximately 50% of pregnancies in the United States are unplanned (Finer & Henshaw, 2006). The importance of preconception health care intervention has been formally recognized by the Centers for Disease Control and Prevention (CDC) with published recommendations. These recommendations address several aspects of women's health related to lifestyle and nutrition, including obesity, diabetes, folic acid deficiency, and alcohol use (Johnson et al., 2006). One of the most important avoidable conditions that can influence a woman's reproductive success is overweight/obesity, affecting over 50% of women in the United States between the ages of 20 and 39 years (Ogden et al., 2006). Obesity can decrease fertility and negatively affect pregnancy outcome, which is discussed further in the Wellness Concerns section of this chapter. Attempted weight loss with nutritionally inadequate or fad diets prior to pregnancy can set the stage for poor nutritional health that can later lead to adverse pregnancy outcomes if not corrected. It is essential that health risks associated with poor pregnancy outcome are addressed before conception in females of childbearing age. For example, adequate folic acid intake is needed to decrease risk of neural tube defects, a birth defect that affects brain and spinal cord development, yet intake of this vitamin is often inadequate

among females of childbearing age (American Dietetic Association [ADA], 2008). Iron and calcium intake are also often suboptimal. Box 13-1 outlines factors for the nurse to consider when discussing preconception nutritional health.

Nutritional Needs

Maternal nutrition during pregnancy influences infant health. Adequate nutrition to support fetal development includes sufficient kcalories for needed maternal weight gain. Sufficient macro- and micronutrients intake is a part of the necessary foundation on which to build a healthy pregnancy.

Energy

Energy requirements during pregnancy are based on the kcalories required to support maternal weight gain. Adequate weight gain is essential in order to provide the energy and substrates needed for fetal growth and development, including associated needs such as the placenta, amniotic fluid, and new maternal tissue. The expectant female will require additional dietary intake to develop expanded volumes of blood and extracellular fluid, new uterine and mammary tissue, and fat stores to support the pregnancy, as depicted in Figure 13-1 ■. The combined energy requirement for new protein and fat tissue exceeds 40,000 kcalories in a normal weight female who gains the recommended amount of weight during the pregnancy (Institute of Medicine [IOM], 2005). During the first trimester, kcalorie requirements are not substantially different than for nonpregnant females, but an additional daily intake of 340 kcalories and 452 kcalories are needed during the second and third trimesters, respectively (IOM, 2005). The nurse can use the whole foods approach to ensuring that adequate energy needs are met from a variety of foods while also providing the recommended intake of nutrients. MyPyramid, the Department of Agriculture's interactive Web-based tool for nutrition education, contains a *MyPyramid for Moms* component that is ideal for educating the pregnant female about nutritional needs. Individualized plans can be developed that meet energy and nutrient requirements based on height, weight, age, physical activity level, and pregnancy trimester. Figure 13-2 ■ depicts a sample of this tool.

MyNursingKit MyPyramid for Moms

BOX 13-1	**Preconception Nutritional Health Considerations**

- *Body weight:* Both overweight and underweight can affect fertility and pregnancy outcome. Achievement of a healthy weight is recommended before pregnancy.
- *Folic acid intake:* Recommendation for all females of childbearing age is 400 mcg/day to reduce the risk of neural tube defects that develop very early in pregnancy.
- *Iron intake:* Iron needs increase significantly during pregnancy. Low iron status before pregnancy increases the risk of iron deficiency during pregnancy, which negatively affects the fetus. Females with closely spaced pregnancies should have extra attention paid to iron status, especially if adherence to iron supplementation in the past is in question.
- *Dietary supplement use:* Little is known about the safety of dietary supplements such as herbs and botanicals on fetal development and health during pregnancy. Clients should be advised to only take prescribed vitamins and minerals unless there is demonstrated proof of supplement safety. Excess vitamin A should be avoided.
- *Fad diets:* Restrictive weight loss diets before pregnancy can cause limited food intake and missing nutrients in the diet. For example, a low-carbohydrate diet lacks sufficient grains, fruits, and dairy foods to supply needed B-vitamins, including folic acid, vitamins C and D, and calcium. A diet that contains all food groups or sufficient alternatives is recommended as the foundation of a healthy diet.
- *Alcohol:* Alcohol intake during pregnancy is associated with poor pregnancy outcomes. Abstinence is recommended. Education about alcohol intake during pregnancy should begin before pregnancy. Excessive intake of alcohol before pregnancy can place the mother at increased risk of nutrient deficiencies related to alcohol, such as thiamin and folate.
- *Medical conditions:* Medical conditions that require nutritional intervention should be under optimal control before pregnancy to minimize maternal and fetal health risks. Examples include diabetes mellitus and phenylketonuria.

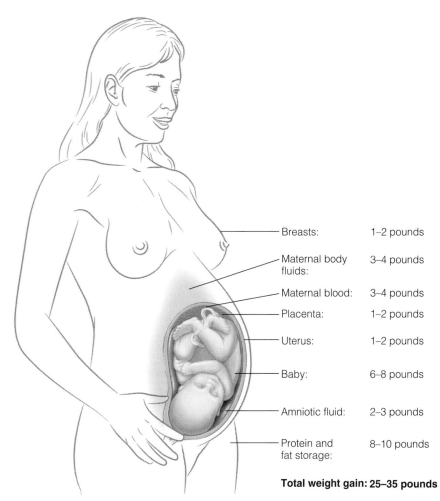

Breasts:	1–2 pounds
Maternal body fluids:	3–4 pounds
Maternal blood:	3–4 pounds
Placenta:	1–2 pounds
Uterus:	1–2 pounds
Baby:	6–8 pounds
Amniotic fluid:	2–3 pounds
Protein and fat storage:	8–10 pounds

Total weight gain: 25–35 pounds

■ FIGURE 13-1 **Pregnancy Weight Gain Distribution.**

Food Group	1st Trimester	2nd and 3rd Trimesters	What counts as 1 cup or 1 ounce?	Remember to...
	Eat this amount from each group daily.*			
Fruits 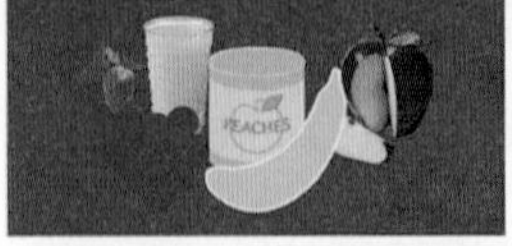	2 cups	2 cups	1 cup fruit or juice ½ cup dried fruit	*Focus on fruits—* Eat a variety of fruits.
Vegetables 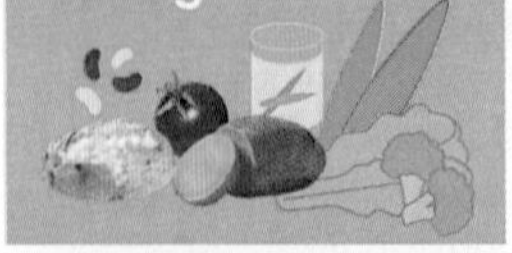	2½ cups	3 cups	1 cup raw or cooked vegetables or juice 2 cups raw leafy vegetables	*Vary your veggies—* Eat more dark-green and orange vegetables and cooked dry beans.
Grains 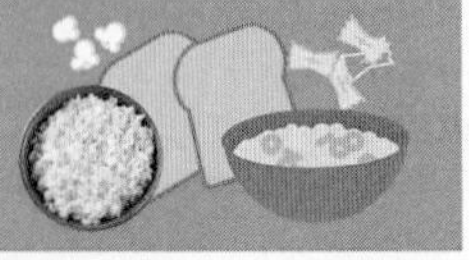	6 ounces	8 ounces	1 slice bread 1 ounce ready-to-eat cereal ½ cup cooked pasta, rice, or cereal	*Make half your grains whole—*Choose whole instead of refined grains.
Meat & Beans 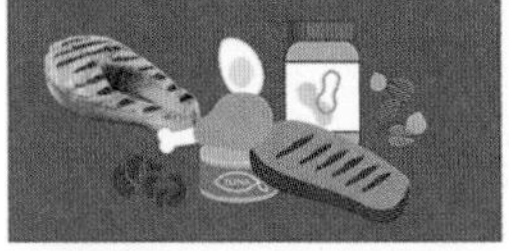	5½ ounces	6½ ounces	1 ounce lean meat, poultry, or fish ¼ cup cooked dry beans ½ ounce nuts or 1 egg 1 tablespoon peanut butter	*Go lean with protein—* Choose low-fat or lean meats and poultry.
Milk 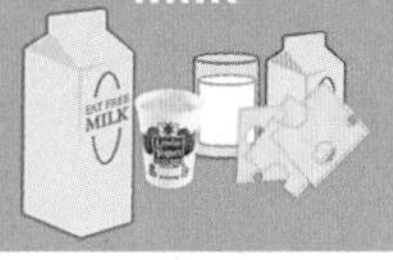	3 cups	3 cups	1 cup milk 8 ounces yogurt 1½ ounces cheese 2 ounces processed cheese	*Get your calcium-rich foods—*Go low-fat or fat-free when you choose milk, yogurt, and cheese.

■ FIGURE 13-2 **MyPyramid for Moms: Pregnancy.**

Source: United States Department of Agriculture, MyPyramid for Moms. Retrieved March 25, 2009, from www.nal.usda.gov/wicworks/Topics/PregnancyFactSheet.pdf

What Is the Recommended Weight Gain?

Weight gain guidelines during pregnancy are based on providing adequate energy and nutrition for a healthy birth weight. Initial recommendations were developed over a decade ago when the primary goal was to avoid a low birth weight and its associated health risks. A more recent increase in birth weight, maternal obesity, and concern about long-term risks of excess weight has brought to light the need to reevaluate long-standing recommendations (IOM, 2009). Excessive prenatal weight gain can lead to postpartum retention of excess weight and risk of large-for-gestational-age infants, postdelivery medical complications in the infant, and overweight later in childhood (ADA, 2008; Mehta, 2008).

Inadequate maternal weight gain remains a health risk despite the more recent concern of excess weight gain and obesity. Inadequate weight gain is associated with small-for-gestational age, or low birth weight, infants. Additionally, low prepregnancy maternal weight is associated with insufficient weight gain, low birth weight, and increased risk of preterm delivery (Cox & Phelan, 2008). Additional risks for inade-

quate gestational weight gain include smoking, low socioeconomic or education status, substance abuse, low dairy intake, anorexia nervosa, domestic violence, unplanned pregnancy, and a short interval between pregnancies (IOM, 2009).

Recommendations for weight gain should be individualized. Factors to consider include prepregnancy weight and risk of a low birth weight infant. Minimal weight gain is necessary during the first trimester. During the second and third trimesters, weight gain approximates 1 lb/week, particularly during weeks 20 to 30 when maternal fat accrual peaks (IOM, 2009). African American and adolescent females are at increased risk of delivering a low birth weight infant compared with the general population and are advised to gain a higher amount of weight during pregnancy. Lifespan Box: Nutritional Needs with Adolescent Pregnancy discusses the issue of adolescent pregnancy and nutritional needs. The recommendations for weight gain during pregnancy are outlined in Table 13-1. No clear-cut guidelines exist regarding weight gain pattern with multiple fetuses. Box 13-2 discusses nutrition and multiple pregnancies.

Lifespan

Nutritional Needs with Adolescent Pregnancy

The pregnant adolescent, especially those age 16 years or younger, has competing nutritional needs to support maternal growth and development along with those for the developing fetus. Ages 12 to 15 years are a period of rapid growth in the female and supporting the additional nutritional needs of a fetus presents a challenge to many. Additionally, the adolescent diet frequently lacks sufficient iron, folic acid, and calcium, which can negatively affect fetal development.

The average birth weight in an adolescent pregnancy is lower than in an older female. Additionally, the risk of miscarriage and premature delivery with associated infant morbidity and mortality are higher in this population.

Nutrition intervention has been reported to improve pregnancy outcome in adolescent pregnancy. The nurse can educate the pregnant adolescent about the importance of adequate weight gain over the course of the pregnancy. Excess weight gain should be minimized because it is associated with retention of that weight gain after pregnancy in the growing adolescent. Up to 50% of pregnant adolescents continue to grow while pregnant and excess weight gain in this group is associated with increased fat deposition. Adolescents who do not meet weight gain guidelines may do so at the expense of both maternal linear growth and infant birth weight. Guidelines used for weight gain during pregnancy are based on adult BMI categories. This issue presents a challenge when assessing weight gain recommendations in the adolescent because BMI assessment is done using percentiles in this age group and adult classification of BMI is not valid. The health care team needs to individually assess the appropriate weight gain for the adolescent rather than solely rely on the adult guidelines.

Micronutrient requirements for the pregnant adolescent mirror those of the pregnant adult female with the exception of calcium. The growing teen requires 1,300 mg of calcium/day because linear height and bone mass gains are crucial in this age span. The nurse can assess intake of calcium along with adherence to iron and prenatal vitamin supplementation to encourage intake of adequate micronutrients to support the needs of both the adolescent and fetus.

Sources: ADA, 2008; Cox & Phelan, 2008; Pencharz, 2005; Wallace et al., 2006.

Protein, Carbohydrate, and Fat

The increase in energy needs during pregnancy should come from a variety of macronutrients in order to provide needed kcalories as well as building blocks for new tissue using protein, fat, and carbohydrate. The dietary reference intake (DRI) for protein increases by 25 gm during pregnancy (IOM, 2005). In general, this increase is easily met using the whole foods approach outlined in MyPyramid for Moms (ADA, 2008). Lean meats, poultry, fish, and legumes provide protein as well as needed iron. Dairy proteins such as milk, yogurt, and cheese provide needed calcium as well.

Table 13-1 Weight Gain in Pregnancy

Body Mass Index (BMI)	Recommended Weight Gain (lb)
Less than 18.5	28–40
18.5–24.9	25–35
25.0–29.9	15–25
Greater than 29.9	11–20
Twins	35–45
Adolescents and African American females	Weight gain should be at the upper range for body mass index (BMI)

Source: IOM, 2009.

Carbohydrate intake is essential during pregnancy to meet the need for glucose by both the mother and fetus. A minimum of 175 gm/day of carbohydrate is needed during pregnancy in contrast to the 130 gm/day minimum for non-pregnant females (IOM, 2005). The nurse should stress the importance of this minimum as a necessary intake to provide glucose for the fetal brain, especially with a client who has a history of following a low-carbohydrate diet.

Fat is an essential component of the diet during pregnancy just as it is throughout the lifespan. Essential fatty acids are needed for cell membranes and are crucial during growth and development. Of particular interest is docosahexaenoic acid (DHA), an omega-3 fatty acid, which is used for growth and function of nervous and visual tissue. DHA is

BOX 13-2	**Nutrition with Multiple Pregnancies**

Nutritional health during multiple pregnancies is crucial because of the risk of premature birth and low birth weight. Although no widespread recommendations exist for any difference in nutrient intake, weight gain recommendations are different for multiple pregnancies, and sufficient energy is required to achieve weight goals. It is recommended that weight gain for twins target 35–45 lb and triplets target 50 lb with a 1.5 lb/week gain starting early in the pregnancy. A general practice is to recommend an additional 150 to 500 kcals/day above normal pregnancy needs for twins to achieve adequate weight gain at week 28 of pregnancy, a weight gain pattern that is associated with optimal pregnancy outcomes. Research is lacking regarding the need for vitamins and minerals during multiple pregnancies. Iron deficiency is more common with multiple pregnancies and is associated with preterm delivery. The nurse can urge adherence to iron supplementation and use of a prenatal vitamin in addition to a well-balanced diet to optimize nutrient intake.

Sources: Klein, 2005; Marcason, 2006; Rosello-Soberon, Fuentes-Chaparro, & Casanueva, 2005.

synthesized from the essential fat linolenic acid and is also found in the foods we eat; thus the amount of DHA in a mother's diet determines how much DHA is available to a fetus. DHA is accrued during gestation in brain cells and retinal membranes, especially during the last trimester of pregnancy (Jensen, 2006). Reduced DHA may be associated with impairments in cognitive and behavioral performance, effects that are particularly important during brain development. Higher maternal intake of DHA during pregnancy is reported in some, but not all, studies to be associated with modest improvements in visual acuity and neurodevelopment in infants (Cetin & Koletzko, 2008; Jensen, 2006). The conversion of linolenic acid to DHA is increased during pregnancy. This change provides DHA to the developing fetus and a source of the fat in breast milk (Innis, 2005). No spe-

cific evidence-based recommendation exists regarding the daily amount of DHA needed in the diet, though the inclusion of two deep, cold-water fish meals per week is believed to provide the 200 to 300 mg/day suggested by many (Cetin & Koletzko, 2008; Jensen, 2006).

Vitamins and Minerals

Intake of several vitamins and minerals has been demonstrated to be inadequate in females of childbearing age as well as those who are pregnant or lactating. Calcium, folic acid, and iron intakes, all important during pregnancy, are among those identified as suboptimal in this population (ADA, 2008). It is important for the nurse to assess intake of these nutrients during prenatal health care and to offer advice on improving intake when indicated. In particular, the nurse

---

BOX 13-3	Vegetarianism during Pregnancy and Lactation

A well-planned vegetarian diet can support the needs of pregnant and lactating females and result in healthy outcomes for the mother and infant. A vegan diet, where no animal products are consumed, can result in similar positive outcomes but requires more attentive planning to include some potentially limited nutrients that are crucial for the developing fetus and breastfed infant. The nurse should assess the intake of the following nutrients in a pregnant or lactating female who follows a vegetarian or vegan diet:

Vitamin B_{12}

Vitamin B_{12} is only found in foods of animal origin. Many case reports exist of infants developing neurological symptoms from deficiency of the vitamin within months after birth related to poor maternal intake during pregnancy or lactation. Growth failure, anemia, and developmental abnormalities can follow. The vitamin B_{12} available to the fetus and breastfed infant is related more to maternal intake of the vitamin than maternal stores. Thus, a reliable, current dietary source of intake is needed throughout pregnancy and breastfeeding. Sources include foods fortified with the vitamin, such as cereals and soy products; multivitamin or synthetic B_{12} supplement; and nutritional yeast. Vegetarians who consume eggs, milk, and other dairy foods are getting a reliable source of vitamin B_{12} in those foods.

Vitamin D and calcium

Adequate vitamin D and calcium intake is essential for fetal and maternal needs during pregnancy and lactation. Traditional sources of vitamin D include fortified milk and sun exposure. A vegan diet does not contain any natural source of vitamin D and must rely on a dietary supplement or vitamin D-fortified foods, such as some soy milks, juices, and cereals, for a dietary source of the vitamin. Calcium sources in the vegan diet include kale, bok choy, collards, and calcium-fortified soy products. The high oxalate and phytate content of plant sources of calcium limit the bioavailability of the mineral for absorption from many

other plant foods. Vegetarians who consume three servings of milk, yogurt, or cheese daily have adequate intake of calcium. Vitamin D needs can be met if milk or fortified yogurt is consumed, but fortification of cheese is not common practice. A multivitamin would provide the recommended vitamin D. All infants, including those who are breastfed by vegetarian or vegan females, need a supplemental form of vitamin D because of the low vitamin D content of breast milk and unfortified infant formulas. The vitamin D content of breast milk is insufficient for the infant even with maternal supplementation. Mothers who have inadequate vitamin D intake during pregnancy are at highest risk of having an infant develop rickets soon after birth.

Iron

Although iron needs are increased during pregnancy and plant-based sources of iron are less well absorbed than animal sources, the prevalence of iron deficiency in vegetarians is not significantly different than among all pregnant females. The same recommendation exists for iron supplementation in pregnant vegetarian females as in those who consume animal products. Consumption of a vitamin C source along with plant-based iron can boost iron absorption. Examples include tomato sauce, orange juice, and green leafy vegetables. Plant-based iron sources include iron-fortified cereals, legumes, dried fruit, and whole grains.

Essential fatty acids

DHA is found primarily in animal sources. Vegetarian and vegan females need to consume the precursor to this essential fatty acid, linolenic acid, in order to obtain a preliminary source of this fat touted for its effects on brain and retina development. Breast milk of vegetarian and vegan females has less DHA than nonvegetarians but increases with improved intake. Flaxseed, canola oil, walnuts, and soy are sources of linolenic acid. Some females choose to take a vegetarian dietary supplement of DHA made from microalgae.

Sources: ADA, 2003; Dror & Allen, 2008; Misra, Pacaud, Petryk, Collett-Solberg, & Kappy, 2008; Penney & Miller, 2008.

should note any restrictive eating patterns that have the potential to limit nutrient intake. Examples include a history of prenatal dieting, therapeutic diets for a medical condition, and vegetarianism. Box 13-3 discusses the specific nutrients that may be of concern with a vegetarian diet.

Folate and Folic Acid

Folate needs increase during pregnancy because of the role that the vitamin plays in cell division, specifically involving nucleic acid synthesis and the increase in red blood cell volume of the mother and fetus. The recommended dietary allowance (RDA) for folate during pregnancy is 600 mcg/day, an increase from the 400 mcg/day recommendation for females of childbearing age (IOM, 1998). The *Dietary Guidelines for Americans* also recommends an intake of 600 mcg/day, urging that it be consumed as the synthetic form of the vitamin, folic acid, which is more bioavailable than folate (United States Department of Agriculture [USDA], 2005). Folic acid is found in supplements and fortified foods, whereas folate is the natural form of the vitamin present in food. Folate is found in green leafy vegetables, oranges, and legumes such as dried beans.

Adequate folic acid intake is associated with a protective effect against neural tube defects, malformations associated with birth defects such as spina bifida and anencephaly where the neural tube that forms the spinal cord and brain fails to close properly during fetal development. Folic acid fortification of white flour began in the United States in 1998 as part of a public health initiative aimed at reducing neural tube de-

fects. Since mandatory folic acid fortification began, maternal blood folate levels were initially increased and rates of neural tube defects were decreased but not eliminated (Cox & Phelan, 2008). More recently, plasma folate levels have fallen in females of childbearing age, especially among non-Hispanic black women (ADA, 2008). The nurse should stress the importance of adherence to folic acid supplementation when advising the female of childbearing age about diet. A multivitamin or fortified food containing 400 mcg/day should be part of the diet until conception, when the need for increased intake quickly occurs. The nurse can instruct the client to check the nutrition fact panel on foods and supplements to determine the folic acid content. Figure 13-3 ■ is an example from a vitamin label. Neural tube defects occur early in pregnancy, hence the broad recommendation to all females of childbearing age to consume adequate intake of the vitamin before pregnancy occurs and then especially in the first trimester of pregnancy (USDA, 2005). The Client Education Checklist: Folate and Folic Acid Intake outlines advice that the nurse can offer when educating a client about folate and folic acid intake.

Vitamin D and Calcium

Adequate intake of vitamin D and calcium during pregnancy is essential for the development of fetal bones and teeth. However, the DRIs for these nutrients do not increase during pregnancy because of increased absorption of calcium, especially during the last two trimesters of pregnancy when calcium transfer to the fetus is increased (IOM, 1997; Kovacs, 2008). In the absence of adequate calcium intake or poor absorption of the mineral because of inadequate vitamin D status, calcium is mobilized from the maternal skeleton during pregnancy to meet the needs of the developing fetus. Low maternal vitamin D plasma levels are associated with low birth weight infants, premature labor, and infants born with poor vitamin D stores (Misra et al., 2008). Rickets can develop in weeks to months in the infant with poor vitamin D status (Kovacs, 2008). The recommended intake for calcium is 1,000 mg/day in adults age 19 to 50 years, and 1,300 mg/day in adolescents (IOM, 1997). Vitamin D intake should be 5 mcg/day (IOM, 1997).

The nurse should assess intake of both calcium and vitamin D in the pregnant female and note risk factors for poor status of these nutrients. Lactose intolerance with avoidance of dairy foods, a vegan diet, and other types of restrictive eating can limit intake of both vitamin D and calcium. Additionally, limited exposure to the sun should be noted whether from cultural practices such as veiling for religious purposes, use of high SPF sunscreen, living in northern latitudes, or remaining indoors. Limited sun exposure lessens vitamin D synthesis by the skin. Vitamin D deficiency is more common among darker skin individuals than those with lighter skin because of decreased synthesis of the vitamin from the sun, and this risk is found among pregnant females as well (Misra et al.,

Supplement Facts
Serving Size: 1 tablet

Amount Per Serving		% Daily Value
Vitamin A	5000IU	100
Vitamin C	60mg	100
Vitamin D	400IU	100
Vitamin E	30IU	100
Thiamin	1.5mg	100
Riboflavin	1.7mg	100
Niacin	20mg	100
Vitamin B$_6$	2mg	100
Folic Acid	400mcg	100
Vitamin B$_{12}$	6mcg	100
Biolin	30mcg	10
Pantothenic Acid	10mg	100
Calcium	162mg	16
Iron	18mg	100
Iodine	150mcg	100
Magnesium	100mg	25
Zinc	15mg	100
Selenium	20mcg	100
Copper	2mg	100
Manganese	3.5mg	175
Chromium	65mcg	54
Molybdenum	150mcg	200
Chloride	72mg	2
Potassium	80mg	2

Find **folic acid.** Choose a vitamin that says "400 mcg" or "100%" next to folic acid.

■ **FIGURE 13-3 Folic Acid on a Label.**

CLIENT EDUCATION CHECKLIST	Folate and Folic Acid Intake
Intervention	**Example**
Assess intake of folate and folic acid.	Folate is the form of the vitamin found in foods, such as green leafy vegetable, oranges, and legumes. Folic acid is the supplemental form of the vitamin found in fortified foods and white flour products.
Educate the client about the role of folic acid in prevention of birth defects.	Folic acid is involved in cell division. Adequate intake is associated with a decreased risk of neural tube defects, birth defects that result from incomplete development of the brain or spinal column.
Outline the need for folic acid.	All females of childbearing age are recommended to consume 400 mcg/day of folic acid from a fortified food or supplement. The need increases to 600 mcg/day during pregnancy. Folate intake can supplement this level of folic acid intake.
Offer specific recommendations for folic acid sources.	Folic acid is present in multivitamins, fortified cereals, and in all products made from white flour.

2008). Chapters 5 and 6 Client Education Checklists outline pointers for the nurse to use when teaching about vitamin D and calcium.

Iron

Iron needs increase substantially during pregnancy because of the increased maternal blood volume and red blood cell mass and the iron needs of the fetus, placenta, and umbilical cord. The RDA for iron during pregnancy is 27 mg/day compared with the 18 mg/day recommended for a nonpregnant female age 19 to 50 years (IOM, 2000). Supplementation is recommended because this amount of dietary iron is difficult to obtain on a daily basis (ADA, 2008). Chapter 6 reviews dietary sources of iron and contains a Client Education Checklist that the nurse can use when offering advice to the pregnant female about improving iron intake and absorption. Additionally, those individuals who consume both a calcium and an iron supplement should be mindful of the interaction between the two nutrients when consumed together. Practice Pearl: Calcium and Iron Supplements discusses this interaction.

When insufficient iron intake occurs during pregnancy, transfer of iron continues to the fetus at the expense of the mother's iron stores. However, iron deficiency and iron-deficiency anemia during pregnancy affect both the mother and fetus. Low birth weight, preterm delivery, and infant mortality risk are all increased as a result of maternal iron deficiency (ADA, 2008; Milman, 2008). Iron deficiency affects about 25% of pregnant females with a higher prevalence found among minority and low-income populations (ADA, 2008; Cox & Phelan, 2008; Milman, 2008). Pregnant adolescents have the highest prevalence of iron deficiency among all populations of pregnant females (American College of Obstetricians and Gynecologists [ACOG], 2008). Poor adherence to supplementation, poor quality diet, multiple pregnancies, and short intervals between pregnancies increase the risk for iron deficiency.

PRACTICE PEARL

Calcium and Iron Supplements

Pregnant females often take both a calcium supplement and an iron supplement. Calcium needs during pregnancy are 1,000 mg/day, which some females take in supplement form. The body does not efficiently absorb more than 500 mg of calcium in a single dose, so these supplements should be taken at separate times of the day. To complicate matters, iron and calcium share some mechanisms of absorption and should not be taken together in supplement form or iron absorption will be diminished. The nurse can brainstorm with the pregnant female appropriate dosing of these supplements to avoid these absorption issues. Many females find it easy to remember to take a supplement when timing is linked to an existing activity, such as brushing teeth, or a meal that occurs at home, such as breakfast.

Assessment of iron intake should be included in the nursing assessment of the pregnant female.

Pica, the consumption of nonfood items, can be found during pregnancy and is often associated with iron deficiency. It is under debate whether the deficiency leads to pica or if the nonfood substances eaten cause iron deficiency. Most likely it is a combination of these two mechanisms, depending on the substances eaten. Pica can also be a cultural practice that may be unrelated to iron status. Because of the embarrassment often associated with practicing pica, it often goes unreported. Cultural Considerations Box: Pica discusses pica during pregnancy and contains suggestions on discussing this practice with the client.

When reviewing laboratory values, the nurse should remember that the expanding maternal blood volume causes hematocrit and hemoglobin levels to decrease during the second trimester, a finding that is related to hemodilution and

MyNursingKit Fetal Alcohol Spectrum Disorders Center for Excellence

Cultural Considerations

Pica

Pica is practiced around the world and has been for centuries with records of this practice found in ancient civilizations. Pica is classified according to the substance eaten. **Geophagia** is the consumption of soil, dirt, or clay or baked clay. Consumption of laundry starch, corn starch, and other similar starches is called **amylophagia**. **Pagophagia** is the consumption of ice and freezer frost. Other substances eaten include ashes, burnt match tips, baking soda, and earthen items such as sand, charcoal, stones, dust, and mortar. Some individuals consume more than one category of nonfood items.

The exact reason that pica occurs is not understood. In some cultures, the eating of nonfood substances is considered abnormal, whereas in others it is commonplace and may be especially linked to beliefs about fertility, childbirth, treatment of pregnancy symptoms, or femininity. In the United States pica is practiced more commonly among African American or Mexican American females than among whites. Those living in rural areas or who have a family history of pica are also more likely to engage in pica. In some cultures, consuming clay is felt to help treat diarrhea. Baked clay is available for purchase in some ethnic food markets. Others consume starches to quell nausea from morning sickness and as a source of kcalories when food is scarce.

Depending on what nonfood substance is eaten, pica can have negative health consequences. Some types of soil and clay can bind important minerals, including iron, and prevent absorption when present in the intestinal tract along with food. Heavy metal poisoning, such as lead, can occur with contaminated soil. Parasites, protozoa, and other infectious organisms can be ingested from soil. Intestinal obstruction has also been reported. Consumption of starches can cause excess weight gain because of the kcalorie content of these carbohydrate sources. Reports of elevated blood glucose have also been made. When corn or laundry starch replaces dietary sources of nutrients, malnutrition can occur because the starches contain only carbohydrate. Pagophagia can lead to dental problems from cracked teeth or damaged enamel. Consuming freezer frost can expose the mother to food contaminants present in the freezer. Excessive baking soda consumption is associated with a high-sodium content and altered blood pH to an alkaline range, called metabolic alkalosis.

An assessment of pica practices should occur with each prenatal visit, especially in females with anemia. A nonjudgmental approach is essential. Embarrassment is felt by many in association with practicing pica and perception of a judging attitude by the nurse could cause some individuals to withhold information about pica. Cultural reasons for pica should be explored so that they can be understood when formulating any needed intervention. Not all pica associated with iron deficiency disappears when the deficiency is treated. The client should be educated about any health concerns related to pica and offered alternatives to any craving-related reasons for it. For example, those who consume ashes or burnt match tips may choose burned toast instead. Coarse dry cereals can be substituted for dirt. The nurse can help the client brainstorm alternatives by exploring if there are any taste preferences that guide pica choices.

Sources: Corbett, Ryan, & Weinrich, 2003; Mills, 2007; Stokes, 2006.

not necessarily diminished iron status. Measurement of serum ferritin stores is a sensitive measure of iron deficiency in clients with anemia with values below 10 to 15 mcg/L that accompany a hematocrit of less than 33% in the first and third trimesters or 32% in the second trimester considered indicative of anemia (ACOG, 2008).

Special Concerns

The nutritional focus during pregnancy is concentrated on both providing adequate nutrients and limiting exposure to substance that are harmful to the developing fetus, called **teratogens**. Alcohol, caffeine, methylmercury, and some dietary supplements are examples of dietary substances that are cause for concern during pregnancy.

Alcohol

Abstinence from alcohol is recommended during pregnancy because of the demonstrated teratogenic effects on the fetus. Alcohol passes from the mother's blood and into that of the fetus, where it is more slowly metabolized than in an adult, exerting its damaging effects for a longer amount of time. Although all organs are affected, detrimental effects on the brain are most noted (Mengel, Searight, & Cook, 2006). Additionally, alcohol constricts blood vessels, limiting blood flow to the placenta and fetus (U.S. Department of Health and Human Services, 2007). Alcohol intake at any time in pregnancy can lead to fetal alcohol spectrum disorder, a condition that causes a range of physical defects and mental and behavioral disabilities. A safe threshold of alcohol intake is not known. Consuming one or more drinks per day or binge drinking places the fetus at highest risk (U.S. Surgeon General, 2005). Permanent brain damage, central nervous system defects, facial anomalies, learning disabilities, problems with language, social skills, and impulse control are lifelong impairments that are part of this disorder (Mengel et al., 2006). A more severe form of this disorder that causes growth retardation and specific facial anomalies is called fetal alcohol syndrome (FAS). Facial anomalies that the nurse may note in a child exposed to prenatal alcohol who has FAS include low-set ears, low nasal bridge, short upturned nose, and abnormal eyelid folds, called epicanthal folds. Figure 13-4 ■ depicts these findings. Screening for prenatal alcohol intake should occur at each prenatal visit using any of the available screening tools and interviewing the client. Assessment of alcohol intake by a health care clinician has been reported to reduce alcohol consumption during pregnancy (Mengel et al., 2006). Additionally, education about the risks associated with fetal exposure to alcohol is essential.

Caffeine

The ADA recommends that pregnant females limit caffeine intake to 300 mg/day because of health risks associated with intake higher than that amount (ADA, 2008). Delayed conception, miscarriage, and low birth weight are linked with high

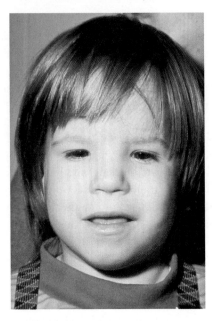

FIGURE 13-4 Fetal Alcohol Syndrome.

Source: Streissguth, A. P., Landesman-Dwyer, S., Martin, J. C., & Smith, D. W. (1980). Teratogenic effects of alcohol in humans and laboratory animals. *Science, 209,* 353–361.

intake of caffeine. Both variation in caffeine metabolism among individuals and difficulty with accurate reporting of caffeine intake have caused inconsistent outcomes in studies investigating caffeine safety during pregnancy. The effect of caffeine on fetal growth is strongest among females consuming more than 300 mg/day compared with those who consume less than 100 mg/day (CARE Study Group, 2008). A small coffee, tea, or soda has less than 100 mg of caffeine, whereas strongly brewed coffee and larger servings can exceed that amount. Additionally, the nurse can remind the pregnant female that the absorption of iron is inhibited when iron-containing foods are consumed along with coffee or tea. Chapter 7 discusses caffeine and caffeine-containing foods in more detail.

Dietary Supplement Use

The use of dietary supplements during pregnancy is not well studied. Herbs and other botanicals especially have not been well researched regarding safety. Some botanical supplements are characterized as uterine stimulants or lead to altered blood clotting, which are dangerous complications during pregnancy (Dugoua, Mills, Perri, & Koren, 2006). Some dietary supplements, especially botanicals, may be teratogens or mutagens (Woolf, 2003). Adequate vitamin A status is essential during pregnancy because of its role in embryonic development and epithelial cell integrity. Hypovitaminosis A is a worldwide health problem. However, supplementation with vitamin A should be used only under health care guidance because the vitamin is considered a teratogen when consumed in excess of 5,000 mcg/day in the active form retinol or retinoic acid (IOM, 2000). Likewise, the acne medication isotretinoin, which is biochemically similar to vitamin A, must be avoided during pregnancy.

An assessment of dietary supplement use that includes vitamins, minerals, botanicals, and any other type of dietary remedy should be included in the nursing assessment of the pregnant female. Because research is so limited in this area, the client should be advised that lack of reports of health concerns for any one supplement should not be misconstrued as evidence of efficacy or safety. The nurse can collaborate with the client and the health care team to determine what dietary supplements are safe versus harmful for the individual client.

Food Safety

Avoidance of foodborne illness and toxins in food is crucial during pregnancy. Pregnant females are at increased risk of developing foodborne illness, especially with listeria, salmonella, and toxoplasma species (ADA, 2008). Safe food handling practices, such as those outlined in Chapter 10, can be incorporated into the educational goals during prenatal health care. Deli meats and hot dogs should be reheated by steaming. Avoidance of soft cheeses; unpasteurized milk; raw sprouts; and raw or undercooked meats, poultry, fish, and eggs is advised in addition to general safe food handling practices (USDA, 2005). Additionally, limiting exposure to methylmercury is recommended to decrease the negative effects of this element on brain development. The Food and Drug Administration (FDA) and the Environmental Protection Agency (EPA) have issued guidelines for the safe consumption of fish for females of childbearing age and children, which are outlined in Client Education Checklist: Methlymercury and Fish. Further information is available online from the agency, including assessment of methylmercury levels in specific bodies of water throughout the country that the nurse can use when counseling those who consume fish caught in local waters.

Symptom Management

Normal symptoms of pregnancy can affect nutritional health if self-prescribed treatment includes altered intake or home remedies that interact with food and nutrient absorption.

Nausea and Vomiting

Nausea and vomiting are symptoms that occur in the first trimester of pregnancy, though they may persist longer. Also called hyperemesis, and commonly called morning sickness, these symptoms can occur at any time of day and affect up to 80% of pregnant females (Bryer, 2005). Hormones are thought to be the cause. The nurse can advise that the client avoid greasy or fatty foods and strong cooking odors. Liquids can be saved for between meals to lessen gastric volume during a meal. Some individuals find that dry carbohydrates consumed in small amounts are helpful. Examples include saltines and other light crackers, dry toast, rice, and plain noodles. The use of ginger to alleviate nausea during pregnancy is a common practice. Research studies have demonstrated its usefulness in treating the symptom while also being safe; ginger acts directly on the digestive tract and avoids the central nervous system side

MyNursingKit Environmental Protection Agency and Mercury: Fish Advisories

| CLIENT EDUCATION CHECKLIST | ✓ | Methylmercury and Fish |

By following these 3 recommendations for selecting fish or shellfish, women and young children will receive the benefit of eating fish and shellfish and be confident that they have reduced their exposure to the harmful effects of mercury.

3 Safety Tips

1. Do not eat
   - Shark
   - Swordfish
   - King Mackerel
   - Tilefish

They contain high levels of mercury.

2. Eat up to 12 ounces (2 average meals) a week of a variety of fish and shellfish that are lower in mercury.
   - Five of the most commonly eaten fish that are low in mercury are shrimp, canned light tuna, salmon, pollock, and catfish.

- Another commonly eaten fish, albacore ("white") tuna has more mercury than canned light tuna. So, when choosing your two meals of fish and shellfish, you may eat up to 6 ounces (one average meal) of albacore tuna per week.

3. Check local advisories about the safety of fish caught by family and friends in your local lakes, rivers, and coastal areas.

   If no advice is available, eat up to 6 ounces (one average meal) per week of fish you catch from local waters, but don't consume any other fish during that week.

   Follow these same recommendations when feeding fish and shellfish to your young child, but serve smaller portions.

Sources: Environmental Protection Agency (EPA) and Food and Drug Administration (FDA), n.d.

effects associated with antinausea medications (Bryer, 2005). Ginger tea, ginger syrup, crystallized or candied ginger, and ginger ale have all been used. Common dosing of ginger during pregnancy is 250 mg up to four times or 1 gm total/day (Bryer, 2005; White, 2007). Persistent vomiting can lead to dehydration and warrants medical attention. When fluid and food intake is chronically compromised, some clients require hospitalization for repletion.

Constipation

Constipation can affect up to 25% of females during pregnancy (Bradley, Kennedy, Turcea, Rao, & Nygaard, 2007). Limited fiber intake, diminished physical activity, and, in some, iron supplementation are often to blame. Those with a past history of constipation are more likely to experience constipation during pregnancy (Bradley et al., 2007). Tolerance to iron supplementation is often related to dose (Cox & Phelan, 2008). Intolerance, such as with constipation, can lead to poor supplement adherence. The nurse can explore alternative forms of iron or alternative dosing schedule with the health care team to improve this symptom and supplement adherence. Adequate fluid and fiber should be included in the diet. The nurse can use *MyPyramid for Moms* to educate the pregnant female about improving fiber intake by choosing whole grains and fruits and vegetables with edible skins or seeds. Chapter 2 has a Client Education Checklist on improving fiber intake.

Wellness Concerns

Some diseases and conditions carry increased risk of poor pregnancy outcome. Obesity, diabetes, and eating disorders are among some of the conditions that are treated with nutrition interventions that can lessen the pregnancy-associated

health risks. A registered dietitian should be part of the health care team when a pregnant female has high-risk conditions for which nutrition intervention is indicated. Ideally, nutrition intervention should begin before conception to set the stage for optimal control of the disease during pregnancy.

Obesity

Obesity is associated with many gestational complications that can be diminished by achieving weight loss prior to conception. The risks include those that affect the mother as well as the fetus. Fetal mortality; congenital malformations, including neural tube defects; preterm delivery; and **macrosomia,** an abnormally large size body, are all increased with infants of obese mothers (ACOG, 2005; ADA, 2008; Mehta, 2008). Obesity is associated with an increased risk of infertility, often because of polycystic ovary syndrome (PCOS) (Mehta, 2008). Although the etiology of PCOS and appropriate management of symptoms are under investigation, it is known that weight loss is a safe and often effective method used to treat infertility associated with this condition (Brassard, AinMelk, & Baillargeon, 2008). Spontaneous abortion risk is elevated in both the obese female undergoing infertility treatment and in those who conceive naturally (ACOG, 2005; Mehta, 2008). Obese females have a higher risk of gestational hypertension and diabetes and a higher rate of cesarean delivery and surgical complications associated with delivery (ACOG, 2005). During pregnancy and delivery, obesity causes difficulty in monitoring fetal development and heart rate (ACOG, 2005). In females planning a pregnancy, weight loss prior to conception is recommended to decrease risk of complications and poor outcome (Weintraub et al., 2008). The ACOG recommends that all obese pregnant females be offered nutrition consultation during and after the pregnancy with the goal of weight loss prior to a subsequent pregnancy (ACOG, 2005). Bariatric surgery is a weight loss alternative that is used in those who are morbidly obese (BMI greater than 40). Pregnancy following bariatric surgery presents unique challenges to nutritional health and concerns regarding pregnancy outcome. Hot Topic Box: Pregnancy and Bariatric Surgery discusses pregnancy in the postoperative bariatric client.

Diabetes Mellitus and Gestational Diabetes Mellitus

An assessment of diabetes risk should be included in the first prenatal visit, especially in females at high risk of developing diabetes such as those who are obese, have a family history, or have delivered a previous large-for-gestational age infant (ADA, 2008). Uncontrolled diabetes during pregnancy is associated with increased risk for miscarriages, stillbirth, macrosomia, obstetric complications, and intrauterine developmental and growth abnormalities (Owens, Kieffer, & Chowdhury, 2006). Diabetes that develops during pregnancy is called gestational diabetes mellitus (GDM) and carries pregnancy health risks similar to other types of diabetes. Laboratory screening for elevated blood glucose in a nondiabetic female is done between 24 and 28 weeks' gestation (ADA, 2008). Intervention to normalize blood glucose control before and during pregnancy is paramount. A carbohydrate-controlled diet is advised. The diet is not low carbohydrate. Adjustments can be necessary to distribute the carbohydrate over the course of a day in a pattern that avoids excessive carbohydrate in the morning when blood glucose can be elevated during pregnancy because of hormonal influences (Marcason, 2005). Careful attention to maintaining adequate weight gain is needed. In the female with GDM, the nurse should monitor the client for overrestriction of energy or carbohydrate intake as a means to avoid insulin therapy. Poor weight gain and positive urinary ketones can be indicative of deliberate or unintentional undereating (Reader, 2007). The amount of kcalories and carbohydrate in the diet is individually managed depending on blood glucose control and maternal weight. The DRI for carbohydrate of 175 gm/day during pregnancy remains a minimum for the client with diabetes (ADA, 2008; Reader, 2007). The nurse can collaborate with the client and the health care team to develop appropriate goals for physical activity since exercise is associated with acutely decreasing blood glucose levels (Reader, 2007). Chapter 19 also discusses diabetes during pregnancy.

Eating Disorders

Females with a history of anorexia nervosa or bulimia nervosa are at increased risk of poor pregnancy outcomes. Bulimia nervosa increases the risk of miscarriage, whereas anorexia nervosa is associated with low birth weight infants (Micali, Simonoff, & Treasure, 2007a). Those with a past history or current eating disorder are also more likely to develop hyperemesis and are at higher risk of cesarean delivery (Zerbe, 2007). The nurse can be involved in screening for symptoms

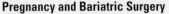

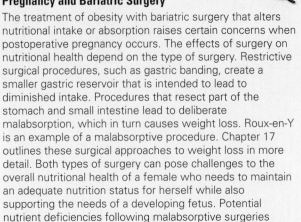

hot Topic

Pregnancy and Bariatric Surgery

The treatment of obesity with bariatric surgery that alters nutritional intake or absorption raises certain concerns when postoperative pregnancy occurs. The effects of surgery on nutritional health depend on the type of surgery. Restrictive surgical procedures, such as gastric banding, create a smaller gastric reservoir that is intended to lead to diminished intake. Procedures that resect part of the stomach and small intestine lead to deliberate malabsorption, which in turn causes weight loss. Roux-en-Y is an example of a malabsorptive procedure. Chapter 17 outlines these surgical approaches to weight loss in more detail. Both types of surgery can pose challenges to the overall nutritional health of a female who needs to maintain an adequate nutrition status for herself while also supporting the needs of a developing fetus. Potential nutrient deficiencies following malabsorptive surgeries include iron, folic acid, vitamin B_{12}, and calcium. Thiamine deficiency can also occur because of vomiting, a potential side effect of restrictive procedures. These consequences of bariatric surgery can place a female at risk for nutrition deficits that need to be corrected before conception.

It is essential that excellent preconception and prenatal nutritional monitoring occur with the client who has had bariatric surgery. Current guidelines recommend that females wait 1 year postoperatively before conception to avoid a pregnancy during the rapid weight loss phase that occurs during the first 12 to 18 months after surgery. Despite this recommendation, pregnancies are reported in this early postoperative time span. Improved fertility with weight loss and potentially poor absorption of oral contraceptives following surgery are often cited. Studies of outcomes of early postoperative pregnancies have demonstrated varying results ranging from normal to small-for-gestational-age infants despite close monitoring, warranting further study before conclusions can be drawn that would change the current recommendation on pregnancy timing.

Despite the potential for nutritional deficits at the time of conception and during pregnancy, overall, the risk of gestational complications associated with obesity is diminished following bariatric surgery. Pregnancy-associated hypertension and gestational diabetes mellitus are decreased following bariatric surgery compared with pregnant obese females who have not had surgery. Neonatal outcome is also improved compared with infants born to obese females. Risk of macrosomia in the infant is lessened. Reports exist that maternal noncompliance with vitamin supplementation, which includes folic acid, is associated with higher than expected rates of neural tube defects in the postsurgical client. Additionally, bariatric surgery is considered a risk factor for cesarean delivery.

The nurse working with clients who have had bariatric surgery should routinely include an assessment of nutritional status and adherence to vitamin and mineral supplementation as part of the nursing assessment. It is essential that the pregnant female begin the pregnancy with an optimized nutritional status. During pregnancy, a chewable or liquid prenatal vitamin and mineral supplement can replace the standard postoperative supplement in order to provide appropriate intake of folic acid and iron in particular. Clients who have had a restrictive procedure using adjustable gastric bands may have the band adjusted during the pregnancy to allow for adequate intake or to alleviate nausea and vomiting associated with pregnancy.

Sources: Karmon & Sheiner, 2008a and 2008b; Maggard et al., 2008; Weintraub et al., 2008; Xanthakos & Inge, 2006.

of eating disorders during pregnancy in order to facilitate needed intervention to improve fetal outcome. Eating disorder symptoms tend to lessen during pregnancy but not entirely and not in all cases and then can worsen during postpartum (Crow, Agras, Crosby, Halmi, & Mitchell, 2008; Micali, Simonoff, & Treasure, 2007b). The nurse can collaborate with the health care team to provide appropriate intervention, focusing on educating the pregnant female about appropriate nutrition and weight gain for fetal development. Postpartum follow-up is crucial because of the risk of increased symptoms. In addition to postpartum concerns for the mother, maternal eating disorders are associated with difficulty in feeding infants and young children (Zerbe, 2007). Chapter 17 discusses eating disorder symptoms and treatment in more detail.

Phenylketonuria

Phenylketonuria (PKU) is a genetic disorder that results in elevated blood levels of the essential amino acid phenylalanine because of a missing enzyme responsible for metabolism of the amino acid to tyrosine, another amino acid. Infants exposed to high maternal phenylalanine levels during pregnancy are at high risk of being born with growth retardation, developmental delay, and congenital heart disease, among other effects. Phenylalanine crosses the placenta and leads to higher levels in the fetus than the mother (Maillot, Cook, Lilburn, & Lee, 2007). Maintenance of maternal phenylalanine levels within an acceptable range during pregnancy is associated with greatly diminished risk of poor infant outcomes (Maillot, Lilburn, Baudin, Morley, & Lee, 2008). It is highly recommended that a female with PKU have controlled blood phenylalanine before conception for optimal outcome. However, the majority of pregnancies in those with PKU begin without maternal dietary control of phenylalanine levels (Gambol, 2007). Traditionally, low phenylalanine diets are followed during infancy and childhood but not into adulthood except during pregnancy. The nurse plays a crucial role in educating adolescent and adult females of childbearing age of the essential nature of a phenylalanine restriction during pregnancy to ensure that dietary adherence begins before conception, or in the case of an unplanned pregnancy, as soon as possible after conception. This education should be provided at any well visit where reproductive health is discussed. In addition to the diet, blood phenylalanine levels are monitored and maintained within a target range to provide essential nutrition to the mother and fetus while limiting exposure to high phenylalanine levels. Box 13-4 outlines the recommendations for phenylketonuria during pregnancy.

Gestational Hypertension

Hypertensive disease occurs in up to 20% of pregnant females and, of those, 25% may go on to develop preeclampsia, a condition associated with protein loss in the urine (ADA, 2008). In addition to hypertension, risk factors for preeclampsia in-

---

BOX 13-4	Phenylketonuria and Pregnancy

In females who have phenylketonuria (PKU), a phenylalanine-restricted diet is crucial to lessen the exposure of the fetus to damagingly high phenylalanine levels in the blood. The diet is a low-protein diet because phenylalanine is an essential amino acid and is present in most protein-containing foods. A commercial product is consumed that provides adequate protein without excessive phenylalanine. Carbohydrate and fat-containing foods comprise the rest of the kcalories and nutrients in the diet. Guidelines for managing PKU over the course of pregnancy include:

- Control of blood phenylalanine with diet before conception or, if not possible, as soon as pregnancy is known. Critical body systems are developing in the first 8 weeks of pregnancy and high phenylalanine levels are teratogenic.
- Provision of adequate nutrients and kcalories to promote maternal weight gain. Energy intake should be adjusted if weight gain goals are not met.
- Because of the high risk of maternal nutrient deficiencies on this diet, referral to a registered dietitian is recommended.
- Beginning in the second trimester, diet is liberalized because of increased fetal need. Monitoring of maternal blood phenylalanine levels continues.

Sources: Gambol, 2007: Maillot et al., 2007; Maillot et al., 2008.

---

clude obesity, maternal age greater than 40 years, diabetes, and multiple fetuses (Leeman & Fontaine, 2008). Growth retardation and preterm delivery are fetal risks of preeclampsia (ADA, 2008). Dietary interventions for gestational hypertension and preeclampsia include calcium supplementation, especially in females with high risk of preeclampsia or low-calcium intake (ADA, 2008; Leeman & Fontaine, 2008). It is unclear whether limiting sodium intake has an impact on outcome in this population (Duley, Meher, & Abalos, 2006). Fish oils have been investigated for a possible role as prostaglandin precursors and vasodilators, but findings are inconclusive and warrant larger study (ADA, 2008; Makrides, Duley, & Olsen, 2006). In the meantime, the nurse can suggest consumption of deep, cold-water fish following the guidelines outlined in Client Education Checklist: Methlymercury and Fish.

Lactation

Exclusive breastfeeding, or lactation, during the first 6 months of life and breastfeeding along with the introduction of complementary foods from age 6 months to 1 year is considered the optimal method for feeding infants (ADA, 2005). Breast milk contains proteins in the form of caseins, lactalbumin, and immunoglobulins among other forms that are ideal for infants. Lactose, glucose, and galactose provide needed sources of carbohydrate energy. Fats, vitamins, minerals, and water are

MyNursingKit U.S. Department of Health and Human Services. Breastfeeding: Best for Baby, Best for Mom

BOX 13-5	**Maternal and Infant Benefits to Breastfeeding**

Infant Benefits

Optimal nutrient composition

Antibodies in milk offer protection against some bacterial and viral infections

Decreased lower respiratory illnesses

Decreased rate of sudden infant death syndrome

Increased maternal bonding

Decreased risk of childhood obesity

Maternal Benefits

Lower rate of breast and ovarian cancer

Decreased postpartum bleeding

Faster uterine shrinking (involution)

Decreased cost of infant feeding versus formula

Time saved from preparing formula

Infant bonding

Sources: ADA, 2005; Department of Health and Human Services, 2005; Gartner et al., 2005.

also present. The content of breast milk adapts over time to the nutritional needs of the developing infant and provides nutrients in easily absorbed forms that make breast milk the ideal method to nourish an infant (ADA, 2005). There are numerous benefits to breastfeeding for both the infant and the mother. Nutritional and other health benefits are outlined in Box 13-5. The nurse is ideally situated to promote and support the decision to breastfeed among individuals and to participate in initiatives to increase the prevalence of breastfeeding. Chapter 14 discusses the benefits of breast milk on infant health, the role of the nurse in promotion of breastfeeding, and initiatives to increase breastfeeding. This chapter discussion focuses on the maternal nutritional needs during lactation and the effect on breast milk.

Nutritional Needs

The nutritional content of breast milk reflects the nutritional status of the mother for some nutrients while for others it is unaffected (Kent, 2007). The macronutrients, carbohydrate, protein, and fat, are less affected by the mother's diet than are the vitamins and minerals in breast milk. The nurse should encourage a well-balanced diet to ensure intake of a wide variety of foods and nutrients. *MyPyramid for Moms* contains advice on nutrition and breastfeeding in an interactive format that focuses on whole foods as the way to consume all the needed nutrients during lactation. Figure 13-5 ■ depicts an example of *MyPyramid for Moms* during breastfeeding.

Energy

The average amount of breast milk produced daily is approximately 750 mL, which requires 630 kcal to produce (Kent, 2007). The recommendation for energy intake during lactation incorporates the individualized needs of the mother, the energy cost of milk output, and the mobilization of fat stores

toward milk synthesis. During the first 6 months after birth, the energy cost for milk output is estimated as an extra 500 kcalories/day after accounting for maternal fat stores to contribute almost 200 additional kcalories/day toward that need (IOM, 2005). That amount decreases to 400 kcalories/day after 6 months of lactation. Too restrictive a diet in an attempt to quickly achieve prepregnancy weight can lead to a shortfall of crucial nutrients in the diet. The nurse should assess overall energy intake in the lactating female and educate the client about the importance of a well-balanced diet during breastfeeding.

Vitamins and Minerals

The amount of most vitamins and minerals in the mother's diet is reflected in the composition of breast milk. Vitamins A, B_{12}, D, and E; thiamin; riboflavin; and pyridoxine, selenium, and iodine in breast milk are related to maternal diet (Kent, 2007). Even with adequate intake, the vitamin D content of breast milk is insufficient to meet the needs of the infant, and dietary supplementation of the infant is recommended beginning at age 2 months (Misra et al., 2008). Supplementation of the mother's diet with additional vitamin D does not markedly increase the vitamin D content of breast milk (Kovacs, 2008). Insufficient vitamin D status at birth can lead to development of rickets in the infant within months. The recommended intake for vitamin D by a lactating female is unchanged from prepregnancy recommendations.

Maternal stores of vitamin B_{12} do not cross the placenta during fetal development; instead the vitamin B_{12} in fetal and breastfed infants is derived from current maternal intake of the vitamin. Lack of adequate maternal intake can lead to neurological problems in the infant because of negative effects on myelin development. Box 13-3 discusses the need for vitamin B_{12} supplementation or intake of fortified foods by vegan lactating females who have no dietary source of the vitamin because of restricting intake of animal foods.

Breast milk does not contain high amounts of iron and the needs of the breastfed infant are met with iron supplementation or iron- fortified cereal by age 6 months. The maternal need for iron returns to prepregnancy amounts. Recommendations for intake of most other nutrients remain close to those during pregnancy or return to prepregnancy recommendations. Often the difference in recommendation is small and not easily translated to changes in food intake. Instead of focusing on individual specifics about these nutrients, the nurse can collaborate with the client and brainstorm ways to improve overall intake in accordance with MyPyramid guidelines to meet overall nutrient needs during lactation.

Fluids

Fluid intake during lactation can be met by consuming a variety of nonalcoholic fluids and watery foods to account for the production of approximately 750 mL of breast milk/day

Food Group	Breastfeeding only	Breastfeeding plus formula	What counts as 1 cup or 1 ounce?	Remember to...
	Eat this amount from each group daily.			
Fruits 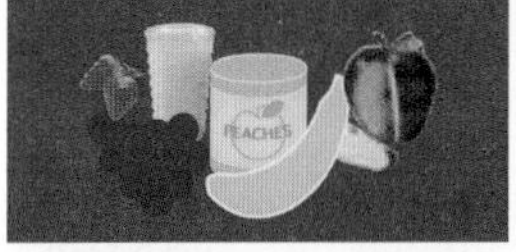	2 cups	2 cups	1 cup fruit or juice ½ cup dried fruit	*Focus on fruits—* Eat a variety of fruits.
Vegetables 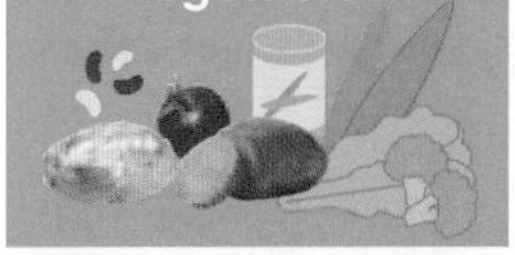	3 cups	3 cups	1 cup raw or cooked vegetables or juice 2 cups raw leafy vegetables	*Vary your veggies—* Eat more dark-green and orange vegetables and cooked dry beans.
Grains 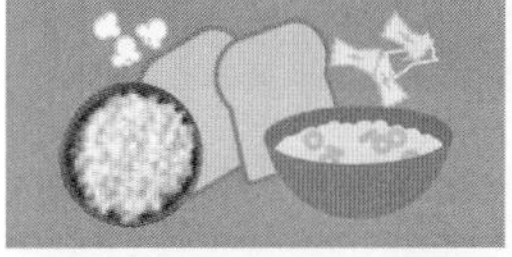	8 ounces	7 ounces	1 slice bread 1 ounce ready-to-eat cereal ½ cup cooked pasta, rice, or cereal	*Make half your grains whole—* Choose whole instead of refined grains.
Meat & Beans 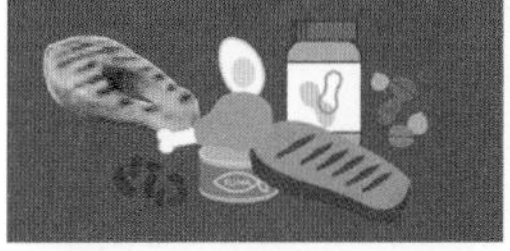	6½ ounces	6 ounces	1 ounce lean meat, poultry, or fish ¼ cup cooked dry beans ½ ounce nuts or 1 egg 1 tablespoon peanut butter	*Go lean with protein—* Choose low-fat or lean meats and poultry.
Milk 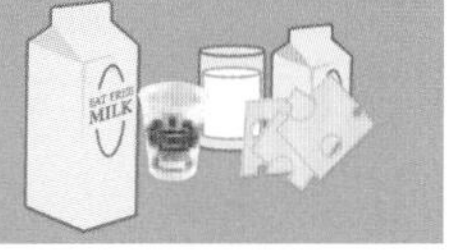	3 cups	3 cups	1 cup milk 8 ounces yogurt 1½ ounces cheese 2 ounces processed cheese	*Get your calcium-rich foods—*Go low-fat or fat-free when you choose milk, yogurt, and cheese.

FIGURE 13-5 MyPyramid for Moms: Breastfeeding.

Source: United States Department of Agriculture, MyPyramid for Moms. Retrieved March 25, 2009, from www.nal.usda.gov/wicworks/Topics/BreastfeedingFactSheet.pdf

along with baseline fluid needs. The recommendation for fluid intake during lactation is 3.1 liters of drinking fluid or 3.8 liters of total fluid/day (IOM, 2004).

Wellness Concerns

Breast milk is considered a safe source of nutrition for the infant. However, under certain circumstances, contamination of breast milk with environmental contaminants, disease, or drugs can affect the safety of breast milk. Box 13-6 outlines medical contraindications to breastfeeding. In addition to the circumstances listed, the nurse should consult with a pharmacist regarding the safety of medication use during breastfeeding. This inquiry should include questions about the safety of dietary supplements as well. Little to no research has been conducted regarding dietary supplements, especially herbs and other botanicals, on the safety of breast milk and infant health.

Methylmercury is an environmental contaminant that can be found in breast milk because of maternal exposure.

BOX 13-6   Contraindications to Breastfeeding

Infant has galactosemia, a genetic metabolic disorder.

Mother has been infected with:
- Human immunodeficiency virus (HIV)
- Human T-cell lymphotrophic virus type I or II
- Active, untreated tuberculosis

Mother is taking any of the following:
- Antiretroviral medications
- Illicit drugs
- Chemotherapy drugs that alter DNA replication or cell division

- What resource can the nurse use to learn whether additional medications are a contraindication to breastfeeding?

Source: CDC, 2007.

Breastfeeding females should be educated about the risks of mercury on infant development. Client Education Checklist: Methlymercury and Fish can guide the nurse in advising the lactating female about reducing intake of high-mercury seafood.

Alcohol is passively diffused into breast milk from maternal blood within 1 hour of ingestion (Giglia & Binns, 2008). Infant exposure to alcohol can affect the brain during this crucial time of development. Although some believe that drinking alcohol helps with relaxation and milk production, alcohol can result in decreased production of breast milk (Gartner et al., 2005; Giglia & Binns, 2008). Abstinence from alcohol during lactation is advised. If an occasional al-

coholic beverage is consumed, it is advised that breastfeeding not occur for 2 hours after the drink is finished (Gartner et al., 2005).

The increasing development of food allergies in children has led some to believe that early exposure to allergens through breastfeeding might be responsible for some food allergies. The nurse should take care to explain to a nursing mother that current guidelines do not support that philosophy under most circumstances. The Evidence-Based Practice Box: Can manipulation of the prenatal diet or breastfeeding prevent or delay the onset of allergies? discusses the role of maternal diet, breastfeeding, and development of allergic disease.

EVIDENCE-BASED PRACTICE RESEARCH BOX

Can manipulation of the prenatal diet or breastfeeding prevent or delay the onset of allergies?

Clinical Problem: The incidence of allergic diseases in children has been increasing. Is there sufficient research evidence that allergic diseases in infants or young children can be prevented or delayed either by manipulation of the mother's diet during pregnancy or by breastfeeding?

Research Findings: Breastfeeding is strongly recommended by health care providers for its multiple benefits for mother and child. It had long been suggested that breastfeeding reduces the incidence of food allergies, eczema, and asthma, particularly in children who might have a familial predisposition to development of those conditions.

Duncan and Sears (2008) examined numerous studies that compared cohorts of breastfed infants over various periods. They could find no evidence suggesting that breastfeeding for a specific length of time offered either protective or preventive effects of the development of allergies. Literature reviews conducted by Heine and Tang (2008) suggested that exclusive breastfeeding and delaying the introduction of solid foods until 6 months was associated with decreased incidence of respiratory allergies and eczema, but it did not reach the level of statistical significance. Evidence for the prevention of food allergies was less definitive.

A group of researchers examined the prenatal maternal diets of 2,641 children when they reached 2 years of age. They found weak associations with maternal intake of n-3 polyunsaturated fatty acids and a decreased risk of development of eczema and food allergies in the children (Sausenthaler et al., 2007). Greer and colleagues (2008) reviewed the evidence on maternal dietary restrictions and the development of allergies and concluded that current evidence is not strong enough to

recommend restrictions on maternal diets. In addition, there is only limited or weak evidence to suggest that specific infant formulas or breastfeeding or the timing of the introduction of solid food has significant effect on the development of allergies. Similar reviews of additional American and European literature reached the same conclusions (Wahn, 2008; Zeiger, 2003).

The American Academy of Pediatrics' most current recommendations are that maternal diets not be restricted as a means to prevent allergic diseases. Further, infants who can be identified as high risk may benefit from at least 4 months of exclusive breastfeeding; however, there is insufficient evidence to suggest that delaying solid foods beyond 4–6 month of age is associated with prevention or delay of allergies (Thygarajan & Burks, 2008).

All researchers suggest that extensive additional studies are needed that examine such factors as maternal age, environmental exposure, maternal smoking status, and allergies in families. In addition, more data are needed that compare breastfed and formula-fed infants and allergies in both groups.

Nursing Implications: There is inadequate evidence to recommend that the maternal prenatal diet be manipulated in a specified manner to prevent development of allergies in infants or children. There is also insufficient evidence to recommend breastfeeding as the ideal means to prevent or delay the onset of allergies in infants or children. Breastfeeding can still be recommended, however, as the ideal food for infants.

CRITICAL THINKING QUESTION:

1. How could the nurse respond to the pregnant woman who says that she has a 4-year old nephew who has lots of allergies and that she will do anything she can to avoid problems with her own baby?

NURSING CARE PLAN Adequate Weight Gain and Pregnancy

CASE STUDY

Katherine is a 30-year-old systems analyst for a governmental agency. She says she is 6 weeks pregnant and has come for her first prenatal visit. This pregnancy is her first. She has been married for 5 years and she and her husband, an elementary school teacher, have just bought a small house in a large urban area. The pregnancy was planned and they are thrilled that she got pregnant so quickly. She describes her overall health as "excellent" with no known chronic health problems or genetic conditions on either side of the family. Her usual health practices include eating organic foods, jogging 5 miles 3 days a week with her husband, and working out at a fitness center 3 evenings a week for about an hour at a time. She tells the nurse that she has had some morning sickness for several weeks but generally feels better by late morning. Now she wants to know about the best dietary plan to limit weight gain so she can have an "easy labor" and have less weight to lose after the baby is born. She plans to breastfeed but will also return to work 6 to 12 weeks after the birth.

Applying the Nursing Process

ASSESSMENT

Height: 5 feet 6 inches Weight: 122 pounds
   (unchanged from prepregnancy) BMI: 20
BP 112/66 P 64 R 14
Hgb 13.4 Hct 40

DIAGNOSIS

Readiness for enhanced nutrition related to planned pregnancy evidenced by requests for information about dietary requirements for pregnancy

EXPECTED OUTCOMES

Weight gain during pregnancy of 25 to 35 pounds
Katherine will articulate reasons for the importance of weight gain during pregnancy
Diet will be modified to include increased caloric intake
Katherine will express positive feelings about pregnancy and weight gain

INTERVENTIONS

Provide written materials about need for increased nutrients and calories during pregnancy and lactation
Using a diagram, explain distribution of pregnancy weight gain that goes to the baby, placenta, fat stores, breasts, increased blood volume, and other needs
Explain importance of increasing consumption of nutrient-dense foods as a source of increased calories
Explain the importance of increased fat stores and continued need to maintain higher caloric intake for successful breastfeeding
Discuss importance of maintaining regular physical activity during pregnancy
Dispel myths about weight gain and the ease of labor and the birth process
Share strategies to deal with morning sickness

EVALUATION

Katherine returned to the clinic a month later for a prenatal visit. Her weight was 123.5 pounds and she said she still felt fine. Fatigue was her biggest problem at this time so she was not working out or running as much as before she got pregnant. Morning sickness was no worse and she felt that by eating small amounts during the day she keeps nausea at a minimum. She and her husband have started to plan space in their house for the baby and are focused on having a healthy baby. She says they know that she will have plenty of time after the birth to lose weight because she cannot imagine having anything but a physically active lifestyle. For the time being, she is drinking 2 glasses of skim milk a day, something she has never done, and will try yogurt and some nuts as snacks as she feels better. Figure 13-6 ■ outlines the nursing process for this case.

Critical Thinking in the Nursing Process

1. How should the nurse respond to the pregnant woman who says that she does not want to gain much weight during pregnancy because she has had many friends who have gained weight and been unable to lose it afterward?

(continued)

Adequate Weight Gain and Pregnancy *(continued)*

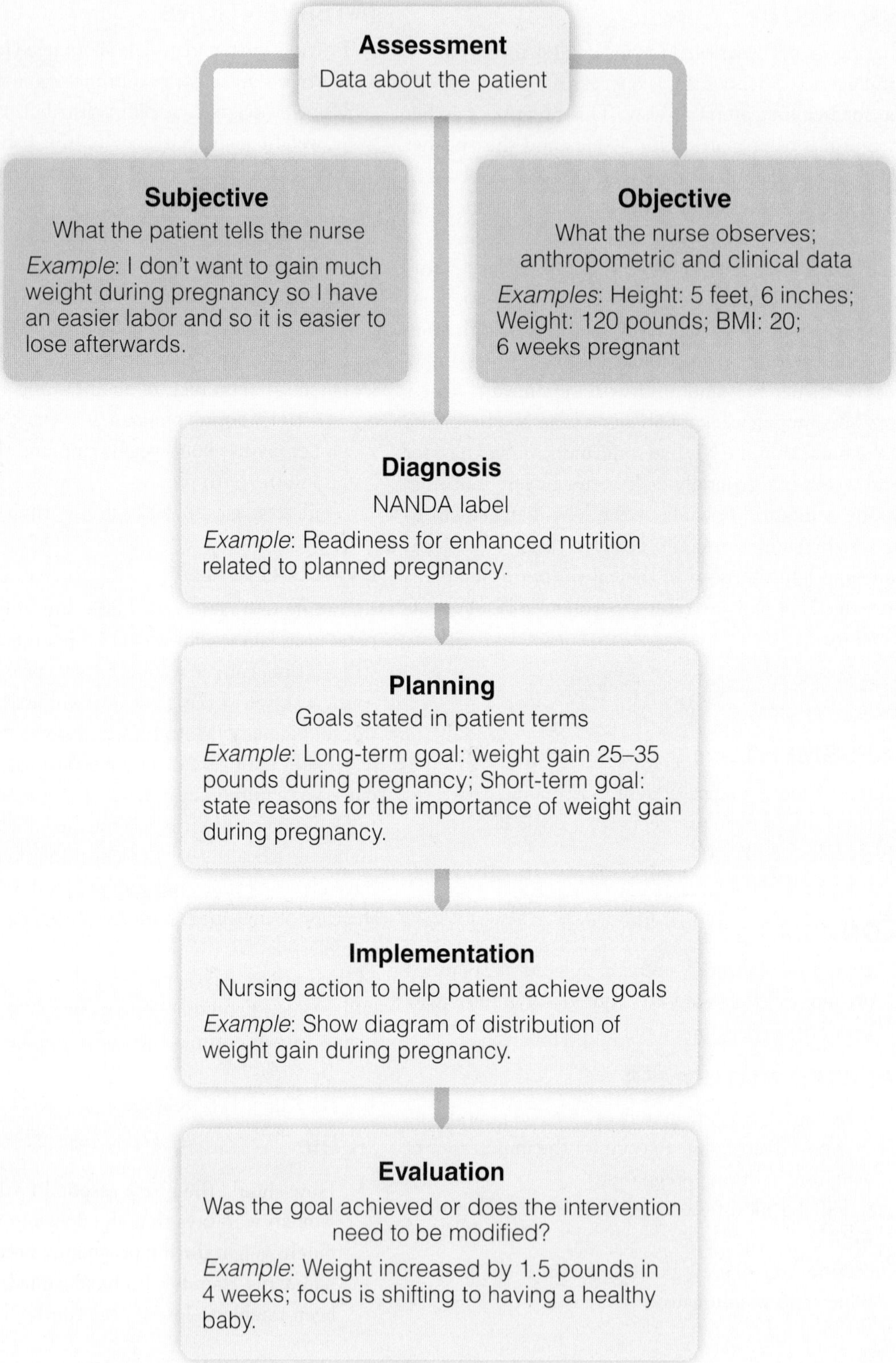

NURSING CARE PLAN

Assessment
Data about the patient

Subjective
What the patient tells the nurse

Example: I don't want to gain much weight during pregnancy so I have an easier labor and so it is easier to lose afterwards.

Objective
What the nurse observes; anthropometric and clinical data

Examples: Height: 5 feet, 6 inches; Weight: 120 pounds; BMI: 20; 6 weeks pregnant

Diagnosis
NANDA label

Example: Readiness for enhanced nutrition related to planned pregnancy.

Planning
Goals stated in patient terms

Example: Long-term goal: weight gain 25–35 pounds during pregnancy; Short-term goal: state reasons for the importance of weight gain during pregnancy.

Implementation
Nursing action to help patient achieve goals

Example: Show diagram of distribution of weight gain during pregnancy.

Evaluation
Was the goal achieved or does the intervention need to be modified?

Example: Weight increased by 1.5 pounds in 4 weeks; focus is shifting to having a healthy baby.

■ FIGURE 13-6 **Nursing Care Plan Process: Adequate Weight Gain and Pregnancy.**

CHAPTER SUMMARY

- Preconception nutritional status can affect fertility and early pregnancy fetal development.

- Energy needs during pregnancy are based on recommended weight gain patterns and are determined individually.

- Requirement for folic acid is increased in pregnancy to decrease the risk of neural tube defects.

- Iron needs during pregnancy increase significantly and often require supplementation instead of just dietary sources of the mineral.

- Alcohol intake during pregnancy can result in neurological damage and developmental delay.

- Pregnant and lactating females need to limit intake of high-mercury seafood because of the negative effect of this metal on brain development.

- Obesity during pregnancy increases maternal and infant health risks. It is recommended that weight loss needs be addressed before pregnancy to improve outcome.

- Medical conditions such as phenylketonuria, eating disorders, diabetes, and others require a collaborative team approach to prenatal care.

- The nutritional needs of a lactating female are based on the energy and micronutrients required for breast milk production. Breast milk contains ideal amounts and forms of most nutrients. Breast milk does not contain adequate vitamin D or iron, and supplementation of the infant is recommended.

EXPLORE **PEARSON mynursingkit™**

MyNursingKit is your one stop for online chapter review materials and resources. Prepare for success with additional NCLEX®-style practice questions, interactive assignments and activities, web links, animations and videos, and more!

Register your access code from the front of your book at www.mynursingkit.com.

NCLEX® QUESTIONS

1. How should the nurse respond to the woman who is 12 weeks pregnant and tells the nurse that she is going to take calcium supplements during pregnancy so she does not gain as much weight by drinking milk and can "use" the extra calories elsewhere in her diet?
   1. "That is a reasonable way to get the calcium you need."
   2. "Milk provides many nutrients in addition to calcium, and if you are concerned about calories and weight gain you could drink skim milk."
   3. "You should drink milk during pregnancy to make sure that your baby develops strong bones."
   4. "A positive pregnancy outcome is more likely when milk is consumed, so you should strongly consider drinking milk every day."

2. The nurse is counseling a client with a BMI of 28 during her first prenatal visit. Which statement by the client indicates that the nurse needs to reinforce dietary teaching?
   1. "I was worried I would be told I couldn't gain weight during pregnancy."
   2. "I will do whatever I need to do to have a healthy baby."
   3. "If I gain only a few pounds I won't have as many problems losing weight afterward."
   4. "I need to take the prenatal vitamin and mineral supplement as directed."

3. A breastfeeding woman may need to take iron supplements to:
   1. Prevent iron deficiency in her infant
   2. Replace her body's iron stores
   3. Add oxygen carrying capacity for her infant
   4. Prevent fluid volume deficit

4. A new mother asks the nurse about effective strategies to ensure successful breastfeeding. Which of the following would be a good suggestion?
   1. Get adequate rest and continue a balanced diet.
   2. Eat about 4,000 calories per day to produce enough milk.
   3. Drink an extra glass of water in the morning.
   4. Take a calcium supplement to fortify the milk.

5. A 17-year-old comes to the clinic for her first prenatal visit and is found to be 4 months pregnant. Dietary teaching for this client should be focused on:
   1. Developing a plan for optimal weight gain
   2. Recommending a suitable vitamin and mineral supplement
   3. Suggesting foods that are high in protein
   4. Assessing the adequacy of her current diet

REFERENCES

American College of Obstetricians and Gynecologists (ACOG). (2005). ACOG Committee Opinion 315: Obesity in pregnancy. *Obstetrics and Gynecology, 106,* 671–675.

American College of Obstetricians and Gynecologists (ACOG). (2008). Practice Bulletin No. 95: Anemia in pregnancy. *Obstetrics and Gynecology, 112,* 201–207.

American Dietetic Association (ADA). (2003). Position of the American Dietetic Association and Dietitians of Canada: Vegetarian diets. *Journal of the American Dietetic Association, 103,* 748–765.

American Dietetic Association (ADA). (2005). Position of the American Dietetic Association: Promoting and supporting breastfeeding. *Journal of the American Dietetic Association, 105,* 810–818.

American Dietetic Association (ADA). (2008). Position of the American Dietetic Association: Nutrition and lifestyle for a healthy pregnancy outcome. *Journal of the American Dietetic Association, 108,* 553–561.

Bradley, C. S., Kennedy, C. M., Turcea, A. M., Rao, S. S., & Nygaard, I. E. (2007). Constipation in pregnancy. *Obstetrics & Gynecology, 110,* 1351–1357.

Brassard, M., AinMelk, Y., & Baillargeon, J. P. (2008). Basic infertility including polycystic ovary syndrome. *Medical Clinics of North America, 92,* 1163–1192.

Bryer, E. (2005). A literature review of the effectiveness of ginger in alleviating mild to moderate nausea and vomiting of pregnancy. *Journal of Midwifery and Women's Health, 50,* e1–e3.

CARE Study Group. (2008). Maternal caffeine intake during pregnancy and risk of fetal growth restriction: A large prospective observational study. *British Medical Journal, 337,* a2332.

Centers for Disease Control and Prevention (CDC). (2007). *When should a mother avoid breastfeeding?* Retrieved December 1, 2008, from http://www.cdc.gov/breastfeeding/disease/contraindicators.htm

Cetin, I., & Koletzko, B. (2008). Long-chain w-3 fatty acid supply in pregnancy and lactation. *Current Opinion in Clinical Nutrition and Metabolic Care, 11,* 297–302.

Corbett, R. W., Ryan, C., & Weinrich, S. P. (2003). Pica in pregnancy: Does it affect outcomes? *American Journal of Maternal Child Nursing, 28,* 183–189.

Cox, J. T. & Phelan, S. T. (2008). Nutrition during pregnancy. *Obstetrics and Gynecology Clinics of North America, 35,* 369–383.

Crow, S. J., Agras, W. S., Crosby, R., Halmi, K., & Mitchell, J. E. (2008). Eating disorder symptoms in pregnancy: A prospective study. *International Journal of Eating Disorders, 41,* 277–279.

Department of Health and Human Services, Office of Women's Health. (2005). *Benefits of breastfeeding.* Retrieved December 1, 2008, from http://www.4woman.gov/Breastfeeding/index.cfm?page=227

Dror, D. K., & Allen, L. H. (2008). Effect of vitamin B_{12} deficiency on neurodevelopment in infants: Current knowledge and possible mechanisms. *Nutrition Reviews, 66,* 250–255.

Dugoua, J., Mills, E., Perri, D., & Koren, G. (2006). Safety and efficacy of St. John's Wort (hypericum) during pregnancy. *Canadian Journal of Clinical Pharmacology, 13,* e268–e276.

Duley, L., Meher, S., & Abalos, E. (2006). Management of pre-eclampsia. *British Medical Journal, 332,* 463–468.

Duncan, J. M., & Sears, M. R. (2008). Breastfeeding and allergies: Time for a change in paradigm. *Current Opinion in Allergy and Clinical Immunology, 8,* 398–405.

Environmental Protection Agency (EPA) and Food and Drug Administration (FDA). (n.d.). *What you need to know about mercury in fish and shellfish.* Retrieved March 25, 2009, from http://www.epa.gov/waterscience/fish/files/MethylmercuryBrochure.pdf

Finer, L. B., & Henshaw, S. K. (2006). Disparities in rates of unintended pregnancy in the United States, 1994 and 2001. *Perspectives on Sexual Reproductive Health, 38,* 90–96.

Gambol, P. J. (2007). Maternal phenylketonuria syndrome and case management implications. *Journal of Pediatric Nursing, 22,* 129–138.

Gartner, L. M., Morton, J., Lawrence, R. A., Naylor, A. J., O'Hare, D., Schanler, R. J., et al. (2005). American Academy of Pediatrics

Policy Statement: Breastfeeding and the use of human milk. *Pediatrics, 115,* 496–506.

Giglia, R. C., & Binns, C. W. (2008). Alcohol, pregnancy and breastfeeding: A comparison of the 1995 and 2001 National Health Survey data. *Breastfeeding Review, 16,* 17–24.

Greer, F. R., Sicherer, S. H., Burks, A. W., and the Committee on Nutrition and Section on Allergy and Immunology. (2008). Effects of early nutritional interventions on the development of atopic disease in infants and children: The role of maternal dietary restriction, breastfeeding, timing of introduction of complementary foods, and hydrolyzed formulas. *Pediatrics, 121*(1), 183–191.

Heine, R. G., & Tang, M. L. K. (2008). Dietary approaches to the prevention of food allergy. *Current Opinion in Clinical Nutrition and Metabolic Care, 11,* 320–328.

Innis, S. M. (2005). Essential fatty acid transfer and fetal development. *Placenta, 26,* S70–S75.

Institute of Medicine (IOM), Food and Nutrition Board. (1997). *Dietary Reference Intakes for calcium, phosphorus, magnesium, vitamin D, and fluoride.* Washington, DC: National Academies Press.

Institute of Medicine (IOM), Food and Nutrition Board. (1998). *Dietary Reference Intakes: Thiamin, riboflavin, niacin, vitamin B_6, folate, vitamin B_{12}, pantothenic acid, biotin, and choline.* Washington, DC: National Academies Press.

Institute of Medicine (IOM), Food and Nutrition Board. (2000). *Dietary Reference Intakes for vitamin A, vitamin K, arsenic, boron, chromium, copper, iodine, iron, manganese, molybdenum, nickel, silicon, vanadium and zinc.* Washington, DC: National Academies Press.

Institute of Medicine (IOM), Food and Nutrition Board. (2004). *Dietary Reference Intakes for water, potassium, sodium, chloride, sulfate.* Washington, DC: National Academies Press.

Institute of Medicine (IOM), Food and Nutrition Board. (2005). *Dietary Reference Intakes for energy, carbohydrate, fiber, fat, fatty acids, cholesterol, protein, and amino acids.* Washington, DC: National Academies Press.

REFERENCES *(continued)*

Institute of Medicine (IOM), Food and Nutrition Board, Board on Children, Youth, and Families. (2009). *Weight gain during pregnancy: Reexamining the guidelines.* Washington, DC: National Academies Press.

Jensen, C. L. (2006). Effects of n-3 fatty acids during pregnancy and lactation. *American Journal of Clinical Nutrition, 83,* 1452S–1457S.

Johnson, K., Posner, S. F., Biermann, J., Cordero, J. F., Atrash, H. K., Parker, C. S., et al. (CDC/ATSDR Preconception Care Work Group, Select Panel on Preconception Care). (2006). Recommendations to improve preconception health and health care—United States. A report of the CDC/ATSDR Preconception Care Work Group and the Select Panel on Preconception Care. *Morbidity and Mortality Weekly Report, 55,* 1–23.

Karmon, A., & Sheiner, E. (2008a). Pregnancy after bariatric surgery: A comprehensive review. *Archives of Gynecology and Obstetrics, 277,* 381–388.

Karmon, A., & Sheiner, E. (2008b). Timing of gestation after bariatric surgery: Should women delay pregnancy for at least 1 postoperative year? *American Journal of Perinatology, 25,* 331–333.

Kent, J. C. (2007). How breastfeeding works. *Journal of Midwifery and Women's Health, 52,* 564–570.

Klein, L. (2005). Nutritional recommendations for multiple pregnancies. *Journal of the American Dietetic Association, 105,* 1050–1052.

Kovacs, C. S. (2008). Vitamin D in pregnancy and lactation: Maternal, fetal, and neonatal outcomes from human and animal studies. *American Journal of Clinical Nutrition, 88,* 520S–528S.

Leeman, L., & Fontaine, P. (2008). Hypertensive disorders of pregnancy. *American Family Physician, 78,* 93–100.

Maggard, M. A., Yermilov, I., Li, Z., Maglione, M., Newberry, S., Suttorp, M., et al. (2008). Pregnancy and fertility following bariatric surgery: A systematic review. *Journal of the American Medical Association, 300,* 2286–2296.

Maillot, F., Cook, P., Lilburn, M., & Lee, P. J. (2007). A practical approach to maternal phenylketonuria management. *Journal of Inherited Metabolic Disorders, 30,* 198–201.

Maillot, F., Lilburn, M., Baudin, J., Morley, D. W., & Lee, P. J. (2008). Factors influencing outcomes in offspring of mothers with phenylketonuria during pregnancy: The importance of variation in maternal blood phenylalanine. *American Journal of Clinical Nutrition, 88,* 700–705.

Makrides, M., Duley, L., & Olsen, S. F. (2006). Marine oil and other prostaglandin precursor supplementation of pregnancy uncomplicated by preeclampsia and intrauterine growth retardation. *Cochrane Database Systematic Review, CD003402.*

Marcason, W. (2005). What is the appropriate amount and distribution of carbohydrates for a woman diagnosed with gestational diabetes mellitus? *Journal of the American Dietetic Association, 105,* 1673.

Marcason, W. (2006). What are the calorie requirements for women having twins? *Journal of the American Dietetic Association, 106,* 1292.

Mehta, S. H. (2008). Nutrition and pregnancy. *Clinical Obstetrics and Gynecology, 51,* 409–418.

Mengel, M. B., Searight, R., & Cook, K. (2006). Preventing alcohol-exposed pregnancies. *Journal of the American Board of Family Medicine, 19,* 494–505.

Micali, N., Simonoff, E., & Treasure, J. (2007a). Risk of adverse perinatal outcomes in women with eating disorders. *British Journal of Psychiatry, 190,* 255–259.

Micali, N., Simonoff, E., & Treasure, J. (2007b). Eating disorder symptoms in pregnancy: A longitudinal study of women with recent and past eating disorders and obesity. *Journal of Psychosomatic Research, 63,* 297–303.

Mills, M. E. (2007). Craving more than food: The implications of pica in pregnancy. *Nursing for Women's Health, 11,* 266–273.

Milman, N. (2008). Prepartum anaemia: Prevention and treatment. *Annals of Hematology, 87,* 949–959.

Misra, M., Pacaud, D., Petryk, A., Collett-Solberg, P. F., & Kappy, M. (2008). Vitamin D deficiency in children and its management: Review of current knowledge and recommendations. *Pediatrics, 122,* 398–417.

Ogden, C. L., Carroll, M. D., Curtin, L. R., McDowell, M. A., Tabak, C. J., & Flegal, K. M. (2006). Prevalence of overweight and obesity in the United States, 1999–2004. *Journal of the American Medical Association, 295,* 1549–1555.

Owens, M. D., Kieffer, E. C., & Chowdhury, F. M. (2006). Preconception care and women with or at risk for diabetes: Implications for community intervention. *Maternal Child Health Journal, 10,* 137–141.

Pencharz, P. B. (2005). Special problems of nutrition in the pregnancy of teenagers. *Nestle Nutrition Workshop Series Pediatric Program, 55,* 213–220.

Penney, D. S., & Miller, K. G. (2008). Nutrition counseling for vegetarians during pregnancy and lactation. *Journal of Midwifery and Women's Health, 53,* 37–44.

Reader, D. M. (2007). Medical nutrition therapy and lifestyle interventions. *Diabetes Care, 30,* S188–S193.

Rosello-Soberon, M. E., Fuentes-Chaparro, L., & Casanueva, E. (2005). Twin pregnancies: Eating for three? Maternal nutrition update. *Nutrition Reviews, 63,* 295–302.

Sausenthaler, S., Koletzko, S., Schaaf, B., Lehmann, I., Borte, M., Herbarth, O., et al. (2007). Maternal diet during pregnancy in relation to eczema and allergic sensitization in the offspring at 2 y of age. *American Journal of Clinical Nutrition, 85,* 530–537.

Stokes, T. (2006). The earth-eaters. *Nature, 444,* 543–544.

Thygarajan, A., & Burks, A. W. (2008). American Academy of Pediatrics recommendations of the effects of early nutritional interventions on the development of atopic disease. *Current Opinions in Pediatrics, 20,* 698–702.

United States Department of Agriculture (USDA). (2005). *Dietary Guidelines for Americans.* Retrieved November 24, 2008, from http://www.health.gov/dietary guidelines/dga2005/document/default.htm

United States Department of Health and Human Services, Substance Abuse and Mental Health Services Administration, (2007). *Effects of alcohol on a fetus.* Retrieved November 24, 2008, from http://www .fasdcenter.samhsa.gov/documents/wynk_ effects_fetus.pdf

United States Surgeon General. (2005). *U.S. Surgeon General releases advisory on alcohol use in pregnancy.* Retrieved November 24, 2008, from http://www.surgeongeneral.gov/ pressreleases/sg02222005.html

Wahn, H. U. (2008). Strategies for atopy prevention. *The Journal of Nutrition, 138,* 1770S–1772S.

Wallace, J. M., Luther, J. S., Milne, J. S, Aitken, R. P., Redmer, D. A., Reynolds, L. P., et al. (2006). Nutritional modulation of adolescent pregnancy outcome—A review. *Placenta, 27,* S61–S68.

Weintraub, A. Y., Levy, A., Levi, I., Mazor, M., Wiznitzer, A., & Sheiner, E. (2008). Effect of bariatric surgery on pregnancy outcome. *International Journal of Gynecology and Obstetrics, 103,* 246–251.

White, B. (2007). Ginger: An overview. *American Family Physician, 75,* 1689–1691.

Woolf, A. D. (2003). Herbal remedies and children: Do they work? Are they harmful? *Pediatrics, 112,* 240–246.

Xanthakos, S. A., & Inge, T. H. (2006). Nutritional consequences of bariatric surgery. *Current Opinion in Clinical Nutrition and Metabolic Care, 9,* 489–496.

Zeiger, R. S. (2003). Food allergen avoidance in the prevention of food allergy in infants and children. *Pediatrics, 111,* 1662–1671.

Zerbe, K. J. (2007). Eating disorders in the 21st century: Identification, management, and prevention in obstetrics and gynecology. *Best Practice & Research Clinical Obstetrics & Gynecology, 21,* 331–343.

Julie Stefanski

14 Infants, Children, and Adolescents

WHAT WILL YOU LEARN?

1. To examine the growth and development patterns occurring during infancy, childhood, and adolescence.

2. To compare the normal nutrient requirements for each stage of growth.

3. To distinguish between the special nutrition issues facing each age group.

4. To evaluate the potential effects of nutrient insufficiency on growth and development.

5. To formulate nursing interventions that target improved nutritional health in this lifespan group.

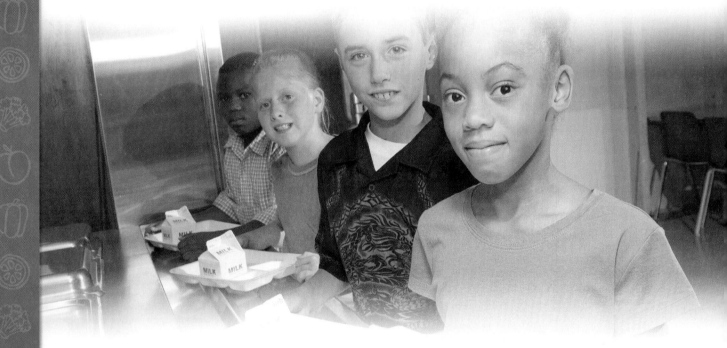

DID YOU KNOW?

▶ One of the most important decisions a mother can make for an infant's health is the choice to formula-feed or breastfeed.

▶ A child may have to try a food 8 to 10 times before finding it familiar or even liking it.

▶ Less than 25% of schoolchildren eat the recommended servings of fruits and vegetables.

▶ Almost half of adolescents regularly skip breakfast.

KEY TERMS

From birth to adulthood, food choices build the pattern for a lifetime of healthy eating. Although the amounts of nutrients required change across the lifespan, the essential nutrients remain the same. The development of a healthy relationship with food is built on important lessons involving both physical and psychological requirements. The foundation of good nutritional health that is built in childhood can set the stage for lifelong healthy lifestyle habits and reduced disease risk.

Nutrition for Infants

The most dramatic growth changes occur during the first year of life. By a child's first birthday, weight will triple and length will double. Infants have very specific nutritional needs to support this rapid growth rate. When considering the nutritional needs of infants, it is inappropriate to use most of the national guidelines designed as blanket recommendations for the nutrient needs of adults. Infants and children have unique nutritional requirements to support growth and development.

Nutrient Needs

When considering the nutrient needs for infants, it is crucial to utilize recommendations specifically established for this population. Rapid growth and ongoing brain development require adequate intake of calories and fat along with additional nutrients.

Energy

Energy requirements during infancy are high. Infants require more calories than adults per kilogram of body weight. In addition to the calories required for rapid growth, an infant's metabolic rate is higher than an adult's because of higher heart and respiratory rates coupled with a relatively higher body surface area in proportion to weight that drives up energy expended to maintain core body temperature. The average newborn infant requires 108 kcalories/kg of body weight/day for the first 6 months of life or an average of 450 kcalories/day. In comparison, the average female adult requires 2,000 kcalories, or about 25 kcalories/kg/day (Institute of Medicine [IOM], 2002). During the second 6 months of life, the amount of kcalories decreases to 98 kcalories/kg/day, but because an infant's weight increases, the average kcalories required increases to 1,000 per day by 1 year of age (IOM, 2002).

Fat is the main source of energy in the diet of an infant and is extremely important in both the development of brain and organ tissue and the construction of adequate energy stores. Development of the central nervous system requires a high-fat intake in comparison to that recommended for an adult. Specifically, the fatty acids docosahexaenoic (DHA) and arachadonic acids are required. Infants who receive these important fats through breast milk or supplemented infant formula are reported to have small but measurable increase in mental and psychomotor development scores than infants who do not consume adequate sources of these fatty acids (Birch et al., 2007; Uauy & Dangour, 2006). Additionally, these two fatty acids play a central role in the development of optimal vision function during infancy (Koletzko et al., 2008). A low-fat diet is inappropriate in children less than 2 years of age because of the crucial requirement for fat in brain and nervous system development.

Protein

Protein is a significant component of an infant's dietary intake. Adequate protein ensures continued rapid growth and development. Protein needs of 2.2 grams/kg/day during the first 6 months and 1.6 grams/kg/day during the second 6 months of age are based on the intake and growth changes of healthy, breastfed infants (IOM, 2002). Excess protein will not benefit a normal infant's growth. Protein intake in excess of recommended amounts cannot be processed properly by an infant's immature kidneys and can overexert them, potentially leading to dehydration or impaired kidney function. The forms of protein in breast milk include casein and whey, whereas infant formulas can contain these proteins or soy-based isolates. Cow's milk also has casein and whey but in different proportions than breast milk or infant formula and is not recommended for the infant's immature kidneys and gastrointestinal tract until after age 1 year. Consumption of cow's milk is associated with intestinal blood loss in infants, which in turn can contribute to risk of anemia (Fernandes, de Morais, & Amancio, 2008).

Fluid

Water is one of the most important nutrients for maintaining life. Infants receive sufficient water through appropriate amounts of breast milk or formula. Offering plain water to an infant is not recommended because water volume can displace important nutrients normally received through breast milk or formula consumption (American Academy of Pediatrics [AAP], 2004).

Vomiting and diarrhea, despite the cause, can lead to dehydration. Infants and young children can become dehydrated more rapidly than older children or adults because of a greater body surface area relative to weight, contributing to insensible water losses, lower water reserves in the body, and dependence on others for fluid (Centers for Disease Control and Prevention [CDC], 2003). The best choice of fluid for correcting mild to moderate dehydration is an oral rehydration solution, which is an electrolyte fluid mixture formulated for children (Diggins, 2008). In extreme fluid loss, repletion with intravenous fluids is necessary. An oral rehydration beverage can be used to replace fluid losses in bottle-fed infants or older children. Liquids such as juice, broth, soda, or some sports beverages can make diarrhea more profuse because the high concentration of these drinks draws water into the intestine; the body always tries to keep fluid concentration even on both sides of a cell membrane. For breastfed infants, continued breastfeeding is appropriate. It is recommended that children return to age-appropriate foods and liquids as soon as rehydrated (CDC, 2003; Diggins, 2008).

Vitamin D

Adequate intake of calcium and vitamin D is essential in childhood for mineralization of bones and teeth. Infants receive vitamin D from infant formula, breast milk, or sun exposure. Infants with dark pigmented skin synthesize less vitamin D when exposed to sunlight than do lighter skinned infants. Although breast milk contains vitamin D, the amount is insufficient to meet the needs of the infant, and supplementation is needed to reach the recommended levels of intake. The AAP recommends that all children from infancy receive 10 mcg or 400 international units/day of vitamin D in contrast to the older Dietary Reference Intake (DRI) recommendation of 5 mcg or 200 international units, which many feel is inadequate to prevent poor vitamin D status (IOM, 1997; Wagner, Greer, & Section on Breastfeeding, Committee on Nutrition, 2008). There is demonstrated widespread vitamin D insufficiency and deficiency among children in the United States (Rovner & O'Brien, 2008). This issue is discussed in Chapter 5.

Vitamin K

Vitamin K is produced by intestinal bacteria. At birth infants have insufficient stores of vitamin K, and because of the sterility of the newborn's intestinal tract, adequate vitamin K has not been produced. Vitamin K is needed for the production of prothrombin, an important constituent of blood clotting. It is a recommended practice for infants to receive an intramuscular injection of vitamin K at birth to prevent vitamin K deficiency bleeding (AAP, 2003). After feeding is initiated, infants receive vitamin K from breast milk or infant formula, in addition to the population of beneficial bacteria that develop in the intestine (AAP, 2003). The DRI for infants less than 6 months of age is 2 mcg and 2.5 mcg between the age of 6 and 12 months (IOM, 2001).

Iron

Iron-deficiency anemia affects over 2 million children in the United States and is one of the most common nutrient insufficiencies (Brotanek, Gosz, Weitzman, & Flores, 2007). Iron is important for adequate development and growth. Deficiencies in infancy and early childhood have been connected with delays in cognitive and motor development that are not always reversible (Beard, 2008). The adequate intake for infants under the age of 6 months is 0.27 mg. After 6 months of age the recommendation is 11 mg/day (IOM, 2001). When mothers consume sufficient iron during pregnancy, the fetus develops stores of iron to draw from during the first 4 to 6 months of life. By 6 months of age, infants need a dietary source of iron. The AAP (1999) recommends that all healthy formula-fed infants receive an iron-fortified formula from birth. Although the iron in breast milk is present in a highly absorbable form, the amount is insufficient to meet the infant's needs and additional supplementation is needed (Ziegler, Nelson, & Jeter, 2009). Iron-fortified rice cereals are among the first foods used to meet increased iron needs.

Fluoride

Fluoride is essential for mineralization of bones and teeth. Fluoride is found in soil and is naturally occurring in some water sources, plants, and animals. Many municipalities choose to add supplemental fluoride to their water supply. The fluoride content of household water varies throughout the United States. Infants over the age of 6 months who are breastfed or formula-fed and who live in communities without fluoridated water may need a fluoride supplement. Routine fluoride supplementation is not recommended. Instead, children should be individually assessed for risk of dental caries or limited intake of fluoride from the water supply before the decision is made regarding supplementation (AAP, 2008). Oral fluoride supplements should only be used if prescribed by a dentist or pediatrician. Care should be taken to avoid oversupplementation from sources such as toothpaste that children may swallow or supplements when used in conjunction with fluoridated water (American Dietetic Association [ADA], 2007).

Excess fluoride intake can cause fluorosis, a cosmetic condition that results from mottled tooth enamel. The tolerable upper limit for infants less than 6 months of age is 0.7 mg/day. Infants between the age of 6 and 12 months should not receive more than 0.9 mg/day (IOM, 1997).

Infant Feeding Decisions

Parents and caregivers of young children have important decisions to make regarding how to best provide adequate nutrition for the child. Whether to breastfeed or provide an infant formula is an early decision that has to be made; later when and how to introduce complementary foods into the diet becomes an important issue.

Breastfeed or Bottle Feed: What Is Best?

A woman's decision to breastfeed or bottle feed her newborn infant is one of the most important decisions she must make as a new mother (AAP, 2005; ADA, 2005). This decision is typically made during the pregnancy or even before a woman has become pregnant. Research has shown that women are greatly influenced by the attitudes of their partner and family in making the decision to breastfeed (Scott, Binns, & Aroni, 1997). Box 14-1 outlines some suggestions that the nurse can make to involve the woman's partner in the feeding process.

Benefits of Breastfeeding

According to the AAP and the ADA, breastfeeding is the ideal source of nutrition for all healthy, full-term infants because of nutritional, immunological, psychological, and even economic benefits (AAP, 2005; ADA, 2005). The World Health Organization, AAP, American College of Obstetricians and Gynecologists, and many other organizations recommend exclusive breastfeeding for the first 6 months of life (AAP, 2005). Continued breastfeeding with the addition of iron-rich foods is recommended by most health care organizations into the first year of life and longer if desired by mother and child (AAP, 2005).

BOX 14-1	Assisting the Breastfeeding Mother: Ideas for the Partner

There are many ways that the partner of a nursing mother can help take care of a new infant other than feeding the infant.
  The mother's partner can:
- Get the mother of the baby a drink of water while she is nursing the baby.
- Help the mother get comfortable by getting her a pillow or footstool for proper positioning.
- Play with other children while the mother nurses the infant.
- Change the baby's diaper.
- Bathe the baby.
- Get the baby and bring him or her to the mother for night feedings.

Breastfeeding can be established within the first hour after birth. An infant can display readiness by displaying a rooting reflex, opening and shutting the mouth, cooing, or other signs of early hunger. Nurses or other health care workers who specialize in lactation can assist with the baby's proper positioning and latching-on to the breast so that the feeding relationship gets started without stress for the infant or mother.

Colostrum is the milk first produced by the mother immediately after birth. This yellow fluid is high in antibodies that a newborn infant can absorb and use to fight infection. Colostrum, or "liquid gold" as some lactation experts have named it, is higher in protein, vitamins, and minerals than mature breast milk.

After initiating breastfeeding, breast milk will change over to mature milk, which is lower in protein than colostrum, but remains high in antibodies, vitamins, and minerals needed for adequate growth. The amount and types of proteins in breast milk match an infant's needs perfectly. Casein, the major protein in breast milk, facilitates increased absorption of calcium in the breastfed infant. Breast milk is digested more rapidly and more efficiently than formula, and thus breastfed children may need to eat more often than formula-fed infants. After birth, an infant should be breastfed whenever hungry, which can be from 8 to 12 times per day.

Infants should nurse on demand to promote breast milk production and adequate nutrition. Infants will be able to go for longer periods without breastfeeding as they become more adept at taking larger amounts of milk per feeding and as their stomach capacity increases. Women should be encouraged to allow an infant to nurse on a single breast until the baby is satisfied and to then switch to the second breast. Nursing for an extended period on one breast allows the baby to extract milk that is higher in fat and calories, known as **hind milk** (Anderson, 1989). The more an infant nurses from the mother, the more milk will be produced for the infant. Excessive use of a pacifier or formula supplementation is not recommended because both interfere with the infant's natural desire to suckle and can impact breastfeeding success (Cinar, 2004; Santo, de Oliveira, & Giugliani, 2007).

Breastfed infants have bowel movements that are very soft, yellow, and seedy in appearance. Infants younger than 1 month typically have more than four bowel movements daily. After 1 month, this number may decrease. After the first 3 or 4 days of life, infants will have six or more wet diapers daily. The nurse can advise mothers of breastfed infants to track the number of feedings and wet or soiled diapers a baby produces in a day (Lawrence & Lawrence, 2005). Significantly notable changes in feeding or diapers should be communicated to the primary health care provider.

Infants require a high-quality source of fat in their diet to provide sufficient calories for growth and important fatty acids for development. Breast milk is an important source of fatty acids such as alpha-linolenic acid, arachadonic acid (ARA), docosahexaenoic acid (DHA), and eicosapenaenoic acid (EPA). Breast milk is also a good source of cholesterol, which promotes development of the nervous system and, most specifically, the brain, where it is a component of myelin. The main carbohydrate in breast milk and infant formula is lactose. Lactose is easy for infants to digest and facilitates calcium absorption.

Breast milk, in contrast to formula, offers an infant unique protection from disease. Human milk contains antibodies that can be used by an infant to fight infection and disease. This prepackaged immunity is passed from mother to infant. Breast milk also contains substances that enable the presence of beneficial bacteria in an infant's digestive tract. One type of bacterium, *Lactobacillus bifidus*, can help to protect infants from the overgrowth of harmful bacterial agents. Infants who are breastfed are less likely to suffer from ear infections, diarrhea, or constipation (Ip et al., 2007).

Long-Term Benefits of Breastfeeding   Babies can taste flavor differences in their mother's milk. This early exposure to a variety of tastes is reported to positively influence food choices later in life (Beauchamp & Mennella, 2009).

Several studies have demonstrated a reduction in risk for certain diseases when infants have been breastfed. Connections between breastfeeding and type 1 diabetes mellitus, lymphoma, asthma, Crohn's disease, ulcerative colitis, obesity, and allergies both to food and the environment have been investigated (AAP, 2005). Breastfeeding also offers a tremendous number of benefits for the mother. These benefits are outlined in Chapter 13.

No matter the duration anticipated, there are benefits to initiating breastfeeding. Mothers who intend to return to work outside the home can still initiate breastfeeding and maintain lactation once returning to work. Several quality manual and electric breast pumps are available for mothers to provide breast milk when they are unable to breastfeed. Breast milk can be frozen and used when a mother is not available to breastfeed an infant. In many states, employers are required to allow a mother time to utilize a breast pump in order to provide milk for her infant.

Contraindications to Breastfeeding
Breastfeeding is not recommended in certain situations, such as when a mother has untreated tuberculosis, has human immunodeficiency virus (HIV), or is taking certain medications or illegal substances (CDC, 2007). Mothers should discuss use of medications with a pharmacist or the prescribing physician before taking any prescription or over-the-counter medication. It is also not recommended that women use tobacco products or drink alcohol while breastfeeding. Smoking decreases breast milk production. Babies who are breastfed within 2 hours of a mother who has consumed alcohol can receive a high concentration of alcohol via the breast milk (AAP, 2005).

Formula Options

If a mother is medically unable or chooses not to breastfeed, standard infant formulas that have soy or cow's milk as a base are specially manufactured for infant tolerance, and most are fortified with iron. Infant formula production is regulated in the United States by the Food and Drug Administration. The composition of infant formulas is based on the structure of human breast milk. Formula is created to be higher in iron and vitamin D than breast milk because infants absorb these nutrients less efficiently from formula than breast milk.

Frequent use of soy formulas has been investigated because of the presence of plant isoflavones, which are similar in structure to estrogen. It is unknown whether consumption of these substances in high amounts has any harmful effects on growing infants. No identifiable negative problems have been documented. The AAP recommends use of soy formulas only when other available cow milk formulas are not tolerated (AAP, 1999). Other specialty formulas are available for premature infants or those with allergy or other medical conditions. A dietitian specializing in pediatric nutrition should be consulted when such specialty formulas are indicated.

Regular unmodified cow's, goat's, rice, or soy milk is inappropriate for infants less than 1 year of age because of inappropriate amounts of protein. Additionally, these milks do not contain the needed amounts of vitamins and minerals. Cow's milk is a common food allergen, and it has been suggested that delaying its introduction into the diet until age 1 year is a strategy to prevent food allergy. However, the effect is inconclusive (Heine & Tang, 2008).

Formulas are available as ready-to-feed (most expensive), concentrate, or powdered (least expensive). The nurse should instruct the caregiver that all reconstituted or opened ready-to-feed formulas should be discarded after 48 hours because of risk of food borne illness. Formulas must be mixed with the proper amount of clean water. Formulas that are mixed with too much water will not provide the appropriate amount of nutrition. Insufficient water in a formula can lead to dehydration or kidney damage. Caregivers must evaluate whether water being used to reconstitute formula needs to be boiled and the method of sterilizing the nipples and bottles used for feeding. Formula manufacturers and the AAP recommend boiling water for several minutes and cooling before reconstituting infant formula (Kleinman, 2004). Some practitioners do not feel that boiling is necessary if the water comes from a reputable water source. Health care providers should take into account whether the source of water requires boiling based on the health of the infant's immune system and the source of the water (Samour & King, 2005).

When and How Should Solid Foods Be Introduced?

Most infants can move from diets fully consisting of breast milk or formula to a gradual addition of semiliquid consistency foods

MyNursingKit U.S. Department of Health and Human Services (USDHHS) Growth Charts

between 4 and 6 months of age. This period is a unique window of time in which infants become developmentally and physically ready to consume solid foods. Infants who are ready to experience solid foods will show several signs of readiness. An infant tasting solid food for the first time should be able to sit up with some support and demonstrate increased tongue and jaw control. A **tongue extrusion reflex,** or tongue thrust, in which a baby pushes items out of the mouth with the tongue, should be diminished.

An infant's digestive tract is immature in comparison to that of an adult. Foods offered too early in life may lead to an immune response to certain foods, including a food allergy. Introduction of complementary foods into the diet is recommended at age 4 to 6 months because this timing may be a window of time when enhanced immune tolerance exists (Heine & Tang, 2008). Delaying the introduction of solid foods beyond 6 months of age has not been associated with a reduction in later food allergies (Zutavern et al., 2008). Infant rice cereal is typically the first food offered because of its low allergy potential. After it has been established that no immune response such as digestive upset, respiratory distress, or skin rash has occurred, second grains such as barley and oats can be offered. Wheat cereal is offered as a later option because of a higher prevalence of allergy to this grain than others. A 3-day waiting period without offering any new foods is a common recommendation to identify allergenic foods.

Infants should not be offered honey or corn syrup before the age of 1 year because of increased risk of being exposed to the spores that cause botulism. After age 1 year, the gastrointestinal tract can destroy the bacterium found in those foods. Table 14-1 outlines the introduction of solid foods to the infant's diet.

Parents can choose from a wide variety of premade infant foods or make their own baby food from nutritious whole foods. Baby desserts have little role in a healthy infant diet. To a baby, strained fruit is a sweet treat that also contributes to a good foundation for a lifetime of healthy eating. Infants should not be offered large amounts of fruit juice because it can lead to diarrhea and replace other needed foods in the diet. Only 2 to 4 ounces of 100% fruit juice offered no more than twice daily is an adequate amount for infants over the age of 6 months.

Tracking Pediatric Growth

If infants consume sufficient amounts of breast milk or infant formula, practically all required vitamin and mineral needs will be met. Changes in weight and height throughout childhood are tracked closely to verify adequate nutritional intake. Nurses accurately access gains in development by utilizing growth charts developed by the National Center for Health Statistics (NCHS). Growth charts can be used as a tool in the overall clinical assessment of a child. Height (or length under the age of 2), weight, head circumference, and body mass index are plotted in comparison to other children of the same age and gender on a growth curve. On-line resources are available for the nurse to learn the proper use of these tools.

Wellness Issues in Infancy

Developmental delays and disabilities as well as special health care needs require comprehensive care that includes nutrition intervention. Infants, children, and adolescents can benefit from nutrition-related nursing interventions formulated to target improved nutrition health. Wellness issues that may begin in the infant are outlined here. Table 14-2 outlines further issues.

Growth Failure

Carefully monitoring a child's growth can identify when gains in weight or length are not occurring as expected. A child who is not growing appropriately may be classified with **failure to thrive.** Poor growth is most often a result of not consuming or not retaining adequate calories. Weight below the fifth percentile on the CDC growth chart or weight that decreases over subsequent office visits can indicate a need for further evaluation of dietary intake. The most important use of growth charting is monitoring individual trends over time. A deviation from a child's own previously established growth pattern, whether in weight or height, can indicate growth failure.

The treatment for true growth failure is best completed with a multidisciplinary approach including a nurse, a pediatrician, a registered dietitian, and if quality of life or behavioral issues exist, a psychologist and social worker. A thorough dietary recall examining the timing of feedings, amounts of nutrition consumed, common procedures when mixing formula, and presence of undesirable food or liquids needs to be completed. Consumption of excess fruit juice can take the place of more nutritious foods in an infant's diet. Fruit juice should be limited to 2 to 4 ounces per day to allow an appetite for other foods (AAP, 2001). The method with which a caregiver mixes and administers formula needs to be discussed in depth to ensure that an infant is receiving the proper concentration of nutrition. Formula that is overdiluted provides excess water with insufficient calories. Observing a feeding session with the primary caregiver can reveal any dysfunctional interactions such as withholding nourishment or poor emotional interaction that can affect the amount of nutrition the infant receives. Once the primary issue has been discovered, interventions can include more frequent or more specific timings of feedings, a calculated change in the caloric concentration of infant formula, or behavioral techniques at mealtimes.

Food Allergies and Intolerances

True **food allergies** are less common than **food intolerances.** A food allergy, or a hypersensitivity to a particular food, is caused when the immune system responds to consumption of a food. A wide range of reactions can occur including rash; itching; vomiting; diarrhea; or swelling of

Table 14-1   Introduction of Solid Foods

Age	Food Item	Amounts	Comments
Birth to 4 months	Breast milk or iron-fortified formula	8–12 nursings 18–32 oz of formula depending on age	Water in addition to breast milk or formula is not needed.
4 to 6 months	Breast milk or iron-fortified formula	4–6 nursings 27–45 oz of formula depending on age	Cereal should be introduced between 4 and 6 months.
	Iron-fortified infant cereal (rice cereal first)	2–3 tbsp	Decrease of the tongue extrusion reflex allows the infant to take food from a spoon.
6 to 8 months	Breast milk or iron-fortified formula	3–5 nursings or 24–32 oz of formula	Breast milk or formula is still needed until after age 12 months. Better ability to bite and chew as teeth erupt.
	Fruits, plain, smooth such as banana, pears, applesauce, or peaches	3–4 tbsp	Sources of vitamin A and vitamin C become more important. Avoid added sugar.
	Vegetables, plain, strained such as avocado, well-cooked carrots, squash, and sweet potato	3–4 tbsp	A good time to introduce new flavors.
	Meats, plain, strained	1–2 tbsp	Meats provide iron, protein, and B vitamins.
	Grain foods such as crackers, unsweetened cereals, or toast	1 serving	Helps with teething and increasing manual dexterity.
	Iron-fortified infant cereal	4–6 tbsp	Should be prepared with breast milk or infant formula.
	Unsweetened fruit juices	2–4 oz	Avoid acidic juices like orange or tomato.
9 to 10 months	Breast milk or iron-fortified formula	3–4 nursings or 24–32 oz of formula	Cow's milk should not be introduced until after age 1 year. Intake of formula/breast milk will start to decrease as solid food increases.
	Fruits, plain, smooth	6–8 tbsp	Avoid added sugar versions.
	Vegetables, plain, strained	6–8 tbsp	Continue to offer new and different vegetables even if baby dislikes the first time.
	Soft meats, cottage cheese, egg yolks, fish, poultry, yogurt	4–6 tbsp	
	Grain foods such as crackers, unsweetened cereals, or toast	1–2 small servings	Avoid very hard biscuits or cookies because they are a choking risk.
	Iron fortified infant cereal	4–6 tbsp	Cereals may include infant rice cereal, oatmeal, or whole grain baby cereals.
	Unsweetened fruit juices	2–4 oz	Do not offer excess juice.
11 to 12 months	Breast milk or iron-fortified formula	3–4 nursings or 24–32 oz of formula	Cow's milk should not be introduced until after age 1 year. Intake of formula/breast milk will start to decrease as solid food intake increases.
	Fruits, plain, soft	2–4 oz	Small, soft pieces of fruits and vegetables can be picked up by baby.
	Vegetables, plain, well cooked	2–4 oz	
	Soft meats, cottage cheese, egg yolks, fish, poultry, yogurt	2–4 oz	Egg whites should be avoided until after age 1 year.
	Grain foods such as crackers, unsweetened cereals, or toast	1–2 servings	Small bites of crackers and O-shaped or other low sugar cereals can be picked up and eaten.
	Iron-fortified infant cereal	2–4 oz iron-fortified cereal	Continue to prepare with infant formula or breast milk until age 1 year.
	Unsweetened fruit juices	3–4 oz	Avoid excess fruit juice. Citrus juice can be introduced after age 1 year.

C̲T̲? How could the nurse explain the need for advancing food textures to the parent who is still feeding an older baby pureed baby foods?

Table 14-2 Special Health Care Needs in Infants, Children, and Adolescents

Developmental Disabilities

Reportedly up to 90% of children under age 3 with developmental disabilities have one or more risk factors for poor nutrition (ADA, 2004). Cognitive and physical disabilities in children can impair feeding skills, cause underweight and overweight, and increase risk for other conditions such as cardiovascular disease. Down syndrome, Prader-Willi syndrome, and spina bifida are all developmental disabilities that increase the risk of obesity in the individual because of altered muscle tone, short stature, or similar characteristics. Other conditions, such as cerebral palsy, can lead to growth issues. Disabilities that lead to feeding dysfunction are associated with poor growth and inadequate fat stores (ADA, 2007). A comprehensive team approach is needed to coordinate nutrition interventions that are customized for the individual. Such interventions can involve altered feeding practices, assistive feeding equipment, assessment for drug and nutrient interactions, modified diet, and enteral nutrition support.

Cystic Fibrosis

Cystic fibrosis is a genetic disorder that causes pancreatic insufficiency that leads to fat and protein malabsorption. Additionally, changes in mucus can cause frequent lung infections. Treatment of this disease requires pancreatic enzyme replacement and close monitoring of nutritional status because slowed growth and weight loss can be common. In children older than age 2 years, energy intake should be up to twice that recommended for a healthy child (Stallings et al., 2008). When growth or weight deficits are apparent, intervention with an oral liquid nutrition supplement is recommended (Stallings et al., 2008). Improved nutrition and growth status is associated with improved markers of pulmonary function and survival in this population (Stallings et al., 2008).

Seizures

Pharmacological therapy is the primary treatment for seizure disorders. However, some children remain symptomatic and require further medical intervention that can include use of a ketogenic diet. Ketogenic diets are low in carbohydrate and high in fat to promote production of ketone bodies, which may have anticonvulsant effects (Wiznitzer, 2008). Such diets are used only with drug-resistant seizure disorders because there are negative consequences that must be balanced when the decision is made to treat with diet. Constipation, metabolic acidosis, dehydration, vomiting, hyperlipidemia, and poor energy level have all been reported (Neal et al., 2008; Wilong, 2007). Close monitoring of the nutritional health of children on a ketogenic diet is crucial to ensure that needed nutrients are obtained on this highly restrictive diet.

the lips, tongue, or face that can lead to respiratory distress. A food intolerance, which does not involve the immune system, causes a physical reaction such as gastrointestinal upset. Lactose intolerance is an example of food intolerance. See Chapter 10 for further discussion of food allergies and intolerances, including the issue of whether manipulation of the maternal or child's diet affects later development of food allergies. On-line resources are available for

the nurse working with children with food allergies and include action plans that the school nurse can utilize. Lactose intolerance is reviewed in Chapter 20.

The nurse should assess the overall adequacy of the diet in infants and children with known food allergies to ensure that sufficient intake is occurring and that unnecessary restrictions have not been placed on the diet by a well-meaning caregiver. Restrictive intake because of real or suspected food allergies or intolerances can place an infant at risk for malnutrition. Children with multiple food allergies should be referred to a registered dietitian experienced in treating this population for guidance in dietary adherence while obtaining adequate nutrition to support growth and development.

Baby Bottle Tooth Decay

Decay of the primary teeth of infants is an unfortunate side effect of inappropriate feeding practices. Allowing a child to fall asleep with a bottle of juice, breast milk, formula, or other sweetened liquids can lead to a pooling of liquid around a child's teeth. The sugary liquid forms a medium for bacterial growth and the creation of acids that cause breakdown of dental enamel. This process, known as **baby bottle tooth decay,** can cause increased discomfort for the infant, intolerance to warm or cold foods, and early tooth loss, leading to misaligned adult teeth. Parents and caregivers should be encouraged to gently use a soft washcloth to cleanse an infant's gums and move on to the use of a soft, infant toothbrush as new teeth erupt (ADA, 2007). The nurse should stress that when a child is allowed to take a bottle to bed, it should only contain water (AAP, 2008). Figure 14-1 ■ depicts baby bottle tooth decay.

Inappropriate Feeding Practices

Inappropriate feeding practices are those that pose a safety or health risk to the infant. Feeding practices vary among cultures and what may be a common practice in one culture may not be viewed the same way in another. When assessing the infant for use of inappropriate feeding practices, the nurse should reserve judgment about practices that are unfamiliar

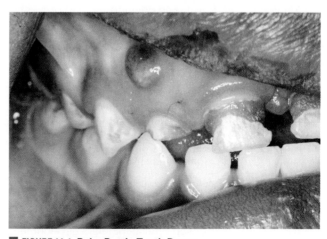

■ **FIGURE 14-1 Baby Bottle Tooth Decay.**
Source: Custom Medical Stock Photo, Inc.

yet pose no safety or health risk. When educating parents or caregivers about unsafe or unhealthy practices, the nurse should determine the basis of what led to such practices to best provide appropriate intervention. Box 14-2 and Practice Pearl: Common Feeding Myths outline some inappropriate feeding practices and myths.

Early Childhood—Toddlers

Between the ages of 1 and 3 years, children often desire more control and an increased sense of independence. A toddler most often asserts the desire for autonomy in areas of toileting, dressing, or self-feeding. Toddlers may be characterized as defiant or suffering from "the terrible twos," but parents need to be aware that an increased desire for control is a normal part of human development.

Meals and snacks provided on a regular basis can help to provide a consistent framework for meeting nutrient needs. Young children benefit from a quiet, safe environment in which they are encouraged to practice feeding themselves. As children's fine-motor skills develop, they will naturally progress from using their hands for eating to eventually using a spoon or other utensil at a later age. Table 14-3 outlines developmental readiness in relation to feeding.

PRACTICE PEARL

Common Feeding Myths

Myth—I think my baby needs cereal in his bottle to sleep through the night. If I cut the nipple to make a bigger hole he can drink it.

Fact—Studies have not shown that giving cereal at night will increase sleep. In actuality giving a baby cereal before the gastrointestinal tract is ready can lead to food allergies and intolerances.

Myth—I only want my baby to have organic foods so I've been using honey in her cereal.

Fact—Honey should not be given to infants less than 1 year of age because of increased chance of botulism. After age 1 year, honey can be added safely.

Myth—I'm worried that my 1-year-old is getting too fat. I've started to cut back on the fat in her food.

Fact—Infants under age 2 need good sources of fat to meet their calorie needs. Babies come in different sizes. A pediatrician or registered dietitian should evaluate whether the child is getting the appropriate amount of nutrition for his or her size.

Nutrient Needs

During early childhood, growth and development progress but at a slower rate than during infancy. Nutritional needs mirror

---

BOX 14-2	Inappropriate Feeding Practices

The following are a list of practices that are inappropriate when feeding children or infants:

- Placing liquids in a bottle other than breast milk, formula, or water. Young children should not be offered iced tea, fruit punch-type drinks, or soda. These liquids replace important foods in a child's diet.
- Not breastfeeding an infant on demand. Limiting the number or duration of feedings to prevent "spoiling" a child or creating a schedule for parental convenience can limit appropriate nutrition and interfere with milk production.
- Preparing formula not according to package directions. Nurses should monitor for inappropriately diluted formula. Watering down formula to prevent stomach upset or to stretch food dollars leads to insufficient nutrition for normal growth.
- Propping a bottle for a baby. This practice deprives infants of nurturing touch and security. Physical contact contributes to appropriate social development. Propping a bottle can also lead to baby bottle tooth decay due to liquids pooling around developing teeth. Infants should not be put to bed with a bottle.
- Putting baby cereal in a baby bottle and cutting the nipple off to make the hole bigger so baby can drink the cereal. This practice has not been shown to enable infants to sleep longer and they may become overweight. It is also a choking hazard. Solid foods should not be added to a bottle except under the direction of a physician.
- Using formulas not appropriate for infant development. Homemade formulas are missing significant amounts

of vitamins and minerals. Inappropriate formulas can lead to failure to thrive and even death.
- Continuing bottle feeding beyond 15 months in a child with a normal progression of development.
- Putting honey on a pacifier or offering honey at less than 1 year of age.
- Giving hard, round, or sticky foods prior to age 2 years.
- Allowing toddlers to make all food decisions. Children should be offered healthy choices from which to pick. They do not have the mental capacity to recognize the importance of healthy food choices.
- Limiting fat in infants less than 2 years of age can lead to malnutrition due to insufficient calories and insufficient fat for brain development.
- Not using proper hand washing when preparing formula or food for infants and children.
- Knowing better than a child whether he or she is hungry or full.
- Offering a reward for eating a certain food.
- Trying to coerce children into eating something when they state they are not hungry.
- Allowing children excessive hours of television viewing, video games, or computer usage because of the association with obesity risk.

- How should the nurse start a conversation with a parent who is mixing formula and cereal in a baby bottle and cutting the nipple to allow the baby to drink the mix?

Table 14-3   Developmental Milestones and Feeding Readiness

At Birth
Sucking, rooting, and swallowing reflexes are present

By 3 Months
Tongue extrusion reflex is still present. Most appropriate food still only liquids

At 4 to 6 months
Able to move tongue from side to side
Cannot swallow lumpy foods, but able to start with smooth textures
Begins to hold bottle if bottle fed

At 7 to 9 months
Pincher grasp begins to develop
Self-feeding begins to develop
Increased ability to bite

At 10 to 12 months
Increased ability to pick up small objects
Begins to be able to pick up a spoon
Wants to self-feed

Between 12 and 18 months
The tongue can move from side to side
Rotary chew develops rather than up-and-down motions
Increased ability to handle soft table food
Refined pincher grasp helps with picking up small food objects to put in the mouth
Can use a spoon but not extremely well

18 to 24 months
Increased ability to use the tongue to clean food residue from the lips
Improved rotary chew, well enough to handle meats, raw fruits, and other textures

this pace of growth and include adequate calories and fat for brain development that is still occurring at this age.

Energy

Children between the ages of 1 and 3 years require an average of 1,000 to 1,300 kcalories/day. With increased growth comes a greater need for protein. The recommended daily amount of protein, 16 grams, can be met through two to three servings of a dairy food and meat or meat substitute offered twice per day (IOM, 2002). Children under the age of 2 years require a higher percentage of fat from the calories consumed in comparison to adults. Fat provides an important source of energy because children have a limited stomach capacity. Children who have a restriction of fat before age 2 years may have difficulty meeting their calorie needs and the requirement of fat for brain development. After age 2 years, a gradual reduction in the calories provided from fat is appropriate (ADA, 2008). Common changes can be to switch from whole milk to reduced-fat milk or using leaner meat choices.

Children age 2 to 3 years should consume 1 to 1.5 cups of fruit, 1 to 1.5 cups of vegetables, 3 to 5 ounces of grains, 2 to 4 ounces of meat or meat substitutes, 2 cups of milk or milk substitute, and 3 to 4 tablespoons of vegetable oils over a day's time. At least half of the grains should come from whole grain sources such as whole wheat, brown rice, barley, oats, or cornmeal. Box 14-3 depicts a sample menu that meets the needs of a 3-year-old child.

Fluids

Fluids such as iced tea, soda, or even large amounts of juice or milk should not replace more nutritious foods in a child's diet. Meeting a toddler's daily calcium requirement of 500 mg can be completed through two to three half-cup servings of milk each day. Even 100% fruit juice should be limited to 4 to 6 fluid ounces daily (AAP, 2001). Children should not be permitted to drink large amounts of sugared liquids via bottles or "sippy" cups because of the effect on both appetite and tooth enamel (Harnack, Stang, & Story, 1999).

Development of the Feeding Relationship

The feeding relationship between caregivers and children is one based on love, patience, and mutual respect for each participant's role in eating. According to Ellyn Satter, a registered dietitian and licensed social worker, caregivers have specific roles in the feeding relationship. Parents are responsible for *what* foods are prepared for meals and *when* the meals or snacks are provided. Children are responsible for choosing *how much* they eat and *if* they decide to try foods or not (Satter, 1987).

BOX 14-3	Sample Menu for a 3-Year-Old

Breakfast
1/2 cup 2% milk
1/2 cup O-shape cereal
1/4 cup blueberries
1/2 slice whole wheat toast
1 tbsp peanut butter

Midmorning Snack
1/2 cup small graham cookies
1/2 cup vanilla yogurt

Lunch
1/2 cup 2% milk
1/2 sliced turkey sandwich on wheat bread
1/4 cup cooked carrots
1/2 cup applesauce

Midafternoon Snack
1/2 cup grape juice
1/2 banana
1 tbsp peanut butter

Supper
1/2 cup 2% milk
1/2 cup cheese ravioli with tomato sauce
1/4 cup cooked green beans
1/2 cup gelatin with peaches

Evening Snack
1/2 cup pudding

In addition to the early exposure to tastes in utero or through breast milk, children experience foods through touch, smell, taste, and sight. Fluctuations in growth can be frustrating for parents because a child may display varied degrees of hunger and disinterest in eating. **Food jags** occur when young children repeatedly request the same food and have little interest in eating a variety of foods. Parents should continue to offer a variety of foods and allow the child to consume the single food in which the child has a great interest. On a short-term basis, overall nutritional status will not be affected. The nurse can encourage the parent to involve the child in some of the meal preparations or shopping decisions to foster an interest in a variety of foods over time. For example, a parent can ask a 3-year-old to be in charge of choosing a vegetable in the grocery store or to help stir a dish being made at home. Helping with age-appropriate tasks during meal preparation also builds fine-motor skills in this age group.

Forcibly insisting that certain foods be eaten does not lead to increased interest or compliance. Toddlers are influenced by many factors in their food selections. Even remaining seated while eating can have a positive effect on the quality of a toddler's nutritional intake (Hoerr, Horodynski, Lee, & Henry, 2006). Children who are encouraged to eat by involving them in food selection and preparation are more likely to try new foods than when caregivers provide negative reinforcement (Satter, 1987). Overly controlling feeding behaviors that may arise because of concerns about overweight or underweight has been demonstrated to contribute to eating in the absence of hunger or overeating and undereating or fussy eating habits, respectively, later in childhood, making such practices counterproductive (Farrow & Blissett, 2008).

Wellness Concerns in Childhood

Toddler nutrition can present some normal nutrition challenges, such as food jags, appetite changes, and development of self-feeding skills. The nurse should assess overall intake, especially if growth or development rates have changed for the individual child. Specific attention should be given to iron status because of the negative effects of iron deficiency on cognitive function. Fortified cereals, developmentally appropriate portions of animal protein, and legumes such as soy, other beans, and split peas along with a vitamin C source to facilitate iron absorption are toddler sources of dietary iron.

Choking Risks

Young children are at great risk for choking on food. Children should be supervised when eating so that they are not running or jumping while eating or putting large quantities into their mouths (AAP, 2007). In addition, some foods

Table 14-4 Decreasing Choking Risk

Children should always be seated and monitored when eating. The following foods can increase the risk of choking.

Food Item	Ways to Decrease Choking
Raw carrots	Can be grated
Whole grapes	Should be cut in half
Whole cherries	Should be cut in half
Whole nuts	Monitor very closely
Peanut butter	Spread thinly
Popcorn	Monitor closely or do not offer
Whole beans	Mash beans
Hot dogs	Should be sliced in half and then cut in small pieces
Large marshmallows	Cut into small pieces
Gum	Do not offer
Hard candies	Do not offer

have more of a choking risk than others. Table 14-4 lists choking hazards for young children.

Lead Hazards

Peeling paint, foreign-made toys, and, in some areas, dirt can all be sources of hazardous amounts of lead. The presence of lead in a child's body can lead to slow growth or iron-deficiency anemia. Lead toxicity can also lead to learning disabilities, behavior problems, and even mental retardation (CDC, 2005).

A child who breathes in dust from a home with lead-based paint or an infant who eats particles of paint or drinks contaminated water are at high risk for lead toxicity. It has been estimated that over a quarter of homes with children under the age of 6 years may have a lead-based paint danger (Jacobs et al., 2002). The impact of poverty on children becomes apparent because lead toxicity is more common among those living in low-income housing and is often coupled with iron deficiency. Children with subadequate intakes of iron, calcium, and zinc often absorb lead more readily because of the lack of competition for absorption that occurs with normal intake of these minerals. The CDC recommends that children consume a diet with adequate dietary calcium and iron along with two servings of fruit per day for vitamin C to promote iron absorption (CDC, 2002).

Preventing lead exposure is easier than treating the problem. When lead has been inhaled or ingested it quickly becomes a part of the skeletal system. Blood levels of lead help physicians to determine treatment for the exposure. The CDC recommends inspection of the home environment and

MyNursingKit Lead Poisoning

MyNursingKit MyPyramid for Preschoolers

PRACTICE PEARL

Teaching Caregivers about Decreasing Lead Exposure

The nurse can teach the caregiver the following ways to decrease lead exposure:

- Ensure that children consume a well-balanced diet containing adequate amounts of iron and calcium.
- Prevent children from eating dirt or paint.
- Monitor recalls of toys and children's jewelry that contain lead.
- Remove flaking or peeling paint from older homes.
- Help children wash their hands and face before eating and sleeping.
- Clean all floors, countertops, and tabletops with a high-phosphate detergent.
- Do not offer children herbal or folk remedies that may contain lead.
- Do not use decorative pottery as a food or beverage container.
- Do not store food in open cans.
- Use cold water from the tap for drinking or cooking.

Source: Centers for Disease Control and Prevention (CDC), (2005).

remediation of any lead content for all children with blood levels greater than 15 mcg/dL (CDC, 2002). Siblings and classmates should also be tested for lead exposure. The family should be educated on sources of lead and exposure prevention. In severe exposure cases, chelation therapy, the use of intravenous agents that attach to lead in the body and help to decrease levels may need to be utilized. Practice Pearl: Teaching Caregivers about Decreasing Lead Exposure outlines advice for the nurse counseling caregivers on the reduction of lead exposure.

Later Childhood—the Preschooler

To coincide with continued growth and development, energy needs for preschoolers increase to 1,800 kcalories/day. Protein needs increase to approximately 24 grams/day (IOM, 2002).

Beyond providing guidelines for the amounts and types of food that children should consume, *MyPyramid for Preschoolers* adapts the latest U.S. dietary guidelines into appropriate recommendations for preschool children and includes many on-line resources for the parents and educators of young children. The key points to help parents maximize their children's health through nutritional intake and movement include:

- Being physically active every day
- Choosing healthy foods from each food group
- Eating more servings from certain food groups like grains, fruits, and vegetables
- Developing healthy habits one step at a time

As children enter the ages between 3 and 5 years, meals often include those served at day care centers, preschools, or other homes outside their own. It is important for parents to continue to offer a variety of foods at meals to expose children to healthy foods and to model healthy eating behaviors. Studies have demonstrated that a mother's food preferences can have a great impact on the food likes and dislikes of their children. Whether a mother eats fruits, vegetables, or dairy products influences a child (Skinner, Carruth, Bounds, & Ziegler, 2002). Research has shown that children may need repeated exposure to healthy foods before learning to accept them (ADA, 2008; Birch & Marlin, 1982). The nurse working with children may note that those involved in gardening-based nutrition activities are more likely to try a variety of fruits and vegetables than their nongardening peers (Robinson-O'Brien, Story, & Heim, 2009).

Parents may ask the nurse whether it is appropriate to hide healthy foods in recipes for familiar meals. Entire cookbooks have been created utilizing this strategy. Children in one study who were fed pasta dishes with or without blenderized vegetables included in the sauce showed no preference for either dish. The pasta dish containing vegetables had lower calories and a higher vitamin and mineral content compared to the vegetable-free entrée (Leahy, Birch, Fisher, & Rolls, 2007). Parents should use caution in incorporating food items that are potential allergens to visiting children. Continuing to offer recognizable foods along with new foods can help children to sample new foods while feeling contented with established preferences.

The amount of food offered to small children does not have to be as large as an adult portion. The appetite of a child is not the same as the appetite of an older person. A smaller stomach may need to be filled several times per day to meet the growth needs of a preschooler. Portion sizes that are larger than appropriate for children can lead to overconsumption at meals (ADA, 2008; Fisher, Liu, Birch, & Rolls, 2007). A common rule that nurses can teach caregivers is to offer 1 tablespoon of a food for each year of age. A 3-year-old can be offered 3 tablespoons of peas to start a meal with more being offered based on the child's appetite.

School-Age Children

As children enter the years between age 5 and 12 years, growth slows in comparison to earlier jumps in stature and weight. Nutrient intake can be difficult to assess as children enter the later stage of this period when they begin to spend more time eating away from home at school and social activities. Snacking can contribute significantly to nutritional health but may also contribute "empty" calories and fat devoid of nutritional value if unhealthy choices occur frequently.

Energy needs for the school-age child between 7 and 12 years old are between 2,000 and 2,200 kcalories/day. Protein

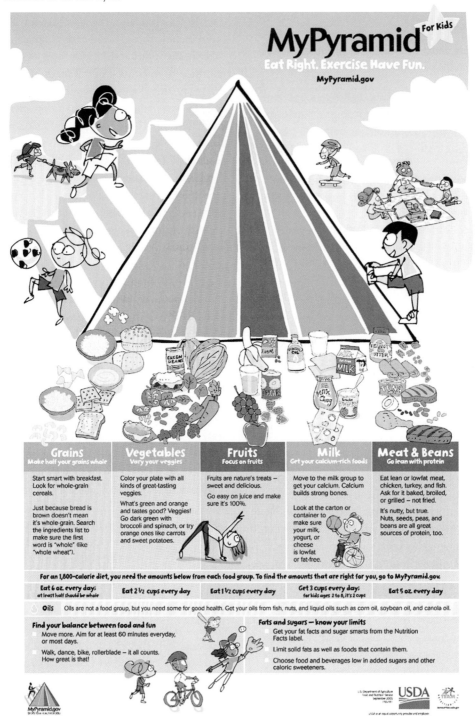

■ FIGURE 14-2 **MyPyramid for Kids.**

Source: United States Department of Agriculture, MyPyramid.gov

needs increase as children's bodies prepare for puberty. An average of 28 to 46 grams is needed depending on age and gender (IOM, 2002). Figure 14-2 ■ depicts the *MyPyramid* that is specifically designed to meet the needs of school-age children. Emphasis is on choosing a variety of foods that are low in fat; meet calcium needs; and contain whole grains, fruits, and vegetables. Children are encouraged to participate in enjoyable physical activity at least 60 minutes on most, if not all, days of

the week (U.S. Department of Agriculture, 2005). A variety of on-line resources is available for the parents and health educators working with school-age children.

Mealtime Nutrition Influences

With the increase in meals and snacks eaten away from home, it is essential that the home and school environment provide a positive model for healthy eating practices.

Breakfast's Influence

Breakfast provides important nutrients for growing children and adolescents. In addition to having an overall more healthful diet than those who skip the meal, eating breakfast has been linked with desirable outcomes in memory, attentiveness, vocabulary, test results, and improved attendance at school (Benton & Jarvis, 2006; Rampersaud, 2009). Anywhere from 10% to 30% of children skip breakfast, with females, overweight, and older children more likely to miss the meal than others (Rampersaud, 2009). The nurse can suggest that caregivers help children to make time to eat breakfast or become involved in the school breakfast program (Affenito, 2007). The nurse can help the parent and child strategize some quick breakfast ideas if lack of time is a barrier to breakfast consumption. It is important that parents be encouraged to model healthy eating behavior, including breakfast consumption, because of the influence that parental actions have on the child's (Pearson, Biddle, & Gorely, 2009). The evidence-based practice box discusses the impact of breakfast on the health of children and adolescents.

Similar to the guidelines for lunch, the school breakfast program is designed to provide one-fourth of the Recommended Dietary Allowance (RDA) by providing milk, fruit, juice, or a vegetable, and one to two servings of grain-based or protein-rich food. Although the nutrition benefits of school breakfast programs have clearly been demonstrated, less than 60% of students typically participate (Gross & Cinelli, 2004).

Children's Lunch Choices

Criteria for school lunch programs encourage schools to provide at least one-third of the RDA for calories, protein, vitamins A and C, iron, and calcium (U.S. Department of Agriculture, 1998.) The National School Lunch program is overseen by the U.S. Department of Agriculture and the Department of Education in each state. After passage of the Healthy Meals for Healthy Americans Act, nutrition

---

EVIDENCE-BASED PRACTICE RESEARCH BOX

Is breakfast the most important meal of the day for children and adolescents?

Clinical Problem: Breakfast has often been called the most important meal of the day. What is the evidence that children and adolescents who skip breakfast have more problems with weight control and academic performance than those who do not skip breakfast?

Research Findings: Several studies have examined the frequency of breakfast consumption and such variables as BMI, obesity, weight change, and school performance. Rampersaud, Pereira, Girand, Adams, and Metzl (2005) reviewed and summarized 47 studies that examined the association of breakfast consumption with nutritional adequacy, weight, and academic performance in children and adolescents. The combined evidence suggested that those who ate breakfast regularly were less likely to be overweight and have better cognitive function, though not all studies supported the general findings. A study by Berkey, Rockett, Gillman, Field, and Colditz (2003) analyzed data from a cohort of 14,000 children aged 9 to 14 years over a 3-year period. They found that skipping breakfast was associated with overweight, and that those normal-weight children who never ate breakfast gained more weight over the study period than the children who ate breakfast. In addition, they found that children who ate breakfast had higher self-reported academic achievement than those who did not eat breakfast.

A Canadian study examined the association between breakfast consumption and weight status in preschool children (Dubois, Girard, & Potvin Kent, 2006). They found that skipping breakfast nearly doubled the odds of being overweight in low-income families. A study of 3,275 school-age children in New Zealand examined the relationship between breakfast consumption and BMI (Utter, Sccragg, Mhurchu, & Schaaf, 2007). They found that children who skipped breakfast were significantly more likely to be socioeconomically deprived and have a higher BMI.

A study using data from 2,516 teens who participated in Project EAT (Eating Among Teens) found that female adolescent dieters had a significantly decreased breakfast consumption, and that adolescent male dieters had a trend toward decreased breakfast consumption (Neumark-Sztainer, Wall, Haines, Story, & Eisenberg, 2007a). One of two studies using data from the 5-year National Longitudinal Study of Adolescent Health (n = 9,919) found that skipping breakfast during the transition to young adulthood was positively associated with weight gain (Niemeier, Raynor, Lloyd-Richardson, Rogers, & Wing, 2006). The other study found that the prevalence of obesity (BMI greater than 30) nearly doubled during the transition to adulthood (Gordon-Larson, Adair, Nelson, & Popkin, 2004).

Nursing Implications: Data demonstrate that breakfast is an important factor in the long-term health of children and adolescents. Skipping breakfast due to socioeconomic factors or self-restriction is associated with weight gain, obesity, and diminished academic achievement. Obesity that begins in childhood is carried over into adulthood.

CRITICAL THINKING QUESTION:

1. What guidance can the nurse give the mother of school-age children who relates that no one in the family eats breakfast because the morning routine is too hectic with everyone getting ready for school and work?

standards for school lunch and breakfast programs were mandated to follow the Dietary Guidelines for Americans. Some school districts are still moving toward reducing the amount of fat and sodium in their meal offerings.

School breakfasts and lunches are provided to families at a minimal cost, at a reduced cost, or free depending on the income of the family (U.S. Department of Agriculture, 2007). Despite the quality of the meals provided, it is important for students to have adequate time to consume their lunch (Conklin, Lambert, & Anderson, 2002). On average, students at all age levels require approximately 7 to 10 minutes to just consume lunch at school. It has been recommended that students have at least 20 minutes to focus on eating their lunch once seated at the school lunch table. Some students, especially boys, may benefit from having recess scheduled prior to the midday lunch period (American Academy of Family Physicians et al., 2000; Bergman, Buergel, Joseph, & Sanchez, 2000). The school nurse should be part of the team that makes decisions that affect the timing of meals offered at schools.

Impact of Family Meals

Children who eat evening meals together with the family have a more balanced nutritional intake than those children who prepare food on their own or eat in front of the television (Gillman et al., 2000; Neumark-Sztainer, Hannan, Story, Croll, & Perry, 2003). Children are also influenced by the food preferences of the person who prepares the meals for a family. The more meals a child shares with the food preparer, the stronger the connection between the child's intake and that of the food preparer's (Hannon, Bowen, Moinpour, & McLerran, 2003).

Wellness Concerns

Nutritional concerns in this age group include the prevention and treatment of childhood overweight and obesity. Additionally, children with special health care needs require additional nutrition intervention to promote good nutritional health. Table 14-2 outlines some of these health care concerns in addition to those discussed.

Self-Prescribed Diets and Supplements

When conducting a nursing assessment for a child of any age, the knowledge and skills of the caregiver regarding food and nutrition should also be assessed. In particular, the use of self-prescribed diets or dietary supplements should be evaluated, especially in children with medical conditions because use of these supplements is much higher in this population than among well children (Ball, Kertesz, & Moyer-Mileur, 2005). Dietary supplements include vitamins, minerals, herbs, and weight loss and sports nutrition products. A study of clients in a pediatric clinic found that over half had used some type of complementary medicine, including herb therapies and home remedies, in the previous year, with almost half of those taking prescription medications si-

multaneously (Jean & Cyr, 2007). Almost 60% of physicians did not know of their clients' use of alternative medicine. Chapter 25 outlines concerns regarding use of dietary supplements.

Some caregivers choose to pursue modification of the diet as a method for treating some conditions. The nurse should evaluate this practice in a nonjudgmental way to ensure that nutritional needs are being met in a safe manner. Hot Topic: Diet and Attention-Deficit Hyperactivity Disorder outlines an example of such dietary practices used by some for treating attention-deficit hyperactivity disorder.

Childhood Overweight

The focus of issues in nutrition for many children has shifted from prevention of nutrient deficiencies to nutrient excess, specifically overweight in children. Overweight in children is defined as the 85th to 94th percentile for body mass index (BMI), whereas obesity is *greater than* 95th percentile (Spear et al., 2007). The number of children who are overweight has recently doubled in those 2 to 5 years of age and tripled among 6- to 11-year-olds (ADA, 2008). Health care professionals should be concerned about monitoring children's weight because obesity is associated with high blood cholesterol, high blood pressure, type 2 diabetes mellitus, asthma, sleep apnea, and negative social interactions (Whitlock, Williams, Gold, Smith, & Shipman, 2005). Early issues such as a high BMI, large waist circumference, high plasma glucose level, low serum high-density lipoprotein (HDL) level, and a high blood triglyceride level as a child can lead to a higher incidence of cardiovascular disease as an adult (Morrison, Friedman, & Gray-McGuire, 2007). The possibility that an overweight preschooler or school-age child will remain overweight into adolescence is high (Nader et al., 2006).

What Is Causing the Increase in Childhood Obesity?

The development of obesity in children is a multifaceted issue involving genetics, metabolism, environmental impact, and psychosocial influences. Over the past years, there has been a shift in energy intake to food sources from outside the home, such as fast-food and other restaurants. Eating out, especially fast food and fried foods, is associated with adiposity and poor intake of dairy, fruits, and vegetables in children and adolescents (Spear et al., 2007). Soft drinks and fruit drinks, fried foods, and salty snacks comprise an increasing proportion of energy intake by children than in prior decades (ADA, 2008). Sugar-sweetened beverages provide little in the way of lasting satiety compared to a solid food of equal calories and also add extra calories that are often not compensated for during the rest of the day (Malik, Schulze, & Hu, 2006). The food that most children consume in the United States does not meet the recommended guidelines of the Food Guide Pyramid. Specifically, intake of fruits and

hot Topic

Diet and Attention-Deficit Hyperactivity Disorder

Attention-deficit hyperactivity disorder (ADHD) has been theorized to affect up to 18% of children and is more common among boys than girls. ADHD often involves difficulty concentrating, forgetting items just reviewed, and poor completion of tasks. Impulsive behavior and overactivity are also common occurrences.

Parents of children with hyperactivity may seek out treatment in the form of nutritional therapies or other alternative approaches. Diet approaches can focus on the elimination of certain foods or ingested substances or the addition of foods, vitamins, or minerals. Limiting sugar, caffeine, food colorings, or additives have been suggested as the key to reducing undesirable behaviors. Several studies have found no link between behavior and sugar intake.

As the commonly consumed diet has shifted from homegrown, whole food options to processed meal and snack choices, several theories have focused on additives, food preservatives, and colors as causes of hyperactivity. The most familiar option among these diets is the Feingold approach. This diet is built on the theory that some children are extremely sensitive to artificially added colors, flavors, preservatives, and other man-made ingredients. Caregivers are instructed to totally eliminate these ingredients from a child's intake in order to improve behavior. Research in this area has been criticized for poor design and is largely inconclusive. Some believe that salicylates found in foods may contribute to symptoms.

Some caregivers manipulate the amount or types of carbohydrates consumed by their children. Parents may initiate elimination of any concentrated sugar, believing that the change will improve concentration and hyperactivity. This association has also not been proven in clinical trials. Many theories exist that hypothesize a connection between altered mood, overactivity, and aggression, but further research is required to establish whether this connection exists.

The possibility of food intolerance contributing to symptoms occurs to some parents; specifically gluten or casein intolerance is cited. All wheat, barley, or rye products are eliminated on a gluten-free diet and only gluten-free oat products are utilized. Dairy products are also eliminated in an attempt to remove any offending agents. No consensus regarding these approaches has been reached.

Nutrient supplementation is based on the hypothesis that nutrients in the diet are not being provided in sufficient amounts to prevent hyperactivity. Megadoses of vitamins or minerals have not been shown to benefit these children and can, in fact, harm children if given in doses exceeding the recommended upper limit.

Other studies have focused on deficiencies of specific fatty acids and possible benefits of omega-3 fatty acid supplementation because of the important role that these fats play in brain and nervous system function. In particular, it has been noted that some children with ADHD have lowered levels of these fatty acids compared to others. Docosahexaenoic acid (DHA) and eicosapentaenoic acid (EPA) have been specifically targeted as the subjects of much research. Supplementation with these fatty acids has reportedly led to subjective improvements in some children, especially those with demonstrated low levels prior to supplementation. Further research is needed before routine supplementation can be advised. Parents considering DHA or EPA supplementation should be encouraged to discuss this issue with the child's primary health care provider.

Sources: Colter, Cutler, & Meckling, 2008; Marcason, 2005; Ramakrishnan, Imhoff-Kunsch & DiGirolamo, 2009; Sinn, 2008.

vegetables by most children is low (Gidding et al., 2006). The average daily intake of fruits and vegetables is 2 and 2.2, respectively (Cook & Friday, 2004).

Lack of physical activity leads to decreased energy expenditure that can cause weight gain when dietary intake remains the same. Once weight gain has occurred, it may perpetuate inactivity if exercise, play, or sport participation becomes more difficult. Overweight children may be embarrassed to participate in team games or sports out of fear of teasing or bullying. Children need to be active every day to develop physical strength and flexibility and to maintain a healthy body weight.

Television viewing and media messages may also play a role in calorie imbalance. Excessive "screen time" or time spent sitting in front of a television, computer game, or the like is considered a behavioral risk for overweight (Spear et al., 2007). In addition to the sedentary nature of television viewing, advertising that targets children and adolescents may influence food choices. Foods that are highly promoted during children's television programs often include breakfast cereals, candy, snack foods, and menu items at fast-food restaurants. The majority of the food products advertised to children are high in sugar, fat, or sodium (Powell, Szczypka, Chaloupka, & Braunschweig, 2007). In some countries, advertising of any nature that is geared toward children is strictly controlled. In the United States several major companies have made strides to redirect advertising away from children. Results in 2006 showed that children and adolescents watched an average of over 3 hours of television daily (TV Bureau of Advertising, 2007). There is evidence that for both children and adolescents increased television viewing is associated with increased body mass (Jackson, Djafarian, Stewart, & Speakman, 2009).

Changes in School Environment

The increasing concern regarding weight gain in children has caused many school districts to evaluate the school environment, including the effect of **competitive foods** on the consumption of prepared school lunches. Competitive foods are those that are not part of the government-funded lunch program and that are available anywhere in the school, such as vending machines, snack bars, fundraisers, and the cafeteria. The availability of foods such as cakes, cookies, and snack foods that can be purchased during the school day can offset students' intake of fruits, vegetables, and protein-rich foods.

The Child Nutrition Reauthorization Act of 2004 required school districts that take part in government-funded lunch programs to develop local wellness policies by the year 2007. These policies address nutrition education, physical activity, and standards for all foods available on school campuses and should involve the entire school community (ADA, 2008). The American Heart Association recommends that schools target both education and the school environment to improve access to healthy foods, physical activity initiatives, classroom education, and farm-to-school nutrition programs (Gidding et al., 2009). The school nurse should be an integral part of any school district wellness policy.

Prevention of Childhood Obesity

Prevention of childhood overweight and obesity targets behaviors believed to contribute significantly to the development of this public health problem. It is felt that prevention behaviors should be instituted early in life to avoid more difficult treatment interventions later in childhood (Barlow, & The Expert Committee, 2007). Overall balanced intake that includes all food groups should be encouraged while limiting intake of sugar-sweetened beverages. Other energy-dense foods, such as those found in many restaurants, should also be moderated. Family meals and daily breakfasts are recommended as routine practices because of their respective associations with reduced prevalence of obesity. Additionally, physical activity is encouraged through the recommendation to limit television viewing to 2 hours daily. Available data and expertise led to the recommendation that 1 hour of moderate to vigorous physical activity should be promoted daily (Spear et al., 2007).

Nurses can promote healthy eating habits by educating children and caregivers about a well-balanced diet that includes all food groups. Although no single food should be labeled as forbidden, the majority of regularly consumed snacks should contain needed nutrients, such as the suggestions outlined in Table 14-5.

Parents should not force children to eat when they are not hungry, but instead allow children to respond to internal cues of hunger and fullness (Johnson & Birch, 1994). Restrictive eating behaviors such as skipping meals should not be pursued. Family members should be encouraged not to tease a child or focus excessively on body weight or physical appearance. Negative comments and teasing about size can

BOX 14-4	Fun Suggestions for Increasing Physical Activity
Jump rope	Throw a ball
Dance	Play Twister
Play tag	Play basketball
Cycle	Jump on a trampoline
Rollerskate	Play Frisbee
Hula hoop	Play Ping-Pong

impact the psychological well-being of the child or adolescent and contribute to risk of overweight or binge eating later in life (Neumark-Sztainer et al., 2007b; Taylor et al., 2006).

Physical activity is a necessity in preventing excessive weight gain. Increasing physical activity in schools by offering recess for younger children and mandatory physical education at all grade levels is a fundamental step in ensuring that children get activity throughout the day. Aerobic fitness may help to reduce comorbidities in children even when body mass is above recommended guidelines (DuBose, Eisenmann, & Donnelly, 2007). The nurse can assess the child for barriers to increasing physical activity and encourage physical activity in enjoyable ways, such as those outlined in Box 14-4.

Treatment of obesity requires an interdisciplinary approach, which is most effective when all family members are involved. Efforts focusing on prevention are important because obesity is difficult to treat once the problem develops. Table 14-6 lists suggestions that the nurse can make that involve family behaviors. Client Education Checklist: Preventing Childhood Overweight and Obesity outlines target areas for nursing interventions in the prevention of obesity. Treatment of overweight or obesity in children is approached individually. Generally, the goal is maintenance of body weight to allow a deflection in BMI percentile as growth occurs rather than a specific plan for weight loss (Spear et al., 2007). If weight loss does occur following healthy lifestyle changes, it should be limited to 1 pound/month in obese children under age 11 years and no more than 2 pounds/week in an obese adolescent (Spear et al., 2007). It is recommended that a registered dietitian with expertise in pediatric obesity provide the nutrition intervention along with the primary care provider (Spear et al., 2007). Chapter 17 outlines the specifics of treatment of overweight and obesity.

Adolescent Nutrition

Rapid growth often begins after age 11 years for girls and between the ages of 12 and 13 years for boys. The average boy will add 8 inches to his height during puberty. In comparison, the average girl will grow 6 inches. After the initial growth period, adolescents will most often continue to grow taller but at a much slower rate.

Table 14-5 Healthy Snacks Ideas

- Fresh fruits such as sliced apples, bananas, oranges, blueberries, strawberries, or melons
- Dried fruit such as raisins or cranberries
- Fruit leather with no added sugar
- Raw vegetables with low-fat dip, bean dip, or hummus
- Yogurt
- String or mini cheese
- Sunflower or pumpkin seeds or spreads made with these seeds
- Dry cereal mixed with small amounts of raisins and other dried fruit, mini chocolate chips, or peanuts (if no allergy)
- Mini wheat bagels topped with seed, nut, or peanut butter; low-fat cheese; or lean lunch meat
- Whole-grain pita rolled up with cheese or nut butter
- Popcorn
- Rice or popcorn cakes

| Table 14-6 | Improving Nutritional Health for the Whole Family |

- Turn off television to decrease distractions and make mealtimes enjoyable
- Be responsible for what, when, and where children eat
- Do not use foods to bribe, reward, or punish a child
- Involve children in purchasing food and preparing meals and snacks
- Start a family garden or grow vegetables or fruits in containers
- Be a positive role model by practicing healthy eating behaviors
- Provide age-appropriate portions on child-sized plates and cups
- Offer a variety of healthy foods and encourage healthy choices
- Serve meals and snacks at a regular time of day with enough time between to develop a healthy appetite
- Provide healthy breakfast choices (example: whole grain, low-sugar cereal)
- Offer a variety of color and texture choices and arrange attractively on plate
- At the grocery store talk about the names, shapes, colors, or how fruits and vegetables grow while in the produce department
- Use kid-friendly recipes and allow children to help prepare parts of the recipe
- Offer water as the drink of choice between meals
- Expect that children will develop food preferences and possibly food jags

Sources: Patrick, Spear, Holt, & Sofka, 2001. The Produce for Health Foundation 2008; Satter, 1987.

Nutrient Needs

The guidelines for recommended nutrient intake for teenagers reflect a growing difference between males and females as the changes created by puberty set in. Prior to puberty, males and females have a similar breakdown of body fat and muscle. After onset of menarche, females develop appropriately needed fat stores in areas of the breasts, hips, and buttocks. In comparison, males increase their lean body tissue and muscle composition. This increase in muscle mass is reflected in higher protein needs per kilogram in males than in females.

Energy

Female adolescents on average require 2,200 kcalories and 45 grams of protein daily (IOM, 2002). Activity levels, height, and weight factor into these requirements. A very active, tall female can need more than 2,200 kcalories to support growth. Guidelines for males are higher to support maintenance of muscle mass. Male teenagers require more than 2,500 kcalories/day. Some adolescents need to consume more than 3,000 kcalories/day to support needs during sports or rapid growth periods. In addition, daily protein needs in-

crease to approximately 50 grams for the typical male adolescent (IOM, 2002).

The dramatic increase in calorie and nutrient needs is impacted by a teenager's changing psychological and social outlook. Most adolescents strive to become more independent with greater time spent with peers in social, school, or work settings. Due to these changes in day-to-day activities and attitudes toward health, all of the increased nutrient needs may not be met. A preoccupation with outward appearance can also affect overall physical and nutritional status.

Calcium and Vitamin D

The need for calcium in a teenager is triple the amount needed by a preschooler. Unfortunately, although adolescence is the critical time for calcium retention and achievement of peak bone mass, intake of calcium often decreases. Soft drinks are more often the chosen beverage than milk or calcium-fortified fruit juice. Without consumption of dairy products it can be difficult for adolescents to meet calcium and other nutrient needs (Gao, Wilde, Lichtenstein, & Tucker, 2006). A minimum of 1,300 milligrams of calcium per day is recommended to support adequate bone growth during the preteen and teenage years (IOM, 1997). Missing the critical goal of contributing significantly to peak bone mass during adolescence can put adults at higher risk of developing osteoporosis. Parents can assist in helping teens to consume enough calcium by serving milk with meals, by having low-fat cheese available for snacks, and by purchasing nondairy sources of calcium such as broccoli, kale, almonds, fortified cereals, soy foods, and calcium-fortified foods such as juices.

In addition, adequate vitamin D is necessary for bone mineralization. Almost 15% of adolescents have vitamin D deficiency, with females, darker-skinned children, and the obese at highest risk (Saintonge, Bang, & Gerber, 2009). Children living in the upper latitudes of the United States are at higher risk for vitamin D deficiency than those living farther south (Hanley & Davison, 2005). The AAP recommends intake of 10 mcg or 400 international units of vitamin D in all children.

Iron

The iron needs of adolescents also increase in order to meet the demands of growing muscles and loss of iron through menstruation in females. Teenage males require 11 mg/day, whereas females require 15 mg/day (IOM, 2001). Foods such as lean meats, including beef, chicken, or fish, can provide well-absorbed iron sources. Teens who adopt a vegetarian lifestyle should be encouraged to consume iron-rich foods such as beans, dried fruits, and fortified breakfast cereal with a vitamin C source such as citrus fruit at the same meal to improve iron absorption.

CLIENT EDUCATION CHECKLIST	Preventing Childhood Overweight and Obesity
Intervention	**Example**
Assess caregiver's knowledge of the impact of childhood overweight on the body.	Obesity is associated with high cholesterol and high blood pressure, type 2 diabetes mellitus, asthma, sleep apnea, and negative social interactions. Healthy habits can be incorporated into daily activities while avoiding excessively restrictive interventions.
Assess caregiver's knowledge of appropriate beverage choices for children.	Infants and young children should not be offered soda, iced tea, fruit punch, or other sweetened beverages. 100% fruit juice should be limited to 4 to 6 fluid ounces daily.
Assess caregiver's knowledge of appropriate portions for children.	Portion sizes that are larger than appropriate for children can lead to overconsumption at meals. *MyPyramid for Kids* outlines age-appropriate portions. For young children, a tablespoon per year of age can be used as a guide for solid foods.
Assess frequency of breakfast consumption.	Breakfast provides important nutrients for growing children and adolescents. Studies have found that even though the quality of breakfast varies among children, those who ate breakfast on a regular basis had better overall nutrition than others who regularly skipped breakfast. Encourage caregivers to offer children breakfast every day. Strategize breakfast options when barriers such as time exist.
Assess frequency of fruit and vegetable intake.	Children should consume five or more servings of fruits and vegetables daily.
Assess frequency of meals eaten outside the home. Assess knowledge of healthy food options at restaurants.	Parents can select healthy food choices at fast-food restaurants such as baked potatoes, salads with low-calorie dressing, lean cuts of meat and seafood, and foods that have been baked, broiled, grilled, or steamed. Avoid oversized portions of food and beverages.
Assess frequency of snack consumption and types of items offered.	Schedule snacks around the same time each day. Offer snack choices based on fruits, vegetables, dairy foods, and whole grains. Do not use food or snacks as a reward.
Assess mealtime environment at home.	Children who eat evening meals together with their family have a more balanced nutritional intake than those children who prepare food on their own or eat in front of the television. Suggest to caregivers that being a healthy role model is important. Children watch and imitate caregivers to learn eating habits.
Assess knowledge of caregiver regarding time spent on computer, television, or video games.	Being inactive can contribute to a sedentary lifestyle. Frequent use of screen time adds to a lifestyle based on inactivity. Childhood overweight is impacted by physical inactivity and overconsumption of calories. Activities that mainly involve sitting such as TV, computer, and video games should be limited to less than 1 or 2 hours per day.
Assess caregiver's knowledge of importance of daily physical activity.	Children need to be active every day to develop physical strength and flexibility and to maintain a healthy body weight. Children age 2 and older should participate in at least 60 minutes of physical activity every day.

Adolescent Choices

Desiring to fit in with peers may override any interest in a balanced diet in this age group. Young adults are greatly influenced by the food choices of their peers. Even celebrities and their beverage or food choices can steer an adolescent toward healthy or unhealthy choices. Growing physical changes and increased independence can lead to experimentation with behaviors that impact health, such as alcohol or tobacco use.

Adolescent perceptions of their caregiver's interest in healthy eating, especially their mother, can help them make healthy choices. Sharing parental beliefs regarding the importance of healthy food choices can positively impact adolescents (Boutelle, Birkeland, Hannan, Story, & Neumark-Sztainer, 2007). Adolescents should be encouraged to choose fruits and vegetables as part of their snacks and school lunches. Eating the recommended five to six servings per day can contribute to total vitamin and mineral needs. Adolescents can be active participants in the food choices and food preparation for the family by selecting meals and recipes for the coming week, assisting in grocery shopping, and even selecting coupons to reduce the cost of food purchases.

Up to 50% of teens eat at least five times or more during the day. Snacking can either help adolescents reach important nutrient goals or add more sugar, fat, and sodium to their daily intake depending on snack choices. Caregivers can purchase snacks that are low in fat and sugar and try to encourage teens to choose items that help increase calcium, iron, and vitamin intake. Options like cereal with low-fat milk, part-skim cheese and whole grain crackers, fresh fruit or vegetables with dip, and calcium-fortified cereal bars or juices are healthy choices.

The nurse should assess the teenager for nutrition knowledge and beliefs and use of dietary supplements and fad diets. Switching to a vegetarian diet is common in this age group and the nurse should evaluate the reason for this choice to ensure that it is not an attempt to mask an eating disorder under the guise of healthy eating. Hot Topic: Vegetarian Diets

hot Topic

Vegetarian Diets in Children

A well-planned vegetarian diet has been recognized by health organizations as compatible with meeting the needs of growing children and adolescents. Families may choose a vegetarian lifestyle for cultural or religious reasons or concern for the environment, health, or animal rights. In 2000, a poll revealed that nearly 6% of children between the ages of 6 and 17 years do not eat meat. Lesser numbers follow a more restrictive diet, limiting eggs and dairy in addition to meat. Types of vegetarian diets vary based on the extent to which animal products are avoided. Properly planned vegetarian diets often have more fruits, vegetables, and fiber and less saturated fat and cholesterol than diets including animal foods. The greatest risk from a poorly planned vegetarian diet occurs during periods of rapid growth when nutrient needs are at their highest. The intake of the following nutrients should be monitored to ensure adequate nutrition.

Energy

Some vegetarian meals and snacks provide lesser calories in an increased volume. Toddlers and young children may not be able to meet their energy needs before their stomach is filled to capacity. Vegetarian children may need to have at least three meals and three snacks per day to meet energy, protein, vitamin, and mineral needs. Good-quality plant fats are an important component of the vegetarian diet for young children to provide essential fatty acids.

Protein

Most plant foods, with the exception of soy, typically are low in one or more essential amino acids. When a wide variety of plant foods is consumed, all essential amino acids can be provided in sufficient amounts. Vegetarian

children who consume dairy, eggs, or soy products in recommended amounts can meet protein needs for adequate growth. Other sources of protein include legumes, grains, and nuts.

Iron

Vegetarian children may be at greater risk for iron-deficiency anemia than their meat-eating peers. Heme iron in animal products is better absorbed than iron in plant foods, known as nonheme iron. Offering a food or beverage at the same meal containing a high amount of vitamin C can boost absorption of the nonheme iron. Foods such as citrus fruits, strawberries, tomatoes, and broccoli are good choices.

Zinc

Zinc is necessary for growth and development. The recommended intake for zinc increases during childhood. Sources of zinc include peas, beans, brown rice, spinach, nuts, tofu, and other soy products.

Calcium

Vegan and vegetarian diets may not contain sufficient calcium if not properly planned. In addition to dairy sources of calcium, plant sources include fortified soy milk, fortified orange or other juice, tofu fortified with calcium, blackstrap molasses, sesame seeds and sesame butter (known as tahini), almonds, and almond butter. For older children, dark green vegetables such as broccoli, mustard and collard greens, okra, and kale can provide a good source of calcium. For younger children the quantity needed to meet calcium needs may be difficult to consume. The nurse should advise that food labels be checked for nutrient fortification because not all fortified foods contain the same level of nutrients.

Vitamin D

Food sources of vitamin D include some brands of soy milk, fortified rice milk, some dry cereals, and fortified juices. For lacto-ovo vegetarians, cow's milk and egg yolks can provide vitamin D. Vitamin D-fortified foods or supplements are needed for children who have no source of vitamin D in their diet.

Vitamin B$_{12}$

Children following a vegan diet need to consume a vitamin B$_{12}$ supplement or foods fortified with the vitamin because it is only found in foods of animal origin. These foods include some brands of soy milk, soy products, nutritional yeast, and some breakfast products. Vitamin B$_{12}$ supplements derived from plant sources are not bioactively available for absorption and should not be recommended. Synthetic vitamin B$_{12}$ is well absorbed and the recommended form. Vegetarian children consuming some dairy products would be provided with a source of vitamin B$_{12}$.

Dietary Fiber

Caregivers of young children need to be careful to avoid large amounts of dietary fiber. Dietary fiber can inhibit absorption of certain vitamins and minerals, such as iron and zinc.

The nurse plays an important role in assessing the diet of vegetarian children and referring the caregiver to a registered dietitian when concerns exist about the adequacy of the diet. The nurse should advise those following a vegan diet that food labels be checked for nutrient fortification because not all fortified foods contain the same level of nutrients. Vitamins B$_{12}$ and D and calcium fortification should be specifically evaluated.

Sources: American Dietetic Association, 2003; Mangels, & Messina, 2001; Messina, Mangels, & Messina, 2004; Vegetarian Resource Group, 2009.

in Children outlines the importance of good planning when children are following a vegetarian diet. Unhealthy preoccupation with body size or a dysfunctional body image can lead to eating behaviors that are detrimental to a teen's emotional and physical health. Disordered eating patterns may manifest themselves in serious conditions such as anorexia nervosa, bulimia nervosa, binge eating disorder, or chronic dieting syndrome. Eating disorders may occur in either gender or any socioeconomic class. Nutrition intervention in the management of eating disorders is thoroughly covered in Chapter 17.

NURSING CARE PLAN Nutrition and the Overweight Child

CASE STUDY

Will, age 8, has come to the clinic with his mom for a checkup. He has been seen regularly since birth and all immunizations are up to date. He has had no significant illness other than several episodes of otitis media treated with antibiotics when he was a toddler. Mom is concerned that he is quite heavy and seems to be gaining weight. She mentions that she is especially concerned that he doesn't seem to have many friends and that his teacher reports that he doesn't engage in activity during recess, preferring to stand around and watch other children play. At home, he watches a lot of television or plays computer games, something he does well. Mom reports that he is an average to good student and does not present any particular discipline problems. Mom further states that her dad, age 54 years, is overweight and has type 2 diabetes; she has heard that overweight children can develop this problem. She is also worried that she might develop diabetes because she knows she has a weight problem.

Upon questioning, Will tells the nurse that he knows he is "fat" and wishes other kids wouldn't tease him. He doesn't like recess because he never gets picked to be part of any teams so he just stays away from the other kids. His favorite foods are pepperoni and sausage pizza, root beer, and ice cream. He says he eats these things three or four times a week with his parents and younger sister. He says he wishes he wasn't "fat," but everyone in his family is and he likes his family.

Applying the Nursing Process

ASSESSMENT

Height: 49 inches Weight: 85 pounds BMI: 25 (exceeds 97th percentile) BP 128/80 P 70 R 16

1 year ago: Height: 46 inches Weight: 70 pounds BMI: 23.2

DIAGNOSES

Imbalanced nutrition: more than body requirements related to consumption of excess nutrients and insufficient activity evidenced by BMI exceeding 97th percentile for age

Readiness for knowledge related to concern for weight management evidenced by request for guidance

Activity intolerance related to sedentary lifestyle evidenced by lack of participation in playground activity

EXPECTED OUTCOMES

Maintenance of current weight or small weight loss
Identification of healthy snacks
Increased activity with family or peers
Participation in food choices and meal preparation

INTERVENTIONS

24-hour food recall
Food diary
Meet with a dietitian to identify specific age-appropriate nutrient needs
Teach mom how to read food labels
Limit pizza to one time per week and try toppings that are lower in fat and calories
Make fruit readily available for snacks
Plan one family outing per week that involves physical activity; increase frequency after 1 month
Involve Will in grocery shopping and meal preparation

EVALUATION

Two months later, Will weighs 81 pounds. Mom says that each day is a struggle to make good choices. She recognizes that they have eaten lots of high-fat and high-carbohydrate foods, and they have not eaten good foods like fruit and vegetables; she regrets not having done a better job of feeding her family. It has been fun fixing some meals as a family and doing grocery shopping, but it is also more time consuming than getting carry-out food for dinner. They try to take a walk every day, but everyone thinks of lots of other things to do instead of spending time together. Will is proud of losing 4 pounds but still doesn't play with anyone at recess. He is trying not to spend so much time on the computer, but because he doesn't have many friends it is hard to think of other things to do. He hopes that if he loses more

Nutrition and the Overweight Child *(continued)*

Assessment
Data about the patient

Subjective
What the patient tells the nurse

Example: "I know I am fat; other kids tease me; I never get picked to be on teams at recess; I am good at computer games."

Objective
What the nurse observes; anthropometric and clinical data

Examples: 85 pounds; 49 inches; BMI: 25 (exceeds 97th percentile); 15 pound weight gain in 1 year

Diagnosis
NANDA label

Example: Imbalanced nutrition more than body requirements related to excess intake and insufficient physical activity

Planning
Goals stated in patient terms

Example: Long-term goal: maintain weight; Short-term goal: develop list of healthy after-school snacks; identify 1 physical activity to engage in at least twice per week

Implementation
Nursing action to help patient achieve goals

Example: Teach how to read food labels; identify acceptable healthy snacks

Evaluation
Was the goal achieved or does the intervention need to be modified?

Example: 4 pound weight loss in 2 months; family struggling with making healthy food choices

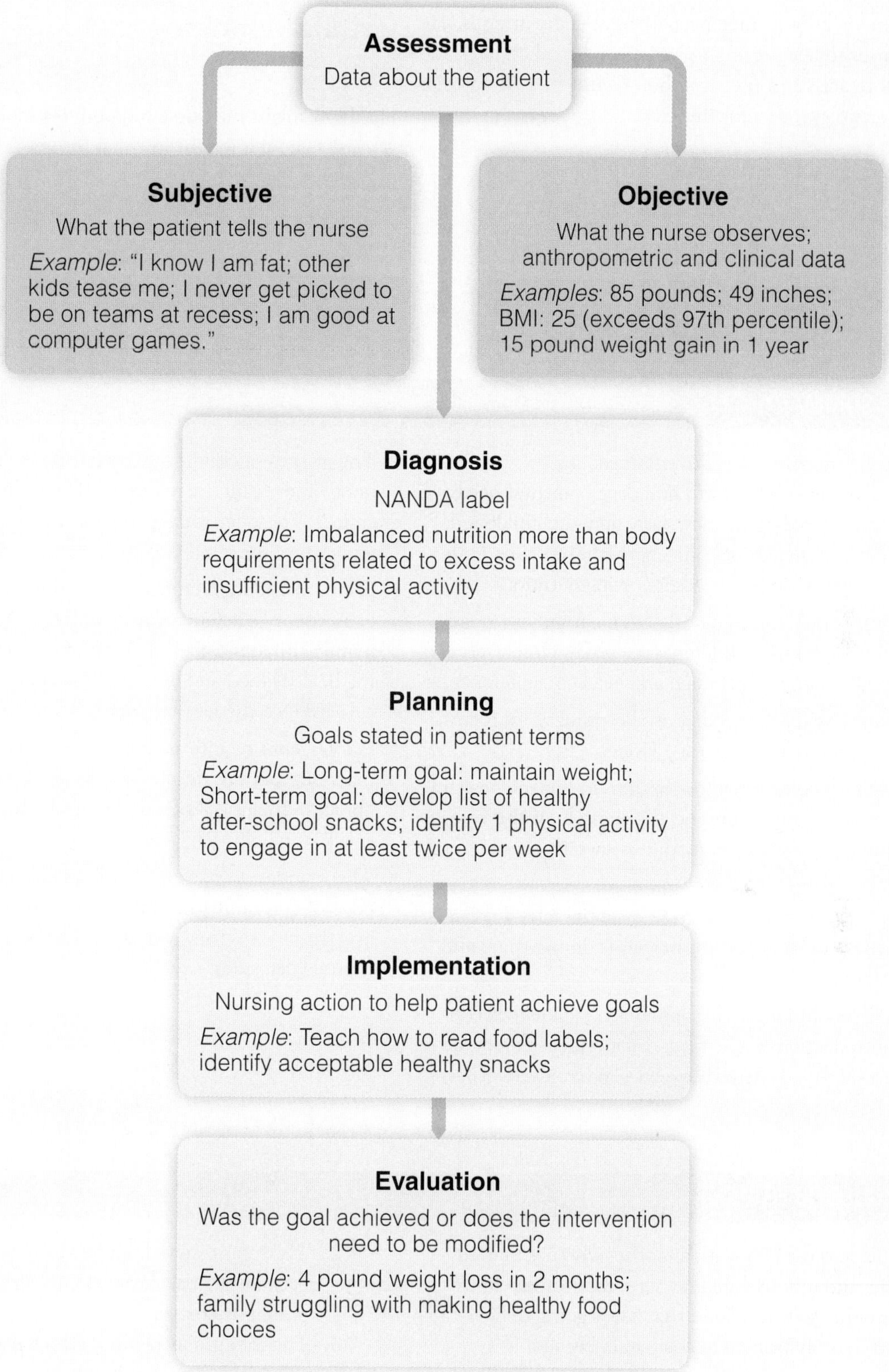

■ FIGURE 14-3 **Nursing Care Plan Process: Nutrition and the Overweight Child.**

(continued)

Nutrition and the Overweight Child *(continued)*

weight or grows taller he will have more friends. He promises to keep trying to make good food choices and be more active in nice weather. Figure 14-3 ■ outlines the nursing process for this case.

Critical Thinking in the Nursing Process

1. **How might the nurse respond to a mother who asks about a weight-loss diet for her school-age son?**

CHAPTER SUMMARY

- The specific nutrients needed throughout life vary in amounts determined by growth and developmental needs. These stages, including infancy, early and late childhood, and adolescence, require specific approaches to meet both physical and psychological needs involving nutrition.

- Infants grow faster than any other human growth stage. The nutritional status of children is tracked by closely monitoring weight; length, or stature; and head circumference.

- Breastfeeding is recommended as the primary source of nutrition for all infants up to age 1 year.

- Infant formulas come in various options to suit the health and digestion of the infant and the lifestyle of the caregivers. Pure cow's milk or unmodified soy milk should not be offered until after age 1 year.

- Infants must receive a diet high in essential fatty acids to provide energy and important nutrients during this rapid growth period.

- Caregivers should follow their physician's guidelines concerning introduction of solid foods. Infant rice cereal should be the first solid food offered between 4 and 6 months of age.

- The growth of children slows during early and late childhood and again increases more rapidly during adolescence. These growth patterns determine the specific amounts of nutrients required.

- Focus on childhood nutrition has shifted from prevention of nutrient deficiencies to avoidance of nutrient excess, mainly childhood obesity. A multifaceted approach including healthy food and lifestyle choices and increased physical activity is the sensible approach in treating this disorder.

- Adolescents require increased amounts of nutrients but may not always meet these goals because of lifestyle choices. Inclusion of family meals and nutrient-dense snacks can help teenagers reach vitamin and mineral goals.

- The foundation of a healthy lifestyle necessitates knowledge of good nutrition on both the part of the caregiver and the child as they learn to make good food choices and lifestyle decisions.

NCLEX® QUESTIONS

1. The nurse is working with a mother who has limited income and is bottle-feeding her 6-month-old child. The mother tells the nurse that she is going to have to switch from formula to cow's milk because it is cheaper. What should the nurse tell the client about the use of cow's milk for infant feeding?
   1. Because the infant is of average weight and has no allergies, this is an acceptable plan.

2. The infant should not be switched to cow's milk because the risk of developing an allergy to milk protein increases.
3. The infant may be fussy for a few days due to the change in taste, but it will not be a problem after the infant adjusts to cow's milk.
4. It will not be a problem as long as whole milk is used.

2. The nurse is discussing the introduction of solid foods with the mother of a 4-month-old infant. Which of the following statements by the mother demonstrates to the nurse that her teaching has been effective?
   1. "If I add a small amount of rice cereal to the bottle-feeding, my baby will adjust to solids more rapidly."
   2. "I should puree a small amount of whatever we are eating and feed the baby at the same time we eat."
   3. "Pureed fruit is most easily accepted and digested by an infant so it should be the first solid food."
   4. "Each new food should be tried for a few days before introducing a new one."

3. Which of the following strategies can the nurse suggest to caregivers of a school-age child to encourage healthy eating habits?
   1. The child should finish eating before going to play.
   2. Allow only a small portion of dessert if the main meal is not completely eaten.
   3. Encourage the child to help in meal preparation.
   4. Do not allow snacking.

4. The adolescent who eats a hamburger, french fries, and cola for lunch can be advised to help balance nutrient intake by making which of the following choices for dinner?
   1. Steak, baked potato, water
   2. Spaghetti, garlic bread, milk
   3. Pork chop, broccoli, milk
   4. Chili, crackers, apple juice

5. A mother reports to the nurse that her toddler refuses to drink milk. Which nutrients are the nurse most concerned will be deficient in the child's diet?
   1. Iron and calcium
   2. Folic acid and vitamin C
   3. Vitamin K and iron
   4. Calcium and vitamin D

EXPLORE PEARSON mynursingkit™

MyNursingKit is your one stop for online chapter review materials and resources. Prepare for success with additional NCLEX®-style practice questions, interactive assignments and activities, web links, animations and videos, and more!

Register your access code from the front of your book at
www.mynursingkit.com.

REFERENCES

Affenito, S. G. (2007). Breakfast: A missed opportunity. *Journal of the American Dietetic Association, 107,* 565–569.

American Academy of Family Physicians, American Academy of Pediatrics, American Dietetic Association, National Hispanic Medical Association, National Medical Association, U.S. Department of Agriculture (USDA). (2000). Prescription for change: Ten keys to promote healthy eating in schools. In *USDA Food and Nutrition Service, Changing the scene: Improving the school nutrition environment.* Washington, DC: Author.

American Academy of Pediatrics (AAP), Committee on Nutrition. (1999). Iron fortification of infant formulas. *Pediatrics, 104,* 119–123.

American Academy of Pediatrics (AAP), Committee on Nutrition. (2001). The use and misuse of fruit juice in pediatrics. *Pediatrics, 107,* 1210–1213.

American Academy of Pediatrics (AAP), Committee on Fetus and Newborn. (2003). Controversies concerning vitamin K and the newborn. *Pediatrics, 112,* 191–192.

American Academy of Pediatrics (AAP). (2004). Statement of endorsement: Managing acute gastroenteritis among children: Oral rehydration, maintenance, and nutritional therapy. *Pediatrics, 114,* 507.

American Academy of Pediatrics (AAP), Work Group on Breastfeeding. (2005). Breastfeeding and the use of human milk. *Pediatrics, 115,* 496–506.

American Academy of Pediatrics (AAP). (2007). Choking prevention and first aid for infants and children [Brochure HE50419]. Elk Grove, IL: Author.

American Academy of Pediatrics (AAP), Section on Pediatric Dentistry and Oral Health. (2008). Preventative oral health interventions for pediatricians. *Pediatrics, 122,* 1387–1394.

American Dietetic Association. (2003). Position of the American Dietetic Association and Dietitians of Canada: Vegetarian diets. *Journal of the American Dietetic Association, 103,* 748–765.

American Dietetic Association. (2004). Position of the American Dietetic Association: Providing nutrition services for infants, children, and adults with developmental disabilities and special healthcare needs. *Journal of the American Dietetic Association, 104,* 97–107.

American Dietetic Association. (2005). Position of the American Dietetic Association: Promoting and supporting breastfeeding. *Journal of the American Dietetic Association, 105,* 810–818.

American Dietetic Association. (2007). Position of the American Dietetic Association: Oral health and nutrition. *Journal of the American Dietetic Association, 107,* 1418–1428.

REFERENCES *(continued)*

American Dietetic Association. (2008). Position of the American Dietetic Association: Dietary guidance for healthy children ages 2 to 11 years. *Journal of the American Dietetic Association, 108,* 1038–1047.

Anderson, G. C. (1989). Risk in mother-infant separation postbirth. *Image: Journal of Nursing Scholarship, 21,* 196–199.

Ball, S. D., Kertesz, D., & Moyer-Mileur, L. J. (2005). Dietary supplement use is prevalent among children with a chronic illness. *Journal of the American Dietetic Association, 105,* 78–84.

Barlow, S. E., & The Expert Committee. (2007). Expert committee recommendations regarding the prevention, assessment, and treatment of child and adolescent overweight and obesity: Summary report. *Pediatrics, 120,* S164–S192.

Beard, J. L. (2008). Why iron deficiency is important in infant development. *Journal of Nutrition, 138,* 2534–2536.

Beauchamp, G. K., & Mennella, J. A. (2009). Early flavor learning and its impact on later feeding behavior. *Journal of Pediatric Gastroenterology & Nutrition, 48,* S25–S30.

Benton, D., & Jarvis, M. (2006). The role of breakfast and a mid-morning snack on the ability of children to concentrate at school. *Physiology & Behavior, 90,* 382–385.

Bergman, E. A., Buergel, N. S., Joseph, E., & Sanchez, A. (2000). Time spent by schoolchildren to eat lunch. *Journal of the American Dietetic Association, 100,* 696–698.

Berkey, C. S., Rockett, H. R., Gillman, M. W., Field, A. E., & Colditz, G. A. (2003). Longitudinal study of skipping breakfast and weight change in adolescents. *International Journal of Obesity and Related Metabolic Disorders, 27,* 1258–1266.

Birch, E. E., Garfield, S., Castañeda, Y., Hughbanks-Wheaton, D., Uauy, R., & Hoffman, D. (2007). Visual acuity and cognitive outcomes at 4 years of age in a double-blind, randomized trial of long-chain polyunsaturated fatty acid-supplemented infant formula. *Early Human Development, 83,* 279–284.

Birch, L. L., & Marlin, D. W. (1982). I don't like it; I never tried it (effects of exposure on two-year-old children's food preferences). *Appetite, 3,* 353–360.

Boutelle, K. N., Birkeland, R. W., Hannan, P. J., Story, M., & Neumark-Sztainer, D. (2007). Associations between maternal concern for healthful eating and maternal eating behaviors, home food availability, and adolescent eating behaviors. *Journal of Nutrition and Education Behavior, 39,* 248–256.

Brotanek, J. M., Gosz, J., Weitzman, M., & Flores, G. (2007). Iron deficiency in early childhood in the United States: Risk factors and racial/ethnic disparities. *Pediatrics, 120,* 568–575.

Centers for Disease Control and Prevention (CDC). (2002). *Managing elevated blood lead levels among young children: Recommendations from the Advisory Committee on Childhood Lead Poisoning Prevention.* Atlanta, GA: Author. Retrieved March 30, 2009, from http://www.cdc.gov/nceh/lead/CaseManagement/caseManage_main.htm

Centers for Disease Control and Prevention (CDC). (2003). Managing acute gastroenteritis among children: Oral rehydration, maintenance, and nutrition therapy. *Morbidity and Mortality Weekly Report, 52,* 1–16.

Centers for Disease Control and Prevention (CDC). (2005). *Preventing lead poisoning in young children.* Atlanta, GA: Author.

Centers for Disease Control and Prevention (CDC). (2007). *When should a mother avoid breastfeeding?* Retrieved March 29, 2009, from http://www.cdc.gov/breastfeeding/disease/contraindicators.htm

Cinar, A. D. (2004). The advantages and disadvantages of pacifier use. *Contemporary Nursing, 17,* 109–112.

Colter, A. L., Cutler, C., & Meckling, K. A. (2008). Fatty acid status and behavioral symptoms of attention deficit hyperactivity disorder in adolescents: A case-control study. *Nutrition Journal, 7,* 8.

Conklin, M. T., Lambert, L. G., & Anderson, J. B. (2002). How long does it take students to eat lunch? A summary of three studies. *Journal of Child Nutrition Management,* Retrieved March 30, 2009, from http://docs.schoolnutrition.org/newsroom/jcnm/02spring/conklin/

Cook, A. J., & Friday, J. E. (2004). Nutrient intakes by pyramid food groups. From farm to food—Practical applications for food consumption data. 28th National Nutrient Databank Conference, June 23–26, 2004, Iowa City, Iowa.

Diggins, K. C. (2008). Treatment of mild to moderate dehydration in children with oral rehydration therapy. *Journal of the American Academy of Nurse Practitioners, 20,* 402–406.

Dubois, L., Girard, M., & Potvin Kent, M. (2006). Breakfast eating and overweight in a pre-school population: Is there a link? *Public Health Nutrition, 9*(4), 436–442.

DuBose, K. D., Eisenmann, J. C., & Donnelly, J. E. (2007). Aerobic fitness attenuates the metabolic syndrome score in normal-weight, at-risk-for-overweight, and overweight children. *Pediatrics, 120,* e1262–e1268.

Farrow, C. V., & Blissett, J. (2008). Controlling feeding practices: Cause or consequence of early child weight. *Pediatrics, 121,* e164–e169.

Fernandes, S. M., de Morais, M. B., & Amancio, O. M. (2008). Intestinal blood loss as an aggravating factor of iron deficiency in infants

aged 9 to 12 months fed whole cow's milk. *Journal of Clinical Gastroenterology, 42,* 152–156.

Fisher, J. O., Liu, Y., Birch, L. L., & Rolls, B. J. (2007). Effects of portion size and energy density on young children's intake at a meal. *American Journal of Clinical Nutrition, 86,* 174–179.

Gao, X., Wilde, P. E., Lichtenstein, A. H., & Tucker, K. L. (2006). Meeting adequate intake for dietary calcium without dairy foods in adolescents aged 9 to 18 years (National Health and Nutrition Examination Survey 2001–2002). *Journal of the American Dietetic Association, 106,* 1759–1765.

Gidding, S. S., Dennison, B. A., Birch, L. L., Daniels, S. R., Gillman, M. W., Lichtenstein, A. H., et al. (2006). Dietary recommendations for children and adolescents: A guide for practitioners. *Pediatrics, 117,* 544–559.

Gidding, S. S., Lichtenstein, A. H., Faith, M. S, Karpyn, A., Mennella, J. A., Popkin, B., et al. (2009). Implementing American Heart Association pediatric and adult nutrition guidelines: A scientific statement from the American Heart Association Nutrition Committee of the Council on Nutrition, Physical Activity and Metabolism, Council on Cardiovascular Disease in the Young, Council on Arteriosclerosis, Thrombosis and Vascular Biology, Council on Cardiovascular Nursing, Council on Epidemiology and Prevention, and Council for High Blood Pressure Research. *Circulation, 119,* 1161–1175.

Gillman, M. W., Rifas-Shiman, S. L., Frazier, A. L., Rockett, H. R., Carmago, C. A., Field, A. E., et al. (2000). Family dinner and diet quality among older children and adolescents. *Archives of Family Medicine, 9,* 235–240.

Gordon-Larson, P., Adair, L. S., Nelson, M. C., & Popkin, B. M. (2004). Five-year obesity incidence in the transition period between adolescence and adulthood: The National Longitudinal Study of Adolescent Health. *American Journal of Clinical Nutrition, 80*(3), 569–575.

Gross, S. M., & Cinelli, B. (2004). Coordinated school health program and dietetics professionals: Partner in promoting healthful eating. *Journal of the American Dietetic Association, 104,* 793–798.

Hanley, D. A., & Davison, K. S. (2005). Vitamin D insufficiency in North America. *Journal of Nutrition, 135,* 332–337.

Hannon, P. A., Bowen, D. J., Moinpour, C. M., & McLerran, D. F. (2003). Correlations in perceived food use between the family food preparer and their spouses and children. *Appetite, 40,* 77–83.

Harnack, L., Stang, J., & Story, M. (1999). Soft drink consumption among U.S. children and

REFERENCES *(continued)*

adolescents: Nutritional consequences. *Journal of the American Dietetic Association, 99*, 436–441.

Heine, R. G., & Tang, M. (2008). Dietary approaches to the prevention of food allergy. *Current Opinion in Clinical Nutrition and Metabolic Care, 11*, 320–328.

Hoerr, S. L., Horodynski, M. A., Lee, S. Y., & Henry, M. (2006). Predictors of nutritional adequacy in mother-toddler dyads from rural families with limited incomes. *Journal of the American Dietetic Association, 106*, 1766–1773.

Institute of Medicine (IOM), Food and Nutrition Board. (1997). *Dietary reference intakes for calcium, phosphorus, magnesium, vitamin D and fluoride.* Washington, DC: National Academy Press.

Institute of Medicine (IOM), Food and Nutrition Board. (2001). Dietary reference intakes for vitamin A, vitamin K, arsenic, boron, chromium, copper, iodine, iron, manganese, molybdenum, nickel, silicon, vanadium, and zinc. Washington, DC: National Academy Press.

Institute of Medicine (IOM), Food and Nutrition Board. (2002). *Dietary reference intakes for energy, carbohydrate, fiber, fat, fatty acids cholesterol, protein, and amino acids.* Washington, DC: National Academy Press.

Ip, S., Chung, M., Raman, G., Chen, P., Magula, N., Devine, D., et al. (2007). Breastfeeding and maternal and child health outcomes in developed countries. *Evidence Report/Technology Assessment, 153*, 1–186.

Jackson, D. M., Djafarian, K., Stewart, J., & Speakman, J. R. (2009). Increased television viewing is associated with elevated body fatness but not with lower total energy expenditure in children. *American Journal of Clinical Nutrition, 89*, 1031–1036.

Jacobs, D. E., Clickner, R. P., Zhou, J. Y., Viet, S. M., Marker, D. A., Zeldin, D. C., et al. (2002). The prevalence of lead-based paint hazards in US housing. *Environmental Health Perspective, 110*, A599–A606.

Jean, D., & Cyr, C. (2007). Use of complementary and alternative medicine in a general pediatric clinic. *Pediatrics, 120*, e138–e141.

Johnson, S. L., & Birch, L. L. (1994). Parents' and children's adiposity and eating style. *Pediatrics, 94*, 653–661.

Kleinman, R. E. (Ed.). (2004). *Pediatric nutrition handbook* (5th ed.). Elk Grove, IL: American Academy of Pediatrics.

Koletzko, B., Lien, E., Agostoni, C., Bohles, H., Campoy, C., Cetin, I., et al. (2008). The roles of long-chain polyunsaturated fatty acids in pregnancy, lactation and infancy: Review of current knowledge and consensus recommendations. *Journal of Perinatal Medicine, 36*, 5–14.

Lawrence, R. A., & Lawrence, R. M. (2005). *Breastfeeding: A guide for the medical profession* (6th ed.).St. Louis, MO: C. V. Mosby.

Leahy, K. E., Birch, L. L., Fisher, J. O., & Rolls, B. J. (2007). How do energy density and portion size of an entrée influence preschool children's energy intake? *FASEB Journal, 21*, 367.1.

Malik, V. S., Schulze, M. B., & Hu, F. B. (2006). Intake of sugar-sweetened beverages and weight gain: A systematic review. *American Journal of Clinical Nutrition, 84*, 274–288.

Mangels, A., & Messina, V. (2001). Considerations in planning vegan diets: Infants. *Journal of the American Dietetic Association, 101*, 670–677.

Marcason, W. (2005). Can dietary intervention play a part in the treatment of attention deficit and hyperactivity disorder? *Journal of the American Dietetic Association, 105*, 1161–1162.

Messina, V., Mangels, R., & Messina, M. (2004). *The dietitian's guide to vegetarian diets* (2nd ed.). Sudbury, MA: Jones & Bartlett.

Morrison, J. A., Friedman, L. A., & Gray-McGuire, C. (2007). Metabolic syndrome in childhood predicts adult cardiovascular disease 25 years later: The Princeton Lipid Research Clinics Follow-Up Study. *Pediatrics, 120*, 340–345.

Nader, P. R., O'Brien, M., Houts, R., Bradley, R., Belsky, J., Crosnoe, R., et al. (2006). Identifying risk for obesity in early childhood. *Pediatrics, 118*, e594–e601.

Neal, E. G., Chaffe, H., Schwartz, R. H., Lawson, M. S., Edwards, N., Fitzsimmons, G., et al. (2008). The ketogenic diet for the treatment of childhood epilepsy: A randomised trial. *Lancet Neurology, 7*, 500-506.

Neumark-Sztainer, D., Hannan, P., Story, M., Croll, J., & Perry, C. (2003). Family meal patterns: Associations with sociodemographic characteristics and improved dietary intake among adolescents. *Journal of the American Dietetic Association, 103*, 317–322.

Neumark-Sztainer, D., Wall, M., Haines, J. I., Story, M., & Eisenberg, M. E. (2007a). Why does dieting predict weight gain in adolescents? Findings from project-EAT-II: A 5-year longitudinal study. *The Journal of the American Dietetic Association, 107*, 448–455.

Neumark-Sztainer, D. R., Wall, M. M., Haines, J. I., Story, M. T., Sherwood, N. E, van den Berg, P. A. (2007b). Shared risk and protective factors for overweight and disordered eating in adolescents. *American Journal of Preventive Medicine, 33*, 359–369.

Niemeier, H. M., Raynor, H. A., Lloyd-Richardson, E. E., Rogers, M., & Wing, R. R. (2006). Fast food consumption and breakfast skipping: Predictors of weight gain from adolescence to adulthood in a nationally representative sample. *Journal of Adolescent Health, 39*(6), 842–849.

Patrick, K., Spear, B., Holt, K., Sofka, D. (2001). *Bright futures in practice: Physical activity and nutrition.* Arlington, VA: National Center for Education in Maternal and Child Health.

Pearson, N., Biddle, S. J., & Gorely, T. (2009). Family correlates of breakfast consumption among children and adolescents: A systematic review. *Appetite, 52*, 1–7.

Powell, L. M., Szczypka, B. A., Chaloupka, F. J., & Braunschweig, C. L. (2007). Nutritional content of television food advertisements seen by children and adolescents in the United States. *Pediatrics, 120*, 576–583.

The Produce for Health Foundation. (2008). *Fruits and veggies, more matters.* Retrieved March 30, 2009, from http://www.fruitsandveggiesmorematters.org/

Ramakrishnan, U., Imhoff-Kunsch, B., & DiGirolamo, A. M. (2009). Role of docahexaenoic acid in maternal and child mental health. *American Journal of Clinical Nutrition, 89*, 958S–962S.

Rampersaud, G. C. (2009). Benefits of breakfast for children and adults: Updated recommendations for practitioners. *American Journal of Lifestyle Medicine, 3*, 86–103.

Rampersaud, G. C., Pereira, M. A., Girand, B. L., Adams, J., & Metzl, J. (2005). Breakfast habits, nutritional status, body weight, and academic performance in children and adolescents. *Journal of the American Dietetic Association, 105*, 743–760.

Robinson-O'Brien, R., Story, M., & Heim, S. (2009). Impact of garden-based youth nutrition intervention programs: A review. *Journal of the American Dietetic Association, 109*, 273–280.

Rovner, A. J., & O'Brien, K. O. (2008). Hypovitaminosis D among healthy children in the United States: A review of the current evidence. *Archives of Pediatric and Adolescent Medicine, 162*, 513–519.

Saintonge, S., Bang, H., & Gerber, L. M. (2009). Implications of a new definition of vitamin D deficiency in a multiracial U.S. adolescent population: The National Health and Nutrition Examination Survey III. *Pediatrics, 123*, 797–803.

Samour, P. Q., & King, K. (2005). *Handbook of pediatric nutrition.* Sudbury, MA: Jones and Bartlett.

Santo, C. C., de Oliviera, L. D., & Giugliani, E. R. (2007). Factors associated with low maintenance of exclusive breastfeeding in the first six months. *Birth, 34*, 212–219.

Satter, E. (1987). *How to get your kids to eat—but not too much.* Palo Alto, CA: Bull.

Scott, J. A., Binns, C. W., & Aroni, R. A. (1997). The influence of reported paternal attitudes on the decision to breast-feed. *Journal of Paediatrics and Child Health, 33*, 305–307.

Sinn, N. (2008). Nutritional and dietary influences on attention deficit hyperactivity disorder. *Nutrition Reviews, 66*, 558–568.

Skinner, J. D., Carruth, B. R., Bounds, W., & Ziegler, P. J. (2002). Children's food preferences. *Journal of the American Dietetic Association, 102*, 1638–1647.

Spear, B. A., Barlow, S. E., Ervin, C., Ludwig, D. S., Saelens, B. E., Schetzina, K. E., et al. (2007). Recommendations for treatment of child and adolescent overweight and obesity. *Pediatrics, 120*, S254–S288.

Stallings, V. A., Stark, L. J., Robinson, K. A., Feranchak, A. P., Quinton, H., & Clinical Practice Guidelines on Growth SubComitee. (2008). Evidence-based practice recommendations for the nutrition-related management of children and adults with cystic fibrosis and pancreatic insufficiency: Results of a systematic review. *Journal of the American Dietetic Association, 108*, 832–839.

Taylor, C. B., Bryson, S., Celio Doyle, A. A., Luce, K. H., Cunning, D., Adascal, L. B., et al. (2006). The adverse effect of negative comments about weight and shape from family and siblings on women at high risk for eating disorders. *Pediatrics, 118*, 731–738.

TV Bureau of Advertising. (2007). *Media trends track. Trends in television: Time spent viewing.* Retrieved March 30, 2009, from http://www.tvb.org/rcentral/MediaTrendsTrack/tvbasics/09_TimeViewingPersons.asp

Uauy, R., & Dangour, A. D. (2006). Nutrition in brain development and aging: Role of essential fatty acids. *Nutrition Reviews, 64*, S24–S33.

U.S. Department of Agriculture. (1998). *National school lunch program regulations.* Retrieved March 30, 2009, from http://www.fns.usda.gov/cnd/lunch/

U.S. Department of Agriculture. (2005). *Physical activity recommendation from the Dietary Guidelines for Americans, 2005.* Retrieved March 30, 2009, from http://www.health.gov/dietaryguidelines/dga2005/document/html/chapter4.htm

U.S. Department of Agriculture. (2007). *School meals.* Retrieved March 30, 2009, from http://www.fns.usda.gov/cnd/

Utter, J., Sccragg, R., Mhurchu, C. N., & Schaaf, D. (2007). At-home breakfast consumption among New Zealand children: Associations with body mass index and related nutrition behaviors. *The Journal of the American Dietetic Association, 107*(4), 570–576.

Vegetarian Resource Group. (2009). *Vegetarian kids and teens.* Retrieved March 30, 2009, from http://www.vrg.org/family/kidsindex.htm

Wagner, C. L., Greer, F. R., & Section on Breastfeeding, Committee on Nutrition. (2008). Prevention of rickets and vitamin D deficiency in infants, children, and adolescents. *Pediatrics, 122*, 1142–1152.

Whitlock, E. P., Williams, S. B., Gold, R., Smith, P. R., & Shipman, S. A. (2005). Screening and interventions for childhood overweight: A summary of evidence for the US Preventative Services Task Force. *Pediatrics, 116*, e125–e144.

Wilong, A. A. (2007). Complications and consequences of epilepsy surgery, ketogenic diet, and vagus nerve stimulation. *Seminars in Pediatric Neurology, 1*, 201–203.

Wiznitzer, M. (2008). From observations to trials: The ketogenic diet and epilepsy. *Lancet Neurology, 7*, 471–472.

Ziegler, E. E., Nelson, S. E., & Jeter, J. M. (2009). Iron supplementation of breastfed infants from an early age. *American Journal of Clinical Nutrition, 89*, 525–532.

Zutavern, A., Brockow, I., Schaaf, B., von Berg, A., Diez, U., Bote, M., et al. (2008). Timing of solid food introduction in relation to eczema, asthma, allergic rhinitis, and food and inhalant sensitization at the age of 6 years: Results from the prospective birth cohort study LISA. *Pediatrics, 121*, e44–e52.

Adult and Older Adult 15

WHAT WILL YOU LEARN?

1. To relate nutritional health goals for the adult and older adult.
2. To examine nutritional issues specific to men's health and women's health during adulthood.
3. To analyze the potential effects of normal aging on nutrition status.
4. To differentiate between changes in nutritional health because of normal aging and health conditions.
5. To summarize the nutritional recommendations that are unique for older adults.
6. To assess risk factors for poor nutritional health in the older adult.
7. To formulate nursing interventions for maintaining or improving nutritional health in the older adult.

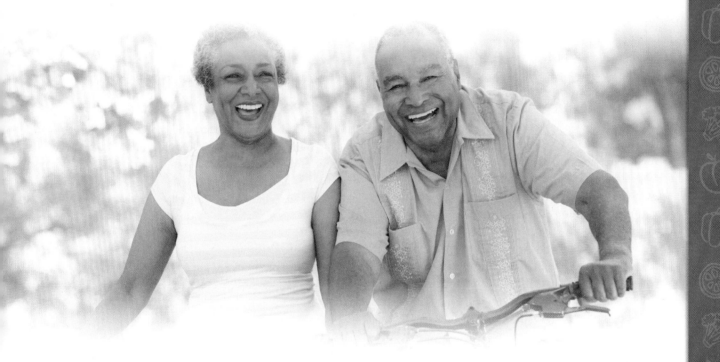

DID YOU KNOW?

▶ Over 75% of females older than age 20 years do not consume the recommended amount of calcium.

▶ An array of dietary supplements are marketed to adults for improved reproductive health, but conclusive research is lacking that supports the safety or effectiveness of most of these products.

▶ Females of childbearing age have increased iron needs and about 15% have iron-deficiency anemia.

▶ Total body water and thirst acuity decrease with age, leaving the older adult vulnerable to dehydration.

▶ Up to 60% of institutionalized or hospitalized older adults are malnourished.

KEY TERMS

anorexia of aging, *333*

atrophic gastritis, *332*

dysphagia, *338*

edentulism, *332*

food insecurity, *334*

phytoestrogens, *330*

sarcopenia, *332*

xerostomia, *332*

Nutritional Health in the Adult and Older Adult

Nutritional habits and lifestyle choices influence health across the lifespan. During adulthood, nutritional health is influenced by the foundation of lifestyle habits and nutritional intake built during childhood, adolescence, and young adulthood. Maintenance and improvement of nutrition status remain a health priority into adulthood. Adequate intake of essential nutrients is needed to help avoid both undernutrition and overnutrition. For example, inadequate calcium and vitamin D status can lead to osteoporosis. Poor intake of iron contributes to risk of iron-deficiency anemia. Nutrition influences the development of chronic diseases that may begin in adulthood. Cardiovascular disease, hypertension, and type 2 diabetes mellitus are examples of chronic diseases that are influenced by overnutrition. Excessive intake of saturated fat and calories can lead to overnutrition that leads to disease risk. The prevention and treatment of overweight and obesity across the lifespan has a positive influence on avoidance of these chronic diseases. The nurse should be involved in educating adults about the role that nutrition plays in preventing chronic disease and the importance of weight management. When working with the older adult, the nurse should be aware that the prevalence of undernutrition is high, especially in hospitalized or dependent older adults, and that the role of the nurse is pivotal in screening for undernutrition and facilitating nutritional intervention when needed.

Nutrition in the Adult

Although linear growth is completed by early adulthood, adequate nutrition remains essential for maintenance and repair of body tissues. The dietary reference intakes (DRIs) for adults between 19 years and 50 years do not change significantly from adolescence with the exception of the recommendations for calcium, phosphorus, and iron. Daily calcium recommendations decrease to 1,000 mg from 1,300 mg as an adolescent, and phosphorus recommendations drop to 700 mg from 1,250 mg (Institute of Medicine [IOM], 1997). At age 50 years, the rec-

ommended intake of both calcium and vitamin D increases to 1,200 mg and 10 mcg, respectively (IOM, 1997). Adequate vitamin D intake is essential to support intestinal absorption of calcium (Heaney, 2008). These recommendations are based on available research outlining the mineral intake needed for achieving and maintaining bone mass in young and middle adulthood (IOM, 1997).

Iron recommendations increase in the adult female, whereas they decrease in the male compared with those recommended during adolescence. The adult male requires only 8 mg/day of iron compared with the 11 mg/day needed during adolescence to support increases in lean body mass and blood volume (IOM, 2001). Iron recommendations for the adult female increase to 18 mg daily from 15 mg daily in adolescence to support iron lost during menses (IOM, 2001). Table 15-1 outlines the significant DRIs that are unique to the adult between 19 and 50 years of age and food sources for those nutrients.

Preventive Nutrition in the Adult: What Are the Concerns?

Health promotion and disease prevention education are essential for the adult in midlife. Successful aging in later life relies on good health. The nurse can take a central role in assisting the adult to reduce risk of chronic disease and optimize health. A healthy diet is one lifestyle aspect central to the prevention of many chronic diseases encountered in midlife and later. Higher levels of body mass index (BMI) are associated with risk of death from cardiovascular disease, diabetes, and kidney disease (Flegal, Graubard, Williamson, & Gail, 2007). Additionally, an increased waist circumference along with an increased BMI increases risk of death compared with those with a distribution of excess adipose that is not as centralized in the abdominal area (Pischon et al., 2008). Overall daily energy intake has increased in adults in the United States since the 1970s (Centers for Disease Control and Prevention [CDC], 2004a), despite the well-researched association between chronic disease and overweight. The food industry in the United States produces an average of 3,900 kcalories/day per person, which is an amount that far

Table 15-1 Dietary Reference Intakes in the Adult and Older Adult

Nutrient	Adults 19–50 Years	Adults Greater Than Age 50 Years	Good Food Sources
Calcium	1,000 mg	1,200 mg	Milk, yogurt, cheese, fortified juice and soy milk, sardines, kale, mustard greens
Phosphorus	700 mg	700 mg	Dairy foods, eggs, meat, fish, poultry
Vitamin D	5 mcg	10 mcg age greater than 50–70 years; 15 mcg age greater than 70 years	Fortified milk and butter, liver
Iron	8 mg males 18 mg females	8 mg males and females	Meat, fish, poultry, legumes, dried fruit, enriched grains
Vitamin B_6	1.3 mg	1.5 mg females, 1.7 mg males	Whole grains, chicken, fish, eggs, pork
Vitamin B_{12}	2.4 mcg	2.4 mcg of synthetic vitamin B_{12}	Foods of animal origin, fortified foods
Fluid	3.7 liters males 2.7 liters females	3.7 liters males 2.7 liters females	Liquids, watery foods

CT? Older adults are advised to consume synthetic forms of vitamin B_{12}. What sources of synthetic vitamin B_{12} could the nurse suggest?
Sources: Adapted from IOM, 1997; IOM, 1998; IOM, 2001; IOM, 2004.

exceeds the energy needs of most people (Ludwig & Nestle, 2008). Just 50 extra calories of unexpended energy each day equates to an extra 5 pounds of body weight over a year (Kumanyika et al., 2008). Portion sizes both in the home and in restaurants have increased markedly for many common foods, especially those with low food cost and often little nutrient density such as soda and fried foods (Lioret, Volatier, Lafay, Touvier, & Maire, 2007; Young & Nestle, 2007). Many consumers do not consider portions listed on food labels when determining the amount of food to consume (Ueland, Cardello, Merrill, & Lesher, 2009). Less physical energy is being expended because of the effect of automation and technology on work and leisure activities (Kumanyika et al., 2008). Compounding the problem of increased energy intake, 40% of adults in the United States never engage in any type of leisure-time physical activity (CDC, 2007).

In addition to the association among overweight, obesity, and chronic disease, other aspects of the diet have been linked to disease risk. Dietary intake may play a role in the risk for some cancers, but research has yielded little in the way of nutrient-specific advice. Instead, recommendations advise consumption of a variety of foods with plenty of fruits, vegetables, and whole grains while limiting excessive intake of saturated fat, trans fat, and alcohol. The U.S. Dietary Guidelines and Food Guide Pyramid outlined in Chapter 9 can be used as a template for educating the adult about chronic disease risk reduction.

Health education should also focus on the prevention of undernutrition in the adult. The nurse should be mindful of risk factors for undernutrition because many are associated with increased risk of medical conditions. For example:

- *Osteoporosis*—Poor calcium and vitamin D are risk factors for the development of osteoporosis (National

Osteoporosis Foundation [NOF], 2008). More than half of all adults have low plasma levels of vitamin D (Holick, 2007). The average intake of calcium falls short of recommended intake by more than 100 mg/day (United States Department of Agriculture [USDA], 2005). The nurse can advise the client about improving calcium intake by using Chapter 6 Client Education Checklist 6-1.

- *Neural tube defects*— Adequate folic acid intake is associated with a decreased risk of neural tube defects, which are malformations associated with birth defects such as spina bifida and anencephaly where the neural tube that forms the spinal cord and brain fails to close properly during fetal development. Survey data have revealed that 60% of U.S. females age 18 to 45 years report not meeting the recommended 400 mcg/day of folic acid (CDC, 2004b). The nurse can outline sources of folic acid to the client using Chapter 13 Client Education Checklist 13-1.

- *Iron deficiency*—Although iron deficiency does not affect the majority of healthy adults, it is a concern for females of childbearing age. Iron losses because of menses and increased requirements during pregnancy predispose females to risk of poor iron status. Iron-deficiency anemia during pregnancy is associated with an increased risk of preterm delivery and low birth weight (American Dietetic Association [ADA], 2008). The nurse can outline sources of iron-rich foods to the client as contained in Table 15-1 and in Chapter 6 Client Education Checklist 6-3.

The nurse should routinely incorporate a nutritional assessment into the overall evaluation of the adult. Chapter 12 discusses nutrition assessment in detail. Discussion of dietary

MyNursingKit National Center for Complementary and Alternative Medicine, Erectile Dysfunction

Table 15-2 Nutrition Health Promotion Goals for the Adult

Health Promotion Goal	Nutrition Recommendation
Reduction of chronic disease risk, including hypertension, cardiovascular disease, type 2 diabetes, and some cancers	• Weight management • Consumption of a low-fat, moderate-sodium diet with a variety of fruits, vegetables, whole grains, low-fat dairy, and lean protein sources • Moderation in alcohol intake
Maximize bone health	Consumption of adequate calcium and vitamin D
Prevention of neural tube defects in infants	Consumption of adequate folic acid by women of childbearing age

intake and the role of nutrition in health maintenance and disease prevention should be integral to health education efforts by the nurse. Hot Topic: Does Nutrition Affect Reproductive Health? is an example of a subject that the adult client may bring up for discussion with the nurse.

The nurse should offer advice based on established national guidelines, providing tailored examples that could be integrated into the individual's specific cultural and lifestyle context. The nurse should assess the client for existing barriers to healthy eating practices, such as a knowledge deficit regarding nutritional value of foods or health guidelines. Conflicting media reports on nutrition can frustrate and confuse the consumer, making interpretation of specific recommendations a challenge for the client. Other factors such as economic status, lifestyle, and social support should be considered when offering advice. Individuals requiring additional education or nutrition intervention should be referred to a registered dietitian. Table 15-2 outlines nutrition health promotion goals for the adult.

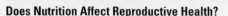

Does Nutrition Affect Reproductive Health?

Many types of dietary supplements and nutritional solutions have been touted in the popular press as treatment for male and female reproductive health symptoms. Some individuals seek dietary alternatives to traditional medical treatment of reproductive health symptoms, whereas others use nutrition intervention as a complement.

In females, diet and dietary supplements have been considered in the management or treatment of a number of obstetric and gynecologic conditions. Much has been written about the nutrition treatment of premenstrual syndrome (PMS) and premenstrual dysphoric disorder (PMDD). Cyclical alterations in calcium homeostasis are felt

to contribute to some of the physical and affective symptoms of these disorders. Calcium supplementation of 1,000 to 1,200 mg has been clinically shown to alleviate many symptoms, including irritability and cramping (American Dietetic Association & Dietitians of Canada, 2004; Pearlstein & Steiner, 2008). The use of vitamin B$_6$ for PMS has been heavily researched and results are variable, though there may be some minor benefit in doses up to 100 mg per day (American Dietetic Association & Dietitians of Canada, 2004; Pearlstein & Steiner, 2008). Other botanical and dietary supplements, such as magnesium, evening primrose oil, and chaste berry, have inconclusive results in the management of PMS (American Dietetic Association & Dietitians of Canada, 2004).

Infertility in males and females is affected by nutritional health. Both overweight and underweight conditions are associated with reduced probability of conception (American Dietetic Association & Dietitians of Canada, 2004; Esposito et al., 2008). The nurse should advise the client seeking advice on nutrition intervention for infertility about the health benefits of attaining a healthy weight. Females with polycystic ovary syndrome should be particularly advised to achieve a healthy weight to improve both fertility and other metabolic symptoms of the disorder, such as insulin resistance (Brassard, AinMelk, & Baillargeon, 2008).

The prescription use of hormone replacement therapy in menopausal females has declined following clinical evidence linking these medications with adverse cardiovascular disease events (Hersh, Stefanik, & Stafford, 2004). Many females are reporting use of alternative medicine, including diet and dietary supplements, to treat menopausal symptoms such as hot flashes. Evidence from clinical trials on most dietary supplements and menopausal symptoms is limited or inconclusive (American Dietetic Association & Dietitians of Canada, 2004; Carroll, 2006). Black cohosh and supplements containing **phytoestrogens**, or weak plant estrogens, such as soy, other beans, flaxseed, red clover, and isoflavones, have shown some promise in treating menopausal symptoms, but questions remain unanswered regarding long-term safety and a possible placebo effect. For example, black cohosh has been reported to cause hepatotoxicity (Mahady et al., 2008). The effect of these types of supplements on estrogenic stimulation of the breast and endometrium is of particular concern, especially in those with reproductive cancer risk, and more research is needed before a recommendation can be given (Carroll, 2006; Rees, 2009).

In males, diet and dietary supplements have been investigated in the prevention and treatment of symptoms of prostate disease and erectile dysfunction. Saw palmetto, derived from a palm tree, has been shown to improve symptoms of benign prostatic hypertrophy such as urine flow when compared with traditional drug treatment in some studies but not others (Bent et al., 2006; Edwards, 2008). Dietary factors that may play a role in prostate cancer prevention include lycopene, a red plant pigment found in tomatoes and other pink or red plant foods (Dahan, Fennal, Kumar, 2008). Long-term studies of vitamin E and selenium taken alone or in combination report no effect on decreased risk of prostate cancer (Lippman et al., 2009).

There is little to no clinical evidence that any dietary supplements improve libido in males (Tamler & Mechanick, 2007). Lifestyle factors, including achievement of a healthy weight, have been linked with maintenance of erectile function in males (Esposito et al., 2008).

The role of diet and dietary supplements in reproductive health is an evolving area of medicine. Currently, research is

MyNursingKit National Center for Complementary and Alternative Medicine, Menopause

too limited to offer the client evidence-based advice regarding most aspects involving dietary supplements and reproductive health. Despite this lack of evidence, many individuals may still self-treat reproductive health symptoms with dietary supplements, believing them to be safe. The nurse working with this population should assess individuals for use of dietary supplements and remain current with the clinical research, conferring with the medical team, including the pharmacist and registered dietitian, when questions arise. Table 15-3 outlines current recommendations for nutrition and reproductive health in males and females.

Table 15-3	Nutrition and Reproductive Health Recommendations
Goal	**Nutrition Recommendation**
Reduction of PMS/PMDD symptoms	1,000 mg–1,200 mg calcium daily
Minimize infertility risk	Weight management
Improvement of symptoms of polycystic ovary syndrome	Weight management
Prevention of neural tube defects in infants	Adequate folic acid intake (400 mcg/day) in all women of childbearing age
Prevention of iron-deficiency anemia in females	Adequate iron intake (18 mg/day) in nonpregnant females
Decrease in menopausal symptoms	Inconclusive results on diet and supplement use in treatment of menopausal symptoms
Decrease in symptoms of benign prostatic hypertrophy	Consult with primary health care provider about use of saw palmetto
Prevention of prostate cancer	Inconclusive; lycopene under study
Improvement of erectile dysfunction	Weight management

Nutrition in the Older Adult

Nutritional health plays an important role in successful aging. In the older adult, nutrition is central to maintaining overall health and functional capacity. Medical nutrition therapy plays a key role in secondary and tertiary prevention strategies by lessening disease risk, slowing disease progression, and minimizing symptoms of chronic disease (American Dietetic Association [ADA], 2005a). A wide spectrum of well-being exists among older adults, presenting the nurse with varied nutritional challenges. Biological changes associated with the aging process, compounded by symptoms and treatment of any chronic diseases, place the older adult at a disproportionate risk of undernutrition compared to other age groups. Overnutrition, specifically in the form of overweight and obesity, is a continued health risk for the older adult, affect-

ing morbidity, mortality, and functional capacity. Dependent older adults in long-term care or those who are hospitalized are at greatest risk of poor nutritional health. The nurse should be aware that any change in the risk factors for poor nutritional health deserves consideration in the older adult.

How Does Aging Affect Nutrition?

Normal aging results in physiological changes to the body that, in turn, have nutritional implications. These changes occur at an individualized pace. The nurse should consider the effects of these biological changes, outlined in Table 15-4, when assessing the nutrition status of an older adult. Physiological changes that result in altered nutritional health should not be dismissed as "just aging," but rather addressed with proper intervention when indicated.

Body Composition Changes

The biological process of aging brings about changes in muscle mass, adipose, bone mineral content, and total body

Table 15-4	Nutrition Implications of Normal Aging Changes
Aging Effect	**Impact**
Altered body composition	↓ Muscle mass ↓ Total body water ↑ Fat Mass ↓ Bone mineral density
Oral and gastrointestinal changes	Altered dentition affects chewing Xerostomia affects taste, swallowing ↑ Cholecystokinin causes ↓ gastric emptying and early satiety ↓ Production of gastric acid alters vitamin B_{12} and iron absorption ↓ Production of intrinsic factor alters vitamin B_{12} absorption
Alteration in sensory perception	Taste and smell impairment Hearing and vision changes affect enjoyment of social dining. Vision can impact meal preparation and seeing food on plate during meal
Altered fluid homeostasis	↓ Total body water and decreased perception of thirst
Socioeconomic changes	Food insecurity from financial constraints or inadequate access to food Social isolation, sadness, bereavement, and depression associated with ↓ intake
Medical conditions or disease	Condition and its treatment, including medications, diet, or hospitalization, can lead to alterations in dietary intake

CT? Which effects cannot be altered with health care intervention? Which effects can have improved outcome with proper nursing intervention?

water. The loss of lean muscle mass in older adults is called **sarcopenia.** Sarcopenia occurs for a number of reasons, some of which are age related and others that are not. Age-related contributors to loss of muscle mass include decreased anabolic hormone production and increased cytokine activity (Rolland et al., 2008). Diminished physical activity and decreased dietary intake can lead to muscle loss as well, regardless of whether these decreases are age associated or a result of a condition or illness. Diminished muscle mass can lead to a cascade of negative consequences for the older person, including loss of strength and endurance that contributes to a functional decline and increased risk of falls (Bischoff, Staehelin, & Willett, 2006; Rolland et al., 2008). Overall energy expenditure decreases with the loss of metabolically active protein tissue (Labossiere & Bernard, 2008). If the older person continues to consume the same amount of calories after muscle loss as beforehand, fat weight gain can ensue if energy expenditure from physical activity is not proportionately increased. This change in body composition can be a challenge to the older adult who has experienced any functional decline. For such clients, the nurse can suggest a referral to a physical therapist for advice on appropriate activity amounts and types to build muscle and increase energy expenditure.

Loss of muscle mass can be masked by a subsequent increase in body fat in older adults. Although the diminished muscle can initially go unnoticed because of weight gain or maintenance, the negative effects on functional status should be evident (Stenholm et al., 2008). For this reason, measurement of body weight alone will not provide a thorough assessment of sarcopenia in the older person. Skinfold thickness can be used, but results are limited because of decreased skin elasticity with aging and diminished distribution of subcutaneous fat (IOM, 2000). Truncal fat and fat deposition around organs increases with age, but these changes are not apparent simply with skinfold measurements. Given these limitations to assessing the older adult, the nurse should obtain serial weights and skinfold measurements, comparing the measurements to prior findings when monitoring for changes in body composition (IOM, 2000).

Almost two-thirds of the water content in the body is found in skeletal muscle. Diminished total body water occurs as a result of muscle loss and places the older adult at increased risk of dehydration and heat stress (Thomas et al., 2008).

Bone mineral density is lost with age and can put the older person at risk for osteoporosis. The nurse should assess the older adult for preexisting risk factors for osteoporosis such as poor calcium or vitamin D status from medications or poor intake that can further compound bone density loss. Bone loss is accelerated following menopause in females, whereas males are at risk for osteoporosis later in life (Cashman, 2007). Older adults with suboptimal bone growth as a child or adolescent are also at risk for osteoporosis. Aging

lessens the ability of the body to manufacture adequate vitamin D from the sun (National Insitutes of Health [NIH], 2008). This change can add to the risk of poor bone health, falls, and fractures (Mosekilde, 2005).

Appetite, Oral, and Gastrointestinal Changes

Aging can lead to alterations in the gastrointestinal tract that foster changes in dietary intake and altered nutrient absorption. The older adult may experience changes in dentition, chewing, and swallowing that can lead to diminished intake and affect nutritional status.

Dentition

Nutrition status can be affected by poor dental health. Missing or loose teeth and poorly fitting dentures can lead to altered dietary intake. **Edentulism,** or missing teeth, affects over one-third of Americans over age 65 years (Labossiere & Bernard, 2008). Practice Pearl: Dental Health stresses the importance of dental health in adulthood. Compromised oral function from defective dentures, no dentures, or loose or occluding teeth is considered a risk factor for malnutrition, morbidity, and mortality in the older person (Padilha, Hilgert, Hugo, Bos, & Ferrucci, 2008). Having fewer or no teeth is associated with an altered selection of foods, leading to poor intake of fiber, vitamins A and C, and folate, among other nutrients (Nowjack-Raymer & Sheiham, 2007).

Xerostomia

Insufficient saliva production, or **xerostomia,** can occur with the aging process. A dry mouth can lead to altered taste perception and difficulty swallowing. Retention of ill-fitting dentures becomes more difficult when there is insufficient saliva production. Dehydration and disease further exacerbate xerostomia. The nurse should be aware that many medications commonly prescribed in this population contribute to diminished saliva production. Examples of drugs that alter saliva production include angiotensin-converting enzyme (ACE) inhibitors and anti-Parkinson's medications.

Atrophic Gastritis

Aging increases the risk of **atrophic gastritis,** a decrease in the size and number of glands and mucous membranes in the stomach. The diminished secretion of hydrochloric acid that

PRACTICE PEARL

Dental Health

The need for good oral hygiene and dental care does not diminish in the elderly. Even in those who have few or no remaining teeth, the nurse should remind the older adult of the need for regular dental checkups to prevent periodontal disease and to check for properly fitting dentures.

occurs affects the digestion and absorption of nutrients that require a more acid medium in the stomach, including vitamin B_{12}, calcium, and iron. Additionally, a decreased secretion of intrinsic factor occurs, further altering vitamin B_{12} absorption. Malabsorption of vitamin B_{12} because of diminished gastric acid is the reason for over one-half of the cases of deficiency found in hospitalized older adults (Dali-Youcef & Andres, 2009). The nurse should also consider the alkalinizing effects of medications such as antacids, proton pump inhibitors, and H_2 receptor blockers because these can alter vitamin B_{12}, calcium, and iron absorption (Dali-Youcef & Andres, 2009; Yu et al., 2008).

Appetite Regulation

The **anorexia of aging** is a term coined to describe the diminished appetite that occurs with aging (Chapman, MacIntosh, Morley, & Horowitz, 2002). Several factors contribute to this effect. Cholecystokinin, a gastrointestinal satiety hormone, has been reported to have increased concentrations with age, which contributes to slowed gastric emptying. Early satiation, because of elevated cholecystokinan, along with changes in other gastrointestinal hormones and central neurotransmitters responsible for the feeding drive, are additional hypotheses given to explain the anorexia of aging (Bhutto & Morley, 2008).

Constipation

Chronic constipation is more likely in older adults than in younger adults despite the fact that there is little change in colon transit time with age (Bhutto & Morley, 2008). Reduced physical activity, medications, and insufficient fluid intake are contributing causes (Muller-Lissner, Kamm, Scarpignato, & Wald, 2005). The nurse should assess the older adult who complains of constipation for adequacy of fluid intake. Adequate fiber, slowly introduced into the diet, is also indicated.

Sensory Changes

Sensory changes that may occur with normal aging can negatively affect nutrition status by altering enjoyment of food, social dining, and by making food preparation difficult or dangerous.

Taste and Smell Changes

Both olfactory perception and taste sensation decline with aging (Bhutto & Morley, 2008). These senses are intertwined and their loss can lead to reduced enjoyment associated with eating. Alteration in the sense of taste and smell is more pronounced in individuals with cognitive impairment and Parkinson's disease (Lafreniere & Mann, 2009; Lang et al., 2006). Many medications commonly prescribed in the older adult further alter taste and smell perception (Hickson, 2006). Additionally, smoking, nasal congestion, and a history of stroke or epilepsy are associated with altered olfaction. The majority of older adults with diminished smell sensation are unaware that this change has occurred (Lafreniere & Mann, 2009).

Taste perception losses that occur with aging are more pronounced because of the effects of medications, which can impart a metallic or bitter taste in the mouth via the saliva (Doty, Shah, & Bromley, 2008). Radiation to the head and neck region can permanently damage taste buds. Older adults may also experience changes in taste thresholds for salty and sweet foods, leading to use of more sweetener or salt in foods in order to perceive those sensations (Bhutto & Morley, 2008).

Diminished ability to taste and smell food can lead to loss of enjoyment of eating and alter the older adult's intake. The nurse can suggest good mouth care when metallic or bitter taste is experienced. Altering the texture of food, adding color to the foods presented, and experimenting with additional flavors and spices may also help.

Vision and Hearing Changes

Poor vision can make the entire food preparation and eating process more difficult or even hazardous. Grocery shopping can be a chore if the ability to read labels is impaired. Food preparation is a challenge when it is difficult to read cooking instructions or accurately see knobs and dials on the stove, microwave, or other cooking equipment. Handling hot liquids is a hazard if the older person cannot discern whether a container is entirely full or pouring is inaccurate. While eating, poor lighting and dishware with either little contrast between the food and plate or busy patterns can make seeing the meal difficult. Visual impairment is associated with poor nutrition status in the older adult (ADA, 2005b).

Hearing loss can leave the older person feeling isolated and lead to diminished enjoyment of social dining. Loud, open dining areas can further frustrate the individual with poor hearing. Some older adults may choose to dine alone as a result of poor hearing. Social dining is important in the older adult and is associated with an increased dietary intake compared to dining in isolation, which is associated with risk of undernutrition (Labossiere & Bernard, 2008; Silver, 2009).

Fluid Balance Changes

Maintaining adequate hydration can be a challenge for some older adults because of diminished total body water that occurs with muscle loss and altered thirst mechanisms. Impaired angiotensin production, decreased renin and aldosterone secretion, and inefficient osmoreceptors in the body contribute to the blunting of the thirst mechanism, leaving the older adult at risk of dehydration (Farrell et al., 2008). Older adults may deliberately self-restrict fluid intake to cope with incontinence or nocturia. Others may restrict fluid to avoid needing assistance with toileting or because of conditions that affect mobility, such as arthritis. Older persons who are dependent on others because of cognitive or physical limitations may have inadequate access to fluids throughout the day, which places them at increased risk of suboptimal hydration. The nurse should be mindful of the risk of dehydration in the older person and monitor for its symptoms. Fever, exudative wounds, and gastrointestinal losses put additional burden on the fluid balance of older adults.

Socioeconomic Changes

Retirement from the workforce can place a financial burden on some older adults. Insufficient funds for both food and other expenses may force some individuals to choose lesser quality or quantity of food. **Food insecurity** from lack of funds or poor access to food affects over 1.4 million households with elderly in the United States (ADA, 2005a). Older adults who experience food insecurity are reported to have insufficient intake of protein, calcium, vitamin A, and many of the B vitamins (ADA, 2006).

Living arrangements also can affect nutrition status in the older adult. Older individuals who do not live with a spouse are reported to have poorer dietary intake than those who do live with a spouse. Social isolation, loneliness, sadness, and bereavement are also linked with risk of undernutrition (Feldblum et al., 2007).

Medical Conditions and Disease-Related Nutrition Changes

Chronic disease or medical conditions place the older adult at increased nutritional risk because of the condition itself or its treatment. Disease pathophysiology may predispose the older adult to altered absorption or utilization of nutrients, such as with some malabsorptive gastrointestinal diseases like inflammatory bowel disease. Functional and cognitive decline can affect nutritional status and make performance of basic activities of daily living difficult. Many over-the-counter and prescription medications are associated with drug-nutrient interactions or side effects that can jeopardize nutritional health. There is a rising trend of dietary supplement use among older adults, increasing the possibility of medication interactions (Wold et al., 2005). Herbal supplements, vitamins, minerals, and other dietary supplements should be considered when assessing for interactions. Therapeutic diets are commonly prescribed as part of medical nutrition therapy of disease but may be too restrictive in some individuals such as the institutionalized older person (ADA, 2005b). Cultural Consideration Box: Therapeutic Diets in the Older Adult points out additional considerations about restrictive diets in the older adult.

Nutrition Recommendations for the Older Adult

Older adults have unique nutritional needs compared with younger adults. The need for energy may decline in those individuals who lose muscle mass and are less active, yet several nutrients have an increased requirement with age. Vitamins B_{12}, B_6, and D and calcium have increased requirements in the adult over age 50 years. Table 15-1 outlines nutrient needs specific to the adult and older adult. The requirement for other

Cultural Considerations

Therapeutic Diets in the Older Adult

Many food preferences that are culturally based do not lend themselves to therapeutic diets without significant modification. For example, refried beans that are prepared with lard are not consistent with a reduced-fat diet, or the use of soy sauce or monosodium glutamate (MSG) is not consistent with a reduced-sodium diet. The nurse needs to be sensitive to cultural preferences while working with clients to determine other culturally acceptable choices. For example, canned low-fat refried beans may be acceptable in place of home-prepared refried beans, or low-sodium soy sauce and elimination of MSG may still provide acceptable taste in some Asian specialties.

nutrients in the older adult remains the same as for the younger adult. A wide spectrum of health among older persons and varying rates of aging make it necessary to consider each person's nutritional needs individually. With age, the variability of nutritional needs becomes wider rather than narrower.

Energy Needs

Energy requirements decline with age largely because of lowered physical activity levels (Lichtenstein et al., 2008). Loss of muscle mass also contributes to declining energy needs, but this effect can be counteracted by maintaining muscle with resistance training (Rolland et al., 2008). A decrease in energy needs in the face of higher nutrient needs presents a nutrition challenge to many older adults. The nurse can make suggestions about nutrient-dense food choices when working with the older adult who is experiencing unwanted weight gain. For example, low-fat or skim milk are good sources of calcium and have less kcalories than whole milk.

Calcium and Vitamin D

Both calcium and vitamin D daily requirements increase with age. Vitamin D requirements double for adults over age 50 years and triple by age 70 years compared with the 5 mcg requirement for younger adults. Vitamin D deficiency is common in older adults because of poor intake, decreased endogenous synthesis, and limited sun exposure, especially in those who are institutionalized (Mosekilde, 2005; NIH, 2008). Up to 90% of older adults do not consume adequate vitamin D (Moore, Murphy, Keast, & Holick, 2004). Medications such as corticosteroids and anticonvulsants can also compromise vitamin D and calcium status. For example, gastric acid-suppressing medications are associated with an increased risk of fractures because of altered calcium absorption (Yu et al., 2008). Muscle weakness and pain from vitamin D deficiency is associated with an increased risk of falls and hip fracture in the older adult (Cauley et al., 2008; Dawson-Hughes, 2008). The Modified MyPyramid for Older

MyNursingKit Modified MyPyramid for Older Adults

EVIDENCE-BASED PRACTICE RESEARCH BOX

What is the recommendation for calcium supplements?

Clinical Problem: Calcium supplements are often recommended to prevent osteoporosis and fractures in postmenopausal and elderly women.

Research Findings: Inadequate dietary intake of calcium and vitamin D has been suggested as a contributing factor in the development of osteoporosis and subsequent fracture of vertebrae and the hip in elderly females. Supplements are frequently recommended as a simple, inexpensive means of increasing calcium intake and prevention of fractures.

Studies of bone marrow density (BMD) show that 500 mg per day of calcium carbonate plus 700 international units of vitamin D when given as supplements to females and males 65 years and older show an increase in BMD and decrease in fractures after 3 years (Dawson-Hughes, Harris, Krall, & Dallal, 1997). The same subjects were followed for an additional 3 years, during which no supplements were given. Endpoint studies of BMD showed no sustained benefit following discontinuance of calcium and vitamin D (Dawson-Hughes, Harris, Krall, & Dallal, 2000).

Postmenopausal women in the Women's Health Initiative Trial who received 1,000 mg of calcium carbonate and 400 international units of vitamin D were followed for 7 years. Women who adhered to the trial had increased

BMD but no significant decrease in hip fracture. They also experienced a small increase in renal calculi (Jackson et al., 2006).

Community-dwelling elderly females who received 600 mg of calcium carbonate twice daily for 5 years showed an increase in BMD and a decrease in hip fractures but only in those who were compliant. A greater benefit was found for institutionalized, frail elderly, probably due to the ability to control compliance (Prince, Devine, Dhaliwal, & Dick, 2006).

Nursing Implications: Studies are equivocal about the benefits of calcium and vitamin D supplements, particularly in community-dwelling elderly who have a balanced diet. There seems to be no sustained benefit if an individual discontinues daily supplements.

CRITICAL THINKING QUESTION:

1. How should the nurse respond to the middle-aged female who says she has heard that calcium supplements will prevent osteoporosis?

2. What could the nurse suggest to the elderly female who says she cannot take the recommended calcium supplements because the pills are too big to swallow?

In Chapter 6, Hot Topic 6-1 discusses how to choose a calcium supplement.

Adults suggests that some older adults should consider a supplement with vitamin D to meet the daily recommendation (Lichtenstein et al., 2008). There is literature to suggest that all ages should get more vitamin D.

Calcium needs increase to 1,200 mg daily in the adult over age 50 years because of accelerated bone loss with age (IOM, 1997). A calcium supplement should be considered in the older adult who is not consuming adequate dietary sources of calcium (Lichtenstein et al., 2008). The Evidence-Based Practice Box: What is the recommendation for calcium supplements? discusses calcium supplements. Sources of dietary calcium are outlined in Table 15-1 and in Chapter 6 Client Education Checklist 6-1.

Vitamin B$_{12}$

The recommendation for daily intake of vitamin B$_{12}$ is modified in adults age 51 years and older because of the effects of poor vitamin B$_{12}$ absorption in this population. The inability to cleave the protein-vitamin B$_{12}$ bond in foods and altered production of intrinsic factor, which are both needed for proper B$_{12}$ absorption, are cited as reasons for poor vitamin B$_{12}$ status in this age group (Allen, 2009; Dali-Youcef & Andres, 2009. The IOM recommends that the recommended daily allowance (RDA) of 2.4 mcg be consumed primarily in the form of synthetic vitamin B$_{12}$ in the older adult (IOM, 1998). This amount does not differ from that recommended

for younger adults; the qualification to consume a synthetic rather than food source of the vitamin is unique to this age population. Synthetic vitamin B$_{12}$ is not bound to protein and, therefore, does not require an acidic gastric environment to initiate its digestion and absorption. Synthetic vitamin B$_{12}$ is found in vitamin supplements and fortified foods, like breakfast cereals, some soy milks, and meal replacement foods.

Symptoms of vitamin B$_{12}$ deficiency are outlined in Chapter 5 and can include macrocytic anemia and neurological symptoms leading to forgetfulness, inability to concentrate, and sensory disturbances. Folic acid supplementation treats the macrocytosis and thus masks that aspect of a vitamin B$_{12}$ deficiency, allowing the neurological symptoms to progress. In the older adult, these symptoms may be overlooked or dismissed as age related. The nurse should urge screening for vitamin B$_{12}$ deficiency in the older adult experiencing related neurological symptoms.

Vitamin B$_6$

Need for vitamin B$_6$ increases slightly with age from the 1.3 mg daily recommended for younger adults. Females over age 50 years require 1.5 mg per day, and males the same age require 1.7 mg daily (IOM, 1998). Unlike vitamins B$_{12}$ and D and calcium, the recommendation for vitamin B$_6$ does not include the suggestion of a vitamin supplement to meet recommended intake levels in the older adult. Foods that contain vitamin B_6 are widely available in the diet from many protein-containing foods, such as meats, poultry, and legumes.

The nurse is often asked for advice about vitamin and mineral dietary supplement use in the adult and older adult. Hot Topic: Who Needs a Multivitamin? summarizes recommendations that are appropriate in these age groups.

hot Topic

Who Needs a Vitamin Supplement?

More than one-third of U.S. adults take a multivitamin and multimineral preparation (NIH, 2006). Often these supplements are self-prescribed for a variety of reasons, including bolstering a poor diet and ensuring adequate intake and a perceived ability of the nutrients to prevent disease. How should the nurse respond when asked by a client about taking a general multivitamin with minerals?

Vitamin and mineral supplements taken to correct a specific nutrient deficiency is standard practice and reasonable. Recommending a supplement in those at risk for malnutrition is also advisable (Wildish, 2004). However, the evidence that a multivitamin prevents disease is under debate with conflicting results. In the older adult, vitamins D and B_{12} and calcium supplements should be considered because of the risk of inadequate status of the nutrients in this population (Lichtenstein et al., 2008). Folic acid is recommended for all women of childbearing age to prevent neural tube defects in infants. Experts are less in agreement about the generic need for a multivitamin-mineral preparation in the adult population. Conclusive evidence that a multivitamin can prevent disease is lacking. For example, there is a lack of strong evidence that multivitamin and multimineral supplements decrease risk of cardiovascular disease or cancer (Huang et al., 2006; NIH, 2006). In the older adult, use of multivitamins is not associated with overall improvement in health benefits in those who have no nutrient deficiencies (Silver, 2009). There is generally no evidence on which to base any recommendation to routinely recommend supplements for disease prevention (Wildish, 2004).

The nurse should not advocate routine use of multivitamins. An assessment of dietary intake and nutritional health should be done before giving advice about supplementation. In certain populations, a multivitamin supplement may be recommended, but every opportunity to promote "food first, supplements second" should be made. Other advice includes the following:

- Multivitamin mineral supplements are not a substitute for a poor diet.
- Supplements should not exceed the RDA amounts, especially for fat-soluble vitamins. High-potency or single-nutrient supplements can increase the risk of excessive nutrient intake.
- Older adults and women of childbearing age should follow specific nutrient supplementation guidelines for their population.
- Individuals who follow restrictive diets, abuse alcohol, or have medical conditions may be at risk for nutrient deficiencies. Universal recommendation of vitamins or minerals should be avoided. Instead, a nutrition

assessment should be conducted before recommending any specific vitamins or minerals.

- The nurse should assess for any oversupplementation or concomitant use of fortified foods that contribute significantly to nutrient intake. For example, an individual may take a high-potency multivitamin containing vitamin C and consume both fortified juices and fortified cereal with vitamin C. Tolerable upper limit recommendations should be observed and include fortified foods and supplements in the calculation. Adults who regularly use multivitamin-multimineral supplements have been reported to have excess intake of iron, vitamin A, niacin, and zinc (Murphy, White, Park, & Sharma, 2007).
- The pharmacist and registered dietitian should be consulted about possible interactions between medications and any dietary supplements, including vitamins and minerals.

Fluid

Specific fluid recommendations exist for the adult over age 50 years. Recommended daily intake of water from all sources is 3.7 L for men and 2.7 L for women (IOM, 2004). Alcohol intake contributes to fluid intake but should not be consumed in excess, as discussed in Box 15-1. The Modified MyPyramid for Older Adults features a foundation composed of fluid to encourage the older person to consume adequate daily fluid (Lichtenstein et al., 2008). In addition to age-related risks for poor fluid status, the nurse should be aware of the presence of risk factors for dehydration, such as fever or exudative wounds, as outlined in Box 15-2. The RDA for fluid is intended for the well population and does not take

BOX 15-1	Alcohol Intake in the Older Adult

Alcohol is referred to as both a tonic and a toxin because of its health benefits and risks. In the older adult, these benefits and risks mirror those found in younger adults when alcohol is consumed in moderation. However, when alcohol is consumed in excess, the negative effects are magnified in the older adult. An age-related change in alcohol dehydrogenase, an enzyme involved in alcohol metabolism, increases the bioavailability of alcohol in this population. This enzyme alteration can lead to increased blood alcohol levels when coupled with the decreased total body water associated with aging. Interactions between alcohol and medications are more likely as well. If alcohol intake is substituted for food, nutritional health can become compromised. The nurse should routinely assess alcohol intake when conducting a nursing assessment. On-line tools, such as the Michigan Alcohol Screening Test—Geriatric version, are available. The nurse can advise the client who has questions about alcohol intake that there are no demonstrated benefits to consuming more than one standard drink/day in females and two/day in males.

Sources: Ferreira & Weems, 2008; Friedlander & Norman, 2006; Lichtenstein, Rasmussen, Yu, Epstein, & Russell, 2008.

BOX 15-2	Symptoms, Risks, and Interventions for Dehydration in the Older Adult

Symptoms of Dehydration

- Decreased urine output
- Darkened urine
- Tenting of skin over the sternum or forehead
- Lethargy and headache
- Confusion
- Dry mucous membranes and axillae
- Long tongue furrows
- Sunken eyes
- Weight loss
- Postural changes in blood pressure and pulse
- Constipation

Risks for Dehydration

- Altered thirst mechanism with aging
- Decreased total body water with aging
- Dysphagia
- Dependency on others with lack of free access to fluids
- Self-restriction of fluid to manage incontinence, nocturia, or difficulty getting to the bathroom
- Increased fluid losses due to exudative wounds, gastrointestinal (GI) losses, fever

Interventions to Prevent Dehydration

- Offer fluids that meet individual personal preferences
- Improve free access to fluids when safety permits
- Verbally prompt to drink throughout the day
- Provide foods with high water content like soups, fruit, sauces
- Provide a person who is self-restricting fluid with a drinking schedule to manage toileting

into account the increased needs that can occur with illness. The nurse needs to carefully monitor fluid balance in the un-well older person by recording intake and output, body weight, and any symptoms related to hydration. Some older adults require prompting to drink throughout the day, especially those with cognitive deficits. Provision of personal preferences for fluid can also increase intake. It is important to allow adequate access to fluids, such as with spill-proof containers at the bedside, in the client who is dependent on others for care but not at risk for aspiration. For those who may be self-restricting fluids to manage toileting, incontinence, or nocturia, the nurse can assist the client with development of a drinking and toileting schedule to accommodate their needs while meeting fluid guidelines.

Protein: Do Older Adults Need More?

Experts do not agree on whether the older adult requires additional protein intake to avoid the loss of muscle mass with age. The RDA for protein remains the same (0.8 mg/kg body weight) for the both the younger and older adult (IOM, 2002). Some researchers agree with this recommendation, whereas others believe this amount to be too low and recommend 1 gm/kg body weight per day, arguing that with limited overall energy intake and average protein intake, protein losses can occur (Campbell, Johnson, McCabe, & Carnell, 2008; Millward, 2008). The nurse should assess the protein intake of the older adult and make suggestions for improved intake when indicated. Financial constraints can lead to limitation of protein-containing foods because of the cost of many of these foods. The nurse can suggest lower cost protein sources, such as peanut butter, tinned meats or tuna, eggs, and powdered milk. Additionally, the nurse should be aware that risk factors such as pressure ulcers, wounds, trauma, burns, sepsis, and malabsorption require increased protein intake.

Nutrition Challenges in the Older Adult

Both overnutrition and undernutrition have health conse-quences in the older person. Quality of life, morbidity, and mortality are negatively affected by poor nutritional status.

Overweight and Obesity

Up to 70% of adults over age 65 years are considered over-weight or obese in the United States (Kruger, Ham, & Prohaska, 2009). Debate exists as to whether overweight and obesity carry the same risk of morbidity and mortality in the older adult as in younger counterparts. Overweight in the older adult may increase survival under certain circumstances, such as following infection or surgery, because of greater nu-tritional reserves (Flegal et al., 2007). Criticism exists that the BMI classification of ideal weight is too restrictive in the older adult because research only supports an association between excess mortality risk and obesity, but not overweight, in this population. Others have reported that overweight and obesity are associated with increased risk of death from any cause, and that this effect is not lessened with age (Ajani et al., 2004).

First, the nurse should assess the dietary intake of the overweight older person because poor quality intake with in-adequate nutrients has been reported in the overweight older adult (Ledikwe et al., 2003). Then the decision to recom-mend weight loss in the overweight older adult should be as-sessed on an individual basis, taking into consideration overall health risks, social support, and diet quality. In addi-tion to risk of cardiovascular disease in particular, the older adult may have diminished quality of life because of the as-sociation of obesity with osteoarthritis, sleep problems, de-pression, fatigue, and other complications (Patterson, Frank, Kristal, & White, 2004). For some, weight loss may be inap-propriate because of risk of subsequent poor nutrition status and quality of life changes. A registered dietitian should be consulted when an older adult requires weight loss to ensure that nutritional health is maintained.

Undernutrition

Poor nutritional health can hasten a decline in the older adult's health status. Unfortunately the prevalence of malnutrition among older adults is high. Close to 60% of hospitalized or institutionalized older persons are malnourished compared with close to 27% of those living in the community (Alibhai, Greenwood, & Payette, 2005). Malnutrition is often manifested in the form of unintentional weight loss in the older person. Weight loss in this population is associated with many negative consequences, including increased risk of hospitalization, in-hospital complications, a decline in functional status, and increased mortality after discharge from the hospital (Alibhai et al., 2005; Locher et al., 2007; Silver, 2009). Poor wound healing, skeletal muscle loss, altered pharmacokinetics, and diminished immune response are all cited as factors resulting from malnutrition that contribute to these risks. Unplanned weight loss is considered to be clinically significant when it reaches 5% or more of body weight over 3 months or 10% or more over 6 months, but any unplanned weight loss is deserving of an assessment.

Why Does Malnutrition Occur in Older Adults?

The nurse should not dismiss weight loss or undernutrition as a natural part of the aging process. Biological factors associated with aging do contribute to the risk of undernutrition, but many additional factors layered on these risks play a significant role in the decline in nutritional health. Left untreated, malnutrition can lead to a sequela of poor outcomes that are difficult to stop once they begin. Undernutrition occurs because of three primary reasons: decreased intake, increased losses of nutrients, or increased nutritional needs that go unmet. In almost 25% to 40% of older adults with unintentional weight loss, no known cause is found (Alibhai et al., 2005). Table 15-5 outlines risk factors for undernutrition in the older adult.

Decreased Intake
Decreased intake of food and fluid can occur for a variety of reasons. Changes in appetite associated with aging can be magnified because of medication side effects, such as sedation, altered taste, and gastrointestinal (GI) symptoms. Pain can cause loss of appetite and make food preparation and eating uncomfortable. Medications to treat pain can in turn affect appetite. Sadness, loneliness, bereavement, and depression contribute to poor appetite and are among the leading causes of unintentional weight loss in the older person (Hickson, 2006). Everyday emotions, both positive and negative, have been shown to affect food intake in the older adult in long-term care (ADA, 2005b).

Physical conditions and disease can lead to diminished dietary intake. Symptoms such as shortness of breath and fatigue leave little energy for the effort of eating. Functional decline from arthritis or other conditions can make shopping, meal preparation, and eating a burden or impossible.

Table 15-5 Risk Factors for Undernutrition in the Older Adult

Decreased Dietary Intake

- Loss of appetite because of pain, medication side effects, GI symptoms, sadness or depression, taste changes, lack of personal preferences in institutional setting, social isolation
- Restrictive diet—therapeutic diet, lack of access to cultural or personal food preferences
- Multiple medications
- Chewing difficulties
- Dysphagia
- Fatigue from shortness of breath, disease symptom, muscle loss, functional decline
- Dependency on others for care
- Improper feeding practices in the dependent client
- Iatrogenic, such as prolonged nothing-by-mouth (NPO) status or reliance on clear liquids
- Functional decline when food shopping, preparation, or self-feeding; examples include muscle loss, neurological conditions, arthritis
- Cognitive impairment

Increased Losses of Nutrients

- Malabsorptive diseases
- Medication and nutrient interactions
- Alcohol
- Chronic diarrhea or vomiting

Increased Nutritional Requirements

- Fever
- Infection or sepsis
- Trauma
- Fracture
- Wounds, pressure ulcers
- Tremor
- Other physiological stress conditions, such as burns or chronic obstructive lung disease

---

Tremors from neurological disease make meal preparation and self-feeding a challenge. Chewing problems from poor dental health or xerostomia can lead to limited intake. In the institutional setting, some texture-altered diets prescribed for chewing difficulties can be visually unappealing and contribute to loss of appetite. **Dysphagia,** or difficulty swallowing, contributes to altered intake when various food consistencies need to be avoided because of aspiration risk. Some older adults may develop an aversion to certain foods or food groups because of an increase in GI symptoms associated with intake of these foods. This effect can lead to overall poorer quality and quantity of intake.

Dependency on others can contribute to inadequate intake and, therefore, malnutrition. Almost 20% of older persons in long-term care are totally dependent on others for feeding and almost 30% require some assistance (ADA, 2005b). It is estimated that between 35 and 40 minutes are needed to feed a dependent nursing home resident (Simmons & Schnelle, 2006). However, it has been reported that less than 10 minutes a meal is spent feeding nursing home residents (Simmons et al., 2008). Additionally, force-feeding has been observed in long-term care (Chang & Roberts, 2008). Other feeding practices that contribute to poor intake include poor positioning of the client, inadequate supervision of intake, and inaccurate recording of amount eaten. Nutrition risk can be overlooked when improper recording of meal intake occurs. Lack of free access to food and fluids can increase risk further in the dependent person.

An older person with cognitive impairment is at risk for diminished intake. Cognitive and behavioral problems can place a roadblock in the eating process when the person has difficulty recognizing mealtime or responding to feeding cues. Busy, overstimulating dining areas, and too many foods on the plate at once can distract the cognitively impaired person. Abnormal eating behaviors are a factor in weight loss in the client with cognitive impairment (Chang & Roberts, 2008). Behavioral responses to feeding such as clenching the jaw shut or expelling food present challenges to the caregiver who is left to interpret the reason for the behavior. The cognitively impaired person may dislike the food, not want to eat more, or not recognize the eating process altogether. The intermittent nature of behavior and feeding challenges in the client with cognitive impairment may contribute to a weight loss that slowly contributes to nutritional decline. A BMI of less than 23 is related to reduced survival in the client with various types of dementia (Faxen-Irving, Basun, & Cederholm, 2005).

In addition to poor feeding practices in the dependent client, other iatrogenic causes of undernutrition exist in the institutionalized person. Lack of food that meets personal, cultural, or religious preferences can contribute to disinterest in eating and poor intake. Cultural Consideration Box: Cultural Issues in Undernutrition of the Older Adult outlines the importance of these considerations in the institutionalized client. Restrictive therapeutic diets are sometimes prescribed based solely on medical diagnoses. Clients in long-term care who have malnutrition are frequently reported to be on a therapeutic diet (ADA, 2005b). Long-term care residents should be on a liberalized diet unless an individualized assessment finds this approach to be contraindicated (ADA, 2005b). In the hospitalized older person, iatrogenic contributors to malnutrition include prolonged nothing-by-mouth (NPO) status and reliance on clear liquid diet or minimal intravenous fluids for nutrition.

In the community-dwelling older adult, food insecurity contributes to poor intake. Lack of funds for food or inadequate access to sufficient food can result in diminished quality and quantity of intake.

Increased Nutrient Losses   Increased nutrient losses contribute to undernutrition when digestion, absorption, and metabolism of nutrients are compromised because of disease, medication, or alcohol. For example, nutrients may be lost from the GI tract because of malabsorptive disease, vomiting, diarrhea, and high-output ostomies. Protein losses can occur because of exudative wounds or nephrotic syndrome, a renal disorder where an abnormal amount of protein is lost in the urine. Medications that alter nutrient absorption or utilization are outlined in Chapter 24. Alcohol can lead to diminished dietary intake in the chronic abuser and poor absorption of a whole host of nutrients, including folate and thiamine.

Increased Nutritional Needs   Unmet increased nutritional needs can jeopardize the nutritional health of the older person. Certain diseases and conditions warrant an increased intake of energy and nutrients because of a hypermetabolic effects. Neurological diseases that result in tremors increase metabolic need for energy because of the increases in physical movement. End-stage cardiopulmonary disease with shortness of breath and labored breathing is an example of a hypermetabolic condition because of the extended physical effort required for breathing. Trauma, fractures, wounds, infection, and fever all contribute to hypermetabolism. Many of these conditions already compromise nutrition status because of the effect of discomfort, pain, or fatigue on appetite. The risk of malnutrition related to normal aging changes becomes magnified when a disease process or physical stressor occurs. Nutrition intervention is essential to avoid the end result of compromised wound healing, diminished immune response, prolonged hospital stay, and other severely negative consequences.

Treatment of Undernutrition in the Older Adult

It is hoped that routine nutritional screening in older adults will lessen the extent of undernutrition in this population. Waiting to screen for nutrition health risk until clients are hospitalized limits the use of screening tools because many individuals are already malnourished (IOM, 2000). Chapter 12 outlines screening and assessment tools for use by the nurse, including specific tools for the older population.

Any amount of unintentional weight loss or change in nutritional status deserves monitoring in the older adult. Waiting until changes meet clinical cutoff points or other criteria can lead to a missed opportunity to improve nutrition status. The nurse should consider all possible contributing causes for the change in nutritional health. Treatment should

Cultural Considerations

Cultural Issues in Undernutrition of the Older Adult
Cultural influences on diet should not be overlooked when assessing and monitoring nutritional health. Every effort should be made to accommodate cultural dietary patterns and food choices to promote nutritional health and quality of life in the institutionalized older adult. The nurse and the dietitian should assess the client for dietary preferences and practices and coordinate appropriate accommodations with the food service department and the client's family. Individualized dietary considerations in an institutional setting can provide the older adult with a sense of care and comfort.

be focused on the cause, when known, as well as the symptoms. Intervention for undernutrition in the older population is multidisciplinary. Nursing collaboration with the registered dietitian, pharmacist, social worker, and physical therapist, among other health care professionals, is essential when indicated. Dysphagia should be evaluated by a speech language pathologist. All aspects affecting dietary intake need evaluation, including medications, physical environment, functional capacity, quality of any feeding assistance, and the diet itself. Table 15-6 outlines intervention examples for a variety of causes of undernutrition in the older adult.

An attractive dining environment with good lighting and minimal distractions may improve intake. Social dining, whether family-style meals in long-term care or congregate meal sites in the community, is associated with improved dietary intake over dining alone (Labossiere & Bernard, 2008; Silver, 2009).

Improvement in feeding assistance is crucial to the nutritional status of the dependent older person. Correct positioning, ample feeding time, and being fed in a caring fashion are essential. The client with cognitive impairment requires special attention and cueing during the feeding process. Often clients with cognitive impairment have improved intake earlier, rather than later, in the day; this tendency should be maximized with nutrient-dense food offered during early meals and at the start of a meal. Table 15-7 outlines feeding assistance hints for these populations.

Milkshake-like dietary supplements are routinely prescribed when weight loss occurs, but concern exists that they cause satiety and diminished intake at mealtime, yielding no

---

Table 15-6 Nursing Interventions for Undernutrition in the Older Adult

Alter diet
- Suggest liberalization of restrictive therapeutic diet.
- Individualize texture modification of foods. Avoid overly modified textures when not indicated.
- Provide personal, cultural, and religious food preferences when possible.
- Optimize flavoring of food to counter altered taste perception.
- Provide nutrient-dense foods with "more calories per bite" for clients with early satiety. For example, cream soup instead of clear soup, ice cream or pudding instead of gelatin, crackers with peanut butter instead of plain.
- Provide between-meal snacks, timing to not interfere with appetite at meals.
- Avoid carbonated beverages and use of straws because swallowing of air will lead to early satiety.
- Optimize intake at best-tolerated meal of the day. In clients with dementia, optimize breakfast and lunch.
- Offer most nutrient-dense food at the beginning of a meal.
- Time liquid supplements at least 1 hour before meals.
- Consult the speech language pathologist for dysphagia evaluation and recommendations for diet consistency modification.

Improve dining environment
- Encourage social dining
- Family-style dining in long-term care
- Adequate lighting without glare
- Soothing mealtime music
- Meals served on chinaware, not disposable ware
- Avoid busily patterned plates with clients who have visual difficulties
- Minimize mealtime distractions and interruptions

Provide assistance with activities of daily living
- Social service consult for home services; referral to congregate meal site or Meals on Wheels
- Physical therapy and occupational therapy consult for rehabilitation or adaptive equipment for meal preparation or feeding

---

Table 15-7 Feeding Assistance

If the client has visual impairment but is capable of eating without assistance
- Avoid use of plates with busy patterns that can make it difficult to see food.
- Use the clock analogy to orient the person to the location of food on the plate: "Your green beans are at 3 o'clock and your baked fish is at 6 o'clock."

General proper feeding technique
- Position the individual with the body at a 90-degree angle to the lap.
- Seat the person in a chair that is a comfortable height to the table surface.
- Sit at eye level to the individual while feeding.
- Ensure that food temperature is not too hot before serving.
- Encourage self-feeding whenever possible. Use assistive devices such as a plate guard, utensils with built-up grip, or suction cup to hold the plate in place as needed.
- Try finger foods with a client who cannot manage utensils but may be able to self-feed.
- Serve only manageable bolus of food at one time to avoid choking.
- Wait until food has been swallowed before offering more food.
- Allow sufficient time for unrushed feeding.

If the client has cognitive impairment
- Follow proper feeding techniques (above).
- Place the food in front of the person one dish at a time to simplify its presentation.
- Offer soothing quiet music, which may have a calming effect during the meal.
- Provide cues to the eating process and match utensil to the dish: "Here is your custard and the spoon to use to eat it." Providing cues by using words and gestures to remind the individual to chew or swallow may be needed.
- Minimize disruptions by others during the meal to avoid distraction.
- Offer the most nutrient-dense items first to maximize intake.

CLIENT EDUCATION CHECKLIST

Nutrition Tips for Improving Intake for Older Adults with Unplanned Weight Loss

1. Educate the client about the importance of both adequate calories and protein in restoring body weight. Adequate calories must be present in the diet to avoid use of dietary protein for energy instead of tissue synthesis.
2. Hints to optimize calorie intake
   Choose nutrient-dense foods with "more calories per bite"
   - Choose nutritional liquids such as milk, smoothies, juices vs. water, coffee, tea, soda
   - Choose cream soup or chowder vs. clear soup
   - Snack on crackers and cheese, nuts, powdered breakfast drinks vs. plain crackers or snack foods
   - Cooked vegetables vs. salads
   - Dried fruit vs. juice
   - Reduced fat or whole fat dairy foods vs. nonfat dairy
   Add supplemental calories to foods
   - Add powdered milk to regular milk
   - Add cheese to casseroles
   - Add creams, sauces, dressings to foods
   - Make hot cereal with milk or half and half vs. water
   - Add cream cheese or peanut butter and jelly to toast
3. Hints to optimize protein intake
   - Animal protein sources
     Dairy: liquid and powdered milk, sliced cheese, cottage cheese, yogurt, ice cream, pudding, custard
     Meats, poultry, fish, eggs: fresh, frozen, or tinned meats, poultry, and fish; fresh or powdered eggs
   - Plant protein sources: canned beans, peanut butter, hummus, lentils, tofu
4. Minimize sources of early satiety
   - Avoid sources of excess swallowed air: straws, gum chewing, carbonated drinks
   - Minimize liquids at meals; save for after or between meals
   - Choose frequent small meals
   - Time snacks and supplements at least an hour before a meal
5. Maximize intake according to stamina level
   - Choose nutrient-dense foods at the start of the meal
   - Optimize intake early in the day before fatigue sets in
   - Choose quick protein sources when there is no energy for meal preparation: peanut butter, canned tuna or chicken, canned beans, cheese
   - Prepare and freeze extra servings of meals when energy level is increased
6. Make appropriate referrals for other health care interventions, targeting the cause of weight loss (social work, speech language pathology, occupational therapist, etc.)

overall benefit. Studies of these oral nutrition supplements have shown benefit in some circumstances, such as following a hip fracture, and not in others (Milne, Avenell, & Potter, 2006; Silver, 2009). When oral nutrition supplements are prescribed, it is best to offer them between meals (Labossier & Bernard, 2008). Small portions of supplements can be provided in place of other liquids when medications are given unless contraindicated because of a drug interaction. Offering a variety of flavors may lessen the chance of taste fatigue. Provision of between meal snacks and nutrient-dense foods should be routine when weight gain is a goal (Silver, 2009; Zizza, Tayie, & Lino, 2007). Client Education Checklist: Nutrition Tips for Improving Intake for Older Adults with Unplanned Weight Loss outlines educational pointers for the nurse to offer to clients or caregivers when attempting to improve nutritional intake. More aggressive nutritional intervention should be in keeping with the client's wishes and advance directives.

Fluid intake should be considered in the client with unplanned weight loss. Dehydration or suboptimal hydration is a health risk and contributes to poor nutritional health when swallowing is affected or lethargy develops. Box 15-2 outlines risks, symptoms, and intervention for dehydration.

When multidisciplinary strategies to optimize intake do not result in improvements, the health care team can determine if a pharmacological approach to appetite stimulation is indicated. Megace, dronabinol, and other medications can be effective in stimulating appetite in some older clients (Labossiere & Bernard, 2008). The medications should be stopped if no effect occurs or if there are side effects, such as delirium.

MyNursingKit Unexplained Weight Loss in the Older Adult

NURSING CARE PLAN | # Nutrition and Unplanned Weight Loss in the Older Adult

CASE STUDY

Laura is a 78-year-old widow who lives alone in a small duplex owned by her daughter. Her three grown children are married and live in cities about 75 miles away. She lives on a modest income consisting of Social Security and a small pension. Her children pay some of her utilities and purchase small extras like a daily newspaper subscription. She gets annual checkups and a year ago started taking alendronate sodium (Fosamax) for osteoporosis. She has had no other health concerns. Lately she has noticed that her appetite is not what it used to be and that she seems to have lost weight. She has also noticed that she seems to tire more quickly. When she goes for her annual checkup she mentions appetite and fatigue and her concern that they will interfere with a planned trip to her granddaughter's college graduation from the same university she graduated from 58 years earlier.

Applying the Nursing Process

ASSESSMENT

Laura is articulate and thoughtful in her communication with the nurse. She has no significant past medical history except for the cesarean birth of her third child 45 years earlier. She acknowledged being increasingly "stooped over" along with back pain that she tries to ignore because she does not want to become dependent on any medication. Nighttime incontinence has occurred occasionally but she says that it has occurred less frequently since she eliminated coffee and other fluids after dinner. She confesses to being "a bit" thirsty.

Laura's vital signs are as follows: T: 97.8 F, P: 74, R: 18, and BP: 118/66. Physical examination reveals marked kyphosis with a 2-inch loss of stature in the past year. She describes her back pain as "nagging" and at "7" on a 1 to 10 scale. Her weight is down 8 pounds from her previous weight of 134 pounds. Her skin is warm and dry and her hair is dry and brittle. The complete blood count reveals a hemoglobin of 10.2 mg/dL and a hematocrit of 30%.

DIAGNOSES

Imbalanced nutrition: less than requirements related to decreased nutrient intake

Deficient fluid volume related to self-imposed restrictions

Pain related to changes in bone mineral density

Risk for falls related to changes in posture

Functional incontinence related to motor and sensory losses

EXPECTED OUTCOMES

Weight will increase on increased intake of nutrient-dense foods

Laura will verbalize food choices reflecting knowledge of nutrient-dense foods that are culturally acceptable

Mucous membranes will be moist and pink

Pain will be relieved with proper use of nonprescription medications

Home environment will be assessed for safety

Referral to a specialist who deals with female incontinence will be given

PLANNING

Obtain a 24-hour food and fluid recall

Weigh weekly and record results

Discuss the possibility of use of the Meals on Wheels program or attendance at a congregate meal site for one meal a day

Consider social services consult to explore adequacy of financial resources and safety of home environment

Begin use of nonprescription medications for pain management, following dosage instructions

Drink at least one 8-ounce glass of water with each meal

Make an appointment with a health care provider who specializes in female urinary incontinence

Teach importance of good oral hygiene and ongoing dental care

Suggest smaller, more frequent meals of nutrient-dense foods

EVALUATION

Laura's weight increases 1.5 pounds in 2 months. She has seen a specialist who deals with incontinence and has learned some techniques to strengthen pelvic floor muscles. There are still episodes of incontinence at night, but they have diminished as she has gotten more proficient at the exercises and has decided to get up once at night to use the bathroom. Laura reported that she is taking an over-the-counter medication for pain with breakfast and before bed; she states that it has reduced her pain level to about "3" most of the time. She has gone to the senior center a few times but does not yet feel comfortable in that setting so she only plans to go if there is an interesting program. She discussed finances with her children at the graduation festivities and they have agreed to help with a few more of her expenses. Figure 15-1 ■ outlines the nursing care process for this case study.

Nutrition and Unplanned Weight Loss in the Older Adult *(continued)*

NURSING CARE PLAN

Assessment
Data about the patient

Subjective
What the patient tells the nurse

Example: I am tired all the time; I don't drink much for fear of being incontinent.

Objective
What the nurse observes; anthropometric and clinical data

Examples: 8-pound weight loss in 1 year; dry mucous membranes; Hgb: 10.2 mg/dL

Diagnosis
NANDA label

Example: Deficient fluid volume related to self-imposed restrictions. Imbalanced nutrition, less than body requires related to decreased intake

Planning
Goals stated in patient terms

Example: Long-term goal: weight returns to 134 pounds; Short-term goal: weight increases 1 pound per month; fluid intake of at least 8 ounces

Implementation
Nursing action to help patient achieve goals

Example: Referral to congregate meal site; 8 ounces of water with each meal

Evaluation
Was the goal achieved or does the intervention need to be modified?

Example: 1.5-pound weight gain in 2 months; increased fluid intake and decreased incontinence

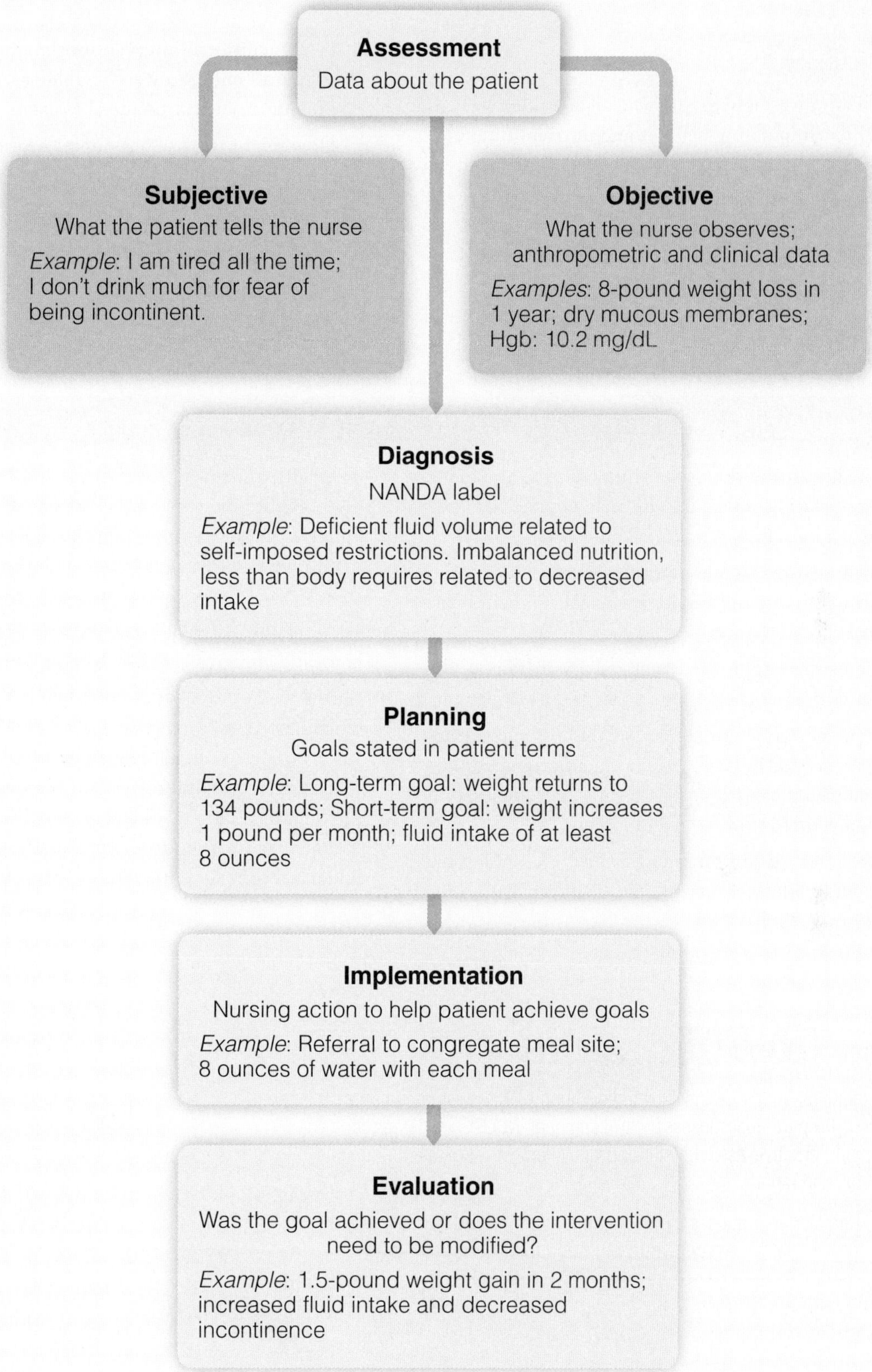

■ FIGURE 15-1 **Nursing Care Plan: Nutrition and Unplanned Weight Loss in the Older Adult.**

(continued)

Nutrition and Unplanned Weight Loss in the Older Adult *(continued)*

NURSING CARE PLAN

Critical Thinking in the Nursing Process

1. Laura was able to gain a small amount of weight by manipulating her diet and nutrient intake. What additional assessment might be indicated if she failed to gain any weight or lost more weight in 2 months?

2. What additional interventions might be necessary if Laura's children were unable or unwilling to provide any extra financial assistance?

3. How might the use of nonprescription pain medications affect Laura's appetite?

4. Even though Laura has episodes of urinary incontinence, the nurse has recommended drinking more water. Why was this recommendation made?

CHAPTER SUMMARY

- Nutritional health in the adult is influenced by the foundation of nutrition intake and lifestyle choices made in childhood, adolescence, and early adulthood.

- Overnutrition and undernutrition affect nutritional health in adulthood. Both conditions can be present in an individual.

- Inadequate intake of iron and calcium is a nutritional concern in the adult female.

- Health promotion efforts should focus on preventing chronic disease with weight management and maintaining a balanced diet with adequate fruits, vegetables, and whole grains that is low in fat and sodium.

- Nutrition intervention for maintenance of reproductive health focuses on weight management and a balanced intake of nutrients.

- The aging process leads to physical alterations that predispose the older adult to poor nutritional health. Changes in body composition, digestion, and absorption of nutrients and altered thirst mechanisms are examples of these alterations.

- Older adults may require dietary supplementation of calcium and vitamins D and B_{12} beyond the amounts present in the diet.

- The nurse plays an important role in providing nutrition intervention to adults. Nutritional screening and assessment are included in the nursing process. The nurse can provide the adult and older adult with guidance and education as part of the team approach to health education and monitoring of nutrition status.

PEARSON

EXPLORE **mynursingkit**™

MyNursingKit is your one stop for online chapter review materials and resources. Prepare for success with additional NCLEX®-style practice questions, interactive assignments and activities, web links, animations and videos, and more!

Register your access code from the front of your book at
www.mynursingkit.com.

NCLEX® QUESTIONS

1. A middle-aged client with osteoarthritis and a BMI of 29 asks the nurse about dietary means to keep the arthritis from getting worse. The nurse should suggest that the client:
   1. Take a calcium supplement twice daily
   2. Increase consumption of foods rich in omega-3 fats
   3. Begin a weight loss program
   4. Increase consumption of protein-dense foods

2. An elderly client complains of difficulty swallowing whole wheat bread, even after chewing it for a long time. Which age-related change will the nurse tell the client is the most likely cause of the problem?
   1. Periodontal disease
   2. Decreased saliva production
   3. Slowed peristalsis
   4. Loss of bone density in the jaw

3. An elderly client is a Seventh Day Adventist and a practicing lacto-ovo vegetarian. The client has been instructed to increase consumption of protein. Which of the following would the nurse suggest to provide the greatest increase in protein?
   1. Brown rice and tofu stir fry
   2. Cheese snack crackers
   3. Cream of mushroom soup
   4. Banana smoothie prepared with juice

4. A young adult client has complained of frequent constipation. When no functional cause is found, the nurse discusses foods high in fiber. Which food choice indicates that the client has understood the teaching?
   1. Applesauce
   2. Black beans
   3. Bananas
   4. Spaghetti

5. How can the nurse who works in a long-term care setting help an elderly client with Alzheimer's disease increase fluid intake?
   1. Put a pitcher of water at the bedside every change of shift.
   2. Ask the client every 2 hours if he is thirsty.
   3. Make sure that the client takes all meals in the dining room.
   4. Give the client a glass of water between each meal.

REFERENCES

Ajani, U. A., Lotufo, P. A., Gaziano, J. M., Lee, I. M., Spelsberg, A., Buring, J. E., et al. (2004). Body mass index and mortality among U.S. male physicians. *Annals of Epidemiology, 15,* 731–739.

Alibhai, S. M. H., Greenwood, C., & Payette, H. (2005). An approach to the management of unintentional weight loss in elderly people. *Canadian Medical Association Journal, 172,* 773–780.

Allen, L. H. (2009). How common is vitamin B-12 deficiency? *American Journal of Clinical Nutrition, 89,* 693S–696S.

American Dietetic Association (ADA). (2005a). Position of the American Dietetic Association: Nutrition across the spectrum of aging. *Journal of the American Dietetic Association, 105,* 616–633.

American Dietetic Association (ADA). (2005b). Position of the American Dietetic Association: Liberalization of the diet prescription improves quality of life for older adults in long-term care. *Journal of the American Dietetic Association, 105,* 1955–1965.

American Dietetic Association (ADA). (2006). Position of the American Dietetic Association: Food insecurity and hunger in the United States. *Journal of the American Dietetic Association, 106,* 446–458.

American Dietetic Association (ADA). (2008). Position of the American Dietetic Association: Nutrition and lifestyle for a healthy pregnancy outcome. *Journal of the American Dietetic Association, 108,* 553–561.

American Dietetic Association & Dietitians of Canada. (2004). Position of the American Dietetic Association and Dietitians of Canada: Nutrition and women's health. *Journal of the American Dietetic Association, 104,* 984–1001.

Bent, S., Kane, C., Shinohara, K., Neuhaus, J., Hudes, E. S., Goldberg, H., et al. (2006). Saw palmetto for benign prostatic hypertrophy. *New England Journal of Medicine, 354,* 557–566.

Bhutto, A., & Morley, J. E. (2008). The clinical significance of gastrointestinal changes with aging. *Current Opinion in Clinical Nutrition and Metabolic Care, 11,* 651–660.

Bischoff, H. A., Staehelin, H. B., & Willett, W. C. (2006). The effect of undernutrition in the development of frailty in older persons. *Journal of Gerontology: Medical Sciences, 61A,* 585–588.

Brassard, M., AinMelk, Y., & Baillargeon, J. P. (2008). Basic infertility including polycystic ovary syndrome. *Medical Clinics of North America, 92,* 1163–1192.

Campbell, W. W., Johnson, C. A., McCabe, G. P., & Carnell, N. S. (2008). Dietary protein requirements of younger and older adults. *American Journal of Clinical Nutrition, 88,* 1322–1329.

Carroll, D. G. (2006). Nonhormonal therapies for hot flashes in menopause. *American Family Physician, 73,* 457–464.

Cashman, K. D. (2007). Diet, nutrition, and bone health. *Journal of Nutrition, 137,* 2507S–2512S.

Cauley, J. A., Lacroix, A. Z., Wu, L., Horwitz, M., Danielson, M. E, Bauer, D. C., et al. (2008). Serum 25-hydroxyvitamin D concentrations and risk for hip fractures. *Annals of Internal Medicine, 149,* 242–250.

Centers for Disease Control and Prevention (CDC). (2004a). Trends in intake of energy and macronutrients—United States 1971–2000. *Morbidity and Mortality Weekly Report, 53,* 80–82.

Centers for Disease Control and Prevention (CDC). (2004b). Use of vitamins containing folic acid among women of childbearing age—United States, 2004. *Morbidity and Mortality Weekly Review, 53,* 847–850.

REFERENCES *(continued)*

Centers for Disease Control and Prevention (CDC), National Center for Health Statistics. (2007). Prevalence of sedentary leisure-time behavior among adults in the United States. Retrieved January 25, 2009, from http://www.cdc.gov/nchs/data/hestat/3and4/sedentary.htm

Chapman, I. M., MacIntosh, C. G., Morley, J. E., & Horowitz, M. (2002). The anorexia of aging. *Biogerontology, 3,* 67–71.

Chang, C., & Roberts, B. L. (2008). Feeding difficulty in older adults with dementia. *Journal of Clinical Nursing, 17,* 2266–2274.

Dahan, K., Fennal, M., & Kumar, N. B. (2008). Lycopene in the prevention of prostate cancer. *Journal of the Society for Integrative Oncology, 6,* 29–36.

Dali-Youcef, N., & Andres, E. (2009). An update on cobalamin deficiency in adults. *QFM, 10,* 17–28.

Dawson-Hughes, B. (2008). Serum 25-hydroxy-vitamin D and functional outcomes in the elderly. *American Journal of Clinical Nutrition, 88,* 537S–540S.

Dawson-Hughes, B., Harris, S., Krall, E. A., & Dallal, G. E. (1997). Effect of calcium and vitamin D supplementation on bone density in men and women 65 years of age and older. *New England Journal of Medicine, 337*(10), 670–676.

Dawson-Hughes, B., Harris, S., Krall, E. A., & Dallal, G. E. (2000). Effect of withdrawal of calcium and vitamin D supplements on bone mass in elderly men and women. *American Journal of Clinical Nutrition, 72*(3), 745–750.

Doty, R. L., Shah, M., & Bromley, S. M. (2008). Drug-induced taste disorders. *Drug Safety, 31,* 199–215.

Edwards, J. L. (2008). Diagnosis and management of benign prostatic hyperplasia. *American Family Physician, 77,* 1403–1410.

Esposito, K., Giugliano, F., Ciotola, M., DeSio, M., D'Armiento, M. D., & Giugliano, D. (2008). Obesity and sexual dysfunction, male and female. *International Journal of Impotence Research, 20,* 358–365.

Farrell, M. J., Zamarripa, F., Shade, R., Phillips, P. A., McKinley, M., Fox, P. T., et al. (2008). Effect of aging on regional cerebral blood flow responses associated with osmotic thirst and its satiation by water drinking: PET study. *Proceedings of the National Academy of Sciences, 105,* 382–387.

Faxen-Irving, G., Basun, H., & Cederholm, T. (2005). Nutritional and cognitive relationships and long-term mortality in patients with various dementia disorders. *Age and Ageing, 34,* 136–151.

Feldblum, I., German, L., Castel, H., Harman-Boehm, I., Bilenko, N., Eisinger, M., et al. (2007). Characteristics of undernourished older medical patients and the identification of predictors for undernutrition status. *Nutrition Journal, 6,* 37.

Ferreira, M. P., & Weems, M. K. (2008). Alcohol consumption by aging adults in the United States: Health benefits and detriments. *Journal of the American Dietetic Association, 108,* 1668–1676.

Flegal, K. M., Graubard, B. I., Williamson, D. F., & Gail, M. H. (2007). Cause-specific excess deaths associated with underweight, overweight, and obesity. *Journal of the American Medical Association, 298,* 2028–2037.

Friedlander, A. H. & Norman, D. C. (2006). Geratric alcoholism. *Journal of the American Dental Association, 137,* 330–338.

Heaney, R. P. (2008). Vitamin D and calcium interactions: Functional outcomes. *American Journal of Clinical Nutrition, 88,* 541S–544S.

Hersh, A. L., Stefanik, M. L., & Stafford, R. S. (2004). National use of postmenopausal hormone therapy. *Journal of the American Medical Association, 291,* 47–53.

Hickson, M. (2006). Malnutrition and aging. *Postgraduate Medicine, 82,* 2–8.

Holick, M. F. (2007). Vitamin D deficiency. *New England Journal of Medicine, 357,* 266–281.

Huang, H., Caballero, B., Chang, S., Alberg, A. J., Semba, R. D., Schneyer, R. F., et al. (2006). The efficacy and safety of multivitamin and mineral supplement use to prevent cancer and chronic disease in adults: A systematic review for a National Institutes of Health State-of-the-Science Conference. *Annals of Internal Medicine, 145,* 372–385.

Institute of Medicine (IOM). (1997). *Dietary reference intakes for calcium, phosphorus, magnesium, vitamin D and fluoride.* Washington, DC: National Academies Press.

Institute of Medicine (IOM). (1998). *Dietary reference intakes for thiamine, riboflavin, niacin, vitamin B-6, folate, vitamin B-12, pantothenic acid, biotin and choline.* Washington, DC: National Academies Press.

Institute of Medicine (IOM). (2000). *The role of nutrition in maintaining health in the nation's elderly.* Washington, DC: National Academies Press.

Institute of Medicine (IOM). (2001). *Dietary reference intakes for vitamin A, vitamin K, arsenic, boron, chromium, copper, iodine, iron, manganese, molybdenum, nickel, silicon, vanadium, and zinc.* Washington, DC: National Academies Press.

Institute of Medicine (IOM). (2002). *Dietary reference intakes for energy, carbohydrate, fiber, fat, fatty acids cholesterol, protein, and amino acids.* Washington, DC: National Academies Press.

Institute of Medicine (IOM). (2004). *Dietary reference intakes for water, potassium, sodium, chloride, and sulfate.* Washington, DC: National Academies Press.

Jackson, R. D., LaCroix, A. Z., Gass, M., Wallace, R. B., Robbins, J., Lewis, C. E.et al. (2006). Calcium plus vitamin D supplementation and the risk of fractures. *New England Journal of Medicine, 354*(7), 669–683.

Kruger, J., Ham, S. A., & Prohaska, T. R. (2009). Behavioral risk factors associated with overweight and obesity among older adults: The 2005 National Health Interview Survey. *Prevention of Chronic Disease, 6.* Retrieved February 2, 2009, from http://www.cdc.gov/pcd/issues/2009/jan/07_0183.htm

Kumanyika, S. K., Obarzanek, E., Stettler, N., Bell, R., Field, A. E., Fortmann, S. P., et al. (2008). Population-based prevention of obesity: The need for comprehensive promotion of healthful eating, physical activity, and energy balance. *Circulation, 118,* 428–464.

Labossiere, R., & Bernard, M. A. (2008). Nutritional considerations in institutionalized elders. *Current Opinion in Clinical Nutrition and Metabolic Care, 11,* 1–6.

Lafreniere, D., & Mann, N. (2009). Anosmia: Loss of smell in the elderly. *Otolaryngology Clinics of North America, 42,* 123–131.

Lang, C. J., Leuschner, T., Ulrich, K., Stobel, C., Heckmann, J. G., & Hummel, T. (2006). Taste in dementing diseases and Parkinsonism. *Journal of the Neurological Sciences, 248,* 177–184.

Ledikwe, J. H., Smiciklas-Wright, H., Mitchell, D. C., Jensen, G. L., Friedmann, J. M., & Still, C. D. (2003). Nutrition risk assessment and obesity in rural older adults: A sex difference. *American Journal of Clinical Nutrition, 77,* 551–558.

Lichtenstein, A. H., Rasmussen, H., Yu, W. W., Epstein, S. R., & Russell, R. M. (2008). Modified MyPyramid for older adults. *Journal of Nutrition, 136,* 5–11.

Lioret , S., Volatier, J. L., Lafay, L., Touvier, M., & Maire, B. (2007). Is food portion size a risk factor of childhood overweight? *European Journal of Clinical Nutrition,* doi:10.1038/sj/ejcn/1602958.

Lippman, S. M., Klein, E. A., Goodman, P. J., Lucia, M. S., Thompson, I. M., & Ford, L. G. (2009). Effect of selenium and vitamin E on risk of prostate cancer and other cancers. *Journal of the American Medical Association,* doi:10.1001/jama.2008.864.

Locher, J. L., Roth, D. L., Ritchie, C. S., Cox, K., Sawyer, P., Bodner, E. V., et al. (2007). Body mass index, weight loss, and mortality in community-dwelling older adults. *Journal of Gerontology Medical Sciences, 12,* 1389–1392.

Ludwig, D. S., & Nestle, M. (2008). Can the food industry play a constructive role in the obesity epidemic? *Journal of the American Medical Association,* 1808–1811.

Mahady, G. B., Low Dog, T., Barrett, M. L., Chavez, M. L., Gardiner, P., Ko, R., et al. (2008). United States Pharmacopeia review of black cohosh case reports of hepatotoxicity. *Menopause, 15,* 628–638.

REFERENCES   *(continued)*

Millward, D. J. (2008). Sufficient protein for our elders? *American Journal of Clinical Nutrition,* 88, 1187–1188.

Milne, A. C., Avenell, A., & Potter, J. (2006). Meta-analysis: Protein and energy supplementation in older people. *Annals of Internal Medicine, 144,* 37–48.

Moore, C., Murphy, M. M., Keast, D. R., & Holick, M. F. (2004). Vitamin D intake in the United States. *Journal of the American Dietetic Association, 104,* 980–983.

Mosekilde, L. (2005). Vitamin D and the elderly. *Clinical Endocrinology, 62,* 265–281.

Muller-Lissner, S. A., Kamm, M. A., Scarpignato, C., & Wald, A. (2005). Myths and misconceptions about chronic constipation. *American Journal of Gastroenterology,* 100, 232–242.

Murphy, S. P., White, K., Park, S., & Sharma, S. (2007). Multivitamin-multimineral supplements' effect on total nutrient intake. *American Journal of Clinical Nutrition, 85,* 280S–284S.

National Institutes of Health (NIH). (2006). NIH State of the Science conference statement on multivitamin/mineral supplements and chronic disease prevention. *NIH Consensus State of the Science Statements, 23,* 1–30.

National Institutes of Health (NIH), Office of Dietary Supplements (ODS). (2008). *Dietary supplement fact sheet: Vitamin D.* Retrieved January 30, 2009, from http://ods.od.nih.gov/factsheets/cc/vitd.html

National Osteoporosis Foundation (NOF). (2008). *Clinician's guide to the prevention and treatment of osteoporosis.* Retrieved December 19, 2008, from http://nof.org/professionals/NOF_Clinicians_Guide.pdf

Nowjack-Raymer, R. E., & Sheiham, A. (2007). Numbers of natural teeth, diet, and nutritional status. *Journal of Dental Research, 86,* 1171–1175.

Padilha, D. M., Hilgert, J. B., Hugo, F. N., Bos, A. J., & Ferrucci, L. (2008). Number of teeth and mortality risk in the Baltimore Longitudinal Study of Aging. *Journal of Gerontology Biological Science and Medical Sciences, 63,* 739–744.

Patterson, R. E., Frank, L. L., Kristal, A. R., & White, E. (2004). A comprehensive examination of health conditions associated with obesity in older adults. *American Journal of Preventative Medicine, 27,* 385–390.

Pearlstein, T., & Steiner, M. (2008). Premenstrual dysphoric disorder: Burden of illness and treatment update. *Journal of Psychiatry & Neuroscience, 33,* 291–301.

Pischon, T., Boening, H., Hoffman, K., Bergmann, M., Schulze, M. B., Overvad, K., et al. (2008). General and abdominal adiposity and risk of death in Europe. *New England Journal of Medicine, 359,* 2105–2120.

Prince, R. L., Devine, A., Dhaliwal, S. S., & Dick, I. M. (2006). Effects of calcium supplementation on clinical fracture and bone structure: Results of a 5-year double-blind, placebo-controlled trial in elderly women. *Archives of Internal Medicine, 166(8),* 869–875.

Rees, M. (2009). Alternative treatments for the menopause. *Best Practice & Research Clinics Obstetrics and Gynecology, 23,* 151–161.

Rolland, Y, Czerwinski, S., Abellan Van Kan, G., Morley, J. E., Cesari, M., Onder, G., et al. (2008). Sarcopenia: Its assessment, etiology, pathogenesis, consequences and future perspectives. *The Journal of Nutrition, Health, & Aging, 12,* 433–450.

Silver, H. (2009). Oral strategies to supplement older adults' dietary intakes: Comparing the evidence. *Nutrition Reviews, 67,* 21–31.

Simmons, S. F., Keeler, E., Zhuo, X., Hickey, K. A., Sato, H., & Schnelle, J. F. (2008). Prevention of unintentional weight loss in nursing home residents: A controlled trial of feeding assistance. *Journal of the American Geriatric Society, 56,* 1466–1473.

Simmons, S. F., & Schnelle, J. F. (2006). Feeding assistance needs of long-stay nursing home residents and staff time to provide. *Journal of American Geriatric Society, 54,* 919–924.

Stenholm, S., Harris, T. B., Rantanen, T., Visser, M., Kritchevsky, S. B., & Ferruci, L. (2008). Sarcopenic obesity: Definition, cause, and consequences. *Current Opinion in Clinical Nutrition and Metabolic Care, 11,* 693–700.

Tamler, R., & Mechanick, J. I. (2007). Dietary supplements and neutraceuticals in the management of andrologic disorders. *Endocrinology Metabolic Clinics of North America, 36,* 533–552.

Thomas, D. R., Cote, T. R., Lawhorne, L., Levenson, S. A., Rubenstein, L. Z., Smith, D. A., et al. (2008). Understanding clinical dehydration and its treatment. *Journal of the American Medical Directors Association, 9,* 292–301.

Ueland, O., Cardello, A. V., Merrill, E. P., & Lesher, L. L. (2009). Effect of portion size information on food intake. *Journal of the American Dietetic Association, 109,* 124–127.

United States Department of Agriculture (USDA). (2005). What we eat in America, NHANES, 2001–2002: Usual nutrient intakes from food compared with DRIs. Retrieved December 19, 2008, from http://www.ars.usda.gov/SP2UserFiles/Place/12355000/pdf/usualintaketables2001-02.pdf

Wildish, D. E. (2004). An evidence-based approach for dietitian prescription of multiple vitamins with minerals. *Journal of the American Dietetic Association, 104,* 779–786.

Wold, R. S., Lopez, S. T., Yau, C. L., Butler, L. M., Paroe-Tubbeh, S. L., Waters, D. L., et al. (2005). Increasing trends in elderly persons' use of nonvitamin, non-mineral dietary supplements and concurrent use of medication. *Journal of the American Dietetic Association, 105,* 54–63.

Young, L. R., & Nestle, M. (2007). Portion sizes and obesity: Responses of fast-food companies. *Journal of Public Health Policy, 28,* 238–248.

Yu, E. W., Blackwell, T., Ensrud, K. E., Hillier, T. A., Lane, N. E., Orwoll, E., et al. (2008). Acid-suppressive medications and risk of bone loss and fracture in older adults. *Calcified Tissue International, 83,* 251–259.

Zizza, C. A., Tayie, F. A., & Lino, M. (2007). Benefits of snacking in older Americans. *Journal of the American Dietetic Association, 107,* 800–806.

Section 4

Clinical Nutrition and Diet Therapy

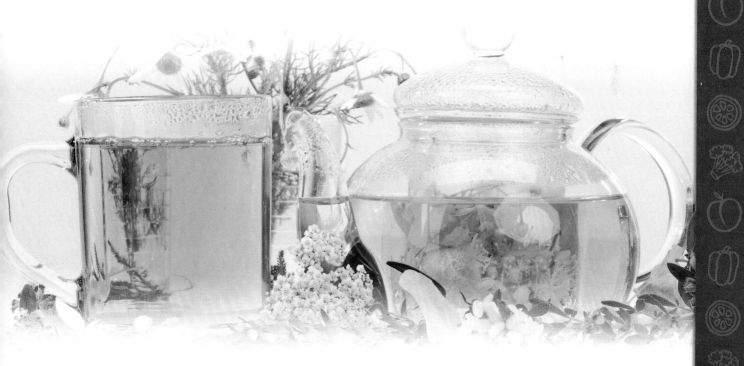

Nutrition Care and Support 16

WHAT WILL YOU LEARN?

1. To categorize components of standard and texture-modified hospital diets and summarize the indication for their use.

2. To formulate nursing interventions for the hospitalized client with malnutrition.

3. To differentiate between the indications, risks, and benefits for enteral and parenteral nutrition support.

4. To relate the role of the nurse in providing palliative nutrition care.

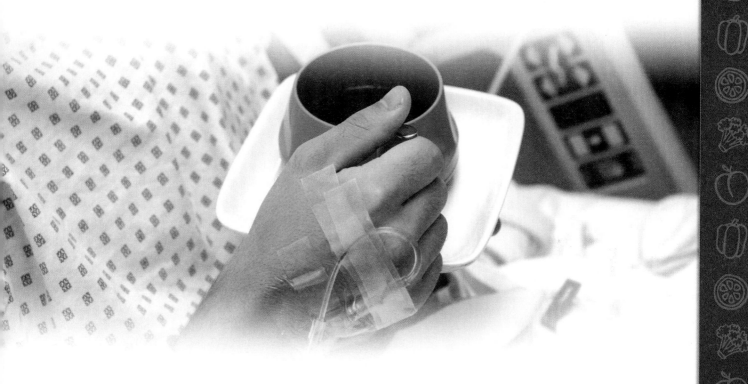

DID YOU KNOW?

▶ A clear liquid diet is inadequate in all nutrients and should not be used for more than a few days.

▶ Some malnutrition that occurs in the hospitalized client is because of the medical process.

▶ The once common practice of using blue food dye in feeding formulas could cause skin, organ, and body fluid discoloration and was associated with death in some clients.

▶ A liter of intravenous 5% dextrose (D5W) only contains 170 calories.

▶ The loss of appetite in a terminally ill client is reported to not contribute to suffering or discomfort.

KEY TERMS

advance directive, *359*

early satiety, *356*

elemental formulas, *361*

enteral nutrition, *359*

hypertonic, *361*

iatrogenic malnutrition, *353*

isotonic, *361*

medical nutrition therapy, *352*

modular formulas, *361*

osmolality, *361*

palliative nutrition, *367*

paralytic ileus, *365*

parenteral nutrition, *359*

polymeric formulas, *361*

refeeding syndrome, *356*

short bowel syndrome, *365*

The Nutrition Care Process in Acute and Subacute Care

The process of nutrition care involves the assessment of an individual's nutrition status followed by the planning, implementation, and monitoring of customized goals and objectives that are targeted at optimizing health as outlined in Chapter 1. The nutrition care of a client in acute, subacute, or long-term care follows this same process and includes goals that are aimed at the role nutrition plays in any acute process occurring during hospitalization as well as long-term goals. Nutrition care that encompasses the assessment and treatment of any disease, condition, or illness is referred to as **medical nutrition therapy.** Treatment can include nutrition therapy with a modified diet, nutrition education, and provision of specialized nutrition support with oral nutrition supplements, tube feedings, or intravenous nutrition. In health care institutions, the nurse collaborates with the nutrition professional to ensure that optimal nutritional care is provided.

Hospital and Long-Term Care Nutrition Services

Health care institutions vary in the type and availability of nutrition services provided. Both clinical and food service aspects of nutrition care fall under the umbrella of nutrition services in the health care setting. Acute care facilities have full-time nutrition professionals on staff to provide clinical nutrition expertise to the health care team. Typically, these professionals include registered dietitians (RDs) and dietetic technicians, registered (DTRs), who are responsible for the assessment of nutrition status and planning of nutrition care. The nurse also has an integral role in this process because of the central nursing position on the health care team and the concentrated involvement of the nurse in direct client care.

In long-term or home health care, the RD generally acts as a consultant to the health care team, whereas the nurse plays a more central role in overseeing nutrition care than occurs in acute care. Nutrition care is part of the nursing process in all health care settings.

As with clinical nutrition services, food service varies among health care institutions. Services range from hotel-style room service to traditional predetermined meals served at specific times with little client choice. A selective menu is offered by many health care institutions, allowing the client to choose among foods permitted by the diet prescription. Although this practice is of benefit to most clients, Practice Pearl: Menu Assistance outlines a sometimes overlooked aspect of this menu style. In most acute care settings, clients are served a meal at the bedside among all the trappings of their medical care, which can have a negative effect on appetite and intake. Clients requiring any mealtime assistance must wait for available staff before consuming a meal. Busy mealtimes and staffing issues may result in untimely assistance that can negatively impact intake. In a study of hospitalized older adults, meal trays left out of reach or the need to wait

PRACTICE PEARL

Menu Assistance

Selective menus help optimize intake by allowing the client to make food choices. The nurse should assess whether a client has any barriers that could interfere with filling out this type of menu, such as vision difficulties, illiteracy, or inability to understand the language used on the menu. Cultural food practices could leave some clients unable to decipher unfamiliar foods offered. Appropriate assistance should be provided. Some food service departments have menus available in a variety of languages to assist in meal selection.

for help opening containers or using cutlery resulted in meal delays of up to 43 minutes (Xia & McCutcheon, 2006). Dining room style service is being used in some acute and long-term care settings to encourage improved intake with uninterrupted mealtime in a pleasant, supervised eating environment (Wright, Hickson, & Frost, 2006). This style of food service also affords the health care team an opportunity to provide ready assistance if needed and the ability to monitor intake on a regular basis.

The nurse can find an outline of nutrition services and detailed information on normal and therapeutic diets available by referring to the institution's diet manual. Some institutions refer to the diet manual as a nutrition practice manual, reflecting the evolution in health care to evidence-based practices (Chima, 2007). Hospital protocols for nutrition practices, such as specialized nutrition support, would be included in the manual.

Therapeutic Diets in Acute and Long-Term Care

A variety of normal and therapeutic diets are prescribed in acute and long-term care. A regular or house diet does not restrict intake of any nutrient, food group, or consistency of food. Other types of diets can alter the texture and types of foods provided based on a client's nutritional or physical needs. Table 16-1 outlines common hospital diets that are modified in texture or food consistency. Therapeutic diets that are prescribed as part of medical nutrition therapy are outlined in the respective chapters on illnesses and conditions that follow.

The nurse should be mindful and intervene if a client receives an overly modified diet. Diminished or inadequate intake for any reason places a client at risk for malnutrition, which can negatively impact health outcomes. Prolonged use of clear liquids does not provide adequate energy or nutrients but merely serves as oral hydration. The prescription of clear liquids postoperatively for uncomplicated surgery is a common practice but is not based on evidence-based research. Additionally, the routine use of clear liquids following acute pancreatitis instead of progressing to a soft or light diet is under debate (Thomson, 2008). Clear liquids should not be used as the sole source of nutrition for more than 72 hours (Hancock, Cresci, & Martindale, 2002). Oral nutrition supplements containing additional energy and protein are available that comply with clear liquid restrictions. A nutrition consult is indicated when prolonged clear liquids are required. When texture modification is needed, such as with chewing or swallowing difficulties, the client should receive the consistency of food that matches assessed need. Offering a client applesauce or pureed meat when simply chopping an apple or avoiding tough meats is sufficient can lead to diminished appetite and intake. Older adults in long-term care should have therapeutic diets liberalized to optimize intake

unless there is a strong medical contraindication (American Dietetic Association [ADA], 2005). Collaboration with the registered dietitian and other members of the health care team will ensure that an appropriate diet is provided to the client.

Malnutrition of the Hospitalized Client

Malnutrition occurs in the hospital and in subacute and long-term care at a surprisingly significant rate. Depending on the nutrition assessment parameters used to define malnutrition, up to 50% of adults in health care institutions have protein-calorie malnutrition (Bavelaar et al., 2008; Norman, Pichard, Lochs, & Pirlich, 2008). The occurrence of malnutrition in older adults is disproportionately higher than in other age groups (Norman et al., 2008). Lifespan Box: Malnutrition and the Older Adult discusses malnutrition in the older adult.

Malnutrition is associated with negative health outcomes that further jeopardize the well-being of the client. In addition to an increased length of stay and associated economic costs, malnutrition is linked to increased infection rates, disease complications, poor wound healing, altered pharmacokinetics, and, ultimately, increased mortality rates (Norman et al., 2008). These detrimental effects occur because malnutrition eventually affects all systems and tissues in the body (National Institute for Health and Clinical Excellence [NICE], 2006). Box 16-1 outlines the effects of malnutrition in more detail.

Despite the known negative consequences, continuing research highlights the poor job that primary care professionals are doing at recognizing and intervening when malnutrition exists. Several studies have reviewed medical records of hospitalized adults and reported that only about one-half of malnourished clients had documentation by a physician or nurse regarding an accurate assessment of nutrition status (Bavelaar et al., 2008; Singh, Watt, Veitch, Cantor, & Duerksen, 2006; Suominen, Sandelin, Soini, & Pitkala, 2009).

The nature of the presenting disease or condition places many clients at risk of malnutrition before hospitalization occurs. For example, liver or gastrointestinal diseases affect nutrient absorption or metabolism. For others, malnutrition occurs or worsens during hospitalization. Poor intake, malabsorption and nutrient losses, and increased metabolic needs are the primary reasons that malnutrition occurs. These are further delineated in Box 16-2. Malnutrition that occurs because of health care practices or treatment is called **iatrogenic malnutrition.** Examples of health care practices that foster poor nutritional health include failure to identify clients at risk for poor nutrition, prolonged use of clear liquid diets, missed or interrupted meals or tube feedings because of medical testing or procedures, treatment and medication side effects that diminish appetite, and lack of adequate feeding assistance. Preoperative routines can contribute to nutritional

Table 16-1 Common Texture-Modified Diets

Diet	Use	Foods Allowed	Foods Not Allowed	Nutritional Adequacy and Advice
Regular or House	General diet for those not requiring texture or nutrient modification	All	None	Adequate if consumed as offered.
Clear Liquids	Hydration Bowel preparation for some procedures Transition to solid food from nil per os (NPO)	See-through items liquid at room temperature Clear juices—cranberry, apple, grape Clear drinks—fruit punch, sodas (ginger ale, lemon-lime, etc.), plain tea, black coffee Broth, bouillon Gelatin Popsicles, ices Hard candy, honey	Opaque liquids Solid food	Inadequate in all nutrients and low in energy. Consider nutrition supplementation to diet in at-risk clients. Monitor length of time on diet and consult nutrition team if 5 days or more.
Full Liquids	Chewing or swallowing difficulties	Foods liquid or pourable at room temperature Juices Dairy or dairy alternative—beverages, ice cream, yogurt Custard, pudding Hot cereal Liquid oral nutrition supplements All clear liquid items	Solid foods Liquid at room temperature foods with added solids (e.g., ice cream w/nuts or fruit)	Nutritionally adequate when supplements consumed. If dysphagia and aspiration risk are present, consult speech language therapist for swallowing evaluation and safety recommendations on food texture. High lactose content can be lowered w/use of dairy alternatives. High-fat and low-fiber content for prolonged use.
Mechanical or Dental Soft	Chewing or swallowing difficulties	Liquids Minced, soft, chopped or ground food: Proteins—poultry, fish w/o bones, cooked beans, eggs, chopped or cut meats w/o casings or grizzle, sauces added for moisture as needed Grains—all except as noted Fruit and vegetables—soft, peeled, cooked, or canned as tolerated Desserts on full liquid diet or as tolerated	Whole nuts Seeds Meat with casings (hotdogs, sausage) Tough meats Hard crusted bread Fruits/vegetables with edible skin Raw vegetables	Nutritionally adequate if all food groups consumed; can be low fiber. Customize texture modification to minimum amount that meets client needs. Avoid overmodification. If dysphagia and aspiration risk are present, consult speech language therapist for swallowing evaluation and safety recommendations on food texture.
Pureed	Advanced chewing or swallowing difficulties	Blenderized or pureed foods Any food allowed that can be pureed to a custard-like consistency w/o solids remaining Liquids can be added to yield desired consistency	Whole nuts Seeds Hard bread/rolls Dried fruit Fruits/vegetable skin Any food that cannot be pureed to a smooth consistency	Nutritionally adequate. Customize texture modification to minimum amount that meets client needs. Avoid overmodification. Essential food is presented in attractive manner to stimulate appetite (e.g., molds, garnishes, parfait presentation). Refrain from commenting on unappealing appearance of diet if providing feeding assistance.

BOX 16-1	Effects of Malnutrition

Altered Protein Status: Loss of Somatic and Visceral Protein

Poor wound healing

↓ Immune response

Loss of muscle strength, endurance

Loss of respiratory muscle

↓ Plasma proteins and altered fluid balance because of change in oncotic pressure

↓ Organ tissue with protein loss

Altered pharmacokinetics with loss of plasma proteins for drug binding

Altered Fluid and Electrolyte Balance

Loss of electrolytes w/tissue wasting

Loss of plasma proteins and effect of albumin on fluid balance

Altered Reproductive Health

Infertility

Bone loss with ↓ estrogen production

Altered Functional Status

Skeletal muscle loss w/ ↓ strength, ↑ risk of falls, ↓ functional capacity

Altered mental health—apathy, listlessness, poor concentration

Fatigue

Hypothermia

Delayed recovery from illness

↑ Risk of morbidity and mortality

---

risk. In addition to missed meals, prolonged fasting or intake of only clear liquids that are common before and after surgery, and false reliance on intravenous dextrose as a significant source of calories can jeopardize nutrition status. One liter of 5% dextrose has only 170 kcalories. Preoperative fasting is not indicated in most cases and may contribute to diminished glycogen stores postoperatively (Weimann et al., 2006). The practice of fasting before surgery to avoid aspiration risk has been replaced by allowing clear liquids and solids up to 2 and 6 hours, respectively, preoperatively (Weimann et al., 2006). Every attempt should be made to screen each client for malnutrition risk factors on admission and to provide ongoing monitoring of nutrition status while hospitalized. This screening process is part of the nursing assessment. The registered dietitian should be consulted to perform a more in-depth assessment when an individual is believed to be at risk for malnutrition. Nutrition assessment is outlined in Chapter 12.

Lifespan

Malnutrition and the Older Adult

Although malnutrition is an unfortunately common occurrence in the hospitalized older adult, it should never be dismissed as acceptable or "*just a part of aging.*" The older adult is at risk for malnutrition because of physical changes that do occur with aging. This risk is compounded when illness and its treatment further compromise nutritional health, as outlined in detail in Chapter 15. Involuntary weight loss that occurs in hospitalized older adults places them at risk for in-hospital complications, prolonged length of stay, and increases post-hospital mortality risk for up to 3 years (Kagansky et al., 2005; Neumann, Miller, Daniels, & Crotty, 2005; Thomas, 2005).

Whether weight loss or altered nutritional status occurs because of aging, a medical condition, or treatment, intervention is essential to prevent poor health outcomes. The nurse should collaborate with the health care team to prevent malnutrition from occurring in the hospital, when possible, and to intervene early when malnutrition risk is suspected.

CT? What recommendation could the nurse make about a restrictive therapeutic diet prescribed for an older adult who is eating poorly? What causes of malnutrition from Box 16-2 are a concern in the older adult?

How Is Malnutrition Treated?

Treatment of malnutrition is determined by the etiology of this condition. Whether malnutrition stems from decreased intake, malabsorption and nutrient losses, or unmet increased needs, the priority is optimizing intake to compensate for these deficits while also addressing appropriate interventions that target the cause. Treatment of malnutrition as only a nutritional problem while overlooking its etiology will not result in a successful outcome. A team approach is often necessary to fully address the problem. For example, contributors to malnutrition such as medication side effects, psychosocial and economic issues, self-care limitations, and dysphagia require the collaborative advice of other health care professionals to brainstorm solutions. An individual should be encouraged to consult with a religious leader if religious fasting practices negatively impact nutrition status as outlined in Cultural Considerations Box: Religious Fasting.

In clients with a functional gastrointestinal tract who are able to safely consume oral intake, optimized intake of nutrient-dense foods is recommended. The nurse can suggest ways to increase the nutrient content and amount of food as outlined in Client Education Checklist: Optimizing Oral Intake. The

BOX 16-2	Etiology of Malnutrition

Decreased Intake

Loss of appetite

Lack of availability of personal or cultural food preferences

Pain

Medication side effects: sedation, tremor, intestinal symptoms, fatigue, anorexia, dysphagia

Gastrointestinal symptoms: nausea, vomiting, diarrhea, constipation, bloating

Poor dental health: loose teeth, missing teeth, ill-fitting dentures, caries

Sensory changes: poor vision, diminished smell or taste ability

Physical disability: limited ability to shop, cook, or feed

Diminished cognitive state: dementia, sedation, altered consciousness

Psychosocial issues: loneliness, depression, bereavement, sadness, anxiety

Food insecurity: lack of funds or access to food

Dieting or restrictive eating, food faddism

Alcohol or drug abuse

Dependency on others

Increased Nutrient Losses

Malabsorptive conditions or disease: short bowel syndrome, inflammatory bowel disease, liver disease

Drug-nutrient interactions

High-output enteric fistula, vomiting, diarrhea

Increased urinary nutrient loss

Alcohol abuse

Exudative wound

Increased Metabolic Needs

Trauma

Wounds and fractures

Fever

Infection/sepsis

Hypermetabolic conditions: burns, end-stage obstructive lung disease, surgery

Conditions w/involuntary movements: Parkinson's disease, tremor

Increased physical activity

Iatrogenic

Any medically caused reason for ↓ intake, ↑ nutrient losses, ↑ metabolic needs as above

Prolonged use of clear liquids or NPO status

Insufficient delivery of tube feedings or oral supplements

Insufficient delivery of parenteral nutrition

Inadequate assistance with feeding

Interrupted meals

client with poor appetite should be encouraged to consume foods with high rather than low nutrient content at the start of the meal to avoid unnecessarily filling up on foods with little nutritional value. Offering nutrient-dense meals and snacks more frequently is helpful for those who get full too

quickly, a condition called **early satiety.** Provision of proper feeding assistance is crucial in the client who is unable to self-feed. Box 16-3 highlights such feeding techniques.

During recovery from malnutrition, clients should be monitored for **refeeding syndrome.** Refeeding syndrome occurs with the reintroduction of energy into the diet. The resulting uptake and metabolism of glucose by cells also causes shifts in potassium, magnesium, and phosphorus that can lead to lethal alterations in fluid and electrolytes (Panteli & Crook, 2009). This syndrome can occur with all types of nutrition therapy, including an oral diet, tube feedings, and intravenous nutrition. Treatment includes the slow reintroduction of energy in those felt to be at risk for refeeding syndrome, including the severely malnourished, alcoholics, those who have fasted or taken minimal nutrition for greater than 7 days, and individuals with eating disorders. Alterations in plasma potassium, magnesium, and phosphorus are treated pharmacologically in most cases (Stanga et al., 2008).

Cultural Considerations

Religious Fasting

The practice of fasting is a traditional part of many religions. The voluntary abstention from all or some foods can be part of a religious ritual or act of repentance. For example, the fast of Ramadan is part of the Fourth Pillar of Islam. Followers fast from dawn to dusk during the 30 days of Ramadan. Fasting is traditionally practiced during observance of Yom Kippur in the Jewish faith as well as on other holy days by the strictly observant. Greek and Coptic Orthodox Christians fast in varying degrees over 150 days a year. Most religions that practice fasting exempt pregnant or nursing females and the ill from fasting obligations. However, the decision to forgo fasting is a personal one and some elect to fast despite exemption. Hospitalized clients who are at risk of malnutrition and are observant of fasting practices should be respectfully encouraged to consult with a religious leader and the health care team when making this decision.

Oral Nutrition Supplements

Oral liquid nutrition supplements are often used to supplement calorie and protein intake. These products fall into the category of enteral nutrition formulas, which are outlined in Table 16-2. Intake of these liquid supplements can provide a much needed source of additional nutrients, but care should

BOX 16-3	Providing Feeding Assistance

Ready Client for Meal

Eyeglasses on

Adequate lighting

Dentures in

Clean table or bedside tray top

Position client properly: head and torso at 90-degree angle to lap

Provide Appropriate Level of Assistance

Position meal, utensils, client to maximize independent feeding

Physical assistance as needed. Examples include:
- Open containers, uncover plates, set up cutlery, cut food, pour liquids
- Guide client in getting food onto utensil if able to self-feed
- Provide finger foods if not able to use cutlery but able to self-feed
- Adaptive equipment to assist in self-feeding (built-up utensils, scoop dish, etc.)

- Full feeding assistance with hand feeding. Allow ample time and pace. Sit and face client when feeding. Introduce pleasant conversation. Ask family or friends about client's interests if conversation is difficult. Communicate with staff client preferences for feeding routine. Do not mix together foods on plate.

Verbal guidance as needed. Examples include:
- Cueing for clients with altered cognition who may not realize meal process. Clients may need cue to chew or swallow. Cues may be verbal or play acted. Match utensil to food and provide cue (*"Here is your ice cream and a spoon to use to eat it"*).
- Describing foods and location on tray/plate for clients w/poor vision (*"I have opened the ice cream cup for you and put it at the 2 o'clock position on your tray."*)
- Encouragement to try a food or fluid or to consume more

be taken that they do not simply replace existing intake or interfere with mealtime appetite. A review of research trials that tested the usefulness of this practice in older adults found that oral supplements improved overall intake and lessened medical complications in those who were already undernourished (Milne, Avenell, & Potter, 2006; Volkert et al., 2006). No effect on outcome was seen when supplements were routinely used in well-nourished older adults. Providing oral nutrition supplements is associated with increased weight gain in adults with illness-related malnutrition, but no evidence is available on the effect of this practice on long-term survival (Baldwin, Parsons, & Logan, 2007). In a study

Table 16-2   Enteral Nutrition Formulas

Category	Feature	Use	Nursing Considerations
Polymeric	Intact (whole) proteins, fat, and carbohydrate	General needs	Isotonic if 1 kcal/mL Available in ↑protein or calorie versions w/1.5 to 2 kcal/mL Varying fiber content Lactose-free available Oral versions flavored
Elemental	Protein as amino acids or dipeptides and tripeptides Simple sugars Minimal fat	Malabsorptive conditions Feeding into jejunum	Hypertonic—monitor tolerance as rate/concentration advance Can be flavored for oral intake
Modular	Single component of carbohydrate, protein, or fat	Supplemental source of nutrient to mix with other formula or create one when standard choices fail to meet need	Alone does not provide full nutrition
Specialty	Combination of nutrients specifically recommended for condition or disease	Specific diseases w/unique nutritional recommendations (e.g., modified protein in renal or liver disease) that cannot be met with standard formula	More expensive than standard formulas May be isotonic or hypertonic

PRACTICE PEARL

Improving Intake of Oral Nutrition Supplements

The taste of oral liquid nutrition supplements does not appeal to all clients. Flavors can be limited, leading to taste fatigue and then decreased intake. Ample fortification with vitamins and minerals lend these products an organic smell and taste that overpowers some taste buds. The nurse should consider the following ideas to foster intake:

- Serve the liquid supplement cool or cold. Room temperature supplements have a strong taste.
- Supplements can be served instead of juice or water with a medication pass if there are no drug–supplement interaction contraindications.
- Alternate flavorings or mix-ins can be used to avoid taste fatigue from repetitive flavors. Chocolate syrup, instant hot cocoa powder, pasteurized eggnog, and eggnog or peppermint flavoring are possible ideas, among others.
- Avoid offering liquid supplements within an hour of mealtime or appetite may be affected.

of oral nutrition supplement use in nursing homes, it was reported that the frequency and amount of intake was increased when staff were given specific prescribing parameters about exactly when to offer the supplement rather than generic "between meals" type of direction (Simmons & Patel, 2006). Practice Pearl: Improving Intake of Oral Nutrition Supplements provides advice on improving intake of oral supplements.

Nutrition Support: Enteral and Parenteral Nutrition

Some individuals are unable to safely take adequate oral nutrition or do not have a functioning gastrointestinal tract and as a result the use of specialized nutrition support may be indicated. Timely nutrition support is especially crucial in the critically ill client, those expected to not tolerate oral nutrition for 3 to 5 days or more, and those with existing risk of malnutrition (ASPEN, 2002; Heyland et al., 2003; Kreymann et al., 2006; NICE, 2006). Early nutrition therapy within 24 to 48 hours of hospitalization is advised in the critically ill

---

CLIENT EDUCATION CHECKLIST	Optimizing Oral Intake
Intervention	**Example**
Increase "calories-per-bite" of intake.	Add calories to existing dishes: sauces, butter, gravy, dressings, dried fruit. Add protein to existing dishes: cheese, powdered milk, peanut butter, nuts. Substitute high-calorie foods for low-calorie versions: whole vs. skim milk, cream vs. clear soup, juice or milk vs. water.
Encourage nutrient-dense foods.	Consume higher calorie foods at start of meal before fullness occurs. Follow guidelines for increasing calories-per-bite. Try ↑protein desserts made w/dairy or egg: pudding, custard, ice cream.
Offer more frequent meals and snacks.	Decrease time between meals and snacks. Combine foods with protein for snacks: peanut butter or cheese and crackers, yogurt, trail mix w/dried fruit and nuts.
Conserve physical energy needed for the meal.	Consume more nutritious meals earlier in the day when energy level is best. Consume more nutritious food earlier in the meal when energy level is better. Have ready-to-eat foods on hand for when fatigue prevents meal or snack preparation: microwavable or frozen meals, fortified cereal w/nuts and whole milk, canned milk shakes or smoothies, breakfast bars.
Limit foods that cause early satiety and have little nutritional value.	Eat most nutritious foods first in meal. Watch mealtime liquids, especially carbonated drinks, broth-type soups. Monitor intake of bulky vegetables, raw foods, excess fiber.
Improve the eating environment.	Increase sensory appeal of food w/flavoring, color, texture, aroma. Assess for medications that alter taste sensation. Avoid smoking before meals. Eat in social setting w/others.
Use oral liquid nutrition supplements.	Take at specific times. Drink cool or cold, not at room temperature. Mix into other foods (pudding, cocoa, etc.). Take instead of water or juice w/medications if no drug-supplement interaction.

client because of the associated increased metabolic demands and the link between poor nutrition status and morbidity and mortality (Jones & Heyland, 2008). The decision to pursue aggressive nutrition support should be in keeping with the client's self-determined health care goals or **advance directive.** *Advance directive* is a term for the legal document that outlines an individual's health care wishes and is referred to in the event that a client becomes unable to communicate.

Nutrition support that utilizes the gastrointestinal tract is called **enteral nutrition.** Alternatively, **parenteral nutrition** refers to intravenous nutrition, based on the derivation from *par* (near or equal to) and *enteral* (intestinal). Both types of nutrition support can supply adequate energy and nutrients to meet metabolic requirements. Evidence points to the health and economic benefits of enteral nutrition over parenteral nutrition in clients who have a functional diges-

tive tract (Heyland et al., 2003; Kreymann et al., 2006; Pritchard, Duffy, Edington, & Pang, 2006). Hyperglycemia and sepsis are more frequent complications in the client population receiving parenteral nutrition than in those receiving enteral nutrition (Jeejeebhoy, 2007). Theories exist that overfeeding practices and possible translocation of intestinal bacteria when the gut is not used contribute to these parenteral nutrition complications (Jeejeebhoy, 2007). Bacterial translocation can occur during critical illness because the gastrointestinal tract becomes more permeable, allowing bacteria to travel in the peritoneum and internal organs as depicted in Figure 16-1 ■. Use of the intestine with enteral nutrition is associated with maintenance of the intestinal barrier and immune function (Guzy et al., 2009).

The initial choice of feeding method is dependent on the level of intestinal function. Enteral nutrition is recommended

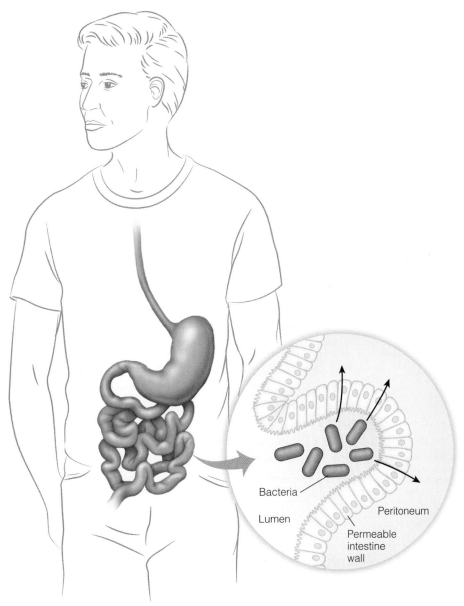

■ FIGURE 16-1 **Bacterial Translocation.**

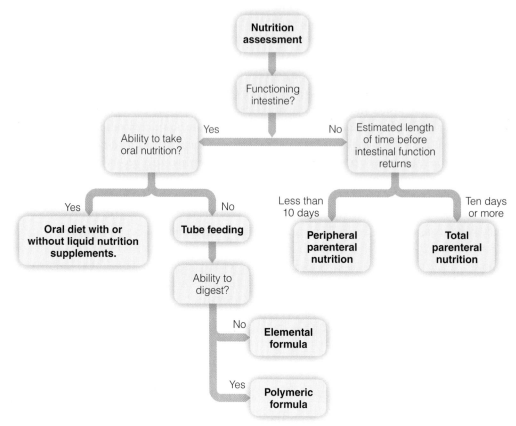

■ FIGURE 16-2 **Treatment Algorithm for Nutrition Support.**

in clients with at least some ability to digest and absorb nutrients via the digestive tract. In the past, parenteral nutrition was routinely used for conditions such as pancreatitis and short bowel syndrome because of the diminished digestive and absorptive capability associated with these diagnoses. Now enteral nutrition with modified formulas has been shown to be an effective route of nutrition support in many of these clients (Louie et al., 2005; McClave, Chang, Dhaliwal, & Heyland, 2006). Use of a decision tree or algorithm is helpful in determining which route of nutrition support is indicated for a client. Figure 16-2 ■ is an example of a nutrition support algorithm.

The nurse is a central member of the health care team responsible for implementing and monitoring nutrition support in clients. In some in-patient settings, a formal nutrition support team, which includes a nurse, dietitian, physician, and pharmacist, is responsible for overseeing nutrition support in that institution. Nutrition support protocols dictate the role of each team member and the evidence-based practices associated with the delivery of enteral and parenteral nutrition. In other institutions, the client's nurse holds primary responsibility for the nursing role in nutrition support. The nurse is involved in the delivery and monitoring of specialized nutrition support, including care of parenteral catheters and feeding tubes. Additionally, client education

and psychosocial support are important nursing roles. Lifespan Box: Nutrition Support and the Pediatric Client outlines an example of such client education in the pediatric client. In the home care setting, nurses are involved in overseeing both enteral and parenteral nutrition in the client on long-term nutrition support.

Enteral Nutrition

Enteral nutrition support can involve the use of oral liquid nutrition supplements or tube feedings depending on the client's capacity to safely take oral nutrition. Tube feeding is indicated in clients who cannot safely take adequate oral nutrition.

Lifespan

Nutrition Support and the Pediatric Client

Children may require specialized nutritional support in the form of enteral or parenteral nutrition for short- or long-term periods. The placement of a feeding tube or intravenous line can be a frightening experience for a pediatric client. The nurse is instrumental in providing the child with an age-appropriate explanation of the procedure, the equipment, and its purpose. Allowing the child to see the equipment set up ahead of time and demonstrating feeding with a doll or stuffed animal can be helpful.

Examples of this include clients at risk of aspirating oral intake and those who are unconscious, experiencing significant anorexia, or are unable to consume adequate intake to match increased metabolic demands. Some clients take a combination of oral and tube feedings, such as burn clients with excessive metabolic demands or clients transitioning back to oral intake from tube feeding.

Tube Feedings

The choice of tube feeding formula and delivery method is customized for each client depending on medical condition, gut function, and length of time estimated for nutrition support. The nurse should be knowledgeable about the enteral product formulary available and the indication for each product. Additionally, it is essential that the nurse is proficient in the delivery of feedings, monitoring client tolerance, and assessing for complications.

Enteral Nutrition Formulas

A variety of enteral nutrition formulas is available with an array of nutrient mixes and forms. Table 16-2 outlines the various categories of formulas. In the client with full digestive and absorptive function, a formula with intact macronutrients is recommended. These formulas are also referred to as **polymeric formulas.** Intact nutrients are those in a whole, undigested form such as soy protein and the milk proteins casein and whey versus proteins already broken down to amino acids or peptides. Intact nutrients require gastrointestinal enzymes and secretions in order to be fully digested and absorbed. Conditions such as pancreatitis or other malabsorptive diseases can require a formula with predigested macronutrients, such as amino acids or simple sugars, because of limited gastrointestinal enzyme secretion or reduced absorptive capability. Predigested formulas are referred to as **elemental formulas.** Other types of formulas, called **modular formulas,** can be used to mix with polymeric or elemental formulas to increase the nutrient content. A modular formula can contain just a protein, fat, or carbohydrate source. Additionally, specialized formulas are marketed to target disease-specific use when unique recommendations exist for feeding with certain diagnoses. Examples include higher fat formulas designed for respiratory clients and formulas enriched with certain amino acids like glutamine, felt to benefit the client during physiological stress. Disease-specific feeding needs are discussed in the respective disease chapters.

The **osmolality** of formulas differs and can affect client tolerance to the feeding. Osmolality is the number of dissolved particles with an ionic charge in 1 liter of a solution. Elemental formulas have more particles per liter because the whole version of macronutrients has been broken down to the smaller parts. For example, large protein molecules are broken down to contain many small amino acid molecules, which results in more charged particles per liter. Additionally, high-calorie or high-protein formulas have a high osmolality because they contain more nutrients and

charged particles per liter than do standard polymeric formulas containing 1 kilocalorie/mL. Higher osmolality can affect formula tolerance because the body always seeks to keep an equal concentration of particles on each side of any membrane, including the gut wall, and does so by shifting water. The osmolality of body fluids is almost 300 mOsm/L. Enteral formulas that are **hypertonic,** or have an osmolality greater than that of the body, can cause water to shift into the intestines in an attempt to equalize the high particle concentration on either side of the intestinal wall. The result can be diarrhea. Formulas that are **isotonic,** or approximate the body's osmolality, are less likely to cause this problem. Isotonic formulas tend to be those that are polymeric formulas and have approximately 1 kilocalorie/mL. The effect of formula choice on feeding tolerance is discussed further in the section on complications of tube feeding.

Formula Delivery

The choice of feeding tube site and the pattern of formula delivery depend on several factors. Consideration should be given to risk of aspiration, duration of nutrition support needed, and medical diagnoses.

Feeding Tube Choices   Feeding tubes can be temporary, as in a nasogastric tube, or surgically placed for long-term use. Figure 16-3 ■ depicts the different types of feeding tubes. Surgically placed feeding tubes are used when it is estimated

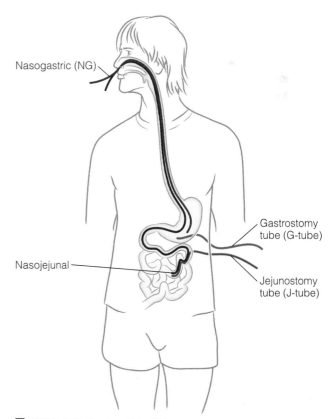

Nasogastric (NG)

Nasojejunal

Gastrostomy tube (G-tube)

Jejunostomy tube (J-tube)

■ **FIGURE 16-3 Feeding Tube Sites.**

that the need for nutrition support will extend beyond a month or more (ASPEN, 2002). Permanent feeding tubes provide the client with some relief from the quality of life issues associated with nasogastric tubes, such as nasal irritation, tube presence in the line of vision, and easy dislodgment of the tube that then requires replacement. Gastrostomy tubes (called PEG or G-tubes) and jejunostomy tubes (J-tube) are surgically placed tubes that deliver formula directly from outside the body to the stomach and jejunum, respectively. A J-tube would be placed when feeding into the upper digestive tract is contraindicated, such as following surgical removal of the upper small intestine or stomach or because of obstruction. Typical nasogastric feeding tubes (NG tubes) are inserted through the nose and reach the stomach. Longer length tubes are used when the client is at risk of aspiration or when feeding into the small intestine rather than the stomach is indicated. These tubes can reach the duodenum or jejunum depending on tube length. Postpyloric placement of a feeding tube delivers feedings directly into the small intestine but is no guarantee against pulmonary aspiration of intestinal contents. However, bypassing the stomach eliminates the contribution of high gastric residuals of formula to aspiration risk. Use of longer tubes is associated with reduced incidence of pneumonia in critically ill clients compared with those receiving gastric feeding (Heyland et al., 2003). Longer tubes are also used in conditions such as partial upper intestinal obstruction, where distal delivery of formula bypasses the site of the stricture or obstruction. Nasojejunal tubes are indicated with pancreatitis to bypass the site of pancreatic enzyme secretion and minimize stimulation of the pancreas, as outlined in Chapter 20. When feedings are delivered directly to the jejunum, an elemental formula must be used because the sites of active digestion and enzyme secretion have been bypassed. The nurse should consult with the pharmacist when caring for a client with a jejunal tube to assess for medication compatibility with this delivery method via a small-bore tube, any interactions with the enteral formula, and for site of drug absorption. Jejunal delivery of some medications can bypass the site of the drug's absorption.

Feeding Administration   Enteral feedings can be delivered continuously, intermittently, or in several bolus feedings depending on the condition of the client. Aspiration risk, gastric emptying, and tube length dictate how a feeding is administered. Continuous feedings deliver the feeding over the full course of the day. Use of a feeding pump or a gravity drip system delivers the prescribed volume of formula per hour. A feeding pump is generally preferred over gravity drip with continuous feeding to avoid the risk of an accidental bolus with the gravity system. Box 16-4 outlines the method for determining feeding delivery rates and beginning feeding. Continuous feeding is recommended to reduce intolerance and risks associated with delivery of larger volumes. Clients with slowed gastric emptying and those at risk for pulmonary aspiration should be fed continuously to minimize the chance of large gastric residuals, which contribute to intolerance and aspiration risk. Feedings delivered directly to the small intestine with a postpyloric tube or a J-tube benefit from continuous formula delivery because of a lack of any intestinal reservoir to hold larger volumes and the resultant chance of intolerance to a bolus of hypertonic formula. Other patterns of formula delivery can be used in the client who is not at risk of aspiration and are seen more commonly in clients receiving long-term gastric feeding. Intermittent feedings deliver formula over the course of approximately a half hour or more at a faster rate than is done with continuous feeding, resulting in a larger volume delivered in a shorter amount of time. Intermittent feeding schedules are variable but generally occur every 4 to 6 hours, mimicking the eating process. Box 16-4 outlines this prac-

---

BOX 16-4	**Calculating Feeding Delivery Goals**

The registered dietitian makes volume recommendations for a total amount of enteral nutrition formula ultimately needed to meet a client's estimated nutritional requirements. Follow these steps to calculate the delivery rate of formula needed with varying methods of administration.

   An estimate is made that a client needs 3,600 kilocalories using a polymeric formula with 1.5 kilocalories/mL.

1. Determine the final volume needed to provide 3,600 kilocalories: 3,600 kilocalories ÷ 1.5 kilocalories/mL = 2,400 mL or 2.4 L goal
2. Determine the goal administration rate for the appropriate method of delivery
   - Continuous delivery: 2,400 mL needed ÷ 24 hours/day = 100 mL/hour
   - Intermittent delivery: 2,400 mL needed ÷ 4 to 6 feedings/day = 400 mL to 600 mL/feeding
   - Bolus delivery: 2,400 mL needed ÷ 4 to 6 feedings/day = 400 mL to 600 mL/feeding
3. Feedings start at a low volume and advance over hours or days depending on client tolerance. Concentration of hypertonic formulas can be diluted temporarily if diarrhea occurs or is likely.

   ▪ What are the advantages and disadvantages to each of these methods of delivery? Why might a client be switched to another method?

tice. Bolus feedings occur at the frequency of intermittent feedings but deliver the formula over fewer minutes and can utilize a syringe for delivery. Less time is devoted to bolus feeding than with other methods, which is a quality of life benefit, but quick delivery of large volumes is not well tolerated by all clients. Nausea, fullness, and cramping can result.

Complications and Monitoring of Enteral Nutrition

Enteral nutrition support is not without associated risks and, therefore, requires diligent monitoring. Common complications and nursing interventions are outlined in Table 16-3. Many complications are avoidable with proper feeding practices that observe client positioning, medication administration, and delivery of the prescribed volume.

The nurse should strictly follow guidelines for administration of medication via the feeding tube and routinely consult with the pharmacist about compatibility of enteral formula with drugs. Some medications, such as proton pump inhibitors, phenytoin, warfarin, and fluoroquinolones, present timing and incompatibility challenges. Others, such as enteric coated or extended release drugs should not be crushed. Hypertonic and sorbitol containing drugs can cause diarrhea that frequently gets blamed on the tube feeding for-

mula. Hypertonic medications include liquid versions of chloryl hydrate, acetaminophen, and potassium chloride. Sorbitol containing drugs include many liquids, elixirs, and syrups. The amount of sorbitol in medications has a cumulative effect (Williams, 2008). Chapter 24 outlines this topic further.

Proper client positioning with the head of the bed at a 30- to 45-degree angle is crucial in prevention of aspiration. Unfortunately, adherence to this guideline is frequently a problem and often for no known reason (Miller, Grossman, Hindley, Macgarvie, & Madill, 2008). Monitoring the client for aspiration with the use of blue food dye is no longer considered appropriate as outlined in the Evidence-Based Practice Box: Is blue dye safe as a method for detecting pulmonary aspiration in clients receiving enteral therapy? and Hot Topic: Preventing Bronchial Aspiration of Tube Feedings.

The nurse is instrumental in assisting the client who is transitioning back to oral intake with advice and encouragement about nutrient-dense foods to consume. Tube feedings should not be discontinued entirely until the client is meeting a significant portion of his or her nutritional needs orally. Intermittent or bolus feedings can be helpful in this transition to allow oral intake in the absence of concomitant formula feeding. In addition to providing clinical monitoring of

Table 16-3 Enteral Nutrition Complications and Nursing Interventions

Complication	Recommendations and Nursing Interventions
Aspiration	Keep head of bed up at 30–45-degree angle. Avoid intermittent or bolus feeding. Consider postpyloric or permanent feeding tube. Avoid use of blue food dye to signal aspiration.
Clogged tube	Flush tube before and after each medication is administered. Flush tube every 4 hours and when feedings are temporarily stopped. Flush tube after checking for gastric residuals. Limit use of acid pH fluids in tube.
Diarrhea	Assess contribution of formula osmolality, concentration, or rate to symptom. Avoid intermittent or bolus feeding. Consider medical conditions: bowel impaction or obstruction, intestinal disease, bacterial infection, hyperthyroidism. Consider medications associated with side effect (antibiotics, hypertonic or sorbitol-containing drugs, magnesium, phosphorus). Hypertonic drugs can be diluted with water during delivery. Maintain safe feeding handling practices.
Drug–formula interaction	Consult with pharmacist. Some medications are incompatible with enteral formula use. Flush feeding tube with 30 mL of water before and after each medication is administered.
Foodborne illness	Wash hands before handling formula or equipment. Wipe off container top before opening. Refrigerate open formula no greater than 24 hours. Observe limited 8–12-hour hang time for formula at room temperature. Change feeding setup daily.
Gastric residuals	Monitor for gastric residuals and hold if greater than 250 mL. Consider use of longer tube for small intestinal feeding beyond ligament of Trietz. Consider use of promotility agent. Follow guidelines for aspiration prevention.

EVIDENCE-BASED PRACTICE RESEARCH BOX

Is blue dye safe as a method for detecting pulmonary aspiration in clients receiving enteral therapy?

Clinical Problem: Blue dye has been used for many years to color enteral feedings as a means of detecting aspiration of formula. Is there sufficient evidence to continue the practice?

Research Findings: Nurses have long been concerned about detecting aspiration in clients who receive enteral feedings. It has been thought that when pulmonary suctioning is performed and blue-tinted secretions are obtained, it is evidence of pulmonary aspiration. Aspiration pneumonia can have life-threatening consequences in compromised individuals, so early detection of aspiration can lead to effective treatment.

Evidence has emerged that instillation of blue dye in enteral feedings can have serious effects for some clients. Skin discoloration was reported in one pediatric client (Zillich, Kuhn, & Petersen, 2000). Two cases of colored colons found at autopsy have been reported (Boutilier, Murray, & Walley 2000; Granville & Finch, 2001). In each case, the client had been treated with enteral feedings in which blue dye was used to detect potential aspiration. Lucarelli, Shirk, Julian, and Crouser (2004) reported two cases in which critically ill clients who were at high risk for aspiration were started on enteral feedings to which blue dye was added. Both clients eventually required hemodialysis, and blue-green discol-

oration was subsequently found in the dialysate. Both clients died. Although a cause and effect relationship could not be established, the writers recommended that alternative methods of detecting aspiration be used.

Researchers reported that an animal study they conducted showed that dye was visible less than 50% of the time when suctioned secretions were examined. Each subsequent suctioning decreased visibility. The researchers concluded that because dye is not visible in suctioned secretions, it is not reliable enough to recommend its continued use (Metheny et al., 2002). The U.S. FDA (2003) summarized reports of client complications related to the use of blue dye in enteral feedings, as did Sanko (2004).

Nursing Implications: There is no research evidence to support the use of blue dye (or any other dye) in enteral feedings to detect pulmonary aspiration. There is evidence to suggest that its use places clients at risk for complications; therefore, use of food dye should no longer be a standard nursing practice.

CRITICAL THINKING QUESTION:

1. How should the new nursing graduate respond to the long-standing practice of putting blue dye in the enteral feedings at the long-term care facility where she has begun her first professional position?

hot Topic

Preventing Bronchial Aspiration of Tube Feedings

Bronchial aspiration of gastric contents is a complication associated with tube feedings. Large volume aspiration and less noticeable microaspiration both place the client at increased risk of pulmonary injury and aspiration pneumonia. Frequently, clients receiving enteral nutrition support are already at risk for aspiration because of underlying medical illness and associated treatment. Prevention of aspiration by modifying controllable risk factors can be accomplished with nursing interventions. First, it is essential to recognize the associated risk factors for aspiration, which include:

- Supine position
- Delayed gastric emptying
- Large volume gastric residuals
- Sedation or altered consciousness

In the past, the focus was on detecting aspiration in the absence of evidence-based practice recommendations for preventing aspiration. For years blue food dye was used to detect the presence of bronchial aspiration of tube feedings. The dye was routinely added to the enteral formula as a marker. The presence of a blue aspirate from the lung was indicative of formula aspiration into the respiratory tract. Now the use of blue food dye is contraindicated following case reports of skin discoloration, blue-green tinting of organs and urine, and interference with pH and occult blood testing. Reports of bacterial contamination of multiple-use dye containers added to the negative effects of this practice. Further, unexplained metabolic acidosis and death

has been associated with the use of blue food dye, especially in clients already at risk for altered gastrointestinal permeability or sepsis, such as with celiac disease, renal failure, burns, and trauma.

Current recommendations regarding pulmonary aspiration of tube feedings focus on prevention of this occurrence using interventions as outlined:

- *Confirmation of feeding tube placement*—Radiographic confirmation of tube placement is the gold standard. There is no definitive bedside method to detect whether a tube has been placed in the stomach, small intestine, or lung. Auscultation and pH testing of the tube aspirate are unreliable. Once placement is confirmed, marking the tube where it exits the body and monitoring the external length of the tube to detect movement are recommended.

- *Client positioning*—A semirecumbent position with the head of the bed at a 30- to 45-degree angle is associated with decreased risk of aspiration. Research has pointed to a habitual overuse of the supine position without medical indication for it.

- *Management of gastric residuals*—Delayed gastric emptying can occur because of hyperglycemia, medications, and medical conditions such as diabetes and thyroid disease. Improved blood glucose control and minimization of sedative medications are medical interventions to target. Additionally, a promotility agent for gastric emptying should be considered. Postpyloric placement of a feeding tube will reduce large volume gastric residuals. Holding feedings when gastric residuals exceed 250 mL is indicated, though some recommend a lower volume threshold for temporarily stopping feedings.

Sources: Adapted from Bowman et al., 2005; Food and Drug Administration (FDA), 2003; Metheny, 2006.

MyNursingKit Oley Foundation: Home Parenteral and Enteral Nutrition Support

the client on long-term or permanent enteral feeding, the nurse can provide needed psychosocial support. Body image issues and adjustment to a lifestyle that does not involve eating can be difficult. Loss of social contacts and deprivation of the pleasure of eating have a negative effect on quality of life (Bozzetti, 2008). Local and on-line support groups exist to support clients who are on home enteral nutrition.

Parenteral Nutrition

Parenteral nutrition is indicated when a client requires specialized nutrition support and the gastrointestinal tract is not functioning. Intestinal obstruction, bowel ischemia, lack of gut peristalsis (**paralytic ileus**), and loss of significant absorptive surface (**short bowel syndrome**) are examples of conditions that can warrant parenteral nutrition support. A combination of parenteral and enteral nutrition support can be used when tolerance to enteral nutrition is limited (de Aguilar-Nascimento & Kudsk, 2008).

Parenteral Formulas

Parenteral nutrition is comprised of carbohydrates, protein, and lipids. Vitamins, minerals, and electrolytes are also included. In certain cases, medications such as insulin can be added by the pharmacist when preparing the solution. The prescription for parenteral nutrition is customized to meet the unique nutritional and metabolic needs of a client.

Nutrient Content

The macronutrient content of parenteral nutrition must be in the most basic form because the solution bypasses the digestive and absorptive processes and is infused directly into the bloodstream. Dextrose is the intravenous name for glucose, which is the carbohydrate used in parenteral solutions. This form of simple carbohydrate has 3.4 kcalories/gm. It is available in solutions from 5% dextrose in water (or D5W) and higher. Box 16-5 outlines sample calculations that the nurse could do to assess the energy contribution of intravenous dextrose. The nurse should be mindful that provision of dextrose alone is not considered nutrition support and does not contribute significant energy toward the client's needs. Dextrose solutions over 10% must be infused via a central vein because of the hypertonic concentration that results in water shifts into the vein, a consequence that would have a negative outcome in a small peripheral vein. The liver has a limited ability to handle metabolism of high glucose loads. If the recommended threshold of 4 mg glucose/kg body weight/minute is exceeded, hyperglycemia and its consequences can develop in the short term; fatty liver is a long-term risk (Ukleja & Romano, 2007).

Protein in parenteral solutions is in the form of amino acids. Solutions vary in concentration from 3% to 15%. Amino acids contain 4 kcalories/gm but seldom do clinicians consider this nutrient for its energy contribution when calculating the needs of the critically ill client because its purpose is for protein synthesis, not fuel. The nutrition support team determines the protein needs of the client as well as the indication for any specialized amino acids formulas, such as those with extra glutamine or arginine. These amino acids and others may have some beneficial effects in the critically ill client, though research results vary (Todd, Gonzalez, Turner, & Kozar, 2008). Chapter 22 discusses this concept. The protein needs for various medical conditions, such as renal disease, burns, and sepsis, are discussed in the respective chapters on those disorders.

Lipids are available in solutions of 10% or 20% concentration and contain 1.1 kcalories/mL or 2 kcalories/mL, respectively. In addition to contributing to fuel needs, lipids provide essential fatty acids to the client unable to meet those needs enterally. Soybean oil has been used traditionally in lipid solutions, but recent developments favor solutions made from coconut, olive, or fish oils for their improved effect on immunity and the inflammatory response (Gawecka, Michalkiewicz, Kornacka, Luckiewicz, & Kubiszewska, 2008; Wanten & Calder, 2007). Lipid emulsions are isotonic and, therefore, can be delivered through a peripheral vein or along with the peripherally or centrally administered dextrose/amino acid solution without affecting the osmolality.

BOX 16-5	Calculating Energy from Dextrose Solutions

Peripheral intravenous infusion of dextrose is limited to 5–10% solutions. Follow these steps to calculate the contribution of dextrose to a client's overall energy needs.

An order is written for 2 L/day of D5W.

1. D5W = 5% dextrose in water or 5 gm dextrose/100 gm water
2. 5 gm dextrose/100 gm water = 50 gm dextrose/1,000 gm water (or 1,000 mL water because the density of water is 1 gm/mL)
3. If 50 gm dextrose/1,000 mL, then 100 gm dextrose in prescribed 2,000 mL (2 L)
4. 100 gm dextrose × 3.4 kcalories/gm = 340 kcalories in 2 L D5W

- Follow these same steps and calculate the amount of energy in 3 L of D10W. What conclusion do you find about the energy provided by this solution when it is not accompanied by any other source of nutrition (oral, enteral, or parenteral) as can be a common occurrence?

Electrolytes, vitamins, and minerals are added to the parenteral solution in accordance with medical standards and client need. Electrolytes are adjusted based on the client's laboratory indices. Vitamin additives may or may not contain vitamin K, a fact that should be monitored in the client on anticoagulant therapy as outlined in Chapter 24. Some health care institutions utilize standardized parenteral nutrition formulas, whereas others use customized formulas that are compounded by the pharmacist. Others use a combination of both types.

Administration Route and Rate

The route and rate of parenteral solution delivery depends on the condition and assessed nutrient needs of the client.

Peripheral Parenteral vs. Total Parenteral Route

The estimated course of nutrition support will dictate the type of parenteral nutrition used, as noted in Figure 16-1. Parenteral nutrition via a peripheral vein is used in cases where the need for nutrition support is estimated to be short term and the client is able to handle the fluid volume of the solution (ASPEN, 2002). When it is likely that parenteral nutrition will be needed for more than 10 days, or the client is fluid restricted, total parenteral nutrition (TPN) utilizing a central vein is indicated (ASPEN, 2002). Peripheral parenteral nutrition (PPN) solutions must be approximately isotonic because vein collapse or phlebitis will result from hypertonic solution in a small vein. As a result of this requirement, PPN dictates the need for a lower dextrose concentration, with resultant lower calories, compared with TPN. The propensity to develop peripheral thrombophlebitis over time, coupled with the limited calorie content of peripheral solutions, illustrates its appropriateness for short-term rather than long-term use (Culebras, Martin-Pena, Garcia-de-Lorenzo, Zarazaga, & Rodriguez-Montes, 2004). Hypertonic solutions found in TPN are tolerated by the large central veins, such as the subclavian vein depicted in Figure 16-4 ■, used to deliver this type of nutrition.

Administering Parenteral Nutrition

Like enteral nutrition, parenteral nutrition is begun gradually with careful monitoring of client tolerance. High dextrose content and alterations in endogenous insulin production warrant close attention to blood glucose initially and then throughout the course of treatment. The nurse should be familiar with the institution's nutrition support protocol that outlines parameters for beginning parenteral nutrition and recommended volume limitations to avoid glucose intolerance or adverse reactions to intravenous lipids. Likewise, the protocol should outline a standard for tapering parenteral nutrition when indicated. Sudden cessation of high dextrose solutions, whether inadvertent or emergent, can lead to hypoglycemia because of circulating insulin in the bloodstream. TPN should be tapered over a minimum of several

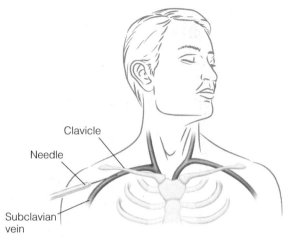

FIGURE 16-4 Subclavian Line.

hours to allow adjustment of endogenous insulin, or when necessary, peripheral dextrose should be administered to compensate for abrupt cessation.

Complications and Monitoring of Parenteral Nutrition

Parenteral nutrition requires diligent monitoring for short- and long-term complications. In particular, administration of high dextrose solutions using central venous access warrants close attention because of the accompanying septic and metabolic risks. Reports of the negative effects of hyperglycemia in the critically ill have further reinforced the need for close monitoring of blood glucose levels. Hyperglycemia in hospitalized clients is considered an independent risk factor for poor health outcomes, including infectious complications, poor wound healing, and dehydration; thus avoidance of iatrogenic contribution to this risk is urged with clients receiving parenteral nutrition (Balasubramanyam, 2009; Nasraway, 2006). Additional complications include catheter-related infections and electrolyte disturbances, which includes refeeding syndrome. Complications and monitoring advice are outlined in Table 16-4. The nurse working in a hospital, long-term care, or home care should be fully knowledgeable about the respective institution's protocol for monitoring parenteral nutrition and the responsibilities of the nurse in the meticulous care of the intravenous line.

In addition to monitoring the clinical tolerance to parenteral nutrition, the nurse is instrumental in providing the client with needed psychosocial support. In a review of quality of life issues in clients on home parenteral nutrition, problems such as depression, anxiety, sleep disruption, and altered social life were cited as common (Huisman-de Waal, Schoonhoven, Jansen, Wanten, & van Achterberg, 2007). Both local and on-line social support groups exist for home parenteral nutrition clients and caregivers.

Table 16-4   Parenteral Nutrition Complications and Nursing Intervention

Complication	Recommendations and Nursing Interventions
Altered fluid status	Monitor daily weight and intake and outputs (I & Os). Monitor lab values. Observe for signs of fluid excess or dehydration (edema, thirst, heart rate, urine output).
Altered metabolic status • Acid-base disturbances • Hyperglycemia • Hypertriglyceridemia • Refeeding syndrome	Monitor laboratory values. Formula can be altered by nutrition team. Avoid exceeding maximum recommended glucose delivery rate. Insulin may be added to solution with prescription. Avoid exceeding maximum recommended lipid delivery rate. Assess for overfeeding of dextrose or lipid. Consider cyclical lipid infusion vs. continuous. Increase feeding rate slowly to achieve goal in clients at risk (prolonged poor intake, low weight). Monitor fluid status, laboratory values for potassium and phosphorus. Replace as needed.
Catheter infection or malfunction	Follow institutional protocol for aseptic technique in caring for catheter and dressing. Monitor site for signs of infection. Maintain dedicated line for parenteral solution.
Drug–parenteral solution interaction	Catheter for parenteral nutrition should not be used for drug delivery. Consult with pharmacist on compatibility of medications given through Y-injection site near solution infusion.
Hepatobiliary disease (long-term complication)	Monitor liver function tests. Avoid overfeeding—minimize hyperglycemia/hypertriglyceridemia.
Metabolic bone disease (long-term complication)	Monitor for symptoms of bone disease (pain, atraumatic fractures). Underlying medical condition may predispose to risk. Consult with nutrition team for alternate supplementation of calcium, vitamin D, or formula change.

Palliative Nutrition and End-of-Life Care

Aggressive provision of specialized nutrition support is not always indicated. In cases such as the terminally ill client or those with advanced dementia, the health care team and the client or proxy should evaluate the benefits and burdens of nonoral feeding, whether by feeding tube or parenteral route (ADA, 2008; Hoffer, 2006). **Palliative nutrition,** or nutrition meant to aid in relief of symptoms or discomfort rather than cure, may be indicated in some clients. The decision whether or not to pursue active provision of nutrition and hydration is a multidisciplinary one with the client's wishes at the center. When clients are unable to express a decision about medical care, their advance directive should be consulted. An alternative decision-maker or legally designated health care proxy may also be involved. For the informed client with decision-making capacity, the bioethical principle of autonomy should be central in medical care choice, accompanied by doing no harm (nonmaleficence), doing good (beneficence), and justice (ADA, 2008). The cultural contribution to decisions about providing nutrition during the end of life is outlined in Cultural Consideration Box: Palliative Nutrition Decision Making.

Cultural Considerations

Palliative Nutrition Decision Making

Cultural beliefs, especially those that are religious, play an important role in an individual's regard for life and philosophy about life-prolonging treatments during terminal illness. Some religions recognize the need for an individualized "benefit vs. burden" approach to providing aggressive nutrition or hydration, whereas others dictate that there is a moral obligation to continue treatment once it has begun (ADA, 2008). Deep-rooted cultural and religious beliefs lead some to consider the withholding of nutrition support as deliberate starvation (Casarett, Kapo, & Caplan, 2005). It is essential that the health care team explore and respect the effect of any cultural or religiously held beliefs and values on the client's decision making.

If the decision is made to not pursue active nutrition support, providing oral hydration and nutrition can be implemented to client tolerance. The nurse should assess the client for symptoms, including any discomfort, and collaborate with the client to determine what and how much they wish to consume. In the terminally ill client, loss of appetite is common and not felt to negatively impact on overall comfort or suffering (ADA, 2008). Thirst can be alleviated with liquids as tolerated, ice chips, mouth care, and lubricating the lips (ADA, 2008; Casarett, Kapo, & Caplan, 2005). When dehydration and its metabolic consequences occur, a sedative effect results along with reduction in oral secretions, urination, and bronchial congestion—all of which may lessen client suffering (ADA, 2008; Truog & Cochrane, 2005). In a world of high technology, medical advances, and profound personal beliefs, it can be a difficult process for the clinician to be involved in decision making regarding the withholding of nutrition support. An understanding of the ethical, legal, medical, and personal components contributing to how such decisions are made is essential for the nurse involved in end-of-life care.

NURSING CARE PLAN Nutrition and Home Enteral Feedings

CASE STUDY

Hiram is an 82-year-old man who had a cerebral vascular accident (CVA), or stroke, 6 months ago. He lives with his elderly wife, Rebecca, who is his primary caregiver. Until the time of his CVA he had been independent and loved traveling. He now has significant right-sided weakness and dysphagia. A home care aide comes in three times a week to assist with bathing and to allow his wife to get out of the house for awhile. He has a bolus enteral feeding that his wife administers with a syringe through a PEG tube. His two married sons come at least once weekly, but they have college-age children and are busy professionals so find it hard to spend much time with their parents. Both provide some financial assistance by paying utility bills and for lawn care services. They express concern about learning any of the physical care. Hiram is due for a checkup with his primary care provider so Rebecca calls ahead to share some of her concerns with the nurse. She said she is getting worn out with the physical care of her husband who uses a walker but moves very slowly. She also mentions that he has become incontinent due to frequent episodes of diarrhea. He seems to be more depressed and gets angry very easily, something he never did in the past. She asks if there is any hope he will ever eat again; he is so thin.

Applying the Nursing Process

ASSESSMENT

Weight: 128 pounds Height: 5 feet 8 inches BMI: 19.5
Weight 1 month ago: 133.5 pounds
T 97.8 P 76 R 14 BP 126/68
Right-sided weakness; unable to shake hands or grasp a ball
Requires assistance to stand or sit
PEG tube in place; site is dry without redness or swelling
Bowel sounds are very active
Wearing adult incontinence pads
States: "I am disgusting and feel dirty all the time."

DIAGNOSES

Imbalanced nutrition: less than body requirements related to inadequate balance of intake and output
Fecal incontinence related to enteral feeding
Impaired body image related to incontinence, weight loss, and loss of mobility
Impaired mobility related to neurological dysfunction
Family stress related to role changes

EXPECTED OUTCOMES

Weight gain of 1 pound in 2 weeks
Plan for additional help with caregiving
No additional episodes of fecal incontinence
Additional assistive devices to improve mobility
Expressed improvement in appearance

INTERVENTIONS

Discuss enteral feedings with Rebecca: specific formula, rate and time of administration
Determine if there is a pattern to diarrhea episodes
Consult with pharmacist regarding whether any prescribed medications are hypertonic or contain sorbitol
Referral to speech therapy to reassess dysphagia and determine possibility of oral feedings
Social service referral for home safety assessment and level of possible family involvement in care
Physical therapy referral for reassessment of mobility level and need for additional assistive devices

EVALUATION

Hiram and Rebecca return to the clinic 2 weeks later. Hiram has gained 1.5 pounds. They now have a pump that is used for intermittent feedings. Both of them have learned to set it and have confidence that the slower rate for the feeding has diminished the diarrhea. They have used the pump for 10 days and he has had diarrhea only three times since they started using it. No medications were felt to contribute to the diarrhea. They stated that the near-elimination of diarrhea has been the biggest improvement. They had home visits from the speech and

Nutrition and Home Enteral Feedings *(continued)*

physical therapists. The speech therapist stated that no improvement was expected and that enteral feedings would be required for the foreseeable future. The physical therapist will visit three times weekly for strengthening exercise and recommended a lift device and a chair that rises electronically. In consultation with their sons and so-cial service, they are beginning to explore assisted living facilities. They do not want to leave their home, but Rebecca acknowledges that she does not know how much longer she can continue to provide the level of care Hiram now requires. Figure 16-5 ■ outlines the nursing process for this case.

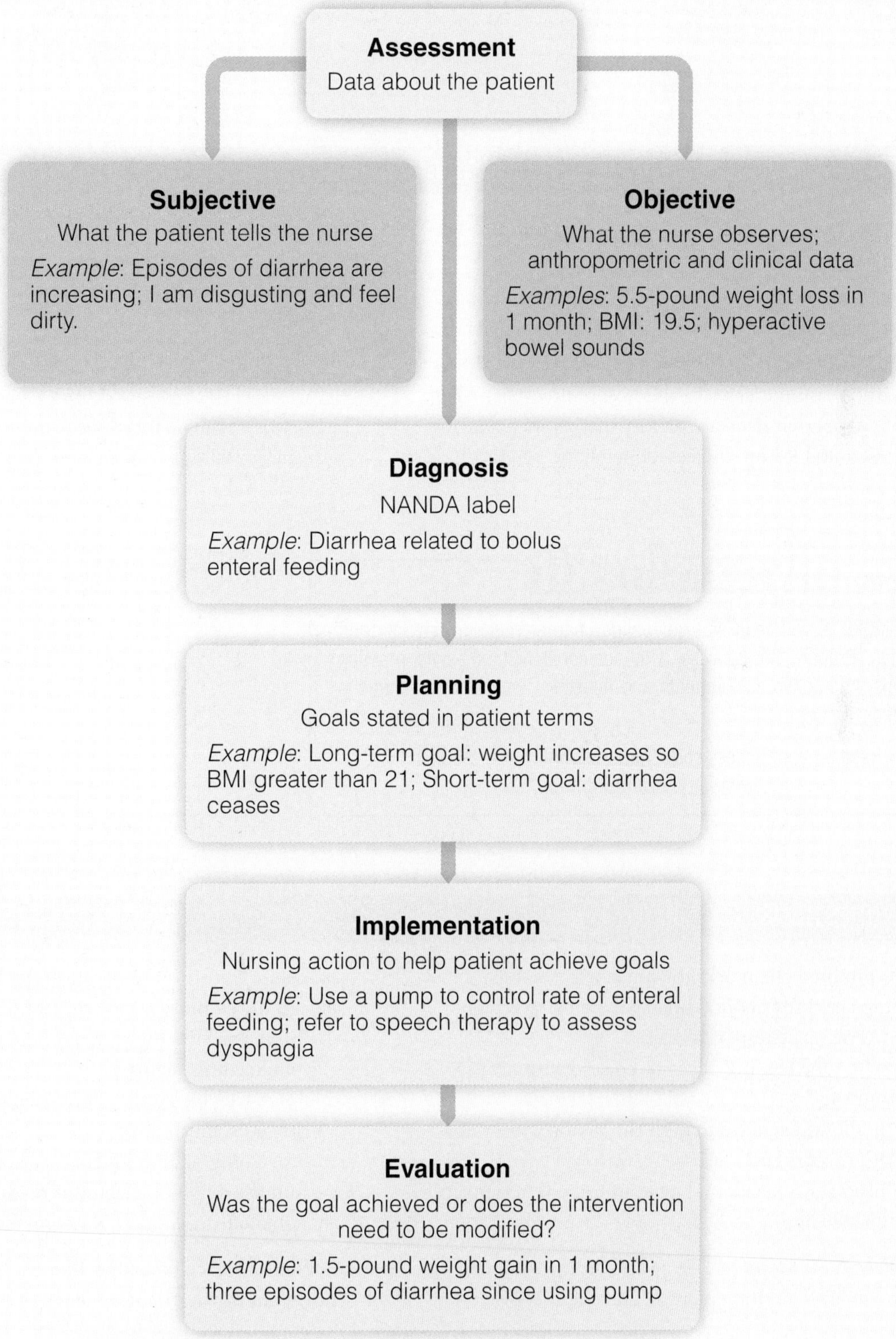

Assessment
Data about the patient

Subjective
What the patient tells the nurse
Example: Episodes of diarrhea are increasing; I am disgusting and feel dirty.

Objective
What the nurse observes; anthropometric and clinical data
Examples: 5.5-pound weight loss in 1 month; BMI: 19.5; hyperactive bowel sounds

Diagnosis
NANDA label
Example: Diarrhea related to bolus enteral feeding

Planning
Goals stated in patient terms
Example: Long-term goal: weight increases so BMI greater than 21; Short-term goal: diarrhea ceases

Implementation
Nursing action to help patient achieve goals
Example: Use a pump to control rate of enteral feeding; refer to speech therapy to assess dysphagia

Evaluation
Was the goal achieved or does the intervention need to be modified?
Example: 1.5-pound weight gain in 1 month; three episodes of diarrhea since using pump

■ **FIGURE 16-5 Nursing Care Plan Process: Nutrition and Home Enteral Feedings.**

(continued)

Nutrition and Home Enteral Feedings (continued)

Critical Thinking in the Nursing Process

1. What assessment data should the nurse request from a client who develops diarrhea while receiving home enteral therapy?

2. What can the nurse suggest to the client and family members who express concern about being able to manage enteral feedings at home?

CHAPTER SUMMARY

- *Medical nutrition therapy* is the term used to indicate the nutritional care of any medical illness or condition.

- The nutrition care of the hospitalized client includes both the clinical nutrition services of medical nutrition therapy and the provision of food service.

- Malnutrition risk increases in the hospitalized client because of factors that decrease dietary intake, increase nutrient losses, and lead to increased metabolic needs.

- The provision of specialized nutrition support in the form of enteral or parenteral nutrition should be done after careful consideration of the indications, risks, and benefits of treatment.

- Palliative nutrition care involves providing hydration and nutrition in accordance with client-centered decisions.

- The nurse is a vital member of the interdisciplinary health care team providing nutrition support and care.

PEARSON
EXPLORE mynursingkit™

MyNursingKit is your one stop for online chapter review materials and resources. Prepare for success with additional NCLEX®-style practice questions, interactive assignments and activities, web links, animations and videos, and more!

Register your access code from the front of your book at
www.mynursingkit.com.

NCLEX® QUESTIONS

1. A hospitalized client asks the nurse why the tube feeding lasts only about 6 hours before being replenished. The nurse responds that:
   1. "The tube feeding needs to be cold while it is running."
   2. "It allows the nurse to flush the tubing with water."
   3. "It prevents bacterial overgrowth."
   4. "It prevents accidental rapid infusion of too much tube feeding."

2. A client had extensive surgery and during recuperation needed TPN for a month. The client is going to make the transition to oral feeding. What will be included in the nurse's plan of care?
   1. Stop the TPN infusion at 0800 on the morning oral feeding begins.
   2. Give ice chips until client tolerance for oral feeding is established.
   3. Give only small frequent meals during the day and run the TPN for 8 hours at night.
   4. Gradually reduce TPN as oral feedings increase.

3. A client is placed on a mechanical soft diet. The nurse knows the client understood dietary teaching

when the client states which of the following foods should not be eaten?

1. Hot dogs
2. Apricot nectar
3. Macaroni and cheese
4. Canned tuna

4. A family member examined the bag of TPN and asked the nurse why it contained insulin because the client was not diabetic. The nurse responded that:
   1. "A recent diagnosis of type 2 diabetes had been made and that insulin was necessary to treat the client."
   2. "The TPN contains a high concentration of sugars and extra insulin is needed to help break down the sugars until the client's pancreas gets used to the load."
   3. "This way the client will not need daily injections."
   4. "I will verify this order with the physician."

5. The spouse of an elderly client receiving home enteral therapy calls to tell the nurse that diarrhea has become a big problem. In order to assess the situation, what should the nurse first ask the spouse?
   1. "What is the name of the feeding solution and how fast is it running?"
   2. "What is the reason for the enteral feeding?"
   3. "Does the client have edema or increased thirst?"
   4. "When was your last consultation with the dietitian?"

REFERENCES

American Dietetic Association (ADA). (2005). Position of the American Dietetic Association: Liberalization of the diet prescription improves quality of life for older adults in long-term care. *Journal of the American Dietetic Association, 105*, 1955–1965.

American Dietetic Association (ADA). (2008). Position of the American Dietetic Association: Ethical and legal issues in nutrition, hydration, and feeding. *Journal of the American Dietetic Association, 108*, 873–882.

ASPEN Board of Directors and the Clinical Guidelines Task Force. (2002). Guidelines for the use of parenteral and enteral nutrition in adult and pediatric patients. *Journal of Parenteral and Enteral Nutrition, 26*, 1SA–126SA.

Balasubramanyam, A. (2009). Intensive glycemic control in the intensive care unit: Promises and pitfalls. *Journal of Endocrinology & Metabolism, 94*, 416–417.

Baldwin, C., Parsons, T., & Logan, S. (2007). Dietary advice for illness-related malnutrition in adults. *Cochrane Database Systematic Review, 1*, CD 002008.

Bavelaar, J. W., Otter, C. D., van Bodegraven, A. A., Thijs, A., & van Bokhorst-de van der Schueren, M. A. E. (2008). Diagnosis and treatment of disease-related in-hospital malnutrition: The performance of medical and nursing staff. *Clinical Nutrition, 27*, 431–438.

Boutilier, R. G., Murray, S. K., & Walley, V. M. (2000). Green colon: An unusual appearance at autopsy. *Archives of Pathology and Laboratory Medicine, 124*(9), 1397–1398.

Bowman, A., Greiner, J. E., Doerschug, K. C., Little, S. B., Bombei, C. L., & Comried, L. M. (2005). Implementation of an evidence-based feeding protocol and aspiration risk reduction algorithm. *Critical Care Nursing Quarterly, 28*, 324–333.

Bozzetti, F. (2008). Quality of life and enteral nutrition. *Current Opinion in Clinical Nutrition and Metabolic Care, 11*, 661–665.

Casarett, D., Kapo, J., & Caplan, A. (2005). Appropriate use of artificial nutrition and hydration—Fundamental principles and recommendations. *New England Journal of Medicine, 353*, 2607–2612.

Chima, C. S. (2007). Diet manuals to practice manuals: The evolution of nutrition care. *Nutrition in Clinical Practice, 22*, 89–100.

Culebras, J. M., Martin-Pena, G., Garcia-de-Lorenzo, A., Zarazaga, A., & Rodriguez-Montes, J. A. (2004). Practical aspects of peripheral parenteral nutrition. *Current Opinion in Clinical Nutrition and Metabolic Care, 7*, 303–307.

de Aguilar-Nascimento, J. E., & Kudsk, K. A. (2008). Early nutritional therapy: The role of enteral and parenteral nutrition. *Current Opinion in Clinical Nutrition and Metabolic Care, 11*, 255–260.

Food and Drug Administration (FDA), Center for Food Safety and Applied Nutrition (2003). *FDA Public Health Advisory: Reports of blue discoloration and death in patients receiving enteral feedings tinted with the dye, FD&C blue1.* Retrieved April 1, 2009, from http://www.cfsan.fda.gov/~dms/col-ltr2.html

Gawecka, A., Michalkiewicz, J., Kornacka, M., Luckiewicz, B., & Kubiszewska, I. (2008). Immunologic properties differ in preterm infants fed olive oil vs. soy-based lipid emulsions during parenteral nutrition. *Journal of Parenteral and Enteral Nutrition, 32*, 448–453.

Granville, L. A., & Finch, C. (2001). Blue colon at autopsy. *Archives of Pathology and Laboratory Medicine, 125*(5), 599.

Guzy, C., Schirbel, A., Paclik, D., Wiedenmann, B., Dignass, A., & Sturm, A. (2009). Enteral and parenteral nutrition distinctively modulate intestinal permeability and T cell function in vitro. *European Journal of Nutrition, 48*, 12–21.

Hancock, S., Cresci, G., & Martindale, R. (2002). The clear liquid diet: When is it appropriate? *Current Gastroenterology Reports, 4*, 324–331.

Heyland, D. K., Dhaliwal, R., Drover, J. W., Gramlich, L., Dodek, P., & the Canadian Critical Care Practice Committee. (2003). Canadian clinical guidelines for nutrition support in mechanically ventilated critically ill patients. *Journal of Parenteral and Enteral Nutrition, 27*, 355–373.

Hoffer, L. J. (2006). Controversy: Tube feeding in advanced dementia: The metabolic perspective. *British Medical Journal, 333*, 1214–1215.

Huisman-de Waal, G., Schoonhoven, L., Jansen, J., Wanten, G., & van Achterberg, T. (2007). The impact of home parenteral nutrition on daily life—A review. *Clinical Nutrition, 26*, 275–288.

Jeejeebhoy, K. N. (2007). Enteral nutrition versus parenteral nutrition – the risks and benefits. *Nature Clinical Practice: Gastroenterology & Hepatology, 4*, 260–265.

Jones, N. E., & Heyland, D. K. (2008). Implementing nutrition guidelines in the critical care setting: A worthwhile and achievable goal? *Journal of the American Medical Association, 300*, 2798–2799.

Kagansky, N., Berner, Y., Morag-Koren, N., Perelman, L., Knobler, H., & Levy, S. (2005). Poor nutritional habits are predictors of poor outcome in very old hospitalized patients. *American Journal of Clinical Nutrition, 82*, 784–791.

Kreymann, K. G., Berger, M. M., Deutz, N. E. P., Hiesmayr, M., Jolliet, P., Kazandjiev, G., et al. (2006). ESPEN guidelines on enteral nutrition. *Clinical Nutrition, 25*, 210–223.

REFERENCES *(continued)*

Louie, B. E., Noseworthy, T., Hailey, D., Gramlich, L. M., Jacobs, P., & Warnock, G. L. (2005). Enteral or parenteral nutrition for pancreatitis: A randomized controlled trial and health assessment. *Canadian Journal of Surgery, 48,* 298–306.

Lucarelli, M. R., Shirk, M. B., Julian, M. W., & Crouser, E. D. (2004). Toxicity of Food Drug and Cosmetic Blue No. 1 dye in critically ill patients. *Chest, 125*(2), 793–795.

McClave, S. A., Chang, W. K., Dhaliwal, R., & Heyland, D. K. (2006). Nutrition support in acute pancreatitis: A systematic review of the literature. *Journal of Parenteral and Enteral Nutrition, 30,* 143–156.

Metheny, N. A. (2006). Preventing respiratory complications of tube feedings: Evidence-based practice. *American Journal of Critical Care, 15,* 360–369.

Metheny, N. A., Dahms, T. E., Stewart, B. J., Stone, K. S., Edwards, S. J., Defer, J. E., et al. (2002). Efficacy of dye-stained enteral formula in detecting pulmonary aspiration. *Chest, 122*(1), 276–281.

Miller, C. A., Grossman, S., Hindley, E., Macgarvie, D., & Madill, J. (2008). Are enterally fed ICU patients meeting clinical practice guidelines? *Nutrition in Clinical Practice, 23,* 642–650.

Milne, A. C., Avenell, A., & Potter, J. (2006). Meta-analysis: Protein and energy supplementation in older people. *Annals of Internal Medicine, 144,* 37–48.

Nasraway, S. A. (2006). Hyperglycemia during critical illness. *Journal of Parenteral and Enteral Nutrition, 30,* 254–258.

National Institute for Health and Clinical Excellence (NICE). (2006). *Nutrition support in adults: Full report.* Retrieved April 1, 2009, from http://www.nice.org.uk/guidance/index.jsp?action=download&o=29981

Neumann, S. A., Miller, M. D., Daniels, L., & Crotty, M. (2005). Nutritional status and clinical outcomes of older patients in reha-

bilitation. *Journal of Human Nutrition & Dietetics, 18,* 129–136.

Norman, K., Pichard, C., Lochs, H., & Pirlich, M. (2008). Prognostic impact of disease-related malnutrition. *Clinical Nutrition, 27,* 5–15.

Panteli, J. V., & Crook, M. A. (2009). Refeeding syndrome still needs to be recognized and managed properly. *Nutrition, 25,* 130–131.

Pritchard, C., Duffy, S., Edington, J., & Pang, F. (2006). Enteral nutrition and oral nutrition supplements: A review of the economics literature. *Journal of Parenteral and Enteral Nutrition, 30,* 52–59.

Sanko, J. S. (2004). Aspiration assessment and prevention in critically ill enterally fed patients: Evidence-based recommendations for practice. *Gastroenterology Nursing, 27*(6), 279–285.

Simmons, S. E., & Patel, A. V. (2006). Nursing home staff delivery of oral liquid nutritional supplements to residents at risk for unintentional weight loss. *Journal of the American Geriatric Society, 54,* 1372–1376.

Singh, H., Watt, K., Veitch, R., Cantor, M., & Duerksen, D. R. (2006). Malnutrition is prevalent in hospitalized medical patients: Are housestaff identifying the malnourished patient? *Nutrition, 22,* 350–354.

Stanga, Z., Brunner, A., Leuenberger, M., Grimble, R. F., Shenkin, A., Allison, S. P., et al. (2008). Nutrition in clinical practice—the refeeding syndrome: Illustrative cases and guidelines for prevention and treatment. *European Journal of Clinical Nutrition, 62,* 687–694.

Suominen, M. H., Sandelin, E., Soini, H., & Pitkala, K. H. (2009). How well do nurses recognize malnutrition in elderly patients? *European Journal of Clinical Nutrition, 63,* 292–296.

Thomas, D. R. (2005). Weight loss in older adults. *Reviews in Endocrine & Metabolic Disorders, 6,* 129–136.

Thomson, A. (2008). Nutritional support in acute pancreatitis. *Current Opinion in Clinical Nutrition and Metabolic Care, 11,* 261–266.

Todd, S. R., Gonzalez, E. A., Turner, K., & Kozar, R. A. (2008). Update on postinjury nutrition. *Current Opinion in Critical Care, 14,* 690–695.

Truog, R. D., & Cochrane, T. I. (2005). Refusal of hydration and nutrition. *Archives of Internal Medicine, 165,* 2574–2576.

Ukleja, A., & Romano, M. M. (2007). Complications of parenteral nutrition. *Gastroenterology Clinics of North America, 36,* 23–46.

Volkert, D., Berner, Y. N., Berry, E., Cederholm, T., Coti Bertrand, P., Milne, A., et al. (2006). ESPEN guidelines on enteral nutrition: Geriatrics. *Clinical Nutrition, 25,* 330–360.

Wanten, G., & Calder, P. C. (2007). Immune modulation by parenteral lipid emulsions. *American Journal of Clinical Nutrition, 85,* 1171–1184.

Weimann, A., Braga, M., Harsanyi, L., Laviano, A., Ljungquist, O., Soeters, P., et al. (2006). ESPEN guidelines on enteral nutrition: Surgery including organ transplant. *Clinical Nutrition, 25,* 224–244.

Williams, N. T. (2008). Medication administration through enteral feeding tubes. *American Journal of Health-Systems Pharmacy, 65,* 2347–2357.

Wright, L., Hickson, M., & Frost, G. (2006). Eating together is important: Using a dining room in an acute elderly medical ward increases energy intake. *Journal of Human Nutrition and Dietetics, 19,* 23–26.

Xia, C., & McCutcheon, H. (2006). Mealtimes in hospital-who does what? *Journal of Clinical Nursing, 15,* 1221–1227.

Zillich, A. J., Kuhn, R. J., & Petersen, T. J. (2000). Skin discoloration with blue food coloring. *The Annals of Pharmacotherapy, 34*(7-8), 868–870.

Weight Management 17

WHAT WILL YOU LEARN?

1. To relate the assessment parameters used in formulating nursing nutritional interventions for overweight clients and those with eating disorders.
2. To analyze risk factors for the development of overweight and eating disorders.
3. To formulate a treatment plan using lifestyle management for overweight.
4. To examine nutritional concerns following bariatric surgery.
5. To define and differentiate between the clinical parameters and treatment approaches of each type of eating disorder.

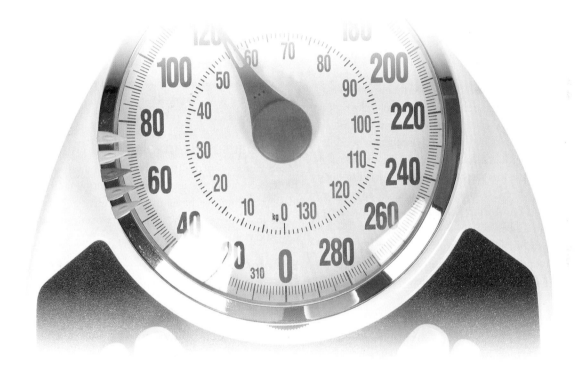

DID YOU KNOW?

- Two-thirds of dieting high school students are already at a normal weight.
- Restaurant portion sizes have increased between two- to eightfold in the last decade.
- Some forms of weight loss surgery cause lifelong malabsorption.
- The risk of developing an eating disorder is increased with participation in certain sports, such as wrestling, cross country, and gymnastics.
- Binge eating disorder is included in the category of eating disorders even though overweight is generally the outcome.

KEY TERMS

abdominal obesity, *374*

anorexia nervosa, *391*

bariatric surgery, *386*

binge eating disorder, *394*

bulimia nervosa, *393*

disordered eating, *388*

empty calorie foods, *378*

hunger-obesity paradox, *376*

lanugo, *391*

morbid obesity, *376*

orthorexia, *391*

night eating syndrome (NES), *394*

refeeding syndrome, *392*

What Is Weight Management?

The prevalence of weight management issues is increasing across the lifespan. The nurse working in most settings should be well versed in current treatment approaches to this expanding problem. The rise in overweight and obesity has been labeled an epidemic by some, encompassing all population and age groups. In contrast, the Western cultural obsession with thinness has generated a lucrative diet industry of books, products, and diet programs. Sixty percent of adolescent females have attempted to diet in the last year when less than 30% are overweight. Of those, almost 12% use fasting for 24 hours as a weight loss method and almost 5% use laxatives or vomiting to try controlling weight (Centers for Disease Control and Prevention [CDC], 2008a). Unhealthy or severe dieting practices are one risk factor for the development of eating disorders (Neumark-Sztainer et al., 2006). Weight management encompasses nutrition interventions for overweight, obesity, and eating disorders.

Overweight and Obesity

Overweight and obesity are defined as the accumulation of excess body fat. Body mass index (BMI) is used as a measure to determine weight status although it does not specifically measure body fat. A BMI *greater than or equal to* 25 is considered overweight, and a BMI *greater than or equal to* 30 denotes obesity. Waist circumference and waist-to-hip ratio are used as adjunct tools to define **abdominal obesity,** the accumulation of excess fat around the midsection of the trunk versus the hips. Abdominal obesity is a risk factor for cardiovascular disease (Mahabadi et al., 2009). Chapter 12 outlines the methods used in the measurement of BMI and waist circumference.

Over 60% of adults in the United States are overweight or obese, an almost twofold increase in obesity since the 1980s (CDC, 2008b). Lifespan Box: Overweight and Obesity outlines the prevalence of overweight and obesity across the lifespan, illustrating the importance of weight management

intervention. Further, certain ethnic populations have a greater prevalence of overweight as outlined in Cultural Considerations Box: Overweight among Ethnic Groups. In particular in both adults and adolescents, the highest prevalence of obesity is found among black females, especially those with lower income and less education (Ogden, 2009). However, the greatest increase in the prevalence of obesity is found among high-income groups for all race-ethnic populations (Ogden, 2009).

What Causes Overweight and Obesity?

Many factors contribute to the development of overweight. Biology, including genetics; environmental factors; and medications are among the many reasons cited as possibly playing a role in why overweight and obesity occur in some individuals and not in others.

Biology

Genetic and metabolic influences predispose some individuals to overweight. Body weight is regulated through a variety of endocrine hormones and the hypothalamus. Metabolic disorders, such as hypothyroid disease, can affect metabolism and body

---

Lifespan

Overweight and Obesity

Who is overweight in the United States?

12.4% of children age 2–5 years

17% of children age 6–11 years

17.6% of adolescents age 12–19 years

66.9% of adults age 20 years and over are overweight or obese.

34% of adults age 20 years and over are obese.

33% of adults age 65 years or over are obese.

Extreme obesity (BMI greater than 40) exists in 2.8% men and 6.9% of women.

Source: CDC, 2008b.

Cultural Considerations

Overweight among Ethnic Groups

Children age 2–19 years:

24% of non-Hispanic black females and 18.6 % of males are overweight.

19.7% of Mexican American females and 27.5% of males are overweight.

14.4% of non-Hispanic white females and 15.5 % of males are overweight.

Adults 20 years and older:

80.5% of non-Hispanic black females and 72.1% of males are overweight (over 50% of females are obese).

74.4% of Mexican American females and 77.3% of males are overweight (over 40% females are obese).

57.4% of non-Hispanic white females and 72.1% of males are overweight (over 30% are obese).

Source: CDC, 2008b.

weight. Hormones that affect appetite and satiety, such as peptide YY, ghrelin, cortisol, and leptin are being investigated for potential links to obesity (Kushner, 2008). Leptin is believed to be responsible for exerting a feedback signal to the body when fullness occurs. Obese individuals have elevated plasma leptin levels in proportion to excess fat, yet some exhibit leptin resistance exhibited by a failure to exert the satiety signaling effect of the hormone (Bellar, Jarosz, & Bellar, 2008). The leptin gene code as well as several others may be involved in the genetic expression of obesity and are the subject of ongoing research. The effect of stress and sleep deprivation on appetite regulation is another evolving area of research. Cortisol and other components of the hypothalamic-pituitary-adrenal axis are altered with both stress and lack of sleep and may, in turn, foster a false hunger cue to the body (Lamberg, 2006). The Evidence-Based Practice Box: Does stress lead to the consumption of additional food and consequent weight gain? discusses the research relating to this aspect of weight management. Despite the interest

EVIDENCE-BASED PRACTICE RESEARCH BOX

Does stress lead to the consumption of additional food and consequent weight gain?

Clinical Problem: Many people report that stress causes them to eat more and then they gain weight. What research has been done that shows a link between stress and weight gain in adults?

Research Findings: Many working adults experience varying degrees of stress in the workplace. Just as there can be many causes of stress, there can be many responses to that stress, one of which is a reported tendency to eat more and experience subsequent weight gain. There have been some studies seeking to determine the relationship between stress and weight gain. A team of researchers studied a cohort of more than 6,700 female Danish nurses who participated in a longitudinal health study. The researchers studied psychological workload (busyness in the job, job speed, job influence), lifestyle, and familial predisposition to obesity. They found over a course of 6 years that high psychological workload and familial predisposition to obesity were significantly predictive of weight gain (Overgaard, Gamborg, Gyntelberg, & Heitmann, 2004, 2006). Another study of Danish males examined the relationship between BMI and psychological demands at work. The researchers found that in the presence of stress, weight increased among obese employees and decreased among employees with a lower BMI (Hannerz, Albertson, Nielsen, Tuchsen, & Burr, 2004).

A group of researchers examined data from a 5-year study of British civil servants (5,547 males, 2,418 females). They attempted to determine if job stress and initial BMI influenced weight gain or loss. Findings showed that among men, job stress was significantly associated with baseline BMI; those with the highest BMI gained weight and those with the lowest BMI lost weight. Similar findings were not present with women (Kivimaki et al., 2006). A weak association between baseline BMI and work stress was found in

a study of 45,810 male and female employees in Finland (Kouvonen, Kivimaki, Cox, Cox, & Vahtera, 2005). Another study of almost 8,000 Finnish men and women showed only a weak association with work stress and weight gain. However, BMI was not a variable in this study (Lallukka, Laaksonen, Martikainen, Sarlio-Lahteenkorva, & Lahelma, 2005).

A study of a random sample of Australian male and female workers examined psychosocial working conditions and their influence on BMI. No longitudinal data were available and all data were self-reported. Researchers found that for males working long hours was positively associated with a higher BMI, and high physical demand (activity) was associated with a lower BMI. Similar results were not found with women (Ostry, Radi, Louie, & LaMontagne, 2006).

Another small study (308 subjects) of British civil servants examined the association of work stress and the risk of developing metabolic syndrome. Researchers found that over the 14 years for which data were available, employees with chronic stress at work were significantly more likely to have developed metabolic syndrome than those with low work stress (Chandola, Brunner, & Marmot, 2006).

Nursing Implications: There is some evidence that work-related stress is associated with weight gain. However, it seems that weight gain may be most closely associated with initial BMI, such that those with a higher BMI, especially males, are more likely to gain weight.

CRITICAL THINKING QUESTIONS:

1. How can the nurse respond to the middle-age client who recognizes weight gain and attributes it to eating in response to stress and sitting at a desk most of the day at work?

2. What food suggestions can the nurse give a client who says that a chocolate bar is good for stress relief and is a real comfort food?

in this fascinating area of biological influences on body weight, it is still felt that environmental influences must be present to lead to the genetic expression of obesity (American Dietetic Association [ADA], 2009; Bouchard, 2008).

Environment

Environmental influences that cause a change in energy balance can lead to weight gain. Factors that foster an increased consumption of calories and decreased expenditure of energy affect the calorie balance equation. Calorie-dense foods are widely available and standard portion sizes of many foods have increased. Americans are consuming more food outside the home than in the past. Prepared and restaurant foods often have larger portions, evidenced by serving sizes that are two- to eightfold greater than what the United States Department of Agriculture (USDA) recommends (Fisher & Kral, 2008). Restaurants offer increased portions of inexpensive, high-calorie foods such as sodas and fried food to appeal to the cost-conscious consumer. Research has shown that when larger portions are prepared, even in the home, larger portions are then served, and larger portions are also eaten. This effect is especially found to be true with foods that lack a specific shape that would denote a portion (Fisher & Krall, 2008). Further, food is widely available at all hours of the day and in nonfood venues such as gas stations and bookstores. Sweetened beverages, such as soda, are particularly targeted as contributors to obesity because such drinks contain excess kcalories and do not affect satiety (Bachman, Baranowski, & Nicklas, 2006). The sweeteners themselves are not felt to possess physiological or metabolic properties that cause obesity, but rather are a vehicle for intake of excess energy (Melanson et al., 2008).

Technology and a sedentary lifestyle contribute to decreased energy expenditure that offsets energy balance. Energy-saving devices such as remote controls, automatic door openers, power tools, and automated machinery result in less human energy use. Less physical labor and lack of exercise lead to a sedentary lifestyle. Almost 40% of adults in the United States are considered sedentary (CDC, 2008b). Increased "screen time" watching television or playing computer games is associated with obesity (Spear et al., 2007). Lower socioeconomic or educational status and development of built communities that foster automobile use rather than physical activity are additional contributors to a sedentary lifestyle (Spear et al., 2007).

Food insecurity and poverty are associated with overweight in what has been termed the **hunger-obesity paradox** (Tanumihardjo et al., 2007). This scenario is characterized by habitual intake of low-cost, high-fat foods and possible physiological adaptations to periods of episodic hunger from lack of food. The result is a combination of obesity and poor nutrient intake.

Medications and Weight Gain

Some medications have the unfortunate side effect of causing weight gain either by fostering increased appetite or reduced metabolic rate. Psychotropic medications in particular are linked with unintended weight gain. Atypical antipsychotics and some antidepressants and mood stabilizers are associated with weight gain. Medications such as the anticonvulsants valproic acid and carbamazepine, cyprohepatide used for allergy treatment, and corticosteroids also contribute to weight gain (Leslie, Hankey, & Lean, 2007). Cardiovascular medications called beta blockers are reported to slow metabolic rate by up to 12%, which can be clinically significant in some individuals (Dickerson & Roth-Yousey, 2005).

Health Risks of Obesity

Obesity, especially **morbid obesity** (BMI greater than 40), is associated with increased mortality and a shortened lifespan compared with normal weight (Flegal, Graubard, Williamson, & Gail, 2007; Poirier et al., 2006). Overweight may not negatively affect life expectancy to the same extent as does obesity, but it is associated with comorbid illnesses and conditions that affect quality of life. Comorbid illnesses associated with overweight and obesity include the following (Flegal et al., 2007; Kushner, 2007; Spiotta & Luma, 2008; Stothard, Tennant, Bell, & Rankin, 2009):

- Cardiovascular disease, high blood lipids, and hypertension
- Type 2 diabetes and insulin resistance
- Infertility and risk of congenital abnormalities and caesarian delivery with pregnancy
- Certain cancers
- Degenerative joint disease
- Sleep apnea and other chronic respiratory diseases
- Gastroesophageal reflux
- Kidney stone formation
- Gallstone formation
- Nonalcoholic fatty liver disease

In children, overweight and obesity contribute to similar health concerns as in the adult but also sets the stage for additional risks, including the likelihood of adult obesity. Obesity in children promotes advanced maturation, including increased levels of reproductive hormones, which in turn is a risk factor for the development of insulin resistance, polycystic ovary syndrome, growth plate injuries, and low self-esteem (ADA, 2006a; Levitsky, Misra, Boepple, & Hoppin, 2009).

Medical and Nutritional Interventions for Overweight and Obesity

In the United States, the National Heart, Lung, and Blood Institutes (NHLBI) recommends weight loss for obese individuals and those who are overweight and have an increased waist circumference or two or more cardiovascular risk factors (NHLBI, 1998). Although many individuals associate the need to lose weight with an all-or-nothing goal of achieving slimness, nurses should educate their clients that a beneficial improvement in health risks can be accomplished with a 5% to 10% reduction in weight (Poirier et al., 2006). Maintenance of weight loss in excess of 10% of body weight is poor in most groups of dieters, with fewer than 20% of individuals maintaining significant weight loss longer than 5 years (Daniels, 2006). Surgical intervention for severe obesity results in a greater percentage of weight loss than from diet and exercise but carries a risk of short- and long-term complications that must be weighed against outcome.

Assessment

Nursing intervention begins with a thorough assessment to provide the basis for a personalized approach. Providing a client with generalized recommendations for weight reduction along with lists of foods to avoid does not result in successful intervention for most individuals. Strategizing with the client and providing customized advice is preferable. Table 17-1 outlines factors to consider during the assessment of an overweight individual. Chapter 12 outlines specifics on performing the anthropometric measurements and nutrition history. Measurement of both BMI and waist circumference is recommended in adults because of the link between the central deposition of fat and cardiovascular disease (Mahabadi et al., 2009). Before beginning the assessment, resist telling clients that they are overweight. Practice Pearl: Beginning the Assessment provides a gentler approach to starting the assessment.

Treatment Options

Intervention for weight control depends on the results of the assessment. For example, an overweight client who is not ready to focus on losing weight can brainstorm with the nurse strategies to prevent further weight gain. Recommendations regarding lifespan considerations should be population specific, because weight control approaches for the adult do not uniformly apply to groups such as children, pregnant females, and older adults. Lifespan Box: Weight Control in Children, Pregnant Females, and Older Adults addresses lifespan specific concerns.

Weight management goals should be developed in collaboration with the client. Goals should be specific and

PRACTICE PEARL

Beginning the Assessment

Most overweight people know they are overweight. Resist initially *telling* someone that he or she is overweight and listing off all the accompanying health risks. Instead *ask* about the client's feelings regarding his or her body and weight. For example, say, "How do you feel about your weight?" This conversation starter will help later in assessing motivation and readiness for weight control that set the stage for client-centered goal setting. For the client who does not know he or she is overweight or the associated health risks, an initial goal may be to educate the client about body weight and these risks.

Table 17-1 Assessing the Overweight Client before Nutrition Intervention

Assessment Component	Parameters
Physical	• BMI: measure height and weight • Waist circumference • Waist-to-hip ratio • Body fat percentage
Medical History	• Existing comorbidities to overweight • Medical contributors to weight gain: active mental illness, metabolic disorders, limited mobility • Medications that contribute to weight gain • Weight history, pattern of weight gain, contributors/triggers to weight gain or regain after loss, maximum and minimum adult weights, family weight history • Physical activity level and ability
Nutrition	• Nutrition history: diet recall, meal and snack patterns, food preparation methods, skipped meals, meals away from home, time available for meals, dietary supplement use • Dieting history: methods of weight loss (types of diets, programs, products used), success and failures, length weight loss is maintained • Knowledge about nutrition, meal preparation skills, sources of health information
Motivation and Readiness for Change	• Personal reasons for weight control • Personal goals regarding weight and health • Personal readiness and willingness to manage weight (vs. being told by others) • Barriers to success: poor social support system, poor finances, food insecurity, substance abuse, eating disorder (binge eating, bulimia), active mental illness, barriers to physical activity

CT? What measures can the nurse take during the assessment process to avoid making the overweight client feel uncomfortable because of weight issues? What equipment should be available? How should the examination room and office be designed and furnished to be welcoming to all body types?

geared to behaviors and health outcomes in both the short and long term. Barriers to weight control should be specifically addressed in goal setting. Understanding motivation and readiness to address weight management plays a central role in determining goals. Reasonable and achievable goals will promote improved well-being and a sense of accomplishment. Goal setting specific only to cosmetic changes should be de-emphasized (ADA, 2009). A reduction of 10% of body weight is recommended as reasonable and achievable but obviously can be in contrast to a client's goal to achieve ideal weight because of societal influences on weight standards

Lifespan

Weight Control in Children, Pregnant Females, and Older Adults

Weight control guidelines for adults are not always appropriate for other population groups.

Children: Seldom is it appropriate to encourage a strict diet in an overweight child. Instead, lifestyle modifications, including balanced intake, fun physical activity, and family involvement, foster slowed weight gain while promoting normal growth and development is indicated.

Pregnant Female: Weight loss during pregnancy is contraindicated. Appropriate weight gain is essential for a healthy pregnancy. Obese females should gain approximately 11–20 pounds while pregnant.

Older Adults: Age alone does not preclude recommending weight loss. However, because of the high prevalence of undernutrition among older adults, careful evaluation should be made to assess risks and benefits of weight loss. Preservation of lean muscle is essential to avoid a functional decline.

CT? What advice should the nurse give to a pregnant female or child's parent or caregiver who requests a recommendation for a diet book or structured weight loss diet?

(NHLBI, 1998). Client education should focus on the benefits of even modest weight loss and discuss the negative effects of yo-yo weight control, where large amounts of weight are quickly and repeatedly lost and then slowly regained much to detriment of muscle mass and self-esteem. Even small amounts of weight loss can improve a sense of well-being and control of blood pressure, blood glucose, and lipids.

Lifestyle Modifications

Lifestyle modifications for weight loss include diet, physical activity, and behavior modification. Approximately 20% of overweight individuals who lose weight with nonsurgical intervention are successful at maintaining weight loss of at least 10% of body weight for at least 1 year, and attribute success to ongoing attention to diet, engaging in an hour of daily physical activity most days, and behaviors such as weight checks and not skipping breakfast (van Wormer et al., 2009). Figure 17-1 ■ outlines the treatment algorithm for lifestyle modifications for adults in weight control. In children, the American Academy of Pediatrics recommends that nutrition, behavior, and physical activity interventions focus on weight maintenance as the initial step. A more structured approach is not used unless the child continues to gain weight with increases in stature and remains in the 95th percentile or above for BMI (Spear et al., 2007). Weight maintenance interventions should include the whole family and focus on healthful eating, regular physical activity, and reduced screen

time. A more structured approach involves a referral to a registered dietitian for nutrition intervention and regular follow-up by a primary health care provider. Children who are obese and have associated conditions should be referred to a multidisciplinary team experienced with pediatric obesity (Spear et al., 2007). Chapter 14 also discusses the approach to weight management for children.

Diet Clients often ask for an opinion on dietary approaches to weight loss, the latest fringe diet, and dietary supplements that promise no-effort weight loss. There are no miracle cures or hidden secrets about weight loss. Most research shows that weight is lost when the energy balance equation is tipped into negative balance with any combination of decreased calorie intake or increased calorie expenditure. Some diets are touted as a better approach to weight loss than others but on close evaluation are found to work just because they are simply lower calorie. Much research has been devoted to manipulating carbohydrate, protein, or fat content in the diet to promote weight loss, but results have not proven a significant effect of these changes independent of calorie content on long-term weight loss (Kushner, 2007). Improving dietary calcium status with either calcium supplements or high-calcium foods has been implicated by some as beneficial in promoting weight control, especially in those with poor baseline calcium intake, but results of clinical studies have been equivocal and require further study (ADA, 2009; Bortolotti et al., 2008; Clifton, 2008). In the meantime, the nurse can certainly recommend adequate calcium intake to clients inquiring about this research but without a promise that it will result in weight loss.

The majority of diets touted for weight loss manipulate energy intake in one way or another in order to decrease the amount of kcalories consumed. Others alter nutrient composition or food combinations, believing that these changes lead to weight loss. Diets can be generally classified into the following categories:

Low-calorie diets: Low-calorie diets range in level from near starvation to merely subtracting 500 to 1,000 calories from an individual's baseline daily energy needs. Such diets can be in liquid or solid form. Some include purchased meal replacement drinks or packaged foods. The risks and benefits of various low calorie diets are outlined in Table 17-2.

Any diet that yields an energy deficit will result in weight loss. The simplest approach is to brainstorm low-calorie alternatives to high-fat and high-calorie foods that contain little nutrition (called **empty calorie foods**) to achieve a daily deficit of 500 to 1,000 calories, which should foster weight loss of 1 or 2 pounds per week based on the knowledge that 1 pound of fat contains 3,500 kcalories. A careful evaluation of the nutrition history should yield possibilities for achieving this deficit by

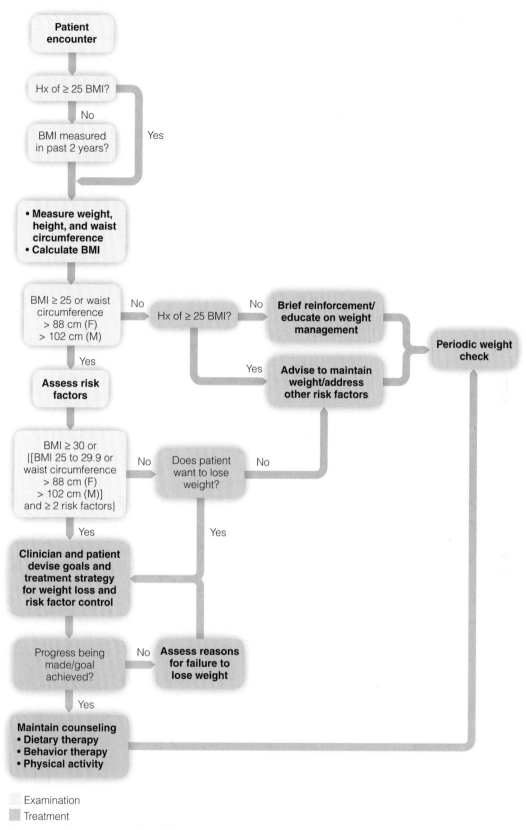

Examination
Treatment

■ **FIGURE 17-1 Treatment Algorithm for Weight Control.**

Source: National Heart Lung and Blood Institute (NHLBI) (1999). Clinical guidelines for the identification, evaluation and treatment of overweight and obesity in adults. The evidence report. Retrieved April 8, 2009, from www.nhlbi.nih.gov/guidelines/obesity/ob_gdlns.pdf page xvii

Table 17-2 Low-Calorie, Altered Nutrient, and Novelty Diets

Diet	Definition	Risks and Benefits
Low calorie		
• Starvation	*Less than or equal to* 200 calories	Loss of fluid and electrolytes, especially potassium Inadequate nutrient intake Muscle loss Not lifestyle management
• Very low calorie	200–800 calories Liquid or solid food Includes formal programs at medical centers and some weight loss centers	Loss of fluid and electrolytes, especially potassium Inadequate nutrient intake Muscle loss may occur Not lifestyle management Used under medical supervision for extreme obesity
• Low calorie	Reduced calorie intake compared with usual Liquid or solid food Includes formal programs at some weight loss centers and meal-replacement drinks and packaged food	Can be nutritionally balanced if all food groups are included Meal replacement drinks and packaged food approach not conducive to learning permanent new food behaviors
Nutrient altered		
• Low carbohydrate	*Less than or equal to* 100 gm carbohydrate/day	Ketosis Often high fat Forbidden foods lead to inadequate nutrient intake Low fiber May or may not be reduced calorie
• Moderate fat, moderate to high carbohydrate	Greater than 50% of calories as carbohydrate and 25–35% as fat	Generally balanced nutrients May or may not be reduced calorie
• Low fat or very low fat	Less than 25% calories as fat and high carbohydrate with high fiber	↑ Carbohydrate can lead to ↑ triglycerides ↑ volume of fiber may ↓ absorption of some nutrients Too ↓ fat can ↓ HDL cholesterol, essential fats May or may not be reduced calorie
Novelty		
• Single food	Focus on specific food as contributing to weight loss (e.g., grapefruit, vinegar, or cabbage soup)	Inadequate nutrient intake if only single food is ingested Boredom and lack of lifestyle management Reduced calorie only because of limiting nature of foods
• Food combining	Foods are eaten in set combinations felt to cause weight loss (e.g., fruit eaten only with proteins and vegetables with grains, specific foods recommended for body or blood type)	Some diets lack food groups and, therefore, are nutritionally inadequate No scientific evidence of magic to food combining Often reduced calorie because of limited intake

using alternative foods or modifying portions. Table 17-3 outlines examples of calorie swaps for achieving reduced calorie intake. Emphasis on portion sizes, consuming a healthful balance of foods, and eating regular meals should be underlined as reviewed in Box 17-1. Cultural

practices should be considered when guiding the client; healthful choices are outlined in Cultural Considerations Box: Healthful Ethnic Food Preparation.

Interactive tools, advice, and structured meal plans based on a set energy intake are available using on-line re-

Table 17-3   Creating a Calorie Deficit

Instead of:	Suggest:	Calories Saved (avg):
1½ cups whole milk	1½ cups skim milk	100
4½ in. bagel	2 English muffin halves	100
1 tbsp oil to sauté	Cooking spray to sauté	100
2 tbsp mayonnaise	2 tbsp low-calorie mayonnaise	100
7 oz pork tenderloin	5 oz pork tenderloin	100
4 vanilla crème sandwich cookies	2 vanilla crème sandwich cookies	100
3 oz fried chicken breast, skin on	3 oz crispy baked chicken breast, skinless	100
1 cup premium ice cream	1 cup soft serve frozen yogurt	100

CT? Where could the client find this type of information when grocery shopping?

Source: United States Department of Agriculture Nutrient Database. Retrieved April 8, 2009, from http://www.nal.usda.gov/fnic/foodcomp/search

sources with MyPyramid. This information can be provided to clients with computer access wishing a more structured approach. Individuals should be referred to a registered dietitian when more extensive advice is needed.

BOX 17-1

Healthful Weight Loss Approaches

The nurse can guide the client toward a healthful approach to weight loss that includes:

- Foods from all food groups:
  Lean proteins: beans, peas, lentils, skinless poultry, fish, lean meat
  Fruits and vegetables and whole grains to supply at least 20 gm fiber/day
  Low-fat and skim milk dairy sources or calcium-fortified dairy alternatives
- Moderate portion sizes: serve smaller portions at home, share large meals or desserts in a restaurant, avoid eating foods right from the container
- Reading food labels to learn portion sizes and calorie content
- Watching liquid calories: limit alcohol, especially cocktails with high-calorie mixers; limit sugary drinks such as soda, excessive juice, sweetened coffee and tea drinks. There are 100–200 calories in a 12 oz beer, 5 oz wine, 1½ oz hard liquor, 12 oz juice, soda, or fruit drink
- Making small substitutions in usual intake to reduce calorie intake: swap high-calorie foods for lower-calorie versions or reduce portion size; use preparation methods that minimize added calories such as baking, grilling, and broiling versus frying or using high-calorie sauces
- Regular meals and snacks to avoid overhungry state: no skipped meals
- Learning to identify true hunger versus other feelings that lead to eating such as boredom, thirst, fatigue, loneliness, or other emotions
- Reducing amount of time spent sitting
- Engaging in enjoyable physical activity

Altered fat, carbohydrate, or protein diets: Evidence is lacking that low-fat, high-protein or low-carbohydrate diets without a calorie restriction work for long-term weight loss any better than low-calorie diets (Kushner, 2007). Reduced kcalorie diets result in weight loss regardless of composition (Sacks et al., 2009). Low-fat diets are the composition of diets most often recommended by health care organization because of the association between low-fat intake and reduced risk of cardiovascular disease and some cancers (ADA, 2009). However, low-carbohydrate diets are a popular approach and are reported to foster a higher initial weight loss during the first 6 months of dieting than a traditional low-fat diet, though the difference between the two approaches disappears after 12 months (ADA, 2009; Eckel, 2008; Hession, Rollard, Kulkami, Wise, & Broom, 2009). Low-carbohydrate, high-protein diets may foster weight loss because of several mechanisms, including the following (ADA, 2009; Katan, 2009; Paddon-Jones et al., 2008):

- The self-limiting nature of the diet that results in eventual lowered calorie intake.
- Increased protein content has satiating power that results in decreased intake of calories because of the perception of fullness.
- The metabolism of protein utilizes more energy than does that of carbohydrate or fat. This energy cost is referred to as the thermic effect.
- Appetite can be diminished with the elevated blood ketones that result from fat breakdown in the absence of carbohydrate.
- Water loss from the depletion of glycogen; glycogen is stored in muscle and liver with accompanying water molecules. The water loss accounts for the larger amounts of weight loss seen early in the course of low-carbohydrate diets.

Cultural Considerations

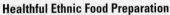

Healthful Ethnic Food Preparation

Most cultures have a wide range of food preparation techniques that vary from high calorie, high fat to low calorie, low fat. The nurse can brainstorm with the client methods to reduce excess calorie intake while maintaining cultural practices by suggesting the following:

Chinese

Jum (poached)

Chu (boiled)

Kow (roasted)

Shu (barbeque)

Hoisin, oyster, spicy, mustard, and light stir-fry sauces

Lean proteins such as fish filet, chicken without skin, lean beef, tofu

Vegetable-based dishes

Steamed vs. fried rice

Japanese

Yakimono (broiled)

Teriyaki sauce

Menrui or soba noodles, cellophane noodles

Tofu or bean curd

Grilled vegetables

Rice

Thai

Basil, lime, fish, hot or chili sauces

Barbeque, broiled, boiled, steamed, or braised dishes

Napa, bamboo shoots, black mushrooms

Ginger, garlic, scallions, onions

Vegetable-based dishes

Italian

Red sauces vs. white or cream sauces

Piccata

Manzanne (eggplant)

Onions, shallots, peppers, mushrooms

Herbs and spices

Grilled fish or vegetables

Mexican

Rice and beans

Salsa and green chili sauce vs. sour cream, guacamole

Picante sauce

Ceviche (fish marinated in lime juice)

Corn or flour soft tortilla vs. hard taco or tortilla

Grilled dishes

Middle Eastern

Chickpeas, fava beans

Spiced ground meat

Smoked eggplant

Garlic or tomato sauces

Tomatoes, onions, green pepper, cucumbers

Couscous, bulgur, rice

Skewered or kabob grilled meats

Meats or vegetables stuffed with rice, spices

Indian

Masala, tikka, or tandoori dishes

Cooking with curry or yogurt

Lentils, chickpeas, split peas (dal)

Basmati rice (pullao)

Spinach (saag)

Matta (green peas)

Chicken or shrimp kebab

Nan bread

Vegetable-based dishes

Source: Adapted from NHLBI, 1998.

In the short-term, low-carbohydrate diets can be considered an alternative to other types of kcalorie restricted diets by most people provided excessive intake of saturated fats is avoided (Gardner et al., 2007; Shai et al., 2008). Although low-carbohydrate diets are reported to have a favorable effect on some blood lipid levels, they are also associated with an unfavorable increase in low-density lipoprotein cholesterol, also called LDL or "bad" cholesterol, and should not be recommended to individuals with high LDL cholesterol (ADA, 2009; Eckel, 2008). Additionally, individuals with kidney disease should avoid this diet because the high-protein content could affect kidney health (ADA, 2009). Clients who choose this diet should be advised about these effects as well as the long-term issues with limiting dietary sources of carbohydrates such as milk, yogurt, fruits, vegetables, and whole grains that contain crucial nutrients such as calcium, folate, vitamins A and C, and fiber. Most studies of low-carbohydrate diets have included a multivitamin, multimineral supplement to compensate for many of the nutrients that are lacking in the diet (Westman et al., 2007). Low-carbohydrate diets are counterproductive for the athlete trying to both lose weight and participate in physical activity because depletion of glycogen stores from insufficient carbohydrate intake impairs athletic performance.

Novelty diets: Novelty diets promise weight loss with magical combinations of foods or ingredients. Combination diets, rotations diets, and diets where certain foods are attributed to cause weight loss are examples outlined in Table 17-2. Often such diets are accompanied by books written by celebrities who have no nutrition background. If such novelty approaches to weight loss really did contain a magical cure for long-term weight loss, obesity statistics would not be increasing as they are.

When approached for an opinion about any diet, the nurse can help the client evaluate the program using Client Education Checklist: Evaluating Weight Loss Programs and Products.

CLIENT EDUCATION CHECKLIST 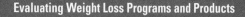 Evaluating Weight Loss Programs and Products

The nurse can advise the client seeking information on weight loss to consider these parameters when making choices about weight management methods:

A weight loss approach is healthy if it:

- Contains foods from all major food groups, emphasizing moderation in saturated fat intake, and encouraging consumption of a variety of nutritious foods
- Does not require intake of dietary supplements to compensate for insufficient intake
- Does not overemphasize or forbid a specific food or food group
- Allows snacking
- Can be followed without interruption of family or social lifestyle
- Fosters no more than 2 lb. weight loss on average/week
- Emphasizes physical activity
- Supports long-term beneficial behavioral changes

- Suggests consultation with a primary health care provider before beginning the plan

A weight loss approach could be quackery if:

- Weight loss results are promised with little or no effort, such as with creams or patches worn on the skin, calorie or fat "trappers" or "blockers" that compensate for overindulgence, pills that build muscle without exercising.
- Miracle or hidden secret to weight loss is touted.
- Mainstream medical care is criticized.
- Pseudomedical jargon is used in marketing to impress consumers and infer scientific expertise.
- Testimonials and anecdotes are used in product promotion instead of solid clinical research.
- Specific food or food group are labeled as poisonous, toxic, or responsible for weight gain.
- Special powers are assigned to a food, food group, or combination of foods.

Physical Activity Inclusion of regular physical activity into lifestyle habits contributes to weight management by increasing energy expenditure and favorably improving energy balance. Regular physical activity assists in weight loss and the prevention of weight gain (ADA, 2009; Donnelly et al., 2009). Cardiorespiratory and other health improvements from exercise are associated with decreased risk of morbidity and mortality even when weight loss is not a result (Eckel, 2008). Collaboration with the client to develop specific achievable activity goals is essential, paying particular attention to current physical fitness level, ability, and barriers to physical activity. For some individuals, a recommendation to increase the number of steps taken per day is a starting point to overcoming sedentary behavior. Less screen time and time spent sitting is good advice for all age groups. Strength training in combination with a reduced kcalorie diet is associated with preservation of lean muscle during weight loss (Donnelly et al., 2009). An increase in activity need not be in large continuous time blocks, but rather can be accumulated over the day in small increments, especially when lack of time to exercise is a barrier to increased activity. Clients who have not exercised in a long time or have poor mobility may feel self-conscious about beginning new activities. Establishing reasonable short-term goals for increased activity, logging time spent in physical activity, and on-line resources that calculate calories expended with activities can be good motivational tools for clients. The American College of Sports Medicine recommends that individuals eventually reach 150 to 250 minutes/week of physical activity for weight management (Donnelly et al., 2009). Box 17-2 depicts examples of moderate amounts of physical activity for the nurse to suggest when setting goals with the client.

Behavior Modification Modification of behaviors that contributed to weight gain is essential for long-term weight

management. New behaviors that result in successful weight loss need to be integrated into long-term lifestyle habits. For example, long-term weight monitoring, a low-fat diet, and regular physical activity are identified as behaviors that contribute to long-term maintenance of successful weight loss (Eckel, 2008). The nurse can assist the client in identifying personal factors that contributed to weight gain or regain and engage in problem-solving solutions. Behavior modification involves identifying triggers for undesired behaviors, such as increased food intake or lack of activity, and then learning, practicing, and rewarding new positive behaviors. Such changes take place over time in a step-by-step process. Some clients can have an all-or-nothing approach to weight loss and expect to alter many behaviors overnight for quick results. The nurse can work with the client to target specific achievable behavior changes in a tiered approach, where a succession of new behavioral goals is built slowly. Small, incremental changes provide the client with a more successful experience rather than short-lived drastic changes (ADA, 2009). Behavioral goals should reflect the client's level of motivation and readiness for change. The client who is only contemplating weight loss would have different goals than the individual who has successfully begun behavior changes and is ready to progress to a new set of goals.

In addition to setting goals, tools used in behavior modification include self-monitoring behaviors, stimulus control, and cognitive restructuring. Table 17-4 outlines these components with specifics given for weight loss.

Medications and Dietary Supplements

Pharmacotherapy for weight loss is only recommended for overweight individuals with a BMI of at least 27 with at least one obesity-related condition or those with a BMI *greater than or equal to* 30 (NHLBI, 1998).

MyNursingKit Energy Calculator

BOX 17-2	Examples of Moderate Amounts of Physical Activity

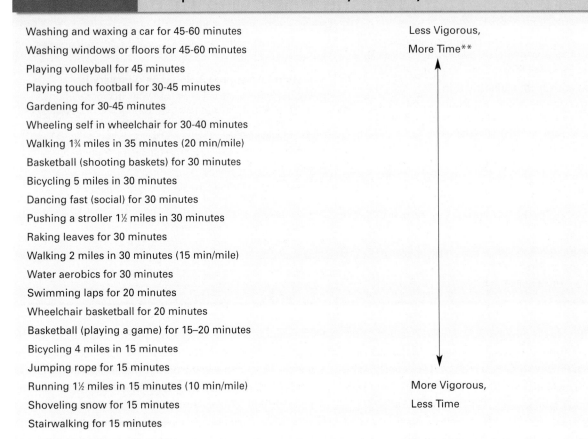

Washing and waxing a car for 45-60 minutes

Washing windows or floors for 45-60 minutes

Playing volleyball for 45 minutes

Playing touch football for 30-45 minutes

Gardening for 30-45 minutes

Wheeling self in wheelchair for 30-40 minutes

Walking 1¾ miles in 35 minutes (20 min/mile)

Basketball (shooting baskets) for 30 minutes

Bicycling 5 miles in 30 minutes

Dancing fast (social) for 30 minutes

Pushing a stroller 1½ miles in 30 minutes

Raking leaves for 30 minutes

Walking 2 miles in 30 minutes (15 min/mile)

Water aerobics for 30 minutes

Swimming laps for 20 minutes

Wheelchair basketball for 20 minutes

Basketball (playing a game) for 15–20 minutes

Bicycling 4 miles in 15 minutes

Jumping rope for 15 minutes

Running 1½ miles in 15 minutes (10 min/mile)

Shoveling snow for 15 minutes

Stairwalking for 15 minutes

Less Vigorous,
More Time**

More Vigorous,
Less Time

* A moderate amount of physical activity is roughly equivalent to physical activity that uses approximately 150 calories of energy per day, or 1,000 calories per week.
** Some activities can be performed at various intensities; the suggested durations correspond to expected intensity of effort.
Source: NHLBI, 1999.

Sibutramine (Meridia) and Orlistat (Xenical and Alli) are two medications approved in the United States for long-term use for weight loss. Sibutramine acts on the central nervous system to lessen hunger and increase satiety. The nurse should be aware that this prescription drug interacts with some antidepressant medications and has cardiovascular side effects, including increased heart rate and blood pressure, which require careful client selection for this therapy (ADA, 2009; Eckel, 2008). Orlistat is taken with meals and acts in the gastrointestinal tract to inhibit the enzyme lipase, decreasing absorption of fat by up to 30% (Kushner, 2008). Practice Pearl: Nursing Recommendations with Orlistat outlines nursing recommendations for the client taking Orlistat. Clinical trials report that an additional 3% to 5% weight loss is attributable to pharmacotherapy when it is combined with lifestyle modifications (Eckel, 2008).

Approximately one-third of adults attempting weight loss have tried a dietary supplement as part of that effort (Pillitteri et al., 2008). The most common dietary supplements used contain a stimulant, such as caffeine or bitter orange (Blanck

et al., 2007). Stimulants such as bitter orange can increase heart rate and elevate blood pressure, which are side effects that have led to reports of fainting, heart attack, and stroke in people taking dietary supplements that contain this ingredient (National Institutes of Health [NIH], 2008). Often, consumers assume that dietary supplements are well-tested and approved by the Food and Drug Administration (FDA) before being marketed and that a natural product must be a safe product (Pillitteri et al., 2008; Rogovik & Goldman, 2009). Both assumptions are false. Dietary supplements are not regulated as medications but as food. Most dietary supplements for weight loss have little clinical evidence to support their use and are lacking in safety data, yet this deficit does not stop clients from seeking a "magic bullet" to manage weight. Many of these products interact with prescription medications or present risks to specific individuals, such as pregnant females or clients with cardiovascular disease. Additionally, the FDA has issued alerts for many dietary weight loss supplements that have been found to be tainted with a variety of medications, including diuretics and sibutramine (FDA, 2009). The use of

Table 17-4   Behavior Modification in Weight Control

Behavior Component	Behavior Example
Self-monitoring: conducting self-checks and keeping records	• Monitoring calorie or fat intake • Keeping a food diary • Monitoring activity level • Logging weight weekly • Measuring portion size of snack foods
Stimulus control: targeting cues to undesired behaviors and controlling them	• Planning meals ahead of time to avoid stopping at fast-food restaurants when pressed for time • Keeping high-calorie foods in the cupboard instead of out in view • Placing fruit in a bowl on the table instead of hidden in the refrigerator • Carrying alternative snack foods in the car or backpack to avoid the vending machine • Eating breakfast to avoid being overhungry and overeating at lunch • Preparing smaller amounts of a recipe to avoid consuming bigger single servings • Having portioned desserts or fatty snacks sitting at the dinner table to avoid absent-mindedly munching in front of the television • Meeting a friend for a walk rather than at the donut shop
Cognitive restructuring: reframing thinking about behaviors and enhancement of self-reliant skills	• Use self-talk, motivational quotes, books, or other meaningful approaches to reinforce idea that weight loss requires practicing new behaviors over time. • Develop problem-solving approach to slip-ups and barriers instead of abandoning efforts or being self-critical. • Collaborate ways to develop new coping skills when poor diet or lack of exercise result from stress, boredom, frustration, or other emotional challenges. • Develop nonweight positive outcomes as part of goal setting. • Brainstorm self-rewards when small and large milestones are reached.

CT? What are some ways the nurse can collaborate on behavior modification approaches with the client who undermines weight loss attempts with negative self-talk? What about the client who has no social support to bolster positive efforts?

PRACTICE PEARL

Nursing Recommendations with Orlistat

- The nurse should warn clients that Orlistat works by causing excretion rather than absorption of about one-third of the dietary fat in a meal. However, a high-fat intake at a single meal leads to oily anal spotting, oily stools, and fecal urgency.
- A daily multivitamin is recommended in clients taking Orlistat to compensate for any decreased absorption of fat-soluble vitamins.
- Dosing of the multivitamin should avoid a 2-hour window before or after taking Orlistat or the fat-soluble vitamins will not be absorbed.
- Orlistat is the only prescription weight loss medication approved for adolescents.

Sources: ADA, 2009; Eckel, 2008; Kushner, 2007; Rogovik & Goldman, 2009.

herbal-based dietary supplements is not recommended for weight loss because of unpredictable ingredients, effects, and safety (NHLBI, 1998). The use of weight loss supplements by children should be avoided (Rogovik & Goldman, 2009).

The nurse should query clients attempting weight loss about use of dietary supplements. An open-ended, nonjudgmental question works well, such as "Tell me about what you have tried as a method of weight control. Have you tried any diets? Over-the-counter pills, supplements, or products?" It is crucial for the nurse to remain up to date on available safety and efficacy of these products in order to provide reliable advice to the client. Box 17-3 outlines examples of dietary supplements

BOX 17-3	Dietary Supplement Ingredients Marketed for Weight Loss*

Stimulants: bitter orange (synephrine or citrus aurantium), guarana (Brazilian cocoa), yerba mate, caffeine with or without willow root, green tea, kola nut

Claim altered metabolism or absorption: chromium, ginseng, fat blockers (chitosan and others), guggul gum (gugulipid), apple cider vinegar, hydroxycitric acid (HCA or garcinia cambogia), conjugated linoleic acid (CLA), pyruvate

Increase sense of fullness: fibrous compounds such as psyllium, guar gum

Diuretics or cathartics: aloe, buckthorn, dandelion, cascara, senna in some dieter's teas

*None of these supplements has substantial significant clinical or safety evidence to support use. Chapter 25 outlines dietary supplements in detail.

 ■ What advice should the nurse offer to the client with hypertension who is taking a stimulant dietary supplement?

Sources: Adapted from: Clifton, 2008; NIH, 2008; Rogovik & Goldman, 2009.

marketed for weight loss. More extensive information on dietary supplements is found in Chapter 25.

Bariatric Surgery

National guidelines regarding surgical intervention for weight loss recommend that this approach be reserved for individuals with a BMI greater than 40 or those with a BMI greater than 35 with accompanying obesity-related conditions (Mechanick et al., 2008). **Bariatric surgery** is the term used that encompasses all types of intestinal surgeries performed to foster weight loss. Candidates for bariatric surgery should have previously tried to lose weight through various means, be well-informed about all aspects of the surgery, and be motivated (NHLBI, 1998). The nurse is included in the extensive team approach to evaluating appropriate candidates for this procedure. All aspects of physical and mental health are considered. Bariatric surgical procedures and associated risks and benefits are outlined in Table 17-5.

Types of Surgery Surgical options for obesity are restrictive or restrictive/malabsorptive in nature. Restrictive procedures reduce the size of the gastric reservoir to 3 oz or less (NIDDK, 2008). Adjustable or permanent banding or staples are placed around the upper portion of the stomach, creating a small pouch and narrow channel into the stomach. The smaller gastric reservoir theoretically limits the total daily volume of food, which in turns leads to weight loss (Tucker, Szomstein, & Rosenthal, 2007). Clients can expect to lose almost 50% of excess body weight, though some regain weight during the initial 3 to 5 years postoperatively (ADA, 2009). Figure 17-2 ■ depicts an example of restrictive surgical procedures. Such sur-

geries are less invasive than malabsorptive procedures and can be reversed if needed (NIDDK, 2008).

Restrictive/malabsorptive procedures include the Roux-en-Y and biliopancreatic diversion surgeries. Roux-en-Y gastric bypass is the most commonly performed weight loss surgery performed in the United States (Tucker et al., 2007). Clients can expect to lose up to 70% of excess weight, depending on the extent of malabsorption caused by the surgery (ADA, 2009). With this procedure, a small gastric pouch is created to reduce food intake and then connected to the lower jejunum to deliberately foster malabsorption of kcalories and nutrients normally absorbed in the duodenum and upper jejunum. In the biliopancreatic diversion, a large portion of the stomach is removed and the remnant is attached to the distal ileum. In some cases, a duodenal switch is also performed and a small portion of the duodenum remains intact. These surgeries promote quicker weight loss than purely restrictive surgeries. More substantial weight loss with these procedures is attributed to the gastric resection, the malabsorptive outcome, and alterations in gastrointestinal hormones. Ghrelin secretion, known to stimulate hunger, is altered by these procedures and lessens hunger (Doucet, 2008). Figure 17-2 outlines examples of these procedures.

Postoperative Nutrition Concerns The nurse should be aware of both short- and long-term nutritional recommendations following bariatric surgery. The nutritional consequences of bariatric surgery depend in part on the type of surgery performed. Both categories of procedures require careful advancement of the diet postoperatively. Vomiting is com-

Table 17-5 Bariatric Surgery Risks and Benefits

Procedure	Risks	Benefits	Nutrition Concerns
Restrictive: gastric banding, adjustable banding	• Less than 1% operative mortality • 5% operative morbidity—leakage, wound infection, failed staple closure • Vomiting w/ ↑ volume intake, stenosis, blockage • Weight regain if frequent calorie intake	• Weight loss up to 50% of excess weight • Restricted volume of food tolerated at one time • Procedure easy to perform • Procedure is reversible	• Vomiting • Hydration • Possible weight regain • Thiamine deficiency w/protracted vomiting
Restrictive/ Malabsorptive • Roux-en-Y • Biliopancreatic diversion (BPD)	• Approximately 1% operative mortality • 5% operative morbidity—intestinal leak, wound infection, staple line failure, incisional hernia, marginal ulcer, stomal stenosis • Dumping syndrome in up to 15% of clients • Malabsorption and diarrhea • Gastric resection portion of procedure not reversible	• More pronounced weight loss vs. restrictive procedures • Weight loss of up to 70% of excess weight • Reversible procedure except gastric resection portion	• Vomiting • Dumping syndrome • Iron deficiency—loss of acid environment and site for absorption • Calcium deficiency and metabolic bone disease long-term • Vitamin B_{12} and folate malabsorption—deficiency in less than 1 year • Thiamine deficiency w/ vomiting and poor intake → Wernicke's encephalopathy • Pellagra and polyneuropathies

Sources: Adapted from: Mechanick et al., 2008; NIDDK, 2008; Tucker, Szomstein, & Rosenthal, 2007.

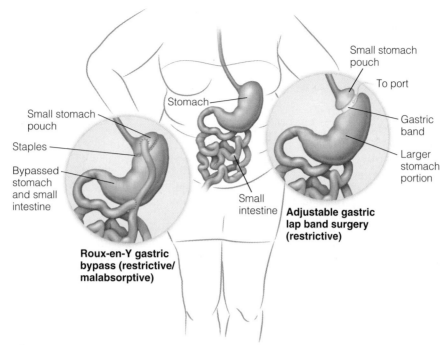

Small stomach
pouch

Stomach

Small stomach
pouch
To port
Gastric
band
Larger
stomach
portion

Small stomach
pouch

Staples

Bypassed
stomach
and small
intestine

Small
intestine

**Adjustable gastric
lap band surgery
(restrictive)**

**Roux-en-Y gastric
bypass (restrictive/
malabsorptive)**

■ **FIGURE 17-2** **Bariatric Surgeries.**

mon initially and can predispose the client to dehydration and protein, kcalorie, and thiamin deficiency (Tucker et al., 2007). The restrictive/malabsorptive procedures are more likely than just a restrictive procedure to result in long-term nutritional deficiencies (NIDDK, 2008). Anemia, metabolic bone disease, and vitamin B_{12} deficiency are common long-term complications, especially when a client does not adhere to recommended vitamin and mineral supplementation advice (Colossi et al., 2008; Tucker et al., 2007). Metabolic bone disease is more likely in those who lose weight more rapidly and had poor vitamin D status before surgery, which is common among obese clients because vitamin D becomes sequestered in adipose and less available to the body (Williams, Cooper, Richmond, & Schauer, 2008). Nutrition status should be assessed every few months following surgery and then annually thereafter, including an evaluation of bone mineral density when indicated (Mechanick et al., 2008). About 10% of clients are unsuccessful at losing weight postoperatively because of frequent snacking, consumption of high kcalorie foods, and lack of physical activity (NIDDK, 2008). Nutrition recommendations are outlined in Box 17-4 and include guidelines for routine vitamin and mineral supplementation. On-line resources are also available.

Bariatric surgery is believed to be equally safe for adolescents as is reported for adults (NIDDK, 2008). In addition to the recommended psychosocial and medical screening that is advised for adults, adolescents having bariatric surgery should meet the following additional criteria: extreme obesity (BMI greater than 40), adult height has been reached, and serious weight-related health problems exist (NIDDK, 2008). The more restrictive/malabsorption procedures such as biliopancreatic diversion

and duodenal switch are not recommended in adolescents because of the high risk of malnutrition and metabolic bone disease associated with those surgeries (Levitsky et al., 2009).

Pregnancy following bariatric surgery results in unique nutritional challenges. Although successful weight loss is associated with improved maternal and neonatal outcomes, careful attention to the unique nutritional needs of both pregnancy and bariatric surgery remains essential (Maggard et al., 2008). These guidelines are found in Hot Topic Box 13-1.

Size Acceptance, Health at Every Size, and Sensitive Care of the Overweight

Varying philosophies exist about the need to manage weight, especially in the overweight individual who has no medical complications associated with excess weight. Clinical studies on the Health at Every Size (HAES) approach have revealed that indeed healthful behavior changes and an intuitive approach to eating improves mental and physical health in obese individuals even without weight loss (Provencher et al., 2007). Clients learn to respond to internal cues for hunger and satiety and move away from a restrictive dieting approach. An appreciation for varying sizes and shapes of bodies is central to size acceptance. The focus is on all aspects of health promotion, including enjoyable eating and exercise, rather than counting calories. HAES programs are reported to have increased long-term maintenance of new health behaviors compared to a diet approach (Bacon, Stern, Van Loan, & Keim, 2005). Traditional weight loss programs that focus on weight alone run the risk of instilling a short-term, quick-fix approach and stigmatizing the overweight

MyNursingKit American Society for Metabolic and Bariatric Surgery

BOX 17-4	Nutrition Recommendations Following Bariatric Surgery

Postoperative

First day: ice chips, frequent small sips of water

First week or two: small frequent clear liquids slowly work up to 64 oz/day; no caffeine

Week 2 or 3: advance to full liquids per surgical team
- Sips, not gulps, of fluid
- Avoid undue fullness

1 month: progress to puree and then soft foods—2 tbsp per meal and ↑ as tolerated

3 months: progress to solids per surgical team

Overall:
- Liquids: avoid high sugar or carbonated.
- No liquids w/meals: wait 60–90 minutes.
- Eat slowly.
- Cut foods to small size and chew well.
- Eat three to five small meals/day.
- Consume at least 60 gm protein daily: soft proteins to initially consume include canned tuna, salmon, and chicken; eggs; nonfat milk, yogurt, cottage cheese; tofu; mashed legumes. Advance to moist, chopped proteins and then regular consistency as directed, chewing well.

Treat dumping syndrome as outlined in Chapter 20

Problem foods: dry, sticky, gummy, or stringy items may cause vomiting, intolerance

Supplements

Daily chewable or liquid multivitamin (some clients benefit from prenatal formula)

Vitamin D and calcium in citrate form (loss of acid environment for absorption; avoid carbonate forms)

Monitor for low iron status and supplement as needed. Malabsorptive procedures likely to cause poor iron status (loss of acid environment and absorption site)

Vitamin B_{12} and folate for malabsorptive procedures

Thiamine if persistent nausea and vomiting

Long term

Malabsorptive procedures are likely to cause more deficiencies than restrictive procedures

Monitor for iron, vitamin B_{12}, and folate status

Ensure adequate calcium and vitamin D to avoid metabolic bone disease

Monitor for excessive vomiting w/ altered hydration and electrolyte status. Ensure adequate thiamine intake

Monitor for signs of protein deficiency w/ complaint of hair loss

Monitor for excessive weight loss or weight regain

Sources: Adapted from: Benson-Davies & Quigley, 2008; Mechanick et al., 2008; Tucker et al., 2007; Williams, Cooper, et al., 2008.

MyNursingKit Weight Bias, The Obesity Society

based on cosmetic appearance (Cohen, Perales, & Steadman, 2005). Advertisements for programs with "before" and "after" pictures are an example. Distorted cultural definitions of normal weight further fuel this weight bias. Instead the focus should be on achieving health, regardless of size.

The nurse should be sensitive to the needs of the overweight client. For many clients, a health care visit is a negative experience because of the physical environment and any perception of insensitive care or weight prejudice (The Obesity Society, 2009). The clinical setting should be welcoming to all clients with wide-based armless chairs to accommodate all body sizes, readily available large-size blood pressure cuffs, appropriate-sized examination gowns, and a scale that can measure clients who weigh more than 300 lb without creating an awkward scene (The Obesity Society, 2009). Additionally, it is important to separate any issues of weight-related problems from any personal opinion about the client (NHLBI, 1998). In a culture where obesity is stigmatized, health care providers need to address any personal size prejudice that may interfere with good client care.

Eating Disorders

Eating disorders are categorized as psychiatric illnesses, but in addition include symptoms and treatment with a medical and nutritional focus. Because of the broad symptomology, treatment of eating disorders is multidisciplinary; the nurse plays

an important role in this approach. Eating disorders occur primarily in adolescents and young adults but are found in individuals across the lifespan. This disease is more prevalent among females, with males comprising only 10% of those with eating disorders (Hudson, Hiripi, Pope, & Kessler, 2007).

What Is an Eating Disorder?

Strict criteria exist for the diagnosis of a clinical eating disorder of anorexia nervosa, bulimia nervosa, and eating disorders not otherwise specified (EDNOS), which includes binge eating disorder. All are characterized by an abnormal relationship with food exemplified by altered eating patterns and distorted thinking about food and weight (ADA, 2006b). Formal criteria for diagnosis are based on the *Diagnostic and Statistical Manual of Mental Disorders, 4th edition* (DSM-4). The medical, nutritional, physiological, and psychological symptoms and consequences of each disorder occur along a continuum and some are not exclusive to one disorder. On one end of the continuum are minor alterations in food-related behaviors or thoughts, whereas on the opposite end are clinical eating disorder diagnoses that meet the strict DSM-4 criteria. Some individuals have a few, but not all, qualifying symptoms for a diagnosis and would be considered to have either EDNOS or a subclinical eating disorder, also called **disordered eating.** Adolescents in particular may not meet the strict criterion for a clinical eating disorder, yet intervention is clearly indicated. Symptoms and other clinical findings are discussed within the respective sections on each disorder in this chapter. No matter where an individual falls on the continuum of symptoms, the nurse has a role in the assessment and intervention developed for the client.

What Causes an Eating Disorder?

Much research and debate surround the discussion on what causes the development of an eating disorder. These complex disorders also have a complex etiology that crosses biological, psychological, and sociocultural influences. Biological causes of eating disorders, such as genetic and neurobehavioral influences, have been postulated as contributors to a predisposition to eating disorder development. Research has found a familial association between traits such as depression, anxiety, perfectionism, and obsessive-compulsive disorder and eating disorders. Molecular genetic and twin studies suggest some heritability of eating disorders but lack consistency as to specifics (Striegel-Moore & Bulik, 2007). There is an association between substance abuse and eating disorders with a high rate of co-occurrence of these conditions in the population with eating disorders. It is felt that the presence of eating disorders increases the risk of substance abuse; in particular, a link between bulimia, impulsivity, and substance abuse is often cited (Halmi, 2009). Other possible biological contributors to the development of eating disorders include altered neuropeptide and neurotransmitter levels (Halmi, 2009; Striegel-Moore & Bulik, 2007).

Psychological risk factors for eating disorders include mood disorders, sexual abuse, and low-self esteem as outlined in Box 17-5. Environmental influences can contribute to eating disorder development, especially in those who have other risk factors. A mother's drive for thinness and a father's perfectionism are associated with a female's risk of developing an eating disorder (Canals, Sancho, & Arija, 2009). Cultural pressure to be thin, media influences, negative comments from others—including teasing about weight—and unhealthful weight control practices, such as severe dieting and use of diet pills, have been cited (Eisenberg & Neumark-Sztainer, 2008; Neumark-Sztainer et al., 2006). Additionally, there is an increased rate of distorted eating patterns found among females who are on lifelong therapeutic diets that require dietary restraint, such as with type 1 diabetes (Goebel-Fabbri, 2009).

Eating disorder prevention programs are effective when they specifically address body acceptance interventions and provide education that empowers those at risk to question the cultural standards that create the thin ideal and a dieting mentality (Shaw, Stice, & Becker, 2008). Other types of programs that focus on education about eating disorders and treatment may contribute to the normalization of these disorders and not serve as a prevention intervention (Schwartz, Thomas, Bohan, & Vartanian, 2007). The school nurse participating in eating disorder prevention education should be mindful of the different outcomes associated with these two types of programming.

Eating Disorder Assessment and Treatment

Careful assessment is needed to diagnose an eating disorder because much of the criteria that determine the diagnosis are gathered during the client interview and physical examination. Laboratory values are generally normal unless the condition is advanced or there has been protracted vomiting or diuretic or laxative misuse. Treatment varies for each type of eating disorder, but all should involve a multidisciplinary approach. No single treatment type of treatment has been

BOX 17-5	Risk Factors for Eating Disorder Development

Personality traits and psychological comorbidities:

Low self-esteem
Difficulty expressing negative emotion
Difficulty in resolving conflict
Perfectionism
Compulsiveness
Depression
Anxiety

Restrictive diet:

Chronic or severe dieting
Chronic restrictive medical diets (e.g., diabetic diet)

Biology/family influence:

Family history of eating disorder, substance abuse, depression, obesity
Early menarche
Genetics
Altered neurotransmitter function (serotonin)

Environment:

Family dieting
Critical comments about body from others
Sport participation with
  • aesthetic pressure to be thin (ballet, gymnastics, cheerleading, figure skating)
  • performance pressure to be thin (track, cross-country, gymnastics)
  • weight class (wrestling, rowing, martial arts, jockey)
Occupational pressure to be thin (modeling, acting)
Overvaluation on weight and appearance by family, peers, and cultural influence

Other factors:

Sexual abuse

■ Which eating disorder risk factors are modifiable? What role can the nurse have in reducing these risks in susceptible populations?

Sources: Adapted from: Halmi, 2009; Nattiv et al., 2007; Striegel-Moore & Bulik, 2007.

MyNursingKit Eating Disorder Prevention Program

found effective for anorexia, bulimia, or binge eating. Each client should have an individual treatment plan based on diagnosis, symptoms, and coexisting conditions. The nurse should be mindful that in the pregnant female with a history of an eating disorder, symptoms may improve during the pregnancy but relapse after childbirth, warranting close postnatal monitoring for this risk (Crow, Agras, Crosby, Halmi, &

Mitchell, 2008). Table 17-6 presents a summary of assessment and treatment features for all three eating disorders.

Anorexia Nervosa

Early diagnosis and intervention for anorexia nervosa and its associated conditions is associated with improved outcome compared with delayed intervention (Papadopoulos, Ekbom,

Table 17-6   Assessment and Treatment of Eating Disorders

	Anorexia Nervosa	Bulimia Nervosa	Binge Eating Disorder
Medical and Psychological Symptoms	Weight loss with BMI *less than or equal to* 17.5 or weight *less than or equal to* 85% ideal Fear of fat/weight gain General appearance: ↓ muscle mass and adipose, brittle hair, alopecia, lanugo Cardiac: ↓ heart rate, ↓ blood pressure, ↓ left ventricular mass, QT elevation Intestinal: delayed gastric emptying, bloating, constipation Skeletal: ↓ bone density, ↓ linear growth Skin: ↓ temperature and cold intolerance, pallor, orange palms from excessive intake of carrots, dry skin Reproductive: irregular menses or amenorrhea, ↓ libido Psychological: insomnia, irritability, anxiety, depression, self-injury, substance abuse, labile mood	Normal or above normal weight Symptoms result of purging method: • Vomiting: dental enamel erosion, gastric reflux and bloating, bloodshot eyes, swollen parotid glands, hoarse voice, callous knuckle, poor or absent gag reflex, cardiomyopathy with ipecac use • Diet pill abuse: central nervous system (CNS) stimulation with ↑ heart rate • Laxatives: dehydration, altered electrolytes • Diuretics: dehydration, altered electrolytes, edema with sudden halt of use • Exercise: overuse injury, low strength or muscle wasting despite level of activity Psychological: depression, anxiety, substance abuse, impulsiveness, self-injury	Weight gain Overweight or obese
Laboratory Values	Usually within normal limits (WNL) ↑ Cholesterol Anemia Altered thyroid function	Dehydration ↓ Potassium w/ vomiting ↓ Chloride w/ laxative or diuretic use	Usually within normal limits (WNL) unless comorbid conditions exist
Nutrition History and Food Behaviors	Restrictive eating, may be under guise of "healthy eating" Food aversions w/ list of "bad" foods Overconsumption of liquids and calorie-free foods Spitting out chewed food Interest in cooking for others Excessive gum chewing and caffeine intake Eating alone Food rituals (e.g., cutting food in small pieces, putting mustard on many foods, eating foods in set order)	Bingeing followed by compensatory purging Restrictive eating when not bingeing List of "good" and "bad" foods Stockpiling food for binges or frequent shopping for items	Bingeing without compensatory purging History of chronic dieting

Table 17-6 Assessment and Treatment of Eating Disorders *(continued)*

	Anorexia Nervosa	Bulimia Nervosa	Binge Eating Disorder
Nutrition Treatment (component of multidisciplinary approach)	Weight restoration: up to 2 lbs./week outpatient and 3 lbs./week inpatient Correct nutritional deficiencies Monitor for refeeding syndrome Educate about nutritional needs Correct nutrition, food and weight misconceptions Address food phobias Reintroduce forbidden foods after overall intake improves Facilitate social dining Contract with client about food-related behaviors Ensure adequate calcium and vitamin D status for bone health	Normalize chaotic eating patterns Avoid overhungry state with regular eating every 3–4 hours Avoidance of finger foods and eating directly from food containers Cognitive behavior therapy: identify food or environmental binge triggers, brainstorm urge delay behaviors to avert a binge, address nutrition misconceptions Educate about side effects of purging: vomiting, laxative and diuretic abuse, excessive exercise, diet pills Contract with client about food- and purging-related behaviors Weight loss prescription contraindicated during treatment of eating disorder	Normalize chaotic eating patterns Avoid overhungry state with regular eating every 3–4 hours Avoidance of finger foods and eating directly from food containers Cognitive behavior therapy: identify food or environmental binge triggers, brainstorm urge delay behaviors to avert a binge, address nutrition misconceptions Inconclusive whether weight loss prescription is effective during treatment for binge eating

Brandt, & Ekselius, 2009). Recognition of the disorder can be obscured because clients often present for nonspecific or unrelated symptoms. For example, some clients will restrict intake under the guise of "healthy eating," which may not arouse suspicion of disordered eating. **Anorexia nervosa** is characterized by a refusal to maintain body weight at a minimal weight for height with an intense fear of gaining weight and an altered self-evaluation of personal weight. Specific findings are outlined in Table 17-6. A careful assessment may yield information on restrictive eating, disturbed eating habits, amenorrhea, or unrealistic expectations regarding body weight or shape. Athletic females presenting with either amenorrhea or a stress fracture should be screened for disordered eating because these three conditions can be associated in that population and are referred to as the Female Athlete Triad as discussed in Chapter 11 (Nattiv et al., 2007). Self-reported vegetarianism can be a marker for disordered eating when individuals use this type of eating to seek a socially acceptable way to mask restrictive eating (Klopp, Heiss, & Smith, 2003). **Orthorexia** is a term used to describe restrictive eating habits that focus to excess on "being healthy," excluding once enjoyable foods because they have what is perceived to be too much fat, kcalories, or another "unhealthy" aspect. Clients with orthorexia may slip into behaviors that closely resemble anorexia nervosa.

Physical symptoms of anorexia nervosa result from malnutrition and its effects on organ systems. Cardiovascular, reproductive, endocrine, and neurological symptoms can occur. Cognitive function can be affected by the loss of gray and white matter from the brain during semistarvation (Yager & Andersen, 2005). Loss of subcutaneous fat leads to poor body

temperature regulation, cold intolerance, and development of **lanugo**, a downy growth of hair meant to preserve body heat. Semistarvation causes the body to conserve energy by lowering heart rate, respiratory rate, and gut transit. Clients may complain of constipation, gastric bloating, and fullness because of delayed gastric emptying. Laboratory values are often normal, unless the condition is quite advanced (Williams, Goodie, & Motsinger, 2008). Thyroid function abnormalities and anemia occur in some individuals. Diminished bone mineral density occurs in relation to the duration of anorexia and amenorrhea because of the negative effect of estrogen deprivation on bone modeling: the longer the duration of anorexia and amenorrhea, the likelihood increases that osteopenia or osteoporosis may occur (Jayasinghe, Grover, & Zacharin, 2008). The nurse should explain the relationship between the eating disorder and any physical or laboratory findings to reinforce the consequences of the behaviors, especially in the client who denies any problem or is unready to pursue treatment. The client with normal laboratory values should learn that normal values are not an indicator of good health when other symptoms are present.

Treatment

The initial goal of intervention for anorexia nervosa is weight restoration and correction of any medical or metabolic symptoms. The choice of inpatient or outpatient management of the client is dependent on the acuity of symptoms. Severely abnormal vital signs (heart rate less than 35–40 beats per minute [bpm] and symptomatic hypotension), cardiac arrhythmia, weight less than 70% to 75% of ideal, electrolyte abnormalities,

CLIENT EDUCATION CHECKLIST — What to Expect with the Refeeding Process

The process of refeeding after starvation or semistarvation can lead to metabolic and physical changes. The nurse can educate the client about the following physiological responses to the reintroduction of adequate nutrition:

- Water weight gain occurs early in the process when glycogen stores improve, because glycogen forms a complex with water in the liver and muscle.
- Weight restoration ultimately should include a healthful body composition with adequate lean muscle and adipose stores. Adipose is essential for organ protection, body temperature regulation, and as a reserve for energy and hormone production.

- Intestinal transit time is slowed with anorexia and bulimia. Constipation and delayed gastric emptying can give a sense of fullness that should not be interpreted as overeating. If delayed gastric emptying is problematic, frequent small meals can help. Carbonated beverages and gum chewing should be avoided to minimize bloating. Adequate fluid and fiber can help constipation. Intestinal symptoms should improve with time and adequate intake.
- Metabolic rate becomes elevated with increased intake following starvation. Physical symptoms can include increased sweating or a feeling of warmth and increased hunger. The recommended level of intake may need to be increased to promote weight gain when this change occurs.

psychiatric emergencies, and nonresponsiveness to outpatient treatment are indications for inpatient treatment (ADA, 2006a; Williams, Goodie, & Motsinger, 2008). Long-term goals include improvement in eating behaviors and psychological and emotional health. Psychological symptoms and obsession with weight and shape generally remit significantly later in recovery than physical symptoms and may relapse or persist in some (Attia & Walsh, 2009). The Maudsley approach to anorexia nervosa treatment in adolescents uses a philosophy that encourages intensive and active family-based intervention in the feeding process and overall treatment. Evidence-based and case report research supports its use in this specific population (Loeb, Hirsch, Greif, & Hildebrandt, 2009). Clinicians using this approach require specific training. On-line resources are available for parents seeking information and providers of this form of treatment.

Weight restoration goals are typically up to 1 to 2 lb/week outpatient and 3 lb/week inpatient (ADA, 2006b; Williams, Goodie, & Motsinger, 2008). A structured meal plan calculated to provide sufficient calories for weight gain is used with the inpatient population. Mealtimes are observed by a member of the health care team and physical activity is limited to ensure a positive energy balance. The client is monitored for the squirreling away of food, after-meal visits to the restroom, and any other food behaviors used to avoid intake. Exercise is limited or completely restricted to optimize weight gain. Clients are weighed daily, usually facing backward to the scale (called *blind weighing*) to buffer any reaction to weight gain. The client should be weighed in a gown and after voiding to avoid any possibility of weighting the scale with hidden objects in clothing or excessive fluid intake. Urine specific gravity should be checked to see if deliberate fluid loading is occurring.

Outpatient clients are given customized nutrition recommendations based on individual weight gain and nutritional goals. The registered dietitian determines with the client and the health care team whether structured or more flexible nu-

trition recommendations are indicated. The gradual addition of approximately 500 extra kcalories/day to the client's present intake should theoretically lead to a 1 lb/week weight gain. However, when successful refeeding begins, the resting energy expenditure has been reported to increase disproportionately and it is not uncommon to require more calories than calculated to foster weight gain (van Wymelbeke, Brondel, Brun, & Rigaud, 2004). After explicitly assessing the client for the possibility of increased exercise or use of diet pills contributing to any lack of weight gain, the nurse can educate the client about this initial metabolic response by the body. The nurse can also educate the client about the body's normal response to refeeding to minimize fear and behavioral noncompliance because of symptoms. Client Education Checklist: What to Expect with the Refeeding Process outlines pointers for the nurse to review with the client.

All clients should be monitored for **refeeding syndrome,** a sequela of symptoms that occurs when sudden adequate calories are supplied to the body after starvation. Uptake of glucose into cells leads to shifts in potassium and phosphorus that can lead to precipitous drops in plasma levels during the first few weeks after intake is increased. Box 17-6 outlines the effects and treatment of refeeding syndrome.

Decreased bone mineral density resulting in osteopenia or osteoporosis is a short- and long-term risk with restrictive eating. Chronic low intake of kcalories and weight loss leads to estrogen deprivation and amenorrhea, which in turn negatively affects bone mineral density. The nurse should educate the client about current recommendations for improving bone health in anorexia nervosa, as outlined in Practice Pearl: Amenorrhea and Bone Health in Anorexia Nervosa.

Bulimia Nervosa

Bulimia nervosa can go undetected if clients are judged by appearance alone because, often, they are of normal weight or are slightly overweight (ADA, 2006b). Approximately

BOX 17-6 Refeeding Syndrome

Refeeding syndrome occurs with significant calorie intake following starvation or semistarvation. Symptoms occur as a result of increased uptake of glucose into cells and can have dangerous results if left unmonitored. The nurse should be alert to the following symptoms of refeeding syndrome:

- Hypophosphotemia
- Hypokalemia
- Hypomagnesemia
- Cardiac rhythm changes
- Edema
- Congestive heart failure

   Treatment is pharmacological correction of electrolyte deficiencies and careful monitoring. When possible, gradual increases in calorie intake rather than abrupt overfeeding can lessen the risk of refeeding syndrome symptoms.

half of all individuals with anorexia go on to develop bulimia (Guarda, 2008). **Bulimia nervosa** is characterized by a binge-purge cycle. The definition of a binge is subjective but generally includes the consumption of a large amount of food in a short interval of time with an accompanying sense of loss of control. Foods consumed during the binge are often those that the individual considers forbidden, such as high-fat or high-kcalorie items. A person with bulimia may plan a binge

PRACTICE PEARL

Amenorrhea and Bone Health in Anorexia Nervosa

Loss of bone mineral density is prevalent in anorexia nervosa. Adolescents with anorexia further jeopardize bone health because peak bone mass has yet to be accrued, increasing the risk of long-term poor bone health. Lack of menses contributes to bone loss without the bone-protecting effects of sufficient estrogen. Often, oral contraceptives are prescribed with the erroneous belief that this approach will provide protection against bone loss. Oral contraceptives have not been shown to increase bone mineral density in anorexia nervosa. To improve bone health, the nurse can educate the client on the following:

- Improvements in bone mineral density occur with weight restoration.
- Natural resumption of menstruation improves bone mineral density.
- Resumption of menses generally occurs at a weight 5# above where amenorrhea occurred.
- Use of oral contraceptives does not improve bone mineral density.
- Adequate calcium and vitamin D intake are needed for bone health.

Sources: Golden, 2007; Jayasinghe et al., 2008; Misra et al., 2008; Vescovi, Jamal, & DeSouza, 2008.

ahead of time or it may be triggered by emotional feelings as a maladaptive coping behavior. Compensatory purging follows the binge and can be in the form of vomiting; misuse of laxatives, diuretics, or diet pills; fasting; or excessive exercise. Most clients with bulimia nervosa have restrictive eating patterns when not bingeing.

Symptoms of bulimia nervosa are associated with the method of purging used. Vomiting can lead to dental enamel erosion, "chipmunk cheeks" from swollen parotid glands, gastrointestinal complaints, and altered electrolyte levels. Russell's sign, a calloused or reddened knuckle of the index finger, occurs from teeth abrading the finger when used to stimulate purging. Use of syrup of ipecac to induce vomiting leads to cardiomyopathy (Williams, Goodie, & Motsinger, 2008). Laxative and diuretic use is ineffective in reducing kcalorie intake but is employed nevertheless and can lead to alterations in fluid and electrolyte status. Specific alterations are outlined in Table 17-6. The use of excessive exercise to compensate for bingeing can go unnoticed until it reaches an extreme because of the social acceptability of this normally healthful behavior. Stress fractures, continued exercising despite an injury, and forgoing other activities in order to exercise are warning signs of this behavior.

Treatment

Nutritional treatment of bulimia nervosa is aimed at correction of chaotic eating patterns. Collaborating with the client to help normalize eating and correct nutritional and weight misperceptions can help the client to separate nutritional contributors to bulimic behaviors from emotional and psychological contributors. It is important that a multidisciplinary team works together to complement client care. Cognitive behavior therapy has been shown to be effective in helping clients develop new coping strategies to combat feelings that lead to bulimic behaviors (Williams, Goodie, & Motsinger, 2008). Often, the client with bulimia nervosa is trying to lose weight and may continue to do so during treatment. However, restrictive eating can contribute to the chaotic eating and binge-purge cycle. The nurse should reinforce the knowledge that simultaneous dieting and recovery from bulimia are incompatible behaviors (ADA, 2006b). Weight loss may be achieved when eating patterns are normalized, but restrictive eating is contraindicated to achieve this goal. A regular pattern of eating with avoidance of excessive hunger is a central part of nutrition intervention. Educational and behavioral advice aimed at changing compensatory purge activities is also warranted. Clients who misuse diuretics or laxatives should be educated about weaning from those behaviors. Treatment guidelines are outlined in Table 17-6.

Binge Eating Disorder and EDNOS

Binge eating disorder falls under the diagnostic category of EDNOS along with other patterns of disordered eating that warrant attention but do not meet the strict criteria for a diagnosis of anorexia or bulimia nervosa. **Binge eating disorder** is characterized by the same bingeing behavior as found with bulimia but without the compensatory purging that follows. Clients with binge eating disorder are often overweight. Additionally, the prevalence of binge eating disorder in males exceeds that found with anorexia or bulimia (Hudson et al., 2007).

Treatment

Treatment of binge eating disorder is multidisciplinary, focusing on any medical complications related to overweight, underlying mental health issues, and normalization of eating patterns similar to the approach for bulimia (Williams, Goodie, & Motsinger, 2008). Much has been made of a possible association between a stress response and binge eating (Gluck, 2006). It is a subject of debate whether weight management for obesity and binge eating disorder can be addressed simultaneously or, as in bulimia, the disordered eating pattern should be addressed first (ADA, 2006b; Williams, Goodie, & Motsinger, 2008). The nurse should be aware that clients with binge eating disorder may present asking for weight management advice and not divulge the presence of bingeing unless asked sensitively about it. Less than half of individuals with bulimia or binge eating disorder seek help for these disorders (Hudson et al., 2007).

Identification of two additional distinct eating related disorders is being recognized. **Night eating syndrome (NES)** and nocturnal sleep-related eating disorder are characterized by eating during normal sleeping hours, but the latter is treated as a sleep disorder because it is associated with other sleep disturbances and individuals are unaware of the nocturnal eating. NES and its treatment are outlined in Hot Topic: Night Eating Syndrome.

hot Topic

Night Eating Syndrome

Night eating syndrome (NES) is found during periods of stress in an individual and is characterized by insomnia and eating a significant portion of calories during normal sleeping hours followed by poor appetite in the morning hours. Clients awaken at least three times a week during the night and consume at least 25% of their energy needs. Unlike bulimia, the eating episodes are not considered binges and there is no compensatory behavior. Obesity is often the result. Treatment is aimed at mediating the stress and mood disorders that are associated with the syndrome. The following is recommended:

- Muscle relaxation techniques.
- Pharmacological treatment (select serotonin reuptake inhibitors).
- There is no sense of loss of control as found with binge eating disorders. Other than ensuring adequate nutrient intake, nutritional intervention for this syndrome is largely unstudied.

Sources: Allison et al., 2008; Goel et al., 2009; Howell, Schenck, & Crow, 2009; Stunkard, Allison, & Lundgren, 2008.

NURSING CARE PLAN Nutrition and the Overweight Adult

CASE STUDY

Caroline is a 29-year-old elementary school teacher who is concerned about her weight and its effect on her life. Most recently, one of her fifth grade students asked her why she taught them about the right foods to eat in health class even though she was "fat." She said she nearly cried and knows that at 209 pounds she is overweight. She related that she has always had a weight problem, just like everyone else in her family. She said she has never had a boyfriend, even though she really wants to get married and have children. She loves the kids in her class and works hard to be a good teacher.

She said she gets too tired at the end of the day to do anything but go home, make dinner, and watch television or play the piano a bit before doing some prep work for the next day's classes. Dieting never seems to work for more than a week or two, when she gets discouraged and gives up if there is not any significant weight loss. Right now she is so tired of being fat that she wants the bariatric surgery she has heard about and hopes her insurance will cover it; otherwise she will take a weekend job to earn some extra money to pay for it. Her last medical visit was for a sinus infection about 5 years ago, so she believes she is in good health because she is never sick.

Nutrition and the Overweight Adult *(continued)*

NURSING CARE PLAN

Applying the Nursing Process

ASSESSMENT

Height: 5 feet 2 inches (158 cm) Weight: 209 pounds (95 kg) BMI: 38

BP 152/92 P 84, regular R 20

Elbow breadth measurement indicates a medium frame size

Hemoglobin: 13.5 gm/dL Hematocrit: 41% Fasting blood glucose: 117 mg/dL

Mother has a history of type 2 diabetes, onset about the age of 48, currently doing well taking an oral antidiabetic agent

Caroline ambulates without difficulty but feels "winded" after a few minutes walking

She eats 3 meals a day and snacks when the students have recess and in the evening

DIAGNOSES

Imbalanced nutrition: more than body requirements related to consumption of calories exceeding energy expenditure (sedentary lifestyle)

Disturbed body image related to embarrassment and negative statements about appearance

Risk for loneliness related to obesity

Activity intolerance related to obesity

Health seeking behavior related to expressed interest in bariatric surgery

EXPECTED OUTCOMES

Weight loss of 10 pounds in 2 months using a diet plan

Fasting blood glucose less than 110 mg/dL

Participation in one weekly evening activity with adults

Able to walk one block without feeling short of breath

States the benefits and drawbacks of bariatric surgery

INTERVENTIONS

Food diary and 24-hour food recall

Teaching about type 2 diabetes

Meet with a dietitian to discuss a weight-reduction diet

Increase daily activity by making small changes such as parking in a more distant parking space at school or stores

Plan one activity each week that involves being with other adults

Share materials about bariatric surgery and encourage discussing it with others who have had the procedure

EVALUATION

Caroline was concerned about some of the potential side effects and complications of surgery so she agreed to try dieting first. After 2 months, she was pleased to have lost 13 pounds but described it as "very difficult." She was always hungry, but enlisted a couple of colleagues at school to gently remind her of her goal. She started eating oatmeal for breakfast but had to put a few chocolate morsels on top to make it palatable. It was easy to take a salad for lunch because her friends would eat with her, and she substituted pretzels for the potato chips she preferred. She had started going outside at recess so she would not eat during that time and actually found she enjoyed talking to the adult playground monitors to keep her mind off food. It was hard to control portions at dinner because she ate alone all the time, but she was trying to make just enough food so there would not be leftovers. She still felt too tired to go out in the evenings and really felt too shy to go anywhere alone. She was pleased that even parking a little farther away could increase her stamina and in nice weather she would walk around the apartment complex where she lived. Because her blood pressure was 148/88 and her glucose was now 112 mg/dL she felt she could keep trying the diet and lifestyle changes and wait to see if she really wanted surgery. Figure 17-3 ■ outlines the nursing process with this case.

Critical Thinking in the Nursing Process

1. How could the nurse respond if Caroline had insisted that surgery was what she really wanted?

2. What are some foods that the nurse could suggest to the client who is trying to lose weight and lower blood glucose?

(continued)

Nutrition and the Overweight Adult *(continued)*

Assessment

Data about the patient

Subjective

What the patient tells the nurse

Example: Weight loss diets don't seem to work; I'm always tired; I want bariatric surgery.

Objective

What the nurse observes; anthropometric and clinical data

Examples: 209 pounds; 62 inches tall; BMI: 38; medium frame size; BP: 162/92

Diagnosis

NANDA label

Example: Imbalanced nutrition: more than body requirements related to excess intake and sedentary lifestyle

Planning

Goals stated in patient terms

Example: Long-term goal: lose 10 pounds in 2 months; Short-term goal: state benefits and drawbacks of bariatric surgery

Implementation

Nursing action to help patient achieve goals

Example: Refer to dietitian; discuss risks and benefits of bariatric surgery

Evaluation

Was the goal achieved or does the intervention need to be modified?

Example: Lost 13 pounds but it was "very difficult;" stamina increasing; stay with diet for now

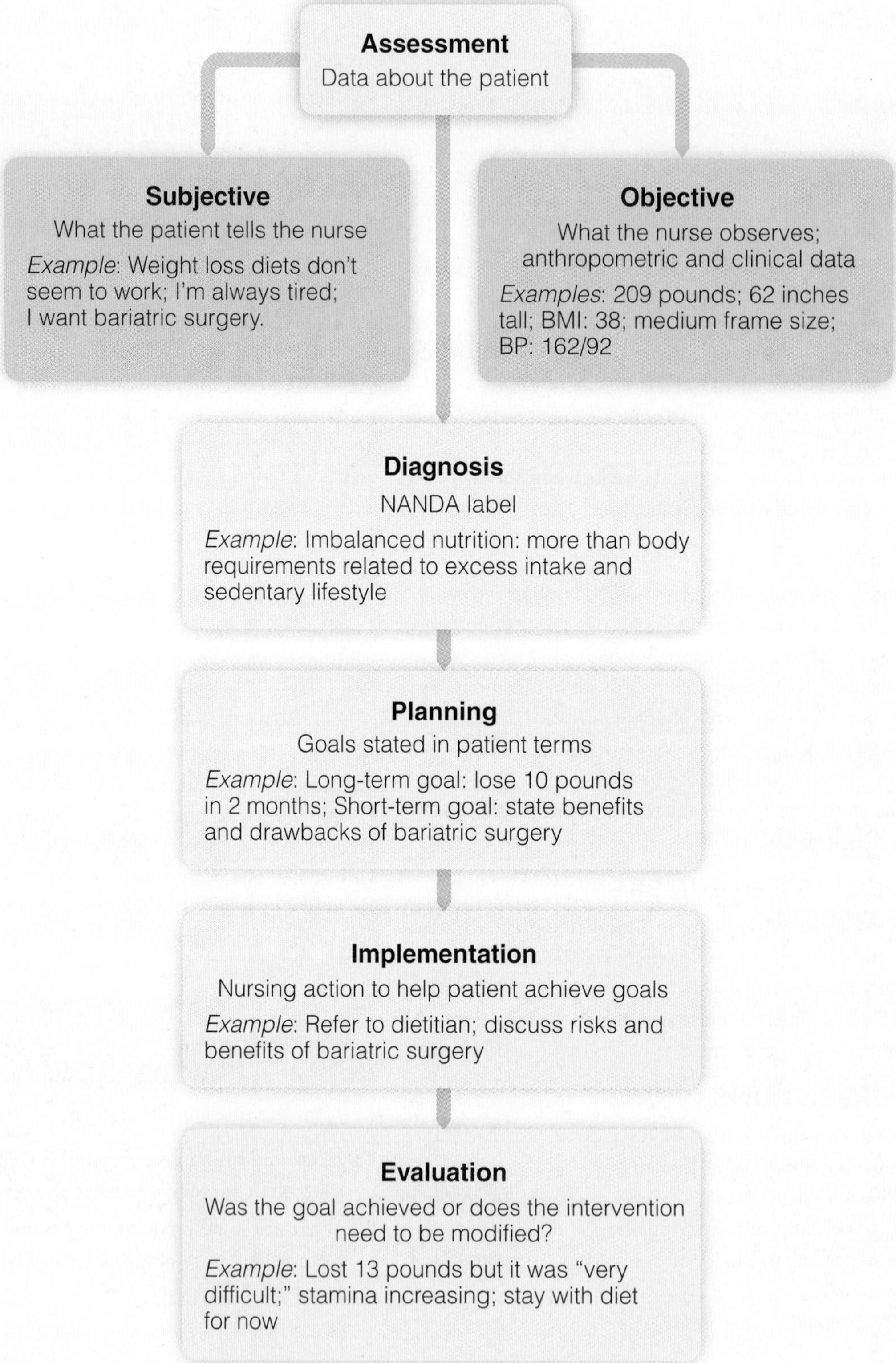

■ FIGURE 17-3 **Nursing Care Process Plan: Nutrition and the Overweight Adult.**

CHAPTER SUMMARY

- Weight management issues are prevalent across the lifespan and include both overweight and underweight.

- Many factors contribute to the increasing prevalence of overweight, including increased calorie intake from larger portions of food, decreased energy expenditure from sedentary lifestyles and biological influences.

- The nurse is a vital member of the health care team providing evidence-based guidance in lifestyle management to the overweight client. Lifestyle management includes diet, exercise, and behavior modification.

- Surgical and pharmacological interventions are reserved for the very obese client, especially those individuals with comorbid conditions resulting from being overweight.

- Use of dietary supplements, fad diets, and unsound nutritional practices are not recommended as methods of weight management.

- Eating disorders are psychiatric diagnoses with physical, medical, and nutritional implications.

- Clients with eating disorders are at risk for short- and long-term nutritional problems. Diminished bone density is a common long-term problem even after recovery occurs.

- The nurse is a vital member of the interdisciplinary health care team, providing intervention for anorexia nervosa, bulimia nervosa, and binge eating.

EXPLORE   mynursingkit™

MyNursingKit is your one stop for online chapter review materials and resources. Prepare for success with additional NCLEX®-style practice questions, interactive assignments and activities, web links, animations and videos, and more!

Register your access code from the front of your book at
www.mynursingkit.com.

NCLEX® QUESTIONS

1. A mother is concerned that her 12-year-old daughter who is 5 feet tall and weighs 115 pounds is going to become obese. How should the nurse respond to this concern?
   1. "Your daughter's adult weight cannot be predicted so a healthy balanced diet and some physical activity are all that is necessary at this age."
   2. "Your daughter is approaching adolescence and as her growth accelerates she will not gain weight."
   3. "A careful nutritional history that includes anthropometric data, nutrient intake, and pattern of activity will help determine if a problem exists."
   4. "This is a serious problem and your daughter should be evaluated for diabetes or a thyroid condition."

2. A client with anorexia nervosa has an initial nursing diagnosis of *Impaired Nutrition: less than body requirements*. Which of the following is a realistic outcome for this client?

   1. Weight gain of 1 pound a week
   2. Limits fluid intake to 1 liter a day
   3. States understanding of a maintenance diet
   4. Requests one snack a day

3. A middle-age client has experienced problems with weight cycling and wants to avoid it after a recent weight loss. What could the nurse suggest to help this client avoid weight gain?
   1. Consume at least 2 liters of fluids a day to maintain a feeling of fullness.
   2. Continue doing whatever helped the weight loss in the first place.
   3. Incorporate daily physical activity and dietary management in a weight maintenance plan.
   4. Avoid increased consumption of simple carbohydrates.

4. The nurse knows the client understands the teaching about orlistat (Xenical) when the client states:
   1. "I need to take a daily multivitamin 2 hours before or after taking the medication."
   2. "I need to increase fiber consumption to prevent constipation."
   3. "The medication aids the absorption of good fats and promotes elimination of bad fats."
   4. "I should call my health care provider every week to report how much weight has been lost."

5. The nurse can be reasonably certain that a client is exhibiting readiness for dietary teaching for weight management when the client states:
   1. "My doctor told me to lose 50 pounds to help get my blood pressure under control."
   2. "I know I have to give up ice cream."
   3. "If I don't lose weight I will not go to my high school reunion in 4 months."
   4. "My knees are starting to hurt so I am going to try to lose some weight and see if that helps."

REFERENCES

Allison, K. C., Engel, S. G., Crosby, R. D., de Zwaan, M., O'Reardon, J. P., Wonderlich, S. A., et al. (2008). Evaluation of diagnostic criteria for night eating syndrome using item response theory analysis. *Eating Behaviors, 9,* 398–407.

American Dietetic Association (ADA). (2006a). Position of the American Dietetic Association: Individual-, family-, school- and community-based interventions for pediatric overweight. *Journal of the American Dietetic Association, 106,* 925–945.

American Dietetic Association (ADA). (2006b). Position of the American Dietetic Association: Nutrition intervention in the treatment of anorexia nervosa, bulimia nervosa, and eating disorders. *Journal of the American Dietetic Association, 106,* 2073–2082.

American Dietetic Association (ADA). (2009). Position of the American Dietetic Association: Weight management. *Journal of the American Dietetic Association, 109,* 330–346.

Attia, E., & Walsh, B. T. (2009). Behavioral management of anorexia nervosa. *New England Journal of Medicine, 360,* 500–506.

Bachman, C. M., Baranowski, T., & Nicklas, T. A. (2006). Is there an association between sweetened beverages and adiposity? *Nutrition Reviews, 64,* 153–174.

Bacon, L., Stern, J. S., Van Loan, M. D., & Keim, N. L. (2005). Size acceptance and intuitive eating improve health for obese, female chronic dieters. *Journal of the American Dietetic Association, 105,* 929–936.

Bellar, A., Jarosz, P. A., & Bellar, D. (2008). Implications of the biology of weight regulation and obesity on the treatment of obesity. *Journal of the American Academy of Nurse Practitioners, 20,* 128–135.

Benson-Davies, S., & Quigley, D. R. (2008). Screening postoperative bariatric patients for marginal ulcerations. *Journal of the American Dietetic Association, 108,* 1369–1371.

Blanck, H. M., Serdula, M. K., Gillespie, C., Galuska, D. A., Sharpe, P. A., Conway, J. M., et al. (2007). Use of nonprescription dietary supplements for weight loss is common among Americans. *Journal of the American Dietetic Association, 107,* 441–447.

Bortolotti, M., Rudelle, S., Schneiter, P., Vidal, H., Loizon, E., Tappy, L., et al. (2008). Dairy calcium supplementation in overweight or obese persons: Its effect on markers of fat metabolism. *American Journal of Clinical Nutrition, 88,* 873–874.

Bouchard, C. (2008). Gene-environment interactions in the etiology of obesity: Defining the fundamentals. *Obesity, 16,* S5–S10.

Canals, J., Sancho, C., & Arija, M. V. (2009). Influence of parent's eating attitudes on eating disorders in school adolescents. *European Child & Adolescent Psychiatry,* doi 10.1007/S00787-009-0737-9.

Centers for Disease Control and Prevention (CDC). (2008a). Youth risk behavior surveillance—United States, 2007. *Morbidity & Mortality Weekly Report, 57,* 1–131.

Centers for Disease Control and Prevention (CDC). (2008b). *Health United States, 2008.* Retrieved April 6, 2009, from http://www.cdc.gov/nchs/data/hus/hus08.pdf#075

Chandola, T., Brunner, E., & Marmot, M. (2006). Chronic stress at work and the metabolic syndrome: A prospective study. *BMJ (Clinical Research Ed.), 332,* 521–525.

Clifton, P. M. (2008). Dietary treatment for obesity. *Nature Clinical Practice: Gastroenterology & Hepatology, 5,* 672–681.

Cohen, L., Perales, D. P., & Steadman, C. (2005). The O word: Why the focus on obesity is harmful to community health. *California Journal of Health Promotion, 3,* 154–161.

Colossi, F. G., Casagrande, D. S., Chatkin, R., Moretto, M., Barhouch, A. S., Repetto, G., et al. (2008). Need for multivitamin use in postoperative period of gastric bypass. *Obesity Surgery, 18,* 187–191.

Crow, S. J., Agras, W. S., Crosby, R., Halmi, K., & Mitchell, J. E. (2008). Eating disorder symptoms in pregnancy: A prospective study. *International Journal of Eating Disorders, 41,* 277–279.

Daniels, J. (2006). Obesity: America's epidemic. *American Journal of Nursing, 106,* 40–49.

Dickerson, R. N., & Roth-Yousey, L. (2005). Medication effects on metabolic rate: A systematic review (part 2). *Journal of the American Dietetic Association, 105,* 1002–1009.

Donnelly, J. E., Blair, S. N., Jakicic, J. M., Manore, M. M., Rankin, J. W., & Smith, B. K. (2009). American College of Sports Medicine position stand: Appropriate physical activity intervention strategies for weight loss and prevention of weight regain for adults. *Medicine & Science in Sports & Exercise, 41,* 459–471.

Doucet, E. (2008). Gastrointestinal peptides after bariatric surgery and appetite control: Are they in tuning? *Current Opinion in Clinical Nutrition and Metabolic Care, 11,* 645–650.

Eckel, R. H. (2008). Nonsurgical management of obesity in adults. *New England Journal of Medicine, 358,* 1941–1950.

Eisenberg, M., & Neumark-Sztainer, D. (2008). Peer harassment and disordered eating. *International Journal of Adolescent Medicine & Health, 20,* 155–164.

Fisher, J. O., & Krall, T. V. E. (2008). Super-size me: Portion size effects on young children's eating. *Physiology & Behavior, 94,* 39–47.

Flegal, K. M., Graubard, B. I., Williamson, D. F., & Gail, M. H. (2007). Cause specific excess deaths associated with underweight, overweight and obesity. *Journal of the American Medical Association, 298,* 2028–2037.

Food & Drug Administration (FDA). (2009). *FDA expands warning to consumers about tainted weight loss pills.* Retrieved April 8, 2009, from http://www.fda.gov/bbs/topics/NEWS/2008/NEW01933.html

Gardner, C. D., Kiazand, A., Alhassan, S., Kim, S., Stafford, R. S., Balise, R. R., et al. (2007). Comparison of the Atkins, Zone, Ornish, and LEARN diets for change in weight and related risk factors among overweight and premenopausal women. *Journal of the American Medical Association, 297,* 969–977.

Gluck, M. E. (2006). Stress response and binge eating disorder. *Appetite, 46,* 26–30.

Goebel-Fabbri, A. E. (2009). Disturbed eating behaviors and eating disorders in type 1 dia-

REFERENCES *(continued)*

betes: Clinical significance and treatment recommendations. *Current Diabetes Report, 9,* 133–139.

Goel, N., Stunkard, A. J., Rogers, N. L., Van Dongen, H. P., Allison, K. C., O'Reardon, J. P., et al. (2009). Circadian rhythm profiles in women with night eating syndrome. *Journal of Biological Rhythms, 24,* 85–94.

Golden, N. H. (2007). Eating disorders in adolescence: What is the role of hormone replacement therapy? *Current Opinion in Obstetrics & Gynecology, 19,* 434–439.

Guarda, A. S. (2008). Treatment of anorexia nervosa: Insights and obstacles. *Physiology & Behavior, 94,* 113–120.

Halmi, K. A. (2009). Perplexities and provocations of eating disorders. *The Journal of Child Psychology, 50,* 163–169.

Hannerz, H., Albertson, K., Nielsen, M.L., Tuchsen, F., & Burr, H. (2004). Occupational factors and 5-year weight change among men in a Danish national cohort. *Health Psychology, 23*(3), 283–288.

Hession, M., Rollard, C., Kulkami, U., Wise, A., & Broom, J. (2009). Systematic review of randomized controlled trials of low-carbohydrate vs. low-fat/low-calorie diets in the management of obesity. *Obesity, 10,* 36–50.

Howell, M. J., Schenck, C. H., & Crow, S. J. (2009). A review of nighttime eating disorders. *Sleep Medicine Review, 13,* 23–34.

Hudson, J. I., Hiripi, E., Pope, H. G., & Kessler, R. C. (2007). The prevalence and correlates of eating disorders in the National Comorbidity Survey Replication. *Biological Psychiatry, 61,* 348–358.

Jayasinghe, Y., Grover, S. R., & Zacharin, M. (2008). Current concepts in bone and reproductive health in adolescents with anorexia nervosa. *British Journal of Obstetrics & Gynecology, 115,* 304–315.

Katan, M. B. (2009). Weight-loss diets for the prevention and treatment of obesity. *New England Journal of Medicine, 360,* 923–924.

Kivimaki, M., Head, J., Ferrie, J. E., Shipley, M. J., Brunner, E., Vahtera, J., et al. (2006). Work stress, weight gain and weight loss: Evidence for bidirectional effects of job strain on body mass index in the Whitehall II study. *International Journal of Obesity (London), 30*(6), 982–987.

Klopp, S. A., Heiss, C. J., & Smith, H. J. (2003). Self-reported vegetarianism may be a marker for college age women at risk for disordered eating. *Journal of the American Dietetic Association, 103,* 745–747.

Kouvonen, A., Kivimaki, M., Cox, S. J., Cox, T., & Vahtera, J. (2005). Relationship between work stress and body mass index among 45,810 female and male employees. *Psychosomatic Medicine, 67*(4), 577–583.

Kushner, R. F. (2007). Obesity management. *Gastroenterology Clinics of North America, 36,* 191–210.

Kushner, R. F. (2008). Anti-obesity drugs. *Expert Opinion on Pharmacotherapy, 9,* 1339–1350.

Lallukka, T., Laaksonen, M., Martikainen, P., Sarlio-Lahteenkorva, S., & Lahelma, E. (2005). Psychosocial working conditions and weight gain among employees. *International Journal of Obesity (London), 29*(8), 909–915.

Lamberg, L. (2006). Rx for obesity: Eat less, exercise more and—maybe—get more sleep. *Journal of the American Medical Association, 295,* 2341–2343.

Leslie, W. S., Hankey, C. R., & Lean, M. E. J. (2007). Weight gain as an adverse effect of some commonly prescribed drugs: A systematic review. *Quarterly Journal of Medicine, 100,* 395–404.

Levitsky, L. L., Misra, M., Boepple, P. A., & Hoppin, A. G. (2009). Adolescent obesity and bariatric surgery. *Current Opinion in Endocrinology, Diabetes, and Obesity, 16,* 37–44.

Loeb, K. L., Hirsch, A. M., Greif, R., & Hildebrandt, T. B. (2009). Family-based treatment of a 17-year-old twin presenting with emerging anorexia nervosa: A case study using the "Maudsley method." *Journal of Clinical Child & Adolescent Psychology, 38,* 176–183.

Maggard, M. A., Yermilov, I., Li, Z., Maglione, M., Newberry, S., Suttorp, M., et al. (2008). Pregnancy and fertility following bariatric surgery: A systematic review. *Journal of the American Medical Association, 300,* 2286–2296.

Mahabadi, A. A., Massaro, J. M., Rosito, G. A., Levy, D., Murabito, J. M., Wolf, P. A., et al. (2009). Association of pericardial fat, intrathoracic fat, and visceral fat with cardiovascular disease burden: The Framingham Heart Study. *European Heart Journal, 30,* 850–856.

Mechanick, J. I., Kushner, R. F., Sugerman, H. J., Gonzalez-Campoy, M., Collazo-Clavell, M. L., Guven, S., et al. (2008). American Association of Clinical Endocrinologists, The Obesity Society, and the American Society for Metabolic & Bariatric Surgery medical guidelines for clinical practice for the postoperative nutritional, metabolic, and nonsurgical support of the bariatric surgical patient. *Endocrine Practice, 14,* 1S–83S.

Melanson, K. J., Angelopoulos, T. J., Nguyen, V., Zukley, L., Lowndes, J., & Rippe, J. M. (2008). High-fructose corn syrup, energy intake, and appetite regulation. *American Journal of Clinical Nutrition, 88,* 1738S–1744S.

Misra, M., Prabjakaran, R., Miller, K. K., Glodstein, M. A., Mickley, D., Clauss, L., et al. (2008). Weight gain and restoration of menses as predictors of bone mineral density change in adolescent girls with anorexia ner-

vosa. *Journal of Clinical Endocrinology & Metabolism, 93,* 1231–1237.

National Heart, Lung, and Blood Institute (NHLBI). (1998). *Clinical guidelines for the identification, evaluation and treatment of overweight and obesity in adults. The evidence report.* Retrieved April 8, 2009, from http://www.nhlbi.nih.gov/guidelines/obesity/ob_gdlns.pdf

National Institute of Diabetes, Digestive and Kidney Disease (NIDDK). (2008). *Bariatric surgery for severe obesity.* Retrieved April 8, 2009, from http://win.niddk.nih.gov/publications/gasurg12.04bw.pdf

National Institutes of Health (NIH), National Center for Complementary and Alternative Medicine (NCCAM). (2008). *Bitter orange.* Retrieved April 8, 2009, from http://nccam.nih.gov/health/bitterorange/

Nattiv, A., Loucks, A. B., Manore, M. M., Sanborn, C. F., Sundgot-Borgen, J., & Warren, M. (2007). American College of Sports Medicine position stand: The female athlete triad. *Medicine & Science in Sports and Exercise, 39,* 1867–1882.

Neumark-Sztainer, D., Wall, M., Guo, J., Story, M., Haines, J., & Eisenberg, M. (2006). Obesity, disordered eating, and eating disorders in a longitudinal study of adolescents: How do dieters fare 5 years later? *Journal of the American Dietetic Association, 106,* 559–568.

Ogden, C. L. (2009). Disparities in obesity prevalence in the United States: Black women at risk. *American Journal of Clinical Nutrition, 89,* 1001–1002.

Ostry, A. S., Radi, S., Louie, A. M., & LaMontagne, A. D. (2006). Psychosocial and other working conditions in relation to body mass index in a representative sample of Australian workers. *BMC Public Health, 6,* 53–58.

Overgaard, D., Gamborg, M., Gyntelberg, F., & Heitmann, B. L. (2004). Psychological workload is associated with weight gain between 1993 and 1999: Analyses based on the Danish nurse cohort study. *International Journal of Obesity and Related Metabolic Disorders, 28*(8), 1072–1081.

Overgaard, D., Gamborg, M., Gyntelberg, F., & Heitmann, B. L. (2006). Psychological workload and weight gain among women with and without familial obesity. *Obesity (Silver Spring, MD), 14*(3), 458–463.

Paddon-Jones, D., Westman, E., Mattes, R. D., Wolfe, R. R., Astrup, A., & Westerterp-Plantenga, M. (2008). Protein, weight management, and satiety. *American Journal of Clinical Nutrition, 87,* 1558S–1561S.

Papadopoulos, F. C., Ekbom, A., Brandt, L., & Ekselius, L. (2009). Excess mortality, causes of death and prognostic factors in anorexia nervosa. *British Journal of Psychiatry, 194,* 10–17.

REFERENCES *(continued)*

Pillitteri, J. L., Shiffman, S., Rohay, J. M., Harkins, A. M., Burton, S., & Wadden, T. (2008). Use of dietary supplements for weight loss in the United States: Results of a national survey. *Obesity, 16*, 790–796.

Poirier, P., Giles, T. D., Bray, G. A., Hong, Y., Stern, J. S., Pi-Sunyer, X., et al. (2006). Obesity and cardiovascular disease: Pathophysiology, evaluation, and effect of weight loss. *Circulation, 113*, 898–918.

Provencher, V., Begin, C., Tremblay, A., Mongeau, L., Boivin, S., & Lemieux, S. (2007). Short-term effects of a "Health-at-Every-Size" approach on eating behaviors and appetite ratings. *Obesity, 15*, 957–966.

Rogovik, A. L., & Goldman, R. D. (2009). Should weight-loss supplements be used for pediatric obesity? *Canadian Family Physician, 55*, 257–259.

Sacks, F. M., Bray, G., Carey, V., Smith, S. R., Ryan, D. H., Anton, S. D., et al. (2009). Comparison of weight-loss diets with different compositions of fat, protein, and carbohydrate. *New England Journal of Medicine, 360*, 859–873.

Schwartz, M. B., Thomas, J. J., Bohan, K. M., & Vartanian, L. R. (2007). Intended and unintended effects of an eating disorder educational program: Impact of presenter identity. *International Journal of Eating Disorders, 40*, 187–192.

Shai, I., Schwarzfuchs, D., Henkin, Y., Shahar, D. R., Witkow, S., Greenberg, I., et al. (2008). Weight loss with a low-carbohydrate, Mediterranean, or low-fat diet. *New England Journal of Medicine, 359*, 229–241.

Shaw, H., Stice, E., & Becker, C. B. (2008). Preventing eating disorders. *Child & Adolescent Psychiatric Clinics of North America, 18*, 199–207.

Spear, B. A., Barlow, S. E., Ervin, C., Ludwig, D. S., Saelens, B. E., Schetzina, K. E., et al. (2007). Recommendations for the treatment of child and adolescent overweight and obesity. *Pediatrics, 120*, S254–S288.

Spiotta, R. T., & Luma, G. B. (2008). Evaluating obesity and cardiovascular risk factors in children and adolescents. *American Family Physician, 78*, 1052–1058.

Stothard, K. J., Tennant, P. W., Bell, R., & Rankin, J. (2009). Maternal overweight and obesity and the risk of congenital anomalies: A systematic review and meta-analysis. *Journal of the American Medical Association, 301*, 636–650.

Striegel-Moore, R. H., & Bulik, C. M. (2007). Risk factors for eating disorders. *American Psychologist, 62*, 181–198.

Stunkard, A., Allison, K., & Lundgren, J. (2008). Issues for DSM-V: Night eating syndrome. *American Journal of Psychiatry, 165*, 424.

Tanumihardjo, S. A., Anderson, C., Kaufer-Horwitz, M., Bode, L., Emenaker, N. J., Haqq, A. M., et al. (2007). Poverty, obesity, and malnutrition: An international perspective recognizing the paradox. *Journal of the American Dietetic Association, 107*, 1966–1972.

The Obesity Society. (2009). *Obesity, bias, and stigmatization.* Retrieved April 8, 2009, from http://www.obesity.org/information/weight_bias.asp

Tucker, O. N., Szomstein, A., & Rosenthal, R. J. (2007). Nutritional consequences of weight-loss surgery. *Medical Clinics of North America, 91*, 499–514.

van Wormer, J. J., Martinez, A. M., Martinson, B. C., Crain, A. L., Benson, G. A., Cosentino, D. L., et al. (2009). Self-weighing promotes weight loss for obese adults. *American Journal of Preventative Medicine, 36*, 70–73.

Van Wymelbeke, V., Brondel, L., Brun, J. M., & Rigaud, D. (2004). Factors associated with the increase in resting energy expenditure during refeeding in malnourished anorexia nervosa patients. *American Journal of Clinical Nutrition, 80*, 1469–1477.

Vescovi, J. D., Jamal, S. A., & DeSouza, M. J. (2008). Strategies to reverse bone loss in women with functional hypothalamic amenorrhea: A systematic review of the literature. *Osteoporosis International, 19*, 465–478.

Westman, E. C., Feinman, R. D., Mavropoulos, J. C., Vernon, M. C., Volek, J. S., Wortman, J. A., et al. (2007). Low-carbohydrate nutrition and metabolism. *American Journal of Clinical Nutrition, 86*, 276–284.

Williams, S. E., Cooper, K., Richmond, B., & Schauer, P. (2008). Perioperative management of bariatric surgery patients: Focus on metabolic bone disease. *Cleveland Clinic Journal of Medicine, 75*, 333–338.

Williams, P. M., Goodie, J., & Motsinger, C. D. (2008). Treating eating disorders in primary care. *American Family Physician, 77*, 187–195.

Yager, J., & Andersen, A. E. (2005). Anorexia nervosa. *New England Journal of Medicine, 353*, 1481–1488.

LeAnne Bloedon

Cardiovascular and Lipid Disorders 18

WHAT WILL YOU LEARN?

1. To summarize the risk factors for coronary heart disease, comparing which factors are amenable to dietary intervention.
2. To differentiate between saturated, monounsaturated, polyunsaturated, and trans fatty acids and accompanying food sources.
3. To relate the parameters of the National Cholesterol Education Program's Therapeutic Lifestyle Changes (TLC) to reduce low-density lipoprotein (LDL) cholesterol.
4. To strategize lifestyle modifications to manage hypertension.
5. To translate the medical nutrition therapy for the client with metabolic syndrome.
6. To analyze and prioritize nutrition-related issues in the client with heart failure.

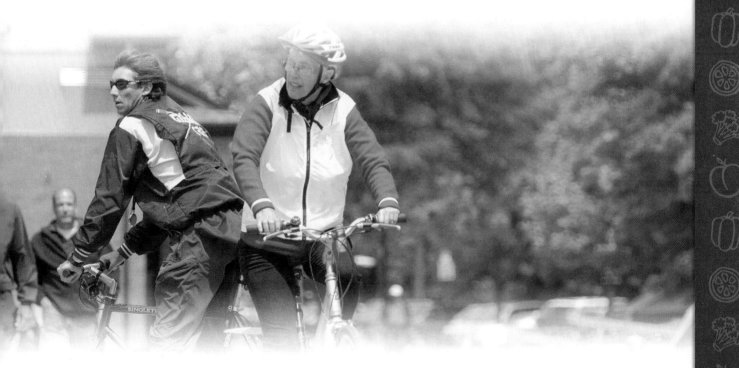

DID YOU KNOW?

► Dietary supplements such as high doses of vitamin E, beta carotene, and selenium are marketed for heart health despite a lack of strong clinical evidence that they work and even some data that suggest potential risk.

► Some types of fat can raise blood cholesterol, whereas other types can lower it.

► Clients with blood pressure that is above normal, but not at the level of hypertension, are at risk for developing hypertension and heart disease and need to be treated with diet and lifestyle modifications.

► Diets rich in fruits, vegetables, and low-fat dairy products are as effective at lowering blood pressure as low-sodium diets. When used in combination, these two lifestyle modifications have a greater effect on reducing blood pressure.

► Clients with heart failure should restrict sodium intake, but rarely need to restrict fluid intake in the outpatient setting if kidney function is normal.

KEY TERMS

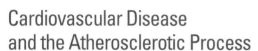

Cardiovascular Disease and the Atherosclerotic Process

Cardiovascular disease (CVD) continues to rank as the number one killer in the United States in both men and women (Centers for Disease Control and Prevention [CDC], 2008a). Cardiovascular disease includes all diseases associated with the heart and blood vessels. **Atherosclerosis,** a main cause of CVD, is a degenerative disease of the lining of the vascular wall leading to narrow, clogged, and hardened arteries. Although there are multiple causes of atherosclerosis, two key factors that nutrition can affect include blood cholesterol and the immune system. Cholesterol is a type of lipid (fat) that is made in the human body as well as obtained through the diet. It is necessary for the synthesis of steroid hormones, vitamin D, and bile acids as well as aids in the structure of cell membranes. Cholesterol travels through the blood within particles called **lipoproteins.** Lipoproteins are made up of both lipids and protein and transport fat-soluble products such as cholesterol, triglycerides, and fat-soluble vitamins in the blood. The classes of lipoproteins include very low-density lipoprotein, intermediate density lipoprotein, low-density lipoprotein (LDL), high-density lipoprotein (HDL), and chylomicrons. Although cholesterol serves a vital role in the body, too much cholesterol in the blood can be detrimental to health because of its relationship to **coronary heart disease (CHD).** CHD is also called coronary artery disease and occurs because of narrowed blood vessels that supply the heart. LDL is the main carrier of cholesterol to peripheral tissues. Numerous studies link elevated total and LDL cholesterol with an increased risk of CHD. For this reason, many consumers refer to LDL cholesterol as "bad" cholesterol. Epidemiological studies reveal that for every 1% decrease in LDL cholesterol, risk of CVD is reduced by 1% (Gaziano, 1996). This statistic can be offered to the client and translated to meaningful numbers to help with motivation when dietary changes are needed to reduce disease risk. For example, a client with a blood LDL level of 150 mg/dL can be told, "if you reduce your LDL to 120 mg/ dL, your risk of cardiovascular disease will decrease by 20%."

When cells receive enough cholesterol from the LDL particle to meet the body's needs, they no longer accept cholesterol and the excess remains in the blood circulating in the LDL particle. LDL cholesterol can become oxidized, which then allows certain cells of the immune system called **macrophages** to bind better to cholesterol. Macrophages have an unlimited capacity for cholesterol uptake. After becoming laden with excess cholesterol, they become white foam cells that can infiltrate the lining of the arteries. This process signals platelets to the area of the macrophage, which, along with other particles, stick to foam cells, releasing factors and attracting more macrophages to the area that repeat this process. Over time, this process involving the immune system and cholesterol can lead to a buildup of plaque within the lining of the blood vessel, narrowing the vessel and increasing the risk of an occlusion, which in turn can lead to a heart attack. Figure 18-1 ■ depicts the development of atherosclerosis.

HDL is the lipoprotein that picks up cholesterol from cells and carries it to the liver for excretion, a process termed **reverse cholesterol transport.** Various types of research have been and are currently being conducted exploring the role of HDL in reducing risk of CVD. Epidemiological studies have consistently shown that high levels of HDL cholesterol are inversely related to risk of CHD (Kwiterovich, 1998). For this reason, many consumers call HDL the "good" cholesterol. Low levels of HDL cholesterol increases risk of CHD independently of LDL cholesterol. A 1% decrease in HDL cholesterol is associated with a 2% to 3% increase in CHD risk (Gordon et al., 1989). Therefore, addressing LDL and HDL cholesterol independently are important for the nurse to consider in assessing risk of CVD and educating the client.

Who Is at Risk for CVD?

In an attempt to better prevent and treat CVD, researchers are constantly searching to identify risk factors in addition to those traditionally accepted. To date the traditional, established risk factors for CVD include the following (National

Normal artery

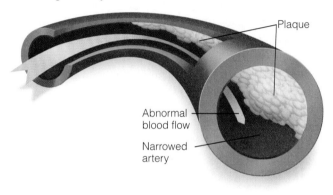

Narrowing of artery

■ **FIGURE 18-1 Progression of Atherosclerosis.**

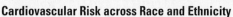

Cultural Considerations

Cardiovascular Risk across Race and Ethnicity

Although the risk of cardiovascular disease increases with age across all races and ethnic groups, certain populations are at greater risk. In particular, the cardiovascular risk factors diabetes and hypertension afflict African Americans more than Caucasians. In the United States, over 10% of the African American adults have diabetes, and one-third of this group is unaware of their condition. The incidence of diabetes among African Americans is 60% greater than in Caucasians. In addition, African Americans have greater complication rates resulting from diabetes compared to Caucasians. For example, African Americans are twice as likely to suffer from lower-limb amputations and diabetes-related blindness.

Hispanic individuals are also at greater risk for diabetes. Currently, almost 10% of Hispanic adults have diabetes. Among this group, 35% have diabetes-related eye complications and are five times more likely to suffer from kidney failure from diabetes as compared to U.S. Caucasian residents with diabetes.

Native Americans and Alaska Natives have the highest prevalence of diabetes in the United States with over 15% of the total Native Americans/Alaska Native population being affected.

Although hypertension affects Caucasian and Hispanic populations at a similar rate, African Americans are about 1.5 times more likely to have hypertension.

Obesity increases the risk of both type 2 diabetes and hypertension. African American and Hispanic children and adults are more likely to be obese compared to Caucasian individuals. Approximately 50% of African Americans and almost 40% of Hispanic adults between the ages of 20 and 39 years are obese. Native American and Alaska Native adults are almost as likely to be obese as African American adults.

Particular attention needs to be given to these populations who are at greater risk for cardiovascular disease in order to screen for early detection and initiate proper management to reduce related risk of disease and death.

Sources: American Diabetes Association, 2008; CDC, 2006; CDC, 2008b; Ogden et al., 2006.

Cholesterol Education Program, Adult Treatment Panel III [NCEP ATP III], 2002):

- Elevated LDL cholesterol
- HDL cholesterol less than 40 mg/dL
- Increased age (greater than or equal to 45 years old, men; greater than or equal to 55 years old, women)
- Diabetes mellitus
- Hypertension (blood pressure greater than 140/90 mm Hg)
- Family history of premature CHD (CHD in male first-degree relative aged less than 55 years and/or CHD in female first-degree relative aged less than 65 years)
- Current cigarette smoker

Risk factors amenable to dietary intervention include elevated LDL cholesterol, low HDL cholesterol, diabetes mellitus, and hypertension in addition to emerging risk factors such as high triglycerides. Risk of CVD is more prevalent in some population groups than others, especially because of increased risk of hypertension or diabetes. Cultural Considerations Box: Cardiovascular Risk across Race and Ethnicity discusses this issue.

Reducing Risk of CVD: Targeting Hypercholesterolemia and Nutrition

In an attempt to reduce morbidity and mortality from CVD in the United States, the National Heart, Lung, and Blood Institute launched the NCEP whose goal is to reduce the in-

cidence of **hypercholesterolemia** (high levels of blood cholesterol). The NCEP regularly issues guidelines to detect, evaluate, and treat hypercholesterolemia. In each of these reports, dietary manipulation is considered to be the cornerstone of management of high levels of LDL cholesterol. Nurses can serve as a vital resource to clients in discussing which factors affect risk of CVD, current guidelines that reduce CVD risk, and educating clients in determining ways to implement needed lifestyle changes to reduce risk.

Reducing elevated LDL cholesterol is the first goal for both **primary and secondary prevention** of CHD (primary prevention refers to delaying or preventing onset of CHD and secondary prevention refers to preventing recurrent coronary events or death in those with existing CHD). Determining a client's LDL cholesterol goal and appropriate

Table 18-1	NCEP's LDL Cholesterol Goals Based on Cardiovascular Risk (ATP III)	
Risk Category	**LDL-Cholesterol Goal**	
CHD and CHD Risk Equivalent*	Less than 100 mg/dL	
Multiple (2+) Risk Factors†	Less than 130 mg/dL	
0–1 Risk Factor†	Less than 160 mg/dL	

C_T? How many risk factors does the following client have and what is the LDL-C goal?

Harris Hebrides is a 59-year-old male who presents today for a routine annual exam. He came in last week for routine labs with the following values: Total cholesterol: 218 mg/dL; LDL-C: 180 mg/dL; HDL-C: 48 mg/dL; and glucose: 92 mg/dL. He has a history of hypertension that is controlled with medication. He reports that there is no history of heart disease on his mother's side, but that his father had a heart attack at age 48 years. He smoked 1 pack per day for 12 years but quit 10 years ago. He does not have any significant medical history other than hypertension.

*CHD: coronary heart disease
CHD Risk Equivalent status refers to other forms of cardiovascular disease, including peripheral artery disease, abdominal aortic aneurysm, and carotid artery disease; diabetes mellitus; and greater than or equal to 2 risk factors with 10-year risk for "hard" CHD greater than 20%.
† Risk factors include current cigarette smoker, hypertension, high-density lipoprotein cholesterol less than 40 mg/dL, family history of CHD, and age as greater than or equal to 45 years for men and greater than or equal to 55 years for women.
Source: Adapted from: NCEP Adult Treatment Panel III, 2002.

therapy is individually assessed based on the client's risk status as described in Table 18-1. Diet recommendations should always be part of the therapeutic regimen for anyone not at LDL goal. Although raising HDL cholesterol via pharmacological means has not been identified as a specific goal, recommendations encourage nondrug therapies that raise HDL cholesterol levels as a part of management of other lipid and nonlipid risk factors.

Dietary Factors That Influence Blood Cholesterol

Dietary fat has the potential to both lower and raise LDL and HDL cholesterol depending on the type and amount of fatty acid in the diet. Dietary cholesterol can also modestly increase LDL cholesterol though to a lesser degree than saturated fat (NCEP ATP III, 2002). Nutritional factors that can lower LDL cholesterol include plant sterols/stanols and viscous (often called "soluble") fiber. Soy has also been explored for its potential use in lowering LDL cholesterol.

Dietary Fat

There are three types of fat found in food: saturated fatty acids (SFAs), monounsaturated fatty acids (MUFAs), and polyunsaturated fatty acids (PUFAs). The fatty acids differ in their physical and chemical properties as well as their effects on blood cholesterol. SFAs have a solid texture at room temperature, whereas both MUFAs and PUFAs are liquid at room temperature. MUFAs are found in food in either a *cis* or *trans* configuration. Trans-MUFAs (often called trans fats) are primarily found in foods such as margarine or shortening whose oils have been purposefully partially hydrogenated to produce a more solid fat at room temperature. Chapter 4 discusses the chemistry of these fats. Food manufacturers find trans fats attractive because they can increase shelf life and flavor in products such as snack foods, candies, crackers, fried foods, baked products, and french fries. Polyunsaturated fatty acids are subdivided into n-6 or n-3 fatty acids (often called omega-6 and omega-3 fatty acids, respectively). There are two polyunsaturated fatty acids that are essential fatty acids, meaning they cannot be synthesized by the body, yet are vital to sustain life. One of these is the n-6 fatty acid, linoleic acid; the other is the n-3 fatty acid, alpha linolenic acid (ALA). Two additional n-3 polyunsaturated fatty acids that have been

Table 18-2	Commonly Consumed Fatty Acids and Accompanying Food Sources	
Fatty Acid	**Type**	**Major U.S. Food Sources**
Lauric	Saturated Fat	Products made with coconut oil, milk, palm oil
Myristic	Saturated Fat	Milk and dairy products, palm oil
Palmitic acid*	Saturated Fat	Beef, pork, milk and dairy products, chocolate, palm oil
Stearic acid*	Saturated Fat	Beef, pork, chocolate
Oleic acid*	Cis-monounsaturated fat	Olive oil, canola oil, meat
Elaidic acid	Trans-monounsaturated fat	Foods made with hydrogenated fats (margarines, french fries, candies, snacks, baked goods)
Linoleic acid*	n-6 Polyunsaturated fat	Sunflower, corn, safflower, soybean oils
α-Linolenic acid	n-3 Polyunsaturated fat	Flaxseed, canola and soybean oil, walnuts
Eicosapentaenoic acid	n-3 polyunsaturated fat	Fatty fish, marine animals
Docosahexaenoic acid	n-3 polyunsaturated fat	Fatty fish, marine animals

*These four fats account for 90% of fatty acids in the U.S. diet.

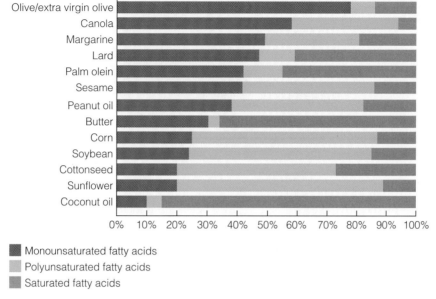

■ FIGURE 18-2 **Fatty Acid Composition of Commonly Consumed Fats and Oils.**

extensively studied in relation to CVD include the fatty acids found in some fish and marine animals, eicosapentaenoic acid (EPA) and docosahexaenoic acid (DHA). Table 18-2 describes the major fatty acids within each subgroup and their accompanying food sources and Figures 18-2 ■ and 18-3 ■ show fatty acid classification and composition of commonly consumed fats and oils.

The Effects of Fatty Acids on Blood Cholesterol Diets high in saturated, polyunsaturated, and monounsaturated fats have overall different, but consistent, effects on LDL and HDL cholesterol as illustrated in Table 18-3. Data show that diets high in SFAs increase LDL cholesterol, whereas those

high in PUFAs decrease LDL cholesterol (NCEP ATP III, 2002). The effects of MUFAs on LDL cholesterol depend on whether the fatty acid is in the cis or trans configuration. Cis-MUFAs like oleic acid in olive oil slightly decrease or do not change LDL cholesterol, whereas trans fats found in margarine, shortening, and products made from these sources increase LDL. The fact that diets high in saturated and trans fats increase LDL cholesterol is an essential message for the nurse to relate when educating an individual about lifestyle modifications.

Diets high in SFAs, PUFAs, or cis-monounsaturated fatty acids have been shown to either produce a modest increase in HDL cholesterol or have no effect. The concern over trans

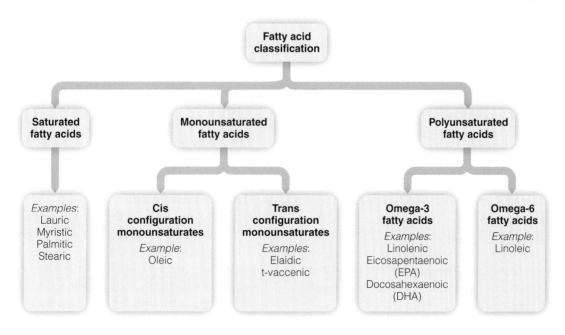

■ FIGURE 18-3 **Classification of Fatty Acids.**

Table 18-3 Effects of Saturated, Polyunsaturated, and Monounsaturated Fat on LDL and HDL Cholesterol

Fat	LDL-Cholesterol	HDL-Cholesterol
Saturated	↑	Modest ↑
Polyunsaturated	↓	Modest ↑ or No change
Cis-Monounsaturated	Modest ↓ or No change	Modest ↑ or No change
Trans-Monounsaturated	↑	↓

Sources: Mensink, 2005; NCEP ATP III, 2002; Woodside & Krombhout, 2005.

fats is that in addition to increasing LDL cholesterol, they also decrease HDL cholesterol—two negative effects.

Regardless of the health benefits from some types of dietary fat, all fat contains 9 kcalories/gm and excess intake can contribute to excess caloric intake and increased weight. As outlined in Chapter 4, total fat intake should not exceed 35% of total kcalories in the diet.

Other Dietary Components and Blood Cholesterol

Phytosterols are plant sterols and stanols that chemically resemble cholesterol (Ostlund, 2004). They are present in a normal diet from fruits and vegetables and are not made by humans. Although not fully understood, it is believed that phytosterols inhibit cholesterol absorption in the intestine and in doing so increase cholesterol synthesis by the liver and clearance of LDL cholesterol from the blood (Jones & AbuMweis, 2009). Several clinical trials reveal that 1 to 3 gm/day of plant stanols are safe and reduce LDL cholesterol up to 15% (Chen, Wesley, Shamburek, Pucino, & Csako, 2005) with the optimal intake being 2 gm/day (Katain et al., 2003). Plant stanols/sterols are available in the United States currently in the form of spreads (Benecol® and Take Control®) that are similar in appearance and taste as margarine or butter but contain negligible amounts of trans fat, are low in saturated fat and cholesterol, and are available in regular or light (lower calorie) versions. In addition, the regular version can be used in baking or frying as an alternative to butter or margarine. Newer products are continually appearing on the market with added plant stanols and sterols, such as yogurts and snack and cereal bars. The nurse can advise that the client read the nutrition facts panel to determine the cumulative amount of these substances in the diet.

Viscous fibers, often referred to as "soluble fibers" can reduce LDL cholesterol, whereas insoluble fibers found in foods such as wheat and corn do not have a significant effect (Anderson & Hanna, 1999). Fibers that have been shown to lower LDL cholesterol include psyllium, pectin, β-glucan, certain gums, mucilage, and lignin, with the first three having the greatest effect. Major food sources that contain one or more of these viscous fibers include oats, barley, fruits (apples, citrus fruits), legumes, and flaxseed. The mechanism by which viscous fibers reduce LDL cholesterol is not completely identified, although the primary hypothesis is by binding to bile acids to increase cholesterol excretion. Because the synthesis of bile acids requires cholesterol, more cholesterol in the blood will be used to create new bile acids, thus lowering serum cholesterol. Incorporating between 5 and 10 grams of viscous fiber may be accompanied by an approximate 5% reduction in LDL cholesterol (Anderson & Hanna, 1999).

Initially, research suggested that a large amount of soy protein in the diet (about 25 gm/day) reduces LDL cholesterol (Anderson, Johnstone, & Cook-Newell, 1995); however, recent information suggests a minimal effect. Reviews of cumulative data on soy on LDL cholesterol and other risk factors for CVD conclude that consuming a large amount of soy protein (about 50 gm/day, which is equivalent to about 6 cups of cooked soybeans) in substitution for animal or dairy protein may slightly reduce LDL cholesterol with no effects on HDL cholesterol or triglycerides (Sacks et al., 2006; Taku et al., 2007). Therefore, consuming large amounts of soy is not significantly effective at reducing LDL cholesterol. Although incorporating soy protein may not significantly affect cholesterol, soy beans and products made from soy, including soy milk, tofu, miso, soy nuts, and soy butter, may help reduce risk of CVD in other ways and are beneficial to overall health. Soy and soy-based products are high in protein but low in saturated fat and contain PUFAs, calcium, potassium, and vitamin K.

The effect of high-protein diets on CVD risk is a matter under debate. Such diets can be high in saturated fat and lead to elevated LDL cholesterol but may also foster weight loss in some clients. The Evidence-Based Practice Box: Are diets low in carbohydrates and high in protein and fat effective in reducing LDL and cardiovascular risk? discusses these diets.

Medical Nutrition Therapy for Hypercholesterolemia

Current guidelines maintain that dietary intervention be incorporated into both primary and secondary prevention of CVD through a multifactorial lifestyle approach termed therapeutic lifestyle changes (TLC). Because control of LDL cholesterol is the primary target, the focus should be reducing daily intake of dietary SFAs and cholesterol to less than 7% of total calories and less than 200 mg, respectively.

EVIDENCE-BASED PRACTICE RESEARCH BOX

Are diets low in carbohydrates and high in protein and fat effective in reducing LDL and cardiovascular risk?

Clinical Problem: Elevated LDL cholesterol and depressed HDL cholesterol levels are indicators of cardiovascular risk. Diets that are high in protein and fat while being low in carbohydrates are promoted for their ability to reduce caloric intake, leading to weight loss, reduction in LDL cholesterol, and improvement in HDL cholesterol and serum triglycerides.

Research Findings: Low-carbohydrate, high-protein/fat diets have been advocated for weight loss and, by association, for reduction of cardiovascular risk. These diets tend to be controversial because they contradict conventional wisdom about the efficacy of a diet low in total calories from fat for weight loss. In addition, there are no long-term studies to support the safety or efficacy of such diets and data reveal no difference between low-carbohydrate/high-fat diets compared to high-carbohydrate/low-fat diets on weight loss greater than 6 months.

Weight reduction and prevention of obesity are important goals in reducing cardiovascular risk. Carbohydrate-restricted diets are based on structured meal plans that are associated with higher intake of protein and total fats because protein is supplied mainly by animal sources. Studies examining the effects of carbohydrate-restricted diets on weight loss and lipid levels and cardiovascular risk have been conducted.

Data were analyzed from more than 80,000 females in the Nurses' Health Study. Using a self-report food-frequency questionnaire, researchers calculated the association between a low-carbohydrate diet score and risk of CHD. They concluded that low-carbohydrate diets were not associated with an increased risk of CVD; however, only when protein came from plant sources was there a suggestion of a decrease in risk (Halton et al., 2006).

In an earlier study, the effects of very low-carbohydrate vs. low-fat diets on lipid levels were examined. The 15 male subjects with an average body mass index (BMI) of 34 each consumed the experimental diets for two consecutive 6-week periods. The researchers found that only the low-fat diet resulted in a significant decrease in LDL cholesterol levels; however, the weight loss was most significant with the low-carbohydrate diet (Sharman, Gomez, Kraemer, & Volek, 2004).

Another study conducted with 100 middle-age, overweight women (mean BMI of 32) compared the effects of a reduced-calorie, low-carbohydrate, high-protein, low-fat diet with an increased-carbohydrate, low-fat diet. Both groups of subjects experienced weight loss and a decrease in serum lipid levels; however, minimal effects in other cardiovascular risk factors were found (Noakes, Keogh, Foster, & Clifton, 2005). Miller et al. (2009) reported that a high-protein, low-carbohydrate, high-fat diet such as the Atkins diet resulted in a higher total and LDL-cholesterol level during the weight maintenance phase of the diet compared with diets that contained less saturated fat and more carbohydrate, changes that were also associated with a decline in endothelial function.

Two recent studies on overweight men examined the effect of low-carbohydrate diets on lipid levels when a soluble fiber supplement was added to the diet. Wood, Volek, Liu, et al. (2006) concluded that weight loss was the variable that accounted for the decrease in LDL cholesterol and increase in HDL cholesterol levels. Additional studies by Wood, Volek, Davis, Dell'ova, & Fernandez (2006) and Wood et al. (2007) concluded that a very low-carbohydrate diet (13% of total calories) and a fiber supplement led to an overall weight reduction and decrease in LDL cholesterol levels. Another group of researchers found similar results but only in diets with 54% carbohydrates compared to one with 26% carbohydrates (Krauss, Blanche, Rawlings, Fernstrom, & Williams, 2006).

Nursing Implications: Low-carbohydrate, high-fat diets should not be promoted for reduction of cardiovascular risk. Current studies fail to demonstrate the long-term value of such diets in lowering LDL cholesterol and weight reduction. Further, low-carbohydrate/high-fat diets are typically high in saturated fat, which research consistently reveals increases risk of CVD. There are no long-term studies assessing the effects of low-carbohydrate/high-fat diets on CVD risk. Increased physical activity, coupled with a diet that is low in saturated and trans fats and high in fiber, are more beneficial in reducing cardiovascular risk.

CRITICAL THINKING QUESTIONS:

1. How should the nurse respond to the obese middle-age client who asks if reducing carbohydrates or fats is better at lowering cholesterol?

2. How would the nurse respond to the middle-age male who has lost 85 pounds on a low-carbohydrate diet and states that his cholesterol, triglycerides, and glucose are in normal ranges and now wants his school-age children to begin the same diet?

Enhancement of LDL lowering can be achieved by adding 2 grams of plant stanols/sterols per day (this amount is equivalent to 4 tbsp of Benecol® spread or 2 to 3 tbsp of Take Control®) and consuming at least 5 to 10 grams of viscous fiber per day. Incorporating viscous fiber at levels up to 25 gm/day may provide additional benefit. NCEP has not made specific quantitative recommendations for trans fats but encourages intake to be low. Recently, the American Heart Association revised its diet and lifestyle recommendations to include a limit of trans fatty acids from hydrogenation to less than 1% of total calories per day (Lichtenstein et al., 2006). As of January 1, 2006, the Food and Drug Administration (FDA) requires food manufacturers to list the amount of trans fatty acids from hydrogenation on the nutrition facts panel if the content per serving is greater than 0.5 gram (FDA, 2003). Nurses should be familiar with the nutrition facts panel on food products and be able to help clients choose foods lower in saturated and trans fats and cholesterol by comparing similar products of the same serving size. Foods higher in saturated and trans fats should be replaced with foods higher in polyunsaturated and monounsaturated fats, which may increase or preserve HDL cholesterol levels. Because all fat is equivalent in calories (9 kcal per gram of fat), clients who need to lose weight or maintain weight may need to be on the lower range of the recommendations for total fat (i.e., 25–30%) and focus on obtaining the majority of these calories from monounsaturated and polyunsaturated fats. As a result, lowering the amount of total fat intake also lowers intake of calories. Key questions that should be asked prior to implementing individual dietary modifications are described in Box 18-1.

The NCEP also recognizes the importance of restoring or maintaining an appropriate body weight and incorporating regular physical activity, which can improve **dyslipidemia** (disorders in lipoprotein metabolism involving high levels of

MyNursingKit National Cholesterol Education Program

Table 18-4	Macronutrient Recommendations for the TLC Diet
Nutrient	**Recommended Intake**
Energy	Adequate calories to lose or maintain weight
Total Dietary Fat	25–35% of total calories
Saturated Fat	Less than 7% of total calories
Polyunsaturated Fat	Up to 10% of total calories
Monounsaturated Fat	Up to 20% of total calories
Carbohydrate	50–60% of total calories
Total Dietary Fiber	20–30 grams per day
Viscous fiber	10–25 grams per day
Protein	Approximately 15% of total calories
Dietary Cholesterol	Less than 200 mg per day

Source: NCEP Adult Treatment Panel III, 2002.

LDL cholesterol, low levels of HDL cholesterol, and high levels of triglycerides). Macronutrient recommendations for the TLC diet are presented in Table 18-4 and Client Education Checklist: Therapeutic Lifestyle Changes Recommendations. Recommendations for weight loss and weight maintenance are discussed in Chapter 17. Adherence to TLC should be assessed every 4 to 6 months in the first year and every 6 to 12 months thereafter. It is estimated that total LDL-cholesterol may be lowered 25% to 30% if all therapeutic options included in TLC are followed. Research studies found that this level of LDL reduction is possible over 1 month (Kendall & Jenkins, 2004). However, when the guidelines are followed for 1 year, average reductions can be half of this level, which still can bring a significant number of clients to goal (Jenkins et al., 2006).

Diet and Risk of CVD: Beyond Hyperlipidemia

Although LDL cholesterol is the primary target of therapy to reduce risk of CVD, there are other risk factors, both traditional and emerging, where nutrition may have an impact and thus warrant discussion.

Omega-3 Fatty Acids

Increasing evidence suggests that n-3 PUFAs play an important role in primary and secondary prevention of CVD. Dietary contributors of these fatty acids include foods and products derived from both marine (EPA and DHA) and plant (ALA) sources.

Marine Sources   The interest in fish and n-3 PUFA from fish originated when an observational study in the 1970s revealed that Greenland Eskimos had a low mortality rate from heart disease. This finding was surprising because the overall diet was not low in total or saturated fat and was relatively high in n-3 polyunsaturated fat (Dyerberg & Bang,

BOX 18-1	**Key Diet Questions for Clients with Hypercholesterolemia**

1. How many times per day/week do you eat the following?*
   a. Meats such as hamburger, steak, duck, hot dogs, bacon, pastrami, corned beef, sausage, and salami
   b. Whole milk and dairy products made from whole milk (cheeses, ice cream, milk shakes, sour cream, creamer or half-half, recipes/dishes where whole milk is used)
   c. Eggs (with yolk)
   d. Butter or margarine
   e. Fruits, vegetables, and oats. How are fruits and vegetables consumed (is the skin peeled off or consumed, are they consumed as raw, steamed, fried, or grilled)?
   f. Fatty fish such as salmon, mackerel, swordfish, shark, tuna, trout, herring, or sardines. How are these prepared (baked, grilled, fried, etc.)?
   g. Candies, pastries, cakes, pies, muffins, cookies salty snacks, and/or french fries
2. What type of fat/oil do you use in cooking?
3. How often do you eat out? What types of foods do you consume and where?
4. When you eat at home, who prepares the meals and snacks?
5. What do you consider are important aspects of eating (e.g., eating with friends/family, convenience, affordable foods, taste, nutrient label, as a way to deal with stress, etc.)?

 ▪ For these questions, it is important to ask about portion sizes.

CLIENT EDUCATION CHECKLIST   ✓   Therapeutic Lifestyle Changes Recommendations

Intervention	Example
Reduce daily saturated fat intake to less than 7%.	• The nutrient label on most food products contains total dietary fat and saturated fat. The percent of saturated fat from total dietary fat should be less than 7%. • Saturated fat is found in fatty cuts of meat and meat drippings/stock, bacon, sausage and processed meats, egg yolks, butter, fat or oil that is solid at room temperature (lard or shortening), coconut, cocoa butter, palm oil, avocado, whole milk and products made from whole milk, cocoa butter, avocados, and desserts, cakes, pies, cookies and other similar snacks. • Meats high in saturated fat should be replaced with meats low in saturated fat such as fish, chicken, and white turkey without the skin. • Low-fat or fat-free dairy products should replace whole milk and products made from whole milk. • Butter, lard, and shortening should be replaced with fats/oils that are lower in saturated fat and higher in monounsaturated and polyunsaturated fats such as olive, canola, or soybean oils or Benecol® or Take Control® spreads made with plant stanols or sterols.
Reduce daily dietary cholesterol intake to less than 200 mg.	• Dietary cholesterol is found in animal meat and animal by-products such as milk, eggs, cheese, and butter. Fruits, vegetables, and grains do not contain cholesterol, but products that have milk, cheese, or butter added to them would also have dietary cholesterol. • Dietary cholesterol has less impact on LDL cholesterol as compared to SFA, but often, these two dietary factors are found in the same foods. • Dietary cholesterol is listed on the nutrient label, and foods with less than 200 mg should be recommended.
Include 2 gm of plant stanol/sterols per day.	• Currently, the two spreads available in the United States with plant sterols/stanols are Benecol® and Take Control®. • Additional products with plant stanols/sterols are being developed.
Include greater than 5–10 gm of viscous fiber per day.	• Foods high in viscous fiber include oats, oatmeal, and oat bran; barley; psyllium seeds; legumes; and various fruits and vegetables. • Legumes provide ~1–3 gm of viscous fiber per ½ cup. • Fruit provides ~1–2 gm of viscous fiber per serving. • Broccoli and carrots provide ~1 gm of viscous fiber per ½ cup*. • Oat products provide ~1 gm of soluble fiber per ½ cup*.

*Source: NCEP ATP III, 2002.

1979). Naturally, EPA and DHA are found primarily in fatty, cold water fish as outlined in Box 18-2. Farm-raised and wild fish do not significantly differ in their EPA and DHA content; however, farm-raised fish contain on average higher levels of saturated and total polyunsaturated fats (Gebauer, Psota, Harris, & Kris-Etherton, 2006). Many studies have consistently shown a protective effect of consuming fish high in EPA and DHA on risk of CVD (Iso et al., 2006; Mozaffarian, 2008). The proposed possible cardioprotective mechanisms of action include reducing triglycerides, inflammation, and platelet adhesion; inhibiting plaque formation; decreasing arrhythmias; and decreasing blood pressure (Psota, Gebauer, & Kris-Etherton, 2006; Riediger, Othman, Suh, & Moghadasian, 2009; Van Horn et al., 2008). Many national, international, and professional organizations have made recommendations for consuming fish as well as the specific fatty acids EPA and DHA. These recommendations are summarized in Box 18-2.

In meeting recommendations, clients need to consider safety concerns such as methylmercury and polychlorinated biphenyls (PCBs). Mercury levels are high in large fish that have lived a long period such as shark, swordfish, king mackerel, and tilefish, whereas PCBs were found to be higher in farm-raised salmon compared to wild salmon (Gebauer et al., 2006). Therefore, it may be best to choose fish high in omega-3 fats that are low in mercury while choosing a variety of wild and farm-raised fish within these species. There are specific fish recommendations for women who may become pregnant, are currently pregnant, or are nursing as well as young children that are described in the Lifespan Box: Fish Recommendations for Pregnant or Lactating Females and Young Children. Practice Pearl: Fish Oil Supplements outlines specific information and concerns about fish oil supplements.

Plant Sources   ALA is the plant-derived omega-3 fatty acid. Recommendations on intake and major sources of

MyNursingKit Fish and Omega-3 Fatty Acids

BOX 18-2	Omega-3 (n-3) Fatty Acid Recommendations

Recommendations for intake of omega-3 fatty acids differ between primary prevention advice and that given to individuals with existing cardiac disease (secondary prevention). The nurse should be mindful of these differences.

Sources

- Marine: Fatty, cold water fish such as salmon, certain species of tuna, mackerel, sardines, herring, and trout. Limit processed versions of marine sources, such as fish sticks, because of high saturated fat content.
- Plant: Flaxseeds, flaxseed oil, walnuts, walnut oil, soybeans, soybean oil, rapeseeds, canola oil.
- Supplements: Eicosapentaenoic acid (EPA) and docohexaenoic acid (DHA) containing supplements available as capsules in varying dosages.

Recommendations

- Primary prevention: Consume 2 fish meals/week (~8 oz fish total) (Lichtenstein et al., 2006; United States Department of Agriculture [USDA], 2005).
- Secondary prevention: 1 gm/day EPA + DHA, which equals to 2–3 oz of fish/day (Lichtenstein et al., 2006).
- Adhere to recommendations targeted to children and pregnant or lactating females on minimizing exposure to methylmercury and PCBs from marine sources (Riediger et al., 2009).
- Adhere to safety recommendations regarding use of omega-3 dietary supplements with anticoagulant or antiplatelet therapy (see Practice Pearl: Fish Oil Supplements).

ALA are outlined in Box 18-2. Research suggests that ALA may be cardioprotective by having positive effects on the inflammatory process of CVD. Clients should be encouraged to replace low ALA oils (corn oil and safflower oil) with canola, soybean, and flaxseed oil. For additional sources of ALA, clients can consider incorporating ground flaxseed and walnuts into their diets; however, clients should be made aware that these foods are high in kcalories, a concern for clients who need to lose or maintain weight.

Lifespan

Fish Recommendations for Pregnant or Lactating Females and Young Children

1. Do not eat shark, swordfish, king mackerel, or tilefish because they contain high levels of mercury.
2. Eat up to 12 ounces (two average meals) a week of a variety of fish and shellfish that are lower in mercury.

   Five of the most commonly eaten fish that are low in mercury are shrimp, canned light tuna, salmon, pollock, and catfish. Another commonly eaten fish, albacore ("white") tuna (often served as tuna steaks), has more mercury than canned light tuna. When choosing your two meals of fish and shellfish, up to 6 ounces (one average meal) of albacore tuna can be consumed per week.
3. Check local advisories about the safety of fish caught by family and friends in your local lakes, rivers, and coastal areas. If no advice is available, eat up to 6 ounces (one average meal) per week of fish you catch from local waters, but do not consume any other fish during that week.

Chapter 13 discusses these recommendations in detail and contains a Client Education Checklist on the subject.

Sources: Food and Drug Administration (FDA) and Environmental Protection Agency (EPA), 2006.

PRACTICE PEARL

Fish Oil Supplements

Most clients with CHD will not be able to eat fish everyday to meet the requirements for secondary prevention, making fish oil supplements a possible option. Most fish oil supplements contain approximately 180 mg EPA and 120 mg DHA per 1,000 mg capsule. Therefore, clients with CHD need ~3 capsules per day to meet this requirement. Although fish oil supplements at this level are generally safe, they can cause nausea, dyspepsia (indigestion), modest increases in LDL cholesterol, and a fishy after-taste.

Theoretically, the use of EPA and DHA supplements may affect platelet aggregation and vitamin K-dependent coagulation factors. There have been several case reports suggesting that fish oil can provide additive anticoagulant effects when given with warfarin (Buckley, Goff, & Knapp, 2004) and antiplatelet effects when given with warfarin and aspirin in combination (McClaskey & Michalets, 2007). Clients taking anticoagulant or antiplatelet medications should consult with their primary health care provider before using fish oil supplements.

Additionally, concerns over mercury or PCB contamination of some fish oil supplements underscore the importance of having access to standardized and regulated dietary supplements. A prescription form of fish oil called Omacor® (Reliant Pharmaceuticals) is now approved by the FDA. Each capsule contains 840 mg of EPA/DHA.

Alcohol and CVD

Population studies indicate that the association between alcohol intake and mortality is represented by a J-shaped curve, meaning that moderate alcohol intake may be beneficial, whereas excess intake may be detrimental (Gronbaek, 2006). Most of the benefit of moderate alcohol consumption is related to reduced risk of CVD, whereas excessive intake is related to cirrhosis, pancreatitis, neurological disorders, certain cancers, as well as addiction and motor vehicle accidents related to impaired decision making. Additionally, clients trying to reduce cardiac risk should know that intake of three or more drinks per day is associated with high blood triglyceride levels, cardiomyopathy, hypertension, and stroke (Saremi & Arora, 2008). Moderate alcohol intake is defined as less than or equal to two standard drinks/day for men and less than or equal to one standard drink/day for women (one standard drink is equivalent to 5 oz of wine, 1.5 oz 80-proof of liquor, or 12 oz of beer). Ethanol in all alcoholic beverages as well as polyphenols found in red wine are believed to be involved in the proposed protective effects on CVD risk. Alcoholic beverages may decrease coagulation, platelet aggregation, thrombosis, and inflammation while increasing HDL cholesterol. Phenolic compounds (flavonoids and nonflavonoids) found in red wine may have additional benefit by improving endothelial function, decreasing LDL oxidation and proliferation of smooth muscle cells (Szmitko & Verma, 2005). There are no available randomized controlled trial data on the impact of alcohol and specifically red wine on CVD risk, and thus it is important for the nurse to recognize that the available data suggest an association, but not a cause and effect. The NCEP recognizes the association between moderate alcohol intake and reduction in CVD risk, but in light of the associated risks does not recommend clients start drinking to prevent CVD risk. Recommendations regarding alcohol intake should be individualized based on overall medical history, disease risks, and health goals (Mukamal & Rimm, 2008).

Dietary Supplements

The nurse should be aware that some clients may choose to take dietary supplements based on a belief that such products prevent CVD. However, little research exists to support this practice. Hot Topic Box: Dietary Supplements for Reducing CVD Risk discusses dietary supplements and prevention of CVD.

Hypertension

Approximately one in four Americans suffers from **hypertension,** defined as systolic blood pressure (SBP) greater than 140 mm Hg or diastolic blood pressure (DBP) greater than 90 mm Hg (Joint National Committee [JNC], 2003). Hypertension is more prevalent in African Americans and older adults than in other population groups. Hypertension is an independent risk factor for CVD. The Joint National Committee (JNC) on the Prevention, Detection, Evaluation and Treatment of High Blood Pressure includes a new category called "pre-hypertension" in its guidelines and defines it as having an SBP of 120 to 139 mm Hg or a DBP of 80 to 89 mm Hg. Clients with blood pressure meeting this criterion are at risk for developing hypertension and thus CVD and are candidates for lifestyle modifications.

Lifestyle modifications should be included in the management of all individuals with high blood pressure, including those defined as having pre-hypertension. Lifestyle factors

hot Topic

Dietary Supplements for Reducing CVD Risk

Various types of research have investigated the effects of novel dietary components on reducing risk of CVD. Both traditional dietary supplements, such as vitamins, and botanical substances have been studied for a possible effect on reduction of blood lipids and prevention of CHD. Early studies showing promise for dietary supplement use based solely on observational research often have not been reproducible when a clinical research is conducted. To date, there is little evidence that any dietary supplement can prevent or treat CVD. For example, a study of long-term use of vitamins E and C reported an increased risk of hemorrhagic stroke associated with vitamin E intake and no overall reduction in cardiac risk from either vitamin (Sesso et al., 2008). High-dose vitamin E supplementation may increase total mortality (Miller et al., 2005). Elevated plasma homocysteine, an amino acid, is associated with risk of CHD (Humphrey, Fu, Freeman, & Helfand, 2008). Adequate levels of folic acid and vitamins B_6 and B_{12} are needed to metabolize homocysteine. Early reports that targeted reduction in homocysteine with supplementation of these vitamins were hopeful that this approach would reduce disease risk. Although supplementation with these B vitamins does lower homocysteine levels, no associated reduction in risk of CVD has been proven (Albert et al., 2008; Bonaa et al, 2006). The dietary supplement guggulipid, a product marketed to reduce LDL cholesterol, was instead shown to increase LDL cholesterol and was associated with a dermatologic hypersensitivity reaction in some clients (Szapary et al., 2003). The use of raw or commercial garlic to treat elevated LDL cholesterol has had mixed research results, with most reports finding little clinical effect (Frishman, Beravol, & Carosella, 2009; Gardner et al., 2007).

Why would there be a discrepancy in observational data compared to clinical trials? First, it is important to remember that observational studies can reveal an *association* between, for example, diet and a condition or disease, but only clinical trials that can control for potential confounders can investigate *cause and effect.* Another important point is that looking at the effects of food containing a certain dietary component vs. extracting that dietary component and providing it in large quantities via a dietary supplement are completely different things. Foods high in a particular antioxidant, for example, are often high in other antioxidants, fiber, and phytochemicals and low in saturated fat and cholesterol. The beneficial effect of the food may be due to several of these components acting together compared to one particular dietary component. Once you take out a particular component of food, you cannot compare the individual component to the food product where it is naturally found. Finally, because dietary supplements do not fall under strict regulatory practices as drugs do, there are no standardized manufacturing regulations; thus comparing different brands of dietary supplements among themselves as well as the food in which the component is naturally found is not appropriate.

Dietary supplements carry some risk and thus the health care team must always weigh risk vs. benefit in determining whether a dietary supplement should be recommended. Because there are many proven nonpharmacological means to reduce CVD risk, at this time there is inadequate data to support recommending any dietary supplements for primary or secondary prevention of CVD other than fish oil capsules if recommendations cannot be met via the diet.

contributing to the development or worsening of high blood pressure include obesity, lack of physical activity, alcohol abuse, and smoking. Nursing interventions should target each of these risk factors in the client with hypertension or pre-hypertension. There is a linear association between excess body weight in obese individuals and severity of hypertension. Weight loss of 10 to 20 lb is associated with a 2.8 to 7 mm Hg reduction in SBP and a 2.5 to 3 mm Hg reduction in DBP (The Trials of Hypertension Prevention Collaborative Research Group, 1997; He, Whelton, Appel, Charleston, & Klag, 2000). Further, weight loss enhances the blood pressure lowering effects of antihypertensive medications. Engaging in regular aerobic physical activity at least 30 minutes per day can reduce blood pressure by 4 to 9 mm Hg (Kelley & Kelley, 2000; Whelton, Chin, Xin, & He, 2002) and assist in restoring and maintaining an appropriate weight. In addition to weight management, clients should be instructed to not consume more than two alcoholic drinks per day for men and no more than one alcoholic drink per day for women. The contribution of alcohol to high blood pressure is associated with the total amount and not affected by type of alcohol. Overall dietary choices should be addressed because a diet low in sodium and rich in fruits, vegetables, and low-fat dairy products has been shown to significantly reduce blood pressure. The Dietary Approaches to Stop Hypertension (DASH) study revealed that a low total and saturated fat diet emphasizing fruits (5 servings per day), vegetables (3 servings per day), and low-fat dairy products (2 servings per day) that included whole grains, poultry, fish, and nuts and limited amounts of red meat and sweets for 8 weeks significantly lowered SBP by 5.5 mm Hg and DBP by 3 mm Hg compared to the average American diet (Appel et al., 1997). Follow-up studies report a decrease in risk of CHD, stroke, and overall mortality in those with hypertension who follow the DASH diet (Fung et al., 2008; Parikh, Lipsitz, & Natarajan, 2009). Reduction in blood pressure reportedly begins within 2 weeks on the diet. Additionally, the researchers reported that reducing sodium to levels less than 2,300 mg/day along with the other aspects of the DASH diet significantly reduced blood pressure in clients with and without hypertension (Sacks et al., 2001).

Limited data suggest that adequate calcium and potassium intake may positively affect blood pressure. In particular, a high-potassium intake fosters renal sodium excretion, which has a beneficial effect on blood pressure (Wexler & Aukerman, 2006). Following the DASH diet should supply adequate levels of both of these nutrients.

The PREMIER trial revealed that adopting current JNC recommendations of weight loss, sodium reduction, inclusion of regular physical activity, and limitation on alcohol consumption significantly reduced blood pressure over 1½ years (Elmer et al., 2006). Adding the DASH diet to these modifications increased consumption of fruits, vegetables, fiber, and minerals and further reduced blood pressure, but differences were not statistically significant.

Medical Nutrition Therapy for Hypertension

Clients with pre-hypertension and hypertension should include lifestyle modifications as part of their therapeutic regimen, whether pharmacological therapy for high blood pressure is included or not (JNC, 2003; Khan et al., 2008). Individuals who are abusing alcohol or currently using tobacco products should be educated about the dangers of these lifestyle habits and their contribution to hypertension. Nurses should work with the treating physician and other health care providers as well as the client to determine an appropriate interventional program to address these concerns. Overweight (body mass index [BMI] greater than or equal to 25 kg/m²) and obese individuals (BMI greater than or equal to 30 kg/m²) should work with a dietitian to implement a plan to attain and maintain an appropriate body weight as described in Chapter 17. Health care providers, including nurses, should educate the client about the importance of physical activity and accompanying health benefits. In addition, the nurse should spend time discussing potential options for exercise with the client based on the client's physical capabilities, past medical history, and logistical concerns. Finally, the client should be educated about reducing sodium intake and incorporating components of the DASH program as outlined in Tables 18-5 and 18-6. Box 18-3 describes the labeling claims for sodium content of foods and

Table 18-5	Sodium Content of Various Foods	
Food	**Serving Size**	**Sodium Content (mg)**
Salt	1 tsp	2,000
Cream of tomato soup	1 can (10.75 oz)	1,800
Tomato soup, condensed	1 can (10.75 oz)	1,680
Soy sauce	1 tbsp	1,000
Ham, roasted	3.5 oz	840
Pizza, pepperoni	1 slice, 12″ pizza	769
Carrots, canned	1 can	687
Hot dog	1	650
Tomato sauce	½ cup	640
Frozen dinner, spaghetti and meatballs	1 serving	548
Cottage cheese (1% fat)	4 oz	460
Turkey breast, deli	3 oz	270
Carrots, raw	1 cup	88
Carrots, frozen	1 cup	84
Cola, diet	12 ounces	57
Cola, regular	12 ounces	15
Apple, raw with skin	1 medium	1

CT? What alternatives to the high-sodium foods could the nurse suggest?

Source: United States Department of Agriculture, 2009.

Table 18-6 Following the Dash Eating Plan

The DASH eating plan shown below is based on 2,000 calories a day. The number of daily servings in a food group may vary from those listed depending on your caloric needs. Use this chart to help you plan your menus or take it with you when you go to the store.

Food Group	Daily Servings	Serving Sizes	Examples and Notes	Significance of Each Food Group to the DASH Eating Pattern
Grains*	6–8	1 slice bread 1 oz dry cereal** ½ cup cooked rice, pasta, or cereal	Whole wheat bread and rolls, whole wheat pasta, English muffin, pita bread, bagel, cereals, grits, oatmeal, brown rice, unsalted pretzels and popcorn	Major sources of energy and fiber
Vegetables	4–5	1 cup raw leafy vegetable ½ cup cut-up raw or cooked vegetable ½ cup vegetable juice	Broccoli, carrots, collards, green beans, green peas, kale, lima beans, potatoes, spinach, squash, sweet potatoes, tomatoes	Rich sources of potassium, magnesium, and fiber
Fruits	4–5	1 medium fruit ¼ cup dried fruit ½ cup fresh, frozen, or canned fruit ½ cup fruit juice	Apples, apricots, bananas, dates, grapes, oranges, grapefruit, grapefruit juice, mangoes, melons, peaches, pineapples, raisins, strawberries, tangerines	Important sources of potassium, magnesium, and fiber
Fat-free or low-fat milk and milk products	2–3	1 cup milk or yogurt 1½ oz cheese	Fat-free (skim) or low-fat (1%) milk or buttermilk, fat-free, low-fat, or reduced-fat cheese, fat-free or low-fat regular or frozen yogurt	Major sources of calcium and protein
Lean meats, poultry, and fish	6 or less	1 oz cooked meats, poultry, or fish 1 egg***	Select only lean; trim away visible fats; broil, roast, or poach; remove skin from poultry	Rich sources of protein and magnesium
Nuts, seeds, and legumes	4–5 per week	⅓ cup or 1½ oz nuts 2 tbsp peanut butter 2 tbsp or ½ oz seeds ½ cup cooked legumes (dry beans and peas)	Almonds, hazelnuts, mixed nuts, peanuts, walnuts, sunflower seeds, peanut butter, kidney beans, lentils, split peas	Rich sources of energy, magnesium, protein, and fiber
Fats and oils**	2–3	1 tsp soft margarine 1 tsp vegetable oil 1 tbsp mayonnaise 2 tbsp salad dressing	Soft margarine, vegetable oil (such as canola, corn, olive, or safflower), low-fat mayonnaise, light salad dressing	The DASH study had 27% of calories as fat, including fat in or added to foods
Sweets and added sugars	5 or less per week	1 tbsp sugar 1 tbsp jelly or jam ½ cup sorbet, gelatin 1 cup lemonade	Fruit-flavored gelatin, fruit punch, hard candy, jelly, maple syrup, sorbet and ices, sugar	Sweets should be low in fat

*Whole grains are recommended for most grain servings as a good source of fiber and nutrients.

**Serving sizes vary between ½ cup and 1¼ cups, depending on cereal type. Check the product's nutrition facts label.

***Because eggs are high in cholesterol, limit egg yolk intake to no more than four per week; two egg whites have the same protein content as 1 oz of meat.

****Fat content changes serving amount for fats and oils. For example, 1 tbsp of regular salad dressing equals one serving; 1 tbsp of a low-fat dressing equals one-half serving; 1 tbsp of a fat-free dressing equals zero servings.

Source: National Institutes of Health (NIH), National Heart, Lung, and Blood Institutes, n.d.

beverages as mandated by the Food and Drug Administration. Key diet history questions for clients with elevated blood pressure are presented in Box 18-4. The nurse can identify which changes listed in the Client Education Checklist: Lifestyle Modifications for Elevated Blood Pressure the client is willing and able to make and collaborate with the client to implement realistic changes that may lower blood pressure. A Client Education Checklist specific to just reducing intake of dietary sodium is contained in Chapter 6.

Metabolic Syndrome

Metabolic syndrome is a cluster of metabolic abnormalities that is characterized by abdominal obesity, insulin resistance, dyslipidemia, and elevated blood pressure (Grundy et al.,

---

BOX 18-3 | **Labeling Claims for the Sodium Content of Food and Beverages**

- Sodium free: Less than 5 mg sodium per serving
- Very low sodium: Less than 35 mg per serving
- Low sodium: Less than or equal to 140 mg sodium per serving
- Reduced or less sodium: Greater than or equal to 25% less sodium than regular product
- Light: Greater than or equal to 50% less sodium per serving compared to regular product
- No salt added or no salt: No salt has been added in the preparation of the product.

Source: FDA, 2008.

2005). It is estimated that one in five Americans has metabolic syndrome in some form and prevalence increases with age (Ford, Giles, & Dietz, 2002). Metabolic syndrome increases the risk of both type 2 diabetes mellitus and CVD (Grundy et al., 2005). The NCEP defines the diagnosis of metabolic syndrome as described in Table 18-7. Waist circumference is an essential parameter to obtain when establishing this diagnosis. Chapter 12 outlines the technique for performing this measurement.

Managing Metabolic Syndrome

The underlying risk factors for metabolic syndrome include overweight or obesity and physical inactivity. The overall goal in clients with metabolic syndrome is to reduce risk of CVD. Therefore, the focus should be on the risk factors for CVD, including elevated LDL cholesterol, hypertension, and diabetes in addition to restoring and maintaining an appropriate body weight and including regular physical activity.

Medical Nutrition Therapy for Metabolic Syndrome

Nutritional goals for metabolic syndrome should include losing or maintaining appropriate body weight and increasing physical activity. For individuals who are overweight or obese, the goal should be to lose 7% to 10% of body weight over 6 to 12 months (Grundy et al., 2005) because this level of weight loss has been shown to prevent diabetes (Knowler et al., 2002). The nurse can use this statistic to encourage the client who might reject the idea of weight management out of false belief that a significant amount of weight loss must be achieved for effect. The client should be encouraged to perform greater than or equal to 30 minutes of moderate-intensity exercise (such as brisk walking) on most, if not all, days of the week (Grundy et al., 2005) based on the client's physical condition and capabilities. Weight loss and physical activity each can directly or indirectly improve LDL and HDL cholesterol levels as well as reduce risk for diabetes and hypertension. The nurse should collaborate with the client to develop a plan for making lifestyle changes that are realistic for the individual. If the client has elevated LDL cholesterol, the TLC diet should be incorporated with energy intake adjusted to support weight loss or maintain weight as required. Because many clients with metabolic syndrome have dyslipidemia characterized by high levels of serum triglycerides and low levels of HDL cholesterol, the percentage of calories from fat should be

---

BOX 18-4 | **Key Diet Questions for Clients with Elevated Blood Pressure**

1. How many alcoholic drinks do you consume per day or week (1 drink = 12 oz beer, 5 oz wine, or 1.5 oz hard liquor)?

2. How many servings of vegetables do you eat per day (inquire about type; whether raw, frozen, or canned; portion size; and how prepared)?
   a. If the client reports eating less than 2 servings per day, ask which vegetables the client likes.
   b. Identify the obstacles to eating more vegetables (e.g., is the issue one of convenience, price, preparation, family, etc.).

3. How many servings of fruit do you eat per day?
   If the client reports eating less than 2 servings per day, ask the same questions as identified under #2.

4. How many servings of milk do you drink per day (8 oz is one serving)?
   a. What type of milk do you drink (e.g., whole, 2%, 1%, 12%, or skim)?

   b. How many servings of other dairy products (cheese, ice cream, yogurt, sour cream, cream cheese, creamer, soymilk, etc.) do you consume per day?

5. Do you use salt at the table (i.e., add it to your foods)?
   If yes, how often and which foods (identify low-sodium products to enhance taste)?

6. How often (and which foods) do you use salt in the preparation of food?

7. How often do you eat salty foods (e.g., chips, pretzels, salted nuts, popcorn, roasted ham, bacon, canned foods, or smoked foods)?

8. Do you look at the sodium content of foods on the nutrient label?

9. How often do you eat out of the home? Which types of foods do you eat when eating out?

CLIENT EDUCATION CHECKLIST — Lifestyle Modifications for Elevated Blood Pressure

Intervention	Example

Encourage the client to engage in regular aerobic physical activity and discuss how to incorporate this into one's day based on individual preferences, lifestyle, past medical history, and logistical factors.	• Regular physical activity can reduce blood pressure, enhance weight loss, improve serum cholesterol, and improve one's quality of life.
	• Ideas for moderate physical activity include:
	  a. Brisk walking or light jogging (during lunch break or with the kids), 30 minutes per day
	  b. Household activities requiring moderate effort, such as raking, mopping, waxing car, vacuuming large areas, 30 minutes per day
	  c. Spend time with the family by swimming, tennis (doubles), golf (walking the course), bicycling

Discuss with the client the importance of restoring and maintaining an appropriate body weight.	• 10–20 pounds can reduce blood pressure significantly in overweight (BMI greater than or equal to 25 kg/m²) and obese (BMI greater than or equal to 30 kg/m²) clients. • Weight loss enhances the effects of blood-lowering medications, improves blood glucose, serum cholesterol, and sense of well-being.
Address lifestyle factors that can worsen hypertension.	• Assess alcohol and tobacco use. • Discuss with the client how reducing alcohol intake and stopping smoking can improve blood pressure and reduce risk of CVD. • Refer the client for further evaluation/treatment when indicated.
Encourage greater than or equal to 5 servings of fruits and vegetables per day.	• Identify which fruits and vegetables the client likes. • Identify obstacles to consuming greater than or equal to 5 servings per day (e.g., lifestyle constraints, economic constraints, issues at the home, etc.) and discuss solutions to increase consumption. • Discuss the data revealing the effect of the DASH diet on lowering blood pressure.
Encourage consuming less than 2,400 mg of sodium per day.	• Identify foods high and low in sodium. • Point out on the nutrition label where sodium content is located. • Discuss low-sodium alternatives to cooking and enhancing the flavor of foods based on client preference.

Table 18-7   Diagnosis of Metabolic Syndrome

Positive diagnosis based on the presence of three or more of the following:

Risk Factor	Defining Level
Abdominal obesity (waist circumference†)	
Men	>102 cm (>40 in)
Women	>88 cm (>35 in)
Triglycerides	≥150 mg/dL
HDL cholesterol	
Men	<40 mg/dL
Women	<50 mg/dL
Blood pressure	≥130/≥85 mm Hg
Fasting glucose	≥100 mg/dL

†Waist circumference criteria for Asian Americans is ≥35 inches in men and ≥ 31 inches in women
Source: NCEP ATP III, 2002.

monitored closely because diets containing less than 25% of total calories from fat may increase triglycerides and lower HDL concentrations by providing too much sugar, whereas diets containing more than 35% of calories from fat often contain too much saturated fat (Grundy et al., 2005). Specific recommendations for reducing hypertriglyceridemia are summarized in Box 18-5. If the client with metabolic syndrome has pre-hypertension or hypertension, consideration should be given to reduction in sodium as well as incorporating the DASH diet. The client with diabetes or pre-diabetes should be encouraged to include viscous and total fiber in the diet at levels described in TLC to improve glucose metabolism (Davy & Melby, 2003; McKeown et al., 2004).

The nurse may need to involve a dietitian for more detailed diet instruction. Involving a dietitian is helpful because this person can translate science into practical suggestions about food, uncover hidden dietary sources of saturated and trans fats, sodium, dietary cholesterol, and kcalories; identify dietary deficiencies; and clarify myths about fad diets.

| BOX 18-5 | **Dietary Treatment of Hypertriglyceridemia** |

Elevated blood triglyceride levels are considered an emerging risk factor for coronary heart disease. Hypertriglyceridemia is treated by pharmacological agents and modification of several aspects of the diet. Niacin in the form of niacinamide can be a component of treatment; the high doses used classify its use as a pharmacological agent rather than a dietary supplement. The following dietary components should be targeted:

Weight management: A moderate weight loss can result in over a 20% reduction of triglycerides. Weight management that follows TLC guidelines is advised.

Alcohol: In clients with a triglyceride level below 500 mg/dL, intake of more than a moderate intake of alcohol should be discouraged because of the effects on triglyceride level and general health. Those with severe hypertriglyceridemia should abstain from drinking alcohol.

Carbohydrate: In some individuals, high-carbohydrate intake, especially in the form of simple sugars, is associated with elevated triglycerides. Recommendations include limiting intake of simple sugars and avoiding a fat intake below 25% of total kcalories that may result in excessive carbohydrate intake to achieve sufficient energy intake. Additionally, too low of a fat intake results in reductions in beneficial HDL cholesterol.

Omega-3 fats: From 2 to 4 gm total EPA and DHA per day are used in treating hypertriglyceridemia with an expected 30% to 50% reduction in triglyceride levels.

Sources: Adapted from: Bunzell, 2007; Oh & Lanier, 2007; Yuan, Al-Shali, & Hegele, 2007.

Heart Failure: Nutritional Concerns and Issues

Heart failure is the leading cause of acute hospitalizations in U.S. residents over the age of 65 years (Azhar & Wei, 2006). The role that diet plays in both the prevention and management of heart failure is increasingly recognized, although currently there are no national medical nutrition therapy recommendations for heart failure (Lennie, 2006). However, because heart failure is characterized by decreased cardiac output, venous stasis, sodium and fluid retention, undernutrition, and multiple organ failure where systemic inflammation plays a key role, it is essential to discuss the role of nutrition in the management of this condition.

Medical Nutrition Therapy for Heart Failure

Medical nutrition therapy for heart failure should focus on promoting a diet to control fluid and sodium retention, attaining and maintaining an appropriate body weight, and ensuring that the diet is adequate in vitamins, minerals, and protein because these nutrients are often needed in increased amounts and may be underconsumed. The client may also need other dietary interventions because of comorbidities such as diabetes, CVD, hypertension, obesity, or renal insufficiency.

Fluid and sodium retention are common physiological consequences of heart failure; thus to assist in diuretic therapy, sodium intake should be restricted (Beich & Yancy, 2008). In clients with preserved or depressed left ventricular ejection fraction, sodium should be restricted to 2 to 3 gm/day. In clients with moderate to severe heart failure, sodium restriction to levels less than 2 gm/day should be considered (Heart Failure Society of America, 2006). In the hospital setting, fluid intake should be restricted to less than 2 L/day in clients with severe hyponatremia (serum sodium less than 130 mEq/L) and should be considered in clients with refractory or advanced heart failure (Ershow & Costello, 2006; Nohria, Lewis, & Stevenson, 2001). Sodium restriction in conjunction with fluid restriction will help maximize diuretic therapy in these extreme cases. The nurse or dietitian should review with the client major sources of dietary sodium and the importance of avoiding adding salt to food. The client should be taught where to find sodium content on the nutrition label of most foods and to choose foods that are low in sodium. Salt substitutes, spices, and low-sodium marinades or sauces may be a good substitution for clients who use salt often at the table, but clients with renal failure or those taking potassium-sparing diuretics should be instructed to look for nonpotassium containing salt substitutes. Poor knowledge about sodium restriction significantly increases the risk of hospital readmission for heart failure, underlining the importance of thorough education of the client (Kollipara et al., 2008). Maintaining a fluid restriction outside of the hospital is generally reserved for advanced heart failure and clients receiving high doses of oral diuretic agents. In clients where fluid restriction is needed, fluid intake can be monitored by daily weight tracking and comparing urine output with fluid consumed, because fluid intake should not be more than the amount of urine produced. Client Education Checklist: Fluid Restriction in the Client with Heart Failure (HF) outlines nutrition intervention for the client with heart failure.

Cardiac cachexia in clients with heart failure is defined as weight loss of more than 6% of the previous normal weight over 6 months associated with heart failure (Flippatos, Anker, & Kremastinos, 2005). Cardiac cachexia is estimated to occur in 10% to 15% of clients with heart failure (Azhar & Wei, 2006). This condition is seen in advanced disease as-

| CLIENT EDUCATION CHECKLIST | Fluid Restriction in the Client with Heart Failure (HF)* |

Intervention	Example
Review how to convert ounces of fluid to liters.	• Point out where the fluid content is located on a label (often in fluid ounces). • 34 fluid ounces = 1 liter. • To convert ounces to liters, divide your fluid in ounces by 34. For example, 12 ounces of fluid is equivalent to 0.35 L fluid ($^{12}/_{34}$ = 0.35).
Review standard serving sizes of commonly consumed beverages.	• 1 can of soda = 12 ounces (0.35 L). • 1 individual bottle of soda = 20 ounces (0.6 L fluid). • Coffee cups typically hold 6 ounces but are often sold in restaurants in 12-, 16-, and 20-ounce (and larger) portions. • Water bottles range in size from 8 ounces (0.2 L) to 51 ounces (1.5 L).
Ensure that daily fluids are compromised from nutrient-dense foods and beverages.	• Limit "empty" calorie beverages such as regular and diet colas, coffee, and tea. • Remember that fluids in foods such as soups, popsicles, ice cream, pudding, and Jello count toward your daily requirement.
Provide suggestions to clients when they feel thirsty.	• Suck on ice chips or hard candy.

*Fluid restriction in the outpatient setting is reserved for advanced heart failure and clients taking high doses of oral diuretics.

sociated with a progressive decline in cardiac performance, resulting in muscle and adipose wasting and undernutrition. Undernutrition is often due to one or a combination of the following: increased nutrient losses, unmet increased nutritional requirements, and decreased nutritional intake. Bowel wall edema because of heart failure can cause malabsorption (von Haehling, Doehner, & Anker, 2007). Dyspnea can lead to increased metabolic needs because of the physical work of breathing. Early satiety and fatigue further compound poor dietary intake. Nutrition alone is not the cause of this condition because hormonal and proinflammatory effects are also seen (von Haehling et al., 2007). Typical clinical features of this condition include upper-body and temporal wasting as well as peripheral edema. Clients with cardiac cachexia should work with a dietitian to ensure that intake of calories and protein is adequate. The client with cardiac cachexia may have decreased nutrient intake because of early satiety from hepatomegaly and ascites; dyspnea and fatigue; lack of desire to eat low-sodium foods; and anorexia, nausea, or vomiting from medications associated with treating heart failure. In these cases, a dietitian can be very helpful in recommending high-protein, high-calorie foods and supplements that are compatible with the client's food preferences, medical issues, and lifestyle factors. Often, dietary intake can become so diminished in these clients that sodium intake is well below the dietary restriction. The dietitian may suggest liberalizing the intake of some moderate sodium foods to increase diet palatability and hence intake while still maintaining the overall sodium restriction. In clients with cachexia who are in negative nitrogen balance, protein intake should be increased to 1.5 to 2 gm/kg/day. Providing smaller portion meals more frequently may improve intake (Heart Failure Society of America, 2006), although enteral feedings may be needed if oral intake cannot provide adequate nutrition. Electrolytes and hydration status should be carefully monitored in these clients because of the effects of a sodium-restricted diet and diuretic therapy, especially in the older client. Because malnutrition may be highly prevalent in clients who do not demonstrate clinical signs of cachexia (Aquilani et al., 2003) all clients with heart failure should be individually assessed for poor nutrition intake. A daily multivitamin-multimineral supplement should be prescribed for clients with cachexia or undernutrition and considered for those reporting poor nutrient intake to ensure adequate intake of micronutrients. In particular, adequate thiamin intake should be addressed. Loop diuretics used to treat heart failure contribute to urinary thiamin loss that can predispose the client to thiamin deficiency (Wooley, 2008). Thiamin deficiency, called beri-beri, can cause symptoms similar to heart failure and exacerbate the underlying disease. There are no data to suggest that dietary supplements providing levels above the recommended amounts are beneficial to the client with heart failure. Before recommending a dietary supplement, the nurse should ask the client about dietary supplement use to ensure that excessive intake does not occur.

NURSING CARE PLAN **Nutrition and Hyperlipidemia**

CASE STUDY

Horace, age 58 years, describes himself as a "meat and potatoes man." He works the day shift at an auto-parts assembly plant, a job he has had for 33 years. He is looking forward to retiring in 2 years, at which time he and his wife of 36 years plan to travel around the country and spend time with their adult children and grandchildren. When his insurance plan changed he had a blood screening that showed an elevated LDL cholesterol level and a mildly elevated blood glucose. He says he has not seen a physician for many years, feels fine, and that his parents are in their 80s and in generally good health. He says he knows he has "good genes" and there is no need to worry about cholesterol levels or anything else. He has come to the clinic as a follow-up to the screening because the insurance company sent him a letter strongly suggesting an appointment with a health care provider. He says he is here only because he does not want to risk getting in trouble with the insurance company because of the coverage it provides for his wife's arthritis.

Applying the Nursing Process

ASSESSMENT

> Height: 5 feet, 10 inches Weight: 212 pounds
>   BMI: 30 BP 148/90 mm Hg P 76 bpm RR 16
> Fasting cholesterol (mg/dL): 290; LDL: 137; HDL: 38;
>   Fasting serum glucose: 128 mg/dL

Horace has central obesity and loose flesh on his upper arms. His skin is smooth and dry with no obvious lesions. Teeth are in good condition. He says he eats "three squares" a day, one of which is the lunch he carries to work. He denies alcohol intake beyond one beer each Friday after work with his friends. He typically glances at the paper and watches TV after eating a dinner prepared by his wife.

DIAGNOSES

> *Imbalanced nutrition; more than body requirements* related to BMI of 30
> *Risk for cardiovascular disease* related to elevated LDL cholesterol and serum glucose, low HDL cholesterol, high blood pressure
> *Alteration in health maintenance* related to knowledge deficit as evidenced by belief in "good genes"
> *Sedentary lifestyle* related to lack of interest in physical activity

EXPECTED OUTCOMES

> Weight loss of 1 pound a week
> Knowledge of risk factors for cardiovascular disease and diabetes
> Participation in 30 minutes of physical activity three times a week
> Meal plans that include increased fruit, vegetables, and fiber; reduced sodium

PLANNING

> 24-hour food recall and 3 days (2 week days and 1 weekend day) of recording food and beverages
> Involve his wife in diet teaching
> Meet with a dietitian to develop acceptable strategy for weight reduction along with cholesterol, glucose, and blood pressure control
> Discuss factors that contribute to the development of cardiovascular disease
> Develop a plan for increasing physical activity
> Monitor serum cholesterol, glucose, and blood pressure after 2 months

EVALUATION

Horace and his wife met with the dietitian and nurse. He expresses gratitude for finding out about his elevated cholesterol because he "wants to be around for the grandkids." Because family is so important, he and his wife are working hard to eat more whole grain products and more vegetables. His wife has begun preparing only the amount of food they will eat at each meal; she gives the example of making only one pork chop for each of them. She also heard about using smaller plates and is doing that as well. Vegetables are not a favorite but she makes sure they eat frozen green beans or a salad two or three times a week. Horace has begun taking turkey sandwiches in his lunch and using mustard instead of mayonnaise for flavoring. He says he is still hungry and cannot stand to give up an afternoon snack, so he tries to eat a few reduced sodium saltine crackers or pretzels instead of cookies. The activity is a challenge because he really feels tired at the end of his shift. In the nice weather he tries to walk around the block, but because his wife has arthritis she cannot always go with him and he does not like to walk alone. His weight is now 201 pounds and he feels that he can continue to work on lowering it. His cholesterol is 262 mg/dL with an LDL of 131 mg/dL and HDL of 40 mg/dL. His glucose is 123 mg. He will continue working on diet and activity and return in 2 months for additional laboratory work. Figure 18-4 ■ outlines the nursing process for this case.

Nutrition and Hyperlipidemia *(continued)*

NURSING CARE PLAN

Assessment
Data about the patient

Subjective
What the patient tells the nurse

Example: I am a meat and potatoes man; I don't worry about cholesterol because I have good genes.

Objective
What the nurse observes; anthropometric and clinical data

Examples: 212 pounds; BMI: 30; serum cholestrol: 290 mg/dL; blood glucose: 128 mg/dL

Diagnosis
NANDA label

Example: Imbalanced nutrition: more than body requirements related to excess nutrient intake

Planning
Goals stated in patient terms

Example: Long-term goal: weight loss of 1 pound per week; Short-term goal: identify foods high in fiber and low in saturated fat

Implementation
Nursing action to help patient achieve goals

Example: Refer to dietitian; discuss factors that contribute to development of heart disease

Evaluation
Was the goal achieved or does the intervention need to be modified?

Example: 11-pound weight loss in 2 months; cholesterol: 262 mg/dL; eating more whole grain bread

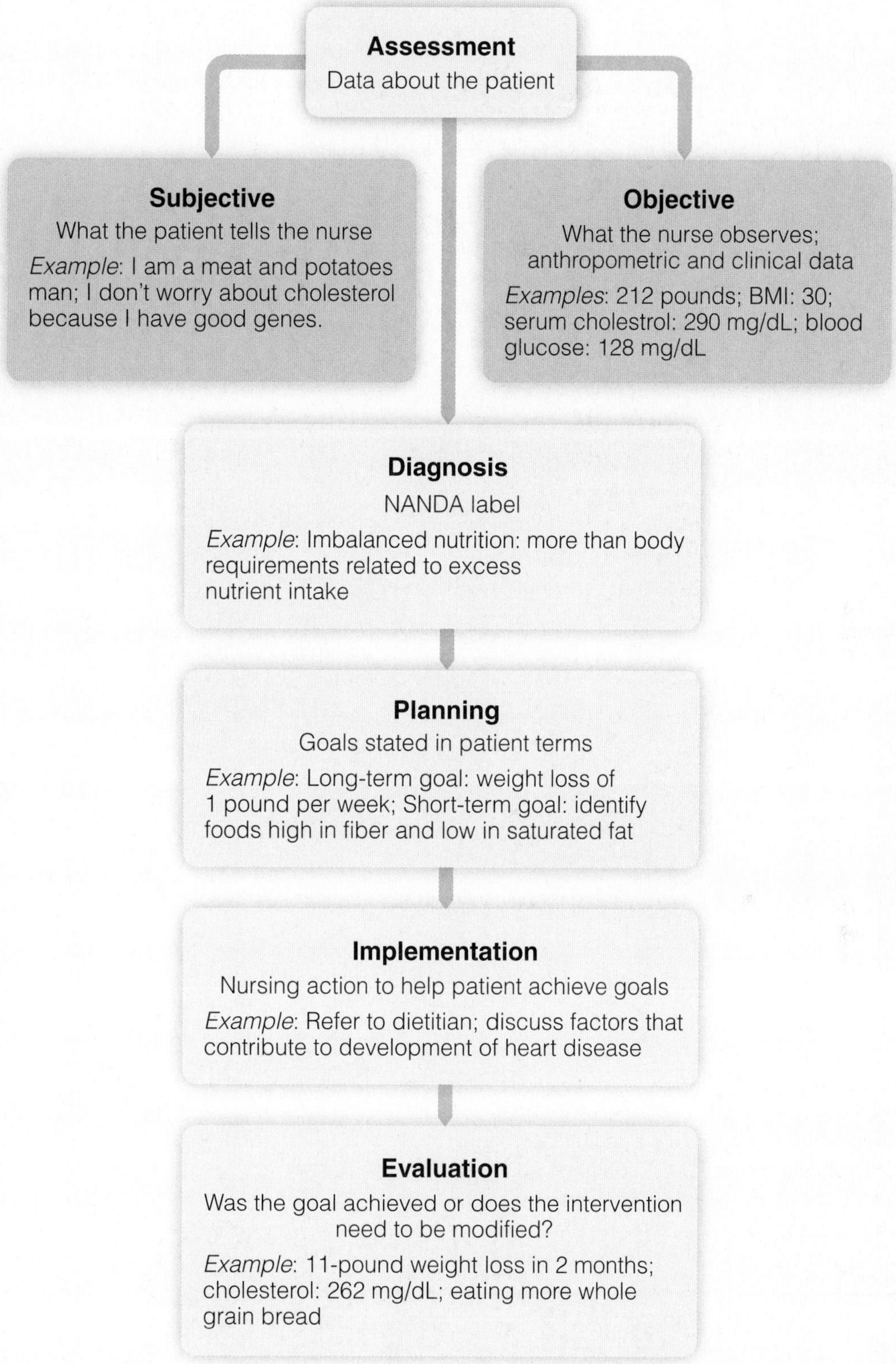

■ FIGURE 18-4   **Nursing Care Plan Process: Nutrition and Hyperlipidemia.**

(continued)

Nutrition and Hyperlipidemia *(continued)*

NURSING CARE PLAN

Critical Thinking in the Nursing Process

1. What are some of the immediate dietary steps a nurse can suggest to a client who presents with an elevated LDL cholesterol level?

2. What are some things a nurse can explain to a client who states that it is no longer necessary to follow dietary interventions because a cholesterol-lowering medication has been started?

CHAPTER SUMMARY

- Nutrition and lifestyle intervention can have a significant impact on primary and secondary prevention for CVD through reducing LDL cholesterol, raising HDL cholesterol, improving glucose metabolism, and reducing elevated blood pressure.

- To reduce risk of CVD, the primary target is reducing LDL cholesterol to goal based on individual risk factors.

- Diet interventions to address hypercholesterolemia include: limiting saturated and trans fats, increasing viscous ("soluble") fiber and plant stanols/sterols, restoring and maintaining an appropriate body weight, and including regular physical activity.

- n-3 polyunsaturated fats including EPA, DHA found in some fatty fish, and ALA found in flaxseed, walnuts, canola and soybean oils, are associated with a reduced risk of CVD.

- For primary prevention of CVD, clients should be encouraged to consume at least 2 servings of fish per week.

- Secondary prevention recommendations include 2 to 3 oz daily consumption of fish or the use of fish oil capsules to supply ~1 gm of EPA and DHA. All individuals, despite risk of CVD, should be encouraged to replace low ALA

fats and oils (butter, safflower, corn oil) with those higher in ALA (canola, soybean, or flaxseed oil).

- Clients with pre-hypertension and hypertension should adapt lifestyle modifications known to improve blood pressure, including weight reduction; regular physical activity; reduction in sodium intake; increase in fruits, vegetables, and low-fat dairy products; and consuming no more than two alcoholic drinks per day for men and one drink per day for women.

- Metabolic syndrome increases risk of both diabetes and CVD. Management of this condition includes restoring and maintaining an appropriate weight, including regular aerobic exercise, and reducing LDL cholesterol to goal if elevated.

- Medical nutrition therapy for heart failure includes reducing sodium and fluid retention; attaining and maintaining an appropriate body weight; and ensuring that the diet is adequate in vitamins, minerals, and protein. Those with cardiac cachexia should require nutrition intervention to ensure that needs are met to improve nutritional health.

EXPLORE **PEARSON mynursingkit™**

MyNursingKit is your one stop for online chapter review materials and resources. Prepare for success with additional NCLEX®-style practice questions, interactive assignments and activities, web links, animations and videos, and more!

Register your access code from the front of your book at
www.mynursingkit.com.

NCLEX® QUESTIONS

1. A middle-age client with mildly elevated serum LDL cholesterol wants to use diet to lower his cholesterol level. The client asks the nurse about what foods, in addition to oatmeal, may help lower cholesterol. The nurse suggests which of the following?
   1. Whole wheat bread
   2. Apples
   3. Cabbage
   4. Corn

2. The nurse knows that teaching about a low-sodium diet has been effective when a client states which of the following food choices would be good to take to work for lunch?
   1. Salami sandwich with whole wheat bread
   2. Ham salad with low-sodium crackers
   3. Shrimp with lettuce and low-fat French dressing
   4. Roast turkey sandwich on white bread

3. A client asks the nurse if becoming a vegetarian is the best way to lower an elevated cholesterol level. The nurse should respond that:
   1. "Yes, vegetarians always have low cholesterol because they do not eat meat."
   2. "No, there are many ways to lower the cholesterol level; a vegetarian diet is only one of them."
   3. "Yes, it is impossible for a vegetarian to have elevated cholesterol."
   4. "No, consuming too little cholesterol can be harmful."

4. A client who is planning a low-fat, low-cholesterol, low-sodium diet wants to know if it possible to have desserts. The nurse responds with which of the following suggestions?
   1. Ice cream with fresh strawberries
   2. Two small chocolate chip cookies
   3. Three gingersnap cookies
   4. Lemon meringue pie

5. Which breakfast selection by a client with hypercholesterolemia indicates to the nurse that additional teaching is not needed?
   1. Orange juice, shredded wheat with low-fat milk, strawberries, coffee
   2. Grapefruit juice, egg omelet, toast with margarine
   3. Tea, canned pineapple, vanilla whole milk yogurt, bagel with margarine
   4. Orange juice, bagel with strawberry cream cheese

REFERENCES

Albert, C. M., Cook, N. R., Gaziano, J. M., Zaharris, E., MacFayden, J., Danielson, E., et al. (2008). Effect of folic acid and B vitamins on risk of cardiovascular events and total mortality among women at high risk for cardiovascular disease: A randomized trial. *Journal of the American Medical Association, 299,* 2027–2036.

Albert, C. M., Hennekens, C. H., O'Donell, C. J., Ajani, U. A., Carey, V. J., Willett, W. C., et al. (1998). Fish consumption and risk of sudden cardiac death. *Journal of the American Medical Association, 279,* 23–28.

American Diabetes Association. (2008). *Diabetes statistics for African Americans.* Retrieved April 27, 2009, from http://www.diabetes.org/diabetes-statistics/african-americans.jsp

Anderson, J. W., & Hanna, T. J. (1999). Impact of nondigestible carbohydrates on serum lipoproteins and risk for cardiovascular disease. *Journal of Nutrition, 129,* 1457S–1466S.

Anderson, J. W., Johnstone, B. M., & Cook-Newell, M. E. (1995). Meta-analysis of the effects of soy protein intake on serum lipids. *New England Journal of Medicine, 333,* 276–282.

Appel, L. J., Moore, T. J., Obarzanek, E., Vollmer, W. M., Svetkey, L. P., Sacks, F. M., et al. (1997). A clinical trial of the effects of dietary patterns on blood pressure. DASH Collaborative Research Group. *New England Journal of Medicine, 336,* 1117–1134.

Aquilani, R., Opasich, C., Verri, M., Boschi, F., Febo, O., Pasini, E., et al. (2003). Is nutritional intake adequate in chronic heart failure patients? *Journal of the American College of Cardiology, 42,* 1218–1223.

Azhar, G., & Wei, J. Y. (2006). Nutrition and cardiac cachexia. *Current Opinion in Clinical Nutrition & Metabolic Care, 9,* 18–23.

Beich, K. R., & Yancy, C. (2008). The heart failure and sodium restriction controversy: Challenging conventional practice. *Nutrition in Clinical Practice, 23,* 477–486.

Bonaa, K. H., Njolstad, I., Ueland, P. M., Schirmer, H., Tverdal, A., Steigen, T., et al. (2006). NORVIT trial investigators. Homocysteine lowering and cardiovascular events after acute myocardial infarction. *New England Journal of Medicine, 354,* 1578–1588.

Brunzell, J. D. (2007). Hypertriglyceridemia. *New England Journal of Medicine, 357,* 1009–1017.

Buckley, M. S., Goff, A. N., & Knapp, W. E. (2004). Fish oil interaction with warfarin. *The Annals of Pharmacotherapy, 38,* 50–53.

Centers for Disease Control and Prevention (CDC). (2006). *Office of women's health: Overweight and obesity.* Retrieved April 27, 2009, from http://www.cdc.gov/women/natstat/overwght.htm

Centers for Disease Control and Prevention (CDC) (2008a). *National Center for Health Statistics fastats: Deaths/mortality.* Retrieved February 15, 2009, from http://www.cdc.gov/nchs/fastats/deaths.htm

Centers for Disease Control and Prevention (CDC). (2008b). *Health United States, 2008.* Retrieved April 27, 2009, from http://www.cdc.gov/nchs/data/hus/hus08.pdf#075

Chen, J. T., Wesley, R., Shamburek, R. D., Pucino, F., & Csako, G. (2005). Meta-analysis of natural therapies for hyperlipidemia: Plant sterols and stanols versus policosanol. *Pharmacotherapy, 25,* 171–183.

Davy, B. M., & Melby, C. L. (2003). The effect of fiber-rich carbohydrates on features of syndrome X. *Journal of the American Dietetic Association, 103,* 86–96.

Dyerberg, J., & Bang, H. O. (1979). Haemostatic function and platelet polyunsaturated fatty acids in Eskimos. *Lancet, ii,* 433–435.

Elmer, P. J., Obarzanek, E., Vollmer, W. M., Simons-Morton, D., Stevens, V. J., Young,

D. R., et al. (2006). Effects of comprehensive lifestyle modification on diet, weight, physical fitness and blood pressure control: 18 month results of a randomized trial. *Annual of Internal Medicine, 144,* 485–495.

Ershow, A. G., & Costello, R. B. (2006). Dietary guidance in heart failure: A prospective on needs for prevention and management. *Heart Failure Review, 11,* 7–12.

Flippatos, G. S., Anker, S. D., & Kremastinos, D. T. (2005). Pathophysiology of peripheral muscle wasting in cardiac cachexia. *Current Opinion in Clinical Nutrition & Metabolic Care, 8,* 249–254.

Food and Drug Administration (FDA). (2003). *Food labeling: Trans fatty acids in nutrition labeling, nutrient content claims, and health claims* (Federal Register - 68 FR 41433 July 11, 2003). Retrieved July 1, 2009, from http://www.fda.gov/OHRMS/DOCKETS/98fr/03-1725.pdf

Food and Drug Administration (FDA). (2008). *A food labeling guide: Appendix A: Definitions of nutrient content claims.* Retrieved April 27, 2009, from http://www.cfsan.fda.gov/~dms/2lg-xa.html

Food and Drug Administration (FDA), Environmental Protection Agency (EPA). (2006). *What you need to know about mercury in fish and shellfish.* Retrieved April 27, 2009, from http://www.epa.gov/waterscience/fish/files/MethylmercuryBrochure.pdf

Ford, E. S., Giles, W. H., & Dietz, W. H. (2002). Prevalence of the metabolic syndrome among US adults: Findings from the Third National Health and Nutrition Examination Survey. *Journal of the American Medical Association, 287,* 356–359.

Frishman, W. H., Beravol, P., & Carosella, C. (2009). Alternative and complementary medicine for preventing and treating cardiovascular disease. *Disease of the Month, 55,* 121–192.

Fung, T. T., Chiuve, S. E., McCullough, M. L., Rexrode, K. M., Logroscino, G., & Hu, F. B. (2008). Adherence to a DASH-style diet and risk of coronary heart diease and stroke in women. *Archives of Internal Medicine, 168,* 713–720.

Gardner, C. D., Lawson, L. D., Block, E., Chatterjee, L. M., Kiazand, A., Balise, R. R., et al. (2007). Effect of raw garlic vs. commercial garlic supplements on plasma lipid concentrations in adults with moderate hypercholesterolemia. *Archives of Internal Medicine, 167,* 346–353.

Gaziano, J. M., Hebert, P. R., & Hennekens, C. H. (1996). Cholesterol reduction: Weighing the benefits and risks. *Annuals of Internal Medicine, 124,* 914–918.

Gebauer, S. K., Psota, T. L., Harris, W. S., & Kris-Etherton, P. M. (2006). N-3 fatty acid dietary recommendations and food sources to achieve essentiality and cardiovascular bene-fits. *American Journal of Clinical Nutrition, 83,* 1526S–1535S.

Gordon, D. J., Probstfield, J. L., Garrison, R. J., Neaton, J. D., Castelli, W. P., Knoke, J. D., et al. (1989). High-density lipoprotein cholesterol and cardiovascular disease: Four prospective American studies. *Circulation, 79,* 8–15.

Gronbaek, M. (2006). Factors influencing the relation between alcohol and cardiovascular disease. *Current Opinion in Lipidology, 171,* 17–21.

Grundy, S. M., Cleeman, J. I., Daniels, S. R., Donato, K. A., Eckel, R. H., Franklin, B. A., et al. (2005). Diagnosis and management of the metabolic syndrome. An American Heart Association/National Heart, Lung, and Blood Institute Scientific Statement. *Circulation, 112,* 2735–2752.

Halton, T. L., Willett, W. C., Liu, S., Manson, J. E., Albert, C. M., Rexrode, K., et al. (2006). Low-carbohydrate-diet score and the risk of coronary heart disease in women. *New England Journal of Medicine, 355* (19), 1991–2002.

He, J., Whelton, P. K., Appel, L. J., Charleston, J., & Klag, M. J. (2000). Long-term effects of weight loss and dietary sodium reduction on incidence of hypertension. *Hypertension, 35,* 544–549.

Heart Failure Society of America. (2006). Nonpharmacologic management and health care maintenance in patients with chronic heart failure. *Journal of Cardiac Failure, 12,* e29–37.

Humphrey, L. L., Fu, R., Freeman, M., & Helfand, M. (2008). Homocysteine level and coronary heart disease incidence: A systemic review and meta-analysis. *Mayo Clinic Proceedings, 83,* 1203–1212.

Iso, H., Kobayashi, M., Ishihara, J., Sasaki, S., Okada, K., Kita, Y., et al. (2006). Intake of fish and n-3 fatty acids and risk of coronary heart disease among Japanese: The Japan Public Health Center-Based (JPHC) Study Cohort I. *Circulation, 113,* 195–202.

Jenkins, D. J., Kendall, C. W., Faulkner, D. A., Nguyen, T., Kempt, T., Marchie, A., et al. (2006). Assessment of the longer-term effects of a dietary portfolio of cholesterol-lowering foods in hypercholesterolemia. *American Journal of Clinical Nutrition, 83,* 582–591.

Jones, P. J., & AbuMweis, S. S. (2009). Phytosterols as functional food ingredients: Linkages to cardiovascular disease and cancer. *Current Opinion in Clinical Nutrition and Metabolic Care, 12,* 147–151.

Katain, M. B., Grundy, S. M., Jones, P., Law, M., Miettinen, T., & Paoletti, R. for the Stresa workshop participants (2003). Efficacy and safety of plant stanols and sterols in the management of blood cholesterol levels. *Mayo Clinical Proceedings, 78,* 965–978.

Kelley, G. A., & Kelley, K. S. (2000). Progressive resistance exercise and resting blood pressure. *Hypertension, 35,* 838–843.

Kendall, C. W., & Jenkins, D. J. (2004). A dietary portfolio: Maximal reduction of low-density lipoprotein cholesterol with diet. *Current Atherosclerosis Reports, 6,* 492–498.

Khan, N. A., Hemmelgarn, B., Herman, R. J., Rabkin, S. W., McAlister, F. A., Bell, C. M., et al. (2008). The 2008 Canadian Hypertension Education Program recommendations for the management of hypertension: Part 2—therapy. *Canadian Journal of Cardiology, 24,* 465–475.

Knowler, W. C., Barrett-Connor, E., Fowler, S. E., Hamman, R. F., Lachin, J. M., & Walker, E. A. (Diabetes Prevention Program Research Group). (2002). Reduction in the incidence of type 2 diabetes with lifestyle intervention or metformin. *New England Journal of Medicine, 346,* 393–403.

Kollipara, U. K., Jaffer, O., Amin, A., Toto, K. H., Nelson, L. L., Schneider, R., et al. (2008). Relation of lack of knowledge about dietary sodium to hospital readmission in patients with heart failure. *American Journal of Cardiology, 102,* 1212–1215.

Krauss, R. M., Blanche, P. J., Rawlings, R. S., Fernstrom, H. S., & Williams, P. T. (2006). Separate effects of reduced carbohydrate intake and weight loss on atherogenic dyslipidemia. *American Journal of Clinical Nutrition, 83* (5), 1025–1031.

Kwiterovich, P. O., Jr. (1998). The antiatherogenic role of high-density lipoprotein cholesterol. *American Journal of Cardiology, 82,* 13Q–21Q.

Lennie, T. A. (2006). Nutritional recommendations for patients with heart failure. *Journal of Cardiovascular Nursing, 21,* 261–268.

Lichtenstein, A. H., Appel, L. J., Brands, M., Carnethon, M., Daniels, S., Franch, H. A., et al. (2006). Diet and lifestyle recommendations revision 2006: A scientific statement from the American Heart Association Nutrition Committee. *Circulation, 114,* 82–96.

McClaskey, E. M., & Michalets, E. L. (2007). Subdural hematoma after a fall in an elderly patient taking high-dose omega-3 fatty acids with warfarin and aspirin: Case report and review of the literature. *Pharmacotherapy, 27,* 152–160.

McKeown, N. M., Meigs, J. B., Liu, S., Saltzman, E., Wilson, P., & Jacques, P. F. (2004). Carbohydrate, nutrition, insulin resistance, and the prevalence of the metabolic syndrome in the Framingham Offspring Cohort. *Diabetes Care, 27,* 538–546.

Mensink, R. P. (2005). Metabolic and health effects of isomeric fatty acids. *Current Opinion in Lipidology, 17,* 27–30.

Miller, E. R., III, Pastor-Barriuso, R., Dalal, D., Riemersma, R. A., Appel, L. J., & Guallar, E. (2005). Meta-analysis: High-dosage vitamin E supplementation may increase all-cause mortality. *Annals of Internal Medicine, 142,* 37–46.

REFERENCES *(continued)*

Miller, M., Beach, V., Sorkin, J. D., Mangano, C., Dobmeier, C., Novacic, D., et al. (2009). Comparative effects of three popular diets on lipids, endothelial function, and C-reactive protein during weight maintenance. *Journal of the American Dietetic Association, 109,* 713–717.

Mozaffarian, D. (2008). Fish and n-3 fatty acids for the prevention of fatal coronary heart disease and sudden cardiac death. *American Journal of Clinical Nutrition, 87,* 1991S–1996S.

Mukamal, K. J., & Rimm, E. B. (2008). Alcohol consumption: Risks and benefits. *Current Atherosclerosis Report, 10,* 536–543.

National Cholesterol Education Program (NCEP) Expert Panel on Detection, Evaluation and Treatment of High Blood Cholesterol in Adults (Adult Treatment Panel [ATP] III). (2002). Third report of the National Cholesterol Education Program (NCEP) expert panel on detection, evaluation and treatment of high blood cholesterol in adults (Adult Treatment Panel III) final report. *Circulation, 106,* 3143–3421.

National Institutes of Health, National Heart, Lung, and Blood Institutes. (n.d.). *Your guide to lowering your blood pressure with DASH—How do I make the DASH?* Retrieved April 27, 2009, from http://www.nhlbi.nih.gov/health/public/heart/hbp/dash/how_make_dash.html

Noakes, M., Keogh, J. B., Foster, P. R., & Clifton, P. M. (2005). Effect of an energy-restricted, high-protein, low-fat diet relative to a conventional high-carbohydrate, low-fat diet on weight loss, body composition, nutritional status, and markers of cardiovascular health in obese women. *American Journal of Clinical Nutrition, 81* (6), 1298–1306.

Nohria, A., Lewis, E., & Stevenson, L. W. (2001). Medical management of advanced heart failure. *Journal of the American Medical Association, 287,* 628–640.

Ogden, C. L., Carroll, M. D., Curtin, L. R., McDowell, M. A., Tabak, C. J., & Flegal, K. M. (2006). Prevalence of overweight and obesity in the United States, 1999–2004. *Journal of the American Medical Association, 295,* 1549–1555.

Oh, R. C., & Lanier, J. B. (2007). Management of hypertriglyceridemia. *American Family Physician, 75,* 1365–1371.

Ostlund, R. E. (2004). Phytosterols and cholesterol metabolism. *Current Opinion in Lipidology, 15,* 37–41.

Parikh, A., Lipsitz, S. R., & Natarajan, S. (2009). Association between a DASH-like diet and mortality in adults with hypertension: Findings from a population-based study. *American Journal of Hypertension, 22,* 409–416.

Psota, T. L., Gebauer, S. K., & Kris-Etherton, P. (2006). Dietary omega-3 fatty acid intake and cardiovascular disease. *American Journal of Cardiology, 98,* 3i–18i.

Riediger, N. D., Othman, R., Suh, M., & Moghadasian, M. H. (2009). A systematic review of the roles of n-3 fatty acids in health and disease. *Journal of the American Dietetic Association, 109,* 668–679.

Sacks, F. M., Lichtenstein, A., Van Horn, L., Harris, W., Kris-Etherton, P., & Winston, P. (American Heart Association Science Advisory for Professionals from the Nutrition Committee). (2006). Soy, protein, isoflavones and cardiovascular health. *Circulation, 113,* 1034–1044.

Sacks, F. M., Svetkey, L. P., Vollmer, W. M., Appel, L. J., Bray, G. A., Harsha, D., et al. (2001). Effects on blood pressure of reduced dietary sodium and the dietary approaches to stop hypertension (DASH) diet. *New England Journal of Medicine, 344,* 3–10.

Saremi, A., & Arora, R. (2008). The cardiovascular implications of alcohol and red wine. *American Journal of Therapeutics, 15,* 265–277.

Sesso, H. D., Buring, J. E., Christen, W. G., Kurth, T., Belanger, C., MacFadyen, J., et al. (2008). Vitamins E and C in the prevention of cardiovascular disease in men: The Physicians' Health Study II randomized controlled study. *Journal of the American Medical Association, 300,* 2123–2133.

The Seventh Report of the Joint National Committee (JNC) on Prevention, Detection, Evaluation and Treatment of High Blood Pressure. (2003). The JNC 7 Report. *Journal of the American Medical Association, 289,* 2560–2572.

Sharman, M. J., Gomez, A. L., Kraemer, W. J., & Volek, J. S. (2004). Very low-carbohydrate and low-fat diets affect fasting lipids and postprandial lipemia differently in overweight men. *Journal of Nutrition, 134* (4), 880–885.

Szapary, P., Wolfe, M. E., Bloedon, L., Cucchiara, A., DeMardoresosian, A., Cirigliano, M. C., et al. (2003). A randomized clinical trial of guggulipid in patients with hypercholesterolemia. *Journal of the American Medical Association, 290,* 765–772.

Szmitko, P. E., & Verma, S. (2005). Antiatherogenic potential of red wine: Clinician update. *American Journal of Physiology, Heart, and Circulatory Physiology, 288,* H2023–2030.

Taku, K., Umegaki, K., Sato, Y., Taki, Y., Endoh, K., & Watanabe, S. (2007). Soy isoflavones lower serum total and LDL cholesterol in humans: A meta-analysis of 11 randomized controlled trials. *American Journal of Clinical Nutrition, 85,* 1148–1156.

The Trials of Hypertension Prevention Collaborative Research Group. (1997). Effects of weight loss and sodium reduction intervention on blood pressure and hypertension incidence in overweight people with high-normal blood pressure. *Archives of Internal Medicine, 157,* 657–667.

United States Department of Agriculture (USDA). (2009). *National Nutrient Database for Standard Reference, Release 21. Sodium, Na (mg) of selected foods per common measure.* Retrieved April 27, 2009, from http://www.nal.usda.gov/fnic/foodcomp/Data/SR21/nutrlist/sr21w307.pdf

U.S. Department of Agriculture, U.S. Department of Health and Human Services. (2005). *Dietary Guidelines Advisory Committee report.* Retrieved February 15, 2009, from http://www.health.gov/dietary guidelines/dga2005/report

Van Horn, L., McCoin, M., Kris-Etherton, P. M., Burke, F., Carson, J. S., Champagne, C. M., et al. (2008). The evidence for dietary prevention and treatment of cardiovascular disease. *Journal of the American Dietetic Association, 108,* 287–331.

von Haehling, S., Doehner, W., & Anker, S. D. (2007). Nutrition, metabolism, and the complex pathophysiology of cachexia in chronic heart disease. *Cardiovascular Research, 73,* 298–309.

Wexler, R., & Aukerman, G. (2006). Nonpharmacologic strategies for managing hypertension. *American Family Physician, 73,* 1953–1956.

Whelton, S. P., Chin, A., Xin, X., & He, J. (2002). Effect of aerobic exercise on blood pressure. *Annals of Internal Medicine, 136,* 493–503.

Wood, R. J., Fernandez, M. L., Sharman, M. J., Silvestre, R., Grene, C. M., Zern, T. L., et al. (2007). Effects of a carbohydrate-restricted diet with and without supplemental soluble fiber on plasma low-density lipoprotein cholesterol and other clinical markers of cardiovascular risk. *Metabolism, 56,* 58–67.

Wood, R. J., Volek, J. S., Davis, S. R., Dell'ova, C., & Fernandez, M. L. (2006). Effects of a carbohydrate-restricted diet on emerging plasma markers for cardiovascular disease. *Nutritional Metabolism, 4,* 3–19.

Wood, R. J., Volek, J. S., Liu, Y., Shachter, N. S., Contois, J. H., & Fernandez, M. L. (2006). Carbohydrate restriction alters lipoprotein metabolism by modifying VLDL, LDL, and HDL subfraction distribution and size in overweight men. *Journal of Nutrition, 136* (2), 384–389.

Woodside, J. V., & Krombhout, D. (2005). Fatty acids and CHD. *Proceedings of the Nutrition Society, 64,* 554–564.

Wooley, J. A. (2008). Characteristics of thiamin and its relevance to the management of heart failure. *Nutrition in Clinical Practice, 23,* 487–493.

Yuan, G., Al-Shali, K. Z., & Hegele, R. A. (2007). Hypertriglyceridemia: Its etiology, effects, and treatment. *Canadian Medical Association Journal, 176,* 1113–1120.

Charlotte Wisnewski

19 Diabetes Mellitus

WHAT WILL YOU LEARN?

1. To differentiate between classifications of diabetes in terms of age of onset, etiology, risks, typical symptoms, and treatment plans.

2. To compare carbohydrate, fat, and protein metabolism occurring in diabetes mellitus to that of normal metabolism.

3. To summarize the specific dietary recommendations across the lifespan for individuals with type 1 or type 2 diabetes, including those with comorbid conditions.

4. To assess cultural and lifespan variations when assisting clients to set goals and manage change in their nutritional patterns.

5. To counsel clients regarding use of sweeteners, alcohol, dietary supplements, and vitamins.

6. To develop nursing interventions to assist the client and family in self-management of diabetes in aspects of nutritional intake, carbohydrate counting, weight loss strategies, maintenance of good health, and food intake during exercise.

7. To relate the strategies for prevention and treatment of hypoglycemia and hyperglycemia.

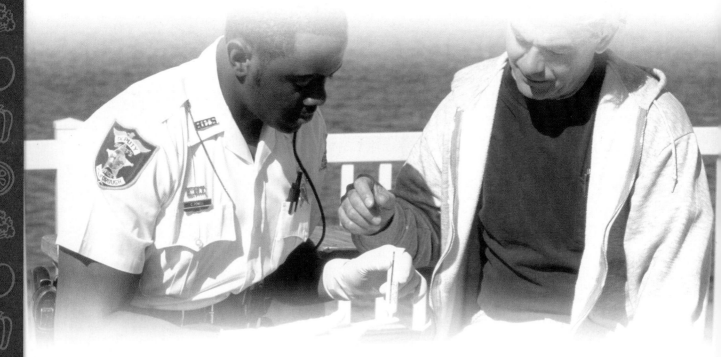

DID YOU KNOW?

▶ The "ADA" diet does not exist, but you may see this label on dietary menus in a hospital.

▶ Sugar (sucrose) is not a forbidden food for people with diabetes.

▶ People with diabetes may drink alcohol within certain guidelines.

▶ Modest weight loss can help prevent type 2 diabetes.

▶ Bariatric surgery has been shown to be very effective in controlling hyperglycemia and diabetes in clients who are obese.

KEY TERMS

endogenous insulin, *426*

euglycemia, *427*

hyperglycemia, *425*

hypoglycemia, *431*

ketones, *428*

polydipsia, *426*

polyphagia, *426*

polyuria, *426*

renal threshold, *428*

What Is Diabetes?

Diabetes mellitus is a chronic disease involving abnormal carbohydrate, fat, and protein metabolism characterized by hyperglycemia. It is not one disease, but several different diseases with varying etiologies resulting from glucose intolerance or high blood glucose, called **hyperglycemia.** The person with diabetes mellitus usually has decreased or absent insulin production from the beta cells of the pancreas. The diagnosis of diabetes is made on the basis of a fasting blood glucose of *greater than or equal to* 126 mg/dL. It is estimated that 8% of the population in the United States has diabetes with more than twice as many at risk of diabetes (Centers for Disease Control and Prevention [CDC], 2008). The incidence of type 2 diabetes is increasing throughout the world at epidemic rates and is partially attributed to the concurrent epidemic rate of obesity. As estimated by the International Diabetes Federation (IDF) (2007), 246 million people currently have diagnosed or undiagnosed diabetes and by the year 2025 that number will have increased to 380 million.

How Is Diabetes Classified?

The American Diabetes Association (ADA) classifies diabetes into four categories: prediabetes, type 1 diabetes, type 2 dia-

betes, and gestational diabetes (ADA, 2009). These classifications and the corresponding names have been changed several times in the past as more is learned about the pathogenesis, risk factors, and etiology of the disease. An overview of the four main types of diabetes is presented in Table 19-1.

Prediabetes

Prediabetes is characterized by hyperglycemia, but glucose levels are not increased to the extent that qualifies for a diagnosis of diabetes. Prediabetes is defined by either impaired glucose tolerance (glucose *greater than or equal to* 140 mg/dL and less than 200 mg/dL) or impaired fasting blood glucose (100–125 mg/dL) (CDC, 2008). The increasing epidemic of overweight and obesity is believed to be linked to the increasing occurrence of prediabetes. Over 57 million people in the United States have prediabetes (CDC, 2008). Although this statistic is of concern for all individuals at risk, it is especially troubling among children and adolescents where it is emerging as a new health care issue. The risk of prediabetes in overweight and obese adolescents is over twice that of healthy weight peers and is linked to the coexisting presence of cardiovascular risk factors (Li, Ford, Zhao, & Mokdad, 2009).

Lifestyle management interventions are recommended for the treatment of prediabetes and for the prevention of

Table 19-1 Classification of Diabetes, Etiology, and Typical Age of Onset

Diabetes Classification	Etiology	Typical Age of Onset
Type 1	Autoimmune beta cell destruction resulting in absolute insulin deficiency	Childhood through young adult (age 30)
Type 2	Progressive insulin secretory defect and insulin resistance; insulin secretion may be low, normal, or increased	Over age 40
Gestational	Diagnosed during pregnancy; may or may not continue after pregnancy (if so will be reclassified as type 2)	Young women of childbearing age
Secondary	Results from certain medications, certain other chemicals, associated with other autoimmune diseases; results from pancreatitis, cystic fibrosis	Usually over age 40 years but can occur at any age

type 2 diabetes, which can be the ultimate result if intervention does not occur (Unger & Moriarty, 2008). Weight loss, a diet that follows recommendations for reducing cardiovascular disease risk, and physical activity are recommended. The American Diabetes Association (ADA) recommends a weight loss of 5% to 10% of body weight and at least 150 minutes/week of moderate activity such as walking (American Diabetes Association, 2009). A variety of dietary approaches have been investigated for an effect on decreasing risk of type 2 diabetes in those with prediabetes. The Diabetes Prevention Study demonstrated that lifestyle intervention, including dietary interventions, prevented one case of diabetes per seven persons treated over 3 years (Knowler et al., 2002). A diet rich in fruits, vegetables, and whole grains with low-fat dairy and minimal alcohol has been linked with reduced risk of diabetes (Brunner et al., 2008). In the Nurses Health Study, a healthy diet high in cereals and polyunsaturated fat while low in trans fats and processed carbohydrate foods was more strongly associated with a lower risk for diabetes among minorities (Blacks, Asians, and Hispanics) than Caucasians (Shai et al., 2006). The nurse can advise the client with prediabetes about the risk of developing type 2 diabetes and the importance of weight management and cardiovascular risk reduction in lessening disease risk. Guidelines outlined in Chapter 17 and Chapter 18 can assist the nurse with these interventions.

Type 1 Diabetes

Although there are several causes of type 1 diabetes, the most common form represents an autoimmune etiology. In type 1 diabetes (previously called insulin-dependent diabetes or juvenile onset diabetes), the pancreatic beta cells in the islets of Langerhans fail to produce insulin because of the autoimmune destruction of the beta cells, leading to an absolute deficiency of insulin. The clinical onset of type 1 diabetes is characteristically very rapid with signs of diabetes appearing in days to a few weeks. The rapid onset of type 1 diabetes is because of the importance of insulin and its critical functions.

Why Does Type 1 Diabetes Occur?

The exact mechanism that leads to the development of type 1 diabetes remains elusive. A series of events that includes a combination of genetic, immunologic, and environmental triggers is felt to result in the destruction in the pancreatic islets responsible for producing insulin (Kim & Lee, 2009). There is no clear dietary cause of these events, but it has been observed that a deficiency of vitamin D is associated with an increased risk of type 1 diabetes (Merriman, 2009). Studies have also focused on the early introduction of cow's milk to the diet as a risk factor, but results are equivocal (ADA, 2008).

Symptoms of Type 1 Diabetes

Type 1 diabetes is characterized by increased thirst **(polydipsia),** increased hunger **(polyphagia),** extreme

PRACTICE PEARL

Diabetic Ketoacidosis

If type 1 diabetes remains untreated or is inadequately treated, the person will begin demonstrating signs of diabetic ketoacidosis (DKA), including hyperglycemia, nausea and vomiting, abdominal pain, acetone breath, and ketone bodies in the urine. Progression to an unconscious state will eventually occur over a several day period. DKA is a medical emergency requiring intravenous (IV) administration of insulin, saline, potassium, and other electrolytes. The nurse should educate people with diagnosed type 1 diabetes to be aware of these symptoms to prevent DKA.

weight loss, and loss of large amounts of water in the form of urine **(polyuria).** Only about 10% of people with diabetes are estimated to have type 1, but because this form of diabetes usually begins in childhood or early adulthood (up to age 30), the person faces a lifetime of managing the disease. Because type 1 commonly occurs in thin individuals, the extreme weight loss is very obvious and weight regain may even be needed. Practice Pearl: Diabetic Ketoacidosis discusses more information about the effects of untreated type 1 diabetes.

Treatment Plan for Type 1 Diabetes

Type 1 diabetes must be treated with insulin. Modification of the diet plan, called medical nutrition therapy (MNT), and prescribed physical activity guidelines are also essential to the control of type 1 diabetes. Oral hypoglycemic agents cannot be used because they affect the insulin produced by the body, called **endogenous insulin;** in type 1 diabetes there is an absolute lack of insulin production. Insulins, including short acting, rapid acting, intermediate, and long acting, are used in various combinations. Rapid-acting insulin may be given before each meal to emulate the function of the pancreas, and long-acting insulin may be given both morning and evening to simulate the basal function of the pancreas, which keeps the blood glucose stable over time. A consistent carbohydrate diet with insulin correction for hyperglycemia before each meal is recommended for those with type 1 diabetes on intensive control and multiple injections (ADA, 2008). Specific dietary guidelines are discussed later in the chapter.

Type 2 Diabetes

Type 2 diabetes is most often diagnosed in overweight people over the age of 40 years. However, there is a form of type 2 diabetes common in overweight children and adolescents that is emerging parallel to the obesity epidemic (Cali & Caprio, 2008). Practice Pearl: Type 2 Diabetes in Children discusses this issue. In addition to overweight, another common characteristic of type 2 diabetes is that by the time the disease is diagnosed, the person may already be beginning to demonstrate evidence of complications of diabetes, such as neu-

PRACTICE PEARL

Type 2 Diabetes in Children

Type 2 diabetes in children was virtually unknown prior to the 1990s. It is believed that the increasing prevalence of overweight and obesity has greatly contributed to the present epidemic. Factors such as excessive consumption of sweetened drinks and fast foods and a sedentary level of activity are felt to significantly contribute to risk of overweight. Nurses should use every opportunity to educate both parents and children about the need for healthy nutrition and physical activity to prevent type 2 diabetes.

ropathy, blindness or increasing visual impairment, coronary artery disease, renal disease, and stroke, among other signs.

Why Does Type 2 Diabetes Occur?

In type 2 diabetes, insulin uptake to glucose-stimulated cells (muscle and adipose tissues) is disturbed. This alteration is labeled insulin resistance. Over time, there can be progressive degeneration of the pancreatic beta cells and diminished insulin production (Gerich & Dailey, 2004). Studies show a correlation between type 2 diabetes, genetics, insulin resistance, and obesity, though obesity plays the most significant role. No set genetic pattern is found to predispose an individual to diabetes (Romao & Roth, 2008).

Symptoms of Type 2 Diabetes

The classical symptoms (polyphagia, polyuria, and polydipsia) found in type 1 diabetes do not occur as frequently in type 2 diabetes because of the continued production of endogenous insulin. The slower onset of type 2 diabetes leads to later diagnosis because the symptoms are not as obvious. Common symptoms include fatigue, visual blurriness, tingling and numbness in the hands and/or feet, recurrent infections in the feet and legs, nails with fungal infections, dry skin, and lesions on the feet and legs that are slow to heal.

Treatment Plan for Type 2 Diabetes

In the early stages of type 2 diabetes, it may be possible to treat the disease effectively with a combination of nutrition and increased physical activity. The dietary interventions should focus on losing weight and heart healthy nutrition. As the disease progresses in intensity and glycemic control becomes more difficult, oral medications are added to the treatment plan. Later, insulin can be added if oral medications are contraindicated or are ineffective in glycemic control. Depending on the level of hyperglycemia and other concomitant conditions, some newly diagnosed individuals may be placed on insulin at the beginning of their treatment regimen. Table 19-2 shows the current blood glucose recommendations for adults with type 1 or type 2 diabetes.

All individuals should be given meal planning and activity guidelines and encouraged to learn more about their

Table 19-2   Glycemic Goals for Adults with Diabetes

Test	Recommended Value for People with Diabetes	Normal Value (Nondiabetes)
Hemoglobin A1C	Less than 7% Less than 6% if safely achieved Adjust in those with frequent history of hypoglycemia, limited life expectancy, or long-standing, extensive disease	4–6%
Preprandial capillary plasma glucose	90–130 mg/dL	Less than 100
Postprandial capillary plasma glucose	Less than 180 mg/dL	Less than 140

Sources: ADA, 2009; Canadian Diabetes Association, 2008; Del Prato, Felton, Munro, Zimmet, & Zinman, 2007.

disease in order to achieve good glycemic control. A multidisciplinary team approach can be used to address medical and pharmacological interventions, diet, and management of any comorbid conditions that result. Dietary interventions are discussed later in this chapter.

Gestational Diabetes

Diabetes when first diagnosed during pregnancy is called *gestational diabetes*. Some women will not have diabetes and hyperglycemia once pregnancy is completed, whereas others will remain with overt diabetes that is then reclassified as type 2 diabetes. Gestational diabetes is treated with dietary interventions and physical activity. Treatment can include insulin if diet and activity do not achieve glycemic goals. Pregnant females must work intensively to attain normal blood glucose, called **euglycemia.** If not well controlled, gestational diabetes can lead to higher rates of mortality and morbidity in women and their babies. High-risk women should have glucose testing as soon as the pregnancy is diagnosed; low-risk women can have testing at 24 weeks of gestational age (ADA, 2009). In order to consider a woman at low risk, she must be younger than 25 years of age and be a member of an ethnic group with a low prevalence of diabetes. Additionally, she must have been of normal weight before pregnancy and have no history of hyperglycemia, diabetes in a close relative, or poor obstetric outcome. The ADA has educational materials available for those working with females with gestational diabetes.

Diabetes and Metabolism

A lack of insulin will affect carbohydrate, fat, and protein metabolism. Under normal circumstances glucose and sodium are

MyNursingKit American Diabetes Association: Gestational Diabetes

together actively transported into certain tissues facilitated by glucose transporters (GLUT 1-5). The insulin hormone is required to transport glucose into muscle, fat, and liver cells. Insulin molecules attach to the surface of the cell membrane, and glucose enters the cells to meet the cellular metabolic energy needs. In diabetes, the altered metabolism of glucose in turn affects the metabolism of fats and proteins as the body attempts to compensate for a lack of glucose uptake into cells.

Carbohydrate Metabolism in Diabetes

A lack of insulin production is devastating because glucose cannot enter the cells from the blood in adequate levels for metabolic needs; hyperglycemia results as more and more glucose accumulates in the blood. Hyperglycemia results in the loss of large amounts of water through the kidneys. As blood glucose rises above a set level for retention of glucose by the kidney, called the **renal threshold,** the kidney begins excreting some of the extra glucose. The concentration of glucose molecules in the urine acts as an osmotic agent and draws significant water into the urine, which leads to polyuria and potential dehydration and electrolyte imbalances.

Fat Metabolism in Diabetes

When energy needs are not being supplied by glucose, fat stores are used in an attempt to meet energy needs. As fat stores are catabolized, the person with undiagnosed or poorly controlled diabetes begins losing large amounts of weight. In the absence of insulin, rapid fat catabolism begins and **ketones,** a by-product of fat metabolism, are produced and accumulate in the blood. The ketones are eliminated by the kidneys but at a rate that is slower than the rate at which they are produced. Ketone levels can be measured in the blood and urine to determine whether fat catabolism is occurring. Large levels of ketones indicate the shift from carbohydrate to fat metabolism and are a marker of uncontrolled diabetes. As ketones accumulate in the blood (ketosis), further metabolic alterations occur, including altered blood pH (acidosis) and dangerous fluid and electrolyte changes that can progress into a comatose state and eventual death if insulin need and metabolic alterations are not addressed.

Protein Metabolism in Diabetes

Protein catabolism also occurs in the absence of insulin. Skeletal muscle is broken down to provide amino acids that can be metabolized to glucose in an attempt to meet energy needs; muscle wasting results when this shift occurs. The presence of insulin and adequate cellular uptake of glucose inhibits this protein catabolism.

Additionally, insulin has many effects on the transcription of numerous genes. Deficiency of insulin decreases gene expression necessary for target tissues to respond normally to insulin such as the GLUT 4 class of glucose transporters (Watson & Pessin, 2001).

Medical Nutrition Therapy for Diabetes

No matter what type of diabetes a person has, MNT is the cornerstone of the lifestyle changes that are recommended. All of the organizations that have an interest in diabetes recommend that MNT teaching be undertaken by a registered dietitian familiar with the treatment plan for diabetes. The nurse's role is to assist the client as needed in understanding the components of the nutrition plan and reinforce the meal planning guide and education provided. In some settings, a dietitian may not be available and the nurse can refer the client to the nearest hospital or diabetes center for more education by certified diabetes educators (CDEs) who are usually registered nurses, dietitians, and, occasionally, pharmacists with expert training in diabetes management. Many hospitals have CDEs on staff to educate those with diabetes about their disease. Box 19-1 outlines general teaching guidelines for meal plan education. See Practice Pearl: Nursing Diet Intervention for a teaching hint when a CDE or dietitian is not available initially.

Carbohydrate Intake Recommendations

The ADA recommends that carbohydrate (CHO) along with monounsaturated fats comprise 60% to 70 % of the total kcalories in the diet (ADA, 2008). No specific CHO amount is given, though a minimum consumption of 130 gm of CHO/day is recommended because of the brain's need for glucose as a crucial energy source (Institute of Medicine [IOM], 2002). In the past, the term "ADA diet" was used

BOX 19-1	**Nursing Interventions for Meal Planning Education**

- Encourage the person with diabetes to make practical, step-by-step changes to achieve the desired goal (Vaughn, 2005).
- Encourage a visit to a registered dietitian for meal planning and formulation of the diet plan.
- Encourage both spouses (significant other, caregiver) to attend the teaching session. Peel (2005) found that men processed dietary management as a family matter, whereas women as an individual concern.
- Use the portion control method by using a lunch plate instead of a dinner plate in those seeking weight management.
- Utilize culturally competent informational sources, such as educational handouts and videos, with people who are similar to the client.
- Encourage a Mediterranean-type diet with high consumption of fiber-rich fruits, legumes, vegetables, increased intake of monounsaturated fats, lean meat, low-fat dairy products, and lowered intake of processed meat (Biesalski, 2004).
- Help the client to prioritize tasks and goals related to diabetes that are most important to the person.

MyNursingKit MyFoodAdvisor American Diabetes Association

PRACTICE ● PEARL

Nursing Diet Intervention

The nurse without immediate access to a registered dietitian or CDE is strongly encouraged to teach the client with diabetes about a "heart healthy meal plan" to decrease the likelihood of the person developing the number one complication of diabetes: coronary heart disease. A low-fat diet with carbohydrates from whole grains, fruits, and vegetables can be stressed until a referral can be made for medical nutrition therapy.

BOX 19-2	Calculating Carbohydrates

A client with diabetes is estimated to need 2,400 kcalories/day. What is the recommendation for carbohydrate intake?

1. **Multiply kcalorie requirement by recommended range of carbohydrate intake:**

   2,400 kcalories × 50% carbohydrate kcalories = 1,200 total carbohydrate kcalories

2. **Divide total carbohydrate kcalories by kcalories/gm carbohydrate:**

   1,200 total carbohydrate kcalories ÷ 4 kcalories/gm carbohydrate = 300 gm carbohydrate

3. **Divide carbohydrate intake over the day into the appropriate amount of meals and snacks:**

   300 gm of carbohydrate can be divided into three meals with 100 gm of carbohydrate each if no snacks are consumed.

   OR

   If two snacks with 30 gm of carbohydrate each are consumed, the amount of carbohydrate/meal is lowered to 80 gm each.

4. **For the client using the "carbohydrate choice," each set portion of food with 15 gm of carbohydrate is one choice. Divide total carbohydrate grams by 15 gm per carbohydrate choice:**

   300 gm total carbohydrate per day ÷ 15 gm carbohydrate per choice = 20 carbohydrate choices/day. These choices should be distributed over the day. The client must know correct portion that equals 15 gm of carbohydrate for each food.

along with a specific calorie level to denote a set distribution of CHO, fat, and protein in the diet that was believed to be ideal for all people with diabetes (ADA, 2008). Current recommendations are individualized based on the client's needs; the term "ADA diet" has become outdated.

A variety of CHO sources from fruits, vegetables, whole grains, legumes, and low-fat milk should be incorporated into the diet. Although the overall recommendation for fiber in the diabetic diet is the same as for the general population, it is recommended that persons with type 2 diabetes specifically choose whole-grain foods more frequently than the lower fiber counterpart (ADA, 2008). Whole-grain foods and fiber each have been associated with improved insulin sensitivity, which can improve glycemic control in those with some endogenous insulin production (ADA, 2008). As part of the nursing assessment, a review of fiber intake can be used to formulate interventions that target improved fiber intake. For example, the nurse can suggest brown rice versus white rice and whole wheat flakes or oatmeal versus cornflakes. Chapter 3 outlines fiber in detail. Sucrose-containing foods are allowed as a part of the overall CHO intake. However, these foods can add to excessive caloric intake and need to be moderated to avoid weight gain. Additionally, excessive substitution can displace more nutritious foods in the diet and compromise nutritional health.

There are several methods utilized when calculating CHO intake. One method involves estimating total energy needs and allotting half of the calories to CHO in the diet. Next, the CHOs are divided between three meals and any snacks. Using the fact that 1 gm of CHO has 4 kcalories, a specific recommendation can be made for total CHO per meal or snack. Box 19-2 outlines an example of these calculations. For individuals who might adhere better to the diet with a more streamlined approach, a swap system is used that allocates 15 gm of CHO for each food serving of CHO. Some refer to this 15 gm CHO portion as a "carbohydrate choice." Figure 19-1 ■ depicts an example of this using a food label. Individuals are taught general portions for each food group that equate to 15 gm of CHO and are given a recommendation for number of CHO choices to have per meal or snack. If snacks are desired or needed because of insulin require-

ments, then several servings of CHO would be subtracted from a meal to allow for one or more snacks such as midmorning, midafternoon, or bedtime. CHO counting can be taught to individuals who are willing and able to learn the number of grams of CHO found in commonly used foods. Client Education Checklist: Teaching Carbohydrate Counting outlines the method of CHO counting. The ADA has on-line tools to assist with CHO counting and general diet recommendations. The consistent CHO diet in which the meal plan has a set number of CHOs per meal is now highly recommended for type 1 diabetes, pregnant females, and anyone who is utilizing intensive insulin regimens (ADA, 2008).

An older method of determining CHO intake utilizes food exchanges and is a good method when weight management is also a goal. The dietitian can calculate the number of grams of total CHO for the day and then establish a dietary plan for the day based on work habits, lifestyle, food preferences, insulin scheduling, and other factors. CHOs may need to be covered by insulin before mealtimes if the person requires insulin management. More intense control of blood glucose levels and correlation to specific CHO intake is a

Plain Yogurt

Nutrition Facts

Serving Size 1 container (226g)

Amount Per Serving

Calories 110   Calories from Fat 0

	% Daily Value*
Total Fat 0g	0%
Saturated Fat 0g	0%
Trans Fat 0g	
Cholesterol Less than 5mg	1%
Sodium 160mg	7%
Total Carbohydrate (15g) ←	5%
Dietary Fiber 0g	0%
Sugars 10g	
Protein 13g	
Vitamin A	0%
Vitamin C	4%
Calcium	45%
Iron	0%

* Percent Daily Values are based on a 2,000 calorie diet. Your Daily Values may be higher or lower depending on your calorie needs:

> One carbohydrate choice

Fruit Yogurt

Nutrition Facts

Serving Size 1 container (227g)

Amount Per Serving

Calories 240   Calories from Fat 25

	% Daily Value*
Total Fat 3g	4%
Saturated Fat 1.5g	9%
Trans Fat 0g	
Cholesterol 15mg	5%
Sodium 140mg	6%
Total Carbohydrate (45g) ←	15%
Dietary Fiber Less then 1g	3%
Sugars 44g	
Protein 9g	
Vitamin A	2%
Vitamin C	4%
Calcium	35%
Iron	0%

* Percent Daily Values are based on a 2,000 calorie diet. Your Daily Values may be higher or lower depending on your calorie needs:

> Three carbohydrate choices

■ **FIGURE 19-1   Carbohydrate Counting on the Food Label.**

Source: Food and Drug Administration (FDA) (2004). How to understand and use the nutrition facts label. Retrieved November 9, 2009, from http://www.fda.gov/Food/LabelingNutrition/ConsumerInformation/ucm078889.htm

CLIENT EDUCATION CHECKLIST	Teaching Carbohydrate Counting
Process	**Rationale**
1. Teach the kinds of foods (fruits, vegetables, cakes, cookies, candy, milk, pasta, bread, etc.) that contain carbohydrate (CHO), including combination foods, such as whole milk, which also contains fat and protein.	Many people do not know what a CHO food is or may think it is simply a "starchy" food.
2. Explain the concept that one CHO serving or "carbohydrate choice" contains 15 grams of carbohydrate.	A serving of CHO is based on the knowledge that total CHO is central and a variety of sources can be consumed.
3. Give a list of common foods and how much one serving may be; e.g., one serving of rice is 1/3 cooked cup; this amount may be different than what is listed on the rice box label.	Food label servings are not necessarily the same size as one CHO choice.
4. Based on the client's insulin dosage and schedule, medication requirements, lifestyle and physical activity, and previous meal patterns, decide on the total amount of CHO (about 50%).	The average person will have about 30% fat and about 20% protein, which leaves about 50% for CHO.
5. Distribute the total amount of CHO between meals, considering dietary patterns, need or desire for snacks, and insulin regimen. For the average person of normal weight, this is about four to five CHO servings per meal.	Snacks are not mandated if the person is on injections before meals or is at low risk for hypoglycemia. Children and active people may require snacks to avoid hypoglycemia and meet nutritional needs.
6. Strive for the same number of CHO servings at each meal day to day. This pattern is termed the *consistent carbohydrate plan*.	Most Americans eat a lighter breakfast, heavier lunch, and then the heaviest meal at night.
7. If the person is motivated, teach the concepts of both grams and servings.	In advanced CHO counting, both concepts are necessary to adjust insulin dosages according to the number of grams being consumed.

Table 19-3	Advanced Carbohydrate Counting
Keep food intake records for several weeks, including the number of carbohydrate grams.	These records should include a "bite of this or that."
Keep blood glucose records, both premeal and 2-hour postmeal, on the same days that food intake is being recorded.	Premeal target is 90–130 mg/dL. Postmeal target is 180 mg/dL (ADA, 2009).
Make changes in food, medication, or physical activity based on glucose patterns.	This process is called pattern management; changes should be made in areas where target glucose levels are not being met. One target should be worked on at a time. For instance, start with fasting blood glucose and get that area into control first; move on to premeal targets and then postmeal.
Calculate insulin-to-carbohydrate ratios.	For meals that the postmeal glucose reading is regularly within range, divide the number of carbohydrate grams in the meal by the number of premeal insulin units administered. This ratio can be used to establish the amount of insulin needed at future meals.

CT? Why must blood glucose levels be well controlled before a client uses advanced carbohydrate counting?

concept covered in advanced CHO counting and is detailed in Table 19-3. A client needs a high level of knowledge and motivation to follow this type of diabetes management.

If **hypoglycemia** occurs, 15 to 20 gm of carbohydrate is the recommended intake (ADA, 2009). Glucose is the preferred treatment, but any food containing sufficient CHO can be used. Blood glucose levels should be rechecked in 15 minutes because it is possible that the correction from CHO intake is only temporary (ADA, 2009). An additional 15 to 20 gm of CHO and continued monitoring may be needed if blood glucose levels remain low.

Glycemic Index and Glycemic Load

The ability of a food to affect the glucose response following consumption varies. Glycemic index and glycemic load are methods used to quantify the body's response to specific foods. *Glycemic index* is a term that has gained a lot of attention over the last decade. In this system, CHOs are rated according to how rapidly the food is digested and metabolized to produce blood glucose during the 2 hours after consumption when compared to an equal amount of CHO from a slice of white bread or 50 gm of glucose. CHO sources that are rapidly digested into glucose and enter the blood quickly have a higher glycemic index than those that are slowly digested and cause gradual glucose increases. A food that has a high glycemic index, such as potato, would cause a higher postprandial (postmeal) glucose response than an equal amount of CHOs from a food such as brown rice, which has a lower glycemic index. Fiber-rich foods tend to have a lower glycemic index because they are digested slowly; glucose moves into the bloodstream at a slower rate than a low-fiber food (American Dietetic Association, 2008). Foods that have a high glycemic index would generate a larger demand for insulin than one with a lower glycemic response. Low glycemic index diets have been associated with a lower post-

prandial glucose and insulin response in clients with diabetes (Riccardi, Rivellese, & Giacco, 2008).

Extensive lists exist that rate the glycemic index of many foods. This information is not mandatory on food labels in North America, though it can be found on some food labels in Australia and the United Kingdom. It takes a highly motivated individual to learn the glycemic index ratings of common foods in the diet. Additionally, although available, the ratings are not universal for each food. It is important to realize that the glycemic index of a single food can vary with different varieties of the same item, preparation methods, or when combined with other foods. For example, a new red potato has a different glycemic index than a russet baked potato or fried potato. Additionally, a 50 gm CHO portion differs widely among foods and often is not similar to the amount commonly consumed. For example, 50 gm of CHO are contained in almost 5 cups of grated raw carrots. The overall glucose effect of a food eaten with a meal will not be the same as when the food is eaten by itself. Other food components such as fat and protein will influence the overall rate of digestion of the meal. All of these variabilities make the use of glycemic index less useful as a single tool for glucose management.

A related term that is less commonly used than glycemic index is *glycemic load*. Glycemic load represents both the quantity and the quality of CHOs and is calculated as the product of the glycemic index of a specific food and the amount of CHO eaten, rather than the set 50 gm CHO portion used in glycemic index calculations.

The ADA reports that monitoring glycemic load and glycemic index may offer a modest benefit over consideration of just total CHO intake (ADA, 2008). This effect is especially seen in those who previously were consuming what amounted to a high glycemic index diet and switched to low glycemic food choices. In observational studies, following a low glycemic index or glycemic load diet is associated with a

MyNursingKit Glycemic Index

reduced risk of type 2 diabetes, but the risk reduction is comparable to that seen with consuming whole grains and fiber (Barclay et al., 2008). When asked for advice about this aspect of CHO intake, the nurse can highlight the benefits of fiber on glycemic control and urge intake of a variety of fiber-rich CHOs, such as whole grains, fruits and vegetables with edible skins or seeds, and legumes. A fiber-rich diet generally contains less energy than a low-fiber diet, an added benefit to those pursuing weight management (American Dietetic Association, 2008). The nurse can educate the client about sources of fiber and how to compare fiber content of products by referring to the nutrition facts panel. Concentrating on just the isolated glycemic index or glycemic load values is not recommended because total CHO, calories, and fiber are important considerations (Riccardi et al., 2008). The nurse should refer a client with diabetes who is interested in pursuing the more complicated glycemic index or glycemic load approach to managing CHO intake to a dietitian or CDE.

Are Nonnutritive Sweeteners Better Than Sugar?

Nonnutritive sweeteners include saccharin, aspartame, sucralose, and acesulfame potassium. The Food and Drug Administration (FDA) has established an acceptable daily intake for any government-approved nonnutritive sweetener that is based on available information regarding health risks associated with chronic consumption. The ADA position regarding these alternatives to sugar states that they are safe for people with diabetes when consumed within recommended intake, but that evidence is lacking regarding any associated long-term improvements on glycemic control or weight management (ADA, 2008).

Sugar alcohols, such as sorbitol and xylitol, are also used as sweeter alternatives to sugar by manufacturers seeking to provide the consumer with a lower CHO version of some sweetened foods. Sugar alcohols provide less calories and a lower glycemic response than sugar because they are not fully absorbed by the intestine (Grabitske & Slavin, 2008). The nurse should urge clients wishing to use these products to carefully read the nutrition facts panel of the label to review the calorie content and total CHO contained in the product. Some individuals mistakenly believe that a lower CHO alternative translates to also include a lower caloric content than the original version of the food, an assumption that is often not true. The client with weight management goals needs to be mindful of the resulting calorie content of any of these foods. Additionally, the client should be advised that sugar alcohols act as laxatives when consumed in large amounts. The Evidence-Based Practice Box: Do clients with diabetes who regularly consume foods with artificial sweeteners have lower energy consumption? discusses nonnutritive sweetener use with diabetes. Chapter 2 discusses these sugar alternatives in more detail.

Fat Intake Recommendations

Dietary fat is a necessary component of the diet for the maintenance of good health. A primary goal for individuals with diabetes is to limit intake of saturated and trans fats to decrease the risk of cardiovascular disease. Diabetes is considered the equivalent of having existing cardiovascular disease when determining cardiac risk. For this reason, the goal for low-density lipoprotein (LDL) cholesterol has been lowered to 100 mg/dL with existing risk such as diabetes and even lower to 70 mg/dL for higher risk clients (Grundy et al., 2004).

The ADA (2008) recommends that monounsaturated fats along with CHOs comprise up to 70% of total energy intake. Cholesterol intake should be less than 200 to 300 mg daily. Furthermore, saturated fats should be limited to no more than 7% to 10% of the total energy intake. Reduction in saturated fat intake is stressed as a method of concurrently reducing calorie intake in those seeking to lose weight (ADA, 2008). If weight reduction is not a goal, saturated fats can be substituted with monounsaturated fats or CHO depending on the client's individual needs. The stricter levels of cholesterol and saturated fat recommendations are for those with elevated LDL cholesterol. Trans fats should be limited to a minimal level. Overall, the recommendations for fat intake mirror those made to reduce risk of cardiovascular disease as outlined in Chapter 18.

Protein Intake Recommendations

The ADA (2008) recommends a protein intake of 15% to 20% of daily caloric intake or at least 0.8 gm/kg/day, the amount recommended for healthy adults. During prolonged hyperglycemia, protein catabolism can contribute to a need for increased protein intake, but consumption of more than 20% of total energy intake as protein is not recommended because of risk of kidney damage (ADA, 2008). If the person has normal renal function, there is insufficient evidence to recommend decreased protein intake. Protein intake is not shown to be an effective treatment of hypoglycemia (ADA, 2008).

Vitamin Supplementation

Routine vitamin supplementation is not recommended for persons with diabetes unless there is an underlying dietary insufficiency or the person is an older adult or pregnant female (ADA, 2008). Chromium supplementation has been studied in diabetes because of a potential role in improving glycemic control, but no benefit has been clearly established in those who are not chromium deficient (ADA, 2008). Large clinical trials investigating dietary supplementation with other vitamin and mineral supplementation have not shown any improvement in diabetes management (ADA, 2008).

Alcohol Intake

For those who drink alcohol, the ADA (2008) recommends that alcohol content be limited to one standard drink for

EVIDENCE-BASED PRACTICE RESEARCH BOX

Do clients with diabetes who regularly consume foods with artificial sweeteners have lower energy consumption?

Clinical Problem: People with diabetes often select foods, especially beverages, that are artificially sweetened. Does this lead to lower total energy consumption, or do they compensate by consuming the "saved" calories in other food choices?

Research Findings: The increased consumption of sugar-sweetened foods and beverages has been linked to increased obesity in children and adults (Bray, Nielsen, & Popkin, 2004; Dubois, Farmer, Girard, & Peterson, 2007; Malik, Schulze, & Hu, 2006; Montonen, Jarvinen, Knekt, Heliovaara, & Reunanen, 2007; Schulze et al., 2004). Weight loss is often a goal, especially in type 2 diabetics, so it logically follows that substitution of artificial sweeteners would lead to decreased calorie consumption and, therefore, a decrease in weight.

Artificial sweeteners have been studied from the perspective of satiety. Because they do not have an energy value, researchers have speculated that individuals who consume them may seek energy from other food sources (Bellisle & Drewnowski, 2007; Cullen et al., 2004; Van Dam & Seidell, 2007; Van Wymelbeke, Beridot-Therond, de La Gueronniere, & Fantino, 2004). The findings consistently demonstrated that individuals, including those with diabetes, who consumed artificially sweetened foods and beverages did not increase consumption of calories. Monsivais, Perrigue, and Drewnowski (2007) also found that there was no difference in calorie consumption between individuals given beverages with artificial sweeteners and sucrose.

The intensity of sweeteners and food consumption was also studied (Appleton & Blundell, 2007; Appleton, Rogers, & Blundell, 2004; Van Wymelbeke et al., 2004). Researchers found that the experience with sweetness was the best predictor of dietary intake; individuals who did not typically use artificial sweeteners had an increase in appetite after eating a food or beverage with intense sweetness.

Binkley and Golub (2007) studied the grocery purchasing patterns of consumers who regularly purchased either diet or regular soft drinks. They found that purchasers of diet beverages made better nutritional choices in most categories, especially with respect to calorie content. They concluded that use of diet soft drinks does not lead to increased consumption of high calorie foods.

Nursing Implications: Artificial sweeteners do not cause replacement of calories with food from other sources. Individuals with diabetes need to be counseled as appropriate about weight loss; products with artificial sweeteners may be part of that plan.

CRITICAL THINKING QUESTION:

1. A middle-age adult with a body mass index (BMI) of 29 was recently diagnosed with type 2 diabetes. He does not like the taste of diet soda and wants to know if he has to give up regular soda.

women and two drinks for men per day. A standard drink is defined as 12 ounces of beer, 5 ounces of wine, or 1.5 ounces of distilled spirits. Alcohol should be consumed with food because of its potential hypoglycemic effect. The hypoglycemic effect is due to the inhibition of gluconeogenesis by alcohol. Further, alcohol intake can inhibit awareness of hypoglycemia (ADA, 2008). Excessive consumption of alcohol is best avoided because alcohol contributes empty calories to the dietary intake and abuse of alcohol can lead to alcohol-related problems, as outlined in Chapter 7. The nurse should remind the client of the calorie content of various drinks, which is outlined in Chapter 7, because this information needs to be incorporated into the diet plan. Nutritious foods should not be eliminated from the diet in order to accommodate the energy content of the alcohol (ADA, 2008).

Do Recommendations Differ for Children, Adults, or Other Groups?

Dietary recommendations that are made for treatment of diabetes are meant for all population groups. However, additional dietary considerations may need to be made for children and adolescents to meet the nutritional needs for growth and development. Other populations deserve attention because of associated increase risk of diabetes among specific cultural groups.

Children and Adolescents: Type 1 Diabetes

The meal plan for children and adolescents is usually developed by a registered dietitian, ideally one who is a CDE. The diet plan must ensure proper nutrition for growth and development without contributing to the risk of obesity. The nursing responsibility is to reinforce the nutrition plan, answer questions, and determine that blood glucose levels are being maintained within the goals outlined by the primary health care provider. The school nurse is the primary provider of diabetes care in the school setting and plays an important role in educating other staff members regarding handling symptoms in the classroom (ADA, 2009). On-line resources are available for the school nurse to assist in the development of a health plan for school use.

Children and adolescents with type 1 diabetes are prone to frequent "highs and lows" in the blood glucose. To prevent lows, the child may eat more frequent snacks than needed because of the fear of the hypoglycemia. The fluctuations in the blood glucose are a complicated phenomenon because of the cardiac and circulatory differences between adults and children and the body's difficulty in adjusting cardiac output to

MyNursingKit American Diabetes Association: For Schools

PRACTICE PEARL

Hypoglycemia in Children
In young children with diabetes, watch for behavior changes to detect signs of hypoglycemia. For example, a child who has been extremely active and suddenly sits down and becomes drowsy is most likely experiencing hypoglycemia.

meet circulatory needs in the younger person (Corigliano, Iazzetta, Corigliano, & Strollo, 2006). When a child participates in sports and other physical activity, a plan to prevent or treat hypoglycemia is needed. Snacks and sport beverages can be used to provide needed CHO, though some children require more than the usual 15 gm CHO portion to treat hypoglycemia if it occurs (Corigliano et al., 2006). In the event of hyperglycemia before exercise, snacks could be reduced in the future but CHO may be needed during the activity to prevent hypoglycemia. Read Practice Pearl: Hypoglycemia in Children to learn more about hypoglycemia in children.

There are numerous issues to consider when educating parents and children with type 1 diabetes about nutrition. Developmental concerns are presented in Table 19-4. For all ages of children and adolescents, the nurse needs to emphasize to parents their responsibility for the coordination of food intake with insulin injections, physical activity, and blood glucose monitoring. The use of an insulin pump can assist the motivated older child and the teenager in managing diabetes without the obvious use of injections. The subcutaneous needle is placed in the subcutaneous tissue of the abdomen and the pump is programmed to continuously deliver a basal dose of short-acting insulin and to deliver bolus doses of insulin just before meals. Glucose monitoring using finger pricking or alternative sites such as the lower arm must still be done, but a continuous blood glucose monitoring device has been introduced to the market that would make the monitoring process more invisible. Adherence to the meal pattern is crucial because hypoglycemia is more likely when receiving a steady continuous dose of insulin without adequate food intake. Some children or teens will find that relief from administering injections is a motivator for diet adherence.

Children and Adolescents: Type 2 Diabetes

Type 2 diabetes in young people as in adults is associated with obesity and insulin resistance. Nutrition interventions should emphasize healthy eating within allowances for growth, development and increased physical activity. Children with type 2 diabetes can be managed on oral agents such as metformin (Glucophage) rather than insulin. The nurse can play an important role in emphasizing the importance of a healthy lifestyle in which the entire family can participate. Modification of the entire family's lifestyle includes both dietary and physical activity changes. The

Table 19-4 Nutritional Developmental Challenges in Children and Adolescents with Type 1 Diabetes Mellitus

Age Range	Nutritional Challenge	Nursing Intervention
Birth to age 3	1. Need for scheduled feedings/meals 2. Maintenance of weight and height trajectory 3. Prevent hyperglycemia and hypoglycemia	• Establish feeding/meal schedule. • For infants, establish nighttime feeding schedule. • Plot weight and height on growth grids at each health visit. • Work with a dietitian for nutrient needs to maintain growth trajectory. • Check blood glucose at established times. • Maintain nutrient balance as established.
Ages 3 to 5	1. Food jags and erratic appetites	• Allow food choices within confines of nutrient needs and dietary balance. • Check blood glucose at established times. • Work with daycare/preschool staff to maintain diet. • Plot weight and height on growth grids.
Ages 6 to 10	1. Influence of peer groups	• Teach child beginning self-management of diet. • Plan for dietary alterations based on participation in sports or strenuous activities. • Allow the child to participate in meal and snack preparation. • Review diet plan with school teachers and staff. • Check blood glucose at scheduled times and as needed.
Adolescence	1. Erratic eating schedules 2. Peer influence	• Assume responsibility for self-monitoring of blood glucose. • Develop ability to plan nutrient intake that accounts for variations in activity and schedules. • Affirm need for social interactions that involve food. • Continue education about healthy food choices.

school nurse can be integral in the team approach to improving the school food environment to include a similar focus on healthy eating and physical activity changes, which is an important step to preventing type 2 diabetes in children and adolescents. Some overweight and obese adolescents resort to unhealthy dieting practices, such as skipping meals or overly restrictive intake, in an attempt to lose weight. Such practices are associated with poor glycemic control (Laurence et al., 2008). The nurse can be instrumental in reinforcing the importance of healthy nutrition habits and weight management strategies.

Mature-onset diabetes of the young (MODY) is a rare form of diabetes caused by a single gene defect that is autosomal dominant (CDC, 2008). The result is decreased insulin secretion that requires diet, exercise, and insulin or oral hypoglycemic agent interventions. Nutrition planning should focus on allowances for growth, health promotion, and restriction of fat intake to prevent cardiac disease as is recommended for type 2 diabetes.

Polycystic ovary syndrome (PCOS) is an endocrine disorder affecting females of reproductive age, including adolescent girls. Individuals with PCOS are typically obese, have insulin resistance, and a high risk of developing type 2 and gestational diabetes. In a review of dietary studies on PCOS, it was noted that weight loss of 5% was associated with improved menstrual cycles and lowered circulating insulin levels (Marsh & Brand-Miller, 2005). Diet studies done in this population are mainly short term, but a diet that is low saturated fat, high-fiber, and low glycemic index CHO has shown weight loss associated with decreased insulin resistance (Colette et al., 2003; Gerhard et al., 2004).

Cultural Considerations

Certain population groups are more susceptible to the development of type 2 diabetes, in part because of an increased prevalence of overweight and obesity (ADA, 2008; Maskarinec et al., 2009). African American, Hispanic, American Indian, and some Asian/Pacific Islander adults have a higher rate of type 2 diabetes compared with other populations. Gestational diabetes and type 2 diabetes in children and adolescents are also increased in these groups (CDC, 2008). Education should focus on the same guidelines for prevention of type 2 diabetes provided to any population but with a specific discussion that underscores the link between the disease and the individual's cultural group.

When diabetes has been diagnosed, the goal of nutritional planning is the same for all populations. The nurse wants to enable the client to normalize blood glucose, attain blood pressure control, optimize lipid levels, attain a desirable weight, and consume an adequate level of nutrients. However, there are differences between groups, including genetic differences, lifestyle practices, and nutritional practices, that all play a role in whether people are able to achieve desired goals.

These differences also influence the educational strategies that the nurse should use to obtain the most effective results.

African Americans

Anderson-Loftin et al. (2005) tested a culturally competent dietary education intervention in a group of rural Southern low-income African Americans. Relevant cultural aspects for this successful group included:

- Importance of food in the African American population. Meals are frequently social events and food preferences are identified with tradition.
- Learning is enhanced when storytelling and other experiential methods are used, especially in a low literacy population.
- Using educators who speak the dialect and idiom of the African American person shows respect for the person and the advice is held in high regard.
- Focusing on only one major dietary intervention (low-fat diet) and using a group family-style environment to prepare and serve the food enhanced the cultural relevance of the teaching technique.

Hispanics

Research has shown that Hispanics face a number of challenges based on their cultural beliefs and traditional practices. The nurse should assess the client for individual traditional practices and beliefs regarding health and diabetes and provide appropriate education to clarify any misinformation. On-line resources are available in Spanish that address both diabetes prevention and treatment. Some of these cultural beliefs about health and diabetes that can also affect dietary practices include the following (Hatcher & Whittemore, 2007; Lipton, Losey, Giachello, Mendez, & Girotti, 1998; Weiler & Crist, 2009):

- Unwillingness to place their own medical needs above the needs of family members
- A distrust of insulin therapy
- A preference for more traditional practices
- A fatalistic acceptance about the course of the disease
- Reliance on informal social networks to meet disease management needs

Asians and Pacific Islanders

Immigrant groups may be at increased risk for type 2 diabetes because of the adoption of Western practices and heightened genetic risks. Abate and Chandalia (2007) have found a gene variant in migrant Asian Indians that causes high insulin resistance and leads to excessive prevalence of diabetes in this population. Cardiovascular disease (CVD) risk has been found to be heightened in many Asian groups at lower body mass indices (BMIs) than in the Caucasian population. A low polyunsaturated fatty acid (PUFA) level has also been associated with CVD risk, leading to the recommendation to

MyNursingKit Spanish Language Diabetes Education

target prevention by dietary practices to increase PUFA intake by eating more fatty fish (Lovegrove, 2007).

There are wide variations in Asians and Pacific Islanders as to dietary practices. People from India are frequently vegetarian, whereas fish is a commonly consumed food in Southeast Asia, such as Vietnam. Dairy products are not commonly used by the Chinese, whereas milk products are extensively used by those from Thailand. The nurse can ask questions to elicit important information regarding dietary practices, meal patterns, and concerns. The nursing assessment should include an evaluation of dietary supplement intake, including herbs. Several plant-based dietary supplements are used in parts of Asia to treat high blood glucose as part of traditional medicine. Cultural Considerations Box: Plant Remedies and Diabetes Management outlines these examples.

Weight Management

The ADA (2009) recommends a modest weight loss of 5% to 10% to decrease the risk of type 2 diabetes. Additionally, weight loss is recommended for the overweight individual with diabetes to achieve a reduction in blood pressure, blood

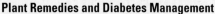

Cultural Considerations

Plant Remedies and Diabetes Management

Several plant-based remedies are used to treat increased blood glucose in the traditional medicines of several Asian countries. Bitter melon, Asian ginseng, and gymnema are examples. The use of bitter melon in dietary supplement form lacks long-term research to determine its efficacy and safety. Consumption of the food form is believed to be safe for most people, but it is unclear whether it affects blood glucose significantly. Caution is given to pregnant females because of a risk of miscarriage associated with bitter melon. Asian ginseng has not been reported to improve blood glucose control over the course of 2 months any better than a placebo. Caution is given for this herb because of a number of drug interactions and its effect on prolonging blood clotting by affecting platelet function. Gymnema lacks significant research, but reports exist of hypoglycemia occurring with its use. The nurse should explore use of dietary supplements when conducting a nursing assessment and be mindful of any known side effects or drug interactions associated with use. Chapter 25 outlines dietary supplement use in detail.

Sources: Geil & Shane-McWhorter, 2008; Intellihealth, 2008; National Center for Complementary and Alternative Medicine, 2008.

glucose, lipid levels, sleep apnea risks, and the overall complications of diabetes.

The nurse can make the same general recommendations for weight loss strategies that are offered to other overweight adults, such as increasing physical activity, decreasing baseline calorie intake by 500 kcalories/day, and brainstorming ways to avoid past barriers to successful weight management. Chapter 17 outlines nutrition intervention for weight loss in more detail. The use of low CHO diets by people with diabetes is discouraged because of the effect of these diets on increasing LDL cholesterol in a population already at risk for CVD (ADA, 2008). The use of bariatric surgery to treat those with type 2 diabetes and morbid obesity is reported to significantly improve health outcome and diminish disease-associated risks when other approaches to weight loss have failed (Cummings, Apovian, & Khaodhiar, 2008).

Hypertension in Diabetes

The diagnosis of hypertension increases the risk of CVD in people with diabetes. Hypertension worsens the existing potential for damage to the microvascular system already associated with hyperglycemia (McGill, 2009). It is crucial that the nurse stress the importance of blood pressure control to lessen risk of complications such as kidney disease, limb amputation, and vision loss that are associated with the combination of diabetes and hypertension. Chapter 18 outlines the dietary intervention for hypertension, which includes weight management, limited sodium intake, and increased intake of high-potassium and high-calcium foods.

Cardiovascular Risk Factors

Medical nutrition therapy in people with diabetes has been shown to prevent or delay onset of cardiac complications, which account for a large percentage of the mortality involving diabetes. Diets that have been found to be helpful are discussed in Hot Topic Box: Eating to Reduce Cardiovascular Risk Factors in Diabetes along with weight loss and physical activity.

Diabetic Nephropathy

Diabetes is the leading cause of kidney failure (CDC, 2008). The ADA (2008) recommends the reduction of protein intake to no more than 0.8 to 1 gm/kg/day in individuals with diabetes and earlier stages of nephropathy (kidney damage due to diabetes) and to 0.8 gm/kg/day in later stages. Ikizler (2007) found that persons with type 2 diabetes who have chronic renal disease have significantly more skeletal muscle

Eating to Reduce Cardiovascular Risk Factors in Diabetes

The number one cause of death in diabetes is cardiovascular disease (CVD). Although medications such as statins, antihypertensives (e.g., beta blockers, calcium channel blockers, and alpha receptor blockers), and low-dose aspirin are prescribed to reduce the risk, nutrition has also been shown to help reduce or at least slow the development of CVD risk. Various diets have been studied to determine their effect on CVD risk factors. However, it is difficult to determine the most effective diet because dietary recall is limited and long-term prospective randomized control trials are difficult and expensive to implement. Also, it is confusing to the public when various diets are recommended for the same objective. Studies have focused on the following:

- Mediterranean-style diet: This diet consists of increasing fresh fruits, vegetables, whole grains, unrefined cereals, olive oil, moderate intake of wine with meals, and moderately high fish intake. Harriss et al. (2007) examined eating patterns of greater than 40,000 Australian men and women over 10 years. Those who ate the most Mediterranean type of foods enjoyed a 30% risk reduction in mortality, including a subset of people with diabetes who had a decreased risk for CVD.

- Dietary Approaches to Stop Hypertension (DASH) diet: This diet emphasizes nine servings of fruits and vegetables per day, whole grains, and low-fat dairy products. DASH study participants lowered their risk of CVD and stroke by following this diet (Law, 2008).

- Low-fat diet. This diet consists of a reduction in caloric intake with an increase in physical activity. Total fat intake should be no more than 30% of total intake and less than 200 to 300 mg of cholesterol/day. Saturated fat intake should be no more than 7% to 10% of total caloric intake, whereas trans fat, found predominantly in baked commercial foods such as cakes, donuts, and cookies, should be minimized. Moderate weight loss (5–10%) will contribute to reduction of blood pressure in most people, especially when combined with the effects of physical activity such as walking (ADA, 2009).

Diet counseling is recommended for everyone with diabetes. Nurses are in a unique position to offer customized advice as part of the team approach to reducing risk of CVD in this population.

protein breakdown compared with matched subjects without diabetes. Type 2 subjects also lose more lean body mass than those without diabetes. In type 1 diabetes, it has been known for many years that without insulin, the body loses large amounts of muscle tissue. However, there is no indication that increasing dietary protein is helpful (Ikizler, 2007).

Diabetic Neuropathies

Up to 70% of people with diabetes experience nerve damage as a result of the disease (CDC, 2008). One of the many complications of diabetes (both type 1 and type 2) is diabetic neuropathy, which is nerve dysfunction due to the hyperglycemia of diabetes. One area that can be affected is the autonomic nervous system of the gastrointestinal (GI) tract. The GI disturbances include gastroparesis, constipation, diarrhea, fecal incontinence, bloating, decreased transit time of food through the stomach, heartburn, nausea, and vomiting. Gastroparesis is associated with hyperglycemia and severe erratic glucose control. In addition to any pharmacological treatment and cessation of smoking, small, frequent meals are indicated with low-fiber, low-alcohol, and low-fat content. Smoking, alcohol, and fat delay gastric emptying (Shakil, Church, & Rao, 2008). High-fiber intake is avoided because of the risk of gastric bezoar formation. Bezoars are undigested food masses that occur when food remains in the intestine too long. Bezoars can result in intestinal blockage if untreated. In some individuals, the use of liquids and pureed foods to replace solid foods is indicated; liquids empty more quickly from the stomach than do solid foods (Patrick & Epstein, 2008).

Peripheral neuropathy leads to loss of sensation and a burning or tingling pain in the hands and feet. Alpha-lipoic acid, a dietary supplement, has been investigated as an adjunct treatment for peripheral neuropathy. Both parenteral and enteral forms of the supplement have demonstrated improvement in symptoms in short-term studies without any evident safety concerns (Foster, 2007; Singh & Jialal, 2008). Long-term studies are needed before this treatment can universally be recommended for diabetic peripheral neuropathy.

Nutrition in Type 2 Diabetes

CASE STUDY

Luis, age 42 years, was diagnosed with type 2 diabetes mellitus 6 months ago. He and his wife of 20 years had two sessions with a certified diabetes educator and dietitian at the time of his diagnosis. They developed a plan for managing his diabetes with oral medication, dietary changes, and activity. Goals were set for slow but steady weight loss of 1 pound a week and engagement in one daily physical activity. He was also taught how to take and record daily blood glucose readings. He made one follow-up clinic visit 1 month after diagnosis. He has come to the clinic now because he is feeling tired a lot of the time and thinks his blood glucose is high. He says he takes his medication as prescribed.

Applying the Nursing Process

ASSESSMENT

Height: 5 feet 8 inches Weight: 224 pounds (weight 5 months ago was 222 lb) BMI: 34

Blood glucose (by finger stick): 188 mg/dL at 0930

BP 164/88 P 82 R 16

Blood glucose record is incomplete because he quit taking readings when supplies ran out; early readings had ranged from 128 to 182 mg/dL

Usually eats three meals a day plus snacks; does not pay much attention to the diabetic meal plan because "it doesn't work for me"

DIAGNOSES

Nutrition imbalanced: more than body requirements related to excess calorie consumption evidenced by BMI of 34

Deficient knowledge of diabetes self-management related to lack of follow-up with diabetic team evidenced by elevated blood glucose, increased weight, and self-reported lack of dietary adherence

EXPECTED OUTCOMES

Blood glucose readings are consistently less than 130 mg/dL

Weight loss of 1 pound per week

Development of a diabetic diet plan that incorporates food preferences and calorie reduction

INTERVENTIONS

24-hour food recall

Begin a food and activity diary

Discuss access to resources for purchase of blood glucose testing supplies

Teach importance of regularly taking and recording blood glucose

Appointment with a certified diabetic educator and dietitian to plan acceptable dietary management

Reinforce importance of taking medication and review side effects

Stress importance of regular follow-up clinic visits

EVALUATION

One month later, Luis is feeling more confident in his ability to manage his diabetes after meeting with the diabetic educator and the dietitian. He now understands the complications that can develop if the blood glucose is not brought under control. Although he admits that he "slips" once in awhile with the diet, he is proud of having lost 5 pounds. He has gotten the whole family involved in planning meals and snacks. His blood glucose the past month has ranged from 126 to 154 mg/dL and he believes that with more attention to his diet, glycemic control will improve even more. Figure 19-2 ■ outlines the nursing process for this case.

Critical Thinking in the Nursing Process

1. How should the nurse respond when the client with diabetes says that it is hard to have a dessert on a diabetic diet?

Nutrition in Type 2 Diabetes (continued)

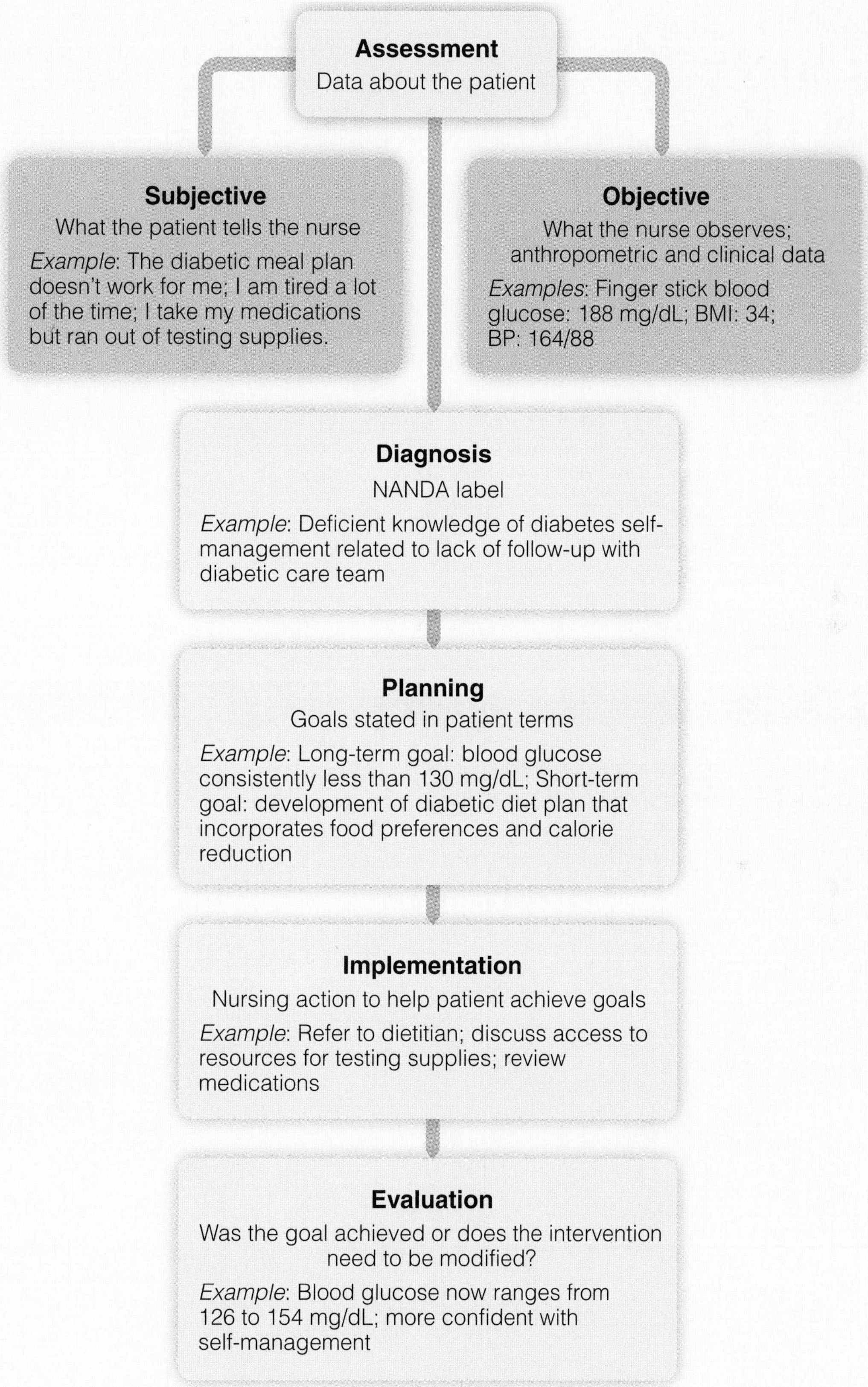

NURSING CARE PLAN

Assessment
Data about the patient

Subjective
What the patient tells the nurse
Example: The diabetic meal plan doesn't work for me; I am tired a lot of the time; I take my medications but ran out of testing supplies.

Objective
What the nurse observes; anthropometric and clinical data
Examples: Finger stick blood glucose: 188 mg/dL; BMI: 34; BP: 164/88

Diagnosis
NANDA label
Example: Deficient knowledge of diabetes self-management related to lack of follow-up with diabetic care team

Planning
Goals stated in patient terms
Example: Long-term goal: blood glucose consistently less than 130 mg/dL; Short-term goal: development of diabetic diet plan that incorporates food preferences and calorie reduction

Implementation
Nursing action to help patient achieve goals
Example: Refer to dietitian; discuss access to resources for testing supplies; review medications

Evaluation
Was the goal achieved or does the intervention need to be modified?
Example: Blood glucose now ranges from 126 to 154 mg/dL; more confident with self-management

FIGURE 19-2   Nursing Care Plan Process: Nutrition in Type 2 Diabetes.

CHAPTER SUMMARY

- People with type 1 diabetes should aim for strict glycemic control. A consistent carbohydrate diet and matching premeal insulin to the number of calories ingested will most effectively assist toward euglycemia.

- People with type 2 diabetes may also use the same approach as for type 1 diabetes but need to focus on losing weight if needed, physical activity, and eating a diet consistent with guidelines aimed at reducing risk of heart disease.

- Children with type 1 diabetes should have strict glycemic control, making certain that nutritional growth needs are met. Snacks can be incorporated into the daily meal pattern to prevent hypoglycemia.

- Women with gestational diabetes need calories for growth of the fetus and tight glycemic control.

- Ethnic minorities are at highest risk for type 2 diabetes and education should be aimed at specific cultural needs.

EXPLORE PEARSON **mynursingkit**™

MyNursingKit is your one stop for online chapter review materials and resources. Prepare for success with additional NCLEX®-style practice questions, interactive assignments and activities, web links, animations and videos, and more!

Register your access code from the front of your book at
www.mynursingkit.com.

NCLEX® QUESTIONS

1. The nurse knows that the client with type 2 diabetes mellitus understands teaching about carbohydrates in the diet when the client states:
   1. "I need to have about half of my daily calories come from carbohydrates."
   2. "I need to be on a low-carbohydrate diet for the rest of my life."
   3. "I should substitute artificial sweeteners for natural sugar when baking."
   4. "I need to learn carbohydrate counting if I want to be successful with my diet."

2. As part of a teaching plan for an adolescent with type 1 diabetes mellitus, the nurse should stress that carbohydrate needs increase during which of the following situations?
   1. An upper respiratory infection
   2. Strenuous physical activity
   3. Studying for final exams
   4. Eating a large holiday meal

3. A middle-age client with a BMI of 31 was recently diagnosed with type 2 diabetes mellitus. The nurse recognizes that dietary teaching has been effective when the client states:
   1. "If I lose 25 pounds, my diabetes will not be as serious."

   2. "If I lose 25 pounds, then I will not have to take any more medication to control my diabetes."
   3. "I can eat everything I like as long as I eat smaller portions."
   4. "I need to follow the meal plan for diabetes from the dietitian."

4. Which of the following dietary instructions about fat intake are appropriate when teaching an adult client with type 2 diabetes mellitus?
   1. "Eat less than 10 grams of fat per meal."
   2. "Eat foods with as little trans fat as possible."
   3. "You may eat any kind of fish several times per week."
   4. "Eggs should only be eaten twice per week."

5. The nurse is preparing to teach the mother of a school-age child who was recently diagnosed with type 2 diabetes mellitus. The focus of the initial teaching session should be:
   1. Weight control
   2. Explaining why the child developed type 2 diabetes mellitus
   3. Developing a culturally acceptable meal plan
   4. Assessing the mother's understanding of type 2 diabetes mellitus

REFERENCES

Abate, N., & Chandalia, M. (2007). Ethnicity, type 2 diabetes, and migrant Asian Indians. *Indian Journal of Medical Research, 125*(3), 251–258.

American Diabetes Association (ADA). (2008). Nutrition recommendations and interventions for diabetes: A position statement of the American Diabetes Association. *Diabetes Care, 31*(Suppl. 1), S61–S78.

American Diabetes Association (ADA). (2009). Standards of medical care in diabetes—2009. *Diabetes Care, 32*, S13–S61.

American Dietetic Association. (2008). Position of the American Dietetic Association: Health implications of dietary fiber. *Journal of the American Dietetic Association, 108*, 1716–1731.

Anderson- Loftin, W., Barnett, S., Bunn, P., Sullivan, P., Hussey, J., & Tavakoli, A. (2005). Soul food light: Culturally competent diabetes education. *The Diabetes Educator, 31*(4), 555–563.

Appleton, K. M., & Blundell, J. E. (2007). Habitual high and low consumers of artificially-sweetened beverages: Effects of sweet taste and energy on short-term appetite. *Physiological Behavior, 92*(3), 479–486.

Appleton, K. M., Rogers, P. J., & Blundell, J. E. (2004). Effects of a sweet and a non-sweet lunch on short-term appetite: Differences in female high and low consumers of sweet/low-energy beverages. *Journal of Human Nutrition and Dietetics, 17*(5), 425–434.

Barclay, A. W., Petocz, P., McMillan-Price, J., Flood, V. M., Prvan, T., Mitchell, P., et al. (2008). Glycemic index, glycemic load, and chronic disease risk—A meta-analysis of observational studies. *American Journal of Clinical Nutrition, 87*, 627–637.

Bellisle, F., & Drewnowski, A. (2007). Intense sweeteners, energy intake and the control of body weight. *European Journal of Clinical Nutrition, 61*(6), 691–700.

Biesalski, H. K. (2004). Diabetes preventive components in the Mediterranean diet. *European Journal of Nutrition, 43*(Suppl. 1), 1/26–1/30.

Binkley, J., & Golub, A. (2007). Comparison of grocery purchase patterns of diet soda buyers to those of regular soda buyers. *Appetite, 49*(3), 561–571.

Bray, G. A., Nielsen, S. J., & Popkin, B. M. (2004). Consumption of high-fructose corn syrup in beverages may play a role in the epidemic of obesity. *American Journal of Clinical Nutrition, 79*(4), 537–543.

Brunner, E. J., Mosdol, A., Witte, D. R., Martikainen, P., Stafford, M., Shipley, M. J., et al. (2008). Dietary patterns and 15-year risks of major coronary events, diabetes, and mortality. *American Journal of Clinical Nutrition, 87*, 1414–1421.

Cali, A. M., & Caprio, S. (2008). Prediabetes and type 2 diabetes in youth: An emerging epidemic disease? *Current Opinion in Endocrinology, Diabetes & Obesity, 15*, 123–127.

Canadian Diabetes Association. (2008). *Clinical practice guidelines.* Retrieved April 13, 2009, from http://www.diabetes.ca/files/cpg2008/cpg-2008.pdf

Centers for Disease Control and Prevention (CDC). (2008). *National diabetes fact sheet.* Retrieved April 13, 2009, from http://www.cdc.gov/diabetes/pubs/pdf/ndfs_2007.pdf

Colette, C., Percheron, C., Pares-Herbute, N., Michel, F., Pham, T. C., Brillant, L., et al. (2003). Exchanging carbohydrate for monounsaturated fats in energy-restricted diets: effects on metabolic profile and other cardiovascular risk factors. *International Journal on Obesity, 27*, 648–656.

Corigliano, G., Iazzetta, N., Corigliano, M., & Strollo, F. (2006). Blood glucose changes in diabetic children. *Acta Bio-medica, 77*(Suppl. 1), 26–33.

Cullen, M., Nolan, J., Cullen, M., Moloney, M., Kearney, J., Lambe, J., et al. (2004). Effect of high levels of intense sweetener intake in insulin dependent diabetics on the ratio of dietary sugar to fat: a case-control study. *European Journal of Clinical Nutrition, 58*(10), 1336–1341.

Cummings, S., Apovian, C. M., & Khaodhiar, L. (2008). Obesity surgery: Evidence for diabetes prevention/management. *Journal of the American Dietetic Association, 108*, S40–S44.

Del Prato, S., Felton, A. M., Munro, N., Zimmet, P., & Zinman, B. (Global Partnership for Effective Diabetes Management). (2007). Improving glucose management: Ten steps to get more patients with type 2 diabetes to glycemic control. *International Journal of Clinical Practice, 157*, 47–57.

Dubois, L., Farmer, A., Girard, M., & Peterson, K. (2007). Regular sugar-sweetened beverage consumption between meals increases risk of overweight among preschool-aged children. *Journal of the American Dietetic Association, 107*(6), 924–934.

Foster, T. S. (2007). Efficacy and safety of α-lipoic acid supplementation in the treatment of symptomatic diabetic neuropathy. *The Diabetes Educator, 33*, 111–117.

Geil, P., & Shane-McWhorter, L. (2008). Dietary supplements in the management of diabetes: Potential risks and benefits. *Journal of the American Dietetic Association, 108*, S59–S65.

Gerhard, G. T., Ahmann, A., Meeuws, K., McMurry, M. P., Duell, P. B., & Connor, W. E. (2004). Effects of a low-fat diet compared with those of a high monounsaturated fat diet on body weight, plasma lipids, and lipoproteins, and glycemic control in type 2

diabetes. *American Journal of Clinical Nutrition, 80*, 668–673.

Gerich, J. E., & Dailey, G. (2004). Advances in diabetes for the millennium: Understanding insulin resistance [Online publication]. *Medscape General Medicine, 6*(3), S11.

Grabitske, H. A., & Slavin, J. L. (2008). Low-digestible carbohydrates in practice. *Journal of the American Dietetic Association, 108*, 1677–1681.

Grundy, S. M., Cleeman, J. I., Merz, C. N., Brewer, H. B., Clark, L. T., Hunninhake, D. B., et al. (2004). Implications of recent clinical trials for the National Cholesterol Education Program Adult Treatment Panel III guidelines. *Circulation, 100*, 227–239.

Harriss, L., English, D., Powles, J., Giles, G. G., Tonkin, A. M., Hodge, A. M., et al. (2007). Dietary patterns and cardiovascular mortality in the Melbourne collaborative cohort study. *American Journal of Clinical Nutrition, 86*, 221–229.

Hatcher, E., & Whittemore, R. (2007). Hispanic adults' beliefs about type 2 diabetes: Clinical implications. *Journal of the American Academy of Nurse Practitioners, 19*, 536–545.

Ikizler, T. A. (2007). Protein and energy intake in advanced chronic kidney disease: How much is too much? *Seminars in Dialysis, 20*(1), 5–11.

Institute of Medicine. (2002). *Dietary reference intakes for energy, carbohydrate, fiber, fat, fatty acids, cholesterol, protein, and amino acids.* Washington, DC: The National Academies Press.

Intellihealth. (2008). *Bitter melon, bitter gourd.* Retrieved April 13, 2009, from http://www.intelihealth.com/IH/ihtIH/WSIHW000/8513/31402/348736.html?d=dmtContent#

International Diabetes Federation. (2007). *Facts and figures.* Retrieved April 13, 2009, from http://www.diabetesatlas.org/content/diabetes-and-impaired-glucose-tolerance

Kim, H. S., & Lee, M. S. (2009). Role of innate immunity in triggering and timing of autoimmune diabetes. *Current Molecular Medicine, 9*, 30–44.

Knowler, W. C., Barrett-Connor, E., Fowler, S. E., Hamman, R. F., Lachin, J. M., Walker, E. A., et al. (2002). Reduction in the incidence of type 2 diabetes with lifestyle intervention or metformin. *The New England Journal of Medicine, 346*(6), 393–403.

Laurence, J. M., Liese, A. D., Lilu, L., Dabella, D., Anderson, A., Impertore, G., et al. (2008). Weight-loss practices and weight-related issues among youth with type 1 or type 2 diabetes. *Diabetes Care, 31*, 2251–2257.

Law, B. M. (2008). DASH dieters show CHD benefit. *(DOC) Diabetes, Obesity, CVD News, 9*.

Li, C., Ford, E. S., Zhao, G., & Mokdad, A. H. (2009). Prevalence of pre-diabetes and its association with clustering of cardiometabolic risk factors and hyperinsulinemia among U.S. adolescents: National Health and Nutrition Examination Survey 2005–2006. *Diabetes Care, 32,* 342–347.

Lipton, R. B., Losey, L. M., Giachello, A., Mendez, J., & Girotti, M. H. (1998). Attitudes and issues in treating Latino patients with type 2 diabetes: Views of healthcare providers. *The Diabetes Educator, 24*(1), 67–71.

Lovegrove, J. A. (2007). CVD risk in South Asians: The importance of defining adiposity and influence of dietary polyunsaturated fat. *Proceedings of the Nutrition Society, 66,* 286–298.

Malik, V. S., Schulze, M. B., & Hu, F. B. (2006). Intake of sugar-sweetened beverages and weight gain: A systematic review. *American Journal of Clinical Nutrition, 84*(2), 274–288.

Marsh, K., & Brand-Miller, J. (2005). The optimal diet for women with polycystic ovary syndrome. *British Journal of Nutrition 94,* 154–165.

Maskarinec, G., Grandinetti, A., Matsuura, G., Sharma, S., Mau, M., Henderson, B.E., et al. (2009). Diabetes prevalence and body mass index differ by ethnicity: The multiethnic cohort. *Ethnicity & Disease, 19,* 49–55.

McGill, J. B. (2009). Improving microvascular outcomes in patients with diabetes through management of hypertension. *Postgraduate Medicine, 121,* 89–101.

Merriman, T. R. (2009). Type 1 diabetes, the A1 milk hypothesis, and vitamin D deficiency.

Diabetes Research and Clinical Practice, 83, 149–156.

Monsivais, P., Perrigue, M. M., & Drewnowski, A. (2007). Sugars and satiety: Does the type of sweetener make a difference? *American Journal of Clinical Nutrition, 86*(1), 116–123.

Montonen, J., Jarvinen, R., Knekt, P., Heliovaara, M., & Reunanen, A. (2007). Consumption of sweetened beverages and intakes of fructose and glucose predict type 2 diabetes occurrence. *Journal of Nutrition, 137*(6), 1447–1454.

National Center for Complementary and Alternative Medicine. (2008). *Asian ginseng.* Retrieved April 13, 2009, from http://nccam.nih.gov/health/asianginseng/

Patrick, A., & Epstein, O. (2008). Gastroparesis. *Alimentary Pharmacology & Therapeutics, 27,* 724–740.

Peel, E. (2005). Taking the biscuit? A discursive approach to managing diet in type 2 diabetes. *Journal of Health Psychology, 10*(6), 779–791.

Riccardi, G., Rivellese, A. A., & Giacco, R. (2008). Role of glycemic index and glycemic load in the healthy state, in prediabetes, and in diabetes. *American Journal of Clinical Nutrition, 87S,* 269S–274S.

Romao, I., & Roth, J. (2008). Genetic and environmental interactions in obesity and type 2 diabetes. *Journal of the American Dietetic Association, 108,* S24–S28.

Schulze, M. B., Manson, J. E., Ludwig, D. S., Colditz, G. A., Stampfer, M. J., & Willett, W. C. (2004). Sugar-sweetened beverages, weight gain, and incidence of type 2 diabetes

in young and middle-aged women. *Journal of the American Medical Association, 292*(8), 927–934.

Shai, I., Jiang, R., Manson, J. R., Stampfer, M. J., Willett, W. C., Colditz, G. A., et al. (2006). Ethnicity, obesity, and risk of type 2 diabetes in women: A 20 year follow-up study. *Diabetes Care, 29*(7), 1585–1591.

Shakil, A., Church, R. J., & Rao, S. S. (2008). Gastrointestinal complications of diabetes. *American Family Physician, 77,* 1697–1702.

Singh, U., & Jialal, I. (2008). Alpha-lipoic acid supplementation and diabetes. *Nutrition Reviews, 66,* 646–657.

Unger, J., & Moriarty, C. (2008). Preventing type 2 diabetes. *Primary Care, 35,* 645–662.

Van Dam, R. M., & Seidell, J. C. (2007). Carbohydrate intake and obesity. *European Journal of Clinical Nutrition, 61*(Suppl. 1), S75–99.

Van Wymelbeke, V., Beridot-Therond, M. E., de La Gueronniere, V., & Fantino, M. (2004). Influence of repeated consumption of beverages containing sucrose or intense sweeteners on food intake. *European Journal of Clinical Nutrition, 58*(1), 154–161.

Vaughn, L. (2005). Dietary guidelines for the management of diabetes. *Nursing Standard 19* (44), 56–64.

Watson, R. T., & Pessin, J. E. (2001). Intracellular organization of insulin signaling and GLUT 4 translocation. *Recent Progress in Hormone Research, 56,* 175–194.

Weiler, D. M., & Crist, J. D. (2009). Diabetes self-management in a Latino social environment. *Diabetes Educator, 35,* 285–292.

Disorders of the Gastrointestinal Tract, Liver, Pancreas, and Gallbladder

20

WHAT WILL YOU LEARN?

1. To analyze the role of nutrition intervention as a central part of managing intestinal disease.
2. To evaluate risk factors for malnutrition that are associated with intestinal diseases.
3. To examine the indications for various therapeutic diets in treating intestinal diseases.
4. To summarize the role of fiber in the treatment of diverticular disease, irritable bowel syndrome, and constipation.
5. To formulate nursing interventions that reduce the symptoms of digestive diseases through dietary alterations.
6. To relate the important role of the nurse in providing nutrition assessment and education to clients who have intestinal diseases and disorders.

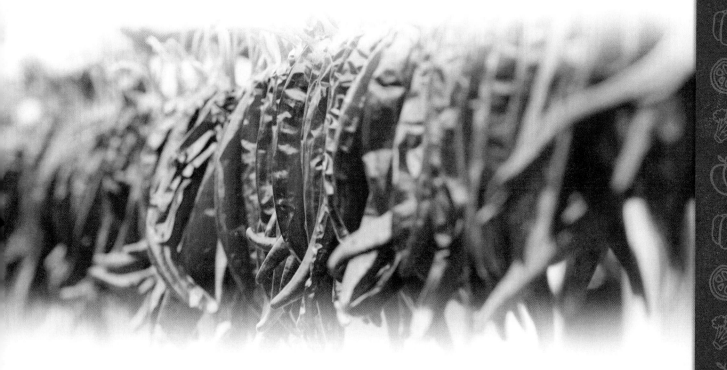

DID YOU KNOW?

► Gluten intolerance and lactose intolerance are not food allergies, although many clients who have these disorders may tell you that they are "allergic" to wheat or milk.

► Yogurt with active cultures can help treat diarrhea from antibiotics or a virus.

► Excessive alcohol intake is a risk factor for a number of intestinal diseases, including ulcer, gastric reflux, pancreatitis, fatty liver, hepatitis, and cirrhosis.

► Over-the-counter and prescription medications that buffer or reduce gastric acid production can decrease iron and vitamin B_{12} absorption.

► Sugar-free foods that contain sorbitol or other sugar alcohols can cause diarrhea.

KEY TERMS

bezoar, *450*

dysphagia, *444*

gluten, *454*

osmolality, *449*

probiotics, *460*

steatorrhea, *452*

How Are Nutrients Digested and Absorbed?

Digestion and absorption begin in the mouth and end in the colon. The intestinal tract and its accessory organs, the liver, gallbladder, and pancreas, orchestrate the digestion and absorption process in a series of coordinated steps involving digestive enzymes and hormones. Muscle contraction within the intestinal wall and various sphincters through the digestive tract control the passage of food and liquids. Foods are mixed beginning with chewing; mixing, or emulsification, continues in the stomach. Chemical breakdown of foods begins in the mouth with the enzyme lingual lipase. The stomach continues the chemical breakdown using pepsin and hydrochloric acid. The small intestine, including the duodenum, jejunum, and ileum, is the site of digestive enzyme secretions from the pancreas and brush border villi. Beginning in the small intestine, carbohydrate, protein, fats, vitamins, and minerals are absorbed after they have been digested into smaller compounds that are present in food. For example, a whole protein found in milk is whey. Whey is broken down by digestive enzymes and absorbed as amino acids or short peptides. Most nutrients are absorbed directly into the bloodstream from the intestine, with the exception of long-chain fatty acids that are absorbed into the lymph system. The large intestine, comprised of the colon, rectum, and anus, is responsible for absorption of fluid and electrolytes. Excretion of cellular waste, undigested fiber, food, and water occurs as the last step in digestion and absorption. Maldigestion and malabsorption alter the delivery and uptake of nutrients by the body. Many disorders of the gastrointestinal tract lead to maldigestion and malabsorption, which are risk factors for declining nutritional health.

Disorders of the Gastrointestinal Tract

Disorders of the gastrointestinal tract include diseases and conditions involving the mouth, esophagus, stomach, small and large intestines, as well as the liver, pancreas, and gallbladder. Figure 20-1 ■ illustrates the entire gastrointestinal system. Individuals with gastrointestinal disease are often at risk for poor nutritional health because of disease symptoms and treatment. Nutrition plays a central role in the management of many intestinal diseases.

Dysphagia

Impaired swallowing is referred to as **dysphagia** and can arise from a number of conditions affecting the upper gastrointestinal tract. The mechanism of swallowing entails oral, pharyngeal, and esophageal phases. Dysphagia can occur because of impairments in one or more swallowing phases from neuromuscular conditions, such as stroke, head injury, dementia, Parkinson's disease, multiple sclerosis; medications, such as anticholinergics and antidepressants; poor or absent dentition; and lack of saliva from medications, disease, or following radiation therapy to the mouth area. Box 20-1 outlines risk factors for dysphagia. Dysphagia is reported more commonly in the older adult because of increased incidence of existing risk factors present in this population (Palmer & Metheny, 2008). Symptoms of dysphagia depend on the affected swallowing phase. The nurse should be aware of these symptoms and refer affected clients for a multidisciplinary swallowing evaluation. The nurse should not rely on the presence or absence of the gag reflex in assessing dysphagia because this finding is not considered an accurate tool. Silent aspiration can occur with little overt symptoms and requires a formal assessment to diagnose (Bottino-Bravo & Thomson, 2008). Generally a speech language pathologist (SLP) is the professional responsible for the formal swallowing evaluation and treatment recommendations.

Unmanaged dysphagia can lead to aspiration pneumonia, dehydration, weight loss, and asphyxiation (Bottino-Bravo & Thomson, 2008; Strowd, Kysima, Pillsbury, Valley, & Rubin, 2008). Clients can become fearful of food sticking in the esophagus, choking, or are embarrassed by drooling and as a result deliberately reduce oral intake. Those who have dysphagia and altered cognition may refuse to take food or spit it out, falsely appearing uncooperative as a result. Dehydration and malnutrition will occur with this diminished intake. Malnutrition can further lead to decompensation in swallowing, causing a downward spiral in health (Leslie, Carding, & Wilson, 2003).

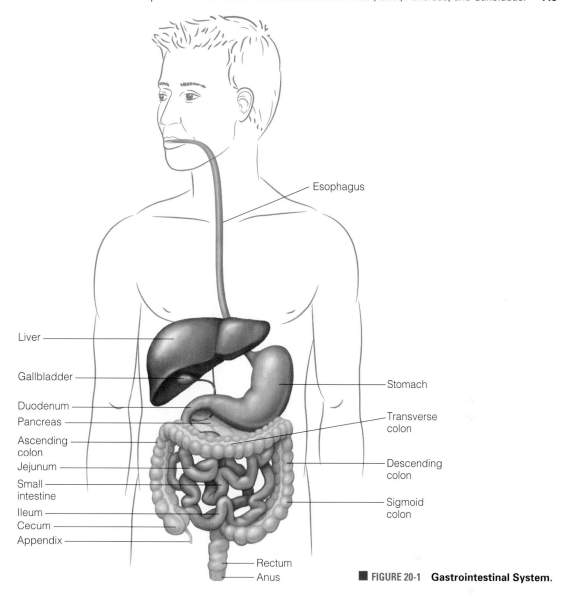

Esophagus

Liver

Gallbladder

Duodenum

Pancreas

Ascending colon

Jejunum

Small intestine

Ileum

Cecum

Appendix

Stomach

Transverse colon

Descending colon

Sigmoid colon

Rectum

Anus

■ **FIGURE 20-1** **Gastrointestinal System.**

| BOX 20-1 | Dysphagia Risks, Symptoms, and Consequences |

Risk Factors for Dysphagia

Neuromuscular conditions: stroke, Parkinson's disease, Huntington's chorea, multiple sclerosis, dementia, amyotrophic lateral sclerosis, myasthenia gravis, scleroderma

Diminished saliva production: postradiation therapy to the head, Sjogren's disease, medications

Poor dentition: loose or missing teeth, ill-fitting dentures

Medications: anticholinergics, antidepressants, sedatives

Head or spinal cord trauma

Obstruction: head or neck tumor, esophageal web, diverticulum, or stricture

Symptoms of Dysphagia

Complaint of difficulty swallowing or food sticking in the throat

Drooling, liquids leaking from the mouth
Refusing to swallow or spitting out of food
Coughing or throat clearing during or after swallow
Multiple swallows for a single bite of food
Food retained in the mouth when next bite is taken
Nasal regurgitation of food or liquid
Voice hoarseness, gurgling, or gravel tone
Lung congestion after meals
Repeated upper respiratory infection
Weight loss

Consequences of Dysphagia

Dehydration
Weight loss and malnutrition
Aspiration pneumonia
Asphyxiation

Nutrition Intervention

The goal of nutrition intervention for dysphagia is to reduce the risk of choking while providing adequate nutrition and a positive eating experience. The SLP will make recommendations to the team about posture during feeding and appropriate food and liquid textures. Modifications to the client's posture can facilitate swallowing or prevent aspiration and include such maneuvers as the chin tuck. Both food and liquid textures should be customized according to the client's swallowing ability. Routine use of a generalized puree or soft diet should be avoided in favor of specific alterations catered to client tolerance. Liquids are categorized as spoon-thick, honey-like, nectar-like, and thin (National Dysphagia Diet Task Force, 2002). Food texture prescriptions range from pureed to regular, but often hard, sticky, and crunchy foods are avoided. Foods and liquids that are more spoon-thick and form a cohesive bolus in the mouth are often attempted first, whereas thin liquids are postponed because of aspiration risk (Dorner, 2002). Commercial powder and gel products are available to thicken liquids and foods to individual tolerance. It is important to shake these products before opening the package to obtain a uniform and properly thickened consistency (Strowd et al., 2008). The nurse should be knowledgeable about the facility's dysphagia diet protocol and learn which foods comprise each transitional stage to lessen risk of aspiration and ensure adherence to texture recommendations. The nurse should monitor the client closely for signs of aspiration and dysphagia. Food pocketing between the gum line and cheek can be discovered after a meal or during mouth care and is indicative of dysphagia. Ongoing assessment of fluid status is needed to avoid dehydration. The nurse may need to assist the client with prescribed postural maneuvers, such as head tipping or chin tuck during swallowing.

When it is determined that oral intake is unsafe because of aspiration risk, enteral nutrition support via a feeding tube can be prescribed. Use of a feeding tube does not eliminate risk of aspiration because of the existing possibility of gastric reflux. Nursing interventions to minimize aspiration risk from tube feedings are outlined in Chapter 16. An overview of nutrition interventions for dysphagia is presented in Table 20-1.

Nausea and Vomiting

Nausea and vomiting are common gastrointestinal symptoms rather than a disease entity. Both symptoms can occur because of a variety of gastrointestinal disorders, such as a virus,

Table 20-1	Nutrition Interventions in Dysphagia Treatment
Intervention	**Intervention Examples**
Ensure proper positioning during meals.	• Position the client with the head and trunk at 90-degree angle to the lap. • Assist with swallowing exercises or posture prescribed by the SLP.
Customize food texture.	Follow prescribed texture recommendations: • Pureed (or pudding-like) • Mechanically altered (foods that are ground, minced, fork mashable, moist, and semisolid) • Advanced (soft, bite-size foods that require some chewing but are not dry, sticky, or hard) • Regular (no restrictions)
Customize liquid texture.	Follow prescribed texture recommendations: • Spoon-thick (pudding-like liquids thickened with commercial thickener, hold shape on a spoon) • Honey-like (liquids that are already the consistency of honey or have thickener added, cannot fit through a straw) • Nectar-like (nectar juices such as peach, pear, apricot, vegetable juices, thin milkshakes or smoothies, hold some shape on a spoon but also fit through a straw) • Thin liquids (water, coffee, tea, milk, clear juice, broths)
Provide a pleasant eating environment.	• Pureed and ground food can be visually unappealing when not presented well. Optimize the eating environment with little distractions to increase pleasantness. When providing feeding assistance, do not mash foods together into a single unattractive mix.
Monitor swallowing safety.	• Ensure that the client is wide awake and alert when eating. • Monitor for signs of aspiration. • Monitor oral hygiene, food pocketing. • When providing feeding assistance: • Allow sufficient time for feeding. • Make sure each bite is swallowed before offering the next bite.
Monitor nutrition and hydration status.	• Advance textures as prescribed. • Communicate with the dietitian regarding overall intake and tolerance to nutrition prescription.

food poisoning, or altered gastric emptying. Additionally, increased intracranial pressure, medications, chemotherapy, motion sickness, and pregnancy, among other conditions, can result in nausea and vomiting. Nutritional health is affected by nausea and vomiting when the symptoms persist and result in insufficient calorie and nutrient intake. When oral intake is safely indicated, the nurse can recommend nutrition intervention as part of overall treatment.

Nutrition Intervention

The goal of nutrition intervention for nausea and vomiting is to promote adequate hydration and nutrition. Carbohydrate-containing liquids and foods are recommended in small amounts throughout the day to avoid queasiness from an empty stomach. Liquids should be consumed separately from foods to minimize gastric distention. High-fat foods should be avoided because these empty more slowly from the stomach and can lead to nausea. Hot foods and foods with strong seasoning or odors can trigger nausea and should be avoided. Clients should be advised to minimize physical movement just before and after eating. Ginger has been shown to be an effective nausea treatment under some circumstances, as outlined in the Evidence-Based Practice Box: Does oral ginger reduce the incidence of nausea and vomiting in postoperative clients? Additionally, Box 20-2 outlines examples of foods to combat nausea.

BOX 20-2	**Nutrition Intervention for Nausea and Vomiting**

Offer small meals and snacks throughout the day.
Drink ample liquids for hydration but not with food to avoid gastric distention.
Offer high-carbohydrate, low-fat foods and liquids.
- Saltines
- Dry toast
- Rice
- Plain pasta
- Cooked cereal
- Dry cold cereal
- Breadsticks
- Pretzels
- Ginger ale and clear sodas—allow carbonation to lessen
- Popsicles
- Gelatin

Avoid:
- Fatty foods such as fried foods, sauces and gravies, heavy meats
- Foods with strong seasoning or odor
- Hot foods
- Large meals
- Physical movement close to time of eating
- Liquids with meals

EVIDENCE-BASED PRACTICE RESEARCH BOX

Does oral ginger reduce the incidence of nausea and vomiting in postoperative clients?

Clinical Problem: Ginger, a spice frequently used in cooking and baking, has a long history of use to treat nausea in pregnancy and for motion sickness. Because nausea and vomiting are common side effects of surgical procedures, there is interest in nonpharmacological agents that can inexpensively treat nausea and vomiting and have minimal side effects.

Research Findings: A meta-analysis conducted by Langmead and Rampton (2001) reviewed four trials in which oral ginger was compared to either a placebo or prescribed antiemetic for postoperative nausea and vomiting. Ginger was statistically superior to the placebo and/or the antiemetic in two studies; however, the other two studies failed to show statistical significance, although there were indications that ginger was more effective. A limitation of the meta-analysis was that the studies that were reviewed used dosages of ginger ranging from 500 mg to 1 gram, given at varied intervals postoperatively.

Nanthakomon and Pongrojpaw (2006) conducted a double-blind random controlled trial with 100 clients in Thailand in which 1 gram of oral ginger or a placebo was given to clients 1 hour preoperatively. Ginger was found to be statistically more likely to decrease postoperative nausea and vomiting than the placebo.

Chaiyakunapruk, Kitikannakorn, Nathisuwan, Leeprakob-boon, & Leelasettagool (2006) reviewed numerous studies in a meta-analysis; however, only five met their inclusion criteria in which at least 1 gram of oral ginger was administered and nausea and vomiting were tracked for 24 hours postoperatively. All but one of the studies involved gynecological surgery. The studies had some limitations, most notably that the majority of clients were Asian with low body mass indices. The studies that were reviewed demonstrated that ginger was statistically significantly better than placebos for preventing nausea and vomiting for at least 24 hours after surgery.

Nursing Implications: Ginger is widely available at low cost and has few side effects; studies show that it may reduce postoperative nausea and vomiting, at least in clients who have had gynecological surgery. However, preoperative administration of an oral supplement may be contraindicated.

CRITICAL THINKING QUESTION:

1. How should the nurse respond to the client who has strong memories of severe nausea and vomiting following surgery 5 years earlier and who is scheduled for orthopedic surgery in 2 weeks and wants to know if there is anything that can be done preoperatively to prevent its occurrence?

Gastroesophageal Reflux, Hiatal Hernia, and Ulcer Disease

Acute inflammation of the esophagus or stomach because of gastroesophageal reflux disease (GERD) or peptic or duodenal ulcer can cause a client to complain of heartburn or stomach pain. A hiatal hernia, a fold in the gastric mucosa above the diaphragm, can contribute to GERD and its symptoms. Pharmacological treatment is the first line of treatment for these disorders of the upper gastrointestinal tract. Nutrition therapy is an adjunct treatment. Nutritional health can be affected by GERD and ulcer disease if individuals overly restrict intake of food while trying to control symptoms. Pain and gastric discomfort also can lead to diminished intake.

Nutrition Intervention

The goal of nutrition treatment of GERD and ulcer disease is reduction in the symptoms through elimination of dietary contributors. Reflux disease occurs because of two main contributors: diminished competence of the lower esophageal sphincter and increased gastric distention or intra-abdominal pressure. Additionally, delayed gastric emptying and increased gastric acid production can contribute to the symptoms. Nutrition interventions are focused on reducing intake of foods known to diminish lower esophageal sphincter pressure.

Additionally, avoidance of foods and behaviors that increase gastric distention are needed. The nurse can also address contributing factors to increased intra-abdominal pressure, such as excess weight and tight clothing. Acidic and spicy foods are avoided by many individuals with GERD or ulcer disease because of the direct irritating nature of these foods on the lower esophagus. Some foods fall into more than one category of contributing factors. For example, alcohol causes increased gastric acid production and decreased low esophageal sphincter pressure and delays gastric emptying (Vemulapalli, 2008). Client Education Checklist: Nutrition Interventions in GERD outlines suggested nutrition intervention for these contributing factors.

Certain populations require additional attention when GERD is an issue. Infants with reflux may vomit feedings, leading to concern about nutritional status during this crucial period of growth. Lifespan Box: Gastroesophageal Reflux in Infants and Children discusses this population. In those with long-standing symptoms, chronic use of acid-suppressing medications can negatively affect absorption of nutrients that require an acid medium for absorption. Practice Pearl: Nutrition and Acid-Suppression Medications discusses this issue. The nurse should include an assessment of this risk when working with clients on these medications.

CLIENT EDUCATION CHECKLIST — Nutrition Interventions in GERD

Assess for Etiology of Symptoms	Intervention
Decreased lower esophageal sphincter pressure	Decrease intake of: • Caffeine (coffee, tea, cola and other sodas [check label], chocolate) • Alcohol • Fatty foods • Carminatives (mints) • Onion and garlic Avoid smoking.
Increased gastric distention or intra-abdominal pressure	• Minimize swallowing of air with carbonated beverages, gum chewing, use of straws, rushed eating. • Consume smaller meals and avoid overeating. • Reduce weight if indicated. • Avoid wearing tight clothing or belts. • Avoid recumbency after eating. Keep the head of the bed elevated with blocks when sleeping.
Gastric contents irritate mucosa	Experiment with tolerance to citrus juices and fruits, tomato products, and red pepper spice (cayenne, hot sauces, hot peppers).
Assess vitamin B_{12} and iron status if acid suppression drugs are used	• Recommend supplemental vitamin B_{12} when indicated. • Optimize iron absorption with concomitant vitamin C intake and avoidance of coffee, tea, and red wine. Outline good sources of dietary iron.
Assess overall nutritional intake	• Some clients will broadly eliminate foods when one food in a group is not tolerated (e.g., eliminating all fruit when only citrus may be an irritant). • Check that alternative sources of nutrients are consumed when certain foods have been eliminated from the diet.

Sources: Adapted from: American Gastroenterological Association (AGA), 2008; National Institute of Diabetes and Digestive and Kidney Diseases (NIDDK), 2007a; Vemulapalli, 2008.

Lifespan

Gastroesophageal Reflux in Infants and Children

Gastroesophageal reflux is common in infants but is self-limiting in most cases and resolves during infancy. Occasionally, GERD and other motility disorders in this population can be related to food allergy and require an evaluation by appropriate allergy and gastrointestinal disease specialists (Ozdemir, Mete, Catal, & Ozol, 2009). When reflux is a concern, the nurse can suggest that the caregiver burp the infant more frequently during feeding and keep the child in an upright position for 30 minutes after feeding (NIDDK, 2007a).Thickened formula is sometimes recommended to reduce the incidence of vomiting (Horvath, Dziechciarz, & Szajewska, 2008). Ongoing reflux with vomiting after feeding, poor weight gain, and a chronic cough or infection require closer evaluation and treatment by pediatric specialists. When GERD occurs in older children, nutrition intervention mirrors that of an adult with customization of advice to include foods found in a child's diet.

What are some sources of caffeine, mints, fatty foods, or acidic foods that children consume?

Dumping Syndrome

Dumping syndrome occurs when rapid gastric emptying results in undigested food being delivered to the small intestine. The high **osmolality** of the food contents draws fluid into the intestine as the body attempts to equalize the concentration gradient between the intestines and the plasma. Osmolality refers to the concentration of particles in a solution, expressed as mmole/kg. Simple sugars found in foods and beverages especially can increase the osmolality of stomach contents. Symptoms of dumping syndrome include abdominal cramping, bloating, and diarrhea typically within an hour following a meal. Late dumping syndrome can occur up

PRACTICE PEARL

Nutrition and Acid-Suppression Medications

Acid-suppression or buffering medications, such as proton pump inhibitors, antacids, and H_2 receptor antagonists, are the frontline therapy in treating reflux and ulcer diseases, but use of these agents is not without nutritional consequences. Vitamin B_{12} and iron require an acid environment in the stomach to initiate digestion and absorption. The nurse should assess the vitamin B_{12} and iron status of clients on long-term treatment for ulcer or GERD to ensure adequacy. Synthetic or supplemental vitamin B_{12} does not require an acid gastric environment and can be recommended for use in this population. Fortified foods and standard multivitamins contain this form of the vitamin. Optimization of iron absorption includes consumption of a vitamin C source concomitant with iron sources and avoidance of coffee, tea, or red wine within an hour of iron intake.

to several hours after a meal with additional symptoms that include hypoglycemia, sweating, and dizziness (NIDDK, 2007b; Tack, 2007). These symptoms occur because of fluid volume shifts and excessive release of insulin in response to the highly concentrated intestinal contents (Tack, 2007). Rapid emptying of the stomach can follow gastric surgeries of many types, including gastric bypass surgery for obesity, vagotomy, and full or partial gastric resection for ulcer disease or neoplasm. Nutritional health is affected with dumping syndrome because of the malabsorption that occurs with the rapid transit of poorly digested food through the gastrointestinal tract.

Nutrition Intervention

The goals of nutrition intervention with dumping syndrome are to prevent rapid gastric emptying and to minimize the hyperosmolar concentration of the stomach contents. Nutrition recommendations include the avoidance of factors that promote quick gastric emptying such as large meals, liquids with meals, carbonated beverages, and extreme food temperatures. Simple sugars, such as juices, sugary desserts, candy, and soda, are best avoided. Little research has been devoted to nutrition treatment of dumping syndrome, and instead most recommendations are based on best practices (Karamanolis & Tack, 2006). Box 20-3 outlines nutrition interventions with dumping syndrome.

Gastroparesis

Gastroparesis is a motility disorder of the stomach that causes delayed gastric emptying. The etiology of the delayed emptying is commonly because of damaged nerves innervating the stomach, especially the vagus nerve (NIDDK, 2007c). Diabetes, smooth muscle disorders, medications, and eating disorders can lead to gastroparesis (Patrick & Epstein, 2008). Symptoms of gastroparesis include nausea and vomiting of undigested food, gastric reflux, and early satiety. In addition

BOX 20-3	Nutrition Intervention for Dumping Syndrome

Minimize Gastric Volume
- Consume small meals.
- Drink fluids between meals, not with meals.
- Avoid carbonated beverages.

Slow Gastric Peristalsis
- Avoid extremely hot or cold foods.
- Choose recumbent position after meals.

Reduce Osmolality of Stomach Contents
- Avoid foods high in simple sugars such as candy, desserts, syrups, excessive fruit.
- Avoid liquids high in simple sugars such as soda, mixed drinks, juices.

to vomiting, nutrition status is affected by early satiety and loss of appetite. Weight loss is common with symptomatic gastroparesis.

Nutrition Intervention

The goal of nutrition therapy with gastroparesis is to promote intake of adequate nutrition in a form that will not further delay gastric emptying. In addition to any pharmacological treatment and cessation of smoking, small, frequent meals are indicated with low-fiber, low-alcohol, and low-fat content. Smoking, alcohol, and fat delay gastric emptying (Shakil, Church, & Rao, 2008). High-fiber intake is avoided because of the risk of gastric **bezoar** formation. Bezoars are undigested food masses that occur when food remains in the intestine too long. Bezoars can result in intestinal blockage if untreated. In some individuals, the use of liquids and pureed foods to replace solid foods is indicated; liquids empty more quickly from the stomach than do solid foods (Patrick & Epstein, 2008). Liquid nutritional supplements and other high-calorie liquids can be recommended with the advice of a registered dietitian to ensure that caloric and nutrient needs are being met. When clients are unable to tolerate adequate nutrition orally, use of a feeding tube placed beyond the stomach is indicated for enteral nutrition support (Patrick & Epstein, 2008).

Lactose Intolerance

Lactose is often called milk sugar because it is the disaccharide found in milk products. Lactose is broken down in the small intestine to the simple sugars glucose and galactose by the brush border enzyme lactase. When the small intestine does not synthesize sufficient lactase, maldigestion of lactose occurs and is referred to as lactose intolerance. In lactose intolerance, undigested lactose reaches the colon where intestinal bacteria digest the sugar and produce glucose, galactose, and gas by-products. When this action occurs, symptoms include bloating, abdominal cramping, and diarrhea. Lactose intolerance occurs along a continuum. Individuals vary in their tolerance to different amounts of lactose, some tolerating lactose when consumed with other foods or in small amounts. Lactose intolerance is common worldwide, affecting 70% of the population. Individuals of Northern European descent have the lowest prevalence of lactose intolerance, whereas Asian populations experience the highest (Eadala, Waud, Matthews, Green, & Campbell, 2009). Secondary lactose intolerance occurs when there is a short- or long-term insult to the brush border villi of the small intestine that produce lactase. Infection, chemotherapy, radiation therapy, inflammatory bowel disease, and celiac disease can cause temporary or permanent lactose intolerance. Diagnosis of lactose intolerance is by a lactose tolerance test or hydrogen breath test. Nutritional health is affected by lactose intolerance if individuals completely eliminate dairy foods from the

diet and fail to consume alternate sources of calcium and vitamin D. Children with lactose intolerance who avoid all milk products consume inadequate calcium and vitamin D to support bone mineralization during this crucial period of growth (Heyman, 2006).

Nutrition Intervention

The goal of nutrition therapy with lactose intolerance is control of gastrointestinal symptoms while promoting adequate intake of calcium and vitamin D. Before counseling an individual about diet and lactose intolerance, the nurse should carefully assess the individual's tolerance to various sources of lactose and be cognizant of dose-dependent and situational variations. It is a general consensus that most people with lactose intolerance are capable of tolerating some lactose in the diet and that tolerance can be improved over time with lactose consumption. Small amounts of lactose consumed with other foods are better tolerated than are larger amounts or consuming a dairy food by itself. Aged, cultured, and fermented dairy products, such as yogurt, aged cheeses, and buttermilk, have reduced lactose content because of the effects of fermentation and advantageous bacteria that produce lactase (NIDDK, 2006). For example, 1 cup of whole milk has 12 gm of lactose, whereas 1 oz of Swiss cheese has only 0.07 mg (Heyman, 2006).

Digestive aids that contain lactase in pill form can be purchased over the counter and added to milk or consumed simultaneously with dairy foods to improve tolerance to lactose. Enzyme-incubated milk can be purchased that already has lactase added. This product has a sweeter taste than standard milk because the lactose is already broken down to glucose and galactose, which are simple sugars.

The nurse should guide the client in assessing the sources of hidden lactose in the diet from processed foods and medications because these can contribute to symptoms. Although lactose intolerance is not a milk allergy, clients can check food ingredient labels for milk allergy warnings and "contains milk" as a way of discovering possible lactose content. Approximately 20% of prescription medications and over 6% of over-the-counter drugs contain lactose (NIDDK, 2006). Medications with lactose include those used to treat intestinal disorders, such as some brands of antispasmodic and antimotility drugs, proton pump inhibitors, and antiemetics (Eadala et al., 2009). A pharmacist can provide the client with more specifics regarding lactose content of medications. Good sources of dietary calcium and vitamin D should be outlined for the client when intake of these nutrients is low. Client Education Checklist: Nutrition Intervention in Lactose Intolerance outlines nutrition intervention guidelines with lactose intolerance.

Inflammatory Bowel Disease

Inflammatory bowel disease includes both Crohn's disease and ulcerative colitis. Both diseases cause inflammation in

CLIENT EDUCATION CHECKLIST	Nutrition Intervention in Lactose Intolerance
Intervention	**Example**
Assess diet and tolerance to lactose.	Assess intake of: • Overall amount of dairy foods • Single doses of dairy foods • Other foods consumed with dairy foods • Hidden lactose in medications, breads, processed meats and mixes, candy, salad dressing • Dietary sources of calcium and vitamin D
Educate on trial-and-error methods for improving lactose tolerance.	Suggest: • Small amounts of dairy foods vs. full portion • Consuming dairy foods with a meal, not alone • Gradually increasing portion of dairy foods as tolerated • Cultured and fermented dairy foods: yogurt with active cultures, buttermilk, aged cheese • Use of oral lactase enzyme tablets, drops, or lactase-incubated milk • Checking ingredient labels for milk and milk by-products listing; processed meats, instant soup, mixes, sauces, baked goods, snacks may reveal hidden lactose • Consult with pharmacist on lactose content of medications
Review nondairy dietary sources of calcium and vitamin D.	If calcium and vitamin D intake is low, suggest: • Calcium-fortified juices • Calcium and vitamin D-fortified soy milk • Fish with edible small bones: sardine, anchovies, canned salmon • Eggs, liver • Leafy green vegetables

CT? What advice should the nurse give regarding calcium or vitamin D supplement use?

the mucosa of the bowel wall. Ulcerative colitis is generally limited in occurrence to the colon, whereas Crohn's disease can occur anywhere in the intestine. In particular, the ileum is a crucial site for nutrient absorption. If clients with Crohn's disease have existing disease in the ileum, absorption of fat, fat-soluble vitamins, vitamin B_{12}, and bile salt reabsorption are diminished. The inflammatory process can lead to gastrointestinal symptoms such as bleeding, pain, poor appetite, abdominal cramping, and diarrhea. Crohn's disease manifests itself through deeper layers of intestinal mucosa than are found with ulcerative colitis and thus is prone to enteric fistula formation, fissures, stricture, and often more severe symptoms. Nutritional health is affected by inflammatory bowel disease because of three factors: diminished intake as a result of symptoms, nutrient losses because of malabsorption and fistulas, and the increased nutritional requirements associated with inflammation and the need to promote mucosal healing and fistula closure. Poor intake can carry over into periods when disease is not active because of ongoing avoidance of foods associated with symptoms that occurred during a disease flare-up. Even when disease is inactive, clients with Crohn's disease are reported to have suboptimal intake of many nutrients, including folate, calcium, and vitamins C and E (Aghdassi, Wendland, Stapleton, & Raman, 2007). Clients

with Crohn's disease are at greater nutritional risk than those with ulcerative colitis because of greater malabsorption related to inflammation and loss of small bowel absorptive surface in addition to the high nutritional requirements for any fistula repair (Jeejeebhoy, 2002a). Bleeding occurs with both types of inflammatory bowel disease and warrants assessment of nutritional parameters for anemias. Risk of osteoporosis is high in inflammatory bowel disease because of malabsorption of calcium and vitamin D that is magnified by the use of corticosteroids as pharmacological treatment of the disease (O'Sullivan, 2009). All of these risk factors for malnutrition are of particular concern in children because of the effect on growth and development, as discussed in Lifespan Box: Inflammatory Bowel Disease in Children.

Nutrition Intervention

The goal of nutrition therapy in inflammatory bowel disease is provision of adequate nutrition to promote tissue healing and optimal nutritional health while not contributing to symptoms. Enteral nutrition should be used unless an intestinal obstruction, perforation, or short bowel syndrome precludes its use. In addition to providing adequate nutrition, enteral nutrition can maintain intestinal integrity, promote healing of inflamed mucosa, and prevent bacterial

Lifespan

Inflammatory Bowel Disease in Children
Growth failure can occur in children with inflammatory bowel disease and requires close attention. Gastrointestinal symptoms can foster decreased intake to a point that there is insufficient intake to meet the increased nutritional needs of the disease and support normal growth and development. Children may avoid foods because of anticipatory pain and further increase nutritional risk. In addition, when growth does occur, bone health can be compromised because of treatment with corticosteroids. Consultation with a registered dietitian who specializes in pediatric medical nutrition therapy is an essential part of treating inflammatory bowel disease and especially when a child is experiencing growth failure.

translocation, a migration of bacteria from the gut to other locations in the body that can cause infection (O'Sullivan & O'Morain, 2006). Low-fat, polymeric, or elemental enteral formulas are used with severe fulminant disease to provide optimal nutrition in an easily digested and absorbed form when oral intake of food and liquids is insufficient. When a disease flare-up is less severe, a low-fiber diet can be recommended. Avoidance of high-fiber fruits, vegetables, grains, nuts, and seeds will decrease fecal residue and stool frequency. In some clients, secondary lactose intolerance can develop with Crohn's disease and modification of lactose intake can alleviate those symptoms. Nutritional supplementation is often needed with Crohn's disease and should be customized based on location of disease. Figure 20-2 ■ depicts the intestinal sites for digestion and absorption of many nutrients. The nurse can use this guide in determining the probability of nutrient malabsorption based on disease location. Disease in the ileum or a resection including the ileocecal valve causes malabsorption of fat, fat-soluble vitamins, and vitamin B_{12}. Vitamin B_{12} indices should be checked annually in those with ileal disease (O'Sullivan & O'Morain, 2006). Fat malabsorption causes fatty diarrhea called **steatorrhea,** which in turn causes malabsorption of calcium. Large losses of intestinal fluid and diarrhea foster loss of zinc from intestinal secretions. It is recommended that zinc be replaced at a rate of 12 to 15mg/L of intestinal output (Jeejeebhoy, 2002b). In addition to replacing malabsorbed vitamins and minerals, a high-calorie, high-protein diet is essential. Oral liquid nutrition supplements are advised to boost intake when food intake is insufficient.

Although no dietary changes are reported to prevent development of inflammatory bowel disease (O'Sullivan, 2009), research has focused on a possible role of omega-3 fats in the reduction of the inflammatory process of inflammatory bowel disease. Clinical trials have yielded mixed results, making it difficult to demonstrate that these fats can be used

to maintain remission of either Crohn's disease or ulcerative colitis (Turner, Steinhart, & Griffiths, 2007; Turner, Zlotkin, Shah, & Griffiths, 2009). Further research is needed before conclusions can be made about the use of omega-3 fats in inflammatory bowel disease treatment.

Short Bowel Syndrome

Short bowel syndrome refers to the loss of intestinal length and the resulting malabsorptive symptoms and poor nutrition status that follow. Surgical resections of the small and large intestine, trauma, disease, and congenital defects contribute to short bowel syndrome (Matarese et al., 2007). Resections for inflammatory bowel disease, bowel infarct, neoplastic disease, and intestinal bypass surgery are some of the surgical contributors to short bowel syndrome. Surgical resections that lead to short bowel can be single or successive surgeries. Individuals with less than 200 cm of remaining small intestine are at risk for short bowel syndrome; those with less than 100 cm remaining will most likely have symptoms, especially if the terminal ileum or colon has been resected or the remaining intestine has disease (AGA, 2003). The terminal ileum is the site of fat, fat-soluble vitamins, vitamin B_{12}, and bile salt absorption. Without a terminal ileum, these substances are delivered to the colon and are poorly absorbed. Colon resection can lead to problems with absorption of fluid and electrolytes. Adaptation in digestive and absorptive function does take place over time. The ileum can adapt to compensate for a jejunal resection, but the jejunum is less able to compensate for a resected ileum (Jackson & Buchman, 2004; Jeejeebhoy, 2002b). Adaptation can take up to 2 years after surgery.

Symptoms of short bowel syndrome are those of malabsorption. Diarrhea, weight loss, growth failure in children, nutrient deficiencies, and fluid and electrolyte imbalance occur. Severe fluid and electrolyte abnormalities are associated with an end-jejunostomy, where the intestinal tract ends with the jejunum because of resection of the ileum and colon (O'Keefe et al., 2006). In long-term short bowel syndrome, cholelithiasis and nephrolithiasis are additional complications. Gallstones occur because of poor reabsorption of bile salts with a diseased or absent ileum; the result is formation of gallstones with low bile salt concentration that are more prone to stone formation (Jeejeebhoy, 2002b). Kidney stones occur when fat malabsorption changes the absorption of oxalates from the diet, contributing to hyperoxaluria and oxalate stone precipitation (Jeejeebhoy, 2002b). Oxalate kidney stones are discussed in Chapter 21.

Nutrition health is greatly affected by short bowel syndrome. Malabsorption of fluid; overall calories; fat; vitamins A, D, E, K, and B_{12}; and minerals such as zinc, magnesium, and potassium put the individual with a short bowel at high risk of malnutrition. Medical management of short bowel syndrome can include use of acid suppression medications that further contribute to vitamin B_{12} and iron malabsorption.

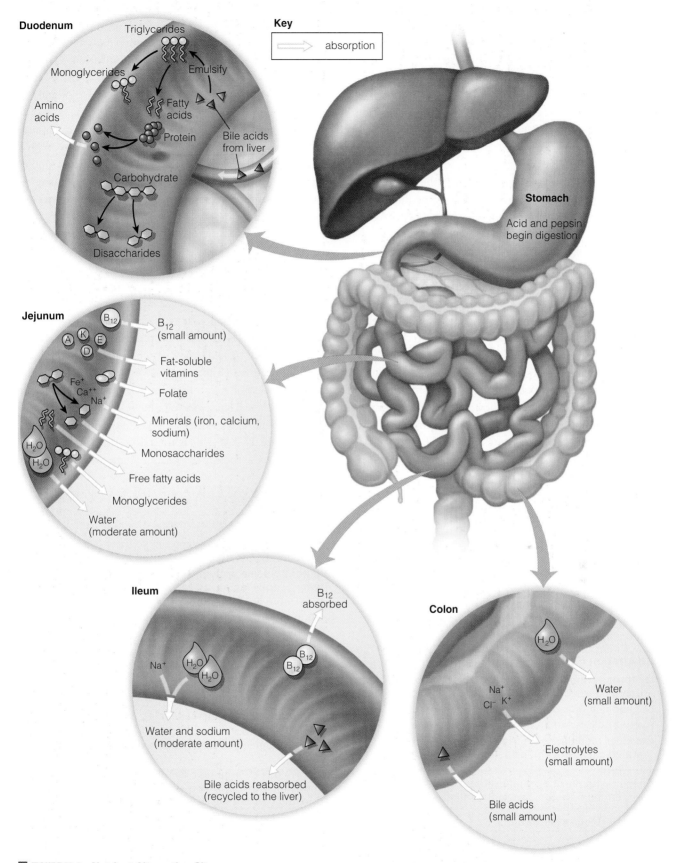

■ FIGURE 20-2   **Nutrient Absorption Sites.**

Nutrition Intervention

The long-term goal of nutrition therapy with short bowel syndrome is to enhance the adaptive process of the intestine to optimize absorption and nutritional health. The ultimate goal is referred to as nutritional autonomy, meaning the client no longer relies on any form of nutrition support from parenteral nutrition or tube feeding. In the short-term, provision of adequate nutrition to improve nutritional health and promote wound healing is essential. The route of initial nutritional support depends on the extent of intestinal loss. Parenteral nutrition is often used at least in the first 10 days postoperatively to provide adequate nutrition, fluids, and electrolytes while intestinal function is assessed (AGA, 2003). Independence from parenteral nutrition takes an extended amount of time for some individuals and never occurs for others, depending on intestinal loss and adaptation. Gradual transition to an isotonic enteral nutrition formula followed by solid food can take months to years. Avoidance of hyperosmolar liquids minimizes diarrhea from fluid shifts that are a result of the body compensating for the high concentration of fluid in the intestine. Box 20-4 outlines guidelines for nutrition intervention in short bowel syndrome. These recommendations can be used, realizing that each client progresses at an individualized rate following intestinal resection.

Intestinal transplantation is indicated with short bowel syndrome when there is intestinal failure and parenteral nutrition complications, such as liver failure, recurrent sepsis, and venous thrombosis that limits intravenous access (Matarese et al., 2007). Parenteral nutrition support is provided following transplant until enteral nutrition formula can be tolerated. Generally, enteral nutrition is begun within a week of surgery. Clients eventually transition to a low-fat, low-lactose diet in the following weeks. Clients are gradually weaned from one form of nutrition support to the next when each successive type is well tolerated in amounts sufficient to meet nutritional needs (Matarese et al., 2007). The nurse should work closely with the nutrition support team when caring for a client with intestinal transplant because close monitoring is essential to ensure that nutritional needs are met.

Celiac Sprue

Celiac sprue, celiac disease, and gluten-sensitive enteropathy are different names for the same autoimmune disease that causes atrophy of intestinal villi when gluten is consumed. Atrophy of the small intestine villi leads to loss of absorptive surface and, therefore, malabsorption. **Gluten** is a protein found in wheat, rye, and barley. Oats can contain some gluten as a result of cross-contamination with other grains during milling or processing. In celiac disease, the presence of gluten in the small bowel causes an immune response with elevated immunoglobulins that directly injure the villi (Niewinski, 2008). Figure 20-3 ■ depicts the villi of the small intestine responsible for absorbing nutrients. Symptoms of celiac sprue

---

BOX 20-4	Nutrition Intervention in Short Bowel Syndrome

Postoperative Nutrition

Provide parenteral nutrition for nutritients, fluid, and electrolytes.

Advance to isotonic enteral formula to minimize diarrhea.

Assess potential nutrient malabsorption based on intestinal loss.

Adaptation Phase

Offer many small, high-calorie meals to maximize energy and nutrient intake.

Consume liquids between meals, not with meals.

Avoid or dilute hyperosmolar beverages.

Consider medium-chain triglyceride supplement for added calories from fat. Tolerance must be monitored.

Consult with nutrition support team on use of glutamine nutrition supplementation.

General Recommendations

Limit lactose.

Avoid sugar alcohols because of laxative effect (e.g., sorbitol, mannitol).

Limit oxalate intake to reduce risk of kidney stones (rhubarb, coffee, tea, cocoa, green leafy vegetables).

Monitor fluid, electrolyte, and vitamin and mineral status, replacing as indicated. Zinc, magnesium, and potassium are commonly required.

Recommend water-miscible form of fat-soluble vitamin supplement and vitamin B_{12} if the ileum was resected or fat malabsorption is present.

Ostomy Diet Recommendations

Chew foods well and avoid high fiber to avoid mechanical obstruction.

Limit foods that may increase odor: asparagus, coffee, garlic.

Consume yogurt or buttermilk, if tolerated, to minimize odor.

Decrease gas by limiting offending foods, gum chewing, drinking with a straw, smoking, and drinking carbonated beverages. Offending foods vary from person to person.

Sources: Adapted from: AGA, 2003; Buchman, 2006; Jeejeebhoy 2002b; Matarese & Steiger, 2006; O'Keefe et al., 2006.

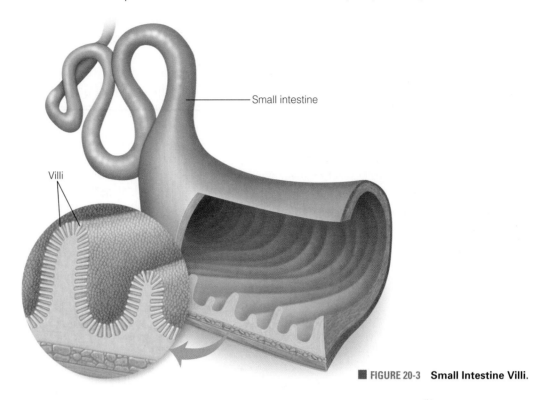

— Small intestine

Villi

■ **FIGURE 20-3 Small Intestine Villi.**

occur along a continuum and many individuals have a silent, atypical presentation that is discovered only with testing following the diagnosis of a family member (Niewinski, 2008). Abdominal pain, bloating, diarrhea or steatorrhea, weight loss, and anemia are symptoms that occur as a result of the disease. In children, growth failure, short stature, irritability, and behavior changes are seen (NIDDK, 2008a). Osteoporosis with bone pain, dermatitis herpetiformis, and infertility are among the complications that occur with untreated celiac disease (Green & Cellier, 2007; Heyman et al., 2009). It has been reported that timing of introduction of gluten in the infant diet may play a role in later diagnosis of celiac disease. Gluten foods introduced early (before age 3 months) or late (not until after age 7 months) is associated with diagnosis of celiac disease in children already genetically at risk for the disease (Green & Cellier, 2007). Celiac sprue is diagnosed by small bowel biopsy or serology for specific elevated immunoglobulins. The nurse should instruct clients being tested for celiac disease to continue with a regular diet before testing to avoid false negative test results (NIDDK, 2008a).

Nutritional health is negatively affected by celiac disease for several reasons. Untreated celiac sprue leads to malabsorption of vitamins, minerals, fat, and overall energy. Weight loss, anemia, and bone disease can result. Nutrition treatment of celiac disease may cause some individuals to restrict intake of B vitamins, fiber, and energy if appropriate food choices are not available. Secondary lactose intolerance occurs when villi producing lactase enzyme are affected and can further restrict dietary intake.

Nutrition Intervention

The goal of treatment of celiac sprue is the optimization of nutritional status through the return of normal intestinal villi morphology and resolution of malabsorptive symptoms. The only known treatment for celiac sprue is lifelong adherence to a gluten-free diet. Avoidance of gluten allows the intestinal villi to heal over time, reducing disease symptoms and malabsorption. Healing occurs within 6 months in children and young adults but can take up to 2 years in older adults (NIDDK, 2008a). Wheat, rye, and barley must be eliminated from the diet entirely. In the United States, elimination of oats is also recommended because testing has shown regular cross-contamination with gluten in the food supply (Thompson, 2004). Oats do not contain gluten and are allowed when a trustworthy, gluten-free source can be ensured (Dickey, 2008). Individuals with celiac disease must be vigilant in the attention given to the diet and label reading in order to avoid gluten intake. Wheat is widely used as a filler or additive in foods and is found in the food supply well beyond the expected flour-based products and cereals. Allergy labeling for wheat can be used to assist the consumer in finding hidden wheat in products. "Gluten-free" product labeling is vague and voluntary in the United States but better defined in Canada and Europe, where "gluten free" translates to less than 20 ppm or 60 mg of gluten (Kupper, 2005; Niewinski, 2008). Barley and rye ingredients are not part of mandated allergy labeling in the United States and must be searched out on the ingredient list. Clients with celiac sprue should be referred to a registered dietitian (RD) for nutrition counseling because of the complicated and

MyNursingKit Celiac Disease, Canadian Celiac Association

Cultural Considerations

Cultural Influences on Intestinal Disease

Certain intestinal diseases are more prevalent in some cultures than in others. Lactose intolerance is common in many populations with up to 75% of African Americans and 90% of Asian Americans experiencing symptoms. In particular, those from Thailand, Indonesia, Korea, and China are more likely to have lactose intolerance (Heyman, 2006). Individuals of Northern European descent have the least incidence of the disorder (Eadala et al., 2009). On the other hand, celiac sprue is more common in Western Europeans and in the United States than in other countries. Prevalence of celiac disease among Irish people is highest, about twice that of the United States (Chand & Mihas, 2006). Celiac sprue is influenced by genetics; over 5% of first-degree relatives of someone with celiac disease will also have the diagnosis (Niewinski, 2008).

MyNursingKit Celiac Sprue Association

life-altering nature of a gluten-free diet. It is recommended that referrals be made specifically to an RD with expert knowledge in celiac disease (NIH, 2004).

The nurse should involve family members in disease and treatment education because of the effect of the disease on lifestyle (Amerine, 2006). Although there is a genetic component to this disease, as discussed in Cultural Considerations Box: Cultural Influences on Intestinal Disease, not all family members will have celiac disease. Quality of life is negatively impacted by a gluten-free diet because of its restrictiveness. Dining out, travel, family meals, and perceived dietary deviance are negatively affected by the nature of the diet (Olsson, Hornell, Ivarrson, & Snyder, 2008; Zarkadas et al., 2006). Nonadherence to the diet is the primary cause of a celiac disease symptoms not responding to treatment (Green & Cellier, 2007). Long-term risks associated with dietary nonadherence include certain intestinal cancers and poor bone mineralization (Green & Cellier, 2007; Heyman et al., 2009).

Gluten-free versions of common foods, such as bread, cereal, and pasta, can be purchased in many grocery stores and on-line, but are often unpalatable, expensive, and not fortified or enriched with the B vitamins and iron found standardly in the gluten-containing versions. When providing follow-up care to clients with celiac disease, care should be taken to assess intake of specialty foods and sources of B vitamins and iron in the diet. Advice should be given on dietary sources of B vitamins and iron when indicated. Use of a gluten-free multivitamin, multimineral supplement may also be indicated. Table 20-2 outlines common sources of gluten in the diet and alternatives to those foods.

Irritable Bowel Syndrome

Irritable bowel is considered a functional disorder and not a disease. Altered intestinal motility and sensitivity cause

symptoms of abdominal bloating and discomfort with either diarrhea or constipation. Medical management of irritable bowel focuses on medications to treat episodic diarrhea or constipation and consideration of psychological treatment. Antianxiety and antidepressant medications along with behavior therapy for stress can prove effective in some clients (Clark & DeLegge, 2008). Nutrition health can be affected by irritable bowel syndrome if it results in the client following an overly restrictive diet in an attempt to self-manage symptoms.

Nutrition Intervention

The goal of nutrition therapy for irritable bowel is relief of gastrointestinal symptoms while providing an adequate diet. Nutrition intervention is largely trial and error (NIDDK, 2007d). The nurse can suggest a symptom diary be kept by the client to better determine any diet or lifestyle factors that are contributing to symptoms. No single food has been reported to universally contribute to this disorder, but the nurse can suggest experimenting with reduction of certain foods and addition of fiber to the diet as outlined in Box 20-5. Guidelines on the addition to fiber to the diet are contained in Client Education Checklist: Fiber in the Diet. Research on treatment of irritable bowel has yielded reports of the placebo effect playing a significant role in symptom reduction in some clients (Clark & DeLegge, 2008).

Diverticular Disease

Diverticulosis is the presence of one or more small pouches, called diverticula, that occur in the colon because of weakened muscle. Diverticulitis is when the diverticula become inflamed and infected. Diverticula form in the muscle layer of the colon wall for complex reasons that include colon structure, genetics, and diet (Salzman & Lillie, 2005). Figure 20-4 ■ depicts diverticula in the colon. Most people with diverticulosis are asymptomatic, but up to 15% experience colicky abdominal pain on occasion (Salzman & Lillie, 2005). Diverticulitis develops in a minority of people with diverticulosis and includes symptoms of acute abdominal pain, fever, nausea and vomiting, and constipation or diarrhea. Diverticulitis is medically managed with antibiotics or surgery, whereas diverticulosis is managed with nutrition intervention (NIDDK, 2008b).

Nutrition Intervention

The goal of nutrition therapy in uncomplicated diverticular disease is intake of sufficient fiber to avoid symptoms. It is common practice to recommend a high-fiber diet in an attempt to decrease intraluminal pressure in the colon; increased pressure is felt to contribute to development of diverticula. The nurse can recommend slowly adding sources of fiber to the diet from varied plant foods such as fruits, vegetables, whole grains, and legumes. Nuts, seeds, and popcorn hulls contain fiber, but some recommend excluding these in

Table 20-2   Gluten-Free Nutrition Guidelines

Eliminate	Examples	Alternatives
Wheat	Wheat flour in: cereals, baked goods, bread, breading, crackers, pasta, snacks, croutons, bread crumbs, stuffing, pizza crust, matzo Mixes such as pancake, baking, cakes, sauces, gravy, cocoa, pudding, seasoning Filler in: food starch, processed meats (cold cuts, sausage, hot dogs), seasoning and seasoned coatings (nuts, french fries), salad dressing, marinades, self-basting poultry, soups and soup base, thickener, sauces (including soy, Worcestershire, teriyaki), baked beans, cream sauces, condiments, nondairy creamer, some ice creams, cream or cottage cheeses, cheese spread, flavored yogurts, imitation crab Bulgur, couscous, durum, semolina, spelt, triticale, wheat germ, wheat bran, farina, kamut, seitan Communion wafers Medications Stamp and envelope adhesive	Corn, rice, potato, soy, and nut flours for cooking or in alternative specialty mixes, snacks, and grain products such as breads, cereal, pasta Use arrowroot, tapioca, cornmeal, or allowed flours as thickeners in cooking Plain meats, poultry, fish, beans, split peas, lentils, eggs, milk, rice, rice noodles, potato, corn and popcorn, vegetables, fruits, plain oils Check labels of rice crackers, rice cakes, corn or rice hot and cold cereals, corn chips, corn tortillas, chocolate milk, yogurts, cheeses to ensure no gluten additives. Dried fruit may be dusted with flour Low-fat and fat-free foods have thickeners added that may contain wheat. Check labels Use wheat allergy labeling to decipher wheat-based fillers, additives Gluten-free wafers Refer to pharmacist for medication assessment of gluten content Wet adhesives with water, not by licking
Rye	Breads, cereal Rye alcoholic beverage	Allowed breads, flours, and cereals
Barley	Barley cereals or in soup Malt beverages (malted milk) Malt extract or syrup Beer and ale	Allowed cereals, beverages: Wine, brandies, tequila, potato vodka do not contain barley. Gluten-free beers are available
Oats	Oat flour in cereals, bread Oat bran, oatmeal	Allowed cereals, flours Oats from trustworthy uncontaminated source allowed
Be aware of controversy on inclusion of some foods in gluten-free diet	Buckwheat, quinoa, amaranth, distilled vinegar, millet, wild rice, wheat starch are allowed by some and not by others	• White, cider, or wine vinegar considered acceptable, but not malt vinegars • Stay up to date on National Celiac Organization guidelines
Monitor nutritional adequacy	Malabsorption of fats, lactose, vitamins, and minerals Restrictive diet eliminates fortified or enriched wheat products and may be low fiber Alternative gluten-free products may not be enriched or fortified	• Follow gluten-free diet to promote mucosal healing • Suggest nongrain sources of B vitamins and iron • Follow recommendations for management of lactose intolerance, checking for good sources of calcium and vitamin D • Suggest alternative whole grains, fruits, and vegetables for fiber • Recommend gluten-free multivitamin

Sources: Adapted from Canadian Celiac Association, 2008; Celiac Sprue Association, 2008; NIDDK, 2008a.

the diet to avoid the risk of their entrapment in a diverticulum and inflammation (NIDDK, 2008b). However, no scientific evidence exists that supports this fear. Recent research suggests that these substances do not contribute to risk of diverticular complications (Marcason, 2008; Strate, Liu, Syngl, Aldoori, & Giovannucci, 2008). Fiber recommendations are outlined in Client Education Checklist: Fiber in the Diet.

When diverticulitis occurs, a high-fiber diet is contraindicated until inflammation has abated and infection is gone (Salzman & Lillie, 2005). Generally, clients follow a clear liquid diet for a few days only. Longer need for a clear liquid diet warrants nutrition attention for alternative calorie and nutrient supplementation. The diet may cautiously be advanced back to a high-fiber diet once the client is improved.

BOX 20-5	Nutrition Intervention in Irritable Bowel Syndrome

Trial of reduced intake of:

- Caffeine (coffee, tea, colas, chocolate)
- Fatty foods
- Sugar alcohols (sorbitol, mannitol, etc.) as dietetic sweetener and in sugar-free and low-carbohydrate foods

No need to avoid lactose unless lactase deficiency is confirmed.

Avoid large meals because overeating can trigger symptoms.

Slowly increase intake of fiber over many days, adding small amounts and assessing tolerance before adding more (see Client Education Checklist: Fiber in the Diet).

Constipation

Constipation has no single definition but may be defined by clients as infrequent or difficult stool passage. Systemic, functional, and neurological disorders are among the multifactorial causes of constipation. Physical inactivity, medications, and medical conditions contribute to constipation in older adults (Hsieh, 2005). Medications such as opiates, anticholinergics, anticonvulsants, and calcium and iron supplements are among the medications that can cause constipation (Fernandez-Banares, 2006). Medical management utilizes medication and encourages nutrition intervention.

Nutrition Intervention

The goal of nutrition therapy in constipation is intake of a high-fiber and adequate-fluid diet to promote normal intestinal transit. Increasing fluid intake appears to be efficacious when dehydration contributes to constipation, but it has questionable merit in well-hydrated individuals (Fernandez-Banares, 2006). The nurse should suggest slowly increasing fiber intake in the diet by 5 gm daily per week until it reaches the recommended 20 gm to 35 gm/day (Hsieh, 2005). Client Education Checklist: Fiber in the Diet outlines advice that the nurse can offer in managing constipation.

Bloating and Intestinal Gas

Gas in the gastrointestinal tract is a normal part of digestion. Clients may complain of increased gas and ask the nurse for advice on symptom relief. Gas originates in the intestines from either swallowed air or digestion of food in the colon by normal gut flora (NIDDK, 2008c). Certain carbohydrates in the diet will produce more gas during digestion than others. Raffinose, lactose, fructose, sorbitol, and some starches and fiber are examples. Box 20-6 outlines advice that the nurse can offer as a trial-and-error approach to treating increased intestinal gas.

Diarrhea

Diarrhea, or loose stool, is a common gastrointestinal symptom and can occur for a number of reasons. Gastrointestinal diseases that cause malabsorption will also cause diarrhea.

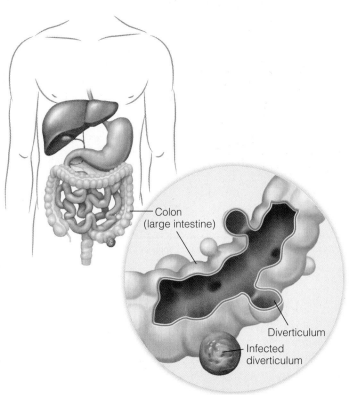

Colon
(large intestine)

Diverticulum

Infected
diverticulum

■ FIGURE 20-4 **Diverticula in the Colon.**

CLIENT EDUCATION CHECKLIST	✓ Fiber in the Diet
Intervention	**Example**
Assess fiber intake.	Conduct brief diet history or food frequency for intake of plant-based foods (grains, vegetables, fruit, nuts, seeds).
Educate on the role of fiber in digestion.	Fiber increases stool weight and promotes laxation.
Educate on target goal for fiber and fluid intake.	Recommendation for fiber intake is up to 38 gm daily for adults. Adequate intake of liquid is essential to avoid constipation and abdominal discomfort.
Advise that fiber be added slowly to minimize bloating side effect.	Add only 5 gm fiber/day each week until goal is reached. Suggestions include: • Swapping refined flour products for whole grains (breads, cereals, crackers) • Consuming plant-based proteins (beans, peas, lentils) • Targeting intake of at least 5 fruit/vegetable servings a day. Whole fruits and vegetables with edible skin have more fiber than juices and peeled produce • Checking ingredient labels of grain products for the word "whole" in the listing (e.g., *whole wheat* vs. *wheat*)

Outline sources of fiber.
Plant foods "closest to the original form" will have more fiber than the processed version of the same food.
	Poor sources of fiber:
	White flour bread, baked goods, pasta and cereals, processed grains, white rice, potato without skin, most juices
	*Animal-based foods contain NO fiber
	2–3 gm fiber/serving:
	    Banana—1
	    Broccoli, raw—1 cup
	    Cantaloupe—1cup
	    Nuts, mixed—1oz
	    Peach with skin—1
	3–4 gm fiber/serving:
	    Almonds—1 oz
	    Apple with skin—1
	    Apricots, dried—10 halves
	    Carrots, raw—1 large
	    Corn, cooked—1 cup
	    Green beans, cooked—1 cup
	    Oatmeal, regular—1 cup
	    Orange—1
	    Pear with skin—1
	    Peas, cooked—1 cup
	    Potato, baked with skin—1
	    Rice, brown—1cup
	    Strawberries—1 cup
	4–5 gm fiber/serving:
	    Figs, dried—2
	    Mini or shredded wheat cereal—1 cup
	    Spinach, cooked—1 cup
	    Whole wheat cereal flakes—1 cup
	Over 5 gm fiber/serving:
	    Beans, kidney, black, cooked—1cup
	    Bran nugget cereal—½ cup
	    Bran flakes—1 cup
	    Bulgur, cooked—1 cup
	    Chickpeas, cooked—1 cup
	    Lentils, cooked—1 cup
	    Raisins—1cup
	    Raspberries or blackberries—1 cup
	    Soybeans, cooked—1 cup

Source: Food values from United States Department of Agriculture, Nutrient Data Laboratory. Retrieved April 27, 2009, from http://www.nal.usda.gov/fnic/foodcomp/search/

BOX 20-6	**Nutrition Intervention for Intestinal Gas**

Decrease amount of swallowed air:

- Refrain from chewing gum.
- Avoid carbonated beverages.
- Eat more slowly.
- Have fit of dentures checked.
- Do not smoke.

Experiment with diet to determine individual contributors. Avoid *excessive* intake:

- Raffinose—in beans, cabbage, broccoli, brussel sprouts, cauliflower. Try digestive enzyme specifically for beans if needed.
- Lactose—in dairy products. Try digestive aids with lactase if needed.
- Fructose—in pears, wheat, fruits in general, additive in some drinks.
- Sorbitol—in sugar-free and low-carbohydrate foods. Watch for other sugar alcohols in foods (all ending in "ol").
- Fiber—soluble fiber in oats, beans, peas, and fruit more likely to contribute than insoluble fiber in wheat and some vegetables.

Source: Adapted from: NIDDK, 2008c.

Pancreatic disease, lactose intolerance, celiac disease, and inflammatory bowel disease are examples. Infections from a virus, bacteria, or parasite are other causes. Prescription and over-the-counter medications, including laxative abuse, can cause diarrhea and should be included in the client assessment. Medical management of diarrhea illness is determined by the cause. Nutrition intervention for acute diarrhea is used to reduce symptoms and optimize hydration. In adults with self-limited diarrhea, the nurse can recommend adequate intake of liquids and temporary avoidance of foods felt to worsen symptoms, such as fatty foods, lactose, and caffeine. Children and older adults with diarrhea who are at risk of dehydration should be given an oral rehydration solution as a beverage. Withholding food for over 24 hours is felt to be inappropriate and does not contribute to improved health (King, Glass, Bresee, & Duggan, 2003) The BRAT diet outlined in Practice Pearl: BRAT Diet is often recommended but

PRACTICE PEARL

BRAT Diet

The BRAT diet has long been recommended as a transitional diet in self-limiting diarrhea illnesses. **B**ananas, **R**ice, **A**pplesauce, and **T**oast will provide pectin, a soluble fiber felt to slow diarrhea, and needed calories when intake is low. This diet can be unnecessarily restrictive and should not be used for any length of time. There is no scientific evidence to support its recommendation.

has little research to support its use (King et al., 2003). Traveler's diarrhea or diarrhea from rotavirus or antibiotic use may benefit from consumption of probiotics in the diet as outlined in Hot Topic: Probiotics Use in Intestinal Disease Treatment.

Chronic diarrhea places an individual at increased nutritional risk because of potential alterations in fluid and electrolyte status as well as malabsorption. Medical management of chronic diarrhea is determined by the cause. Nutrition intervention is used to reduce symptoms while providing adequate nutrition. Diets should be altered as indicated based on the etiology of the symptoms. Altered intake of fat, lactose, caffeine, sugar alcohols, and simple sugar can be tried when a cause is unknown. Intake of excessive sweetened beverages and juices should be assessed because of the osmotic effect of these substances on the gut. In some individuals, many foods are avoided in anticipation of intolerance or symptoms. Overall nutrition status should be monitored when intake is low or lim-

hot Topic

Probiotics Use in Intestinal Disease Treatment

Probiotics are nonpathogenic bacteria that are found in the intestine. Some of these same microbes have been long used in the fermentation process of foods and can be found in yogurt, acidophilus milk, and over-the-counter supplement form. Supplemental forms of probiotics, available as granules, liquids, capsules, and tablets, are considered dietary supplements and, therefore, are not regulated as medications. Lactobacillus and bifidobacterium species are commonly used commercially. More recently, research has focused on the potential beneficial effect that probiotics have on intestinal health by modifying the intestinal flora. Although exact mechanisms remain unclear, varying lactobacillus and bifidobacterium species have demonstrated positive benefits in the treatment of diarrhea from antibiotic use, traveler's diarrhea, and rotavirus in children. Benefit in the management of inflammatory bowel disease, pancreatitis, and lactose intolerance has also been reported. Enhancement of the mucosal barrier and immunomodulating effects from probiotic use are suspected to contribute to these positive effects. Further research must be done before conclusions on use of specific bacteria species and dosing can be made, especially with over-the-counter supplemental probiotics. Meanwhile, the nurse can recommend consumption of yogurt with active cultures as a source of these beneficial bacteria to clients with self-limiting diarrheas, those taking antibiotics, and in clients with bowel disease in whom consumption of dairy foods is not contraindicated. Although treatment with supplemental forms of probiotics is considered generally safe, their use should be avoided by individuals who are immunocompromised. When these products are prescribed as part of medical treatment, the nurse should exercise caution handling the supplements near any open portal, such as a central venous line, because contamination and sepsis have been reported.

Sources: Adapted from: Douglas & Sanders, 2008; Goldin & Gorbach, 2008; Kligler & Cohrssen, 2008; Rhode, Bartolini, & Jones, 2009; Wallace, 2009.

ited in variety. An RD should be consulted when chronic diarrhea leads to weight loss or overly restricted intake.

Liver Disease

Liver disease has a negative effect on nutritional health because the liver functions to metabolize and store many nutrients. Carbohydrate is stored in the liver as glycogen. Fat digestion requires bile that is produced in the liver. Fatty acids and cholesterol are produced in the liver. Plasma proteins responsible for transport of substances, blood clotting, immune status, and maintenance of plasma volume are produced in the liver. The liver activates or stores most vitamins and iron. Hepatic disease can lead to a decline in nutritional status without adequate nutrition intervention. Figure 20-5 ■ depicts the hepatobiliary system responsible for many components of nutrient digestion and metabolism.

Fatty Liver

Fatty infiltration of the liver is considered a health risk because of the potential for it to advance to more severe liver disease, including hepatitis and cirrhosis (Saadeh, 2007). Clients can present with no physical complaints but are found to have an enlarged liver and elevated liver enzyme levels on examination. Generally, the disease is divided into two classifications, nonalcoholic fatty liver disease and alcoholic fatty liver disease, denoting the variant etiologies. Excessive alcohol intake contributes to fatty liver when intake chronically exceeds 20 to 30 gm of alcohol daily (AGA, 2002). One standard drink contains approximately 14 gm of alcohol, as depicted in Chapter 7. Nonalcoholic fatty liver has many contributing factors, some of which are nutritional and cover both extremes of the nutritional health spectrum. Obesity, excessive parenteral nutrition, insulin resistance, diabetes, and hypertriglyceridemia are associated with development of fatty liver. Starvation, rapid weight loss (such as with extreme diets or intestinal bypass surgeries), and small bowel resection also are linked with fatty liver development.

Ingestion of toxic mushrooms and hypervitaminosis A are additional causes (Adams, Angulo, & Lindor, 2005).

Nutrition Intervention

The goal of nutrition therapy with fatty liver disease is to reduce any nutritional risk factors for the disease and its progression. Abstinence from alcohol is indicated in alcoholic fatty liver disease. Treatment of nonalcoholic liver disease should address the suspected etiology. In the overweight or obese individual, slow weight loss is recommended as a best practice. Rapid loss of weight should be avoided because it contributes to fatty liver (Leclercq & Horsmans, 2008). Elevated lipid and glucose levels should be addressed with nutrition intervention and lifestyle management, including exercise (Leclercq & Horsmans, 2008). The prevalence of fatty liver is emerging as a major contributor to liver disease in the Western world and may be linked to the increase in obesity and diabetes prevalence (Adams et al., 2005). The nurse should educate individuals with obesity about the risk of fatty liver and provide lifestyle management guidance on risk reduction through weight management.

Hepatitis

Inflammation of the liver occurs because of viral infection, alcoholic liver disease, or autoimmune disease. Fatty liver can progress to cause inflammation, called steatohepatitis. Symptoms of hepatitis include gastrointestinal complaints, such as abdominal pain, nausea, vomiting, diarrhea, and anorexia. Fatigue, joint pain, and fever further worsen symptoms. Risk of poor nutrition health is increased with hepatitis because of these symptoms and the effects of hepatic inflammation on nutrient metabolism and requirements. Lethargy and gastrointestinal complaints result in diminished oral intake. Metabolism and storage of both macronutrients and micronutrients are affected. Glycogen storage, production of bile, and storage of vitamins and minerals are negatively affected by liver disease. Energy requirements are elevated in hepatitis because of inflammation and fever.

MyNursingKit Hepatitis

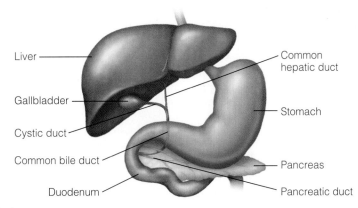

■ **FIGURE 20-5   Hepatobiliary System.**

When alcoholism contributes to the development of hepatitis, nutrition risk is compounded because of the negative effects of chronic alcohol intake on nutrition status. Nutrient intake, metabolism, and storage are affected by alcohol. Oral intake can be chronically compromised when alcohol takes the place of food intake. Metabolic and absorptive loss of vitamins and minerals occurs because of alcohol and nutrient interactions. Chapter 7 outlines these risks further.

Nutrition Intervention

The goal of nutrition therapy with hepatitis is to slow disease progression and foster regeneration of hepatocytes while providing adequate nutrition (Dietitians of Canada, 2003). High intake of calories and protein is needed to provide adequate substrate to promote healing and nutrition restoration. Up to 40% more calories can be required from baseline needs to meet energy requirements (Dietitians of Canada, 2003). Intake of almost twice the recommended dietary allowance of protein is advised. It can be difficult for the client to meet these increased nutritional needs because of symptoms such as nausea, fatigue, and lack of appetite. The nurse can suggest frequent, high nutrient density meals to avoid the abdominal discomfort associated with large meals. Ample high-carbohydrate foods will supply needed glycogen sources while also allaying nausea. Oral liquid calorie supplements can be used to augment intake. Alcohol should be avoided. Supplementation with a multivitamin is indicated if intake is low. Preparations with iron and those with high doses of vitamin A or niacin should be avoided because of potential liver toxicity (Dietitians of Canada, 2003). The nurse should carefully assess the client's use of other nutritional supplements, especially herbals, because some are hepatotoxic. Hot Topic: Complementary Medicine Use in Liver Disease illustrates the importance of including this information in a nursing assessment.

Cirrhosis

Progressive damage to the liver most often occurs because of hepatitis or alcoholism. Inborn errors of metabolism, such as Wilson's disease and hemochromatosis, blockage of the bile duct, and exposure to hepatotoxins, are risk factors for development of cirrhosis (NIDDK, 2008d). As fibrosis replaces hepatocytes, liver function is diminished. Abdominal pain, fatigue, nausea, and weight loss are symptoms that will affect nutritional health. Nutritional health already can be diminished when alcohol is the precipitating cause of the liver disease. If cirrhosis progresses, portal vein hypertension and altered intestinal capillary pressure and permeability cause the third-spacing of fluids in the abdominal cavity known as ascites. Production of plasma proteins, such as albumin, is decreased with advanced liver disease and this reduction contributes to loss of oncotic pressure, worsening ascites. Later, renal involvement impairs free-water excretion and plasma

hot Topic

Complementary Medicine Use in Liver Disease

Survey research has reported that between 12% and 50% of people with liver disease take herbal supplements (Seeff et al., 2008). Little is known about the long-term effects of many of these substances that act like medication in the body. Many over-the-counter botanicals are known to be hepatotoxic. The nurse should advise clients with liver disease to abstain from using the following (Dietitians of Canada, 2003; Seeff, 2007; Stickel & Schuppan, 2007):

- Artemesia
- Cascara
- Comfrey
- Germander (teucrium)
- Horse chestnut
- Jin-bu-huang
- Kava
- Kombucha mushrooms
- Mistletoe
- Pennyroyal
- Sassafras
- Senna
- Shark cartilage
- Skullcap
- Valerian

Several herbal supplements are popular with clients with viral hepatitis. Milk thistle (silymarin) is taken by more than 15% of clients who use herbal medicines and have liver disease (Seeff et al., 2008). Its efficacy is unknown despite some reports of symptomatic improvements (Rambaldi, Jacobs, & Gluud, 2007). Further research is needed on this use of complementary medicine in conjunction with standard antiviral treatment. Licorice root, or glycyrrhizin, is also marketed for liver health and used by those with liver disease for its anti-inflammatory properties, but research is very limited and without conclusion (NCCAM, 2009). Licorice should not be combined with diuretic use because of an associated combined effect on low blood potassium levels (NCCAM, 2008). These examples are good reminders to the nurse to assess use of alternative medicine when conducting client assessments. Further information on complementary medicine and supplements is outlined in Chapter 25.

sodium levels become diluted. Ascites can cause a sense of abdominal pressure and early satiety that lowers oral intake. Portal hypertension is a risk factor for esophageal varices and then bleeding. Alterations in digestion and metabolism further poor nutritional health by limiting substrate storage and production of bile with a fibrotic liver (Tsiaousi, Hatzitolios, Trygonis, & Savopoulos, 2008). Overall, there are multifactorial contributors to the risk of malnutrition in the individual with cirrhosis.

Nutrition Intervention

The goal of nutrition therapy in cirrhosis is enhancement of nutritional status and minimization of disease symptoms.

Adequate calories and protein are essential to avoid weight loss and degradation of plasma and skeletal proteins. An RD should calculate a diet prescription to provide 1.5 gm protein/kg (Dietitians of Canada, 2003; Tsiaousi et al., 2008). Restriction of protein in an attempt to prophylax encephalopathy is contraindicated; chronic intake of low protein will lead to skeletal protein degradation, malnutrition, and elevated by-products of protein breakdown that will tax the metabolic capabilities of the liver. A high-carbohydrate intake is needed because of decreased glycogen storage capabilities. The nurse should suggest a high-carbohydrate snack before bedtime to maintain plasma glucose during the night (Cabre & Gassull, 2005). If steatorrhea is present because of reduced bile production, a trial of a reduced-fat diet is indicated. Decreased fat intake will lessen its contribution to overall energy intake and a proportionate increased intake of carbohydrate calories will be needed. Early satiety can be managed with frequent small meals containing nutrient-dense foods. Liquids should be consumed between meals to avoid gastric distention during a meal. Oral liquid calorie and protein supplements can be used if intake of solid food is poor.

When ascites is present, a sodium restriction is indicated to facilitate diuresis. Commonly, a 2-gm sodium prescription is prescribed. Stricter restrictions are used by some but are poorly tolerated by clients, are impossible to comply with outside the hospital, and are unpalatable. When strict sodium restriction is prescribed, the nurse should assess whether it contributes to poor intake and risk of malnutrition. Malnutrition will result in plummeting plasma albumin and then worsening of ascites. The nurse and the dietitian can work together to assist the client in optimizing oral intake within the parameters of a reduced sodium diet to avoid this risk. A Client Education Checklist for reduced sodium diets is contained in Chapter 6. The nurse should educate individuals with ascites about the importance of complying with a low-sodium diet to minimize ascites and its associated symptoms.

A fluid restriction is indicated in the treatment of ascites only when hyponatremia occurs (DiCecco & Francisco-Ziller, 2006). The level of fluid restriction varies with the magnitude of the hyponatremia and can be as low as 1,000 mL a day. Close attention to intake of nutrient-dense liquids is needed. Wasting precious fluid volume on only water or other calorie-free beverages will provide little in the way of nutrition yet contribute to the sensation of fullness.

Ingestion of raw shellfish should be avoided in liver disease. Infection with the bacteria *Vibrio vulnificus*, harbored in shellfish, is a risk to liver health (NIDDK, 2008d). The nurse should also educate the client about the hazards of using hepatotoxic herbal supplements and large doses of vitamins or minerals.

Hepatic Encephalopathy

Hepatic encephalopathy occurs in advanced liver disease because of decompensation in liver function. Many theories exist as to the cause of the neuropsychiatric symptoms, which range from tremor, incoordination, and mild forgetfulness to somnolence, confusion, and coma. One well-accepted theory is that the advancement of liver disease with portal hypertension leads to development of collateral circulation around the liver, called portosystemic shunting, and that this change in combination with poor metabolic function of the liver results in elevated accumulation of ammonia in the body. Ammonia is a by-product of protein metabolism and in health is converted to urea by the liver and then excreted. Sources of ammonia include dietary protein, breakdown of skeletal protein, blood in the gastrointestinal tract, colonic bacterial metabolism, and the production of the amino acid glutamine by the intestine. Elevated ammonia levels cross the blood-brain barrier, which is felt to be a main cause of encephalopathic symptoms (Blei, Cordoba, & the Practice Parameters Committee, 2001). Medical management of hepatic encephalopathy is aimed at decreasing the presence of precipitating factors, such as gastrointestinal bleeding, and other nitrogenous substances in the gut. Antibiotics and the nonabsorbable sugar lactulose are used to promote catharsis and elimination of offending gut flora (Blei et al., 2001). In the short term, reduction of nutritional sources of proteins is also indicated in the client with moderate to severe encephalopathy (Plauth et al., 2006).

Nutrition Intervention

The goal of nutrition therapy in hepatic encephalopathy is to reduce the contribution of excessive protein metabolism to ammonia production in the short term only. Long-term protein restriction will foster protein catabolism in the body, which will result in increased ammonia production. Additionally, some ammonia is normally taken up by skeletal muscle, but loss of skeletal muscle with prolonged protein restriction will worsen intolerance to protein intake, a vicious cycle that can be avoided with proper diet prescription. Protein can be restricted for a day or two with acute encephalopathy and then reintroduced slowly until up to 1.5 gm/kg are provided (Schulz, Campos, & Coelho, 2008). A starting point for enteral protein intake in acute severe encephalopathy is 0.5 gm/kg/day. Use of plant proteins can improve tolerance in the client who responds poorly to reintroduction of higher amounts of protein because of the effects of the fiber content on intestinal bacteria that contribute to ammonia (Blei et al., 2001). Branched-chain amino acid supplements can also be used in the client who does not tolerate additional protein, but these do not produce results in all clients, are expensive, and often are not palatable (Schulz et al., 2008).

It is imperative that adequate calories are supplied to the client with encephalopathy or skeletal muscle catabolism will result, worsening the ammonia load in the body. The

Table 20-3	Dietary Calculations with Hepatic Encephalopathy

Sources of 7–10 gm of Protein

- Beans, peas, lentils, cooked—½ cup
- Cheese—1 oz
- Egg, whole—1
- Milk or yogurt—8 oz
- Meat, fish, poultry—1 oz
- Nuts, avg—2 oz
- Peanut butter—2 tbsp
- Tofu, firm—1 oz

Sample Calculations of Protein Prescription

1. Initial treatment of acute hepatic encephalopathy calls for 0.5 gm protein/kg/day.
2. After 24–48 hours, advance protein intake by 10 gm/day and monitor tolerance.
3. Goal is up to 1.5 gm protein/kg body weight/day.

Example: Mr. George has end-stage alcoholic liver disease with encephalopathy. He weighs 220 lb (100 kg).

1. Initial treatment calls for 0.5 gm/kg/day or 0.5 gm/day × 100 kg body weight = 50 gm protein/day.
2. After 24–48 hours, Mr. George should be advanced to 60 gm protein/day and monitored.
3. Goal of 1.5 gm protein/ kg/day is 150 grams of protein.

$CT_?$ Calculate a sample daily diet that includes only 50 grams of protein. What will that look like to the client when it is divided into the three meals of the day? What issues might arise with such a low intake?
Source: Food values from United States Department of Agriculture, Nutrient Data Laboratory. Retrieved April 27, 2009, from http://www.nal.usda.gov/fnic/foodcomp/search

route of enteral nutrition depends on the client's level of consciousness. Clients with mild to moderate symptoms will need assistance with feeding because of forgetfulness, confusion, or agitation. Use of a feeding tube is indicated in clients with altered consciousness. Table 20-3 outlines calculations used in determining protein recommendations in hepatic encephalopathy. The nurse should be aware of the sources of protein in the diet when assessing the client's tolerance to nutrition intervention and then diet advancement. The nurse should educate family members about the short-term protein restriction to avoid inadvertent dietary noncompliance from food gifts brought to the hospital.

Pancreatic Conditions

The pancreas has both exocrine and endocrine functions. Endocrine functions include the production of insulin. Exocrine functions affect the digestion and absorption of food. Digestive enzymes lipase and amylase are produced in the pancreas and are involved in the digestion of fats and carbohydrates, respectively. When the pancreas is inflamed or secretions of pancreatic enzymes are obstructed, there are nutritional consequences because of maldigestion and poor ab-

sorption. Pancreatitis and cystic fibrosis are two conditions where altered digestion and absorption occur.

Pancreatitis

Inflammation of the pancreas can occur from chronic alcohol intake or blockage of the common bile duct with gallstones. The result is damage to the organ by the digestive enzymes that it produces and normally excretes into the small bowel. Pancreatitis can be acute or chronic. Symptoms include abdominal pain, nausea, vomiting, and fever. Dehydration and altered electrolyte status are common results. Severe pancreatitis can lead to sepsis and organ failure because of infection. Nutritional health is compromised with both acute and chronic pancreatitis because of diminished pancreatic enzyme excretion into the small bowel. Fat malabsorption in particular is common. Fear of pain associated with eating can cause some individuals to decrease oral intake to manage symptoms. With severe nausea and vomiting, oral intake becomes minimal. Nutritional status can be further challenged because the inflammatory process and fever increase metabolic rate and requirement for energy. Rapid attention to nutritional needs is advised to avoid a downward spiral of nutrition status. Medical management includes pain management and acute fluid resuscitation with correction of electrolyte abnormalities.

Nutrition Intervention

The goal of nutrition therapy in pancreatitis is the rapid provision of adequate nutrition to preserve nutritional status and maintain intestinal function while not contributing to symptoms. Once fluid and electrolyte status is stabilized, enteral nutrition support can begin. In many clients, advancement to a clear liquid, then low-fat, diet is sufficient when pancreatitis resolves in a matter of days. In clients requiring longer than 7 days of inadequate intake, use of an elemental or semi-elemental feeding that reaches distal to the ligament of Treitz is recommended to provide adequate nutrition while not stimulating the pancreas (AGA Institute, 2007). Elemental formulas have no fat and contain protein in the form of amino acids and short peptides and thus do not require pancreatic enzymes for digestion. Most commonly, jejunal placement of a feeding tube is recommended with severe pancreatitis to deliver these formulas and bypass the upper small bowel. Enteral nutrition support has been reported to be preferable to parenteral nutrition support for pancreatic rest because of reduced risks with similar benefits (AGA Institute, 2007). Increased intestinal permeability and bacterial translocation are risk factors for further infection in pancreatitis when the gut is not utilized (Thomson, 2008). Parenteral nutrition does provide adequate nutrition and pancreatic rest at an increased financial cost compared with enteral nutrition but also carries with it a risk of hyperglycemia and sepsis. Parenteral nutrition is indicated when there is intestinal obstruction or enteral nutrition is not tolerated. Hyperglycemia can occur because of the high glucose content of parenteral nutrition and possible diminished endocrine pancreas function. Glucose amounts can be adjusted and insulin prescribed as indicated. Hypertriglyceridemia can also occur with pancreatitis. Triglyceride levels above 400 mg/dL are a contraindication to use of parenteral lipid infusions in the formula (Curtis & Kudsk, 2007). Parenteral nutrition support is outlined in more detail in Chapter 16.

Transition to oral feeding in pancreatitis proceeds to a low-fat diet. When chronic pancreatitis persists with associated symptoms, the low-fat prescription remains in effect. Alcohol is the cause of the majority of cases of chronic pancreatitis and should be avoided (Meier et al., 2006). Loss of exocrine pancreatic function results in diminished pancreatic enzyme production and maldigestion and malabsorption, especially of fat. Clients are prescribed oral pancreatic enzyme replacements to be consumed with food. The nurse should warn clients who are on enzyme replacement to avoid a high-fiber diet because the fiber can render the enzyme replacement unavailable (Giger, Stanga, & DeLegge, 2004). If loss of endocrine pancreatic function occurs, diabetes develops and the client then is prescribed a carbohydrate-controlled diet as outlined in Chapter 19. Replacement of fat-soluble vitamins is indicated if fat malabsorption is chronic. Some clients with chronic pancreatitis require ongoing supplementation with an enteral feeding formula because of persistent pain and inadequate intake.

Cystic Fibrosis and Pancreatic Insufficiency

Cystic fibrosis is a genetic condition that involves a mutation in a protein responsible for transporting ions in epithelial cells. The result is a decreased clearance of mucus that is found on these cells, including those in the pancreas and lung. The result is frequent lung infections, compromised pulmonary function, and insufficient pancreatic enzyme excretion into the small intestine. Salt losses in sweat exceed those of healthy individuals and can lead to acute salt depletion. Nutrition status is affected because of poor digestion and absorption of nutrients and the high metabolic needs associated with infection and labored breathing. Low levels of essential fats and fat-soluble vitamins are reported because of fat malabsorption (Erskine, Lingard, & Sontag, 2007). If the disease affects pancreatic endocrine function, diabetes and its associated health risks are added to the existing risks. Poor growth patterns are common in children with cystic fibrosis, and the majority is found below the 10th percentile for height and weight (Stallings et al., 2008). There is a strong association between survival and nutrition status in this population (Erskine et al., 2007). In addition to medications used to treat pulmonary infections when they occur, routine treatment of cystic fibrosis includes use of pancreatic enzyme replacements. Lung transplantation is used in some clients with severely compromised pulmonary function.

Nutrition Intervention

The goal of nutrition in cystic fibrosis is the achievement and maintenance of adequate nutritional status. In children, this goal includes sufficient nutrition to support normal growth and development. A high-energy diet is needed to meet the increased metabolic needs associated with the disease (Stallings et al., 2008). Oral liquid nutrition supplements can be used in addition to the diet to support weight gain but have no demonstrated benefit over an equal amount of energy from food intake (Smyth & Walters, 2007). Fat intake is not restricted and instead adequate intake of pancreatic enzyme replacements should accompany meals and snacks to facilitate digestion and absorption. Attention must be given to the status of fat-soluble vitamins because of associated malabsorption. In particular, poor blood levels of vitamin D have been reported even with adequate intake (Rovner, Stallings, Schall, Leonard, & Zemel, 2007). A multivitamin that contains adequate fat-soluble vitamins is recommended (Hayek, 2006). Salt should be added to foods to replace that lost in sweat. Children and adults with cystic fibrosis should be monitored by a multidisciplinary team that is expert in the treatment of this disease.

Gallbladder Disease

The gallbladder is the site of bile storage. Bile is secreted from the gallbladder into the small intestine for use in the digestion and absorption of fat and fat-soluble substances, including vitamins A, D, E, and K. Gallstones can form in the gallbladder for a number of reasons, some associated with nutrition. A stone is comprised of cholesterol, bilirubin, and calcium salts that have precipitated from the bile (Cuevas, Miguel, Reyes, Zanlungo, & Nervi, 2004). Symptomatic gallstones cause pain and may block the common bile duct, causing pancreatitis. Although the treatment of gallbladder disease and gallstones is primarily surgical, nutrition has a role in both the prevention and development of gallstones. High-risk populations for cholelithiasis, or gallstone, formation include individuals who are obese or have experienced rapid weight loss or prolonged fasting. Additionally, the use of parenteral nutrition is associated with reduced gallbladder contractions and eventual stone formation (Venneman & van Erpecum, 2006). A high intake of fiber and a low intake of saturated and trans fat are both linked with a lower risk of cholelithiasis (Cuevas et al., 2004; Venneman & van Erpecum, 2006). This association may be related to altered bile composition and increased intestinal transit.

The nurse can advise individuals seeking to lose weight to avoid rapid weight loss because of the associated risk of cholelithiasis. In addition, clients can be encouraged to adhere to the guidelines for a healthy intake of fiber and fat that avoids excessive consumption of saturated and trans fats.

| NURSING CARE PLAN | Nutrition and Irritable Bowel Syndrome

CASE STUDY

Jane is a 48-year-old attorney who was recently diagnosed with irritable bowel syndrome. She relates that she has been troubled her entire adult life with alternating periods of prolonged diarrhea followed by constipation. A recent prolonged bout of diarrhea, accompanied by a 10-pound weight loss and malaise, convinced her to see a physician. She had a general checkup followed by a colonoscopy. Although she expressed "relief that it is not anything serious," she has come to the nurse for guidance on diet and lifestyle management. She is particularly concerned about finding nonpharmacological means to control her symptoms.

Applying the Nursing Process

ASSESSMENT

Height: 5 feet 7 inches Weight: 144 pounds (usual weight is 155) BMI: 22.5
BP 138/76 P 76 R 14
Skin smooth and clear, moist mucous membranes

DIAGNOSIS

Readiness for enhanced knowledge related to request for dietary management
Diarrhea related to altered intestinal motility

EXPECTED OUTCOMES

Absence of diarrhea with regular pattern of defecation
Weight return to normal
Diet plan that is acceptable for client's lifestyle

INTERVENTIONS

Diary that records food intake, bowel elimination pattern, activity, stressful events
Analysis of diary entries

Discussion of foods that seem related to changes in bowel elimination
Development of a meal plan that is balanced and eliminates foods that trigger diarrhea or constipation

EVALUATION

Two months later, Jane reports that she is feeling much better. Using a diary helped her to identify that consumption of coffee- and milk-based beverages from a coffee shop were frequently followed by diarrhea. She also found that on days when she had meetings with the executive team at work, she was more prone to diarrhea. Although she suggested that stress was a contributor to her problem, she did not feel that she could effectively change her work situation. She was adding more fiber to her diet by eating more whole grain bread and a high-fiber cereal in the morning. She related that she had been unwilling to add fiber to her diet for fear that it would increase diarrhea, so she was pleased to find that it added bulk to her stools and did not cause diarrhea. Constipation had not been a problem so she was unable to identify triggers for that. Figure 20-6 ■ outlines the nursing process for this case.

Critical Thinking in the Nursing Process

1. **When a client with irritable bowel syndrome is experiencing constipation, what are some nonpharmacological interventions the nurse can suggest?**

Nutrition and Irritable Bowel Syndrome   *(continued)*

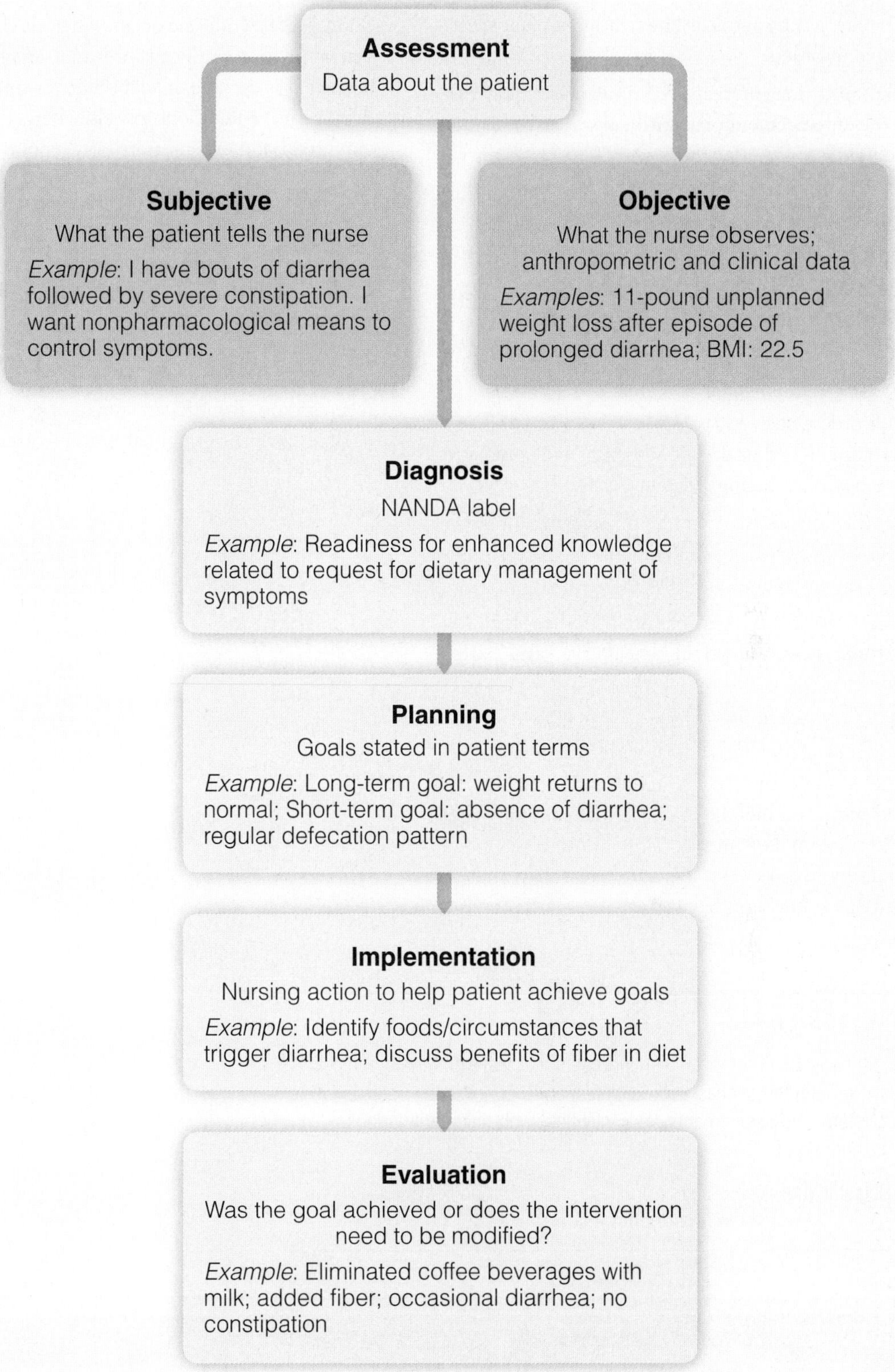

Assessment
Data about the patient

Subjective
What the patient tells the nurse

Example: I have bouts of diarrhea followed by severe constipation. I want nonpharmacological means to control symptoms.

Objective
What the nurse observes; anthropometric and clinical data

Examples: 11-pound unplanned weight loss after episode of prolonged diarrhea; BMI: 22.5

Diagnosis
NANDA label

Example: Readiness for enhanced knowledge related to request for dietary management of symptoms

Planning
Goals stated in patient terms

Example: Long-term goal: weight returns to normal; Short-term goal: absence of diarrhea; regular defecation pattern

Implementation
Nursing action to help patient achieve goals

Example: Identify foods/circumstances that trigger diarrhea; discuss benefits of fiber in diet

Evaluation
Was the goal achieved or does the intervention need to be modified?

Example: Eliminated coffee beverages with milk; added fiber; occasional diarrhea; no constipation

■ FIGURE 20-6   **Nursing Care Plan Process: Nutrition and Irritable Bowel Syndrome.**

CHAPTER SUMMARY

- Nutrition plays a central role in the treatment of most gastrointestinal disorders.

- The goal of nutrition intervention in gastrointestinal disorders is the enhancement of nutritional status while minimizing disease symptoms.

- Dysphagia requires a customized nutrition prescription based on an individual's ability to safely swallow various textures of foods and thicknesses of liquids.

- Gastric reflux disease is treated with nutrition intervention that targets foods that decrease lower esophageal sphincter pressure, minimize gastric pressure, and lessen irritation to the esophagus.

- Motility disorders, such as gastroparesis and dumping syndrome, require diets that do not add excessive volume to the stomach while meeting nutrient needs.

- Lactose intolerance is managed by maximizing intake of lactose-containing foods to the amount tolerated to preserve endogenous lactase synthesis.

- Celiac sprue is treated with a lifelong diet avoiding gluten, which is contained in wheat, rye, and barley products.

- Inflammatory bowel disease can lead to malnutrition because of loss of absorptive surface with inflammation or surgical resection, diminished intake because of symptoms, and increased metabolic needs that go unmet because of limited intake. Nutrition intervention is focused on providing a high-calorie, high-protein intake and replacement of lost nutrients based on the site of the disease.

- Short bowel syndrome occurs when disease or surgical resection leads to reduced intestinal length. The ileum in particular is capable of adapting over time to compensate for absorptive functions lost elsewhere. A combination of parenteral and enteral nutrition support is needed while adaptation occurs.

- A diet with adequate fiber is indicated in the treatment of diverticulosis, constipation, and irritable bowel disease. High-fiber intake should be avoided with diverticulitis or by those using pancreatic enzyme replacements.

- Adequate calories and protein are essential in the treatment of liver disease to promote healing and hepatocyte regeneration. Insufficient intake of protein can lead to a decline in nutritional health and worsened symptoms of ascites and encephalopathy. Ascites is treated with a low-sodium diet.

- Pancreatitis requires a reduction in pancreatic stimulation with either a low-fat diet or elemental enteral nutrition formula, depending on symptoms. Parenteral nutrition support for pancreatitis is not the treatment of choice except in cases of intestinal obstruction or failure of enteral support.

- Cystic fibrosis can result in pancreatic insufficiency and poor digestion and absorption of fat. A diet high in energy with adequate intake of fat-soluble vitamins is essential to maintain nutrition status.

- Risk of gallstones is increased with obesity, rapid weight loss, prolonged fasting, and a high intake of saturated and trans fats.

EXPLORE **PEARSON mynursingkit**™

MyNursingKit is your one stop for online chapter review materials and resources. Prepare for success with additional NCLEX®-style practice questions, interactive assignments and activities, web links, animations and videos, and more!

Register your access code from the front of your book at
www.mynursingkit.com.

NCLEX® QUESTIONS

1. The nurse is teaching a client about prevention of dumping syndrome. The client should be instructed to:
   1. Eat small, frequent meals throughout the day.
   2. Increase consumption of dairy products.
   3. Temporarily increase consumption of simple sugars.
   4. Eat foods that are low in fiber.

2. The nurse is working with a client who has dysphagia as a result of a stroke. Which of the following liquids would be easiest and safest for the client to swallow?
   1. Herbal tea
   2. Pear nectar
   3. Orange juice
   4. Commercial supplements, like Ensure

3. A client has been admitted to the hospital with acute diverticulitis. The nurse expects that the first diet ordered for the client will be:
1. Gluten free
2. High fiber
3. Clear liquid
4. Low fat

4. Which of the following would be a good snack for the client with hepatitis?
1. Banana
2. Jell-O and sugar cookie
3. Carrots and broccoli with cream cheese dip
4. Omelet

5. A child has been diagnosed with celiac disease. When teaching the family, what foods should the nurse be certain are eliminated from the diet plan?
1. Puffed rice cereal
2. Whole wheat bread
3. Peanuts
4. Yogurt

REFERENCES

Adams, L. A., Angulo, P., & Lindor, K. D. (2005). Nonalcoholic fatty liver disease. *Canadian Medical Association Journal, 172,* 899–905.

Aghdassi, E., Wendland, B. E., Stapleton, M., & Raman, M. (2007). Adequacy of nutritional intake in a Canadian population of patients with Crohn's disease. *Journal of the American Dietetic Association, 107,* 1575–1580.

American Gastroenterological Association (AGA). (2002). American Gastroenterological Association medical position statement: Nonalcoholic fatty liver disease. *Gastroenterology, 123,* 1702–1704.

American Gastroenterological Association (AGA). (2003). American Gastroenterological Association medical position statement: Short bowel syndrome and intestinal transplantation. *Gastroenterology, 124,* 1105–1110.

American Gastroenterological Association (AGA). (2008). American Gastroenterological Association medical position statement on the management of gastroesophageal reflux disease. *Gastroenterology, 135,* 1383–1391.

American Gastroenterological Association (AGA) Institute. (2007). AGA Institute medical position on acute pancreatitis. *Gastroenterology, 132,* 2019–2021.

Amerine, E. (2006). Celiac disease goes against the grain. *Nursing, 36,* 46–48.

Blei, A. T., Cordoba, J., & the Practice Parameters Committee of the American College of Gastroenterology. (2001). Hepatic encephalopathy. *American Journal of Gastroenterology, 96,* 1968–1976.

Bottino-Bravo, P., & Thomson, J. (2008). When it's hard to swallow: Dysphagia in home care. *Home Healthcare Nurse, 26,* 244–250.

Buchman, A. L. (2006). Short-bowel syndrome. *Clinical Gastroenterology, 3,* 1066–1070.

Cabre, E., & Gassull, M. A. (2005). Nutrition in liver disease. *Current Opinions in Clinical Nutrition and Metabolic Care, 8,* 545–555.

Canadian Celiac Association. (2008). *The gluten free diet.* Retrieved April 27, 2009, from http://www.celiac.ca/EnglishCCA/egfdiet.html

Celiac Sprue Association. (2008). *Gluten free diet.* Retrieved April 27, 2009, from http://www.csaceliacs.org/#

Chaiyakunapruk, N., Kitikannakorn, N., Nathisuwan, S., Leeprakobboon, K., & Leelasettagool, C. (2006). The efficacy of ginger for the prevention of postoperative nausea and vomiting: A meta-analysis. *American Journal of Obstetrics and Gynecology, 194,* 95–99.

Chand, N., & Mihas, A. (2006). Celiac disease: Current concepts in diagnosis and treatment. *Journal of Clinical Gastroenterology, 40,* 3–14.

Clark, C., & DeLegge, M. (2008). Irritable bowel syndrome: A practical approach. *Nutrition in Clinical Practice, 23,* 263–267.

Cuevas, A., Miguel, J. F., Reyes, M. S., Zanlungo, S., & Nervi, F. (2004). Diet as a risk factor for cholesterol gallstone disease. *Journal of the American College of Nutrition, 23,* 187–196.

Curtis, C. S., & Kudsk, K. A. (2007). Nutrition support in pancreatitis. *Surgical Clinics of North America, 87,* 1403–1415.

DiCecco, S. R., & Francisco-Ziller, N. (2006). Nutrition in alcoholic liver disease. *Nutrition in Clinical Care, 21,* 245–254.

Dickey, W. (2008). Making oats safer for patients with coeliac disease. *European Journal of Gastroenterology and Hepatology, 20,* 494–495.

Dietitians of Canada. (2003). Hepatitis C: Nutrition care. Retrieved March 1, 2009, from http://www.dietitians.ca/resources/HepC_Guidelines_enA.pdf

Dorner, B. (2002, August). Tough to swallow. *Today's Dietitian,* 28–31.

Douglas, L. C., & Sanders, M. E. (2008). Probiotics and prebiotics in dietetics practice. *Journal of the American Dietetic Association, 108,* 510–521.

Eadala, P., Waud, J. P., Matthews, S. B., Green, J. T., & Campbell, A. K. (2009). Quantifying the 'hidden' lactose in drugs used for the treatment of gastrointestinal conditions. *Alimetary Pharmacology Therapeutics, 29,* 677–687.

Erskine, J. M., Lingard, C., & Sontag, M. (2007). Update on enteral nutrition support for cystic fibrosis. *Nutrition in Clinical Practice, 22,* 223–232.

Fernandez-Banares, F. (2006). Nutritional care of the patient with constipation. *Best Practice & Research Clinical Gastroenterology, 20,* 575–587.

Giger, U., Stanga, Z., & DeLegge, M. H. (2004). Management of chronic pancreatitis. *Nutrition in Clinical Practice, 19,* 37-49.

Goldin, B. R., & Gorbach, S. L. (2008). Clinical indications for probiotics: An overview. *Clinical Infectious Disease, 46,* S96–S100.

Green, P., & Cellier, C. (2007). Celiac disease. *New England Journal of Medicine, 357,* 1731–1743.

Hayek, K. M. (2006). Medical nutrition therapy for cystic fibrosis: Beyond pancreatic enzyme replacement therapy. *Journal of the American Dietetic Association, 106,* 1186–1188.

Heyman, M. B. for the Committee on Nutrition. (2006). Lactose intolerance in infants, children, and adolescents. *Pediatrics, 118,* 1279–1286.

Heyman, R., Guggenbuhl, P., Corbel, A., Bridoux-Henno, L., Tourtelier, Y., Balencon-Morival, M., et al. (2009). Effect of gluten-free diet on bone mineral density in children with celiac disease. *Gastroenterologie Clinique et Biologique,* doi: 10.1016/j.gcb.2008.09.020.

Horvath, A., Dziechciarz, P., & Szajewska, H. (2008). The effect of thickened-feed interventions on gastroesophageal reflux in infants: Systematic review and meta-analysis of randomized, controlled trials. *Pediatrics, 122,* e1268–e1277.

REFERENCES *(continued)*

Hsieh, C. (2005). Treatment of constipation in older adults. *American Family Physician, 72,* 2277–2284.

Jackson, C. S., & Buchman, A. L. (2004). The nutritional management of short bowel syndrome. *Nutrition in Clinical Care, 7,* 114–121.

Jeejeebhoy, K. N. (2002a). Clinical nutrition: 6. Management of nutritional problems of patients with Crohn's disease. *Canadian Medical Association Journal, 166,* 913–918.

Jeejeebhoy, K. N. (2002b). Short bowel syndrome: A nutritional and medical approach. *Canadian Medical Association Journal, 166,* 1297–1302.

Karamanolis, G., & Tack, J. (2006). Nutrition and motility disorders. *Best Practice & Research Clinical Gastroenterology, 20,* 485–505.

King, C. K., Glass, R., Bresee, J. S., & Duggan, C. (2003). Managing acute gastroenteritis among children: Oral rehydration, maintenance and nutrition therapy. *Morbidity and Mortality Weekly Review, 52,* 1–16.

Kligler, B., & Cohrssen, A. (2008). Probiotics. *American Family Physician, 78,* 1073–1078.

Kupper, C. (2005). Dietary guidelines and implementation for celiac disease. *Gastroenterology, 128,* S121–S127.

Langmead, L., & Rampton, D. S. (2001). Review article: Herbal treatment in gastrointestinal and liver disease—benefits and dangers. *Alimentary Pharmacology & Therapeutics, 15,* 1239–1252.

Leclercq, I. A., & Horsmans, Y. (2008). Nonalcoholic fatty liver disease: The potential role of nutritional management. *Current Opinion in Clinical Nutrition and Metabolic Care, 11,* 766–773.

Leslie, P., Carding, P. N., & Wilson, J. A. (2003). Investigation and management of chronic dysphagia. *British Medical Journal, 326,* 433–436.

Marcason, W. (2008). What is the latest research regarding the avoidance of nuts, seeds, corn, and popcorn in diverticular disease. *Journal of the American Dietetic Association, 108,* 1956.

Matarese, L. E., Costa, G., Bond, G., Stamos, J., Koritsky, D., O'Keefe, S., et al. (2007). Therapeutic efficacy of intestinal and multivisceral transplantation: Survival and nutrition outcome. *Nutrition in Clinical Practice, 22,* 474–481.

Matarese, L. E., & Steiger, E. (2006). Dietary and medical management of short bowel syndrome in adult patients. *Journal of Clinical Gastroenterology, 40,* S85–S93.

Meier, R., Ockenga, J., Pertkiewicz, M., Pap, A., Milinic, N., MacFie, J., et al. (2006). ESPEN guidelines on enteral nutrition: Pancreas. *Clinical Nutrition, 25,* 275–284.

Nanthakomon, T., & Pongrojpaw, D. (2006). The efficacy of ginger in prevention of post-operative nausea and vomiting after major gynecological surgery. *Journal of the Medical Association of Thailand, 89,* 130–136.

National Center for Complementary and Alternative Medicine (NCCAM). (2008). *Licorice root.* Retrieved February 23, 2009, from http://nccam.nih.gov/health/licoriceroot/

National Center for Complementary and Alternative Medicine (NCCAM). (2009). *CAM and hepatitis C: A focus on herbal supplements.* Retrieved February 23, 2009, from http://nccam.nih.gov/health/hepatitisc/

National Dysphagia Diet Task Force. (2002). *The National Dysphagia Diet: Standardization for optimal care.* Chicago: American Dietetic Association.

National Institute of Diabetes and Digestive and Kidney Diseases (NIDDK), National Institutes of Health (NIH). (2006). *Lactose intolerance.* Retrieved April 27, 2009, from http://www.digestive.niddk.nih.gov

National Institute of Diabetes and Digestive and Kidney Diseases (NIDDK), National Institutes of Health (NIH). (2007a). *Heartburn, gastroesophageal reflux, and gastroesophageal reflux disease.* Retrieved April 27, 2009, from http://www.digestive.niddk.nih.gov

National Institute of Diabetes and Digestive and Kidney Diseases (NIDDK), National Institutes of Health (NIH). (2007b). *Rapid gastric emptying.* Retrieved April 27, 2009, from http://www.digestive.niddk.nih.gov

National Institute of Diabetes and Digestive and Kidney Diseases (NIDDK), National Institutes of Health (NIH). (2007c). *Gastroparesis.* Retrieved April 27, 2009, from http://www.digestive.niddk.nih.gov

National Institute of Diabetes and Digestive and Kidney Diseases (NIDDK), National Institutes of Health (NIH). (2007d). *Irritable bowel syndrome.* Retrieved April 27, 2009, from http://www.digestive.niddk.nih.gov

National Institute of Diabetes and Digestive and Kidney Diseases (NIDDK), National Institutes of Health (NIH). (2008a). *Celiac disease.* Retrieved April 27, 2009, from http://www.digestive.niddk.nih.gov

National Institute of Diabetes and Digestive and Kidney Diseases (NIDDK), National Institutes of Health (NIH). (2008b). *Diverticulosis and diverticulitis.* Retrieved April 27, 2009, from http://www.digestive.niddk.nih.gov

National Institute of Diabetes and Digestive and Kidney Diseases (NIDDK), National Institutes of Health (NIH). (2008c). *Gas in the digestive tract.* Retrieved April 27, 2009, from http://www.digestive.niddk.nih.gov

National Institute of Diabetes and Digestive and Kidney Diseases (NIDDK), National Institutes of Health (NIH). (2008d). *What I need to know about cirrhosis.* Retrieved April 27, 2009, from http://www.digestive.niddk.nih.gov

National Institutes of Health (NIH). (2004). *NIH consensus development conference on celiac disease.* Retrieved April 27, 2009, from http://consensus.nih.gov/2004/2004CeliacDisease118html.htm

Niewinski, M. M. (2008). Advances in celiac disease and gluten-free diet. *Journal of the American Dietetic Association, 108,* 661–672.

O'Keefe, S. J., Buchman, A. L., Fishbein, T. M., Jeejeebhoy, K. N., Jeppesen, P. B., & Shaffer, J. (2006). Short bowel syndrome and intestinal failure: Consensus definitions and overview. *Clinical Gastroenterology, 4,* 6–10.

Olsson, C., Hornell, A., Ivarrson, A., & Snyder, Y. M. (2008). The everyday life of adolescent coeliacs: Issues of importance for compliance with the gluten-free diet. *Journal of Human Nutrition & Dietetics, 21,* 359–367.

O'Sullivan, M. (2009). Session 3: Joint Nutrition Society and Irish Nutrition and Dietetic Institute Symposium on Nutrition and Autoimmune Disease: Nutrition in Crohn's disease. *Proceedings of the Nutrition Society,* doi: 10.1017/S0029665109001025.

O'Sullivan, M., & O'Morain, C. (2006). Nutrition in inflammatory bowel disease. *Best Practice & Research Clinical Gastroenterology, 20,* 561–573.

Ozdemir, O., Mete, E., Catal, F., & Ozol, D. (2009). Food intolerances and eosinophilic esophagitis in childhood. *Digestive Diseases and Sciences, 54,* 8–14.

Palmer, J. L., & Metheny, N. A. (2008). Preventing aspiration in older adults with dysphagia. *American Journal of Nursing, 108,* 40–48.

Patrick, A., & Epstein, O. (2008). Gastroparesis. *Alimentary Pharmacology & Therapeutics, 27,* 724–740.

Plauth, M., Cabre, E., Riggio, O., Assis-Camilo, M., Pirlich, M., & Kondrup, J. (2006). ESPEN guidelines on enteral nutrition: Liver disease. *Clinical Nutrition, 25,* 285–294.

Rambaldi, A., Jacobs, B. P., & Gluud, C. (2007). Milk thistle for alcoholic and/or hepatitis B or C virus liver disease. *Cochrane Database Systematic Review, 17,* CD003620.

Rhode, C. L., Bartolini, V., & Jones, N. (2009). The use of probiotics in the prevention and treatment of antibiotic-associated diarrhea with specific interest in *clostridium difficile-*associated diarrhea. *Nutrition in Clinical Practice, 24,* 33–40.

Rovner, A. J., Stallings, V. A., Schall, J. I., Leonard, M. B., & Zemel, B. S. (2007). Vitamin D insufficiency in children, adolescents, and young adults with cystic fibrosis despite routine oral supplementation. *American Journal of Clinical Nutrition, 86,* 1694–1699.

REFERENCES *(continued)*

Saadeh, S. (2007). Nonalcoholic fatty liver disease and obesity. *Nutrition in Clinical Practice, 22,* 1–10.

Salzman, H., & Lillie, D. (2005). Diverticular disease: Diagnosis and treatment. *American Family Physician, 72,* 1229–1234.

Schulz, G. J., Campos, A. C., & Coelho, J. C. (2008). The role of nutrition in hepatic encephalopathy. *Current Opinion in Clinical Nutrition and Metabolic Care, 11,* 275–280.

Seeff, L. B. (2007). Herbal hepatotoxicity. *Clinics in Liver Disease, 11,* 577–596.

Seeff, L. B., Curto, T. M., Szabo, G., Everson, G. T., Bonkovsky, H. L., Dienstag, J. L., et al. (2008). Herbal product use by persons enrolled in the Hepatitis C Antiviral Long-term Treatment Against Cirrhosis (HALT-C) Trial. *Hepatology, 47,* 605–612.

Shakil, A., Church, R. J., & Rao, S. S. (2008). Gastrointestinal complications of diabetes. *American Family Physician, 77,* 1697–1702.

Smyth, R., & Walters, S. (2007). Oral calorie supplements for cystic fibrosis. *Cochrane Database Systematic Reviews, 24,* CD000406.

Stallings, V.A., Stark, L. J., Robinson, K. A., Feranchak, A. P. & Quinton, H., Clinical Practice Guidelines on Growth and Nutrition Subcommittee, Ad hoc Working Group (2008). Evidence-based practice recommendations for nutrition-related management of children and adults with cystic fibrosis and pancreatic insufficiency: Results

of a systematic review. *Journal of the American Dietetic Association, 108,* 832–839.

Stickel, F., & Schuppan, D. (2007). Herbal medicine in the treatment of liver diseases. *Digestive and Liver Diseases, 39,* 293–304.

Strate, L. L., Liu, Y. L., Syngl, S., Aldoori, W. H., & Giovannucci, E. L. (2008). Nut, corn, and popcorn consumption and the incidence of diverticular disease. *Journal of the American Medical Association, 300,* 907–914.

Strowd, L., Kysima, J., Pillsbury, D., Valley, T., & Rubin, B. R. (2008). Dysphagia dietary guidelines and the rheology of nutritional feeds and barium test feeds. *Chest, 133,* 1397–1401.

Tack, J. (2007). Gastric motor disorders. *Best Practice & Research Clinical Gastroenterology, 21,* 633–644.

Thompson, T. (2004). Gluten contamination of commercial oat products in the United States. *New England Journal of Medicine, 351,* 2021–2022.

Thomson, A. (2008). Nutritional support in acute pancreatitis. *Current Opinion in Clinical Nutrition and Metabolic Care, 11,* 261–266.

Tsiaousi, E. T., Hatzitolios, A., Trygonis, S., & Savopoulos, C. (2008). Malnutrition in end stage liver disease: Recommendations and nutritional support. *Journal of Gastroenterology and Hepatology, 23,* 527–533.

Turner, D., Steinhart, A. H., & Griffiths, A. M. (2007). Omega-3 fatty acids for maintenance of remission in ulcerative colitis. *Cochrane Database Systematic Review,* CD006443.

Turner, D., Zlotkin, S. H., Shah, P. S., & Griffiths, A. M. (2009). Omega-3 fatty acids for maintenance of remission in Crohn's disease. *Cochrane Database Systematic Review,* CD006320.

Vemulapalli, R. (2008). Diet and lifestyle modifications in the management of gastroesophageal reflux disease. *Nutrition in Clinical Practice, 23,* 293–298.

Venneman, N. G., & van Erpecum, K. J. (2006). Gallstone disease: Primary and secondary prevention. *Best Practice & Research Clinical Gastroenterology, 20,* 1063–1073.

Wallace, B. (2009). Clinical use of probiotics in the pediatric population. *Nutrition in Clinical Practice, 24,* 50–59.

Zarkadas, M., Cranney, A., Case, S., Molloy, M., Switzer, C., Graham, I. D., et al. (2006). The impact of a gluten-free diet on adults with coeliac disease: Results of a national survey. *Journal of Human Nutrition & Dietetics, 19,* 41–49.

21 Renal Disease

Cynthia Hoffman

WHAT WILL YOU LEARN?

1. To classify the nutritional and metabolic complications of acute and chronic renal failure.
2. To translate the rationale for the various dietary modifications indicated in the treatment of renal failure.
3. To assess the risk factors for malnutrition in the individual with chronic renal failure and formulate nursing interventions.
4. To differentiate between dietary interventions for renal failure and nephrotic syndrome.
5. To examine the potential consequences of kidney transplant on nutritional health.
6. To develop nursing interventions to reduce the dietary risk factors for kidney stones.
7. To evaluate the current evidence regarding diet influences on risk of urinary tract infection.

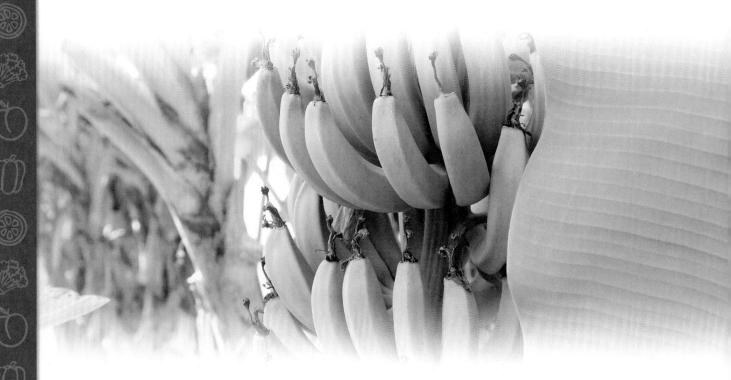

DID YOU KNOW?

▶ Nutrition needs change with renal failure depending on what treatment is used.

▶ Nephrotic syndrome can lead to protein malnutrition.

▶ A low-calcium diet is *not* recommended to prevent calcium-based kidney stones.

▶ Daily intake of cranberry juice may help some individuals lower risk of urinary tract infection.

472

KEY TERMS

acute renal failure (ARF), *474*

anuria, *478*

chronic kidney disease (CKD), *474*

continuous renal replacement therapies (CRRT), *476*

dialysate, *475*

high biological value proteins, *478*

intradialytic parenteral nutrition (IDPN), *484*

maintenance hemodialysis (MHD), *475*

metabolic acidosis, *485*

metabolic bone disease, *479*

oliguria, *478*

peritoneal dialysis (PD), *475*

protein-energy wasting (PEW), *484*

recombinant human erythropoietin, *483*

renal replacement therapy (RRT), *474*

uremia, *474*

Nutrition and Renal Disease

The National Institutes of Health estimate that 26 million Americans have chronic kidney disease, representing a 3% increase over the last 15 years (Coresh et al., 2007). The kidneys have multiple roles in nutrient metabolism, including excreting the end-products of protein metabolism and regulating both fluid and electrolyte balance and micronutrient metabolism. Altered kidney function—whether it is renal failure or other disorders of the kidney, ureter, or bladder—and the various techniques for treating these diseases can impact dietary intake and nutritional health. Because of the complex relationship between kidney disease, nutrient intake, and dietary modifications, a thorough nutrition assessment is an important intervention for individuals with these conditions. In a challenging role, the nurse must work with a registered dietitian to assist in gathering data for a nutrition assessment, provide education regarding dietary modifications, encourage appropriate food choices, and evaluate the adequacy of nutrient intake in this population already at risk for poor nutritional health.

Physiology and Functions of the Kidney

Each kidney is composed of 1 million functioning units called nephrons. The nephron consists of the glomeruli, which produce an ultrafiltrate; the proximal tubules, which reabsorb small nutrients (glucose, amino acids, and vitamins); the distal tubules and loop of Henle, which regulate fluid and electrolytes; and the renal pelvis, which controls the concentration of urine. Figure 21-1 ■ outlines the physiology of the kidney.

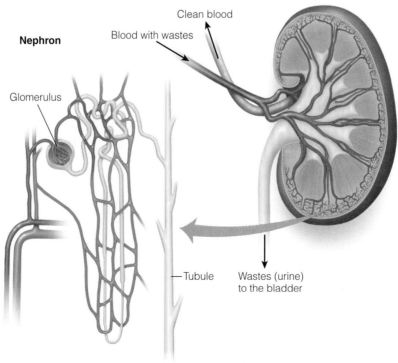

Clean blood

Blood with wastes

Nephron

Glomerulus

Tubule

Wastes (urine) to the bladder

■ **FIGURE 21-1 Normal Kidney Physiology.**

BOX 21-1	Functions of the Kidneys

- Excretion of metabolic end-products of protein metabolism (urea, uric acid, creatinine, and ammonia)
- Excretion of other by-products of metabolism and drugs
- Regulation of electrolyte (sodium, potassium, and chloride), mineral (calcium, phosphorus, and magnesium), and trace element (selenium and zinc) content in the body
- Maintenance of fluid and acid-base balance
- Urine production (concentration or dilution)
- Control of blood pressure
- Regulation of the concentration of extracellular and intracellular fluid
- Maintenance of calcium and phosphorus balance
- Activation of vitamins
- Synthesis of hormones

The main nutrition-related functions of the kidneys are the urinary excretion of end-products of protein metabolism and the reabsorption or excretion as needed of electrolytes, vitamins, minerals, and trace elements. Renal diseases impact specific segments of the nephron. Therefore, the manifestations and nutritional implications of the different diseases reflect the loss of function of that portion of the nephron. The functions of the kidneys are reviewed in Box 21-1.

Renal Failure

Renal failure can occur acutely in response to a sudden compromise to kidney function, such as with a vascular event, or it may occur more slowly and become a chronic condition because of chronic diseases such as hypertension or diabetes. Nutrition intervention is aimed at the resulting metabolic and physiological consequences of renal failure that can vary among clients.

Acute Renal Failure

Acute renal failure (ARF) is a rapid decline in kidney function identified by an increase in blood urea nitrogen (BUN) and creatinine (Cr). Both glomerular filtration and tubular function are reduced. Causes of ARF are categorized as prerenal, postrenal, and renal (intrarenal or intrinsic) and are described in Table 21-1.

ARF results in nutritional and metabolic changes that are a result of the body's response to the physiological stress associated with the condition. These changes include:

- Hypermetabolism
- Protein catabolism with muscle wasting
- Glucose intolerance (hyperglycemia and insulin resistance)
- Fluid and electrolyte imbalances (metabolic acidosis)

Table 21-1   Causes of Acute Renal Failure

Category	Mechanism of Action	Medical Cause
Prerenal	Decreased renal blood flow	Sepsis Hypotension Reduced cardiac output
Postrenal	Obstruction of urine outflow	Ureteral obstruction Bladder outlet obstruction
Renal (intrarenal or intrinsic)	Damage to renal parenchyma	Hypertension Acute tubular necrosis Nephrotoxicity

Because of the critical nature of ARF, nutrition support plays a vital role and potentially affects clinical outcome. The primary goals of nutrition support in ARF are to maintain nutritional status, decrease protein catabolism, and address the metabolic complications of ARF.

Chronic Kidney Disease

Chronic kidney disease (CKD) is a disease characterized by the slow, steady decline in renal function. The decrease in renal function is evaluated by the glomerular filtration rate (GFR) that measures the quantity of ultrafiltrate produced by the nephrons of both kidneys. The progressive decline in renal function with decreasing GFR is permanent, eventually resulting in the development of **uremia,** the accumulation of nitrogenous waste products in the blood. Treatment can involve kidney transplantation or **renal replacement therapy (RRT),** also called dialysis. The National Kidney Foundation (NKF) classifies the severity of kidney disease by stages that are based on the GFR. Stages 1 through 4 are the preliminary stages when the GFR begins to decline. Stage 5 CKD applies to the time when the GFR declines to the degree that RRT must be initiated. Diabetes mellitus and hypertension are the two primary causes of CKD. A complete list of the causes of CKD is found in Box 21-2.

It was first demonstrated over 20 years ago that the restriction of dietary protein intake and control of hypertension can delay the progression of renal failure in animals (Brenner,

BOX 21-2	Causes of Chronic Kidney Disease

- Diabetes mellitus
- Hypertension
- Glomerulonephritis
- Interstitial nephritis
- Hereditary and congenital diseases
- Autoimmune disease

1983; Klahr, Buerkert, & Purkerson, 1983). High-protein diets are associated with microalbuminuria, a loss of small amounts of albumin in the urine considered a risk factor for renal failure (Almeida et al., 2008). More recently, there have been mixed research findings on whether a low-protein diet delays progression of renal failure in those with renal insufficiency. Some have reported that there is a slower decline in GFR after the introduction of a very low-protein diet in those with moderate renal insufficiency (Klahr et al., 1994; Mitch, 2005). In particular, use of plant proteins, such as soy, has been reported to slow the decline in kidney function (Almeida et al., 2008; Bernstein, Treyszon, & Zhaoping, 2007). However, other long-term studies have not shown an overall effect of a low-protein diet on slowing the rate of GFR decline in this population with early signs of renal failure (Bernstein et al., 2007). The need to restrict protein intake to slow the progression of kidney disease remains a controversial topic. Current recommendations suggest that additional, long-term research is necessary to confirm optimal dietary protein intake in renal failure (Fouque, Laville, & Boissel, 2007).

Nutritional therapy is an important component in all stages of CKD. However, when CKD progresses to Stage 5, necessitating dialysis, nutritional therapy is a mandatory part of treatment efforts. Extensive education regarding protein modification and electrolyte restrictions is needed. The nutrition care of the individual receiving dialysis should include frequent assessment of nutritional status and provision of adequate nutrient intake to counter the catabolic effects of both uremia and the protein losses found with dialysis treatments. BUN and Cr are elevated as a result of the nitrogenous by-products of metabolism that are normally excreted by the kidney but instead accumulate in the blood. The physical symptoms of uremia include malaise, weakness, muscle cramps, and itching. Nutritional complications of uremia include nausea, vomiting, and a metallic taste in the mouth. Both the physical symptoms and nutritional consequences of uremia have a negative effect on dietary intake and nutrition status that can put the client at risk for malnutrition.

Treatment

Treatment for renal failure depends on the severity. RRT may be implemented and spans several types of dialysis treatments that function to filter the blood, replacing that function normally done by the kidney. Treatment can also include kidney transplantation. Medical nutrition therapy is an integral part of treatment and aims to slow progression of the disease and alleviate physical and metabolic symptoms.

Renal Replacement Therapies

Dialysis techniques include maintenance hemodialysis (MHD), peritoneal dialysis (PD), and continuous renal replacement therapy (CRRT). Nutritional care is specific to each type of dialysis and based on the impact of the treatment

on caloric needs, intermittent or continuous technique, protein loss into the dialysis fluid, and the extent of the technique on fluid and solute clearance.

Hemodialysis

Maintenance hemodialysis (MHD) is a most common RRT used to treat CKD and acute ARF. A venous catheter or arteriovenous fistula is used for access and blood is pumped through a filter with a semipermeable membrane. The composition of the dialysis fluid, or **dialysate,** is physiologically similar to plasma. The physiological principle of counter-current exchange is utilized to facilitate the removal of waste products, potassium, and, to a lesser degree, phosphorus and magnesium. Fluid removal is accomplished through a pressure gradient between the dialysis fluid and blood. Hemodialysis also clears amino acids, low molecular weight proteins, and some water-soluble vitamins. Such treatments are required three times per week with sessions lasting for 3 to 5 hours.

Medical nutrition therapy for individuals on MHD includes modification of protein and electrolyte intake. Protein intake must be balanced between the need to prevent accumulation of urea and other waste products with a moderate protein restriction yet high enough to prevent protein-calorie malnutrition. Nutrient requirements for adults receiving all types of dialysis are found in Table 21-2.

Peritoneal Dialysis

Peritoneal dialysis (PD) is an effective form of dialysis for CKD and ARF. In PD, a catheter is placed into the peritoneal cavity, utilizing the semipermeable membrane of the peritoneum for removal of solutes and water. A high-dextrose content dialysate is infused into the peritoneum, which removes urea, potassium, and other solutes through the process of diffusion. The dialysate contains a high concentration of dextrose to utilize the principle of osmotic pressure so that water passes from the blood into the dialysate. The dialysate is then withdrawn from the peritoneum and discarded. Intermittent PD treatments last for about 10 to 12 hours, three times per week. In continuous ambulatory peritoneal dialysis (CAPD), four to five exchanges are completed daily with indwelling time of 4 to 6 hours each. CAPD allows a more liberal dietary intake than hemodialysis because the technique provides constant therapy with continual removal of electrolytes. However, amino acid losses are greater with PD than with hemodialysis, causing protein requirements to also be greater. Sodium, potassium, and phosphorus intake are also more liberal than in hemodialysis to adjust for losses into the dialysate. Additionally, there is absorption of glucose from the PD solution, which can provide a significant source of calories and glucose. Practice Pearl: Calorie Contribution of Peritoneal Dialysate outlines how to calculate this contribution to energy intake. A PD solution is available that contains a glucose polymer rather than dextrose (Wolfson,

Table 21-2   Daily Nutrient Recommendations in Renal Disease

	Energy (kcals/kg)	Protein (gm/kg)	Sodium (gm)	Potassium (gm/day)	Phosphorus (mg/day)	Other Nutrients
Chronic Kidney Disease, Stages 1–4 (no dialysis)	30–40	GFR greater than 55: 0.8 GFR 25–55: 0.6	1–3	Based on serum level	800–1000	
Acute Renal Failure (no dialysis)	35–50	0.6–2*	1–3**	2–3**	Based on serum level	
Hemodialysis	35 (less than 60 years of age) 30–35 (greater than 60 years of age)	1.2 (50% HBV)	1–3**	2–3**	800–1000	Supplement with water soluble vitamins intended for dialysis clients. Avoid > 200 mg vitamin C
Peritoneal Dialysis	25–30	1.2–1.3 (50% HBV)	2–4	3–4	1500 mg/day	Supplement with water soluble vitamins intended for dialysis clients. Avoid > 200 mg vitamin C
Renal Transplant	Increased immediate post-transplant Sufficient for weight maintenance after recovery	No restriction Avoid excessive intake	Depends on underlying disease (such as hypertension)	No restriction	No restriction	Monitor for hyperlipidemia or diabetes that require dietary modification
Nephrotic Syndrome	35	0.8 + amount in 24-hour urine collection	2 (individualize depending on edema)	N/A	N/A	Follow guidelines for hyperlipidemia if present

*Protein intake in ARF is individualized based on presence of hypercatabolism, treatment method, and degree of renal failure.
**Electrolyte intake in ARF is individualized based on degree of renal failure, treatment method, and serum level.
Sources: Adapted from: Appel, 2006; Cano et al., 2006; NKF, 2000; Teplan et al., 2009.

Piraino, Hamburger, & Morton, 2002). This glucose polymer is not absorbed and, therefore, does not provide additional glucose calories. This alternative is beneficial for individuals with diabetes mellitus receiving PD. The nutritional requirements for PD are described in Table 21-2.

Continuous Renal Replacement Therapy
Continuous renal replacement therapies (CRRT) are slow, continuous forms of dialysis generally used for hospitalized clients who are unable to tolerate PD or hemodialysis. This form of RRT encompasses a variety of techniques, all using a counter-current exchange similar to standard hemodialysis. However, in hemodialysis a pump provides the hydrostatic pressure necessary for dialysis. Here, either the client's own blood pressure or a pump is used to assist this process, depending on the specific technique. Clearance of fluid and solutes is slower at this low pressure yet is considered adequate because of the continuous process. Because of this slow, continuous clearance, this type of RRT provides a more physiological rate

of fluid and solute removal and is an ideal dialysis technique for the unstable client in a critical care setting.

Clients receiving CRRT are always hospitalized, usually in a critical care setting, and may have other comorbidities that preclude adequate oral intake. As a result, clients may also require enteral or parenteral nutrition support. Standard enteral or parenteral nutrition formulas can be used without the need to restrict fluids or electrolytes because this dialysis technique provides greater fluid and nitrogenous waste removal than with PD or hemodialysis. Likewise, for clients who can take an oral diet, the diet prescription is more liberal than with other types of dialysis. Dialysis solutions used in CRRT may contain dextrose, which is absorbed and therefore provides a source of calories. A 1.5% dextrose dialysate with a flow rate of 1 liter per hour (43% absorption) provides 525 kilocalories. A 2.5% dextrose solution with a 1-liter-per-hour flow rate (45%) absorption provides 920 kilocalories. This solution represents a significant source of calories and should be included in the nutrition prescription. It should be

PRACTICE PEARL

Calorie Contribution of Peritoneal Dialysate

- There is 60% to 70% net absorption of glucose from peritoneal dialysis solutions.
- Dextrose has 3.4 kcalories/gm.
- The nurse can calculate glucose absorption based on dialysate volume and concentration

To calculate the caloric intake from the solution:

1. Multiply the volume per session by number of exchanges/day = Total Volume
2. Multiply Total Volume by the percentage of dextrose in solution = Amount of dextrose (gm)
3. Multiply the grams of dextrose by percent uptake (80%)
4. Multiply the grams of absorbed dextrose by 3.4 (kcal per gram) = total calories absorbed from the solution

Example: Client is receiving continuous peritoneal dialysis 4 times per day using a 2-liter solution of 2.5% monohydrous dextrose

1. 2,000 mL solution × 4 exchanges per day = 8,000 mL dialysis solution
2. 8,000 mL × 0.025 (2.5%) = 200 gm dextrose/day
3. 200 gm dextrose × 0.80 (80% uptake) = 160 gm dextrose
4. 160 gm × 3.4 (calories per gram) = *544 kcal net absorption per day*

emphasized that standard intravenous dextrose solutions, such as D5W (5% dextrose in water) do not provide significant calories. The dextrose calories absorbed from the dialysate during CRRT are so high because of the total volume (24 liters) over a 1 day period.

Medical Nutrition Therapy for Renal Failure

The human body has a remarkable ability to rid itself of unnecessary waste products. The kidney plays a vital role in this process. Because food and liquids are the source of many of these waste products, diet modification plays a very important role when kidney function is diminished. The nutritional management of CKD is designed to maintain BUN within acceptable ranges; regulate sodium, potassium, and phosphorus levels; regulate fluid balance; and prevent the wasting and malnutrition often associated with this disease. Specific nutrient recommendations depend on the degree and type of renal failure, clinical symptoms, and treatment modalities (Beto & Bansal, 2004). The unique nutritional needs of children must also be considered to allow for normal growth and development, as outlined in Lifespan Box: CKD in Pediatric Clients. The diet modifications for all age groups also aim to control the complex interactions among calcium, phosphorus, and vitamin D that lead to bone disease as a long-term complication in this population. Table 21-2 outlines the nutritional recommendations for all types of renal failure.

Lifespan

CKD in Pediatric Clients

CKD can occur at any time of life; however, its impact can be felt most significantly in children. Because growth failure is commonly found in infants and children with renal failure, treatment efforts are focused on normalizing growth and development. Medical management in pediatric clients can include hemodialysis or PD, but a kidney transplant gives the child the best chance for a normal life.

As with adults, a restricted diet and uremic symptoms such as fatigue and anorexia contribute to nutrition challenges. Poor nutritional status ultimately affects bone mineralization and overall growth in pediatric clients. Any change in nutrition status or growth pattern requires aggressive dietary intervention. Some children may require nutrition follow-up as frequently as every 2 to 4 weeks. All children with CKD should have growth and nutrition status assessed twice as frequently as recommended for healthy children the same age.

Nutrition concerns include adequacy of energy intake. Extra calories are required if the child is malnourished or if growth retardation is present. Nutrition supplementation with oral liquid supplements or tube feeding may be indicated if nutritional needs cannot be met with oral intake alone. The restriction of protein intake for pediatric clients is controversial. Adequate protein intake is needed to prevent malnutrition, yet excessive intake should be avoided in order to protect the kidneys from additional damage. The required daily allowance (RDA) for protein is generally the minimum suggested for pediatric clients. Children must also maintain restrictions of sodium, potassium, phosphorus, and fluids. Electrolyte and fluid intake should be individualized according to the specific child's needs.

Control of calcium-phosphorus balance is critical for adequate bone mineralization and growth. Calcium intake from food and supplements provides additional calcium while binding excess phosphorus. Serum vitamin D levels should be measured once a year and supplementation given when values are low. Management of the persistent metabolic acidosis that occurs with CKD is critical to prevent bone demineralization and growth failure. Newer treatments especially beneficial for pediatric clients include recombinant human erythropoietin (rHuEPO) and human growth hormone (rHGH).

The treatment of pediatric CKD is an intense process and mandates a multidisciplinary team of care providers working together to help the infant or child and the family manage this disease. This multidisciplinary team should include a pediatrician, dialysis nurses, a nephrologist, registered dietitian, social worker, and psychologist or counselor. Both the National Institutes of Health and the National Kidney Foundation (NKF) have educational and support Web sites that can be helpful to the child with CKD and their family.

Sources: Kavey et al., 2007; NKF, 2009b; Vimalachandra el al., 2006; Voss, Hodson, & Crompton, 2007.

MyNursingKit National Kidney Foundation—Children

MyNursingKit National Institutes for Health—Children and Renal Failure

Energy

Energy requirements vary greatly in individuals with renal failure. In all forms of renal failure, it is of primary importance to provide adequate energy intake to maintain a healthy body weight. Energy intake must also be sufficient to prevent protein breakdown for use as energy. In Stages 1 through 4 of CKD, there is not an appreciable increase in energy needs that is attributed to renal failure. Factors that normally affect metabolic rate apply to this population as well. However, ARF is a hypermetabolic illness and can require a higher than normal energy intake (Cano et al., 2006). Energy requirements vary greatly; consideration must be given to comorbid illnesses, complications (wound healing, infection), and treatment modality. Energy needs for all stages of CKD and ARF, including different treatment methods, are found in Table 21-2.

Protein

The factors to be considered when determining dietary protein allowance are the type and frequency of RRT and the nutritional status of the individual client. RRTs are a drain on body protein stores because of a loss of amino acids from the blood system into the dialysis fluid, which in turn can result in compromised nutritional health. The amount of amino acids lost in the dialysate varies depending on the type of dialysis and the filter used. Up to 10 gm of amino acids can be lost during hemodialysis with slightly higher losses found during PD (Dukkipati & Kopple, 2009). Protein recommendations have been summarized in Table 21-2. Overall nutritional status, including weight changes and serum BUN and Cr, should be monitored between dialysis treatments and protein allowance adjusted accordingly.

In addition to the amount of protein prescribed, it is recommended that at least 50% of dietary protein come from high biological value sources (NKF, 2006). **High biological value proteins** are those that contain all eight or nine (eight for adults, nine for infants and children) essential amino acids needed to sustain life. Examples include eggs, milk, and meat (including poultry and fish). Soy protein is a plant protein that contains all the essential amino acids. The emphasis primarily on these animal protein sources can be especially difficult because uremia can cause taste alterations that cause meats to seem less palatable. Practice Pearl: Taste Alterations and Protein Foods outlines some advice that the nurse can offer to help with taste alterations. Essential amino acids are reviewed in full detail in Chapter 3.

Lipids

CKD is associated with risk of developing cardiovascular disease (Kaysen, 2009). This risk may be because of the underlying disease state that caused the renal failure or a specific lipid abnormality associated with end-stage renal disease. The hyperlipidemia common in this population is characterized by a high triglyceride level with or without an elevated cholesterol level. Medical and nutrition intervention for el-

PRACTICE ⬤ PEARL

Taste Alterations and Protein Foods

Uremia can lead to taste alterations that cause protein-containing foods to taste metallic. Insufficient protein intake can, in turn, compromise nutritional health. The nurse can suggest that cold proteins rather than hot forms of proteins be tried because often these will taste less metallic. Cold chicken in a salad or sandwich instead of a hot, baked chicken breast is an example.

evated lipid levels mirror that prescribed for any other client diagnosed with hyperlipidemia (Kaysen, 2009). Chapter 18 outlines the dietary treatment of hyperlipidemia.

Fluids

Fluid balance must be closely monitored in all individuals receiving maintenance dialysis. Fluid allowance is based on the presence of **oliguria** or **anuria.** Oliguria is defined as a urine volume of less than 500 mL/day, whereas anuria refers to a urine volume of less than 100 mL/day. Daily fluid intake is generally limited to 1,000 mL, which accounts for insensible fluid losses, plus the daily total volume of any urine output. Weight should be measured daily and weight change between dialysis treatments should be limited to 2 to 3 kilograms to limit the effects of chronic fluid overload on the heart because of high intravascular volume. The nurse should educate clients to measure fluid intake and urine output and observe for signs and symptoms of fluid overload, such as edema. Instructions regarding fluid intake should include an explanation of measuring units, such as milliliters, ounces, and cups, and the conversion between these units. The nurse should also explain to the client that any food that is liquid at room temperature such as ice cream, water ice, Jell-O, needs to be included as part of the fluid restriction. On-line tools exist to help clients with all aspects of the diet, including a fluid restriction. Thirst can be a difficult problem for clients with renal failure and can lead to problems with adherence to a fluid restriction. It is important to provide suggestions on managing thirst without drinking excess fluid. Suggestions for helping clients manage thirst are included in Box 21-3.

Sodium

A major role of the kidney is the regulation of sodium balance and its associated effect on fluid balance. Excess sodium is excreted by the kidneys. In cases of inadequate sodium intake, sodium can be retained by the kidneys. Because of the loss of this balancing ability in renal failure, the majority of clients with chronic kidney disease must limit the amount of sodium in the diet to minimize the negative effects of sodium and fluid retention. Sodium is present in varying levels in almost all foods. The most concentrated source of sodium in the diet

BOX 21-3	Nursing Interventions to Manage Thirst

✓ Limit salt intake. Salt can increase thirst.
✓ Chew on ice cubes rather than drinking water.
✓ Sip beverages slowly.
✓ Use small cups or glasses rather than large ones.
✓ Choose tart flavorings for allowed beverages such as cranberry, lemon, or lime.
✓ Suck on sour or hard candies or chew gum.
✓ Suck on a piece of cold or frozen fruit.
✓ Take medicines with applesauce rather than liquid.
✓ Rinse mouth with water but do not swallow.
✓ Good oral care, including,
  • Brushing teeth regularly
  • Avoiding mouthwash that contains alcohol and can dry oral mucosa

is sodium chloride or table salt. One teaspoon of table salt has 2,300 mg of sodium. Foods that are high in sodium include those that are processed or pickled. Examples include processed meats, such as lunch meats, hot dogs, sausages; cheeses; pickled foods, such as sauerkraut, olives, pickles; canned soups; salted snack foods; and convenience and frozen prepared meals. The NKF recommends a sodium intake of 1 to 3 grams per day in clients receiving hemodialysis and 2 to 4 grams per day for PD (NKF, 2000). Clients with hypertension or edema may require additional sodium restrictions and more careful monitoring of fluid status. Chapter 6 outlines the sodium content of foods in more detail and contains a Client Education Checklist on sodium reduction. Table 21-2 lists sodium requirements for clients with renal failure.

Potassium

The kidneys play a central role in regulating potassium levels in the blood. In CKD, especially when oliguria is present, potassium excretion by the kidney is diminished and serum potassium levels can increase, resulting in hyperkalemia (Palmer, 2008). Clinical symptoms of excessive serum potassium are unspecific and vague yet its consequences can be grave. Hyperkalemia is, therefore, usually diagnosed by blood tests. Serum potassium needs to be carefully monitored because hyperkalemia can precipitate cardiac arrhythmias and cardiac arrest. Severe hyperkalemia is treated emergently with a variety of medical and pharmacological interventions. One treatment involves the use of Kayexalate (polystyrene sulfonate), a cation-exchange resin that can be administered orally or by enema to increase potassium losses from the intestinal tract (Sood, Sood, & Richardson, 2007). However, because of the many negative side effects of this medication, it is generally given only in emergency cases. Potassium is removed during RRT, but it is also critical to control potassium

intake between treatments to prevent episodes of hyperkalemia. For these reasons it is generally necessary to limit potassium intake in most clients with renal failure. However, treatment with CRRTs actually removes significant amounts of potassium and during this specific therapy serum levels must be carefully monitored to prevent low serum potassium levels.

Like sodium, potassium is found in a wide variety of foods. Certain fruits and vegetables have the highest concentration of potassium and intake of these must be carefully controlled to prevent hyperkalemia. Fruits with high-potassium content include bananas, dried fruits, and citrus fruits, including star fruit. Vegetables with high-potassium content are tomatoes, potatoes, and dried peas and beans. Potassium content of vegetables can be lowered by using the leaching process (NKF, 2009a). Raw vegetables are soaked in a large amount of water for at least 2 hours followed by rinsing and cooking in a large amount of new water. Vegetables with a skin such as carrots and potatoes are peeled first. This extensive process also causes loss of water-soluble vitamins. When working with a culturally diverse population, it is important that the nurse be familiar with the high-potassium fruits and vegetables consumed by these groups. Cultural Considerations Box: Potassium in the Diet outlines examples of these foods. Many salt substitutes are potassium based (potassium chloride) and must be eliminated from the diet. The nurse should advise clients to scrutinize the food label of commercially available salt substitutes and only use those that are an herb or spice mix without added potassium or sodium. Foods with high-potassium content are listed in Box 21-4. Client Education Checklist: Potassium Restriction in Renal Failure outlines advice that the nurse can offer to limit potassium intake.

Recommendations for potassium intake are: 2 to 3 grams per day in those treated with hemodialysis and 3 to 4 grams per day with peritoneal dialysis (NKF, 2000). Potassium intake should be spread over the day to avoid an excessive intake at any one time. The individual potassium allowance should be adjusted based on serum levels and on the potassium content of the dialysate. The potassium content of the dialysate can be adjusted to allow changes in the amount of potassium removed during the dialysis treatment. Potassium requirements are shown in Table 21-2.

Calcium and Phosphorus

Metabolic bone disease is a major complication of CKD. It is characterized as an endocrine disorder involving complex interactions among calcium, phosphorus, vitamin D, and parathyroid hormone (PTH). Under normal circumstances, a drop in the serum calcium level causes increased release of PTH, which signals the release of calcium from the bone and increases renal clearance of phosphate. PTH also increases conversion of the inactive form of vitamin D to the active form within the renal tubules through stimulation of the enzyme 1-[alpha] hydroxylase. Vitamin D then acts to

Cultural Considerations

Potassium in the Diet

Renal diet restrictions are complicated and can be difficult to learn and follow under the best of circumstances. Cultural differences and language barriers can make education of the client with CKD a challenge. Research has indicated that the primary determinants of adherence to renal diet restrictions are food lists and other educational materials printed in appropriate foreign languages (Koh & Koo, 2007). Educational materials should also include culturally significant foods. Inclusion of family members in the nutrition education process is important (Morales-Lopez, Burrowes, Gizis, & Brommage, 2007). Educational materials should be appropriate to the literacy level of the client, with pictorial materials available for those who cannot read.

It is also important to assess the intake of cultural foods that may contain increased amounts of potassium, including:

1. *Mexican/Hispanic foods:* Chorizo sausage, frijoles with cheese, garbanzos (chickpeas), refried beans, salsa, flan or matillas (milk-containing custards), platanos (plantains), mangos, apricot nectar, and coconut milk. Other foods such as tacos, enchiladas, and chimichangas may be high in potassium and should be evaluated for specific high-potassium ingredients

2. *Asian:* Bok choy, Chinese radish, lotus root, certain Oriental mushrooms, duck, and soybeans

3. *African American:* Collard greens, kale, mustard greens, spinach, okra, black-eyed peas, and sweet potato pie

---

BOX 21-4	High-Potassium Content Foods

Fruits and Vegetables

Banana
Oranges and orange juice
Nectarines
Tangerines
Fresh peach and pear
Dried fruit, including apricot, raisin, prune, prune juice
Melons
Tomato: fresh or canned
Tomato sauce or juice
Vegetable juice
Dried peas and beans
Pumpkin
Acorn or winter squash
White or sweet potato
Greens
Broccoli

Milk, Other

Milk: limited to 8 ounces per day
Salt substitute
Cheese
Bran: limited to two bran cereal or bread servings per week
Brewed coffee
Nuts or peanut butter

---

promote increased calcium absorption from the gastrointestinal tract, leading to an increase in serum calcium levels. Dietary vitamin D is initially activated by the liver to 25-hydroxyvitamin D and then within the kidney to the active form 1,25 di-hydroxyvitamin D. Figure 21-2 ■ outlines this complex relationship.

In CKD, this complex series of interactions is disrupted at several key points. There is an increased incidence of 25-hydroxyvitamin D and 1,25 di-hydroxyvitamin D deficiency in all stages of the disease. In clients receiving hemodialysis treatment, this incidence is as high as 97% (Gonzalez, Sachdeva, Oliver, & Martin, 2004). Vitamin D deficiency has been attributed to the low-phosphorus diet prescribed in CKD that restricts the intake of milk, a source of vitamin D. Additionally, the enzyme 1-[alpha] hydroxylase is suppressed in uremic states, leading to decreased conversion of vitamin D to its active form by the kidney. As a result, there is increased stimulation of PTH secretion, which causes a release of calcium from the bones. This condition is called secondary hyperparathyroidism. Under these circumstances, calcium becomes bound to the excess phosphorus in the blood that is elevated because of decreased renal excretion. This calcium-phosphate product is deposited into soft tissues

in the body (Thomas, Kanso, & Sedor, 2008); calcification of soft tissues results. Calcification affects the cardiovascular system, which leads to cardiovascular disease. Other areas affected include the eyes, muscle, lung, gastrointestinal tract, and skin.

In certain instances of severe secondary hyperparathyroidism, it is necessary to provide supplementation of the activated form of vitamin D and cinacalcet, a medication that inhibits the secretion of PTH (Block et al., 2004). Recent studies have demonstrated a decrease in mortality in these clients receiving injectable, activated vitamin D (Wolf & Thadhani, 2007).

Medical nutrition therapy includes modifying the intake of both phosphorus and calcium. Phosphorus intake should be low and calcium intake high. This recommendation can be difficult because most high-calcium products, such as milk and milk products, are also high in phosphorus.

The recommended intake of phosphorus in both PD and hemodialysis is 800 to 1,000 mg/day (NKF, 2000). Milk intake must be restricted to one-half cup per day. Intake of meats, fish, poultry, and cheese is limited to 4 to 5 ounces per day. The nurse should advise the client to avoid phosphorus-containing food additives because these have been shown to contribute to

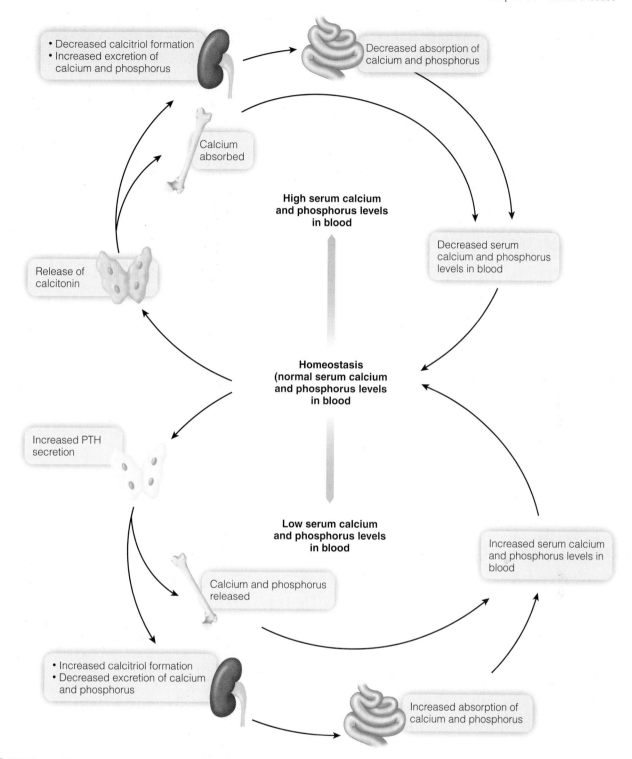

■ FIGURE 21-2 **Vitamin D and Calcium Metabolism**.

hyperphosphatemia in CKD (Sullivan et al., 2009). Such additives are found in processed meats, cheeses, baked goods, dried mixes, and soda and are listed on the ingredient label.

When dietary phosphorus restriction alone does not lower serum phosphorus to an appropriate level, phosphate binders should be prescribed. Calcium-based phosphate binders, such as calcium carbonate and calcium acetate, are initially used as they bind phosphorus and prevent its absorption while provid-

ing supplemental calcium. (NKF, 2003). The total dose of elemental calcium provided by these phosphate binders should not exceed 1,500 mg/day. If calcium-based phosphate binders do not successfully lower phosphorus levels, pharmacological agents can be added. When a magnesium-containing agent, such as MagneBind, is used, serum magnesium must be monitored to avoid hypermagnesemia. Prolonged use of aluminum-based phosphate binders, such as alternaGEL, Alu-Cap,

CLIENT EDUCATION CHECKLIST	Potassium Restriction in Renal Failure
Intervention	**Example**
Assess level of restriction necessary to maintain normal serum potassium level. Consider type and number of dialysis treatments.	Hemodialysis and PD differ in ability to remove potassium and, thus, dietary restriction differs. See Table 21-2 for guidelines.
Educate the client about the consequences of excessive potassium intake on serum potassium and health.	• Severe hyperkalemia can cause cardiac arrest. • Moderate to severe hyperkalemia can create a need for emergency dialysis treatment. • Potassium-lowering medications can be used in urgent situations but have side effects.
Individualize education based on the client's age, educational level, type of dialysis, and other diet restrictions required (e.g., diabetic diet).	• High-potassium foods such as bananas, dried fruit and prune juice, legumes (dried beans, peas, peanuts), melons, oranges, potatoes, spinach, Swiss chard, tomatoes, and whole grains must only be consumed in small portions with limited frequency. Consult a registered dietitian for individualized daily limits in this category. • Potassium intake should be spread throughout the day rather than consumed in one meal. • Consume lower-potassium fluids in place of those with high potassium: lemonade, limeade, cranberry juice, fruit punch, apple juice, coffee, and tea are low in potassium.
Consider possible causes for increased potassium intake.	• Seasonal: Possible increased intake of certain fruits and vegetables with a high-potassium content that are more widely available in summer months. Fresh fruit and vegetables have more potassium than their canned or processed counterparts because potassium is water soluble and some is lost in cooking/processing. • Vegetarian/Vegan diets: Dried peas and beans, a staple of these diets, contain high amounts of potassium. • Salt substitute use: Check the label because some contain potassium chloride.
Advise clients developing weight loss and malnutrition regarding the inclusion of liquid nutritional supplements in their diet in order to increase calorie and protein intake.	Check potassium content of oral liquid nutrition supplements. Consult with a registered dietitian for an alternative if supplement intake results in high-potassium intake overall.

Alu-Tab, Amphojel, and Dialume, can cause aluminum toxicity (Thomas et al., 2008). Use of aluminum-based phosphate binders has been reduced with the introduction of Sevelamer HCl, a binding agent that does not contain calcium, magnesium, or aluminum (Thomas et al., 2008). The nurse should counsel clients receiving phosphate binders to take this medicine with food in order for it to be effective in binding dietary phosphorus and, thereby, controlling serum phosphorus.

The recommended calcium intake is less than 2 grams per day in both predialysis and PD or hemodialysis (NKF, 2000). Calculation of total calcium intake must include any elemental calcium provided by calcium-containing phosphate binders. Foods with high-calcium content are milk and milk products, which must be limited to one-half cup daily because of their high phosphorus content. Unfortunately, the restriction of milk and milk products also limits vitamin D intake because milk is fortified with vitamin D.

Vitamins

Vitamin requirements for clients with CKD are not well established. However, suboptimal intakes of certain vitamins can occur in this population because of limited intake of certain foods because of potassium and phosphorus dietary restrictions. Certain water-soluble vitamins are lost into the dialysate in RRTs. It was previously thought that vitamin supplementation was unnecessary in CKD because water-soluble vitamins are excreted by the kidneys. However, vitamin deficiencies do occur. Common deficiencies include vitamin C, pyridoxine (vitamin B_6), folate, and vitamin D (Kalantar-Zedeh & Kopple, 2003).

The water-soluble vitamins lost into the dialysate during treatment include vitamin C and some of the B-complex vitamins. However, vitamin B_{12} is protein bound and, therefore, not removed during dialysis. Because riboflavin, niacin, biotin, and pantothenic acid are not dialyzable, extra intake of these vitamins is not needed. Supplemental vitamin C in excess of the dietary reference intake (DRI) can help improve absorption of nonheme iron, a beneficial effect in the client with anemia, but serum oxalate levels should be monitored to avoid risk of oxalate deposits and kidney stone development from this product of vitamin C metabolism (Sirover, Siddiqui, & Benz, 2008). The nurse should assess the client for use of any dietary supplements outside of those prescribed to ensure that the client heeds the recommended limit to vitamin C intake outlined in Table 21-2.

It is not necessary to supplement the fat-soluble vitamins in CKD. Because these vitamins are soluble in lipid solutions, they are not affected by dialysis treatments. Vitamin A supplementation in excess of amounts recommended for health should be avoided because hypervitaminosis A can occur more readily in end-stage renal disease (NKF, 2000). Vitamin A is not removed during dialysis and dialysis does not normalize elevated retinol levels. Retinol is the active form of vitamin A. Vitamin D intake should be individualized and, if needed, provided in the activated form.

Multivitamin supplements specifically formulated for individuals with CKD are available. Recent research has demonstrated that a multivitamin supplement is associated with decreased mortality in individuals with end-stage renal disease (Domrose et al., 2007).

Minerals, Trace Elements, and Carnitine

The requirements for minerals and trace elements in renal failure are not well established. The trace elements zinc, selenium, and chromium are excreted by the kidneys. If individuals with renal failure are consuming adequate food, supplementation of these minerals should not be required. Clients should be assessed for risk of a deficiency of iron and zinc. Carnitine deficiency is also reported in this population.

Iron The anemia associated with renal failure is caused by blood loss during hemodialysis, decreased red blood cell survival, and the inability of the kidney to produce erythropoietin (EPO). This anemia is manifested by fatigue and hematological changes. Measurements of serum iron, total iron binding capacity, iron saturation, and ferritin levels are used to assess iron status. In chronic renal failure, anemia is treated with a synthetic form of the hormone EPO, **recombinant human erythropoietin** (Eschbach, Egrie, Downing, Browne, & Adamson, 1987). EPO stimulates the bone marrow to produce red blood cells. Protocols using EPO in combination with adequate iron have been successful in helping clients achieve target hemoglobin levels (Chan, Moran, Hlatky, & Lafayette, 2009).

Oral or intravenous iron supplementation may be prescribed as part of the treatment of anemia. The nurse should remind the client that oral iron should be taken between meals because it can bind with phosphate binders that are taken with meals, rendering the iron unabsorbable.

Zinc Zinc is normally excreted by the kidneys so one might expect normal or elevated levels in those with CKD. However, reduced dietary intake and reduced serum zinc levels have been demonstrated in clients receiving hemodialysis (Navarro-Alarcon et al., 2006; Szpanowska-Wohn, Kolarzyk, & Chowaniec, 2008). Supplementation of the diet with zinc should not occur unless a zinc deficiency has been demonstrated. Unnecessary zinc supplementation should be avoided because of the potential interference with copper absorption, especially in those with marginal copper status.

Carnitine Carnitine is an amino acid derivative necessary for fatty acid transport and mitochondrial energy metabolism. Carnitine deficiency can occur in hemodialysis because of the loss of carnitine into the dialysate (Guarnieri, Bilol, Vinci, Massolino, & Barazzoni, 2007). Carnitine supplementation has been demonstrated to decrease EPO dose, improve exercise tolerance, decrease fatigue, and increase nutritional markers in clients receiving hemodialysis (Duranay et al., 2006; Guarnieri et al., 2007). Routine carnitine supplementation is controversial because of the lack of sufficient controlled trials that examine the effects of carnitine (Handelman, 2006). If carnitine is prescribed, it is administered intravenously three times a week after hemodialysis treatment.

Nutrition Support in Acute and Chronic Renal Failure

Inadequate intake of calories and protein is common in individuals with renal failure, regardless of treatment modality. Physical symptoms, such as anorexia, fatigue, and taste changes, and the restrictive nature of the diet contribute to poor intake. Oral intake can be supplemented in an effort to increase intake. Many liquid energy and protein supplements are available that are specifically formulated to meet nutrition needs in renal failure. Clients need almost continual encouragement from the nurse to maintain a good oral intake. Suggestions for increasing oral intake are included in Box 21-5.

BOX 21-5	**Increasing Oral Intake with CKD**

- Certain protein-containing foods are better tolerated when served at cold temperatures (e.g., cold chicken sandwich rather than hot chicken).
- Cooking odors should be avoided because they can cause nausea. Cooking foods ahead, freezing, and microwaving to reheat can minimize exposure to cooking odors.
- Eating frequent small meals throughout the day ("grazing") rather than eating three larger meals.
- If the client suffers from early satiety or a feeling of fullness, liquids should be taken 1 hour before or 1 hour after the meal instead of with a meal. This recommendation may help lessen early satiety because of the contribution of liquids to fullness.
- Clients with CKD may have a metallic taste in their mouth that can decrease appetite. Maintaining good oral hygiene (especially before meals) by brushing teeth or use of mouthwash can help with this problem.
- Liquid nutrition drinks or supplements specially formulated for CKD can be used to supplement the diet.

When a combination of oral diet and oral liquid supplements is inadequate for an extended period in the outpatient setting or more acutely in the hospitalized client, the initiation of nutrition support should be considered. Chapter 16 discusses the specifics of nutrition support in detail.

Enteral Nutrition   Enteral nutrition should be considered as first-line nutrition support in a client with a functional gastrointestinal tract. Specialized enteral formulas are available to meet the nutritional needs of the client receiving hemodialysis. These formulas are concentrated, containing 1.5 to 2 kcalories/mL that help minimize fluid volume intake compared with the standard 1 kcalorie/mL formulas. Nutrient recommendations for enteral nutrition support in clients with acute or chronic renal failure follow those for an oral diet (Cano et al., 2006). For example, fluid, potassium, and phosphorus may be restricted and appropriate levels of vitamins and minerals are provided. In clients with ARF, the dietitian should assess the client for protein requirements because a catabolic state may require additional protein intake (Moore & Celano, 2005). Clients receiving CRRT may not require specialized renal formulas because of the greater clearance of fluid and electrolytes that this treatment provides. A standard, high-protein formula may be appropriate with this acutely ill population and should be evaluated on an individual basis (Cano et al., 2006). Chapter 16 outlines the particulars of enteral nutrition support and types of formula. Some clients receiving CRRT or PD, such as those with diabetes, may need to have caloric intake modified to adjust for glucose absorption from the dialysate used with these specific treatments.

Parenteral Nutrition   When enteral nutrition alone cannot provide adequate energy and protein intake, parenteral nutrition support should be considered. Parenteral nutrition in the client with renal failure does not differ greatly from that provided for other malnourished individuals. Factors to be considered in the parenteral nutrition prescription include type of renal failure, type of treatment, and presence of hypercatabolism or hypermetabolism. Specialized amino acid solutions containing only essential amino acids are available. Nephramine is an example. These solutions are low in overall protein intake and not necessary for clients receiving dialysis but can be indicated in the client not receiving any RRT. Essential amino acid solutions may be appropriate in certain cases of ARF or in end-stage renal disease when the client is not receiving dialysis treatments. As with enteral nutrition support in this population, clients should be individually assessed to determine overall nutritional needs based on disease, treatment, and nutritional status.

Intradialytic Parenteral Nutrition   Intradialytic parenteral nutrition (IDPN) is a unique method of delivering intravenous nutrition to severely malnourished individuals during hemodialysis treatment. High volume (maximum rate 350 mL/hour during dialysis treatments) hypertonic dextrose,

amino acids, and lipids are infused into the venous blood line during dialysis treatments, providing a significant source of energy and protein. While these nutrients are infused during dialysis, the majority are not lost in the dialysate bath (Cano & Leverve, 2008). The total fluid volume of the formula is included in calculations for target fluid to be removed as part of the dialysis treatment and, therefore, does not need to be included within the fluid restriction prescribed for the client.

The formula prescription must be tailored to the individual client on dialysis, specifically regarding tolerance to dextrose and lipids. Excessive infusion of fats can impair lipid clearance in this population already at risk for hyperlipidemia (Moore, 2008). Glucose infusion rates must be carefully controlled in order to prevent hyperglycemia when treatment is initiated and hypoglycemia when the infusion is discontinued. Blood glucose levels need to be monitored before, during, and after the infusion. Insulin administration may need to be adjusted in clients with diabetes mellitus. A carbohydrate-containing snack can be given during the final 30 minutes of dialysis to prevent hypoglycemia when the formula is stopped with the end of the dialysis session, but circulating insulin levels remain short term (Moore, 2008). In addition to monitoring glucose and lipid tolerance, fluid status is assessed as part of determining the volume of intradialytic parenteral nutrition and fluid removal goals.

The nurse should know that although this type of nutrition support is available, not all clients qualify for Medicare or insurance reimbursement for its cost (Moore, 2008). As a result, alternative routes of nutrition support may have to be sought with some clients.

Malnutrition in Renal Failure

Malnutrition is a complex and challenging complication of renal failure. It is estimated that up to 75% of clients on dialysis are malnourished (Dukkipati & Kopple, 2009). The term **protein-energy wasting (PEW)** has been coined to describe the malnutrition seen in this population (Moore, 2008).

There is a multifactorial etiology to the development of malnutrition in this population. The contributing factors are summarized in Figure 21-3 ■. Inadequate nutritional intake plays an important role in the nutritional decline seen. Multiple nutrient restrictions cause the diet to be difficult to follow and unpalatable. Comorbidities, such as diabetes, require additional dietary restrictions. A fair to poor appetite has been reported to occur in almost 40% of clients receiving hemodialysis (Kalantar-Zadeh, Block, McAllister, Humphreys, & Kopple, 2004). The fatigue associated with dialysis treatments can cause difficulty obtaining and preparing food. Additionally, nutrient losses in dialysis, comorbid illnesses and treatment, and psychosocial issues, such as isolation and depression, further increase the risk of malnutrition (Dukkipati & Kopple, 2009). Megesterol acetate is an appetite stimulant that has

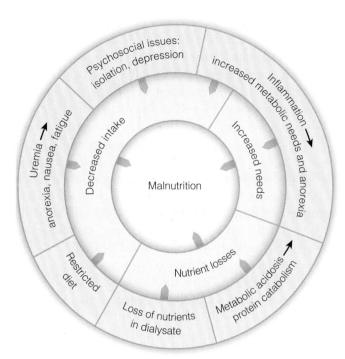

Psychosocial issues: isolation, depression

increased metabolic needs and anorexia

Inflammation

Increased needs

Uremia
anorexia, nausea, fatigue

Decreased intake

Malnutrition

Metabolic acidosis
protein catabolism

Nutrient losses

Restricted diet

Loss of nutrients
in dialysate

■ **FIGURE 21-3** **Development of Malnutrition with Renal Failure.**

been tried in clients with CKD. This medication has been shown to reverse poor appetite in several small studies with a limited number of clients with CKD, but more research is needed before it can be recommended (Chazot, 2009).

The endocrine and metabolic changes associated with uremia are also important factors in the development of malnutrition in renal failure. A common complication of uremia is **metabolic acidosis,** or increased blood pH related to metabolic changes, which causes protein catabolism and decreased synthesis of albumin (Moore, 2008). Endocrine changes can influence appetite and contribute to anorexia. The hormone leptin is found in elevated levels in CKD. Elevated levels of leptin may suppress both appetite and nutrient intake (Mak, Cheung, Cone, & Marks, 2006). A chronic inflammatory state exists and is evidenced by elevated serum levels of C-reactive protein, tumor necrosis factor, interleukin-1, and interleukin-6. These markers of an inflammatory state are associated with anorexia (Chazot, 2009). The combination of these factors contributes to the anorexia and wasting syndrome seen in these clients as well as other disease states. Chapter 22 outlines this effect in more detail.

This very intricate web of interactions between uremia, endocrine changes, and nutrition has been termed the malnutrition–inflammation complex syndrome (MICS). Hypoalbuminemia (serum albumin less than 3.8 gm/dL) is a hallmark of this syndrome and is a strong predictor of morbidity and mortality in individuals receiving hemodialysis (Kalantar-Zedeh et al., 2005). Experts disagree as to the cause of decreased serum albumin in clients with renal failure (Ahuja &

Mitch, 2004). However, whether or not poor nutrition or inflammation is ultimately determined to be the cause of hypoalbuminemia, nutritional interventions that can increase serum albumin are needed. It is estimated that increasing serum albumin to greater than 3.8 gm/dL could reduce deaths in clients receiving hemodialysis by approximately 10,000 per year (Kalantar-Zedeh et al., 2005). Interestingly, obesity is associated with improved survival in the population of those receiving hemodialysis (Schmidt & Salahudeen, 2007).

The client with CKD, whether in the initial stages or in complete renal failure, must have a periodic nutrition assessment to evaluate nutritional status. An important factor in the evaluation of clients receiving dialysis is the documentation of a dry weight. Dry weight refers to the client's weight after a dialysis treatment and will reflect true weight and not the extra fluid that will accumulate in the body between treatments. The dry weight becomes an important baseline measurement and comparisons can be made at later dates to document true weight loss or gain. Other measures of nutrition status, such as the plasma proteins albumin and prealbumin, can be used to assess nutrition status but are affected by any inflammatory processes and so should be used in combination with other assessment parameters rather than as a sole indicator of nutrition status (Cano, Miolane-Debouit, Leger, & Heng, 2009; Thomas et al., 2008). Nitrogen balance studies to determine protein status cannot be done in clients who make little or no urine. Subjective parameters of nutrition status should be regularly assessed to complement anthropometric measurements. Functional status, gastrointestinal symptoms, oral intake, and physical appearance, including muscle and fat stores, can be evaluated.

It is critical for the nurse to continually monitor the dry weight and nutritional status of the client with renal failure. All clients must be encouraged to maintain an adequate oral diet. At the initial signs of deteriorating nutritional status, oral supplements should be considered in an effort to increase intake. If the nutritional status of the client continues to decline, IDPN may be considered. In certain clients who demonstrate all signs of severe malnutrition, an enteral feeding tube may be needed to prevent further deterioration. CKD is a long-term disease process and clients require strong emotional support and continual encouragement from the nurse in order to live successfully with this disease.

Renal Transplantation

Transplantation of the kidney is the most common organ transplant performed (Teplan et al., 2009). Nutrition status plays an important role in both the early and later posttransplant phases. Because of the prevalence of malnutrition in clients with advanced kidney disease, some individuals undergo surgery with poor nutritional health that can negatively affect wound healing, risk of infection, and muscle strength during rehabilitation. The physiological stress of surgery along with the use of high-dose immunosuppressive medications, specifically corticosteroids, increases the immediate postoperative need for calories and protein (Teplan et al., 2009). Protein restriction is not routinely recommended during these weeks because it can lead to protein catabolism and its associated negative consequences (Martins, Pecoits-Filho, & Riella, 2004; Tritt, 2004). A high fluid intake is encouraged to stimulate kidney function and promote urine production (Tritt, 2004). The nurse should carefully monitor fluid balance with daily weights and close attention to intake and urine volume. Table 21-2 summarizes the recommendations for nutrient intake post-transplant.

During the late post-transplant phase, metabolic and nutritional consequences become common and can contribute to morbidity and mortality. Weight gain, hyperlipidemia, hyperglycemia, hypertension, and altered bone health occur because of multifactor contributors. Ongoing use of corticosteroids and other immunosuppressive drugs can cause elevated glucose levels (Tritt, 2004). Up to one-third of those with renal transplant have insulin resistance compared with one-fourth of the general population who are affected (Teplan et al., 2009). Weight gain because of a sedentary lifestyle, medications, and a new-found liberalization of the diet can worsen the risk of developing diabetes post-transplant. Hyperlipidemia is reported in up to 90% post-transplant clients, increasing their risk of cardiovascular disease (Dumler & Kilates, 2007). Hypertension from sodium retention because of medications further contributes to cardiac risk. Bone health is compromised because of long-term corticosteroid use compounding the existing metabolic bone disease found in end-stage renal disease. The risk of fracture in the post-transplant client is four times that of the general population (Palmer, McGregor & Strippoli, 2005). Children who undergo renal transplantation are at risk for the same long-term complications as adults and require close monitoring for risk of weight gain, diabetes, hyperlipidemia, and metabolic bone disease (NKF, 2009b).

The nurse working with the post-transplant population of adults and children can educate the client about lifestyle modifications that can lower risk of long-term metabolic consequences. Weight management with diet and exercise is recommended (Guida et al., 2007; Jezior et al., 2007; NKF, 2009b). A moderate sodium restriction is indicated in those with hypertension. Controlled carbohydrate intake according to established guidelines for diabetes may be needed by some clients with hyperglycemia. Dietary treatment of hyperlipidemia follows guidelines established for the general population (Dumler & Kilates, 2007). Specific recommendations for long-term protein intake are unclear, with some research recommending moderation of intake to not exceed the recommended dietary allowance (RDA) of 0.8 gm/kg body weight/day to avoid burdening the kidney with protein by-products (Bernardi et al., 2003; Martins et al., 2004). Recommendations to improve bone health mirror those used in treating osteoporosis, with a combination of pharmacological and dietary intervention with vitamin D and calcium. Unfortunately, no one specific intervention has been shown to significantly reduce the risk of fracture in this population (Palmer et al., 2005). Of utmost importance in the post-transplant client is the avoidance of grapefruit juice and dietary supplements known to cause a drug interaction with cyclosporines and tacrolimus, which are commonly prescribed to prevent organ rejection. Use of the herb St. John's Wort is associated with unfortunate case reports of organ rejection because of this interaction (Nowack, 2008). Grapefruit juice should be avoided by those on cyclosporines or tacrolimus (NKF, 2009b). In Chapter 22, Box 22-3 covers general post-transplant nutrition concerns that can be applied to the client with renal transplant.

Nephrotic Syndrome

Nephrotic syndrome is a disease caused by damage to the glomerulus, the portion of the kidney that produces an ultrafiltrate and is responsible for reabsorption of proteins. This syndrome has a devastating impact on the normal metabolism of proteins, lipids, and sodium. Although it occurs in both adults and children, it is more prevalent in childhood (Nephrology Channel, 2007).

Nephrotic syndrome is characterized by massive proteinuria, edema, and hyperlipidemia (Appel, 2006). One of the main functions of the glomeruli is the prevention of protein loss into the urine during the ultrafiltration process. Normally albumin and other plasma proteins are reabsorbed with a normal protein excretion not exceeding 150 mg/dL. Damage to the glomerulus, specifically to Bowman's capsule, results in protein excretion into the urine with urine protein levels in clients with nephrotic syndrome reaching in excess of 3.5 gm/day (Appel, 2006). The large loss of protein, primarily albumin, leads to diminished plasma albumin and then edema. Lipid metabolism is also affected by nephrotic syndrome. Through an unknown mechanism, the protein loss and resulting decreased oncotic pressure stimulates hepatic production of lipids. Serum levels of cholesterol, low-density lipoproteins, and very low-density lipoproteins are all increased (Appel, 2006). There is also loss of EPO, resulting in anemia. Urinary loss of vitamin D-binding protein can cause calcium malabsorption and the development of metabolic bone disease. Medical treatment for this syndrome includes management of the underlying disease that caused the nephrotic syndrome. Primary causes of nephrotic syndrome include diabetes mellitus, collagen vascular disease, amyloidosis, glomerulonephritis, IgA nephropathy, toxins, medications, and drug abuse.

Nutrition Intervention

The primary goal of nutrition care for the client with nephrotic syndrome is the provision of adequate calories and protein to prevent malnutrition while decreasing proteinuria and associated symptoms. In the absence of adequate calorie intake, dietary protein is utilized as an energy source, furthering the protein deficit often seen with this condition.

Optimal protein intake in nephrotic syndrome is a controversial topic. In the past, a high-protein intake (up to 1.5 gm/kg/day) was suggested in an effort to prevent hypoalbuminemia and the development of malnutrition. However, subsequent research has demonstrated that high-protein intake can increase proteinuria and contribute to the progression of renal failure. A moderate protein restriction, supported with adequate calorie intake can reduce proteinuria without exacerbating malnutrition (Castellino & Cataliotti, 2002; Maroni, Staffeld, Young, Manatunga, & Tom, 1997). The use of ACE-1 inhibitors can allow for a more liberal protein intake because of the effect of this drug on reducing protein loss into the urine (Appel, 2006; Garini, Mazzi, Allegri, Buzio, & Borghetti, 1996). Current recommendations for protein intake are 0.8 gm/kg/day plus 1 gram of protein for every gram of urinary protein (American Dietetic Association, 2002; McCann, 2002). This calculation equates to the RDA for protein for healthy adults plus an adjustment to replace urinary protein loss. The nurse should stress the importance of adherence to guidelines for the 24-hour urine collection to ensure accurate assessment of protein losses used in the calculation of protein requirements.

A restriction in saturated fat and cholesterol intake is used in conjunction with lipid-lowering medications to decrease hypercholesterolemia (Appel, 2006). Sodium and fluid restrictions are individualized based on the presence and extent of edema. A complete list of nutrition recommendations for nephrotic syndrome is shown in Table 21-2.

Kidney Stones

Kidney stones can be present in the kidneys, ureter, or bladder and are classified according to the compound contained within the stone. Figure 21-4 ■ depicts the location of kidney stones. The most common types of kidney stones are calcium oxalate, uric acid, and cystine stones. Of these three, calcium oxalate stones are the most prevalent (Worcester & Coe, 2008). Stone formation is a complicated process and although all individuals form crystals, only a small percentage convert these crystals to stones. Stones form when the concentration of the solutes, such as calcium oxalate or uric acid in the urine, exceeds the body's ability to hold these particles in suspension. Crystals form from the resulting precipitate and aggregate to form kidney stones.

Prevalence of kidney stones, or nephrolithiasis, is increasing in the United States, which may be related to the

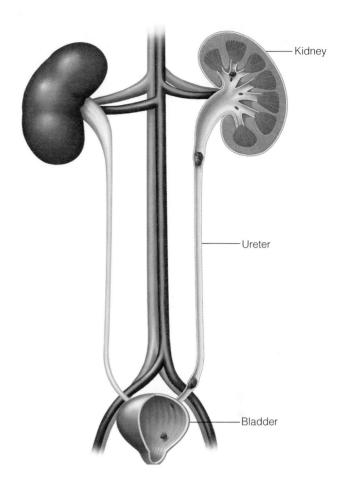

FIGURE 21-4 Kidney Stones.

increased prevalence of obesity, a risk factor for kidney stones (Worcester & Coe, 2008). It is estimated that half of all individuals diagnosed with a kidney stone will have a recurrence within 10 years (Worcester & Coe, 2008). The nurse plays an important role in reducing the rate of recurrent stones through education about lifestyle modifications.

Medical management of kidney stones involves radiographic confirmation of the diagnosis, pain medications, and possibly extracorporeal shock wave lithotripsy, ureteroscopy, or surgical intervention for stone removal (Worcester & Coe, 2008). Subsequent nursing and nutrition intervention for client education are critical in preventing recurrence.

Nutrition Intervention

The primary nutrition intervention to prevent stone formation is increased fluid intake to increase urine volume. Fluid intake is increased because precipitation and aggregation of crystals is less likely to occur in a dilute urine compared with a concentrated one. Avoidance of a supersaturated urine is a key goal for stone prevention. Fluid intake should be sufficient to produce at least 2 liters of urine per day (Krieg, 2005;

Worcester & Coe, 2008). The client should be educated about this goal of urine volume and advised to adjust fluid intake when insensible fluid losses, such as sweating, vomiting, or diarrhea, alter fluid balance and, therefore, urine output. In addition, the fluid intake must occur consistently throughout the day in order to prevent the development of a supersaturated, or concentrated, urine at any given time. Clients can be advised to monitor urine color as a sign of hydration; generally, straw-colored urine indicates better hydration than darker colored urine.

Water is an ideal beverage choice to increase urine volume, but intake of other beverages can also be encouraged. Unlike water, some beverages are capable of changing urine pH, which affects the solubility of crystals in solution and, therefore, stone formation. Some beverages provide substances called crystallization inhibitors. These inhibitors can be beneficial in preventing crystal formation and stone formation. Citrates are one type of crystal inhibitor and can be found in some beverages as well as medication. Potassium citrate, a medication, is often prescribed because it elevates urine pH and urinary citrate levels, which inhibits crystallization of calcium oxalate stones (Worcester & Coe, 2008). The best beverage to prevent kidney stone formation is a subject of debate. Hot Topic: Beverage Intake to Prevent Kidney Stone Formation and Recurrence reviews the effect of beverages on kidney stone formation.

Individuals with a history of calcium oxalate stones should be educated regarding optimum calcium intake. In the past, it was thought that calcium intake should be reduced in this population. However, research has demonstrated that a normal calcium intake is appropriate (Borghi et al., 2002). A long-term reduction in calcium intake places these individuals at risk for the development of osteoporosis and is not associated with a decreased risk of stone recurrence. Additionally, adequate calcium in the diet when dietary oxalate is also present beneficially decreases oxalate absorption by the body (Borghi et al., 2006).

Additionally, those with calcium oxalate stones should limit foods with high oxalate content. Foods to avoid include black tea, chocolate, tree nuts and peanuts, rhubarb, spinach, beets, wheat bran, and strawberries. Boiling high-oxalate vegetables decreases oxalate content (Massey, 2007). High doses of vitamin C should also be avoided, because this vitamin is a precursor to the endogenous production of oxalate. Other causes of increased oxalate include ketogenic diets used to treat epilepsy and fat malabsorption disorders, such as found in pancreatitis and after small bowel bypass surgery for obesity (Lieske, Kumar, & Collazo-Clavell, 2008; Sampath, Kossoff, Furth, Pyzik, & Vining, 2007; Worcester & Coe, 2008). The rationale for oxalate restriction is complicated and not fully

hot Topic

Beverage Intake to Prevent Kidney Stone Formation and Recurrence

The nurse may be asked to advise clients regarding appropriate beverage choices to prevent kidney stone formation and recurrence. Before offering advice, it is critical to know the composition of the kidney stone. Calcium oxalate stones are the most common type of stone. Uric acid stones compromise a minority of kidney stones, whereas brushite and struvite stones are even less common.

What beverages are best at reducing initial stone formation and recurrence? Some beverages offer clear advantages. In particular, those that increase citrate levels are beneficial in the prevention of recurrent calcium oxalate stones associated with low urinary citrate levels. Others, such as cranberry juice and colas, are controversial because of dual effects and may require additional research before definitive statements can be made.

- *Coffee, tea, and cola beverages.* Coffee and tea consumption increases urine volume and, therefore, decrease the risk of stone recurrence. Black tea may need to be avoided because of its high oxalate content. Limited information is available regarding cola beverages. However, it is recommended that they be avoided because they decrease urinary citrate levels and increase urinary oxalate levels.

- *Wine and beer.* Moderate consumption of wine and beer is associated with a decreased risk of stone formation.

- *Lemonade.* Low-sugar lemonade and lemon juice have dual benefits. They can increase urinary citrate level and urine volume, conferring a protective effect against stone recurrence.

- *Grapefruit juice.* Prior recommendations to avoid grapefruit juice were based on studies that observed an increased risk of stone formation in subjects who consumed grapefruit and apple juice. Subsequent research has demonstrated that the citrate content of grapefruit juice increased urinary citrate and increased urine flow, both desirable in preventing stone formation and recurrence. Grapefruit juice contains the most citrate of the fruit juices other than lemon juice.

- *Orange juice.* Orange juice has the positive effect of alkalizing the urine as well as increasing urinary citrate levels. Therefore, orange juice is encouraged as a preventive in stone formation and recurrence.

- *Cranberry juice.* Cranberry juice acidifies the urine. Urine acidification aids in the prevention of brushite and struvite stones. However, an acid urine pH may increase risk of other types of stones when urine volume is low.

- *Black currant juice.* Black currant juice alkalizes the urine and is an ideal beverage to prevent recurrence of uric acid stones.

CT? What overall message should the nurse give to the client who asks about which beverage is best to reduce risk of kidney stone recurrence?

Sources: Adapted from: Aras et al., 2008; Honow, Laube, Schneider, Kebler, & Albrecht, 2003; Kessler, Jansen, & Hesse, 2002; Penniston, Steele, & Nakada, 2007; Trinchieri et al., 2002.

understood. Generally, oxalate is poorly absorbed by the intestine and there is much less oxalate present in the urine compared with calcium. Because of this factor, a high urinary oxalate level has a great influence on the formation of the calcium-oxalate compound. Therefore, reducing dietary oxalate can have a great influence on stone formation (Massey, 2007). Long lists of food oxalate content are available for the curious client to review, but simply restricting intake of those foods highest in oxalate is all that is recommended along with simultaneous intake of calcium to bind dietary oxalate in the intestine and prevent its absorption (Borghi et al., 2006; Massey, 2007). Approximately ½ cup of milk, ice cream, or yogurt or ¾ oz of cheese at a meal containing oxalates is sufficient to bind oxalate (Massey, 2007).

Additional diet adjustments include limiting sodium intake to 2,300 to 3,450 mg/day (NKF, 2009c). This recommendation is because sodium and calcium are both reabsorbed within the renal tubules. The competition at the renal tubule from excessive intake of sodium is associated with decreased calcium reabsorption and subsequent increased calcium excretion in the urine. Chapter 6 contains a Client Education Checklist on reducing sodium intake.

Excessive intake of animal protein should be limited in individuals prone to calcium oxalate and uric acid stones. Animal proteins contain purines, and uric acid is formed in the metabolism of purines. The uric acid is then excreted into the urine where stone formation occurs. Calcium oxalate stone formers should also avoid excessive protein because high-protein intake is associated with increased urinary calcium loss (Worcester & Coe, 2008). Hypercalciuria occurs because the body uses calcium to buffer the acidosis resulting from high-protein intake. Plant-based proteins, such as legumes, do not produce the same urinary effects as animal proteins and are not considered to have the same lithogenic potential (Borghi et al., 2006). The nurse should encourage clients at risk for kidney stone recurrence to limit excessive intake of animal protein, which includes meats, poultry, and fish, and to choose plant-based proteins as a substitute more often. Clients can be advised to choose moderate portions of meats and to consider other protein sources, such as beans, soy products, hummus, or vegetarian burgers, at some meals.

Obesity is a risk factor for development of kidney stones. High circulating insulin or a large body size can alter urinary calcium, oxalate, and uric acid excretion, an effect that is also seen with weight gain or increasing waist circumference

BOX 21-6	Diet Modification for Kidney Stones

- Fluid intake: Adequate to produce greater than 2 liters of urine per day. Adjust intake as needed with changing insensible fluid loss.
- Calcium intake: Adequate intake according to RDA (1,000 mg/day for age 19–50 years).
- Sodium intake: Avoid excessive use of table salt, and processed and convenience foods that are high in sodium.
- Protein intake: Avoid excessive intake of animal protein by consuming less frequently or limiting portion size. Consider choosing more plant-based proteins.
- Calcium oxalate stone formers should limit foods with high oxalate content such as tea, instant coffee, rhubarb, beets, spinach, strawberries, wheat bran, chocolate, and nuts.
- Maintain a healthy weight.

(Taylor, Stampfer, & Curhan, 2005; Worcester & Coe, 2008). The nurse should encourage maintenance of a healthy weight in those at risk for nephrolithiasis. Overall dietary modifications for kidney stones are summarized in Box 21-6.

Urinary Tract Infection

Urinary tract infections occur because of the presence of bacteria in the urine. Most commonly, the source of the bacteria is the individual's own vaginal or fecal microflora (Drekonja & Johnson, 2008). Treatment is pharmacological with no proven nutrition interventions that are effective. However, dietary factors have been implicated in prevention of urinary tract infections in those at high risk for these infections, such as women and children. Research that targets use of dietary components that may change colonic flora, such as fermented dairy products, yogurt with active cultures, and probiotic dietary supplements, has not yielded consistent results to prove a benefit (Barrons & Tassone, 2008; Kontiokari, Nuutinen, & Uhari, 2004). Cranberry juice or its extracts have been more thoroughly investigated for a potential effect on urinary tract infection risk and show more promising results. The Evidence-Based Practice Box: Does cranberry juice prevent urinary tract infections in women? outlines the potential effects of cranberry on occurrence of symptomatic urinary tract infections.

EVIDENCE-BASED PRACTICE RESEARCH BOX

Does cranberry juice prevent urinary tract infections in women?

Clinical Problem Cranberry juice is frequently mentioned as a simple and effective way to prevent urinary tract infections, especially in women. What is the evidence for this frequent recommendation?

Research Findings There is a popular belief that cranberry juice can be used as a home remedy to treat urinary tract infections (UTI). Unfortunately, studies have not shown that cranberries, in any form, have been effective in treating UTIs. There have been studies, however, that examine the question of whether cranberries could prevent UTIs.

Studies have been conducted with cranberries in various forms: juice, concentrate, cocktail, dried berries, and capsules. A pilot study compared dried raisins with dried cranberries to see if UTIs could be prevented in women with a history of frequent UTIs (Greenberg, Newmann, & Howell, 2005). Although the study had only five subjects, the significant difference between the raisins and cranberries led the researchers to conclude that larger studies were needed to see if UTI prevention was indeed possible.

A prospective study by Bailey, Dalton, Joseph-Daughtery, and Tempesta (2007) followed 12 women for 12 weeks, none of whom developed a UTI while taking a 200-mg dose of concentrated cranberry extract. Two years later, eight of the women who continued taking the cranberry extract were free from UTIs caused by *Escherichia coli*. A recent update was conducted for the Cochrane Database by Jepson and Craig (2008). Ten studies with more than 1,000 subjects were reviewed. Various cranberry products were included in the studies. A meta-analysis could be conducted on only four of the studies because of methodological or data issues. The researchers concluded that cranberry juice decreased the incidence of UTIs in women, but the exact dosage or type of other cranberry products could not be determined. It is believed that cranberry juice prevents bacterial adherence to the bladder wall, but the specific component responsible for this effect is uncertain.

Nursing Implications Cranberry products should never be recommended as treatment for UTIs. However, cranberry products, especially juice, may be recommended for prevention of UTIs due to the ease of administration, wide availability, and cost effectiveness. It should be combined with the usual recommendations for adequate fluid intake and proper hygiene.

CRITICAL THINKING QUESTION

1. How should the nurse respond to the client who asks how much cranberry juice she should take to get rid of her UTI?

NURSING CARE PLAN Nutrition and Renal Failure

CASE STUDY

Tim, 61 years old, has a long history of hypertension, type 2 diabetes mellitus, and osteoarthritis. His latest blood work has shown an acceleration of renal failure and he has come to the clinic to discuss additional dietary management with the nurse. He has been faithful in keeping appointments and taking medications, but he frequently jokes with the staff that he is "too far gone" to do much with diet. He has struggled with obesity his entire adult life and says he likes himself the way he is. He retired from being a mail carrier 5 years ago because his knees hurt so badly. Knee replacement surgery was done 3 years ago. His days are filled with reading, watching TV, and visiting with a large extended family. He tells the nurse that he wants to avoid dialysis but cannot envision a diet that he and his wife could follow.

Applying the Nursing Process

ASSESSMENT

Height: 5 feet 9 inches Weight: 263 pounds BMI: 38
BP 158/88 P 82 R 16

Blood glucose (nonfasting finger stick) 210
Blood urea nitrogen (BUN) 35 mg/dL
Creatinine 4 mg/dL
Potassium 5.2 mEq/L

DIAGNOSES

Imbalanced nutrition: more than body requirements related to impaired glucose metabolism and excessive caloric intake evidenced by BMI of 38

Deficient knowledge (dietary) related to stated lack of interest in learning evidenced by frequent statements that he likes himself "as is"

Risk for impaired urinary elimination related to accelerating renal failure and increased potassium

EXPECTED OUTCOMES

Weight loss average of 2 pounds per week

Able to list acceptable foods that have high biologic value protein, are low in potassium, and are low in sodium

Nutrition and Renal Failure *(continued)*

NURSING CARE PLAN

Assessment
Data about the patient

Subjective
What the patient tells the nurse
Example: I am too far gone to change my diet; I like myself the way I am; I don't want dialysis.

Objective
What the nurse observes; anthropometric and clinical data
Examples: 263 pounds; 5 feet 9 inches; BMI: 38; nonfasting blood glucose: 210 mg/dL; potassium: 5.2 mEq/L

Diagnosis
NANDA label
Example: Deficient knowledge related to lack of interest in dietary changes that will help manage renal failure

Planning
Goals stated in patient terms
Example: Long-term goal: renal function remains stable, avoids excessive intake of protein; Short-term goal: identifies foods with low potassium and low sodium content

Implementation
Nursing action to help patient achieve goals
Example: Refer to dietitian; review diabetic diet; outline progression of renal failure

Evaluation
Was the goal achieved or does the intervention need to be modified?
Example: Reduced potassium consumption; continues to express little interest in dietary changes

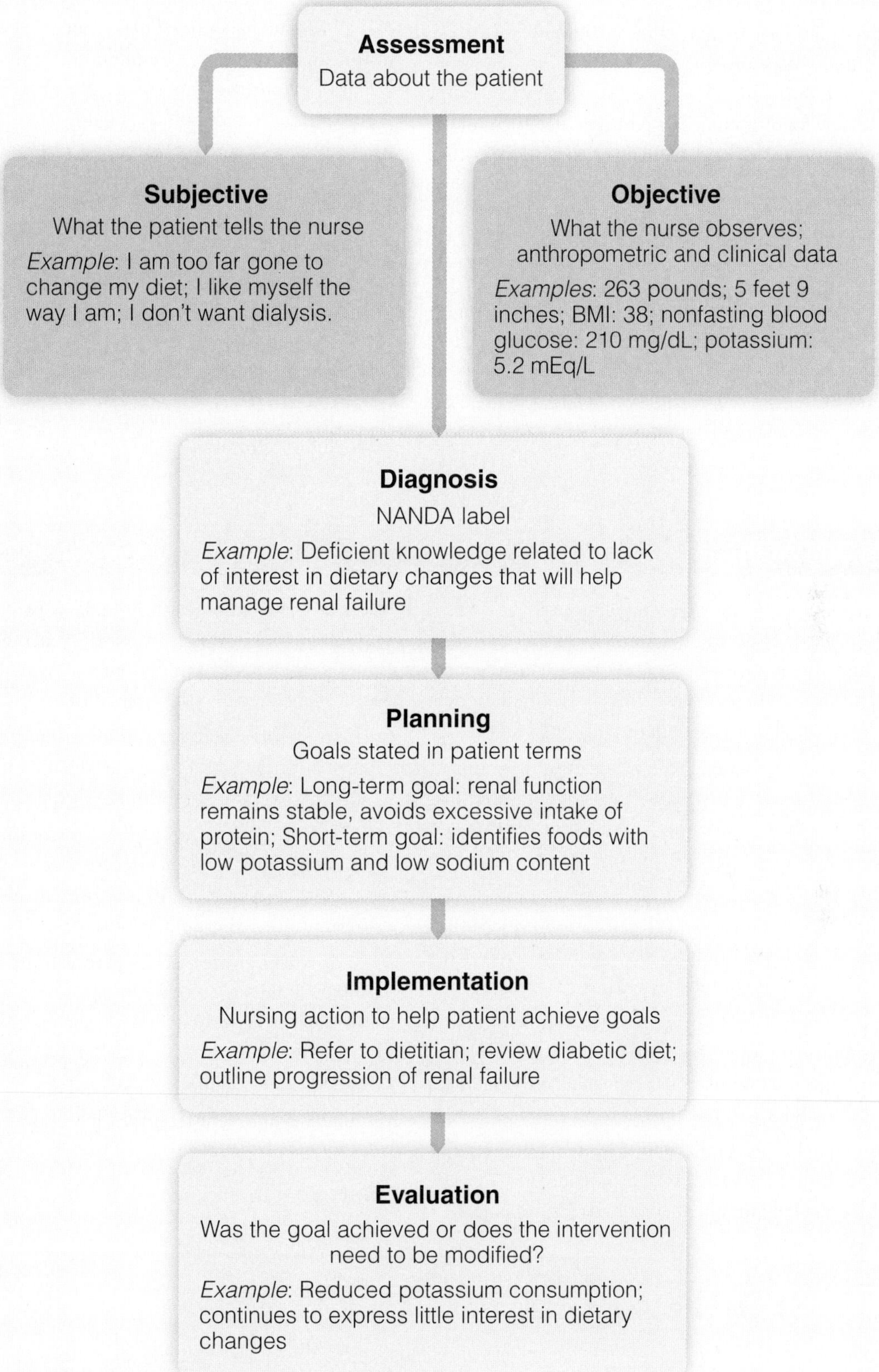

■ FIGURE 21-5 **Nursing Care Plan: Nutrition and Renal Failure.**

(continued)

Nutrition and Renal Failure *(continued)*

NURSING CARE PLAN

INTERVENTIONS

Diet plan that includes limited amounts of high bio-logic value protein and food that are low in potassium and sodium

Review foods included as part of a diabetic diet

Refer to a dietitian specializing in renal nutrition

Review progression of renal failure

EVALUATION

Tim has continued to keep appointments for the past 2 months. His blood glucose remains stable, although elevated. His renal function tests are unchanged. He says that the diet is just not his "style," but that he has made an effort to drink less soda and orange juice. He describes himself as a "meat and potatoes man" and says that he has no interest in making major dietary changes at this point. He has lost 5 pounds but attributes it to taking more walks with his wife. The nurse continues to share information about the importance of using diet to delay progression of renal failure. Figure 21-5 ■ outlines the nursing process for this case.

Critical Thinking in the Nursing Process

1. **When a client with end-stage renal failure and diabetes complains of thirst and has an elevated serum potassium level, what are some suggestions for fluid intake that the nurse can make that lessen potassium intake without increasing carbohydrate intake?**

CHAPTER SUMMARY

• The kidneys play a major role in elimination of waste products from the body and in balancing content of electrolytes and fluids. Loss of the ability to manage waste products, fluids, and electrolytes has severe implications on the diet prescribed for the client with renal failure.

• Renal replacement therapies each have a unique impact on nutritional needs. Nutritional needs of comorbid diseases such as diabetes and cardiovascular disease also need to be considered in the nutrition prescription for the client with CKD.

• Medical nutrition therapy and the nutrition prescription for the client with CKD must address energy intake, protein allowance, lipid content, as well as modifications of sodium, potassium, calcium, and phosphorus.

• Vitamin supplements may be needed by clients receiving hemodialysis. Specific formulations are available that address the unique needs for water- and fat-soluble vitamins.

• Intake of the micronutrients, such as iron and zinc, should be evaluated in clients with CKD. Supplements may be indicated, especially for clients receiving hemodialysis.

• Nutrition support with enteral or parenteral nutrition is occasionally required in cases of acute or chronic renal failure. Special formulations are available to address the needs of clients with renal failure.

• Malnutrition is a common complication of CKD. Nutritional status must be evaluated on a routine basis in order to improve oral intake.

• Nephrotic syndrome is a disease requiring modification of protein, lipid, and electrolyte intake. Nutritional intervention is necessary in an effort to manage proteinuria, edema, and hyperlipidemias associated with this syndrome.

• Individuals prone to kidney stone formation must increase fluid intake and modify intake of the dietary compounds associated with the stone formation.

• Although no nutritional intervention is effective at treating urinary tract infections, regular intake of cranberry juice may prevent recurrent infection.

EXPLORE **PEARSON mynursingkit**

MyNursingKit is your one stop for online chapter review materials and resources. Prepare for success with additional NCLEX®-style practice questions, interactive assignments and activities, web links, animations and videos, and more!

Register your access code from the front of your book at
www.mynursingkit.com.

NCLEX® QUESTIONS

1. A client with renal stones tells the nurse about taking a daily vitamin C supplement. What should the nurse tell this client about vitamin C supplements?
   1. Increase fluid intake to flush any vitamin C residue from the bladder.
   2. Stop taking vitamin C supplements immediately.
   3. Increase vitamin C intake to prevent future stone formation.
   4. Limit vitamin C because it may contribute to formation of calcium oxalate stones.

2. A client with chronic renal failure who has fluid restrictions expresses frustration with an extremely dry mouth. What can the nurse suggest for this client? Select all that apply.
   1. Suck on a hard lemon candy.
   2. Sip 1 ounce of water per hour.
   3. Suck frozen cherries.
   4. Avoid beverages with caffeine.
   5. Chew gum.

3. A client expresses disappointment that bananas are limited as part of the diet plan for chronic renal failure. The nurse explains that:
   1. Bananas have a lot of potassium and that is a nutrient that must be limited in the diet.
   2. The diet emphasizes high biologic value protein and bananas have a lot of carbohydrate.
   3. Bananas have too little fiber for individuals with chronic renal failure.
   4. Bananas frequently cause diarrhea and that contributes to excess fluid loss.

4. Which of the following diet instructions are appropriate when teaching a client in the early stages of chronic renal failure who is not receiving dialysis treatment?
   1. Increase fluid intake to flush the kidneys.
   2. Dietary protein should come from high biologic value sources.
   3. Only sodium found in foods can be consumed.
   4. Vegetables may be eaten as desired.

5. The nurse knows that teaching about dietary methods to prevent urinary tract infections has been effective when the client states:
   1. "I must drink 8 ounces of water every hour I am awake."
   2. "Avoid red meat as a source of protein."
   3. "A daily glass of cranberry juice may be beneficial."
   4. "Avoid carbonated beverages."

REFERENCES

Ahuja, T. S., & Mitch, W. E. (2004). The evidence against malnutrition as a prominent problem for chronic dialysis patients. *Seminars in Dialysis, 17,* 427–431.

Almeida, J. C., Zelmanovitz, T., Vaz, J. S., Steemburgo, T., Perassolo, M. S., Gross, J. L., et al. (2008). Sources of protein and polyunsaturated fatty acids of the diet and microalbuminuria in type 2 diabetes. *Journal of the American College of Nutrition, 27,* 528–537.

American Dietetic Association (ADA). (2002). *Chronic kidney disease medical nutrition therapy protocol. American Dietetic Association medical nutrition therapy evidence-based guides for practice.* Chicago: Author.

Appel, G. B. (2006). Improved outcomes in nephrotic syndrome. *Cleveland Clinic Journal of Medicine, 73,* 161–167.

Aras, B., Kalfazade, N., Tugcu, V., Kemahli, E., Ozbay, B., Polat, H., et al. (2008). Can lemon juice be an alternative to potassium citrate in the treatment of urinary calcium stones in patients with hypocitraturia? A prospective randomized study. *Urology Research, 36,* 313–317.

Bailey, D. T., Dalton, C., Joseph-Daughtery, F., & Tempesta, M. S. (2007). Can a concentrated cranberry extract prevent recurrent urinary tract infections in women? A pilot study. *Phytomedicine: International Journal of Phytotherapy and Phytopharmacology, 14,* 237–241.

Barrons, R., & Tassone, D. (2008). Use of *Lactobacillus* probiotics for bacterial genitourinary infections in women: A review. *Clinical Therapeutics, 30,* 453–468.

Bernardi, A., Biasi, F., Pati, R. T., Piva, M., D'Angelo, A., & Bucciante, G. (2003). Long-term protein intake control in kidney transplant recipients: Effect in kidney graft function and in nutrition status. *American Journal of Kidney Disease, S1,* S146–S152.

Bernstein, A. M., Treyszon, L., & Zhaoping, L. (2007). Are high protein, vegetable-based diets safe for kidney function? A review of the literature. *Journal of the American Dietetic Association, 107,* 644–650.

Beto, J. A., & Bansal, V. K. (2004). Medical nutrition therapy in chronic kidney failure: Integrating clinical practice guidelines. *Journal of the American Dietetic Association, 104,* 404–409.

Block, G. A., Martin, K. J., deFrancisco, A. L. M., Turner, S. A., Avram, M. M., Suranyi, M. G., et al. (2004). Cinacalcet for secondary hyperparathyroidism in patients receiving hemodialysis. *The New England Journal of Medicine, 350,* 1516–1525.

Borghi, L., Meschi, T., Maggiore, U., & Prati, B. (2006). Dietary therapy in idiopathic nephrolithiasis. *Nutrition Reviews, 64,* 301–312.

Borghi, L., Schianchi, T., Meschi, T., Guerra, A., Allegri, F., Maggiore, U., et al. (2002). Comparison of two diets for the prevention of recurrent stones in idiopathic hypercalciuria. *New England Journal of Medicine, 346,* 77–84.

Brenner, B. M. (1983). Hemodynamically mediated glomerular injury and the progressive nature of kidney disease. *Kidney International, 23,* 647–655.

Cano, N., Fiaccadori, E., Tesinsky, P., Tiogo, G., Druml, W., Kuhlmann, M., et al. (2006). ESPEN guidelines on enteral nutrition: Adult renal failure. *Clinical Nutrition, 25,* 295–310.

Cano, N. J., & Leverve, X. M. (2008). Intradialytic nutritional support. *Current Opinion in Clinical Nutrition and Metabolic Care, 11,* 147–151.

Cano, N. J., Miolane-Debouit, M., Leger, J., & Heng, A. (2009). Assessment of body protein: Energy status in chronic kidney disease. *Seminars in Nephrology, 29,* 59–66.

REFERENCES *(continued)*

Castellino, P., & Cataliotti, A. (2002). Changes of protein kinetics in nephrotic patients *Current Opinion in Clinical Nutrition and Metabolic Care, 5,* 51–54.

Chan, K., Moran, J., Hlatky, M., & Lafayette, R. (2009). Protocol adherence and the ability to achieve target hemoglobin levels in hemodialysis patients. *Nephrology, Dialysis & Transplantation,* doi: 10.1093/ndt/gfn780.

Chazot, C. (2009). Why are chronic kidney disease patients anorexic and what can be done about it? *Seminars in Nephrology, 29,* 15–23.

Coresh, J., Selvin, E., Stevens, L. A., Manzi, J., Kusek, J. W., Eggers, P., et al. (2007). Prevalence of chronic kidney disease in the United States. *Journal of the American Medical Association, 298,* 2038–2047.

Domrose, U., Heinz, J., Westphal, S., Luley, C., Neumann, K. H., & Dierkes, J. (2007). Vitamins are associated with survival in patients with end-stage renal disease: A 4-year prospective study. *Clinical Nephrology, 67,* 221–229.

Drekonja, D. M., & Johnson, J. R. (2008). Urinary tract infections. *Primary Care: Clinics in Office Practice, 35,* 345–367.

Dukkipati, R., & Kopple, J. D. (2009). Causes and prevention of wasting in chronic kidney failure. *Seminars in Nephrology, 29,* 39–49.

Dumler, F., & Kilates, C. (2007). Metabolic and nutritional complications of renal transplantation. *Journal of Renal Nutrition, 17,* 97–102.

Duranay, M., Akay, H., Yilmaz, F. M., Senes, M., Tekeli, N., & Yucel, D. (2006). Effects of L-carnitine infusions on inflammatory and nutritional markers in haemodialysis patients. *Nephrology Dialysis Transplantation, 21,* 3211–3214.

Eschbach, J. W., Egrie, J. C., Downing, M. R., Browne, J. K., & Adamson, J. W. (1987). Correction of the anemia of end-stage renal disease with recombinant human erythropoietin. Results of a combined phase I and II clinical trial. *The New England Journal of Medicine, 316,* 73–78.

Fouque, D., Laville, M., & Boissel, J. P. (2007). Low protein diets for chronic kidney disease in non-diabetic adults. *Cochrane Database of Systematic Reviews, 4,* CD001892.

Garini, G., Mazzi, A., Allegri, L., Buzio, C., & Borghetti, A. (1996). Effectiveness of dietary protein augmentation associated with angiotensin-converting enzyme inhibition in the management of the nephrotic syndrome. *Mineral and Electrolyte Metabolism, 22,* 123–127.

Gonzalez, E. A., Sachdeva, A., Oliver, D. A., & Martin, K. J. (2004). Vitamin D insufficiency and deficiency in chronic kidney disease: A single center observational study. *American Journal of Nephrology, 24,* 503–510.

Greenberg, J. A., Newmann, S. J., & Howell, A. B. (2005). Consumption of sweetened dried cranberries versus unsweetened raisins for inhibition of uropathogenic *Escherichia coli* adhesion in human urine: a pilot study. *Journal of Alternative and Complementary Medicine, 11*(5), 875–878.

Guarnieri, G., Bilol, G., Vinci, P., Massolino, B., & Barazzoni, R. (2007). Advances in carnitine in chronic uremia. *Journal of Renal Nutrition, 17,* 23–29.

Guida, B., Trio, R., Laccetti, R., Nastasi, A., Salvi, E., Perrino, N., et al. (2007). Role of dietary intervention on metabolic abnormalities and nutritional status after renal transplantation. *Nephrology Dialysis Transplantation, 22,* 3304–3310.

Handelman, G. J. (2006). Debate forum: Carnitine supplements have not been demonstrated as effective in patients on long-term dialysis therapy. *Blood Purification, 24,* 140–142.

Honow, R., Laube, N., Schneider, A., Kebler, T., & Albrecht, H. (2003). Influence of grapefruit-, orange-, and apple juice consumption on urinary variables and risk of crystallization. *British Journal of Nutrition, 90,* 295–300.

Jepson, R. G., & Craig, J. C. (2008). Cranberries for preventing urinary tract infections. *Cochrane Database of Systematic Reviews,* CD001321.

Jezior, D., Krajewska, M., Madziarska, K., Regulska-Ilow, B., Ilow, R., Janczak, D., et al. (2007). Weight reduction in renal transplant recipients program. *Transplant Proceedings, 39,* 2769–2771.

Kalantar-Zedeh, K., Block, G., McAllister, C. J., Humphreys, M. H., & Kopple, J. D. (2004). Appetite and inflammation, nutrition, anemia, and clinical outcome in hemodialysis patients. *American Journal of Clinical Nutrition, 80,* 299–307.

Kalantar-Zedeh, K., Kilpatrick, R. D., Kuwae, M., McAllister, C. J., Alcorn, H., Kopple, J. D., et al. (2005). Revisiting mortality predictability of serum albumin in the dialysis population: Time dependency, longitudinal changes and population-attributable fraction. *Nephrology Dialysis Transplantation, 20,* 1880–1888.

Kalantar-Zedeh, K., & Kopple, J. D. (2003). Trace elements and vitamins in maintenance dialysis patients. *Advances in Renal Replacement Therapy, 10,* 170–182.

Kavey, R. E., Allada, V., Daniels, S. R., Hayman, L. L., McCrindle, B. W., Newberger, J. W., et al. (2007). Cardiovascular risk reduction in high-risk pediatric patients: A scientific statement from the American Heart Association expert panel on population and prevention science; the councils on cardiovascular disease in the young, epidemiology and prevention, nutrition, physical active and metabolism, high blood pressure research, cardiovascular nursing and the kidney and heart disease; and the interdisciplinary working group on quality of care and outcomes research. *Journal of Cardiovascular Nursing, 22,* 218–253.

Kaysen, G. A. (2009). New insights into lipid metabolism in chronic kidney disease: What are the practical implications? *Blood Purification, 27,* 86–91.

Kessler, T., Jansen, B., & Hesse, A. (2002). Effect of blackcurrant-, cranberry- and plum juice consumption on risk factors associated with kidney stone formation. *European Journal of Clinical Nutrition, 56,* 1020–1023.

Klahr, S., Buerkert, J., & Purkerson, M. L. (1983). Role of dietary factors in the progression of chronic renal disease. *Kidney International, 24,* 579–587.

Klahr, S., Levey, A. S., Beck, G. J., Caggiula, A. W., Hunsicker, L., Kusek, J. W., et al. (1994). The effects of dietary protein restriction and blood pressure control on the progression of chronic renal disease. *New England Journal of Medicine, 330,* 877–884.

Koh, J. C., & Koo, W. (2007). Chinese nutritional educational materials for renal patients. *Journal of Renal Nutrition, 17,* 357–359.

Kontiokari, T., Nuutinen, M., & Uhari, M. (2004). Dietary factors affecting susceptibility to urinary tract infection. *Pediatric Nephrology, 19,* 378–383.

Krieg, C. (2005). The role of diet in the prevention of common kidney stones. *Urologic Nursing, 25,* 451–456.

Lieske, J. C., Kumar, R., & Collazo-Clavell, M. L. (2008). Nephrolithiasis after bariatric surgery. *Seminars in Nephrology, 28,* 163–173.

Mak, R. H., Cheung, W., Cone, R. D., & Marks, D. L. (2006). Leptin and inflammation associated cachexia in chronic kidney disease. *Kidney International, 69,* 794–797.

Maroni, B. J., Staffeld, C., Young, V. R., Manatunga, A., & Tom, K. (1997). Mechanisms permitting nephrotic patients to achieve nitrogen equilibrium with a protein-restricted diet. *Journal of Clinical Investigation, 99,* 2479–2487.

Martins, C., Pecoits-Filho, R., & Riella, M. C. (2004). Nutrition for the post-renal transplant recipients. *Transplantation Proceedings, 36,* 1650–1654.

Massey, L. K. (2007). Food oxalate: Factors affecting measurement, biological variation, and bioavailability. *Journal of the American Dietetic Association, 107,* 1191–1194.

McCann, L. (Ed.). (2002). *Pocket guide to nutrition assessment of the patient with chronic kidney disease.* New York: National Kidney Foundation Council on Renal Nutrition.

Mitch, W. E. (2005). Beneficial responses to modified diets in treating patients with chronic kidney disease. *Kidney International, 94,* S133–S135.

REFERENCES *(continued)*

Moore, E. (2008). Challenges of nutrition intervention for malnourished dialysis patients. *Journal of Infusion Nursing, 31,* 361–366.

Moore, E., & Celano, J. (2005). Challenges of providing nutrition support in the outpatient dialysis setting. *Nutrition in Clinical Practice, 20,* 202–212.

Morales-Lopez, C. M., Burrowes, J. D., Gizis, F., & Brommage, D. (2007). Dietary adherence in Hispanic patients receiving hemodialysis. *Journal of Renal Nutrition, 17,* 138–147.

National Kidney Foundation (NKF). (2000). Kidney disease outcomes quality initiative: K/DOQD clinical practice guidelines for nutrition in chronic renal failure. *American Journal of Kidney Diseases, 35,* S81–S140.

National Kidney Foundation (NKF). (2003). *Clinical practice guidelines for bone metabolism and disease in chronic kidney disease.* Retrieved March 11, 2009, from http://www.kidney .org/professionals/KDOQI/guidelines_bone/ index.htm

National Kidney Foundation (NKF). (2006). *Chronic kidney disease 2006: A guide to select NKF-KDOQI guidelines and recommendations, Section 2: Nutrition, guidelines 15 and 16.* Retrieved March 11, 2009, from http://www .kidney.org/professionals/kls/pdf/ Pharmacist_CPG.pdf

National Kidney Foundation (NKF). (2009a). *Potassium and your CKD diet.* Retrieved March 9, 2009, from http://www.kidney.org/ atoz/content/potassium.cfm

National Kidney Foundation (NKF). (2009b). KDOQI clinical practice guideline for nutrition in children with CKD: 2008 update. *American Journal of Kidney Diseases, 5* (S2), S1–S124.

National Kidney Foundation (NKF). (2009c). *Diet and kidney stones.* Retrieved March 11, 2009, from http://www.kidney.org/atoz/ content/diet.cfm

Navarro-Alarcon, M., Reyes-Perez, A., Lopez-Garcia, H., Palomares-Bayo, M., Olalla-Herrera, M., & Lopez-Martinez, M. C. (2006). Longitudinal study of serum zinc and copper levels in hemodialysis patients and their relation to biochemical markers. *Biological Trace Element Research, 113,* 209–222.

Nephrology Channel. (2007). *Nephrotic syndrome.* Retrieved March 11, 2009, from http://www .nephrologychannel.com/nephrotic

Nowack, R. (2008). Cytochrome 450 enzyme and transport protein-mediated herb-drug interactions in renal transplant patients: Grapefruit juice, St. John's Wort—and beyond. *Nephrology, 13,* 337–347.

Palmer, B. F. (2008). Approach to fluid and electrolyte disorders and acid-base problems. *Primary Care: Clinics in Office Practice, 35,* 195–213.

Palmer, S. C., McGregor, D. O., & Strippoli, G. F. M. (2005). Interventions for preventing bone disease in kidney transplant recipients. *Cochrane Database of Systematic Reviews, 2,* CD005015.

Penniston, K. L., Steele, T. H., & Nakada, S. Y. (2007). Lemonade therapy increases urinary citrate and urine volumes in patients with recurrent calcium oxalate stone formation. *Urology, 70,* 856–860.

Sampath, A., Kossoff, E. H., Furth, S. L., Pyzik, P. L., & Vining, E. P. (2007). Kidney stones and the ketogenic diet: Risk factors and prevention. *Journal of Child Neurology, 22,* 375–378.

Schmidt, D., & Salahudeen, A. (2007). The obesity-survival paradox in hemodialysis patients: Why do overweight hemodialysis patients live longer? *Nutrition in Clinical Practice, 22,* 11–15.

Sirover, W. D., Siddiqui, A. A., & Benz, R. L. (2008). Beneficial hematogic effects of daily oral ascorbic acid therapy in ESRD patients with anemia and abnormal iron homeostasis: A preliminary study. *Renal Failure, 30,* 884–889.

Sood, M. M., Sood, A. R., & Richardson, R. (2007). Emergency management and commonly encountered outpatient scenarios in patients with hyperkalemia. *Mayo Clinic Proceedings, 82,* 1553–1561.

Sullivan, C., Sayre, S. S., Leon, J. B., Machekano, R., Love, T. E., Porter, D., et al. (2009). Effect of food additives on hyperphosphatemia among patients with end-stage renal disease. *Journal of the American Medical Association, 301,* 629–635.

Szpanowska-Wohn, A., Kolarzyk, E., & Chowaniec, E. (2008). Estimation of intake of zinc, copper and iron in the diet of patients with chronic renal failure treated by hemodialysis. *Biological Trace Element Research, 124,* 97–102.

Taylor, E. N., Stampfer, M. J., & Curhan, G. C. (2005). Obesity, weight gain, and risk of kidney stones. *Journal of the American Medical Association, 293,* 455–462.

Teplan, V., Vlakovsky, I., Teplan, V., Stollova, M., Vyhnanek, F., & Andel, M. (2009). Nutritional consequences of renal transplantation. *Journal of Renal Nutrition, 19,* 95–100.

Thomas, R., Kanso, A., & Sedor, J. R. (2008). Chronic kidney disease and its complications. *Primary Care: Clinics in Office Practice, 35,* 329–344.

Trinchieri, A., Lizzano, R., Bernardini, P., Nicola, M., Pozzoni, F., Romano, A. L., et al. (2002). Effect of acute load of grapefruit juice on urinary excretion of citrate and urinary risk factors for renal stone formation. *Digestive and Liver Disease, 34*(Suppl. 2), S160–S163.

Tritt, L. (2004). Nutrition assessment and support of kidney transplant patients. *Journal of Infusion Nursing, 27,* 45–51.

Vimalachandra, D., Hodson, E. M., Willis, N. S., Craig, J. C., Cowell, C., & Knight, J. F. (2006). Growth hormone for children with chronic kidney disease. *The Cochrane Database of Systematic Reviews, 4,* CD 003264.

Voss, D., Hodson, E., & Crompton, C. (2007). Nutrition and growth in kidney disease: CARI guidelines. *Australian Family Physician, 36,* 253–254.

Wolf, M., & Thadhani, R. (2007). Vitamin D in patients with renal failure: A summary of observational mortality studies and steps moving forward. *Journal of Steroid Biochemistry and Molecular Biology, 103,* 487–490.

Wolfson, M., Piraino, B., Hamburger, R. J., & Morton, A. R. (2002). A randomized controlled trial to evaluate the efficacy and safety of icodextrin in peritoneal dialysis. *American Journal of Kidney Diseases, 40,* 1055–1065.

Worcester, E. M., & Coe, F. L. (2008). Nephrolithiasis. *Primary Care: Clinics in Office Practice, 35,* 369–391.

22 Physiological Stress

WHAT WILL YOU LEARN?

1. To analyze how the body's response to physiological stress can lead to risk of malnutrition.
2. To distinguish factors affecting a client's need for calories, protein, vitamins, minerals, and fluid during critical illness.
3. To relate the nutritional care of a perioperative client.
4. To summarize the role of nutrients essential to wound repair, including following trauma, burn injury, or treatment for pressure ulcers.
5. To formulate nursing interventions to optimize the nutrition status of a client with chronic obstructive pulmonary disease or on mechanical ventilation.

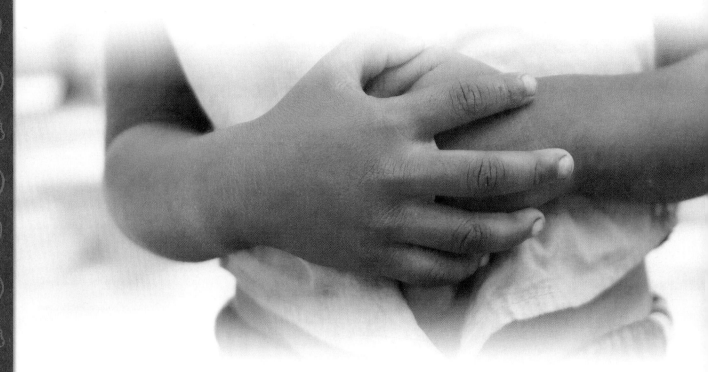

DID YOU KNOW?

▶ The fight-or-flight response during stress is a survival mechanism that involves changes in energy metabolism.

▶ Fever drives up the metabolic rate.
▶ Large wounds can be a source of nutrient loss.

▶ Physiological stress can lead to significant loss of skeletal muscle.

KEY TERMS

acute-phase reactant proteins, *497*

C-reactive protein, *497*

dyspnea, *511*

ebb phase, *497*

exudate, *509*

fight-or-flight response, *497*

flow phase, *497*

hypercatabolism, *497*

hypermetabolism, *497*

ileus, *507*

immunonutrition, *508*

physiological stress, *497*

respiratory quotient (RQ), *511*

What Is Physiological Stress?

Physiological stress is also referred to as metabolic stress. Following a physical insult to the body, such as an injury or surgery, a cascade of reactions involving hormones, inflammatory agents, and the central nervous system results and is categorized as the stress response. This reaction occurs in two phases: ebb and flow. The **ebb phase** is the acute phase, occurring in the early days following the physical insult. The **flow phase** occurs over the following days, weeks, and months until recovery is achieved. During the ebb phase, the body tries to reestablish homeostasis to foster hemodynamic stability and delivery of oxygen to cells. The **fight-or-flight response** hormones, such as catecholamines and cortisol, are triggered in an attempt to provide the body with quick energy in the form of glucose along with stimulation of the central nervous system, all part of the body's defense to respond with "fight or flight." Glucose is generated from glycogen stores in liver and muscle, but these are limited. As a result, skeletal muscle protein is sacrificed to provide a source of glucose using metabolic pathways that catabolize protein into amino acids and shunt them to gluconeogenesis. Fat stores are also mobilized to provide fuel. The increased metabolic rate from central nervous system stimulation leads to **hypermetabolism,** whereas the accelerated protein losses cause **hypercatabolism.** The presence of these two factors together has deleterious health consequences when they persist past the short term.

During the flow phase, two additional responses lead to further protein catabolism as the body copes with the need for fuel and repair. First, inflammation from the injury or infection causes release of cytokines, which results in tissue loss because of the proinflammatory effect (Alberda, Graf, & McCargar, 2006; Wanek & Wolf, 2007). Second, the liver increases production of **acute-phase reactant proteins,** such as **C-reactive protein.** These proteins, which are part of the inflammatory response, are synthesized at the expense of other proteins in the body (Wanek & Wolf, 2007). Skeletal muscle continues to be catabolized to provide substrate for these reactions. Hyperglycemia results as protein catabolism provides substrate for gluconeogenesis, yet insulin resistance limits glucose uptake into liver and peripheral tissue. The effects of hypermetabolism are compounded in the flow phase because of substrate cycling. Substrate cycling is futile cycling of energy metabolism where the body's reaction to physical stress signals varying metabolic pathways that can negate one another, an effect that leads to increased energy expenditure with no benefit (Wanek & Wolf, 2007). Carbohydrate and lipid metabolism is involved in the futile cycling. Figure 22-1 ■ summarizes the effects of the metabolic response to physical stress.

Physical Consequences of the Stress Response

Whereas part of an acute reaction is aimed at survival, accelerated catabolism of protein is thought to be extremely detrimental to recovery (Wanek & Wolfe, 2007). Loss of lean body mass of 10% or more, not uncommon with critical illness, is associated with increased complications, infection, poor wound healing, and development of spontaneous wounds from skin breakdown. A loss of more than 40% of lean mass is associated with mortality (Demling, 2007).

Loss of specific proteins has a direct effect on specific aspects of recovery, especially when malnutrition is a result. Respiratory health is negatively affected by loss of muscle from the diaphragm and auxiliary muscles, leading to diminished contractility and inspiratory muscle strength (Alberda et al., 2006). Such effects can also inhibit sufficient cough or prolong mechanical ventilation needs in some clients (Carli, 2006). The immune system is compromised by such alterations as fewer T-cells, decreased lymphokine production, and decreased antibody affinity (Alberda et al., 2006). Additional risks include susceptibility to infection, poor

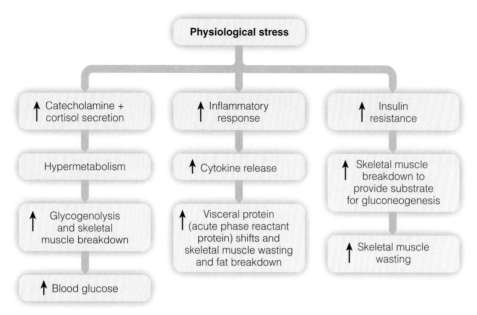

■ FIGURE 22-1 **Metabolic Response to Physical Stress.**

wound healing, and increased rehabilitation needs because of loss of muscle strength.

Hyperglycemia occurs during physiological stress in reaction to the *fight-or-flight* hormone response. High blood sugar has a negative effect on immune function, wound healing, and fluid and electrolyte balance, among many other aspects of critical illness (Inzucchi, 2006). Medications, such as corticosteroids, and overfeeding can contribute further to this negative effect.

The magnitude of the stress response depends on the magnitude of the physical insult and its duration. For example, minor surgery should elicit a lesser stress response than major body burns. Likewise, minor burn injury causes less of a stress response than burns that cover a larger body surface area. Although the fight-or-flight response may be helpful to recover from short-term physical insults to the body, left to continue long term, it becomes an autodestructive process (Demling, 2007).

Because it is established that malnutrition has a negative effect on functional status, recovery time, length of hospital stay, morbidity, and mortality (Norman, Pichard, Lochs, & Pirlich, 2008), it is imperative that timely nutrition support is instituted in the critically ill client. Early introduction of enteral nutrition support is the standard for most critically ill clients with a functioning gastrointestinal tract (Kreymann, 2008).

Assessment of Nutrient Needs

As with any client, a nutrition assessment is needed to provide the foundation on which to build recommendations for nutrition care. Depending on the circumstances, the nurse may or may not be able to gather data about the client's nutritional status before the onset of the physiological stress. Individuals with preexisting risk of malnutrition will be particularly vulnerable to the effects of metabolic stress. Medical conditions and treatment and alcohol abuse are examples. The older adult should be carefully assessed because of the effects of malnutrition on poor health outcome in this population. Lifespan Box: Nutrition and Physiological Stress in the Older Adult outlines these concerns. Additionally, increased nutritional demands for growth and development should be considered in the assessment of infants, children, and the pregnant female.

Anthropometric and laboratory measurements, traditionally a part of a nutrition assessment, are not always reliable indicators of nutrition status during acute critical illness. Dry body weight can be obscured by fluid overload or fluid losses. Visceral proteins are shuttled into action as acute phase proteins in the acute phase of physiological stress and thus are not direct indicators of nutrition status. Nitrogen balance studies are confounded by increased nitrogen excretion despite the presence of catabolism and are not useful if renal failure or uremia occurs. Nitrogen losses from large exudative wounds are difficult to calculate. Instead of relying on hard and fast cut points to define nutrition status in the critically ill client, anthropometric and laboratory measurements should be used to monitor individual trends in clients, using the clients' own values as self-references over time. Additionally, C-reactive protein can be monitored in comparison to visceral proteins, like prealbumin, to determine

Lifespan

Nutrition and Physiological Stress in the Older Adult

Older adults are the most rapidly increasing segment of the population and occupy two-thirds of all intensive care unit beds (Reid & Allard-Gould, 2004). Critical care nurses need to be acutely aware of malnutrition risk in this growing population because of the negative effect it has on health outcomes. A routine nutrition assessment should always be included in a nursing assessment. Even though malnutrition is an unfortunately common occurrence in the hospitalized older adult, it should never be dismissed as acceptable or "just a part of aging." The older adult is at risk for malnutrition because of physical changes that do occur with aging. This risk is compounded when critical illness and its treatment further compromise nutritional health. Older adults found to have existing malnutrition even before the metabolic stress of critical illness takes it toll are already at risk for in-hospital complications, prolonged length of stay, and increased post-hospital mortality (Gariballa & Forster, 2007; Kagansky et al., 2005).

Changes in body composition, including muscle loss associated with aging and declining activity, can leave the older adult with little skeletal muscle reserve during metabolic stress. Alterations in appetite and thirst regulation associated with aging can make optimization of nutrition and hydration status difficult when relying on oral intake. Age-related skin changes compounded by malnutrition predispose an older adult to poor wound healing and risk of pressure ulcer development (Reid & Allard-Gould, 2004). Malnutrition complicates recovery, especially when loss of skeletal muscle limits strength and endurance for rehabilitation. Up to 50% of older adults with hip fracture are already malnourished at the time of injury, and further deterioration of nutrition status continues while hospitalized because of extended hypercatabolism following treatment (Hedstrom & Cederholm, 2006). Poor calcium and vitamin D status further complicate recovery in these clients.

Whether altered nutritional status occurs because of aging, a medical condition, or treatment, intervention is essential to prevent poor health outcomes. The nurse should collaborate with the health care team to prevent malnutrition from occurring in the hospital, when possible, and to intervene early when malnutrition risk is suspected.

whether the acute phase reaction is subsiding. An elevated C-reactive protein indicates that the client is still in the acute phase reaction and visceral proteins should be judged accordingly. Visceral protein status is more indicative of nutrition status when C-reactive protein is decreased provided liver function is normal and, therefore, capable of hepatic protein synthesis. Nutritional status should be evaluated on a regular basis in the critically ill client. Recommendations for energy and nutrient needs evolve over the course of metabolic stress and should be approached based on individual client assessment.

Nutritional Requirements during the Stress Response

Although it is intuitive to most clinicians that nutrition support is essential to combat the effects of metabolic stress and prevent further decline, great controversy surrounds exactly what constitutes adequate nutrition in this physiological state. No blanket recommendation exists that covers the nutritional requirements of all critically ill clients. The body's response to the magnitude and duration of the metabolic insult differs with various types of critical illness and is further altered by individual variations. Individual nutritional needs can shift for an individual over the course of the stress response with periods of increased or decreased needs, depending on the phase of metabolic stress, medical treatment, and rehabilitation. Additionally, debate exists as to whether overly aggressive nutrition support during the first few days of the stress response contributes to poor outcome compared to deliberate underfeeding during that initial time. The general roles of nutrients in physiological stress are outlined in Table 22-1. Concerns specific to the pediatric population are outlined in Lifespan Box: Nutrition and Physiological Stress in the Older Adult.

Energy Needs

Hypermetabolism during physiological stress drives up baseline energy requirements. The registered dietitian generally is responsible for recommending target nutritional needs for the critically ill client. Depending on the medical facility, either predictive formulas or, if available, actual measured energy expenditure using indirect calorimetry are used to determine calorie needs. Chapter 8 outlines these formulas and the use of indirect calorimetry. Both overfeeding and underfeeding critically ill clients can have deleterious effects, necessitating accurate recommendations for energy intake. Overfeeding can lead to hyperglycemia, hyperlipidemia, the development of fatty liver, and excessive production of carbon dioxide, the latter especially of concern in clients with respiratory failure. Although initial underfeeding is recommended by some, chronic underfeeding leads to a cascade of malnutrition risks and poor outcome. The debate surrounding hypocaloric feedings in the early phase of physiological stress is outlined in Hot Topic: The Hypocaloric Feeding Debate.

Although actual measured energy expenditure is considered ideal, metabolic equipment can be costly and thus is not routine in all hospital settings. Box 22-1 outlines the application of common formulas used in critical care, which estimate resting metabolic rate and apply a "stress factor" to the equation based on the estimated degree of hypermetabolism. Such estimates have a subjective nature to them, especially when a client has more than one metabolic stress, such as

Table 22-1 Nutrient Function in Physiological Stress

Nutrient	Function
Protein	Provide amino acids for protein synthesis needed for enzymes, transport of proteins, tissue synthesis, fluid and electrolyte balance, immune function; energy source
Carbohydrate	Source of glucose; energy to spare protein
Fat	Source of essential fatty acids; energy
Vitamin A	Maintenance of epithelial cells, including skin and mucous membranes; involved in immune function and bone development
Thiamine, riboflavin, niacin, pyridoxine	Cofactors and coenzymes in the metabolism of carbohydrate, protein, and fat
Folate	Coenzyme in nutrient metabolism, involved in cell division, formation of red and white blood cells
Vitamin B_{12}	Involved in amino acid and fat metabolism, especially in the intestine, bone marrow, and nerve tissue
Vitamin C	Antioxidant; involved in collagen synthesis, wound repair, synthesis of adrenal cortex hormones; promotes iron absorption when consumed together
Vitamin D	Calcium homeostasis; essential for bone mineralization
Vitamin E	Antioxidant
Vitamin K	Involved in synthesis blood-clotting factors, protein
Calcium	Involved in blood clotting, nerve conduction, smooth muscle contractility; essential for bone mineralization
Copper	Enzyme component; involved in wound repair
Iron	Component of hemoglobin and myoglobin needed for oxygen delivery; essential for normal immune function
Magnesium	Involved in enzyme reactions for protein and glucose metabolism; essential for neuromuscular transmissions
Phosphorus	Provide phosphate source for major cellular energy source, adenosine triphosphate (ATP); component of phospholipids in every cell membrane; involved in acid–base balance, bone mineralization
Potassium	Essential for fluid and electrolyte balance, muscle function
Selenium	Antioxidant
Zinc	Involved in enzyme reactions, including protein, carbohydrate, and lipid metabolism; essential for wound repair
Water	Solvent involved in transport of substances, delivery to and from cells; medium for metabolic reactions; provides structure to cells and vascular volume; plays a role in body temperature regulation; needed for digestion, absorption, and excretion

multiple bone fractures, infection, and wounds, and a personal judgment has to be made about the cumulative effect of those stresses. Medications such as sedatives or inotropics have been shown to alter metabolic rate, yet are not considered in a predictive equation (Faisy, Guerot, Diehl, Labrousse, & Fagon, 2003). Additionally, many equations use present body weight as a factor in the formula, a measurement that can be drastically altered because of fluid overload or obesity in some clients. Predictive equations are known to not widely apply to the critically ill client because of individual differences and should only be considered a starting point in determining an individual client's nutritional needs. Many were developed using healthy adults and

do not correlate well to the needs of the critically ill (Stucky, Moncure, Hise, Gossage, & Northrup, 2008; Weekes, 2007). For example, the long-established and frequently used Harris-Benedict equation was reported to be inaccurate in 39% of critically ill clients when compared with measured energy expenditure using a metabolic cart geared for indirect calorimetry (Boullata, Williams, Cottrell, Hudson, & Compher, 2007). Although this formula is felt to most closely estimate needs compared to other formulas used in the acute-care setting, it is not possible to guess which clients might fall into the almost 40% error zone, driving home the importance of ongoing close monitoring of nutritional status and fine-tuning of recommendations.

Lifespan

Pediatric Concerns with Physiological Stress

The nutritional needs of critically ill pediatric clients are often difficult to determine. Estimation of requirements is often based on equations that are either derived from healthy children or the adult population, making them less accurate in the child experiencing hypermetabolic and hypercatabolic illness. Infants and children who become critically ill are at risk of malnutrition because of existing high metabolic needs in the face of little energy and protein reserves at their young age (Hulst, Joosten, Tibboel, & van Goudoever, 2006; Skillman & Wischmeyer, 2008). Further, existing medical conditions that may be responsible for the current critical illness can have already placed the child at nutritional risk. Almost one-quarter of children admitted to intensive care are reported to have existing malnutrition (Hulst et al., 2004a). Poor nutritional status in infants and children is associated with the same negative health outcomes found in malnourished adults. In the child with a prolonged stay in an intensive care unit, the effects of malnutrition on recovery can persist for an additional 6 months after hospital discharge (Skillman & Wischmeyer, 2008).

It is recommended that actual measured energy expenditure be used to determine calorie requirements in the critically ill pediatric population. Inaccuracies in estimated equations are faulted as contributing to both under- and overfeeding recommendations. Cumulative energy and protein deficits are associated with changes in anthropometric measurements and impaired linear growth in children (Hulst et al., 2004b). It is essential to incorporate physical activity into energy estimations, because it can alter recommendations significantly as the child enters recovery (van der Kulp, de Meer, Westerterp, & Gemke, 2007).

The critical care nurse caring for the pediatric client is faced with many obstacles to providing the client with adequate nutrition. The need for fluid restriction, numerous interruptions to nutrition support because of procedures or gastrointestinal intolerance, and any underprescription of nutrition all lead to accumulating nutritional debt (Hulst et al., 2006). The critically ill child requires close monitoring of nutrition status and frequent adjustment to the nutrition care plan to best provide optimal nutrition to meet the demands of physiological stress, recovery, and later growth catch-up.

hot TOpic

The Hypocaloric Feeding Debate

A debate exists surrounding the effects of intensive nutrition support on critically ill clients during the early days of metabolic stress. One school of thought supports the idea that it may be beneficial to deliberately underfeed individuals by providing a hypocaloric feeding that includes adequate protein. Proponents of hypocaloric feeding cite the negative effects of hyperglycemia during the stress response and feel aggressive institution of full feedings may exacerbate that. Limited research exists to support this idea that shows positive nitrogen balance can be achieved and length of hospital stay and complications are reduced compared with early provision of full calorie and protein needs. Clients are provided 10 to 20 kcalories/kg of ideal or adjusted weight and 1.5 to 2 gm protein/kg. When measured energy expenditure is available to determine calorie requirements, 50% to 90% of measured needs is recommended.

Researchers supporting the practice of providing full energy and protein point to studies that demonstrate increased morbidity in hypocalorically fed clients. It has been reported that the higher the energy debt becomes over the course of days, the higher the number of septic and nonseptic complications found. Further, the length of time that the body can tolerate hypocaloric feedings during metabolic stress is not known because it may be unique for each circumstance and individual.

While unplanned underfeeding can occur in the intensive care unit setting because of poor tolerance to feedings and interrupted or delayed institution of feedings, this results in underfeeding of both calories and protein. Underfeeding both calories and protein is not associated with beneficial outcome; adequate protein was provided in any study that demonstrated a benefit. The fact that so many critically ill clients do not receive the full amount of prescribed nutrition support, regardless of whether it is aimed at adequate or underfeeding, during the first week in the intensive care unit is what makes comparisons between research on either side of the debate difficult to evaluate. Additionally, intravenous dextrose and lipid-based sedatives provide calories that were often not considered in these studies. Last, different methods of determining energy needs were used; some used measured expenditure, while others used estimation formulas that include clinician judgment. Further clinical trials need to be done that carefully consider these factors before a conclusion can be drawn to develop evidence-based recommendations.

Both sides agree that overfeeding the critically ill client is to be avoided. Hyperglycemia, increased lipid levels, fatty liver, and difficulty weaning from mechanical ventilation because of excessive production of carbon dioxide are potential negative effects of overfeeding.

Sources: Adapted from: Berger & Chiolero, 2007b; Boitano, 2006; Hise et al., 2007; Vincent, 2007; Weekes, 2007.

Assessment of energy needs should be an ongoing process with careful attention to medical treatment and trends in measured parameters, such as weight, dietary intake, and laboratory values. The client can be used as a self-reference when making judgments regarding the adequacy of nutrition provided and any need for adjustments. When measured energy expenditure is possible, it should be reevaluated over the course of recovery to provide nutrition that parallels need. For example, the use of barbiturates may lower an otherwise elevated metabolic rate early in the re-

sponse to traumatic brain injury and be followed by periods of increased energy needs when the medication is discontinued or the client begins the physical rehabilitation process. While monitoring the nutritional intake of the critically ill client, the nurse should include an assessment

BOX 22-1	Nutritional Recommendations for Physiological Stress

Calories

Measured energy expenditure is preferred to estimation equations.

Estimation Equations

Use weight in kg, height in cm, and age in years.

Harris-Benedict

1. Determine baseline needs.

Males 66.5 + (13.75 × wt) + (5 × ht) − (6.78 × age)
Females 655.1 + (9.56 × wt) + (1.85 × ht)− (4.68 × age)

2. Estimate *stress factor* and *physical activity* level and multiply with baseline need.
   Stress factors (consider medications, multiple stressors, mechanical ventilation weaning that can alter estimations).
   - Bone fracture: up to 1.3
   - Burns: use Curreri or up to 1.75
   - Multiple trauma: up to 1.6
   - Sepsis, severe infection: up to 1.6
   - Surgery: up to 1.2
   - Traumatic brain injury: up to 1.4

Physical activity level
- Bed rest: 1.2
- Ambulating: 1.3
- Rehabilitation: depends on program

Curreri (for burns): (24 × usual wt) + (40 × % body surface burn)

Protein

Needs range from 1.2 to 2 gm/kg body weight/day depending on condition, loss of skeletal muscle.

Nitrogen balance study can be used as monitoring tool but is invalid in renal failure (see Nutrition Assessment in Chapter 12).

Fluid

Include assessment of fluid balance when determining need. Large losses from vomiting, diarrhea, wounds, sweating or evaporation, and fistula may be difficult to determine. Fluid overload or renal failure will alter these baseline needs.

Adults: 1 mL/kcalorie needed OR 35 mL/kg body weight

Children: 1.5 mL/kcalorie needed OR 50–60 mL/kg in children and 150 mL/kg in infants

Sources: Adapted from: Brain Trauma Foundation, 2007; Curreri, Richmond, Marvin, & Baxter, 1974; Institute of Medicine (IOM), 2004; Kreymann et al., 2006; Prelack, Dylewski, & Sheridan, 2007.

of how closely the delivered amount of nutrition matches that prescribed. Interrupted tube feedings account for the primary discrepancy between prescribed and administered nutrition with enteral nutrition support (van den Broek, Rasmussen-Conrad, Naber, & Wanten, 2009). Alternatives in feeding schedules and formula choice may be indicated when nutritional prescriptions are not being met.

Protein Needs

Hypermetabolism and hypercatabolism contribute to increased protein needs during physiological stress. Box 22-1 outlines general recommendations for protein intake in the critically ill. It is generally assumed that providing increased protein along with adequate calories will spare the body from further protein catabolism and improve outcome. If insufficient protein is available from exogenous sources, such as food, tube feedings, or parenteral nutrition, endogenous protein sources, such as muscle, will be catabolized to meet metabolic needs (Stroud, 2007). Guidelines for daily protein intake range from 1.2 gm/kg body weight up to 2 gm/kg (Frankenfield, 2006; Griffiths & Bongers, 2005; Powell-Tuck, 2007). However, in many cases catabolism has been shown to continue despite high protein and calorie intake because of the metabolic response to injury and inflammation responsible for ongoing mobilization of amino acids from skeletal muscle (Griffiths & Bongers, 2005; Stroud, 2007). Attenuating this stress response and

halting catabolism has been the subject of much research targeting the use of substances such as medications, hormones, and nutritional supplements as potential solutions. Anabolic hormones, such as insulin-like growth factor, testosterone, and human growth hormone, have been used in an attempt to preserve lean body mass, but none is a universal treatment or without side effects (Demling, 2007). Some nonessential amino acids are felt to be conditionally essential during critical illness and may serve as a vehicle for lessening catabolism in some situations. Hot Topic: Amino Acid Supplementation in Critical Illness discusses the use of amino acid supplements in critical illness.

Fluid Needs

Fluid and electrolyte imbalance is a common occurrence during metabolic stress, making estimation of fluid needs a challenge. Fluid overload because of the need for acute resuscitation in some circumstances may be compounded with increased capillary permeability resulting from the inflammatory response and leads to increased interstitial, or third-spacing, of fluid (Lobo, 2004). Large exudative wounds, burn injury, diuretic use, fever, diarrhea, fistula drainage, and vomiting contribute to increased fluid losses. Hyperglycemia causes fluid and electrolyte shifts that further complicate the picture. No specific recommendations exist for fluid requirements in critical illness, though often a rule-of-thumb used is to provide 1 mL of fluid per calorie

MyNursingKit Nutrition and Wound Healing

hot Topic

Amino Acid Supplementation in Critical Illness

Specific amino acids have been the focus of research attention in the nutrition care of critically ill clients. Specifically, glutamine and arginine, two nonessential amino acids, have been deemed conditionally essential because of possibly increased needs during hypermetabolic stress.

Glutamine is one of the most abundant amino acids in the body, yet plasma and muscle levels are reported to drop dramatically during physiological stress. Glutamine is reported to have multiple functions, including:

- Principal fuel of enterocytes, preserving gut integrity
- Principal fuel of leukocytes and macrophages, enhancing immune function
- Antioxidant
- Acid–base homeostasis in the kidney
- Enhancement of heat shock protein expression, managing stress-induced protein changes
- Attenuation of insulin resistance and cytokine production during metabolic stress

Research on the use of glutamine supplementation during critical illness has some promising results in subpopulations of clients. Positive effects have been demonstrated with higher doses and parenteral administration. Specifically, its use in burn and trauma clients is reported to decrease risk of wound infection and length of hospital stay.

Arginine is synthesized from citrulline in a multiple-step process involving the small intestine and renal tubules that normally yields sufficient endogenous production to meet the needs of the body. During critical illness, arginine needs may be increased because of the elevated protein turnover found in metabolic stress. Arginine is reported to have multiple functions, including:

- Intermediary in proline synthesis, essential in wound repair
- Intermediary in polyamine synthesis, needed in cell growth and proliferation, wound repair
- Substrate for production of nitrous oxide (NO), a vasodilator with bacteriostatic effect

Research on the use of arginine supplementation during critical illness has mixed results with a lack of clinical trials examining the effects of arginine alone on outcome. Often, arginine is given with other dietary supplement components such as n-3 fatty acids and nucleotides in mixtures referred to as immunonutrition. Although there have been reports of positive associations between high arginine formulas and reduced infectious complications and improved wound healing, troubling statistics have emerged linking these products with increased mortality in clients with sepsis. Although the exact cause of this increase is unknown, the potential to increase production of NO and its negative cytotoxic effect have been postulated as contributing to this risk. Use of such products is not universally recommended in the critically ill.

Sources: Adapted from: Demling, 2007; Kreymann et al., 2006; Powell-Tuck, 2007; Wischmeyer, 2007; Zhou & Martindale, 2007.

given. Individual differences in fluid balance and renal, cardiac, and liver function necessitate a customized approach to fluid recommendations. The nurse should carefully monitor fluid balance, performing daily weights and taking into consideration fluid losses that are difficult to quantify. Dressings may need to be weighed to estimate fluid loss. The registered dietitian can recommend appropriate nutrition intervention if clients receiving tube feedings or parenteral nutrition require a fluid restriction.

Vitamin and Mineral Needs

Vitamins and minerals serve many important functions in physiological stress. Their role as cofactors and coenzymes in metabolism automatically increases their need when calorie and protein needs are elevated. The healing process requires adequate provision of many vitamins and minerals at each stage of the healing process. Surgical wounds, pressure ulcers, fistula, and burn injuries can benefit from attention to vitamin and mineral status as outlined in Box 22-2 and Client Education Checklist: Nutrition and Wound Healing.

Increased losses of vitamins and minerals can occur during critical illness because of blood loss, diarrhea, fistulas, and exudative wounds (Shenkin, 2006). Water-soluble vitamins and trace minerals are of particular concern, but it is difficult to measure nutrient status during the acute phase of injury or inflammation because of redistribution in plasma and tissue, making laboratory tests of limited value (Berger & Shenkin, 2006). The combination of increased nutrient needs with the potential for increased nutrient losses places clients at particular risk for deficiency. The nurse should be mindful of this combined risk, especially in clients who have preexisting risk factors for malnutrition because of disease, poor dietary habits, or alcoholism. Pregnant females and children are additionally at risk of poor vitamin and mineral status when faced with critical illness because of increased needs to support growth and development. No blanket guidelines exist for providing vitamins and minerals during physiological stress. The recommended dietary allowances (RDA) can serve as a starting point, but these are intended for a healthy population and cannot be extrapolated to address the needs of the critically ill.

Some researchers believe that need for antioxidant vitamins and minerals, such as selenium, and vitamins A and C, is increased because metabolic stress increases production of free radicals that cause oxidative damage; however, evidence is limited that supplementation alters outcome significantly in humans who are not deficient (Berger & Chiolero, 2007a). Studies targeting the use of parenteral antioxidants, in particular selenium, have shown more promise than enteral supplementation, but the limited scale of these findings requires more intensive research before a conclusion can be drawn (Berger & Shenkin, 2006; Heyland, Dhaliwal, Suchner, & Berger, 2005). Of concern is the fact that high-dose supplementation with antioxidants can transform these nutrients into free radicals themselves, potentially worsening the very scenario they were targeted to improve (Berger & Shenkin, 2006).

BOX 22-2 Nutritional Requirements for Wound Healing

Each distinct phase of wound healing requires adequate nutrition. Wound homeostasis, inflammation, proliferation, and remodeling are individual, but overlapping, stages of wound healing with unique requirements for the core nutrients essential to progressive recovery. Although overall nutrition status affects wound healing, core nutrients associated with wound healing include protein, vitamins A and C, zinc, and copper. Adequate hydration is also needed. The role of each nutrient specific to wound healing is outlined below:

- *Protein*—prevents prolonged inflammatory response, provides substrate for tissue synthesis and wound remodeling, contributes to tensile strength of scar.
- *Vitamin A*—enhances early inflammatory response at site, stimulates epithelial cell and bone formation. Clients on corticosteroids with delayed wound healing should have vitamin A status assessed.
- *Vitamin C*—cofactor in collagen formation and other components of intracellular matrix, antioxidant, enhances neutrophil and lymphocyte response.
- *Zinc*—component of over 300 enzymes, including those responsible for protein synthesis, vitamin A transport, cell division, DNA synthesis. Exudative wounds and excessive intestinal losses cause increased loss of zinc.
- *Copper*—cofactor in production of connective tissue and collagen cross-linking.

- *Fluid*—maintains skin turgor, delivers nutrients and oxygen to wound site. Fever, air-fluidized beds, and exudative wounds lead to fluid losses that must be replaced.

Diminished availability of any one of these nutrients can impair wound healing. In the client with metabolic stress, increased demand for nutrients because of the inflammatory response and catabolism can lessen the availability of these nutrients for wound healing purposes. High losses of lean body mass during catabolism limits the amount of protein available for wound repair and when losses exceed 20% of lean body mass, wound repair may cease. Adequate protein intake without adequate calorie intake can shunt protein into use as a calorie source instead of for tissue synthesis.

It is common practice to provide vitamin and trace mineral supplements to clients with large wounds, but this practice is not supported by clinical research unless deficiency is likely or known. In particular, excessive supplementation with zinc can exacerbate a copper deficiency, especially in a client with marginal nutrition status, and excessive vitamin C causes diarrhea. Clients should be discouraged from self-prescribing dietary supplements for wound healing. The nurse should assess the client for use of any herbal dietary supplements that alter blood-clotting or platelet function because this effect can have a negative impact on wound repair.

 ■ What food sources could the nurse recommend to a client to boost intake of the nutrients associated with wound repair?

Sources: Adapted from: Campos, Groth, & Branco, 2008; Keast, Parslow, Houghton, Norton, & Fraser, 2007; Langemo et al., 2006; Posthauer, 2006.

Nutrition Care

The nurse caring for critically ill clients should be knowledgeable about the general nutrition requirements for physiological stress as well as guidelines that are more specific to certain populations. Surgery presents nutritional challenges that can be worsened if malnutrition exists. Wound healing, trauma, burn injury, respiratory failure, and sepsis warrant close attention to nutritional needs and delivery for optimal outcome. Nutrition support in the critically ill can be in the form of food, oral supplements, tube feeding, parenteral nutrition or a combination of approaches. The appropriate route of nutrition support depends on the client's condition and intestinal function. Chapter 16 outlines types of nutrition support in detail. Special attention should be given to those individuals who have had little or no nutrition for many days because they are at risk for refeeding syndrome when feedings are reinstituted. Practice Pearl: Who Is at Risk for Refeeding Syndrome? outlines parameters for the nurse regarding these clients.

PRACTICE PEARL

Who Is at Risk for Refeeding Syndrome?

Refeeding syndrome occurs with significant calorie intake following starvation or semistarvation. Critically ill or postoperative clients who have received little or no nutritional support for over 5 days can be at risk for refeeding. Symptoms occur as a result of increased uptake of glucose into cells when feeding begins and can have dangerous results if left unmonitored. The nurse should be alert to the following symptoms of refeeding syndrome:

- Hypophosphatemia
- Hypokalemia
- Hypomagnesemia
- Cardiac rhythm changes
- Edema
- Congestive heart failure

Treatment is pharmacological correction of electrolyte deficiencies and careful monitoring. When possible, gradual increases in calorie intake rather than abrupt overfeeding can lessen symptom risk.

| CLIENT EDUCATION CHECKLIST | ✓ | Nutrition and Wound Healing |

Intervention	Example
Encourage intake of adequate calories 1. Describe role of calories in healing. 2. List sources of nutrient-dense calories.	1. Adequate intake of calories is needed to spare protein intake for wound repair. Inadequate intake of calories can lead to protein being used for energy rather than tissue synthesis. 2. Foods that provide both calories and nutrients are considered nutrient dense. Examples include high-protein foods (below), grains and vegetables with added calories from sauces, dressings, margarine or spreads, dairy-based desserts.
Encourage intake of adequate protein 1. Describe role of protein in healing. 2. List sources of high-protein foods.	1. Protein is used in synthesis of new tissue, wound remodeling, and maintenance of immune status. 2. Animal proteins include poultry, red meat, fish, eggs, milk, yogurt, and cheese. Plant proteins include soy and other beans, lentils, split peas, nuts, nut butters, and seeds. Clients with diminished appetite may benefit from suggestions in Client Education Checklist: Optimizing Nutrition in the Frail Client with COPD.
Encourage intake of adequate micronutrients 1. Describe role of vitamins and mineral in healing. 2. List dietary sources of vitamins A, C, and zinc.	1. Vitamins and minerals assist the body in each phase of the four-step process of wound healing. Although overall nutrient intake is important, adequate vitamins A and C and zinc intake is needed. 2. Vitamin A: green and orange vegetables, fortified dairy foods, liver. Vitamin C: citrus fruit, green leafy vegetables, tomato. Zinc: high-protein foods also contain zinc.
Encourage intake of adequate fluid 1. Describe role of fluids in healing. 2. List sources of nutrient-dense liquid.	1. Fluid is needed to transport needed nutrients and oxygen to the wound. It also maintains skin integrity and turgor. Large wounds lose fluid that needs to be replaced. 2. Fluids are anything that is liquid at room temperature, including milk or milk substitutes, smoothies, oral liquid nutrition supplements, ice cream, juices, hearty soups, and watery fruit. Milk can be substituted for water when making foods such as hot cereal and cocoa or to reconstitute powdered milk to increase protein.
Explain role of dietary supplements in wound healing	Supplementation with vitamins or minerals beyond the recommended dietary allowance (RDA) is not indicated unless a deficiency is suspected. Some dietary supplements, such as herbs, can alter blood clotting or interact with medications. Use of any dietary supplement should be discussed with the primary health care provider.

Surgery

Perioperative management of the surgical client should include optimization of nutritional intake. Preoperative malnutrition is associated with postoperative complications, such as infection, poor wound healing, and longer hospital stay (Kopp Lugli, Wykes, & Carli, 2008; Sierzega, Niekowal, Kulig, & Popiela, 2007; Sungurtekin, Sungurtekin, Balci, Zencir, & Erdem, 2004). A reverse correlation has been reported between postoperative complications and preoperative albumin levels with worsening outcome as albumin levels decrease below 3.25 mg/dL in clients undergoing gastrointestinal surgery (Kudsk et al., 2003). Existing disease and, in the case of transplant surgery, or-

gan failure can place an individual at risk for poor nutrition status. When feasible, it is suggested that up to 2 weeks of preoperative enteral nutrition support be given to malnourished clients with either a body mass index (BMI) less than 18.5, a greater than 10% unplanned weight loss over 6 months, or an albumin less than 3 mg/dL, even if it means a delay in surgery (Weimann et al., 2006). The specific needs of clients undergoing transplant surgery are outlined in Box 22-3. The nurse working with clients in the preoperative setting should include a nutrition assessment in the presurgical screening and provide appropriate advice on improving nutritional intake where appropriate. Preoperative screening should also include an

BOX 22-3	Nutrition and the Client with Organ Transplant

The optimization of nutrition status before and after transplantation surgery is important. Underlying organ failure and its effects can predispose the transplant candidate to poor nutrition long before surgery. Prolonged waiting lists for surgery can extend this effect but also provides an opportunity to improve nutrition status. Clients awaiting lung transplant often have chronic obstructive pulmonary disease (COPD) or cystic fibrosis, conditions that are associated with malnutrition because of frequent pulmonary infections and increased resting energy expenditure. Chapters on renal, liver, and gastrointestinal diseases outline disease-specific nutritional concerns for the client with renal failure, end-stage liver disease, and short bowel syndrome. No research evidence is available that demonstrates the effect of preoperative nutrition intervention on a living donor participating in transplant surgery. The preoperative nutrition assessment of the client awaiting transplant and, if applicable, the living donor should be conducted using similar guidelines to that of clients awaiting major abdominal surgery.

Following transplant surgery, early nutrition support should begin. Nutritional needs parallel those of a surgical client. The enteral route is preferential. Normal food is tolerated by most, but tube feedings may be required if the client remains on mechanical ventilation or is otherwise unable to be fed orally. Clients undergoing small bowel transplantation require slow reintroduction of enteral nutrition, as outlined in Chapter 20. Young children undergoing intestinal transplant may have been on long-term parenteral nutrition prior to surgery, necessitating the need for development of oral feeding skills after transplantation. Safe food handling practices should be followed because of the risk of food-borne illness in the client on immunosuppressive medications. Long-term nutrition monitoring is essential because of medication side effects, such as hyperglycemia, hyperkalemia, and hypertension from corticosteroids and cacineurin inhibitors. Modifications in potassium or sodium intake can be indicated as well as a carbohydrate-controlled diet. Bone health can be compromised because of the effects of long-term steroids, necessitating close attention to adequate vitamin D and calcium intake. Use of herbal supplements should be discouraged to minimize the risk of drug interactions, as seen with the concomitant use of St. John's Wort and cyclosporines.

■ What are some safe food handling practices that the nurse can review with the transplant client?

Sources: Adapted from: Goulet & Sauvat, 2006; Tynan & Hasse, 2004; Weimann et al., 2006.

assessment of dietary supplement intake to avoid any interactions with anaesthesia, medications, or alterations in blood clotting. Chapters 24 and 25 outline drug, nutrient, food, and dietary supplement interactions in detail with advice specific for the surgical client in Practice Pearl 24-3: Preoperative Assessment.

Preoperative routines can contribute to nutritional risk. Missed meals, prolonged fasting, or intake of only clear liquids provides inadequate nutrition. False reliance on intravenous dextrose as a significant source of calories can jeopardize nutrition status. One liter of 5% dextrose has only 170 kcalories. Preoperative fasting is not indicated in most cases and may contribute to diminished glycogen stores postoperatively (Weimann et al., 2006). The practice of fasting before surgery to avoid aspiration risk has been replaced by allowing clear liquids and solids up to 2 and 6 hours, respectively, preoperatively (Weimann et al., 2006). This practice is reviewed in the Evidence-Based Practice Box: Preoperative Fasting in Pediatric Clients. Carbohydrate loading, not unlike that encouraged with athletes before an event, is being used in oral liquid form before surgery to spare glycogen stores and decrease postoperative metabolic stress and insulin resistance (Kopp Lugli et al., 2008; Martindale & Maerz, 2006).

First postoperative nutritional goals include early reinstitution of feeding, control of plasma glucose, and attenuation of any metabolic stress response (Martindale & Maerz, 2006; Weimann et al., 2006). Second, attention should focus on optimizing nutrition status for healing. Although hyperglycemia has long been considered part of the normal response to metabolic stress, it has been demonstrated that strict glycemic control is associated with improved gut function, reduced infection, and improved morbidity and mortality risk in both medical and surgical clients (Inzucchi, 2006; Martindale & Maerz, 2006; Van den Berghe et al., 2006). In the client with traumatic brain injury, hyperglycemia is associated with detrimental changes in brain tissue and additional injury (Cook, Peppard, & Magnusun, 2008). Providing nutrition via the enteral route with food, oral supplements, or tube feeding is preferred to parenteral nutrition support because of preservation of gut integrity and a reduced risk of infection (Weimann et al., 2006). Traditionally, institution of feeding is withheld until bowel sounds return, indicating the return of bowel motility. More recently that concept has been challenged with several studies reporting that early feedings are generally tolerated and may be associated with a decreased length of hospital stay (Andersen, Lewis, & Thomas, 2006; Charoenkwan, Phillipson & Vutyavanich, 2007). The progression of feedings

Preoperative Fasting in Pediatric Clients

Clinical Problem: Preoperative fasting is often difficult for infants and young children, along with parents who must supervise it. What evidence exists for recommended preoperative fasting times for infants and children?

Evidence: Infants and children who undergo the usual overnight preoperative fast often arrive for surgery hungry, thirsty, dehydrated, and irritable. Parents are the primary caregivers for their fussy, irritable child. A study of 100 infants and children compared those who underwent the usual overnight fast and those who were allowed apple juice in a quantity based on their age, up to 250 mL, between 0600 and 0630 on the day of surgery (Castillo-Zamora, Castillo-Peralta, & Nava-Ocampo, 2005). The researchers found that children who received apple juice were less thirsty and dehydrated than the control group, and they had more positive behavior.

In a review of fasting guidelines, Cook-Sather and Litman (2006) recommended that infants and children be allowed age-appropriate amounts of clear liquids up to 2 hours before surgery. They further recommended that breastfed infants be allowed breast milk up to 3 hours before surgery and formula-fed infants be allowed formula 4 hours before surgery. For the older child, light meals may be acceptable 6 hours before surgery if the surgery is later in the day.

Two studies were conducted with children ages 2 to 10 years who were undergoing ambulatory surgery for tonsillectomy and adenoidectomy (T & A). A descriptive study of 12 children and mothers found that parents had concerns about being able to impose and maintain the fast and that al-lowing fluid as long as permitted improved parents' perceived control of the surgery experience and enhanced postoperative recovery (Klemetti & Suominen, 2008). An additional study of 116 children undergoing T & A examined the effect of preoperative fasting on postoperative pain and nausea and vomiting. The researchers found that children who were allowed preoperative fluids had significantly less pain than the control group, but there were no significant differences in nausea and vomiting, leading them to conclude that more liberal fluid intake led to an improved surgical experience (Klemetti et al., 2009).

A meta-analysis begun in 2005 and extended in 2008 examined 23 studies of various aspects of preoperative fasting, including such variables as gastric pH, irritability, nausea and vomiting, and thirst (Brady, Kinn, O'Rourke, Randhawa, & Stuart, 2005; Jull, 2006). Based on the analysis, they concluded that healthy infants and children should be permitted clear fluids up to 2 hours preoperatively because there were no adverse effects on gastric pH or nausea and vomiting, and that children have a more positive experience in terms of pain, thirst, and hunger.

Conclusions: Sufficient evidence exists for nurses to advocate preoperative fasts not to exceed 2 hours for otherwise healthy infants and children.

CRITICAL THINKING QUESTION:

1. How should the nurse respond to the mother who asks why she had to fast for 12 hours before surgery and her 5-year old can have a small amount of clear liquids until 2 hours before surgery?

following surgery should be adjusted individually for each client with careful attention given to reaching optimal intake. Postoperative **ileus,** or paralytic bowel, is a complication that precludes enteral intake. Manipulation of the intestine during surgery, excessive intraoperative fluids, hyperglycemia, and opioid use can contribute to development of this condition (Martindale & Maertz, 2006). More aggressive nutrition support in the form of tube feedings or parenteral nutrition may be needed in clients who cannot eat for more than 7 days or have insufficient intake for more than 10 days (Weimann et al., 2006). The nutrition support team should be consulted with such clients to determine the appropriate feeding route and formula.

Trauma

Nutrition care of the client with trauma is similar to that of the surgical client but without the opportunity to provide any preoperative nutrition assessment or intervention. Blunt force trauma, bone fractures, and spinal cord and traumatic brain injuries are examples of trauma that results in metabolic stress to the body. Any surgical or medical treatment for trauma will layer those nutritional concerns on top of the challenges from the injury itself. For example, treatment for a fractured mandible with immobilization can preclude any chewing and, therefore, use of liquid and pureed nutrition may be needed for a number of weeks. Abdominal trauma resulting in an open abdomen results in large losses of fluid and electrolytes, along with protein losses of about 2 gm of nitrogen/liter of abdominal fluid output (Cheatham, Safcsak, Brzezinski, & Lube, 2007). Treatment of an open abdomen can include enteral nutrition within the first 4 days following injury, an intervention demonstrated to lead to earlier primary abdominal closure and lower rate of abdominal fistula development than similar clients who received later feeding (Collier et al., 2007). As in other types of metabolic stress, nutrition status should be monitored closely for changing needs, taking into consideration the metabolic demands of wound healing.

Clients with traumatic brain injury may or may not have visible symptoms that signal the elevated nutritional demands that occur with this type of trauma. Some may experience multiple fractures or other injuries, whereas others have a closed head injury without a major visible wound. Hypermetabolism and hypercatabolism result in both scenarios, especially in the early postinjury period and related to the secondary injury that occurs because of brain swelling and cell death (Cook et al., 2008; Krakau et al., 2007). Energy expenditure increases an average of 40% with some clients experiencing an increase that exceeds 100% baseline (Brain Trauma Foundation, 2007). The presence of intermittent muscle contractions following this type of injury further increases energy needs (Cook et al., 2008). Use of corticosteroids to reduce swelling increases this effect, whereas medicinal paralysis or sedation lowers metabolic rate. Institution of nutrition support in this population should begin early after the injury to avoid a mounting nutritional deficit. Evidence to support an exact feeding protocol is limited, but research has demonstrated a trend toward improved outcome when nutrition care is instituted early and adequate intake is reached within the first week following injury (Brain Trauma Foundation, 2007; Perel et al., 2006). Clients with altered gastric emptying require jejunal tube feedings and, in some cases, parenteral nutrition. Depending on the severity of the injury, longer-term tube feeding with a gastrostomy tube can be indicated in clients who persist in a vegetative state. Fluid status must be monitored and feedings adjusted accordingly to avoid fluid overload that could contribute to brain swelling (Cook et al., 2008). As recovery occurs, nutrition care evolves to transitioning to oral intake with varying levels of feeding assistance depending on rehabilitation. In one report of clients with traumatic brain injury, 86% required an initial tube feeding, with 22% gastrostomy tube use. By 6 months postinjury, 92% of clients were taking complete oral nutrition, 84% without assistance (Krakau et al., 2007). Transition to oral feeding can be complicated by dysphagia or facial and dental fractures that make chewing and swallowing difficult. These challenges demonstrate the important point of monitoring nutrition status and intake and utilizing the team approach to nutritional care. Early nutritional needs are high because of the metabolic response to trauma, and the occurrence of weight loss and malnutrition is common in this population. When the metabolic response to stress is lessened during recovery, energy and protein needs can increase again with the physical demands of rehabilitation and the goal of restoring lost muscle mass.

Nutrition care of the client with bone fractures should include an assessment of nutrition status related to bone health. Especially in the older adult, poor nutrition status represents a risk for fractures because of falls or osteoporosis (Cederholm & Hedstrom, 2005). Lifespan Box: Nutrition and Physiological Stress in the Older Adult outlines particular concerns for the older adult and bone fractures.

Infection and Sepsis

Infection causes an inflammatory response that, along with fever, can elevate energy requirements. It is commonly calculated that metabolic rate increases 7% for every 1°F elevation in body temperature above normal. The inflammatory response can be more widespread if sepsis occurs. Sepsis causes a heightened inflammatory response because of the presence of pathogens and their toxins in blood and tissue. When sepsis (or other physiological stressors such as multiple trauma or burns) causes a widespread inflammatory response, the effect is called systemic inflammatory response syndrome (SIRS). SIRS may go on to cause multiple organ dysfunction syndrome (MODS) with hallmark failure of such organs as the kidney, liver, lung, intestine, and heart. One theorized contributor to risk of MODS is bacterial translocation from the intestinal tract. Use of the intestinal tract as a route for nutrition support, either orally or via tube feeding, is recommended to reduce this risk by maintaining gut-associated lymphoid tissue (GALT), an effect that positively influences the systemic immune system (Martindale & Cresci, 2005). In clients who do develop MODS, nutrition care strategies are contingent on an assessment of organ function, because renal or hepatic failure can alter the ability to handle high-protein intake. Additionally, intestinal involvement can cause ileus. The nutrition support team should be consulted when gut function is compromised.

Much research has focused on whether risk of infection in the critically ill client can be altered through nutrition intervention. It has been established that tight glycemic control is associated with reduced risk of infectious complications following surgery (Inzucchi, 2006). Infusion of dextrose with parenteral nutrition should follow established standards, outlined in Chapter 16, to avoid contributing to hyperglycemia. The use of n-3 instead of n-6 fatty acids has been targeted for their anti-inflammatory effect. N-6 fatty acids, commonly found in parenteral nutrition and intravenous sedation medications, are associated with suppression of immune function (Martindale & Cresci, 2005). Nutritional supplementation with arginine and nucleotides is also under investigation, but conflicting results and potentially negative effects of nitrous oxide from arginine metabolism have led to recommendations to avoid these in the critically ill client (Dhaliwal & Heyland, 2005). The use of probiotics and high-dose vitamin and mineral supplementation are other areas of **immunonutrition** that are under investigation.

Burns

Nutrition care following burn injury plays a central role in the treatment of clients. A heightened inflammatory response, direct tissue damage, and increased heat loss place these clients among the most hypermetabolic (Prelack, Dylewski, & Sheridan, 2007). Additional factors compounding the increased nutritional demands include complicating

MyNursingKit Wound Healing and Post-Burn Care

injuries, organ dysfunction, altered fluid homeostasis, and treatment approaches. It can be difficult to ensure an accurate assessment of nutrition status at the time of injury if historical anthropometric values are not available and current body weight and laboratory values are confounded by marked fluid shifts and the acute phase response to the injury. Despite this limitation, weight and laboratory values should be assessed and monitored to establish trends and serve as a base for nutrition recommendations (Prelack et al., 2007).

Estimates of nutritional requirements following a burn injury vary. Energy requirements are driven by the extent of the burn as well as the treatment. Indirect calorimetry is the preferred way to determine energy requirements in this critically ill population, but this technology is not always available. Estimated equations can be used, as outlined in Box 22-1, but are reported to overestimate needs since the advent of early excision and grafting of wounds that result in a diminished hypermetabolic response compared with open wounds (Prelack et al., 2007). Figure 22-2 ■ describes the method for determining burn surface area when using estimation formulas. Other aspects of client management that lower metabolic requirements include sedation, attention to minimizing heat loss with environmental control, and pain control (Prelack et al., 2007). The support of the client with mechanical ventilation affects metabolic requirements, as discussed later in the chapter. Protein and micronutrient recommendations parallel advice given for wound healing. Evidence-based guidelines are lacking for supplementation of vitamins and minerals in the client with burn. Common practice includes provision of a parenteral or enteral multivitamin-multimineral supplement with attention given to zinc, copper, selenium, and vitamin C intake (Graves, Saffle, & Cochran, 2009).

The enteral route of nutrition is preferred for its benefits on preserving gut integrity and avoiding sepsis in the critically ill client. However, in some clients with burn a combination of parenteral and enteral nutrition, or parenteral nutrition alone, may be indicated because of prolonged intolerance to enteral support, ileus, or hemodynamic instability. The increased risk of infection associated with parenteral nutrition is an important consideration in the client with burn injury already at risk for wound infection and sepsis. Glucose control protocols are common in burn centers to minimize the risk of infection and delayed wound healing related to hyperglycemia (Graves et al., 2009). Provision of enteral nutrition support early following injury has shown some promise in blunting the hypermetabolic response found in these clients, but overall evidence is limited and inconclusive as to the best timing to introduce feedings (Wasiak, Cleland, & Jefferey, 2006). Either small bowel or gastric feedings are used, depending on gastric emptying. Use of gastric feedings may help in prevention of Curling's ulcer, a side effect of burn injury (Prelack et al., 2007). Formula with enhanced glutamine content is often used because of a possible benefit in wound healing and should be considered when available (Graves et al., 2009; Kreymann et al., 2006). However, there is insufficient data to routinely recommend the use of other specialty formulas that contain arginine (Kreymann et al., 2006; Prelack et al., 2007).

Pressure Ulcers

Pressure ulcers, also called decubitus ulcers or bedsores, are found in up to 38% of clients in acute and long-term care (Reddy, Gill, & Rochon, 2006). Poor nutrition status is considered a risk factor for development of pressure ulcers, along with other physical risk factors such as immobility (Bluestein & Javaheri, 2008). Current evidence supports the optimization of nutrition status as a strategy in the prevention and management of pressure ulcers. The presence of a pressure ulcer, especially a larger or deeper wound with **exudate,** causes both an inflammatory state leading to hypermetabolism and nutrient losses from catabolism (Keast et al., 2007). Exudate is fluid that seeps from an injury site. Exudative wounds lead to nutrient losses, especially protein, zinc, and fluid. Wound infection worsens these hypermetabolic and hypercatabolic effects. Staging for pressure ulcer definition can serve as a guideline to the nurse concerning the extent of the wound. Stage III and IV pressure ulcers involve full-thickness tissue loss (National Pressure Ulcer Advisory Panel, 2007).

Treatment of an existing pressure ulcer should include attention to advice outlined in Box 22-2. Adequate hydration status, correcting existing nutritional deficiencies, and meeting increased metabolic requirements are central goals. Meeting the increased need for calories and protein with nutritional supplementation from an oral liquid supplement may offer some benefit, though the quantity and quality of research in this area is limited (Reddy et al., 2006). Supplementation with vitamins or minerals is recommended in cases with demonstrated deficiency. Routine use of supplements in the client without demonstrated deficiencies is not recommended (Bluestein & Javaheri, 2008). Commonly, daily doses of up to 50 mg of elemental zinc and 1,000 mg of vitamin C are given short term. This zinc dose exceeds the tolerable upper limit of 40 mg/day and could cause nausea, vomiting, or copper deficiency if administered long term. Clients should be evaluated for side effects and limited to 14 days on this regimen (Posthauer, 2006). Despite its common use, high-dose vitamin C is not proven to accelerate wound healing and large doses can cause diarrhea, an especially undesirable effect in an immobile or incontinent client already at risk for pressure ulcer development (Posthauer, 2007). Best practice guidelines encourage consultation with a registered dietitian for comprehensive nutrition care of these clients (Bluestein & Javaheri, 2008; Keast et al., 2007).

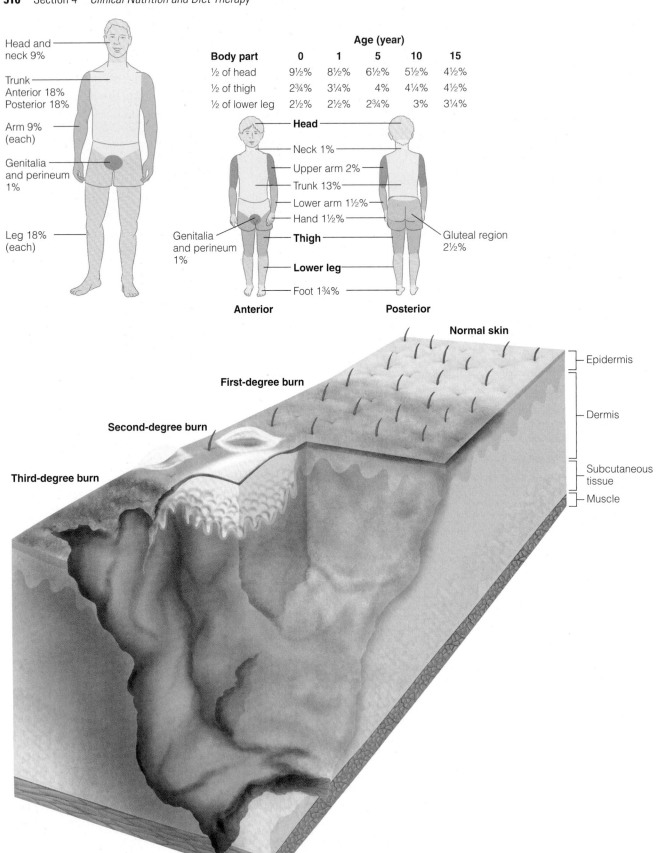

Body part	Age (year)				
	0	**1**	**5**	**10**	**15**
½ of head	9½%	8½%	6½%	5½%	4½%
½ of thigh	2¾%	3¼%	4%	4¼%	4½%
½ of lower leg	2½%	2½%	2¾%	3%	3¼%

Head and neck 9%

Trunk Anterior 18% Posterior 18%

Arm 9% (each)

Genitalia and perineum 1%

Leg 18% (each)

Head

Neck 1%

Upper arm 2%

Trunk 13%

Lower arm 1½%

Hand 1½%

Genitalia and perineum 1%

Thigh

Lower leg

Foot 1¾%

Gluteal region 2½%

Anterior   **Posterior**

Normal skin

First-degree burn

Second-degree burn

Third-degree burn

Epidermis

Dermis

Subcutaneous tissue

Muscle

■ **FIGURE 22-2 Burn Classification and Body Surface Area Estimation.**

Pulmonary Disease and Mechanical Ventilation

Poor nutrition status evidenced by weight loss and low BMI with reduced lean body mass is common in clients with chronic obstructive pulmonary disease (COPD). Between 25% and 40% of individuals with advanced COPD are malnourished with higher incidence occurring in the hospitalized or older client (Anker et al., 2006; Malone, 2004; Odencrants, Ehnfors, & Ehrenberg, 2008). The etiology of the malnutrition is not fully understood and is most likely multifactorial. First, an increase in energy requirements has been demonstrated because of both the increased work of breathing and the inflammatory response to the disease; this effect is compounded by use of medications such as β_2 antagonists (Mallampalli, 2004; Odencrants et al., 2008). Mechanical ventilation is associated with an increase in energy expenditure during the weaning process when clients are physically challenged to breathe on their own. Clients undergoing pulmonary rehabilitation will have increased energy requirements to compensate for increased physical activity. Second, the metabolic response to the inflammatory state can lead to protein catabolism. Medications such as corticosteroids, which may be used acutely or chronically in this population, have a catabolic effect. Additionally, muscle loss occurs with decreased physical activity level. Last, decreased dietary intake occurs because of difficulty breathing, or **dyspnea,** hypoxia during meals, early satiety, and anorexia.

Regardless of the cause of weight loss and malnutrition in this population, poor nutrition status is considered an independent prognostic indicator of mortality in clients with advanced disease (Aniwidyaningsih, Varraso, Cano, & Pison, 2008; Anker et al., 2006; Budweiser et al., 2007). Undernutrition and loss of lean body mass is associated with a decline in pulmonary function demonstrated by diaphragm atrophy, loss of ventilatory muscle strength, and reduced exercise capacity (Aniwidyaningsih et al., 2008). Risk of pneumonia is increased with impaired immune status because of malnutrition. In the client on mechanical ventilation, loss of lean body mass can impede attempts at weaning because of loss of diaphragm and respiratory accessory muscle tissue.

Nutritional care of the client with COPD is targeted at optimizing intake of calories and protein in an attempt to restore lean body mass and provide adequate energy to meet individual needs. Dyspnea during meals and early satiety present challenges to any attempts at increased intake. Practice Pearl: Early Satiety in COPD and Client Education Checklist: Optimizing Nutrition in the Frail Client with COPD outline recommendations for the client with COPD. Use of diet alone, with or without oral liquid nutrition supplements, has not yielded significant results (King, Cordova, & Scharf, 2008). The use of oral liquid nutrition supplements often replaces

PRACTICE PEARL

Early Satiety in COPD
Early satiety can occur from swallowing air, called aerophagia. Labored breathing and dietary habits contribute to aerophagia. The nurse can recommend that clients with COPD and early satiety refrain from chewing gum, drinking carbonated beverages, and using straws, because these practices contribute to swallowed air. Additionally, hurried eating and chewing with an open mouth cause aerophagia.

meal intake and, therefore, fails to result in an overall increase in intake. Improved results have been reported when supplement use is combined with both exercise and anabolic medication use (Anker et al., 2006). In addition to being mindful of calorie and protein intake, the nurse should assess the intake of calcium and vitamin D in clients on steroid treatment because of the negative effect of that treatment on bone health. Appropriate dietary sources of calcium and vitamin D should be recommended as indicated.

When caring for the client who receives tube feedings while on mechanical ventilation, the nurse should be mindful of positioning the client in a semi-recumbent position to reduce the risk of aspiration associated with enteral feedings in these clients (Heyland et al., 2003). The fact that prescribed formula volume often differs greatly from delivered volume in these clients is a subject of nutritional concern. Reports of clients chronically receiving less than 90% of prescribed calories are not uncommon with feeding interruption for procedures or airway management cited most often as the biggest contributor to this deficit (O'Leary-Kelley, Puntillo, Barr, Stotts, & Douglas, 2005; Reid, 2006). Such energy and protein debt can contribute to malnutrition risk in an already vulnerable client.

In clients with COPD or those on mechanical ventilation, increased levels of plasma carbon dioxide can occur because of altered gas exchange. Two components of nutrition support are capable of contributing to that effect: overfeeding and high-carbohydrate feeding. One end-product of macronutrient metabolism is carbon dioxide. Excessive calorie intake can result in increased carbon dioxide production. Additionally, carbohydrates produce more carbon dioxide than do fats or protein when compared as a ratio of oxygen consumed to carbon dioxide produced for metabolism of each macronutrient. This ratio is called the **respiratory quotient (RQ).** The lower RQ for fats prompted the development of high-fat specialty enteral formulas for clients with pulmonary disease. It is unclear whether this theoretical advantage takes on clinical significance if overfeeding is avoided (Anker et al., 2006; Malone, 2004). In clients taking oral nutrition, high-fat supplements can slow gastric emptying, contributing to complaints of early satiety (Anker et al.,

CLIENT EDUCATION CHECKLIST ✓ Optimizing Nutrition in the Frail Client with COPD

Intervention	Example
Encourage intake of nutrient-dense foods 1. Explain the importance of nutritional health with COPD. 2. List foods with "more calories per bite" and those that require little chewing effort to minimize aerophagia and breathing difficulties while eating.	1. Poor nutritional status can lead to loss of muscle that, in turn, decreases functional capacity. Increased lean body mass is associated with improved outcomes. Adequate intake provides needed nutrients to restore lost muscle and provide energy for rehabilitation. 2. High-protein and high-fat foods have "more calories per bite." Examples that are easy to chew include dairy foods, such as milk, yogurt, cheese; dairy-based desserts, such as pudding, custard, ice cream; soft animal proteins, such as canned tuna, other fish, poultry, ground meats, hamburger, eggs; soft plant proteins, such as hummus, peanut butter and nut butters, beans, tofu, lentils, split peas; cream soups and chilis.
Encourage intake of high-fat foods 1. Explain the role of fat intake in COPD. 2. List sources of nutrient-dense high-fat foods.	1. In undernourished clients deliberately being overfed to replete weight, use of high-fat rather than high-carbohydrate intake may lessen the production of carbon dioxide that needs to be expelled. 2. High-fat foods include specialty oral liquid nutrition supplements for clients with pulmonary disease, vegetable oils, fatty fish, peanut butter and nut butters, margarine and butter, dressings, mayonnaise, full-fat dairy foods.
Outline recommendations for clients with early satiety 1. Outline the importance of beginning the meal with the most nutrient-dense foods. 2. Encourage frequent meals and snacks. 3. List dietary practices that contribute to aerophagia. 4. Discourage intake of low-calorie, high-bulk foods.	1. Beginning the meal with the most nutritious foods fosters intake of more calories and protein before satiety sets in than consuming low-calorie but bulky foods, such as broth soups, clear liquids, vegetables, and fruit. 2. Eating small meals or snacking more frequently can result in improved intake over attempting a few large meals that cannot be finished. 3. Swallowing air can cause fullness. Air is swallowed with these habits: using a straw, drinking carbonated beverages, chewing gum, eating quickly, talking while eating, chewing with an open mouth. 4. Low-calorie bulky foods cause satiety only because of their volume and preclude intake of more caloric foods. Liquids, such as coffee, tea, diet soda, broth-type soup, and water are examples. Raw fruits and vegetables provide nutrients but also bulk. Canned fruit, cooked greens, and tomato sauce are alternatives to more bulky raw form.

2006). Manipulating fat and carbohydrate content of meals, supplements, or nutrition support takes a back seat to providing sufficient overall nutrition while avoiding overfeeding. Use of high-fat nutrition may be of benefit in the client who is difficult to wean from the ventilator or the ambulatory client who is being deliberately overfed to foster nutritional repletion (Malone, 2004). High-fat supplements are not indicated in the stable client (Anker et al., 2006).

NURSING CARE PLAN Nutrition and Trauma

CASE STUDY

Ted, 13 years old, was just discharged home after a week in the hospital. He had been in a motor vehicle accident in which he sustained compound fractures of both legs, which required surgery, and numerous lacerations of his face and head, which required more than 50 stitches. The hospitalization included 3 days in critical care and 4 days on the pediatric unit. His hospital stay was complicated by an ileus and the development of a wound infection in his left leg. He lives with his mother and two younger sisters in a small house in which the bedrooms and only bathroom are upstairs. A home health nurse has been assigned to do the initial dressing changes to his wound infection and teach his mother how to do them. Ted tells the nurse that his legs and back will not stop hurting and the lacerations keep itching. He cannot find a way to get comfortable for more than a few minutes. He also tells the nurse that he feels like he is going to "throw up" and is afraid to eat because he could not get to the bathroom if he is sick. His mother says that she gives him the antibiotics

Nutrition and Trauma *(continued)*

NURSING CARE PLAN

Assessment
Data about the patient

Subjective
What the patient tells the nurse
Example: I feel like I am going to throw up and my legs and back hurt.

Objective
What the nurse observes; anthropometric and clinical data
Examples: Open wound on left leg; taking antibiotics and pain medication

Diagnosis
NANDA label
Example: Nausea related to taking medications on an empty stomach

Planning
Goals stated in patient terms
Example: Long-term goal: leg wound healed; Short-term goal: nausea eliminated

Implementation
Nursing action to help patient achieve goals
Example: Allow foods of choice at meals; take antibiotics and pain medications with food

Evaluation
Was the goal achieved or does the intervention need to be modified?
Example: Taking medications with food and drinking daily milk shakes

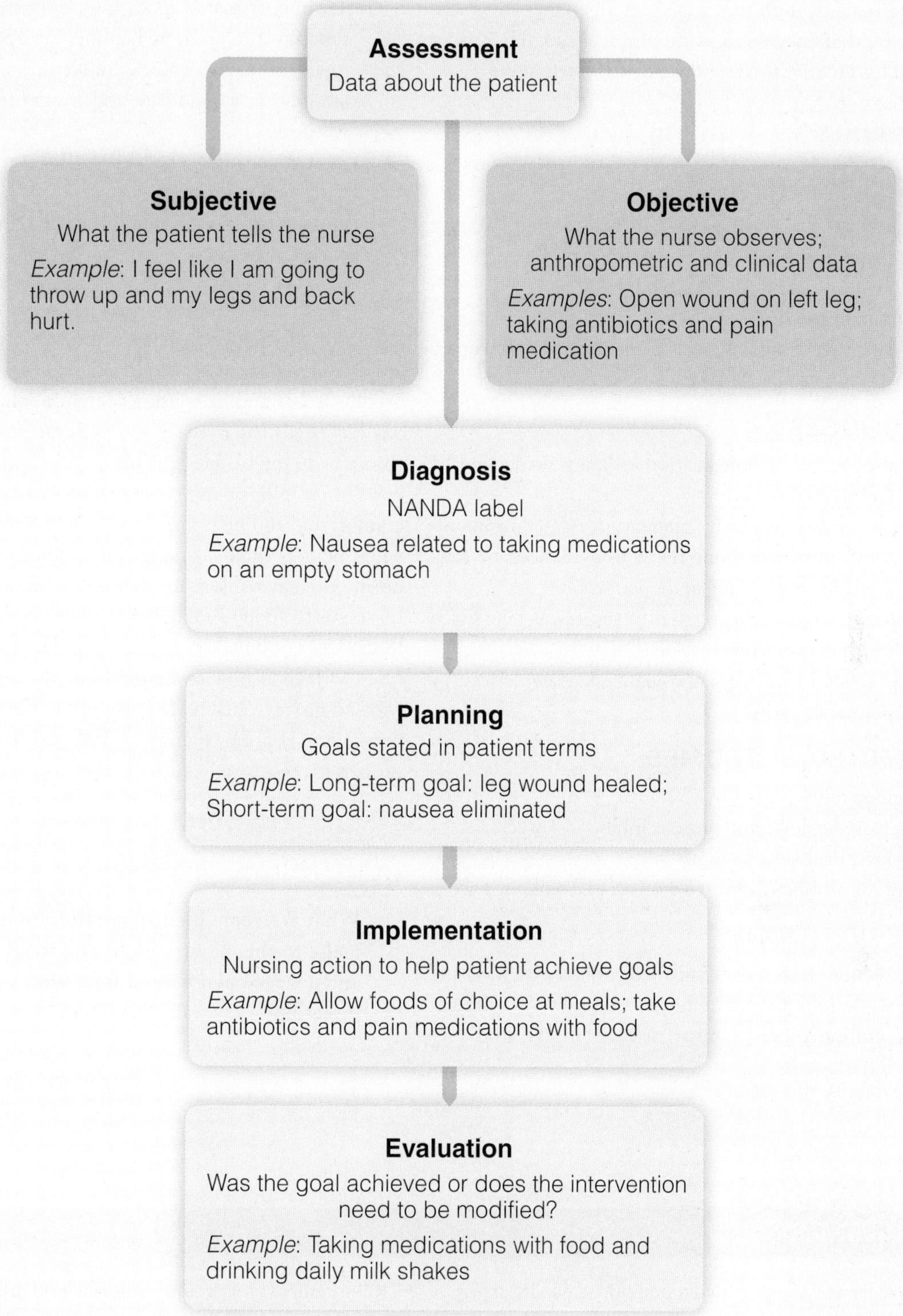

■ FIGURE 22-3 **Nursing Care Plan Process: Nutrition and Trauma.**

(continued)

NURSING CARE PLAN

Nutrition and Trauma *(continued)*

and pain medication that were prescribed, but she keeps worrying that they are making him feel sick. He refuses any of his favorite foods and wants to be left alone.

Applying the Nursing Process

ASSESSMENT

Stated height: 4 feet 10 inches Stated weight: 88 pounds BMI: 38th percentile
BP 84/44 P 102 R 16 T 100.4
Skin pale and dry
Clean, open wound 3 cm × 2 cm on the left lower leg
Rates pain at 7 on 1–10 scale

DIAGNOSES

Nausea related to medication regimen evidenced by feeling like vomiting

Nutrition: less than body requirements related to inability to meet metabolic needs as evidenced by low-grade fever, fracture, and open wound

Impaired skin integrity related to surgery as evidenced by open wound on left leg

Pain related to surgery and leg casts as evidenced by pain scale rating of 7

EXPECTED OUTCOMES

Nausea relieved within 48 hours
Increased caloric and protein intake in 1 week
Wound healed in 1 month
Pain diminishes from 7 to 3 on a 1–10 scale in 1 week

INTERVENTIONS

Stress importance of taking medications with food and water to reduce or eliminate GI upset

Determine usual patterns of food intake and preferred foods

Teach importance of foods high in protein, zinc, and vitamin C to promote healing; incorporate favorite foods to increase caloric intake

Teach mother wound care and require return demonstration

Suggest diversions, like video games, that may help with pain management

Demonstrate use of pillows to maximize comfort with casts

EVALUATION

When the home health nurse returns in 1 week, considerable improvement is noted. Ted reports that his pain is usually at 2–3 and he is using acetaminophen during the day but needs the prescription pain medication to sleep through the night. He and his mother have figured out ways to use pillows in the wheelchair to keep him more comfortable and he is able to transfer himself to the sofa when he gets tired sitting. His grandmother comes over during the day while is mother is at work and she makes his favorite foods, including daily milk shakes, so his mom does not have to cook at night. He takes his antibiotics with food now so he does not have any problems with an upset stomach. The wound remains clean and is now 2.5 × 1.5 cm. Figure 22-3 ■ outlines the nursing process for this case.

Critical Thinking in the Nursing Process

1. **What are some food suggestion the nurse can make to the client who has minimal appetite and a large open wound following a postsurgical infection?**

CHAPTER SUMMARY

- Physiological stress is also called metabolic stress. Injury or infection leads to a hormone and central nervous system response that alters normal metabolism of nutrients.

- Consequences of physiological stress include hyperglycemia, insulin resistance, skeletal muscle breakdown, and weight loss.

- No one set of nutrition recommendations exists for critically ill clients. Instead, each client should be individually assessed and customized nutrition recommendations given.

- Requirements for protein, calories, and micronutrients are increased during physiological stress and may continue to be elevated during rehabilitation.

- Preoperative nutrition assessment can identify clients at risk for poor health outcomes postoperatively because of malnutrition. Nutrition intervention before and after surgery is essential for the surgical client.

- Wound repair requires adequate nutrient status for each of the four stages of healing. Compromised nutrition status limits the availability of crucial nutrients and can delay wound healing.

- Nutritional requirements are increased in clients with end-stage chronic obstructive pulmonary disease, but al-

tered gas exchange, dyspnea, and early satiety often decrease the ability of the client to meet nutritional demands orally.

EXPLORE **mynursingkit**™ PEARSON

MyNursingKit is your one stop for online chapter review materials and resources. Prepare for success with additional NCLEX®-style practice questions, interactive assignments and activities, web links, animations and videos, and more!

Register your access code from the front of your book at
www.mynursingkit.com.

NCLEX® QUESTIONS

1. An elderly client with chronic obstructive pulmonary disease (COPD) has just been transferred to the nursing unit from critical care. What strategy can the nurse suggest to this client who experiences shortness of breath and fatigue during mealtimes?
   1. Eat a large, nutrient-dense breakfast because the client is rested.
   2. Eat small, frequent meals to reduce the energy expended during a meal.
   3. Increase the amount of simple carbohydrates in the diet to provide more energy.
   4. Eat more protein to repair tissue damage.

2. How should the nurse respond to the family members who express concern that their father, who had major surgery 48 hours ago and remains on a ventilator in a critical care unit, will "starve to death" if he does not get something to eat soon. The father has an estimated BMI of 26.
   1. "Your father is getting a sugar solution through the IV line, so he will not starve."
   2. "A person can go a whole week without eating and he will certainly be eating by that time; so we don't have any concerns yet."
   3. "His nutritional status is being evaluated on a daily basis and he may be started on an alternate type of feeding very soon."
   4. "He has more than adequate stores of fat and protein to meet his nutritional needs while in critical care; he will get meals when he is transferred out of the unit."

3. Which of the following clients in the critical care unit would the nurse consider to be at greatest risk for nutritional problems?
   1. A 32-year-old painter who fractured a femur in two places after falling off a ladder and is 6 hours postoperative
   2. A middle-age male with COPD who is admitted for an acute exacerbation of the disease
   3. A 46-year-old obese female with a deep vein thrombosis (DVT) who is receiving heparin
   4. A 70-year-old male who had a myocardial infarction (MI)

4. What is the best way for the nurse to determine the nutritional status of a client with multiple organ dysfunction syndrome (MODS)?
   1. Serum albumin level
   2. Vital signs
   3. Serum electrolytes, blood urea nitrogen, creatinine, and liver function tests
   4. Age and chronic health conditions

5. The nurse is caring for a client who had a liver transplant 2 days ago and continues on mechanical ventilation. What can the nurse expect will be implemented to meet the client's nutritional needs?
   1. Daily liver function tests
   2. A high-protein, low-fat diet will be ordered
   3. Parenteral feeding only
   4. Enteral feeding will be initiated

REFERENCES

Alberda, C., Graf, A., & McCargar, L. (2006). Malnutrition: Etiology, consequences and assessment of a patient at risk. *Best Practice and Research Clinical Gastroenterology, 20*, 419–439.

Andersen, H. K., Lewis, S. J., & Thomas, S. (2006). Early enteral nutrition within 24h of colorectal surgery versus later commencement of feeding for postoperative complications. *Cochrane Database Reviews, 4*, CD004080.

Aniwidyaningsih, W., Varraso, R., Cano, N., & Pison, C. (2008). Impact of nutritional status on body functioning in chronic obstructive pulmonary disease and how to intervene. *Current Opinion in Clinical Nutrition and Metabolic Care, 11*, 435–442.

Anker, S. D, John, M., Pedersen, P. U., Raguso, C., Cicoira, M., Dardai, E., et al. (2006). ESPEN Guidelines on enteral nutrition: Cardiology and Pulmonology. *Clinical Nutrition, 25*, 311–318.

Berger, M. M., & Chiolero, R. L. (2007a). Antioxidant supplementation in sepsis and systemic inflammatory response. *Critical Care Medicine, 35*, S584–S590.

Berger, M. M., & Chiolero, R. L. (2007b). Hypocaloric feedings: Pros and cons. *Current Opinion in Critical Care, 13*, 180–186.

Berger, M. M., & Shenkin, A. (2006). Update on clinical micronutrient supplementation studies in the critically ill. *Current Opinion in Clinical Nutrition and Metabolic Care, 9*, 711–716.

Bluestein, D., & Javaheri, A. (2008). Pressure ulcers: Prevention, evaluation, and treatment. *American Family Physician, 78*, 1186–1194.

Boitano, M. (2006). Hypocaloric feeding of the critically ill. *Nutrition in Clinical Practice, 21*, 617–622.

Boullata, J., Williams, J., Cottrell, F., Hudson, L., & Compher, C. (2007). Accurate determination of energy needs in hospitalized patients. *Journal of the American Dietetic Association, 107*, 393–401.

Brady, M., Kinn, S., O'Rourke, K., Randhawa, N., & Stuart, P. (2005). Preoperative fasting for preventing perioperative complications in children. *Cochrane Database of Systematic Reviews, 2*, CD005285.

Brain Trauma Foundation. (2007). XII. Nutrition. *Journal of Neurotrauma, 24*, S77–S82.

Budweiser, S., Jorres, R. A., Riedl, T., Heineman, F., Hitzl, A. P., Windisch, W., et al. (2007). Predictors of survival in COPD patients with chronic hypercapnic respiratory failure receiving noninvasive home ventilation. *Chest, 131*, 1650–1658.

Campos, A. C., Groth, A. K., & Branco, A. B. (2008). Assessment and nutritional aspects of wound healing. *Current Opinion in Clinical Nutrition and Metabolic Care, 11*, 281–288.

Carli, F. (2006). Postoperative metabolic stress: Interventional strategies. *Minerva Anesthesiologica, 72*, 413–418.

Castillo-Zamora, C., Castillo-Peralta, L. A., & Nava-Ocampo, A. A. (2005). Randomized trial comparing overnight preoperative fasting vs. oral administration of apple juice at 0600–0630 am in pediatric orthopedic surgical patients. *Paediatric Anaesthesia, 15*(8), 638–642.

Cederholm, T., & Hedstrom, M. (2005). Nutritional treatment of bone fracture. *Current Opinion in Clinical Nutrition and Metabolic Care, 8*, 377–381.

Charoenkwan, K., Phillipson, G., & Vutyavanich, T. (2007). Early versus delayed (traditional) oral fluids and food for reducing complications after major abdominal gynecologic surgery. *Cochrane Database of Systematic Reviews, 4*, CD004508.

Cheatham, M. L., Safcsak, K., Brzezinski, S. J., & Lube, M. W. (2007). Nitrogen balance, protein loss, and the open abdomen. *Critical Care Medicine, 35*, 127–131.

Collier, B., Guillamondequi, V., Cotton, B., Donahue, R., Conrad, A., Groh, K., et al. (2007). Feeding the open abdomen. *Journal of Enteral and Parenteral Nutrition, 31*, 410–415.

Cook, A. M., Peppard, A., & Magnusun, B. (2008). Nutrition considerations in traumatic brain injury. *Nutrition in Clinical Practice, 23*, 608–620.

Cook-Sather, S. D., & Litman, R. S. (2006). Modern fasting guidelines in children. *Best Practice & Research, Clinical Anaesthesiology, 20*(3), 471–481.

Curreri, P. W., Richmond, D., Marvin, J., & Baxter, C. R. (1974). Dietary requirements of patients with major burns. *Journal of the American Dietetic Association, 65*, 415–417.

Demling, E. (2007). The use of anabolic agents in catabolic stress. *Journal of Burns and Wounds, 6*, 33–49.

Dhaliwal, R., & Heyland, D. K. (2005). Nutrition and infection in the intensive care unit: What does the evidence show? *Current Opinion in Clinical Nutrition and Metabolic Care, 11*, 461–467.

Faisy, C., Guerot, E., Diehl, J., Labrousse, J., & Fagon, J. (2003). Assessment of resting energy expenditure in mechanically ventilated patients. *American Journal of Clinical Nutrition, 78*, 241–249.

Frankenfield, D. (2006). Energy expenditure and protein requirements after traumatic injury. *Nutrition in Clinical Practice, 21*, 430–437.

Gariballa, S., & Forster, S. (2007). Malnutrition independent predictor of 1 year mortality following acute illness. *British Journal of Nutrition, 98*, 332–336.

Goulet, O., & Sauvat, F. (2006). Short bowel syndrome and intestinal transplantation in children. *Current Opinion in Clinical Nutrition and Metabolic Care, 9*, 304–313.

Graves, C., Saffle, J., & Cochran, A. (2009). Actual burn nutrition care practice: An update. *Journal of Burn Care Research, 30*, 77–82.

Griffiths, R. D., & Bongers, T. (2005). Nutrition support for patients in the intensive care unit. *Postgraduate Medicine Journal, 81*, 629–636.

Hedstrom, M., & Cederholm, T. (2006). Metabolism and catabolism in hip fracture patients. *Acta Orthopaedica, 77*, 741–747.

Heyland, D. K., Dhaliwal, R., Drover, J. W., Gramlich, L., Dodek, P., & the Canadian Critical Care Practice Committee. (2003). Canadian clinical guidelines for nutrition support in mechanically ventilated critically ill patients. *Journal of Parenteral and Enteral Nutrition, 27*, 355–373.

Heyland, D. K., Dhaliwal, R., Suchner, U., & Berger, M. M. (2005). Antioxidant nutrients: A systematic review of trace elements and vitamins in the critically ill. *Intensive Care Medicine, 31*, 321–337.

Hise, M. E., Halterman, K., Gajewski, B. J., Parkhurst, M., Moncure, M., & Brown, J. C. (2007). Feeding practices of severely ill intensive care unit patients: An evaluation of energy sources and clinical outcomes. *Journal of the American Dietetic Association, 107*, 458–465.

Hulst, J. M., Joosten, K., Zimmerman, L., Hop, W., van Buuren, S., Buller, H., et al. (2004a). Malnutrition in critically ill children: From admission to 6 months after discharge. *Clinical Nutrition, 23*, 223–232.

Hulst, J. M., van Goudoever, J. B., Zimmerman, L. J., Hop, W. C., Albers, M. J., Tibboel, D., et al. (2004b). The effect of cumulative energy and protein deficiency on anthropometric parameters in a pediatric ICU population. *Clinical Nutrition, 23*, 1381–1389.

Hulst, J. M., Joosten, K. F., Tibboel, D., & van Goudoever, J. B. (2006). Causes and consequences of inadequate substrate supply to pediatric ICU patients. *Current Opinion in Clinical Nutrition and Metabolic Care, 9*, 297–303.

Institute of Medicine (IOM), Food and Nutrition Board. (2004). *Dietary reference intakes for water, potassium, sodium, chloride and sulfate.* Washington, DC: National Academies Press.

Inzucchi, S. E. (2006). Management of hyperglycemia in the hospital setting. *New England Journal of Medicine, 355*, 1903–1911.

Jull, A. (2006). Review: Children permitted clear fluids < or = to 120 minutes before surgery have similar gastric volumes and pH values as those on standard fasts. *Evidence-Based Nursing, 9*, 11.

Kagansky, N., Berner, Y., Morag-Koren, N., Perelman, L., Knobler, H., & Levy, S. (2005). Poor nutritional habits are predictors of poor outcome in very old hospitalized patients. *American Journal of Clinical Nutrition, 82*, 784–791.

Keast, D. H., Parslow, N., Houghton, P. E., Norton, L., & Fraser, C. (2007). Best prac-

REFERENCES *(continued)*

tice recommendations for the prevention and treatment of pressure ulcers: Update 2006. *Advances in Skin & Wound Care, 20,* 447–460.

King, D. A., Cordova, F., & Scharf, S. M. (2008). Nutritional aspects of chronic obstructive pulmonary disease. *Proceedings of the American Thoracic Society, 5,* 519–523.

Klemetti, S., Kinnunen, I., Suominen, T., Antila, H., Vahlberg, T., Grenman, R., et al. (2009). The effect of preoperative fasting on postoperative pain, nausea and vomiting in pediatric ambulatory tonsillectomy. *International Journal of Pediatric Otorhinolaryngology, 73*(2), 263–273.

Klemetti, S., & Suominen, T. (2008). Fasting in paediatric ambulatory surgery. *International Journal of Nursing Practice, 14*(1), 47–56.

Kopp Lugli, A., Wykes, L., & Carli, F. (2008). Strategies for perioperative nutrition support in obese, diabetic, and geriatric patients. *Clinical Nutrition, 27,* 16–24.

Krakau, K., Hansson, A., Karlsson, T., de Boussard, C. N., Tengvar, C., & Borg, J. (2007). Nutritional treatment of patients with severe traumatic brain injury during the first six months after injury. *Nutrition, 23,* 308–317.

Kreymann, K. G. (2008). Early nutrition support in critical care: A European perspective. *Current Opinion in Clinical Nutrition and Metabolic Care, 11,* 156–159.

Kreymann, K. G., Berger, M. M., Deutz, N. E. P., Hiesmayr, M., Jolliet, P., Kazandjiev, G., et al. (2006). ESPEN guidelines on enteral nutrition: Intensive care. *Clinical Nutrition, 25,* 210–223.

Kudsk, K., Tolley, E., DeWitt, C., Janu, P. G., Blackwell, A. P., Yeary, S., et al. (2003). Preoperative albumin and surgical site identify surgical risk for major postoperative complications. *Journal of Parenteral and Enteral Nutrition, 27,* 1–9.

Langemo, D., Anderson, J., Hanson, D., Hunter, S., Thompson, P., & Posthauer, M. E. (2006). Nutritional considerations in wound care. *Advances in Skin & Wound Care, 19,* 297–301.

Lobo, D. N. (2004). Fluid, electrolytes, and nutrition: Physiological and clinical aspects. *Proceedings of the Nutrition Society, 63,* 453–466.

Mallampalli, A. (2004). Nutritional management of the patient with chronic obstructive pulmonary disease. *Nutrition in Clinical Practice, 19,* 550–556.

Malone, A. M. (2004). The use of specialized enteral formulas in pulmonary disease. *Nutrition in Clinical Practice, 19,* 557–562.

Martindale, R. G., & Cresci, G. (2005). Preventing infectious complications with nutrition intervention. *Journal of Parenteral and Enteral Nutrition, 29,* S53–S56.

Martindale, R. G., & Maerz, L. L. (2006). Management of perioperative nutrition sup-

port. *Current Opinion in Critical Care, 12,* 290–294.

National Pressure Ulcer Advisory Panel. (2007). *Pressure ulcer stages revised by NPUAC.* Retrieved April 27, 2009, from http://www.npuap.org/pr2.htm

Norman, K., Pichard, C., Lochs, H., & Pirlich, M. (2008). Prognostic impact of disease-related malnutrition. *Clinical Nutrition, 27,* 5–15.

Odencrants, S., Ehnfors, M., & Ehrenberg, A. (2008). Nutritional status and patient characteristics for hospitalized older patients with chronic obstructive pulmonary disease. *Journal of Clinical Nursing, 17,* 1771–1778.

O'Leary-Kelley, C. M., Puntillo, K. A., Barr, J., Stotts, N., & Douglas, M. K. (2005). Nutritional adequacy in patients receiving mechanical ventilation who are fed enterally. *American Journal of Critical Care, 14,* 222–231.

Perel, P., Yanagawa, T., Bunn, F., Roberts, I., Wentz, R., & Pierro, A. (2006). Nutritional support for head-injured patients. *Cochrane Database of Systematic Reviews, 4,* CD001530.

Posthauer, M. E. (2006). The role of nutrition in wound care. *Advances in Skin & Wound Care, 19,* 43–52.

Posthauer, M. E. (2007). What is the role of vitamins in wound healing? *Advances in Skin & Wound Care, 20,* 260–264.

Powell-Tuck, J. (2007). Nutritional interventions in critical illness. *Proceedings of the Nutrition Society, 66,* 16–24.

Prelack, K., Dylewski, M., & Sheridan, R. L. (2007). Practice guidelines for nutritional management of burn injury and recovery. *Burns, 33,* 14–24.

Reddy, M., Gill, S. S., & Rochon, P. A. (2006). Preventing pressure ulcers: A systematic review. *Journal of the American Medical Association, 296,* 974–984.

Reid, C. (2006). Frequency of under- and overfeeding in mechanically ventilated ICU patients: Causes and possible consequences. *Journal of Human Nutrition and Dietetics, 19,* 13–22.

Reid, M. B., & Allard-Gould, P. (2004). Malnutrition in the critically ill elderly patient. *Critical Care Nursing Clinics of North America, 16,* 531–536.

Shenkin, A. (2006). Micronutrients in health and disease. *Postgraduate Medical Journal, 82,* 559–567.

Sierzega, M., Niekowal, B., Kulig, J., & Popiela, T. (2007). Nutritional status affects the rate of pancreatic fistula after distal pancreatectomy: A multivariate analysis of 132 patients. *Journal of the American College of Surgeons, 205,* 52–59.

Skillman, H. E., & Wischmeyer, P. E. (2008). Nutrition therapy in critically ill infants and children. *Journal of Parenteral and Enteral Nutrition, 32,* 520–534.

Stroud, M. (2007). Protein and the critically ill: Do we know what to give? *Proceedings of the Nutrition Society, 66,* 378–383.

Stucky, C. H., Moncure, M., Hise, M., Gossage, C. M., & Northrup, D. (2008). How accurate are resting energy expenditure prediction equations in obese trauma and burn patients? *Journal of Parenteral and Enteral Nutrition, 32,* 420–426.

Sungurtekin, H., Sungurtekin, U., Balci, C., Zencir, M., & Erdem, E. (2004). The influence of nutritional status on complications after major intraabdominal surgery. *Journal of the American College of Nutrition, 23,* 227–232.

Tynan, C., & Hasse, J. M. (2004). Current nutrition practices in adult lung transplant patients. *Nutrition in Clinical Practice, 19,* 587–596.

Van den Berghe, G., Wilmer, A., Milants, I., Wouters, P. J., Bouckaert, B., Bruyninckx, F., et al. (2006). Intensive insulin therapy in mixed medical/surgical intensive care units. *Diabetes, 55,* 3151–3159.

van den Broek, P. W., Rasmussen-Conrad, E. L., Naber, A. H., & Wanten, G. J. (2009). What you think is not what they get: Significant discrepancies between prescribed and administered doses of tube feeding. *British Journal of Nutrition, 101,* 68–71.

van der Kulp, M., de Meer, K., Westerterp, K. R., & Gemke, R. J. (2007). Physical activity as a determinant of total energy expenditure in critically ill children. *Clinical Nutrition, 26,* 744–751.

Vincent, J. (2007). Metabolic support in sepsis and multiple organ failure: More questions than answers. *Critical Care Medicine, 35,* S436–S440.

Wanek, S., & Wolf, S. E. (2007). Metabolic response to injury and role of anabolic hormones. *Current Opinion in Clinical Nutrition and Metabolic Care, 10,* 272–277.

Wasiak, J., Cleland, H., & Jefferey, R. (2006). Early versus delayed enteral nutrition support for burn patients. *Cochrane Database Systematic Reviews, 3,* CD005498.

Weekes, E. (2007). Controversies in the determination of energy requirements. *Proceedings of the Nutrition Society, 66,* 367–377.

Weimann, A., Braga, M., Harsanyi, L., Laviano, A., Ljungquist, O., Soeters, P., et al. (2006). ESPEN guidelines on enteral nutrition: Surgery including organ transplant. *Clinical Nutrition, 25,* 224–244.

Wischmeyer, P. E. (2007). Glutamine: Mode of action in critical illness. *Critical Care Medicine, 35,* S542–S544.

Zhou, M., & Martindale, R. G. (2007). Arginine in the critical care setting. *Journal of Nutrition, 137,* 1687S–1692S.

23 Cancer and Human Immunodeficiency Virus (HIV) Infection

WHAT WILL YOU LEARN?

1. To relate current nutrition recommendations for reducing cancer risk.

2. To analyze risk factors for malnutrition that exist in the client with cancer or HIV infection because of the condition or its treatment.

3. To formulate nursing interventions for the prevention or treatment of symptoms and side effects from cancer or HIV infection that negatively impact nutrition status.

4. To examine the recommendations regarding the use of dietary supplements as part of treatment for HIV infection or cancer.

5. To translate the current recommendations for nutrition treatment of metabolic consequences of HIV infection.

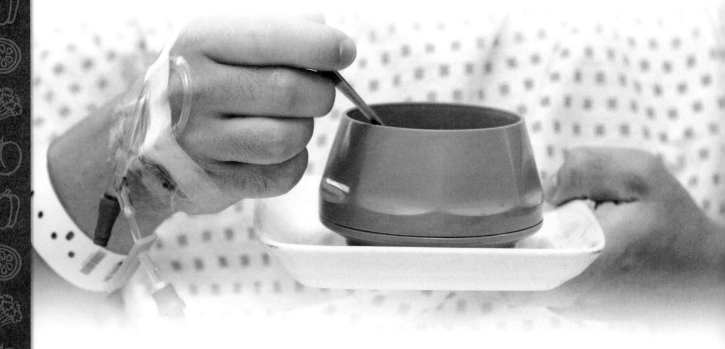

DID YOU KNOW?

▶ The risk of breast cancer increases 25% in women who consume greater than one alcoholic drink/day compared with those consuming *less than or equal to* one drink/day.

▶ Weight loss and wasting, which occur in both HIV infection and cancer, increase risk of death.

▶ Using a straw to drink liquids can minimize oral pain in clients with mouth ulcers or infection.

▶ The herb St. John's Wort interacts with a common class of medications used to treat HIV infection and can jeopardize drug effectiveness.

▶ Some clients stop taking certain antiviral medications that are successfully used to treat HIV infection because the drugs cause altered distribution of body fat.

KEY TERMS

antioxidants, *520*

cachexia, *521*

cacogeusia, *521*

dysgeusia, *521*

HAART, *527*

lipoatrophy, *530*

lipodystrophy, *530*

odynophagia, *521*

phytochemicals, *520*

wasting, *521*

Cancer Prevention and Nutrition

It is estimated that 50% to 75% of cancer deaths in the United States are related to lifestyle behaviors such as smoking, physical inactivity, and poor dietary choices (National Cancer Institute [NCI], 2007). It has been postulated that various dietary components play a role in the prevention of cancer, whereas others have been blamed for fostering its development. It is believed that the risk and course of cancer can be blocked or suppressed at many points along the process and herein lies the potential for nutrition to interact. Conversely, dietary factors may potentiate or trigger the process and increase cancer risk. Laboratory studies have shown that dietary substances can affect cell mutation by inhibiting the uptake or activation of carcinogens. Other substances may slow or stop cancer cell proliferation or progression. These effects are contrasted by dietary components associated with increased cancer risk that act in the opposite fashion, fostering an increase uptake of a carcinogen or potentiating cell division. Despite the wealth of research in this area, little is known about specific roles for most food components in humans. No conclusive evidence exists that any one single dietary component is responsible for either causing or preventing cancer. Box 23-1 outlines a summary of general research findings on diet and cancer risk.

BOX 23-1	**Diet and Cancer: Research Summary**

New studies on the role of nutrition, foods, food component, and nutrients in cancer risk are constantly making the news. When reviewing the latest findings, the nurse should keep in mind the type of study being reported and the existing body of scientific knowledge on the topic. The following is a summary of dietary factors associated with cancer risk:

Alcohol—↑ intake associated with cancer of the mouth, esophagus, pharynx, larynx, liver and breast. Two drinks/day increase the risk of breast cancer in women by 25% compared with one drink/day.

Fats—↑ intake associated with cancer of the colon, prostate, lung, and endometrium. More research needed on types of fat linked with risk. Association may be related to risk associated with obesity rather than dietary fat itself.

Fruits and Vegetables—↓ intake associated with risk of cancer of colon, mouth, pharynx, esophagus, stomach, lung, and, possibly, prostate. Inconclusive and conflicting studies on the risk associated with single components of fruits and vegetables, such as antioxidants, fiber, and plant pigments.

Heterocyclic amines (HCAs)—link between diets high in HCAs, a by-product of high temperature cooking of muscle meats and processed meats, and cancer of the stomach and colon.

Overweight and obesity—prevention of overweight/obesity associated with a decreased risk of colon, postmenopausal breast, uterine, esophageal and renal cell cancer. Approximately 20% to 30% of cancers are related to obesity. Association exists between obesity and breast cancer recurrence.

Soy—limited clinical data on humans that soy consumption over time, especially early in life, may decrease risk of breast cancer. Controversy exists surrounding a possible increase risk of breast cancer with increased intake of soy and soy isoflavones in women at high risk for breast cancer.

Vitamin supplementation—long-term studies have yet to link the use of multivitamin supplements with reduced risk of cancer.

Vitamin D—vitamin D receptors are found in many cells in the body unrelated to bone health or calcium homeostasis. An observational link exists between individuals living in northern latitudes with low plasma vitamin D and increased risk of common cancers.

Sources: Adapted from: Demark-Wahnefried, Rock, Patrick, & Byers, 2008; Fairfield & Stampfer, 2007; Molokhia & Perkins, 2008: Neuhouser et al., 2009.

Much of the research on diet and cancer is based on animal studies, in vitro studies, or epidemiological studies where large populations are observed over time. Animal and in vitro studies have limited application but serve as a starting point to determine possible links between diet and cancer. Epidemiological studies yield associations between diet and disease that are made based on observation—not cause and effect conclusions—thus leaving room for many uncontrolled and unknown factors. For example, comparing the cancer outcome of adults who consume soy and those who do not cannot accurately quantify the possible effect of any soy intake that occurred during childhood and adolescence. Epidemiological evidence should not be equated to experimental evidence. Clinically controlled trials, the gold standard of medical research, are needed to more accurately establish the relationship between diet and cancer risk. The very nature of the disease and the difficulty in singling out potential risk factors over sufficient time are what make sweeping conclusions about diet and cancer difficult to obtain. Observational studies can suggest a link between a diet component and disease, but when the component is isolated and studied, the outcome can change. An example of this finding is illustrated by the famous clinical trial that found increased lung cancer risk among smokers taking beta-carotene supplements when observational studies of a diet high in fruits and vegetables that naturally contain beta-carotene suggested otherwise (Omenn et al., 1996).

Many other substances found in a plant-based diet have been researched for a link to cancer risk. **Antioxidants** and **phytochemicals** are examples. Antioxidants include vitamins E and C and function to neutralize the effects of metabolic and environmental damage to cells. Research on the effect of long-term use of various antioxidant and vitamin supplements has not shown any reduction in cancer risk (Lin et al., 2009; Neuhouser et al., 2009). Phytochemicals are plant chemicals and include flavonoids and many plant pigments, such as lycopene found in tomatoes, and may have an effect on cancer risk. No conclusive evidence exists about the single effect of any of these substances, but the nurse can offer the advice in Practice Pearl: Fruits, Vegetables, and Cancer Risk when asked about this research. Further, conflicting outcomes from different studies make it confusing for those trying to make lifestyle decisions to reduce cancer risk. For example, based on limited evidence the link between increased soy intake, especially early in life, and breast cancer risk is thought to be potentially beneficial to most women but may be harmful to those already at high risk or diagnosed with breast cancer (Guha et al., 2009; Messina & Wu, 2009; Michaud, Karpinski, Jones, & Espirito, 2007a). As a result, the nurse should not recommend excess soy or its derivatives, soy isoflavones, to those at high risk or already diagnosed with breast cancer until more is known (Doyle et al., 2006). National recommendations on diet and cancer do not outline single foods or nutrients and specific cancers because

PRACTICE PEARL

Fruits, Vegetables, and Cancer Risk

No conclusions can be drawn about a specific component of plant foods and cancer risk. The possibility remains that a synergistic effect of the substances in food rather than isolated components influences cancer risk. When asked about fruit and vegetable intake and cancer risk, the nurse can advise the client to eat a variety of fruits and vegetables by varying the colors chosen. Orange, yellow, green, blue, purple, red, and white fruits and vegetables contain different phytochemicals and nutrients. The client can take advantage of any benefit that these substances may have by including a variety of them in the diet, and avoid missing crucial components by resorting to unproven dietary supplement versions.

these relationships are uncertain. Instead, general guidelines advise broader healthy behaviors associated with overall risk reduction. Box 23-2 outlines the current recommendations on diet and cancer.

Nutrition Challenges with Cancer or HIV

Cancer and HIV infection present similar challenges to the nutritional health of the client with either condition. Both diseases share the similarities that disease symptoms and treatments can jeopardize nutrition status. For example, anorexia, altered taste perception, and pain are issues with both diseases. Nausea and diarrhea from radiation therapy or antiviral drugs can lead to diminished intake and cause nutrient losses. A further similarity is that the lack of a universal medical cure for either disease leaves open the possibility that clients may try alternative medicine or dangerous quack-

---

BOX 23-2	**National Recommendations for Cancer Prevention and Diet**

- Consume alcohol only in moderation. Limit intake to less than one drink/day for women and two/day for men.
- Consume five or more servings/day of fruits and vegetables all year round.
- Include a variety of whole grains and legumes in the diet.
- Consume a low-fat diet.
- Maintain a health body weight and avoid excessive weight gain in adulthood.
- Limit consumption of processed meats and red or muscle meats cooked at high temperature (frying, grilling, or broiling well done, barbequing). Limit consumption of charred meats, meat and fish cooked on a direct flame, and cured and smoked meats.

Sources: Adapted from: American Institute for Cancer Research, 2007; Doyle et al., 2006; NCI, 2007.

ery in hope of improved survival. Some alternative treatments are known to jeopardize the success of conventional treatment, such as seen with the concomitant use of the herb St. John's Wort and either protease inhibitors used to decrease viral load with HIV infection or antirejection drugs used in bone marrow transplant for certain cancers (Gardiner, Phillips, & Shaughnessy, 2008).

Weight loss and malnutrition are considered significant independent risk factors for disease progression and mortality with both conditions (Evans et al., 2008; Klustad & Schoeller, 2007). Specifically, weight loss characterized by **cachexia** or **wasting** is classically associated with progression of these diseases. Cachexia and wasting are interchangeable terms that refer to excessive weight loss that is comprised of a significant proportion of muscle compared with the comparative loss of muscle and fat seen in starvation (Evans et al., 2008). It is unclear what contributes to such disproportionate muscle loss; increased inflammatory cell proteins (cytokines), decreased testosterone and insulin-like growth factor, and elevated adrenal hormones have all been postulated as playing a part in the development of cachexia (Tisdale, 2009).

Nutrition care of the client with cancer or HIV infection should begin at diagnosis to optimize health as treatment begins and prevent any decline in nutrition status. The monitoring of nutritional health and provision of appropriate interventions for related symptoms and side effects should be an ongoing part of the medical care of these clients.

Medical Nutrition Therapy and Cancer

The nurse should be aware that risk of weight loss and malnutrition in cancer can occur because of decreased dietary intake, nutrient losses, or unmet elevated nutritional needs that are caused by the disease or its treatment. Significant weight loss and poor nutritional health has been reported in over 50% of clients with cancer at the time of diagnosis (Doyle et al., 2006). Poor nutrition status and weight loss can interfere with completion of cancer treatment, impair healing, increase risk of complications, and diminish quality of life (Doyle et al., 2006). Conversely, some clients with cancer are overweight or obese and remain so over the course of disease treatment. Others gain weight because of treatment side effects. Nutrition therapy for overweight individuals should focus on weight management because of the associated risks between obesity and cancer as well other chronic diseases (Toles & Demark-Wahnefried, 2008).

Disease-Related Nutrition Risk Factors

The nurse should assess the client at the time of diagnosis and at regular intervals for disease-related symptoms that negatively affect nutrition status. Anorexia, taste changes, and pain all can lead to diminished dietary intake. Circulating factors, such as cytokines, produced by the tumor or the body in response to the tumor can directly cause anorexia and early satiety (Tisdale, 2009). Taste changes range from decreased perception to sweetness to an altered threshold for bitter that can cause aversions to meat and other foods. Altered taste perception is called **dysgeusia.** Some clients complain of a persistent metallic or bad taste in the mouth, called **cacogeusia.** During active treatment, up to 50% of clients experience pain, a number that increases with advanced tumor progression (Smith & Toonen, 2007). Depending on the type and location of disease, gastrointestinal symptoms can be present that further predispose the client to weight loss and malnutrition. Tumors involving the gastrointestinal tract, liver, or pancreas can cause difficulties with digestion or absorption or even lead to obstruction. Upper intestinal tumors or those of the head and neck can cause dysphagia and **odynophagia,** or painful swallowing. Psychological response to disease diagnosis exhibited as anxiety or depression can also lead to poor intake. The nurse should be mindful of the cumulative effect of these symptoms occurring in one client.

Weight loss can occur because of any of these described disease symptoms. It may also be unexplained. Unexplained weight loss and tissue wasting in clients with cancer, referred to as cancer cachexia, do not occur with all cancer types. More often, this type of weight loss is seen with solid-type tumors rather than breast cancer or hematological cancers (Tisdale, 2009). In addition to the postulated effects of cytokines on development of cachexia, some tumor cells worsen this wasting effect by fostering futile metabolic changes. Energy inefficient alterations in carbohydrate, lipid, and protein metabolism occur because of excessive lactate produced by tumors, excessive protein breakdown, and decreased fat storage (Tisdale, 2009). The nurse might suspect that unintentional weight loss has occurred because of this wasting effect when a comparison between food intake and assessed energy needs does not correspond with the degree of malnutrition exhibited by the client. A summary of disease-related symptoms that affect nutrition status are outlined in Box 23-3.

Treatment-Related Nutrition Risk Factors

All types of cancer treatment can have profound effects on nutrition status. Chemotherapy, radiation therapy, and surgery each impacts nutritional status. Many clients receive more than one type of treatment, compounding the effects on nutrition, often with little or no recovery time between therapies. Chemotherapy and radiation can occur together in some clients. The side effects of treatment can persist long after treatment is completed. In a review of clients who successfully received chemotherapy and radiation for head and neck cancer, almost one-third still required tube feedings after 1 year because of profound dysphagia following treatment (Shiley, Hargunani, Skoner, Holland, & Wax, 2006). In a study on a similar population, almost one-third of clients were reported to be malnourished at diagnosis and 88% were malnourished when treatment finished (Unsal et al., 2006).

| BOX 23-3 | **Malnutrition Risk Factors of Cancer and Its Treatment** |

Disease and treatment symptoms and side effects will differ depending on the site of disease and treatment agent prescribed.

Disease Effects
Anorexia and early satiety
Cachexia
Dysphagia, odynophagia
Elevated metabolic rate if cachexia is present
Fatigue
Gastrointestinal symptoms—maldigestion, malabsorption
Pain
Psychological stress, anxiety, depression
Taste alterations

Treatment Effects
Chemotherapy
Diarrhea, abdominal pain
Fatigue
Learned aversions
Nausea and vomiting
Neutropenia with risk of food-borne illness

Oral mucositis
Taste changes
Weight gain with some agents

Radiation
Dysphagia, odynophagia
Fatigue
Nausea and vomiting
Diarrhea, abdominal pain
Xerostomia

Surgery
Increased nutritional requirements for healing
Potential for minimal intake before and after surgery
Gastrointestinal surgery site may diminish digestion and absorption

Bone Marrow or Stem Cell Transplant
Combined treatment effects of chemotherapy and radiation
Immunosuppressive therapy increases risk of food-borne illness
If graft-versus-host disease occurs, malabsorption and organ failure are issues

Rapidly dividing cells, such as those in the intestine and bone marrow, are greatly affected by the cytotoxic effects of chemotherapy and radiation. Because of this effect, gastrointestinal side effects occur with a number of chemotherapeutic agents or when radiation therapy involves any area encompassing the intestinal tract. Oral mucositis, nausea, vomiting, abdominal pain, and diarrhea can result, jeopardizing dietary intake and nutritional status. Side effects from chemotherapy depend on the prescribed treatment and the duration and frequency of treatment. Side effects from radiation depend on the area being irradiated and the daily fraction of radiation. Whole body irradiation, high-dose radiation, and radiation that encompasses the abdomen or head and neck area can place the client at risk for malnutrition because of intestinal side effects. Radiation of the head and neck can cause odynophagia and a loss of saliva production, called xerostomia, that makes chewing and swallowing even more difficult. Learned food aversions can occur in clients who have experienced adverse effects of treatment, such as severe nausea and vomiting, and have come to associate those effects with the food consumed at the time. Additionally, repeated treatments resulting in nausea can cause some clients to have anticipatory nausea prior to treatment. Intake can be further diminished because of taste changes, which occur not only from the disease itself, but its treatment. Three-fourths of clients receiving chemotherapy report both taste and smell changes (Bernhardson, Tishelman, & Rutqvist, 2008). Taste changes may gradually improve in

some clients following the cessation of treatment but persist in others (Peregrin, 2006).

The nutritional effects resulting from surgical intervention for cancer are dependent on the tumor site and the extent of surgery. Major surgery with significant nutritional demands for healing can tax the client who may already be at risk for malnutrition. Surgery that involves the gastrointestinal tract can alter digestion and absorption temporarily or more long term. Preoperative testing and postoperative recovery of bowel sounds can leave the client with just clear liquids or nil per os (NPO), failing to meet nutritional needs. Often clients receiving surgical treatment for cancer also have any combination of chemotherapy or radiation therapy before or after surgery, or both. Such clients require close nutrition monitoring and intervention for varying needs, symptoms, and side effects so that a full course of therapy can be completed.

Treatment with a bone marrow or stem cell transplant presents unique nutrition challenges because of the intensity of treatment side effects. High-dose chemotherapy and radiation magnifies the side effects seen with each treatment singly. Severe nausea, vomiting, and oral mucositis occur. Immunosuppressive therapy given after the transplant can increase the risk of developing a food-borne illness in these clients. If an allogenic bone marrow transplant results in graft-versus-host disease, where the donated bone marrow graft rejects the host (body), multiple organ failure can occur that includes profound malabsorptive and digestive prob-

MyNursingKit National Cancer Institute, Eating Hints

lems. Box 23-3 summarizes treatment-related problems that predispose the client to malnutrition.

Nutrition Intervention

For many clients with cancer, preventing weight loss and malnutrition is a vital component of their care. For others, issues of weight management are important. Each client with cancer has individual nutritional needs that are dictated by the type of cancer, the treatment plan, and the accompanying symptoms and side effects. These needs fall along a continuum and can change over the course of the disease, warranting close monitoring and reassessment. Nutrition intervention should be an adjunct to available medical intervention for symptoms or treatment side effects.

Treatment of cancer cachexia is difficult because of the influence of the tumor on appetite and energy metabolism. In addition to supplying adequate calories and protein in the diet or through oral liquid supplements, the use of appetite stimulants has been tried with varying success (Tisdale, 2009). The use of omega-3 fatty acid supplements, which can act as anti-inflammatory agents, has been shown to have a role in treatment of cachexia related to upper intestinal and pancreatic cancers (Colomer et al., 2007; Doyle et al., 2006). In contrast, the Evidence-Based Practice Box: Are omega-3 fatty acids an effective therapy for cancer cachexia? outlines the use of this supplement with other types of cancers.

Nausea and vomiting are common symptoms that can be treated with both medical and nutritional intervention. In addition to pharmacological treatment of these symptoms, further suggestions are outlined in Practice Pearl: Nausea and Hospital Food Service and Box 23-4. Constipation is a common side effect of antinausea and pain medications. Nutrition intervention should include ample fluid and ade-

PRACTICE PEARL

Nausea and Hospital Food Service
Strong food odors can exacerbate nausea. When assisting the hospitalized client with cancer during a meal, the lid covering the meal when it is delivered should be removed away from the client and not directly under the client's nose. This avoids wafting strong food smells trapped under the lid so close to the client.

quate fiber intake as outlined in Chapter 20. Fruits, vegetables, legumes, and whole grains commonly recommended as fiber sources may not be appealing to the client if appetite is poor or if there are other side effects. Blander options can include oatmeal with a small amount of dried fruit or whole-grain cereal flakes mixed in or whole-grain versions of pasta, toast, or crackers. Recommendations for treating other symptoms, including anorexia, diarrhea, taste changes, and fatigue, are included in Boxes 23-5 through 23-11.

Cancer therapy, such as chemotherapy and immunosuppressive therapy, affects the bone marrow and can result in a decreased neutrophil count, or neutropenia. An absolute neutrophil count of less than 1,000/mm^3 is low and 500/mm^3 is considered severe, placing the client at high risk for infection (Smith & Toonen, 2007). Safe food-handling practices are essential to prevent infection from food-borne pathogens. Use of a strict low-microbial or low-bacteria diet has been commonplace in treatment of neutropenia, but this practice lacks strong evidence to support its use and adherence is reportedly difficult (Gardner et al., 2008; Restau & Clarke, 2008). Studies have found that the practice of safe food handling and preparation, including the avoidance of raw fruits

---

EVIDENCE-BASED PRACTICE RESEARCH BOX

Are omega-3 fatty acids an effective therapy for cancer cachexia?

Clinical Problem: Effective treatment for cachexia is desirable to improve a client's nutritional status and to improve body image. Is there a role for omega-3 supplements to treat cachexia?

Research Findings: Cachexia and wasting may occur during treatment with chemotherapy or in later stages of cancer. Nurses are challenged to present clients and their families with effective therapies to deal with this troubling condition. Early studies seemed to indicate that omega-3 supplements would be beneficial.

A recent meta-analysis conducted by Dewey, Baughan, Dean, Higgins, and Johnson (2007) reviewed randomized controlled trials of eicosapentaenoic acid (EPA or omega-3

fish oil) for treatment of cancer cachexia. They were able to locate only five studies that met inclusion criteria of oral EPA compared to a control or placebo group. The studies included a total of 587 subjects. The reviewers analyzed the findings from all five studies and concluded that there were insufficient data to support EPA as superior to a placebo. Data further failed to provide evidence that EPA improved symptoms associated with cachexia (Dewey et al., 2007).

Nursing Implications: There is no research evidence to demonstrate a benefit to adding EPA to other measures when treating clients with cachexia.

CRITICAL THINKING QUESTION:

1. What can the nurse suggest to clients or family members who ask what nonprescription things can be used to diminish the "wasting away" that is occurring?

BOX 23-4	Nausea and Vomiting: Nutritional Treatment

Offer sips of flat ginger ale and dry carbohydrate foods (crackers, rice, pasta, breadsticks, toast).
Avoid empty stomach and greasy or high-fat foods.
Choose bland, odorless, colorless foods to minimize sensory stimulation.
Refrain from favorite foods while symptomatic to avoid learned aversions.
Have others help with meal preparation.
Rest before and after eating to avoid sudden movement.
Time antiemetic medication for full effect during meals.
Avoid liquids with meals.

Sources: Adapted from: NCI, 2006; NCI, 2009a.

BOX 23-5	Diarrhea: Nutrition Intervention

Try low-fat, no caffeine, and low-lactose intake to see if symptoms are relieved.
Avoid extremely hot or cold foods.
Avoid sugar alcohols found in sugar-free or low-calorie foods.
Try soluble fiber foods such as pears, apples, bananas, and barley.
Maintain hydration.
Consider use of sports drinks if hydration or electrolyte intake is poor.

Sources: Adapted from: NCI, 2006; NCI, 2009a.

BOX 23-6	Anorexia and Early Satiety: Nutrition Intervention

Consume small, frequent meals.
Eat nutrient-dense foods at start of a meal and start of the day when appetite may be better.
Maximize calorie and protein intake (see Box 23-11).
Avoid carbonated beverages, gas-forming foods, and excessive liquid at meals because of full feeling that can result.
Try foods with high sensory appeal; that is, colorful, flavorful foods.
Consult with the physician about appetite stimulant.

Sources: Adapted from: NCI, 2006; NCI, 2009a.

BOX 23-7	Dysphagia and Oral Symptoms: Nutrition Intervention

Choose soft, moist foods such as those with gravies, dressings, oatmeal, scrambled eggs, milkshakes, cottage cheese, and macaroni and cheese.
Avoid extremely hot foods.
Use a drinking straw if oral pain is present.
Avoid citrus, tomato, and spicy or pickled foods if mouth sores are present.
Consider an anesthetic mouth rinse, a spray, or lozenges for pain if safety permits. Numb the mouth with ice or popsicles.

Sources: Adapted from: NCI, 2006; NCI, 2009a.

BOX 23-8	Xerostomia: Nutrition Intervention

Consume moist foods, such as those with added sauce, dressing, and casseroles.
Avoid alcohol and alcohol-containing mouthwash.
Consume liquids with meals.
Dunk dry foods in liquids.
Consume tart and sour foods and hard candies because they may stimulate saliva production.
Maintain good mouth care.
Consider use of synthetic saliva.

Sources: Adapted from: NCI, 2006; NCI, 2009a.

BOX 23-9	Taste Changes: Nutrition Intervention

If the client complains of metallic taste, try glass, porcelain, and ceramic cookware and plastic eating utensils to avoid food contact with metal.
Consume cold proteins, such as deli meats, hard-cooked eggs, and canned meats because they have less metallic taste than hot protein foods.
Experiment with altering sweetness and saltiness of foods to taste appeal.
Consume adequate fluids.
Maintain good mouth care.

Sources: Adapted from: NCI, 2006; NCI, 2009a.

BOX 23-10	Fatigue: Nutrition Intervention

Keep ready-to-eat foods on hand for when energy level is low; for example, frozen, boxed, or microwavable entrees, crackers and cheese, soups and stews, sandwich items.
Freeze extra portions of food for later reheating.
Choose nutrient-dense meals and snacks.
Consume smaller meals more frequently if tired before the meal is finished.
Have finger foods to minimize effort of eating.
Maintain hydration.
Try light exercise to increase energy level.

Sources: Adapted from: NCI, 2006; NCI, 2009a.

BOX 23-11	Increasing Calorie and Protein Intake

Increase "calories per bite" with nutrient-dense foods rather than filling up on low-calorie items:
Puddings, tapioca, custard, ice cream
Yogurt, cheese, smoothies
Juice and milk versus water, tea, coffee
Peanut and nutbutters
Non-fat dry milk added to boost recipes
Oral liquid nutrition supplements
Added fats such as cream cheese, butter, margarine, sauces, gravy, dressings

Sources: Adapted from: NCI, 2006; NCI, 2009a.

and vegetables, compared with adherence to a stricter low-microbial diet resulted in no significant differences in positive blood cultures for food-borne pathogens (Demille, Deming, Luinacci, & Jacobs, 2006; Moody, Finlay, Mancuso, & Charlson, 2006). Still others report no difference in rate of infection or fever of unknown origin between a low-bacteria diet, also called a neutropenic or cooked diet, and a diet that does contain raw fruits and vegetables rather than cooked (Gardner et al., 2008). Guidelines on safe food practices with neutropenia are outlined in Box 23-12.

In the United States, the majority of clients with cancer use some form of dietary supplements with almost half trying herbal products (Hardy, 2008). Although data on the use of dietary supplements, including herbs, are limited with regard to cancer treatment, some clients choose to combine this nutrition intervention with conventional treatment. A careful nursing assessment should yield information on any use of dietary supplements so that a discussion can follow about potential consequences. The clinical data concerning use and safety of dietary supplements in cancer occurs along a continuum with some supplements seeming to do no harm—and some, no good—whereas others have potentially dangerous consequences. The nurse should educate the client about known risks associated with certain dietary supplements that either interfere with conventional cancer treatment or have serious side effects. Drug–herb interactions that lower the efficacy of chemotherapy are of significance because of the narrow therapeutic range of most chemotherapy agents. For example, the herb St. John's Wort interacts with chemotherapeutic agents that use the same metabolic enzyme as the herb, causing subtherapeutic levels of chemotherapy. These include irinotecan, taxanes, imatinib, and cyclosporins. Other herbs that interact with some chemotherapies include echinacea, essiac, ginkgo, ginger, and milk thistle (Michaud et al., 2007a; Michaud, Karpinski, Jones, & Espirito, 2007b). Depending on the interaction, the effects of chemotherapy can be diminished or increased, which can lead to drug failure or toxicity, respectively. In addition to altering therapeutic drug levels, other concerns include the following (Lawenda et al., 2008; Michaud et al., 2007a; Michaud et al., 2007b):

- *Altered bleeding.* Some dietary supplements alter platelet function and coagulation, a dangerous effect especially in clients with low platelet counts because of disease or treatment or those on anticoagulant medications. Garlic supplementation is especially cited for this effect.
- *Immunosuppression or stimulation.* Long-term use of echinacea can cause immunosuppression, which is an undesirable effect in those with a depressed immune system because of the disease or treatment. St. John's Wort and garlic may act as immune stimulants and negatively affect antirejection treatment following bone marrow transplant.
- *Antioxidant action.* Antioxidant vitamins, such as A, C, and E, may prevent the oxidizing effect of free radicals deliberately formed by radiation and some chemotherapies, primarily alkylating agents such as cisplatin. Use of antioxidant supplements during treatment has the potential to interfere with the intended effects of many of these treatments and is discouraged.

The nurse should be alert to the fact that unusual side effects or lack of response to effective medications could signal use of dietary supplements during treatment. The client should be encouraged to discuss dietary supplement use at each treatment visit so that a collaborative decision can be made regarding the safety of these products during treatment. Chapters 24 and 25 discuss drug interactions and dietary supplements in more detail. Box 23-13 outlines some questions for the nurse to review with the client considering or using complementary and alternative therapy.

BOX 23-12	Neutropenia and Food Safety Guidelines

- Wash hands before preparing food and after handling raw foods.
- Keep food preparation surfaces, utensils, and storage areas clean.
- Store foods at proper temperature. Refrigerate leftovers within 2 hours. Do not thaw foods at room temperature.
- Wash fruits and vegetables before consuming.
- Take extra care in the handling of raw meat, fish, poultry, and eggs. Keep raw products separate from ready-to-eat foods. Cook to proper temperatures.
- Consume milk and juices that are pasteurized.
- Avoid raw or undercooked food such as sushi, salad bars, raw or undercooked meat, poultry, fish, eggs, and tofu in open bins or containers.
- Observe "sell by" and "use by" dates on foods.
- Avoid foods in packages that are dented, bulging, or swollen before opening.
- Avoid old or moldy fruits and vegetables.

Sources: Adapted from: American Cancer Society, 2008; Doyle et al., 2006; NCI, 2009a.

BOX 23-13	Complementary and Alternative Medicine Use

When a client asks about the use of complementary or alternative medicine or when the nurse learns of existing use, the following questions can be reviewed with the client:

- What benefits can be expected from this therapy?
- What are the risks associated with this therapy?
- Do the known benefits outweigh the risks?
- What side effects can be expected?
- Will the therapy interfere with conventional treatment?

■ How could the nurse respond to the client who is taking dietary supplements but has no knowledge about how to answer most of these questions?

Sources: Adapted from: NCI, 2009b.

Medical Nutrition Therapy and HIV Infection

Medical nutrition therapy is essential throughout the course of HIV infection. Prevention of malnutrition and its associated mortality risk is a central goal of nutritional care in this population. Malnutrition has a negative effect on immune status, independent of HIV infection, and can in turn predispose the body to risk of infection (Colecraft, 2008). Malnutrition and coinfections can have devastating consequences in the client already infected with HIV. Nutrition intervention should target the preservation of body weight, in particular body-protein stores found in muscle and organs, because of the association between maintaining crucial weight and survival with HIV disease (American Dietetic Association [ADA], 2004). As with any disease, the nurse should be aware that risk of weight loss and malnutrition in HIV infection can occur because of decreased dietary intake, nutrient losses, or unmet elevated nutritional needs that are caused by the disease or its treatment.

Virus-Related Nutrition Risk Factors

The nurse should assess the client for the myriad of virus-related symptoms that affect nutritional health in those with HIV infection. An increased viral load and any opportunistic infections that occur because of diminished immunity contribute to elevated energy needs that, in turn, can go unmet because appetite is diminished or gastrointestinal symptoms are present (Chang, Sekhar, Patel, & Balasubramanyam, 2007; Colecraft, 2008). Opportunistic infections can lead to diminished dietary intake because of a host of symptoms from oral lesions and pain, taste changes, and diarrhea to excessive coughing and fatigue. Figure 23-1 ■ illustrates the common oral opportunistic infection candida, which causes pain, taste changes, and diminished intake.

Although highly active antiretroviral therapy **(HAART)** has lessened the incidence of opportunist infections with HIV

infection, complaints of gastrointestinal dysfunction persist. HIV enteropathy is an intestinal condition characterized by chronic diarrhea in the absence of an active pathogenic infection and can lead to risk of malabsorption, weight loss, and dehydration. Chronic diarrhea with HIV infection is defined by the Centers for Disease Control and Prevention (CDC) as two or more loose or watery stools a day for at least 30 days (CDC, 1992). The virus itself as well as mucosal damage to the intestinal immune cells may be to blame for this chronic diarrhea that can cause fat and carbohydrate malabsorption (Colecraft, 2008). Table 23-1 outlines opportunistic infections and other intercurrent disease that can occur with HIV infection and the nutrition-related symptoms.

Clients with HIV infection are at risk for Kaposi's sarcoma and B-cell lymphoma, malignancies that present additional nutritional challenges because of symptoms and treatment side effects. Both types of cancer can cause decreased intake because of oral or gastrointestinal disease involvement. Nutrition intervention should follow recommendations as outlined in the discussion on nutrition and cancer in this chapter.

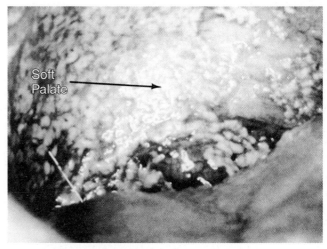

■ FIGURE 23-1 **Oral Candidiasis.**
Source: Centers for Disease Control and Prevention (CDC).

Table 23-1	HIV-Related Symptoms Affecting Nutrition
Opportunistic Infections	**Symptoms**
Campylobacter	Diarrhea
Candidiasis	Oral thrush, mouth pain, altered taste
Coccidioidomycosis	Shortness of breath, fatigue, cough
Cryptococcus	Nausea, vomiting, fever, altered cognition
Cryptosporidiosis	Diarrhea, nausea, vomiting, abdominal pain
Cytomegalovirus	Diarrhea, nausea, vomiting, mouth lesions
Giardia lamblia	Diarrhea, nausea, vomiting
Herpes simplex	Mouth lesions, pain, dysphagia
Isosporiasis	Diarrhea, fever, abdominal pain
Listerosis	Fever, diarrhea, abdominal pain
Microsporidia	Diarrhea, fever, abdominal pain
Mycobacterium avium	Fever, diarrhea, anorexia
Mycobacterium tuberculosis	Cough, fever, fatigue
Oral hairy leukoplakia	Taste changes, oral discomfort
Pneumocystis carinii pneumonia	Shortness of breath, fatigue, cough
Salmonella	Fever, diarrhea, abdominal pain
Shigella	Diarrhea, fever, abdominal pain
Toxoplasmosis of the brain	Fever, altered cognition, nausea, vomiting
Malignancies	
Burkitt's lymphoma	Gastrointestinal involvement possible
Lymphoma	Gastrointestinal involvement possible
Kaposi's sarcoma	Oral lesions, pain, dysphagia
HIV	
Encephalopathy	Altered cognition
Enteropathy	Chronic diarrhea
Myalgia	Muscle pain, weakness
Wasting syndrome	Muscle loss, weight loss, ↑ metabolic rate

Sources: Adapted from: CDC, 1992; Nysoe & Paauw, 2004.

The nurse should include an assessment of the client's psychosocial history when considering nutritional health. Intravenous drug use, poverty, and homelessness are all risk factors for poor nutrition and represent characteristics of those who are underserved by health care and part of the population with increasing case reports of HIV infection (ADA, 2004; Mangili, Murman, Zampini & Wanke., 2006). Food insecurity, because of inadequate funds or access to food, compounds the nutrition risk issues already present with HIV infection. The effects of food insecurity are hard felt in many regions of the world where HIV infection is more prevalent than others. Cultural Considerations Box: HIV and Nutrition in Developing Countries outlines these concerns.

Unintentional weight loss and wasting can be found in up to 10% of adults in the United States with HIV infection (Siddiqui et al., 2009). A higher prevalence of weight loss is found in underdeveloped countries (Berger, Fields-Gardner, Wagle, & Hollenbeck, 2008). Any amount of unplanned weight loss should be investigated and that which exceeds 5% of body weight over 3 months or 10% over 6 months is considered significant, meeting the qualifications to be considered wasting (World Health Organization [WHO], 2005). In addition to the contribution of many factors to the wasting phenomena—including the body's inflammatory response to the virus, the presence of opportunistic infections and other comorbidities, diminished testosterone levels, and psychosocial influences—evidence exists that other more complicated and less well-understood mechanisms are also to blame. Metabolic derangements because of viral effects on the mitochondria

Cultural Considerations

HIV and Nutrition in Developing Countries

In poor and developing countries, food insecurity has been linked to transmission of HIV and poor outcomes associated with the infection. Lack of access to food or insufficient funds predisposes many people to hunger and malnutrition, eroding the foundation that nutritional health provides in decreasing the risk of coinfections. Further, food insecurity worsens in households affected by HIV because of associated health care costs and loss of income. Lack of education regarding normal nutrition needs is also problematic in developing areas, such as Sub-Saharan Africa where the majority of those in the world with HIV infection live with the condition referred to as the "slim disease."

Issues of food insecurity in developing countries can be largely political or economical. The nurse working with this population can assess the barriers to adequate nutrition and customize advice to include recommendations for inexpensive, indigenous foods that contain protein and calories. For example, beans of all types, groundnuts, and cowpeas are protein-containing foods found in Sub-Saharan Africa. White rice, yams, sweet potatoes, cassava, and maize provide carbohydrate-based calories. Reports show that individuals who become engaged in agriculture or have a variety of foods rather than a few in the diet consume increased calories compared to others.

Sources: Adapted from: ADA, 2004; Bukusuba, Kikafunda, & Whitehead, 2007; Tabi & Vogel, 2006; Wiig & Smith, 2007.

can lead to dysfunctional energy production with elevated resting energy expenditure (Chang et al., 2007).

Children and pregnant females with HIV infection have additional nutritional challenges because of the need to provide essential nutrients for growth and development. Lifespan Box: Nutrition and HIV Concerns in Infants and Children outlines these concerns.

Treatment-Related Nutrition Risk Factors

Disease management with pharmacotherapy is a lifelong component for most clients with HIV infection (ADA, 2004). Since the advent of HAART and the reduction in prevalence of opportunistic infections in clients receiving that treatment, nutrition status is affected by medication side effects more commonly than from symptoms of opportunistic infection (Nysoe & Paauw, 2004). Nucleoside reverse transcriptase inhibitors (NRTIs), nonnucleoside reverse transcriptase inhibitors (NNRTIs), and protease inhibitors (PIs) are the commonly prescribed classes of medications that make up HAART. Each class of medication has side effects with potential nutrition implications. Within each class, certain drugs are associated with increased likelihood of causing symptoms compared with others. Often, these medications are used in combination. Food–drug interactions, gastrointestinal side effects, and metabolic derangements are examples of the effects of these medications. Additionally, many antiretroviral drugs have specific food–medication instructions that need to be followed to maintain therapeutic plasma drug levels. Some must be taken with food and others on an empty stomach. Some require a high-fat meal, others warn against it. Alcohol, grapefruit juice, and excessive vitamin E and garlic are known to interact with varying combinations of these drugs. The end result can be a heavy "pill burden" for the client that becomes a barrier to medication adherence or meal intake, or both. Table 23-2 outlines the general side effects associated with HAART medications.

Long-term metabolic complications associated with HAART present unique nutritional challenges to the client taking these medications. In some clients, the secondary consequences that arise from some antiretroviral medications are disturbing enough to foster drug nonadherence as outlined in Hot Topic: Lipodystrophy and HAART. Disturbances in subcutaneous fat distribution with or without fat wasting, insulin resistance, elevated lipid levels, and diminished bone health have been reported. It is essential that clients receiving HAART be monitored to assess for metabolic complications. Body composition should be assessed when possible because changes in fat distribution can mask loss of muscle mass, hiding this negative prognostic indicator.

Some clients choose to explore alternative medicine treatment of HIV infection and its related conditions instead

Lifespan

Nutrition and HIV Concerns in Infants and Children

The nutritional demands of growth and development can be difficult to meet when an infant or child is infected with HIV. Growth stunting and impaired cognitive development occur when disease symptoms prevent adequate intake to meet both the metabolic demands of the infection and normal nutrition in this population. Developmental delays in the infant and young child because of infection-related cognitive changes may affect oral motor feeding skills. Nutrient requirements to provide substrate for catch-up growth following periods of failure to thrive or growth faltering can be difficult to meet, especially if symptoms of infection persist or food insecurity is an issue. Children with HIV infection should be assessed for nutrition status every 6 months at a minimum. More frequent assessment and intervention is needed for those with symptoms or deacceleration of growth velocity.

In addition to the risks of undernutrition in many children, those on antiretroviral therapy are at risk for the development of lipid abnormalities. Up to 50% of children on HAART develop elevated cholesterol levels. Dietary intervention for this population mirrors that for the general population.

HIV-positive mothers who breastfeed their infant face the risk of transmitting the virus to the child. When safe and acceptable replacement feedings are available, these should be encouraged in place of breastfeeding. However, not all mothers have access to safe water sources, funds for feedings, or refrigeration. In such cases, exclusive breastfeeding is recommended. The nurse can play an active role in educating pregnant females with HIV infection about the risks and benefits to the available infant feeding choices.

Sources: Adapted from: ADA, 2004; Bland, Rollins, Coovadia, Coutsoudis, & Newell, 2007; McCrindle et al., 2007.

Table 23-2 Medication Side Effects Affecting Nutrition

Medication	Nutrition-Related Side Effect
NRTIs—Class Effect	**Hepatic Steatosis**
• abacavir	• Nausea, anorexia, cough, dyspnea
• didanosine	• Nausea, diarrhea
• stavudine	• Pancreatitis
• tenofovir	• Nausea, vomiting, diarrhea
• zalcitabine	• Mucosal ulcers, pancreatitis
• zidovudine	• Anemia, headache, nausea
Protease Inhibitors— Class Effect	**Hyperglycemia, Hyperlipidemia, Lipodystrophy**
• amprenavir	• Nausea, diarrhea
• fosamprenavir	• Diarrhea
• indinavir	• Nausea
• lopinavir	• Nausea, vomiting, diarrhea
• nelfinavir	• Diarrhea
• ritonavir	• Nausea, vomiting, diarrhea, taste changes
• saquinavir	• Nausea, diarrhea

Source: Adapted from: Nysoe & Paauw, 2004.

MyNursingKit Medication Adherence

hot Topic

Lipodystrophy and HAART

Lipodystrophy is described as abnormalities in fat distribution and dyslipidemia that occur in persons affected with HIV. This condition is also called fat redistribution syndrome. Up to 70% of clients on HAART exhibit some form of lipodystrophy with up to 50% developing symptoms within 2 years of beginning therapy. Fat abnormalities include two distinct components, which can occur together or alone. **Lipoatrophy** is a term used to describe peripheral fat wasting. Selective loss of fat occurs in the face, extremities, and buttocks. Fat accumulation is the second component and entails increased visceral fat on the trunk. Central fat accumulation and development of enlarged breasts and a dorsocervical fat pad (buffalo or dowager's hump and horse collar) occur. No clinical definition exists to specifically quantify the presence of these changes in subcutaneous fat. Hyperlipidemia is found, especially in those taking protease inhibitors. Triglyceride levels are most commonly elevated, along with cholesterol.

The consequences of lipodystrophy deserve attention. It is believed that hyperlipidemia in this population holds similar risk of cardiovascular disease to the general population and must be treated. Altered body image and quality of life because of fat distribution abnormalities affect self-esteem and, in some cases, medication adherence.

Elevated lipid levels are treated according to established guidelines for the general population, as outlined in Chapter 18. Risk factor and lifestyle modification, including diet, are advised. Often, lifestyle management alone does not reduce lipid levels sufficiently and consideration of pharmacological treatment is made after careful evaluation of possible drug interactions with HAART. In some cases, alternative HAART regimens are prescribed. Use of fish oil supplements has been reported to be beneficial for elevated triglycerides, as in the general population, with no reported effect on HAART.

Distribution of body fat affected by lipodystrophy is difficult to alter. Exercise can be effective for central fat accumulation. Clients should be discouraged from radical dieting to lose fat because lean muscle can be lost, contributing to the potential for wasting syndrome. Some clients resort to cosmetic surgery with liposuction for sites with fat accumulation and injections of fillers for lipoatrophy. These costly approaches may not be covered by health insurance and may only be effective short term.

Guidelines for screening for lipodystrophy include the following:

- Fasting lipid profile before beginning HAART and every 3–6 months thereafter
- Assessment of existing cardiovascular risk factors with encouragement of lifestyle modifications where indicated
- Annual assessment of body composition with waist-to-hip ratio, thigh circumference, skin fold thicknesses where available

Although lipodystrophy can present additional health risks for the client infected with HIV, any management approach, conventional or alternative, should not jeopardize the underlying treatment of the HIV infection.

Sources: Adapted from: Cofrancesco, Freedland, & McComsey, 2009; Fuller, 2008; Marcason, 2009.

of conventional treatment. Others utilize both types of treatment together. The use of dietary supplements, including nonvitamin, nonmineral supplements such as herbs, is reported to be higher in persons with HIV infection than is found in the general population (Hendricks, Sansevero, Houser, Tang, & Wanke, 2007). Habitual intake of select vitamins and minerals in excess of the tolerable upper limits recommended was found in almost 90% of men with HIV infection who were also taking nonvitamin, nonmineral dietary supplements. Such clients were also more likely than not to be taking HAART (Hendricks et al., 2007).

Little long-term scientific evidence exists regarding the use of dietary supplements with HIV infection, but what is known is that St. John's Wort can lead to the therapeutic failure of PI and NNRTIs and that use of garlic or high-dose vitamin C may have similar negative results (Canadian AIDS Treatment Information Exchange [CATIE], 2005). Interactions leading to treatment failure with HAART can cause drug resistance, limiting future treatment options (CATIE, 2005). The use of milk thistle, echinacea, and goldenseal is each being investigated for the potential to increase HAART plasma drug concentrations. Increased plasma drug levels are associated with drug toxicity. Despite the claims that some botanicals work as "immune therapy," no herbal therapy has been proven effective as an antiretroviral treatment (CATIE, 2005).

The many side effects associated with the treatment of HIV infection can be an unmanageable burden to some clients despite the long-term benefits associated with use of antiretroviral therapy. Practice Pearl: Nutrition and Medication Adherence outlines the importance of a nonjudgmental assessment of medication adherence in this population.

PRACTICE PEARL

Nutrition and Medication Adherence

A thorough nursing assessment should include a check on medication compliance in the client with HIV infection. Many nutrition-related factors are affected by HAART and give rise to issues of nonadherence. Complicated food-medication schedules with some drugs can lead to missed dosages or altered drug absorption when instructions are not followed. Suboptimal adherence to dietary instructions related to HAART have been reported in over half of clients studied and can lead to drug resistance and decreased survival (Hermann et al., 2008; Schonnesson, Williams, Ross, Bratt, & Keel, 2007). Gastrointestinal side effects such as nausea and diarrhea can lead some clients to cease taking medications. Interactions between alternative medicine treatments, specifically herbs, and some HAART can alter drug plasma concentration and lead to therapeutic failure, viral resistance, or drug toxicity. The presence of lipodystrophy affects body image in some clients to such a degree that medications are self-discontinued (Fuller, 2008).

Nutrition Intervention

A guiding recommendation to begin nutrition intervention at the time of diagnosis states: "The negative effects of malnutrition are often preventable and are usually not easily reversed" (ADA, 2004). The nutrition care plan should be based on the findings of a careful assessment that considers risk factors for poor nutrition status that are specific to HIV infection and its comorbidities. Box 23-14 outlines parameters that should be included in the nutrition assessment. Particular attention should be paid to obtaining baseline measurements of objective data such as weight and laboratory values for comparison over the course of the disease. When possible, assessment of body composition is helpful to track any changes from lipodystrophy or wasting. Simple measurement of body weight can overlook the shift in body composition that occurs in this population. The strong correlation between weight loss or wasting and poor outcome underlines the need for this monitoring.

Nutrition Intervention for Symptoms and Side Effects

Symptom management should begin with a medical evaluation of the client to determine the cause. Nutrition inter-

vention is aimed at providing symptom or side effect relief and maximizing intake to optimize nutritional status. Clinical stability and nutrition stability often are parallel; thus symptoms can be episodic and lead to episodic declines in nutritional health (Faintuch, Soeters, & Osmo, 2006). In particular, symptoms that are associated with acute weight loss include oral symptoms, difficulty swallowing, and gastrointestinal symptoms (Mangili et al., 2006). Overall, medication side effects are a common contributor to physical complaints made by clients on HAART.

Medical intervention for HIV-associated wasting is the subject of considerable scientific attention. A medical evaluation may or may not reveal the etiology of this classic form of weight loss found in this population. The presence of an opportunistic infection or occult malignancy should be investigated, along with an assessment for endocrine abnormalities, including hypogonadism (Nysoe & Paauw, 2004). In addition to interventions directed at any contributing factors, nutrition treatment can include high-calorie, high-protein intake with liquid nutrition supplements when needed (Leyes, Martinez, & Forga Mde, 2008). Box 23-11 outlines advice on increasing calorie and protein intake.

MyNursingKit USDA HIV Nutrition Resources

| BOX 23-14 | Nutrition Assessment of the Client with HIV Infection |

The nutrition assessment of the client with HIV infection should include the standard components of an assessment. Particular attention should be paid to include the following:

Nutrition History

General diet history

Note baseline nutrition knowledge and sources of information

Cultural influences on nutrition and diet

Note any issues of food insecurity

Dietary supplement use, including vitamins, mineral, herbs, and other natural products

In infants, note maternal HIV status and source of infant feeding: formula or breastfeeding

Physical Exam

Height and weight

Weight history

Body composition measurements: circumference measurements, waist-to-hip ratio, body fat assessment

Visual assessment for lipodystrophy: note subcutaneous fat pattern, presence of temporal or extremity fat loss, existence of central fat accumulation

Laboratory Values

Plasma proteins

Indices for anemia

Lipid levels

Testosterone, if wasting is apparent

Fasting glucose

Bone density, if metabolic bone disease is suspected from HAART

Medical History

Presence of opportunistic infections: note symptoms, treatment, and side effects

Presence of comorbid conditions: malignancies, metabolic disease

Presence of anxiety, depression, altered cognition, or other psychoneurological symptoms

Over-the-counter and prescription drugs: note any food–medication instructions, interactions with food, dietary supplements or nutrients

Self-prescribed treatment for any medical symptoms

Psychosocial History

Alcohol intake

Use of illicit drugs, substance abuse

Body image

Living arrangements

Ability for self-care

 ▪ How would the presence of food insecurity affect prioritizing the goals of nutrition intervention?

Although immune-modulating enteral nutrition supplements and tube feeding formulas are available, conflicting results exist regarding any benefit to these products over standard formulas in treating clients with HIV infection (Okenga et al., 2006). Medical treatment of wasting includes appetite stimulants, anabolic agents such as testosterone replacement and growth hormone, and cytokine antagonists. No one medical intervention has been proved superior or without consequence, leaving much room for further study.

Common complaints that interfere with adequate intake are categorized in Box 23-15. Nutrition intervention for these symptoms and side effects are found in Box 23-4 through Box 23-11. A team approach with psychosocial expertise is needed when issues of food insecurity, altered cognition, substance abuse, or depression-type symptoms are the reason for poor intake. The nurse can assist the client with complicated food–medication schedules by suggesting use of a medicine schedule, pill chart, or other reminder system that suits the client's style.

Food safety education is an important component of nutrition intervention starting at the time of diagnosis. A compromised immune status leaves the client with HIV infection more susceptible to food-borne illness. Some foods are riskier than others because of processing, handling, or storage practices common to the product. Examples include unpasteurized dairy products, cold deli meats, and raw seafood such as sushi. Safe food handling and storage is essential to minimize risk of illness. Good hand washing and use of clean food preparation surfaces and utensils are needed. Observation of proper storage and cooking temperatures helps to lessen the possibility of microbial growth. Salmonellosis, campylobacteriosis, *Mycobacterium avium intracellulare*, listeriosis, and *Vibrio vulnificus* are among the food-borne illnesses presenting an increased risk to those with HIV infection compared with the general population (Hayes, Elliott, Krales, & Downer, 2003). *Cryptosporidium* is one parasite that can be found in water sources and presents a pathogen risk to the person with HIV infection. Clients should be advised against drinking water from lakes or streams, swallowing water while swimming, and consuming water or ice when traveling in foreign countries. Client Education Checklist: Preventing Food-Borne Illness in HIV Infection outlines the components of safe food handling, drinking water safety, and guidelines for safe food while traveling.

Nutrition Intervention for Metabolic Consequences

As clients with HIV infection have improved survival, longer-term consequences have emerged primarily as a result of treatment. Lipodystrophy, outlined in Hot Topic: Lipodystrophy and HAART, is one class of metabolic consequences seen in this population. Additionally, elevated fasting glucose, blood lipids, and insulin resistance are being reported. Management of insulin resistance follows the same lifestyle advice for the non-HIV-infected population, as outlined in Chapter 19. Weight loss, diet modification, and increased exercise are advised for dyslipidemias, as outlined in Chapter 18.

Bone disorders in the form of osteopenia and osteoporosis have been reported in up to 28% of clients not on HAART and up to 50% of those who have received that therapy, which are statistics that exceed those of the general adult population (Morse & Kovacs, 2006). The nurse should assist the client in modifying risk factors for low bone density, such as smoking, low weight, and poor diet, and encourage adequate intake of calcium and vitamin D. Management of low bone mineral density in people with HIV infection mirrors that of the general population; no specific recommendations exist for this population (Morse & Kovacs, 2006; Spach, 2004).

BOX 23-15	Malnutrition Risk Factors of HIV Infection and Its Treatment

↓ Intake

Poor appetite: pain, myalgia, depression, pruritus

Lack of energy to prepare, eat meals: fatigue, persistent cough, headache, muscle loss

Early satiety

Oral and esophageal pain, lesions, dysphagia

Taste changes

Nausea, vomiting, diarrhea

Altered cognition

Complicated food–medication schedule

Food insecurity

Substance abuse

Malabsorption/Nutrient Loss

Diarrhea/enteropathy

Medication interactions

Unmet ↑ Nutritional Needs

Fever

Wounds

Elevated resting energy expenditure

CLIENT EDUCATION CHECKLIST	Preventing Food-Borne Illness in HIV Infection
Intervention	**Example**
Assess the client's knowledge on food safety and HIV infection. Educate about risk of food-borne illness because of HIV infection.	• Discuss the reason for increased risk of food-borne illness. • List symptoms of food-borne illness: fever, chills, diarrhea, abdominal pain, nausea, vomiting, and headache.
Educate on overall safe food practice to prevent food-borne illness, identifying critical points in food safety for risk of infection: purchasing, storage, preparation.	• Purchasing: Separate raw meats, poultry, or fish in the grocery cart by placing in plastic bag and storing on the lower part of the cart. Observe "sell by" dates on products. Avoid open, dented, or damaged packages. • Storage: Store raw meats, poultry, and fish below, away from other food to avoid dripping juices. Check the refrigerator thermometer to ensure that the temperature is less than 40°F. Refrigerate leftovers within 2 hours or 1 hour if in hot weather. Keep the refrigerator clean. Observe "use by" dates on food. • Preparation: Wash hands before preparing food and after touching raw meats, poultry, fish, or eggs. Always use clean surfaces, utensils, and cutting boards. Use a separate or a cleaned cutting board for raw meats, fish, and poultry. Wash fruits and vegetables and peel them. Do not add marinades used on raw products to cooked products. Fully cook meat, poultry, fish, and eggs. Use a thermometer to check temperature. Eggs should be firm and not runny. Reheat leftovers to 165°F.
Educate about risky foods to avoid.	Avoid: • Unpasteurized milk or juice • Soft cheeses such as feta, brie, camembert • Raw sprouts • Ready-to-eat deli foods such as meats, spreads, hot dogs, smoked seafood • Raw or undercooked eggs in eggnog, Caesar dressing, raw dough
Educate about safe drinking water.	• Avoid drinking water from lakes, streams, springs, swimming pools. • Check with local public health authorities about local water safety. • Boil water when indicated, including water used to make ice or to reconstitute beverages. • Bottled water is considered safe.
Educate about safe practices when eating out or traveling.	Observe general recommendations for safe food. Additionally, • Order foods that are thoroughly cooked and eat these while still hot. • Do not eat food from street vendors. • Do not consume fruits or vegetables unless you peel them yourself. • Avoid water and ice in areas with questionable water safety. Instead, consume hot tea, coffee, or canned drinks. • Avoid salad bars and buffets.

Sources: Adapted from: CDC, 2007; USDA, 2006.

NURSING CARE PLAN Nutrition during Chemotherapy

CASE STUDY

Nick, age 48, is an office manager for a small accounting firm. He was diagnosed and treated for colon cancer 4 years ago. His treatment consisted of surgery followed by chemotherapy. At his most recent follow-up visit he was found to have recurrence and will begin chemotherapy in 2 days. He and his wife are meeting with the nurse to discuss the treatment plan and answer questions. Nick says that his most lasting memory of the chemotherapy last time was how sick he got. He related that he had lost 30 pounds and the nausea seemed unending. He had no energy and felt depressed. His children, who were teenagers then, had a hard time coping and he was worried about them having to go through this again. Nick and his wife tried to have the family eat the evening meal together as much as possible; one of their main concerns was finding a way to control or prevent nausea so they could have some "normal" time together.

Applying the Nursing Process

ASSESSMENT

Weight: 162 pounds Height: 6 feet BMI: 22
Hgb 13.8 Hct 41
Weight prior to initial diagnosis 170 pounds
No problems with nausea, diarrhea, constipation, or gas
Skin pale and dry

DIAGNOSES

Readiness for enhanced nutrition related to requests for information about diet recommendations
Risk for impaired nutrition: less than body requirements related to treatment protocol

EXPECTED OUTCOMES

Weight loss of less than 10% of pretreatment weight
Nick and his wife identify four things that can be done to prevent or control nausea

INTERVENTIONS

Dietary strategies to deal with nausea: avoid foods with strong odors, maintain good oral hygiene, avoid an empty stomach yet eat small portions, avoid greasy or fried foods
Take antiemetic medication as prescribed
Rest before eating
Have foods with highest protein and calorie content when experiencing least nausea
Consider using oral liquid nutrition supplements
Have pleasant conversations at mealtime; avoid stressful topics or discussions

EVALUATION

One month later Nick has had two rounds of chemotherapy. His weight is 154 pounds and he feels exhausted; everything "takes so much energy." He works mornings because that is when he feels best but needs to nap in the afternoons. Nick says that he and his wife have tried everything the nurse suggested and that some seem to work better than others. He tries to eat an egg and toast every morning, but finds he cannot eat meat at dinner. His children love beef and chicken but the sight of it upsets his stomach, so his wife lets the children eat while he is resting. They will come to the table for a little conversation while Nick and his wife eat, but they are always eager to leave. Nick says that he knows he has a tough road ahead with six more treatments, but that as long as they can keep the nausea and weight loss in check they will make it. Figure 23-2 ■ outlines the nursing process for this case.

Critical Thinking in the Nursing Process

1. What are some nutritional suggestions that a nurse can offer a client who has started chemotherapy and has already lost 10% of pretreatment weight?

Nutrition during Chemotherapy *(continued)*

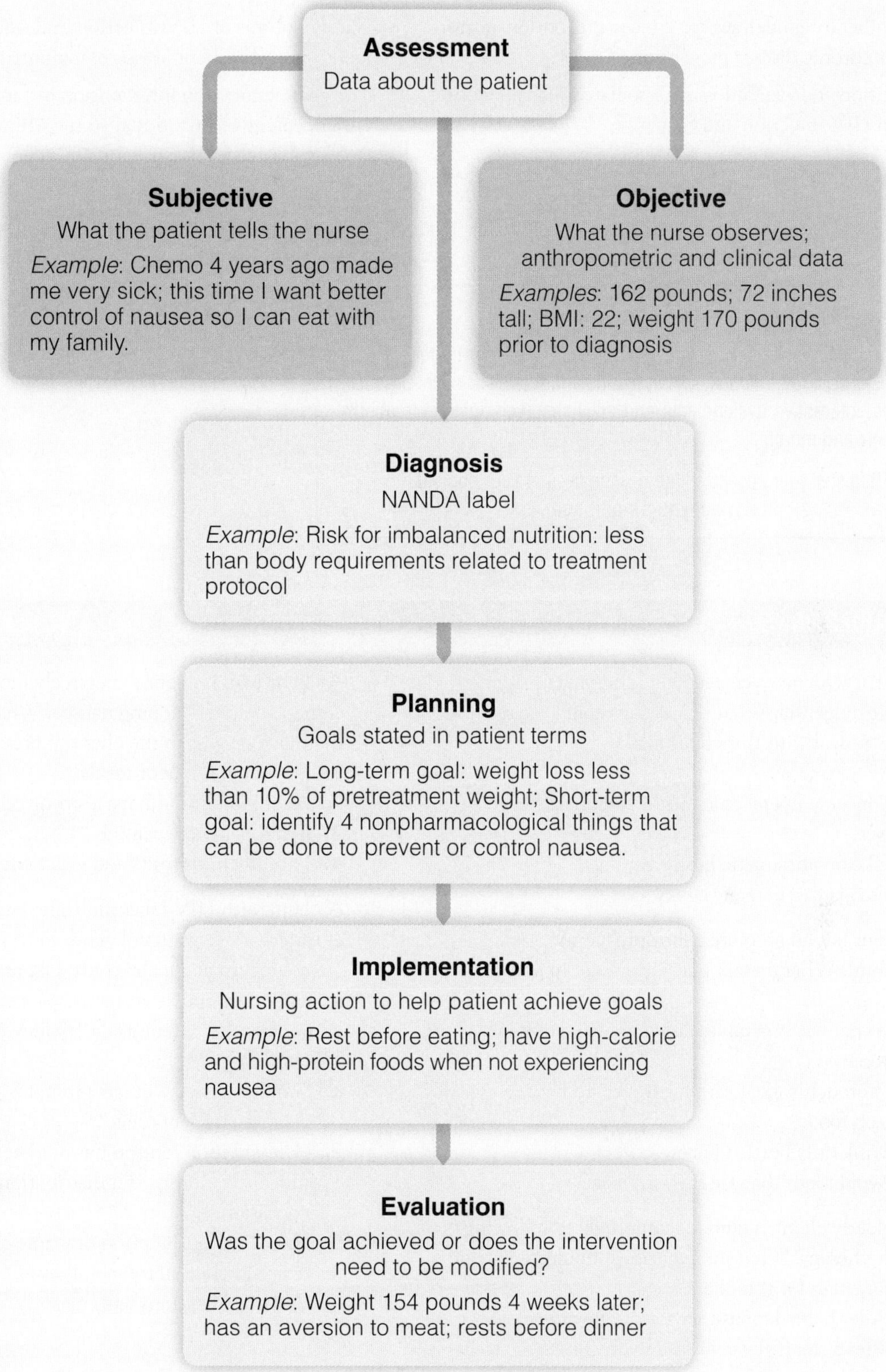

Assessment
Data about the patient

Subjective
What the patient tells the nurse
Example: Chemo 4 years ago made me very sick; this time I want better control of nausea so I can eat with my family.

Objective
What the nurse observes; anthropometric and clinical data
Examples: 162 pounds; 72 inches tall; BMI: 22; weight 170 pounds prior to diagnosis

Diagnosis
NANDA label
Example: Risk for imbalanced nutrition: less than body requirements related to treatment protocol

Planning
Goals stated in patient terms
Example: Long-term goal: weight loss less than 10% of pretreatment weight; Short-term goal: identify 4 nonpharmacological things that can be done to prevent or control nausea.

Implementation
Nursing action to help patient achieve goals
Example: Rest before eating; have high-calorie and high-protein foods when not experiencing nausea

Evaluation
Was the goal achieved or does the intervention need to be modified?
Example: Weight 154 pounds 4 weeks later; has an aversion to meat; rests before dinner

■ FIGURE 23-2 **Nursing Care Plan Process: Nutrition during Chemotherapy.**

CHAPTER SUMMARY

- General dietary guidelines for cancer prevention mirror those for chronic disease prevention.

- Malnutrition and weight loss are associated with poor outcomes in HIV infection and cancer.

- The symptoms of cancer and side effects of treatment place the client at risk of malnutrition.

- The symptoms of HIV infection and side effects of treatment place the client at risk of malnutrition.

- The goal of nutrition intervention in cancer or HIV is the enhancement of nutritional status while minimizing disease symptoms and treatment side effects.

EXPLORE **mynursingkit** PEARSON

MyNursingKit is your one stop for online chapter review materials and resources. Prepare for success with additional NCLEX®-style practice questions, interactive assignments and activities, web links, animations and videos, and more!

Register your access code from the front of your book at
www.mynursingkit.com.

NCLEX® QUESTIONS

1. A client who has received chemotherapy is experiencing dysgeusia. What suggestions could the nurse make to deal with this condition?
   1. Avoid spices and salt.
   2. Consume liberal amounts of carbonated beverages.
   3. Take an antiemetic before eating.
   4. Use glass or ceramic cookware.

2. A client has an absolute neutrophil count of 500/mm³. What dietary precautions are important for this client?
   1. Do not eat vegetables unless they have been frozen.
   2. Thoroughly clean the cutting board between each food.
   3. Drink only bottled juices.
   4. Avoid foods that are high in fiber.

3. An elderly client is immunocompromised following chemotherapy. What interventions should be part of the care plan for this client?
   1. Order pureed foods to make swallowing easier.
   2. Offer a small glass of water every 2 hours to treat dehydration.
   3. Ensure that all hot foods are thoroughly cooked to reduce bacteria.
   4. Limit intake of sugar-sweetened beverages to maintain blood glucose.

4. A client who is about to begin chemotherapy is concerned about developing nausea. What actions can the nurse suggest to the client to prevent nausea?
   1. Eat small, frequent meals.
   2. Avoid foods that have a strong odor.
   3. Thoroughly chew foods.
   4. Eat only fresh fruits and vegetables.

5. A client with HIV takes multiple medications as part of the HAART protocol. The client now expresses great concern about the central fat accumulation from lipodystrophy that has developed and wants to know what diet alterations can alleviate this problem. The nurse replies that:
   1. "Limiting intake of fats promotes weight loss and decrease in symptoms."
   2. "Dietary intervention has not been shown to significantly alter the fat distribution found in this condition."
   3. "Increase consumption of whole grains and fiber to speed cholesterol metabolism."
   4. "Take medications with meals."

REFERENCES

American Cancer Society (2008). *Infections in people with cancer.* Retrieved April 17, 2009, from http://www.cancer.org/docroot/ETO/content/ETO_1_2X_Infections_in_People_with_Cancer.asp

American Dietetic Association (ADA). (2004). Position of the American Dietetic Association and Dietitians of Canada: Nutrition intervention in the care of persons with human immunodeficiency virus. *Journal of the American Dietetic Association, 104,* 1425–1441.

American Institute for Cancer Research. (2007). *Diet and health guidelines for cancer prevention.* Retrieved April 19, 2009, from http://www.aicr.org/site/PageServer?pagename5dc_home_guides

Berger, M. R., Fields-Gardner, C., Wagle, A., & Hollenbeck, C. B. (2008). Prevalence of malnutrition in human immunodeficiency virus/acquired immunodeficiency syndrome orphans in the Nyanza province of Kenya: A comparison of conventional indexes with a composite index of anthropometric failure. *Journal of the American Dietetic Association, 108,* 1014–1017.

Bernhardson, B., Tishelman, C., & Rutqvist, L. E. (2008). Self-reported taste and smell changes during cancer chemotherapy. *Support Care Cancer, 16,* 275–283.

Bland, R. M., Rollins, N. C., Coovadia, H. M., Coutsoudis, A., & Newell, M. L. (2007). Infant feeding counselling for HIV-infected and uninfected women: Appropriateness of choice and practice. *Bulletin of the World Health Organization, 85,* 289–296.

Bukusuba, J., Kikafunda, J. K., & Whitehead, R. G. (2007). Food security status in households of people living with HIV/AIDS in a Ugandan urban setting. *British Journal of Nutrition, 98,* 211–217.

Canadian AIDS Treatment Information Exchange (CATIE). (2005). *A practical guide to herbal therapies for people living with HIV.* Retrieved April 19, 2009, from http://www.catie.ca/pdf/PG_Herb/HERBAL_guide_english_2005.pdf

Centers for Disease Control and Prevention (CDC). (1992). Revised classification system for HIV infection and expanded surveillance case definition for AIDS among adolescents and adults. *Morbidity and Mortality Weekly Report, 41,* 1–19.

Centers for Disease Control and Prevention (CDC). (2007). *Safe food and water.* Retrieved April 19, 2009, from http://www.cdc.gov/hiv/pubs/brochure/food.htm

Chang, E., Sekhar, R., Patel, S., & Balasubramanyam, A. (2007). Dysregulated energy expenditure in HIV-infected patients: A mechanistic review. *Clinical Infectious Diseases, 44,* 1509–1517.

Cofrancesco, J., Freedland, E., & McComsey, G. (2009). Treatment options for HIV-associated central fat accumulation. *AIDS Patient Care and Standards, 23,* 5–18.

Colecraft, E. (2008). HIV/AIDS: Nutritional implications and impact on human development. *Proceedings of the Nutrition Society, 67,* 109–113.

Colomer, R., Moreno-Nogueria, J. M., Garcia-Luna, P. P., Garcia-Peris, P., Garcia-de-Lorenzo, A., Zaraga, A., et al. (2007). N-3 fatty acids, cancer, and cachexia: A systematic review of the literature. *British Journal of Nutrition, 97,* 823–831.

Demark-Wahnefried, W., Rock, C. L., Patrick, K., & Byers, T. (2008). Lifestyle interventions to reduce cancer risk and improve outcomes. *American Family Physician, 77,* 1573–1578.

Demille, D., Deming, P., Luinacci, P., Jacobs, L. A. (2006). The effect of the neutropenic diet in the outpatient setting: A pilot study. *Oncology Nursing Forum, 33,* 337–343.

Dewey, A., Baughan, C., Dean, T., Higgins, B., & Johnson, I. (2007). Eicosapentaenoic acid (EPA, an omega-3 fatty acid from fish oils) for the treatment of cancer cachexia. *Cochrane database of Systematic Reviews,* Issue 1. Art. No.: CD004597. DOI:10.1002/14651858.CD004597.pub2.

Doyle, C., Kushi, L., Byers, T., Courneya, K. S., Demark-Wahnefried, W., Grant, B., et al. (2006). Nutrition and physical activity during and after cancer treatment: An American Cancer Society guide for informed choices. *CA Cancer Journal for Clinicians, 56,* 323–353.

Evans, W. J., Morley, J. E., Argiles, J., Bales, C., Baracos, V., Guttridge, D., et al. (2008). Cachexia: A new definition. *Clinical Nutrition, 27,* 793–799.

Faintuch, J., Soeters, P., & Osmo, H. G. (2006). Nutritional and metabolic abnormalities in pre-AIDS HIV infection. *Nutrition, 22,* 683–690.

Fairfield, K., & Stampfer, M. (2007). Vitamin and mineral supplements for cancer prevention: Issues and evidence. *American Journal of Clinical Nutrition, 85,* 289S–292S.

Fuller, J. (2008). A 39-year-old man with HIV-associated lipodystrophy. *Journal of the American Medical Association, 300,* 1056–1066.

Gardiner, P., Phillips, R., & Shaughnessy, A. F. (2008). Herbal and dietary supplement-drug interactions in patients with chronic conditions. *American Family Physician, 77,* 73–78.

Gardner, A., Mattiuzzi, G., Faderl, S., Borthakur, G., Garcia-Manero, G., Pierce, S., et al. (2008). Randomized comparison of cooked and noncooked diets in patients undergoing remission induction therapy for acute myeloid leukemia. *Journal of Clinical Oncology, 26,* 5684–5688.

Guha, N., Kwan, M. L., Quesenberry, C. P., Wletzien, E. K., Castillo, A. L., & Caan, B. J. (2009). Soy isoflavones and risk of cancer recurrene in a cohort of breast cancer survivors: The life after cancer epidemiology study. *Breast Cancer Research and Treatment,* doi: 10.1007/s10549-009-0321-5.

Hardy, M. L. (2008). Dietary supplement use in cancer care: Help or harm? *Hematology Oncology Clinics of North America, 22,* 581–617.

Hayes, C., Elliott, E., Krales, E., & Downer, G. (2003). Food and water safety for persons infected with human immunodeficiency virus. *Clinical Infectious Diseases, 36,* S106–S109.

Hendricks, K. M., Sansevero, M., Houser, R. F., Tang, A. M., & Wanke, C. A. (2007). Dietary supplement use and nutrient intake in HIV-infected persons. *AIDS Reader, 17,* 211–216.

Hermann, S., McKinnon, E., John, M., Hyland, N., Martinez, O. P., Cain, A., et al. (2008). Evidence-based, multifactorial approach to addressing non-adherence to antiretroviral therapy and improving standards of care. *Internal Medicine Journal, 38,* 8–15.

Klustad, R., & Schoeller, D. A. (2007). The energetics of wasting diseases. *Current Opinion in Clinical Nutrition and Metabolic Care, 10,* 488–493.

Lawenda, B. D., Kelly, K. M., Ladas, E. J., Sagar, S. M., Vickers, A., & Blumberg, J. B. (2008). Should supplemental antioxidant administration be avoided during chemotherapy and radiation therapy? *Journal of the National Cancer Institute, 100,* 773–783.

Leyes, P., Martinez, E., & Forga Mde, T. (2008). Use of diet, nutritional supplements and exercise in HIV-infected patients receiving combination antiretroviral therapies: A systematic review. *Antiviral Therapy, 13,* 149–159.

Lin, J., Cook, N. R., Zaharis, E., Gaziano, J. M., Van Denburgh, M., Buring. J. E., et al. (2009). Vitamins C and E and beta carotene supplementation and cancer risk: A randomized controlled trial. *Journal of the National Cancer Institute, 101,* 14–23.

Mangili, A., Murman, D. H., Zampini, A. M., & Wanke, C. A. (2006). Nutrition and HIV Infection: Review of weight loss and wasting in the era of highly active antiretroviral therapy from the Nutrition for Health Living cohort. *Clinical Infectious Diseases, 42,* 836–842.

Marcason, W. (2009). What does the term HIV-associated lipodystrophy mean? *Journal of the American Dietetic Association, 109,* 364.

McCrindle, B. W., Urbina, E. M., Dennison, B. A., Jacobson, M. S., Steinberger, J., Rocchini. A. P., et al. (2007). Drug therapy of high-risk lipid abnormalities in children and adolescents: A scientific statement from the American Heart Association. *Circulation, 115,* 1948–1967.

REFERENCES *(continued)*

Messina, M., & Wu, A. H. (2009). Perspectives on the soy-breast cancer relation. *American Journal of Clinical Nutrition, 89,* 1S–7S.

Michaud, L. B., Karpinksi, J. P., Jones, K. L., & Espirito, J. (2007a). Dietary supplements in patients with cancer: Risks and key concepts, part 2. *American Journal of Health-System Pharmacy, 64,* 369–381.

Michaud, L. B., Karpinksi, J. P., Jones, K. L., & Espirito, J. (2007b). Dietary supplements in patients with cancer: Risks and key concepts, part 1. *American Journal of Health-System Pharmacy, 64,* 467–480.

Molokhia, E. A., & Perkins, A. (2008). Preventing cancer. *Primary Care Clinics in Office Practice, 35,* 609–623.

Moody, K., Finlay, J., Mancuso, C., & Charlson, M. (2006). Feasibility and safety of a pilot randomized trial of infection rate: Neutropenic diet versus standard food safety guidelines. *Journal of Pediatric Hematology/Oncology, 28,* 126–133.

Morse, C. G., & Kovacs, J. A. (2006). Metabolic and skeletal complications of HIV infection. *Journal of the American Medical Association, 296,* 844–854.

National Cancer Institute (NCI). (2006). *Eating hints for cancer patients.* Retrieved April 19, 2009, from http://www.cancer.gov/cancertopics/eatinghints.pdf

National Cancer Institute (NCI). (2007). *Cancer trends: Progress report.* Retrieved April 17, 2009, from http://progressreport.cancer.gov

National Cancer Institute (NCI). (2009a). *Nutritional implications of cancer therapies.* Retrieved April 17, 2009, from http://www.cancer.gov/cancertopics/pdq/supportivecare/nutrition/HealthProfessional/117.cdr#Section_117

National Cancer Institute (NCI). (2009b). *Questions and answers about complementary medicine in cancer treatment.* Retrieved April 17, 2009, from http://www.cancer.gov/cancertopics/pdq/cam/cam-cancer-treatment/patient/page2#Section_43

Neuhouser, M. L., Wassertheil-Smoller, S., Thomson, C., Aragaki, A., Anderson, G. L., Manson, J. E., et al. (2009). Multivitamin use and risk of cancer and cardiovascular disease in the Women's Health Initiative. *Archives of Internal Medicine, 169,* 294–304.

Nysoe, T. E., & Paauw, D. S. (2004). Symptom management. In *A guide to primary care of people with HIV/AIDS.* Retrieved April 17, 2009, from http://www.hab.hrsa.gov/tools/primarycareguide

Okenga, J., Grimble, R., Jonkers-Schuitema, C., Macallan, D., Melchior, J. C., Sauerwein, H. P., et al. (2006). ESPEN guidelines on enteral nutrition: Wasting in HIV and other chronic infectious diseases. *Clinical Nutrition, 25,* 319–329.

Omenn, G. S., Goodman, G. E., Thornquist, M. D., Balmes, J., Cullen, M. R., & Glass, A. (1996). Risk factors for lung cancer and for intervention effects in CARET, the beta-carotene & retinol efficacy trial. *Journal of the National Cancer Institute, 88,* 1550–1559.

Peregrin, T. (2006). Improving taste sensation in patients who have undergone chemotherapy or radiation therapy. *Journal of the American Dietetic Association, 106,* 1536–1540.

Restau, J., & Clarke, A. P. (2008). The neutropenic diet. *Clinical Nurse Specialist, 22,* 208–211.

Schonnesson, L. N., Williams, M. L., Ross, M. W., Bratt, G., & Keel, B. (2007). Factors associated with suboptimal antiretroviral therapy adherence to dose, schedule, and dietary instruction. *AIDS Behavior, 11,* 175–183.

Shiley, S. G., Hargunani, C. A., Skoner, J. M., Holland, J. M., & Wax, M. K. (2006). Swallowing function after chemoradiation for advanced stage oropharyngeal cancer. *Otolaryngology-Head and Neck Surgery, 134,* 455–459.

Siddiqui, J., Phillips, A. L., Freedland, E. S., Sklar, A. R., Darkow, T., & Harley, C. R. (2009). Prevalence and cost of HIV-associated weight loss in a managed care population. *Current Medical Research and Opinion,* doi: 10.1185/03007990902902119.

Smith, G. F., & Toonen, T. R. (2007). Primary care of the patient with cancer. *American Family Physician, 75,* 1207–1214.

Spach, D. (2004). Metabolic complications of antiretroviral therapy. In *A guide to primary care of people with HIV/AIDS.* Retrieved April 17, 2009, from http://www.hab.hrsa.gov/tools/primarycareguide

Tabi, M., & Vogel, R. L. (2006). Nutrition counseling: An intervention for HIV-positive patients. *Journal of Advanced Nursing, 54,* 676–682.

Tisdale, M. J. (2009). Mechanisms of cancer cachexia. *Physiological Reviews, 89,* 381–410.

Toles, M., & Demark-Wahnefried, W. (2008). Nutrition and the cancer survivor: Evidence to guide oncology nursing practice. *Seminars in Oncology Nursing, 24,* 171–179.

United States Department of Agriculture (USDA). (2006). *Food safety for persons with AIDS.* Retrieved April 17, 2009, from http://www.fsis.usda.gov/Fact_Sheets/Food_Safety_for_Persons_with_AIDS/index.asp

Unsal, D., Mentes, B., Akmansu, M., Uner, A., Oguz, M., & Pak, Y. (2006). Evaluation of nutrition status in cancer patients receiving radiotherapy: A prospective study. *American Journal of Clinical Oncology, 29,* 183–188.

Wiig, K., & Smith, C. (2007). An exploratory investigation of dietary intake and weight in human immunodeficiency virus seropositive individuals in Accra, Ghana. *Journal of the American Dietetic Association, 107,* 1008–1013.

World Health Organization (WHO). (2005). *Interim WHO clinical staging of HIV/AIDS and HIV/AIDS case definitions for surveillance.* Retrieved April 19, 2009, from http://www.who.int/hiv/pub/guidelines/clinicalstaging.pdf

Food, Nutrient, and Drug Interactions

24

WHAT WILL YOU LEARN?

1. To classify mechanisms responsible for drug interactions with food and nutrients.
2. To examine the potential negative effects of certain medications on nutrition status.
3. To distinguish clients at increased risk for clinically significant drug, food, and nutrient interactions.
4. To provide education about drug additives to clients with related food insensitivities.
5. To delineate classes of medications and specific drugs associated with food or nutrient interactions.
6. To formulate nursing interventions to prevent or treat common drug, food, and nutrient interactions.

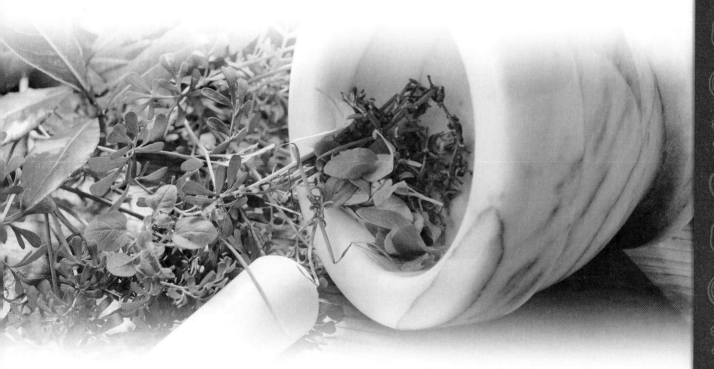

DID YOU KNOW?

▶ Some food interactions can lead to increased circulating levels of a drug and eventual drug toxicity; other interactions can result in treatment failure.

▶ The chance of a drug interaction increases with each added medication used, including dietary supplements and over-the-counter medications.

▶ Lactose is a filler used in some medications, which can present a problem to the unknowing lactose-intolerant client.

▶ Medications that cause intestinal symptoms or altered sense of taste or smell that lead to reduced food intake can contribute to poor nutritional health.

▶ Over-the-counter medications, dietary supplements, and herbs should

not be overlooked when considering drug interactions. For example: ginger, ginkgo, ginseng, garlic, and vitamin E can potentiate the effects of anticoagulant drugs and lead to prolonged bleeding.

▶ Mixing medications with enteral nutrition products can lead to an interaction and clogs a feeding tube if a precipitate forms.

KEY TERMS

MyNursingKit Food & Drug Administration

Drug interactions with food or nutrients can have serious health consequences. Drug effectiveness and nutritional health can be compromised. In addition to traditional drug interactions, the increased use of multiple medications, dietary supplements, and self-medication with over-the-counter drugs are risk factors for a drug interaction. Assessing and educating clients about drug interactions with dietary components is an essential nursing intervention.

How Do Drugs Interact with Food or Nutrients?

It is important for the nurse to be aware that the interactions between medications and food or nutrients can alter normal drug action. Interactions occur at any point in drug absorption, distribution, metabolism, or excretion, otherwise referred to as **pharmacokinetics.** Additionally, the intended action, or **pharmacodynamics,** of a medication may be further affected by a dietary substance that enhances or competes with the intended effect of the drug. Clinically relevant interactions are of highest concern because they can lead to treatment failure, adverse drug effects, or drug toxicity. Interactions that alter nutritional health are also important, but generally the effects are less immediate. Nutrition status can be affected when a medication alters the absorption, metabolism, or excretion of a nutrient or causes side effects that lead to reduced dietary intake. The nurse should assess the client for the potential for both short- and long-term effects of drug interactions with food and nutrients. Table 24-1 outlines nutrients affected by drug interactions. Table 24-2 outlines drugs according to medication class and corresponding food or nutrient interactions.

Alteration in Bioavailability

Interactions that affect drug or nutrient **bioavailability** occur by either fostering or inhibiting their digestion and absorption, altering the amount of the drug or nutrient available to the body. Certain components of food, such as fat or minerals, can change the bioavailability of a drug by either fostering or inhibiting drug absorption. Likewise, drugs can alter nutrient bioavailability. There are several points in the process of digestion and absorption that impact bioavailability. The rate of gastric emptying, gastric pH, the presence of bile, intestinal enzymes, and the physical and chemical characteristics of the drug or food affect bioavailability in the intestinal tract.

The potential for an interaction begins as soon as medication and food are combined, either in the mouth or when mixed together before administration. A food-drug complex can occur between food substances such as fiber or minerals and a medication. For example, digoxin bioavailability is reduced when consumed with a high-fiber food or dietary supplement because of drug-fiber binding. The reduction in digoxin absorption when taken with the fiber supplement psyllium illustrates this combination (Ulbricht et al., 2008). Iron supplements also bind with a high-fiber-content meal. **Chelation** is a specific type of binding that occurs between a metal ion, such as calcium, magnesium, or other mineral, and another molecule, which results in reduced bioavailability (Lentz, 2008). Although it has long been advised that dairy foods or antacids be avoided with drugs like the antibiotic tetracycline because of mineral chelation that reduces bioavailability of the antibiotic, the advent of calcium-fortified foods and common use of dietary supplements have opened a new chapter in the scope of advice that the nurse should provide to avoid this type of interaction. Hot Topic: Drug Interactions with Fortified Foods and Supplements outlines new concerns about calcium chelation with medications.

Administering medications to a client with a feeding tube should be done following proper technique to avoid drug binding and precipitate formation. If the medication is administered incorrectly, medication delivery may be altered or the tube may become clogged. Box 24-1 outlines nursing concerns with the tube-fed client. Practice Pearl:

Table 24-1 Nutrients Affected by Drugs

Nutrient	Nutrient Effect	Affecting Drug
Calcium	↓ Absorption Urinary loss	Acid-suppressing drugs, corticosteroids, tetracycline antibiotics Caffeine, corticosteroids, loop diuretics
Folate/Folic acid	↓ Absorption Altered metabolism Urinary loss	Alcohol, metformin, pancreatin, sulfasalazine Methotrexate, oral contraceptives, phenytoin, trimethoprin Aspirin
Iron	↓ Absorption ↑ Absorption	Acid-suppressing drugs, calcium and magnesium supplements, cholestyramine, tetracycline antibiotics Concurrent vitamin C
Magnesium	Urinary loss	Alcohol, cisplatin, loop and thiazide diuretics
Potassium	Urinary loss	Corticosteroids, loop and thiazide diuretics
Pyridoxine (vitamin B₆)	Altered metabolism	Isoniazid, oral contraceptives, penicillamine, theophylline
Thiamine (vitamin B₁)	↓ Absorption Urinary loss	Alcohol Loop diuretics
Vitamin A	↓ Absorption	Bile acid sequestrants, mineral oil
Vitamin B₁₂	↓ Absorption	Acid-suppressing drugs, colchicine, metformin
Vitamin C	Urinary loss	Aspirin, corticosteroids
Vitamin D	↓ Absorption Altered metabolism	Bile acid sequestrants, mineral oil Phenobarbital, phenytoin
Vitamin E	↓ Absorption	Bile acid sequestrants, mineral oil
Vitamin K	↓ Absorption Altered metabolism	Bile acid sequestrants, mineral oil Antibiotics destroy gut flora that produce vitamin K

Mixing Medications with an Enteral Nutrition Formula offers advice regarding the mixing of drugs and enteral formula. Additionally, mixing drugs with parenteral nutrition formula should follow protocol as outlined in Practice Pearl: Mixing Drugs and Parenteral Nutrition to avoid incompatibility and adverse interactions.

In the stomach, food affects the rate and amount of drug absorption through alterations in drug solubility, gastric pH, and gastric emptying. The amount and speed of drug absorption can be affected by the presence (or absence) of food; hence, medication guidelines that advise "take with food" or "take on an empty stomach." When

Table 24-2 Common Important Drug Interactions with Diet and Nutrients

Drug Class	Nutritional Interaction
Alcohol	↓ Absorption of folate, thiamine, urinary loss of magnesium
Anticoagulant warfarin, dicumerol	See Client Education Checklist: Warfarin Interactions with Food, Nutrients, and Supplements for warfarin
Anti-infective • Protease inhibitors • Antibiotics—tetracyclines and quinolones	↓ Drug effectiveness w/St. John's Wort Calcium and vitamin C supplements affect plasma levels of some brands Grapefruit interaction Follow specific advice on consumption with or without food depending on agent Chelation between drug and calcium, magnesium, iron, zinc in supplements, fortified foods, dairy
Anti-inflammatory corticosteroids	↓ Calcium absorption and urinary losses, urinary potassium loss Blood glucose

(continued)

Table 24-2 Common Important Drug Interactions with Diet and Nutrients *(continued)*

Drug Class	Nutritional Interaction
Cancer	Cisplatin causes magnesium loss Consult with physician about use of antioxidant supplements during radiation or chemotherapy because these may alter treatment effects See Chapter 23
Cardiac Amiodorone	Grapefruit interaction Vitamin B_6 increases photosensitivity effect
Calcium channel blockers	Grapefruit interaction with some agents
Digoxin	Avoid high-fiber intake with dose High-magnesium intake ↓ drug absorption
Diuretics: loop	Urinary loss of calcium, magnesium, potassium, thiamine
Diuretics: thiazide	Urinary loss of magnesium, potassium
Dietary Supplements	See Chapter 25 Avoid use of high-mineral potency supplement with medications warning against dairy or antacid use with drug
Enteral Nutrition	Follow protocol for administering drugs via feeding tube. See Box 24-1 and Practice Pearl: Mixing Medications with an Enteral Nutrition Formula
Gastrointestinal Antacids	Monitor for effects of ↓ phosphate absorption
Acid-suppressing drugs	↓ Absorption of calcium, iron, and food sources of vitamin B_{12}
Herbal	See Chapter 25
Neurological Anticonvulsants: carbamosepine, phenytoin, valproic acid	Monitor calcium, vitamin D status ↓ Absorption of folic acid Avoid phenytoin interaction with enteral formula
Parenteral Nutrition	Do not add drugs to parenteral mix Consult with pharmacist about drug use in multilumen catheters
Psychiatric Lithium	Keep sodium intake constant
MAOI	Follow low tyramine diet Refer to Client Education Checklist: Monoamine Oxidase Inhibitors (MAOI) and Tyramine
Other Antiacne (acitretin, isotretinoin, tretinoin)	Avoid vitamin A supplement
Cyclosporines	St. John's Wort diminishes drug effect Grapefruit interaction
Levodopa	Iron ↓ drug absorption Vitamin B_6 alters drug effectiveness
Levothyroxine	Drug chelates with calcium and iron supplements or fortified foods
Penicillamine	Drug absorption ↓ with calcium, magnesium, iron, zinc supplements

hot Topic

Drug Interactions with Fortified Foods and Supplements

It has long been advised that dairy products and antacids should not be taken at the same time as certain medications, such as the thyroid replacement hormone levothyroxine or certain antibiotics in the fluoroquinolone or tetracycline family. Calcium decreases the absorption of fluoroquinolones by up to 75% and the resulting decreased drug levels can contribute to treatment failure and antibiotic resistance. Now with the advent of heavily fortified foods and the popularity of dietary supplements, this advice needs to be taken to a whole new level. Initial nutrition recommendations for these drugs were aimed at avoiding the binding of calcium, magnesium, or aluminum in foods and antacids with the medication. This binding leads to poor drug absorption. The nurse should advise clients on these medications that the same interaction occurs when the drugs are consumed along with calcium supplements, calcium-fortified foods (like juices, breakfast cereals, or meal replacement bars) or high-potency multimineral supplements. High iron or magnesium content also causes chelation with these drugs.

CT? What other foods are fortified with calcium, iron, or magnesium and might be a concern?

Sources: Adapted from: Cohen, Lautenbach, Weiner, Synnestvedt, & Gasink, 2008; Wallace & Amsden, 2002; Williams, 2008.

food increases the absorption of a drug by more than 25%, it is referred to as a **positive food effect**. If the result is decreased drug absorption by more than 20%, it is called a **negative food effect** (Marasanapalle, Crison, Ma, Li, & Jasti, 2009). A common example of this effect is the drugs

PRACTICE PEARL

Mixing Medications with an Enteral Nutrition Formula

Prevention of a drug–food interaction in the tube-fed client begins by avoiding contact between formula and medication in the tube or feeding setup. When drugs must be administered via the feeding tube, the nurse should:

- Flush the feeding tube with at least 30 mL of warm water before, between, and after administering drugs.
- Liquid medications are preferred with tube feeding administration. Consult with the pharmacist to determine whether crushing a medication is recommended. Sustained release, enteric coated, effervescent, and sublingual drugs should not be crushed. Some drugs are irritants or lose bioavailability when crushed.
- Longer length tubes or jejunal tubes can bypass the site of drug absorption. Check with the pharmacist about the absorption site of medications.
- Phenytoin, warfarin, fluoroquinolone, and tetracycline antibiotics and theophylline have clinically significant interactions with enteral nutrition formula. The nurse should work with the entire medical team to determine whether an alternative route of drug administration or alternative feeding schedule is needed to ensure therapeutic response to the medication and adequate nutrition are provided. Close monitoring of plasma drug levels is essential in this population.

CT? Why flush the tube between each individual drug?

Sources: Adapted from: British Association for Parenteral and Enteral Nutrition (BAPEN), 2006; Phillips & Nay, 2008; Williams, 2008.

BOX 24-1	Drug Interactions with Enteral Feedings

Direct contact between enteral nutrition formula and many drugs will result in a drug–food interaction that could alter the bioavailability of the medication or clog the feeding tube, or both. Although visual inspection of the mixture might reveal formation of a precipitate or creaming effect, some interactions leave no detectable evidence. Drug preparations containing alcohol or syrups with low pH are likely to precipitate when combined with an enteral formula, especially one with a high-protein content. Even when careful flushing protocol is followed for administering medications through a feeding tube, the presence of enteral formula in the stomach negatively affects the bioavailability of certain drugs, such as phenytoin, warfarin, and the fluoroquinolone and tetracycline antibiotics. Feedings must be held for up to 2 hours before and after administering these medications, resulting in diminished delivery of prescribed formula volume. Issues regarding drug administration in the tube-fed client include:

- Reduced drug bioavailability for some medications if in contact with formula in the stomach
- Need to withhold feedings to administer some drugs
- Precipitate formation and tube clogging from inadequate tube flushing or medication combined directly with a formula
- Tube placement site may bypass drug absorption site (longer tubes, J-tubes)
- Liquid versions of medications often are hyperosmotic or contain sorbitol, both of which contribute to diarrhea that is commonly blamed on the feeding

The nurse should follow protocol for drug administration as outlined in Practice Pearl: Mixing Medications with an Enteral Nutrition Formula. The pharmacist should be consulted for any special recommendations regarding drug administration in the tube-fed client, including the need to withhold feedings for any length of time, liquid alternatives to solid pills, and the effectiveness and safety of crushing medications when no liquid version is available.

Sources: Adapted from: Heineck, Bueno, & Heydrich, 2009; Phillips & Nay, 2008; Williams, 2008.

MyNursingKit Indiana University School of Medicine P450 Interactions

PRACTICE PEARL

Mixing Drugs and Parenteral Nutrition

Once parenteral solutions leave the pharmacy, no drugs should be directly admixed to the solution. Medications that are given intravenously to the client receiving parenteral nutrition should be delivered either using peripheral access or through a separate lumen of a multilumen catheter. Parenteral nutrition should be delivered through venous access dedicated for that purpose to minimize contamination risk.

alendronate and risedronate used to slow bone loss with osteoporosis. These medications must be taken on an empty stomach or absorption is greatly reduced (Tanno et al., 2008). Foods can increase the absorption of some medications as in the case of combining drugs that are lipophilic along with a fatty meal (Genser, 2008). The fat content of the meal and the presence of bile to digest the fat facilitate the absorption of the lipophilic drug. Food, especially fatty food, increases the absorption of the chemotherapeutic agent lapatinib compared with a fasted state. Because of this effect and the variability between absorption with an average meal, a fatty meal, and fasting, it is recommended that lapatinib dosing occur in the fasted state to maintain a consistent rate of absorption (Koch et al., 2009). For other medications, the increased absorption with food is desirable. In addition to the effects of fatty food on lipophilic drug absorption, slowed gastric emptying and changes in gastric pH contribute to the effect with other types of drugs (Genser, 2008; Lentz, 2008; Marasanapalle et al., 2009). The nurse should reinforce the reason and importance of following medication label advice regarding food practices and timing.

Drugs, such as alcohol, can directly decrease absorption of nutrients, such as folate and thiamine. Mineral oil, a laxative, has been reported to decrease absorption of fat-soluble vitamins, which can be problematic with chronic use (Gal-Ezer & Shaoul, 2006). Medications that diminish or buffer gastric acid, such as antacids and proton pump inhibitors, will reduce absorption of nutrients requiring an acid medium in the stomach. Calcium, iron, and vitamin B_{12} are examples. Box 24-2 outlines long-term concerns about these medications and nutrient status. Table 24-2 outlines further interactions between medications and nutrient absorption.

The small intestine is a site where drug–drug and food–drug interactions can be significant. The cytochrome P450 3A4 enzyme system in the intestinal wall (and in the liver) metabolizes many drugs, altering them for excretion. Over 50 enzymes are involved, but just 6 of them are responsible for metabolizing over 90% of medications. CYP3A4 and CYP2D6 are the most significant of the enzymes (Lynch & Price, 2007). This enzyme process is called first-pass metabolism or presystemic clearance and results in a reduction in the amount of drug actively available to the body. When more than one drug or a drug and food affect this enzyme system simultaneously, the result is altered drug absorption. Commonly prescribed drugs that use this enzyme system and, therefore, are prone to interactions include statins, antiseizure medications, warfarin, some antidepressants, protease inhibitors, calcium channel blockers, and amiodorone (Lynch & Price, 2007). Some dietary supplements and juices, especially St. John's Wort and grapefruit juice, are metabolized by this enzyme system as well. Some substances cause **inhibition** of the enzyme system and thus foster increased drug absorption because less of the drug is degraded before entering the circulation. An example of this interaction is grapefruit juice, which

BOX 24-2	Long-Term Nutritional Effects of Acid Buffering or Suppressing Drugs

Both older and newer therapies directed at alleviating the symptoms of gastritis and ulcers have been identified as contributing to poor bone health when used long term. Older forms of antacids, such as aluminum and magnesium hydroxides, bind phosphate in the gut. Lack of adequate phosphate absorption has been associated with the development of osteomalacia with case reports across the lifespan.

Newer proton pump inhibitors work to decrease production of hydrochloric acid in the stomach. The resulting hypochlorhydria alters the absorption of calcium. This effect is most pronounced with long-term use of these drugs and in the older adult. Long-term use of proton pump inhibitors at the upper dose limit is associated with an increased risk of hip fracture.

Calcium supplements in the citrate form rely less on an acid environment in the stomach than those that are in the carbonate form.

In addition to alterations in calcium absorption, long-term suppression of acid production can decrease the absorption of iron and food sources of vitamin B_{12}. Supplemental forms of vitamin B_{12} are not affected because no acid is required to cleave the vitamin molecule bound to protein as occurs in food sources. Fortified foods and multivitamins with B_{12} are examples.

The nurse should assess any client on a long-term acid-altering drug regimen for risk factors for poor bone health or anemia. The availability of these medications over the counter and the tendency to self-medicate could let this health risk go unnoticed.

Sources: Adapted from: McColl, 2009; Sivas, Gunesen, Ozoran, & Alemdaroglu, 2007; Targownik et al., 2008; Wright, Proctor, Insogna, & Kerstetter, 2008.

hot Topic

Juices and Cytochrome P-450 System Drug Interactions

The interaction between grapefruit juice and medications was a serendipitous discovery when grapefruit juice was used in a clinical study to mask the taste of a medication and ended up altering the response to the drug. It is now understood that grapefruit juice inhibits the cytochrome P450 3A4 enzyme system responsible for "first-pass metabolism" of many drugs. The inhibition of the enzyme allows more drug to be absorbed than normally would occur, elevating plasma drug levels. It is not entirely clear which component of grapefruit juice is responsible for the effect. Whole grapefruit and Seville oranges also affect the enzyme system. More recently, pomegranate juice and lime juice have been reported to exert similar effects.

The nurse should be aware of the following recommendations regarding this interaction:

- Many drug classes are affected, especially those with a narrow therapeutic range. These include statin drugs, certain antiarrythmics, immunosuppressives, calcium channel blockers and some protease inhibitors.
- Consumption of grapefruit and grapefruit juice should be avoided because the inhibitory effect can last up to 72 hours. Citrus sodas that contain grapefruit (Fresca, Sun Up, for example) do not seem to cause a clinically significant interaction.
- Magnitude of the interaction effect can differ among clients because of genetic variations in the P450 system.
- When continued consumption of grapefruit juice is definitive, alternative brands of a medication in the same drug class may be considered because not all versions are affected for most classes.
- Commonly cited drugs that interact with grapefruit juice include amiodorone, buspirone, carbamazepine, cisapride, cyclosporine, lovastatin, nifedipine, saquinavir, simvastatin, and tacrolimus, among others.

Sources: Adapted from: Genser, 2008; Kiani & Imam, 2007; Nowack, 2008; Ulbricht et al., 2008.

exerts its inhibitory effects on the enzyme system for up to 72 hours (Genser, 2008). **Induction** is the reverse of inhibition, and enzyme action is boosted, lessening absorption of active drug. Many drug–drug interactions are because of induction. Hot Topic: Juices and Cytochrome P-450 System Drug Interactions outlines juices associated with inhibition of the cytochrome P-450 3A4 system. The effect can be significant for clients who take medications using this enzyme system, especially drugs with a narrow therapeutic range. Genetic variants in the enzymes can predispose some individuals to greater drug sensitivities than is found in other people (Lynch & Price, 2007).

Alteration in Metabolism

Interactions that affect drug or nutrient metabolism occur after the digestive and absorptive processes are complete and the substances are in circulation, being transported or distrib-uted to target tissues. Both drug and nutrient levels can be adversely affected by this form of interaction.

Many drugs are bound to plasma proteins while in circulation. The anticoagulant warfarin is an example. Malnutrition that leads to low plasma protein levels reduces the availability of the proteins, specifically albumin, used for drug-binding transport. Drugs that are bound to protein are not active. Without adequate albumin, more free drug is in circulation. This effect increases the amount of active drug distributed and can lead to adverse drug effects and toxicity if left unchecked. The older adult is particularly vulnerable to this effect because of the use of many drugs, called **polypharmacy,** which increases the likelihood of drug interactions even when plasma proteins are within normal limits. Drug interactions that lead to delirium are reported in the older adult with low plasma proteins and polypharmacy (Culp & Cacchione, 2008). Checking plasma levels of drugs and modifying dosage for the malnourished client are methods used to prevent this occurrence.

The liver is the site of both drug and nutrient metabolism, leading to the potential for interactions when metabolic paths intersect. Interactions because of the cytochrome P 450 enzyme system discussed earlier occur in the liver as well as the intestine. Additionally, drugs may alter nutrient metabolism in the liver. Several anticonvulsants, including phenytoin, cause induction of hepatic enzymes that affect folic acid and vitamins D and K, leading to decreased levels of these vitamins. The effect on folic acid status is particularly important in the pregnant female on antiseizure medications because of the association between poor folic acid status and neural tube defects in the fetus. Antiepileptic drugs are already associated with the development of congenital abnormalities and the link may be influenced by folic acid (Kjaer et al., 2008). Folic acid supplementation is recommended. Likewise, these drugs increase the risk of poor bone mineral density, fracture, and osteoporosis because of the negative effects on vitamin D. Adequate intake of both calcium and vitamin D with regular monitoring of bone density is recommended for those taking antiseizure medications (Pack, 2008). Table 24-1 outlines other drugs associated with altered nutrient metabolism.

Another important interaction in this category occurs with the drug class of monoamine oxidase inhibitors (MAOIs) that are used to treat depression. By inhibiting the enzyme monoamine oxidase, the drug also blocks the normal metabolism of tyramine, a substance found naturally in aged or cured foods, such as cheese. When large amounts of tyramine accumulate in the blood, a hypertensive crisis can occur because of tyramine's vasoconstrictor effect. Client Education Checklist: Monoamine Oxidase Inhibitors (MAOI) and Tyramine outlines advice that the nurse should provide to the client prescribed an MAOI drug.

CLIENT EDUCATION CHECKLIST	Monoamine Oxidase Inhibitors (MAOI) and Tyramine
Intervention	**Example**
• Assess client knowledge about how MAOI drugs work and the effect on diet. • Educate on basics of diet–drug interaction.	• Monoamine oxidase is an enzyme present in the digestive tract that normally metabolizes dietary tyramine. • MAOIs block the action of the enzyme, resulting in increased absorption of tyramine into the bloodstream. • Excess tyramine acts as a "pressor" and drives up blood pressure. Symptoms include headache, visual disturbances, confusion, and hypertensive crisis.
Educate the client on a low-tyramine diet.	Tyramine is naturally occurring in some foods and a product of aging and processing in others. Tyramine is found in foods that are aged, fermented, spoiled, or cured. The following foods must be avoided immediately when the drug is begun and continuously until 3–4 weeks after drug discontinuation: • Aged cheeses • Air-dried sausage meats—pepperoni, salami, pastrami, summer sausage • Fermented soy products—soy sauce, teriyaki, soybean paste, tofu, miso, natto, tamari, shoyu, tempeh • Pickled foods in brine—sauerkraut, kim chee • All tap beers • Fava beans, banana peel, marmite yeast extract Encourage intake of foods that are bought and cooked fresh. Avoid prolonged storage of meats (keep less than 4 days) and cheese (keep less than 3 weeks).
Outline additional dietary recommendations with MAOI.	• Monitor intake of stimulants. Caffeine intake should be less than 500 mg/day to avoid intensification of any reaction. • All other alcohol consumption is at the discretion of the prescribing physician.

C_T? Which foods that are high in tyramine might be common food choices in a culturally diverse population?

Source: Adapted from National Institutes of Health (NIH), 2003a.

Alteration in Excretion

Metabolic by-products of medications and nutrients are generated by the liver and kidney before they are excreted. Interactions between drugs and nutrients in the kidney can cause increased excretion or, conversely, reabsorption of the substance. For example, alcohol fosters urinary losses of magnesium. Excess intake of sodium fosters urinary losses of the antipsychotic drug lithium, whereas a sodium restriction can foster increased drug reabsorption and toxicity (Thomsen & Shirley, 2006). Loop diuretics used to treat fluid overload or hypertension cause the beneficial loss of sodium in the urine, but also lead to losses of thiamin, potassium, and calcium. Thiamin losses are particularly significant in the client with congestive heart failure who may be on a loop diuretic, because the deficiency can impair cardiac function and its symptoms mimic those of heart failure (Wooley, 2008). The intake of these clients should be monitored to prevent thiamin deficiency from occurring. The Evidence-Based Practice Box: Do individuals with congestive heart failure (CHF) who are being treated with loop diuretics need thiamine (vitamin B_1) supplementation? discusses this issue in

further detail. Other examples of nutrients affected by medications are outlined in Table 24-1.

Pharmacodynamic Effects

Pharmacodynamic drug interactions occur when a second substance has either similar or counter effects to that of the medication. This effect is not a direct interaction with the drug itself, but rather one that can potentiate or offset the intended therapeutic action of the medication because of the substance's own independent physiological effect. Significant examples of this type of effect include:

- Antiplatelet or anticoagulant medications and dietary supplements with the same or opposite effect
- Immunosuppressant or immunostimulant drugs and dietary supplements with the same or opposite effect
- Sedatives, antidepressant, or antianxiety medications and dietary supplements with similar effects

Dietary supplements that should be avoided with sedative, antidepressant, or antianxiety medications include St. John's Wort and valerian. Echinacea should be avoided by those

EVIDENCE-BASED PRACTICE RESEARCH BOX

Do individuals with congestive heart failure (CHF) who are being treated with loop diuretics need thiamine (vitamin B₁) supplementation?

Clinical Problem: Individuals with congestive heart failure (CHF) typically are treated pharmacologically with long-term diuretic therapy. Loop diuretics are frequently the drug of choice. The increased urine output caused by the diuretics is associated with increased loss of water-soluble vitamins.

Research Findings: Thiamine (vitamin B₁) is a water-soluble vitamin found in pork, whole or enriched grains, enriched rice, and legumes. Thiamine deficiency is associated with beriberi, the wet form of which is manifested by a rapid heart rate, edema, and disrupted cardiac function that may weaken the heart muscle, all symptoms of CHF. Long-term diuretic therapy plays a major role in the medical management of CHF. Researchers are interested in the effect that loop diuretics have on thiamine balance in clients with CHF or if thiamine deficiency plays a role in the development of CHF (Suter & Vetter, 2000).

A study of the vitamin status was conducted on 149 elderly clients hospitalized for CHF. The researchers found that vitamin B₁ levels decreased during hospitalization and the only significant predictor was use of diuretics during the hospital stay (Suter & Vetter, 2000). Zenuk et al. (2003) assessed the thiamine status of inpatient and outpatient adults with CHF who were treated with at least 40 mg/day of furosemide in either single or divided doses. They found that

higher doses were associated with significantly higher levels of thiamine deficiency. Another study assessed the relationship between diuretic therapy and dietary intake of thiamine in a sample of 342 homebound elderly. Researchers found that diuretic users had thiamine intake that was less than the recommended daily allowance (RDA) and less than nondiuretic users (McCabe-Sellers, Sharkey, & Browne, 2005). An additional study determined the prevalence of thiamine deficiency in 100 subjects hospitalized with CHF and compared findings to 50 controls. The researchers found that subjects with CHF had greater urine thiamine loss and less supplementation than the control group; however, they did not find a significant relationship between diuretic use and thiamine deficiency (Hanninen, Darling, Sole, Barr, & Keith, 2006). Summarizing the research findings, Sica (2007) concluded that clients taking diuretics have increased loss of thiamine and are at increased risk of developing a deficiency.

Nursing Implications: Clients receiving long-term diuretic therapy for CHF should have a careful dietary history at each nursing contact and teaching about thiamine-rich foods. Supplementation that includes adequate water-soluble vitamins should be considered.

CRITICAL THINKING QUESTION:

1. A client with CHF is receiving long-term diuretic therapy, among other medications, and is on a low-fat, reduced calorie diet. What foods that are rich in thiamine could the nurse suggest?

---

taking any medications that affect the immune system, such as drugs used to prevent organ transplant rejection as discussed in Chapter 23. Many dietary supplements alter platelet or clotting function and could interfere with the intended effect of anticoagulant therapy. For example, warfarin and ginkgo biloba each alter blood clotting and when used together that effect is potentiated, leading to lengthened bleeding time. Other dietary supplements that have an effect on blood clotting are discussed in Practice Pearl: Preoperative Assessment and in Chapter 25. The interaction between warfarin and increased intake of vitamin K also alters warfarin pharmacodynamics because of the role that vitamin K plays in the synthesis of clotting factors; in this case the result is decreased warfarin action and diminished international normalized ratio (INR), a laboratory test for bleeding time. The effect of increased vitamin K intake can last for days, increasing the risk of forming a blood clot in these clients who are on anticoagulants because of the risk of blood clot formation (Kamali, 2009). Both types of interactions described can have serious consequences for the client prescribed anticoagulant therapy. Client Education

Checklist: Warfarin Interactions with Food, Nutrients, and Supplements outlines the important dietary advice that is compulsory for the client on warfarin. Surprisingly, more than one-third of clients taking warfarin report that they have not received education about an interaction between the medication and specific dietary supplements (Wittkowsky, 2008).

Drug Effects and Dietary Intake

In addition to the described effect that malnutrition has on drug metabolism, many medications have side effects that have a negative impact on nutrition status. Although not considered a true drug interaction, side effects such as nausea, vomiting, diarrhea, altered taste or appetite, and excessive sedation can ultimately jeopardize nutritional health. The nurse should consider drug side effects when assessing nutritional status, especially in the client already at risk for poor nutrition. The nurse should also assess the client for any self-prescribed remedies for the side effects because these, too, can alter drug or nutrient status. For example, some individuals use ginger to quell nausea or bicarbonate of soda (baking

MyNursingKit National Center for Complementary and Alternative Medicine

CLIENT EDUCATION CHECKLIST ✓	Warfarin Interactions with Food, Nutrients, and Supplements
Intervention	**Example**
• Assess knowledge about the interaction between dietary habits and warfarin. • Educate on the basic mechanism to the diet–drug interaction.	Anticoagulant is prescribed to ↓risk of developing a blood clot with certain medical conditions by interfering with vitamin K role in development of certain clotting factors in the liver. Result is prolonged INR.
Educate the client on basic diet recommendations.	Maintain steady and adequate intake of vitamin K to keep an even effect on anticoagulant efforts. Otherwise: • ↓Vitamin K ↑drug effect • ↑Vitamin K ↓drug effect Avoid dietary supplements, including herbs, with similar anticoagulant or antiplatelet effects because of bleeding risk when combined with warfarin.
List specific high vitamin K foods to keep constant and dietary supplements to avoid.	Significant sources of vitamin K include: green leafy vegetables (kale, spinach, turnip and collard greens, Swiss chard, raw parsley, broccoli, endive, romaine, Brussels sprouts). Monitor vitamin K in vitamins, meal replacement drinks, and enteral nutrition formula. Supplements with anticoagulant or antiplatelet effects are outlined in Practice Pearl: Preoperative Assessment.

Source: Adapted from: NIH, 2003b.

PRACTICE PEARL

Preoperative Assessment

A careful diet and drug history is always important. In the preoperative client, undetected interactions between drugs and dietary factors can lead to dangerous alterations in blood clotting or anaesthesia effects. Of particular concern are herbal sedatives or supplements that have either antiplatelet or anticoagulant effects. It is generally recommended that herbal supplements be discontinued up to 3 weeks preoperatively, depending on the product. The nurse should be mindful of the following supplements when assessing the preoperative client:

Supplements with antiplatelet or anticoagulant properties:

Arnica	Inositol
Bilberry	Licorice
Butcher's broom	Meadowsweet
Cat's claw	Motherswort
Danshen	Papaya
Dong quai	Pau d'arco
Feverfew	Red clover
Fish oil	Sweet clover
Flaxseed	Sweet woodruff
Forskolin	Turmeric
Garlic	Vitamin E
Ginger	Wheat grass
Ginkgo	Willow bark
Horse chestnut	

Supplements with sedative effects:

Kava	Valerian

Sources: Adapted from: Gardiner, Phillips,& Shaughnessy, 2008; Kumar, Allen, & Bell, 2005; Messina, 2006; Ulbricht et al, 2008.

soda) for upset stomach. Excessive ginger alters platelet aggregation and baking soda contains significant sodium, two undesired effects for a client with heart failure who is taking anticoagulant medication. Box 24-3 outlines examples of drugs with side effects that impact nutrition status.

Who Is at Risk for a Drug Interaction?

The prevention and management of drug interactions requires careful screening for risk factors that contribute to this prob-

BOX 24-3	Medication Side Effects and Nutrition

Medications can have a negative effect on nutrition status without directly causing any type of drug interaction with food or nutrients. Drug side effects can lead to diminished dietary intake for a number of reasons, including:

- Altered taste/smell—includes diminished taste and bad residual tastes
- Decreased production of saliva or dry mouth
- Anorexia
- Diarrhea or constipation
- Nausea or vomiting
- Gastrointestinal irritation, bloating, or cramping
- Inflamed oral mucosa (glossitis, cheilosis, stomatitis, mucositis)
- Sedation, drowsiness, confusion
- Tremors, shakiness, dizziness, agitation
- Increased blood glucose or lipids
- Increased appetite leading to overeating
- Diuresis that may prompt self-prescribed fluid restriction to avoid frequent urination

MyNursingKit Office of Dietary Supplements

Lifespan

Drug Interactions in the Older Adult

Older adults are at high risk of drug interactions with other drugs and with food or nutrients. The aging process leads to alterations in both pharmacokinetics and pharmacodynamics, causing changes in drug absorption, metabolism, and excretion. Diminished production of gastric acid, decreased intestinal blood flow, and alterations in body composition such as total body water and lean mass all affect drug pharmacokinetics (Genser, 2008). Medical conditions and polypharmacy increase the risk of an interaction with each additional medication taken. The use of over-the-counter medications and dietary supplements adds to the risk of polypharmacy. In a survey of nonvitamin/nonmineral dietary supplement use in adults over age 60 years, almost half of the supplements were found to interact with medications taken by this group (Wold et al., 2005). A careful diet and medication history by the nurse is essential is this population group.

lem. Polypharmacy is a well-accepted risk factor for drug interactions. The greater the number of prescription and over-the-counter medications used by the client, the greater the risk of interaction. Use of self-remedies and the existence of multiple prescribers can cause the potential for an interaction to go unnoticed. Lifespan Box: Drug Interactions in the Older Adult outlines this problem in the older adult. Individuals who have a chronic illness are at risk of drug interactions for multiple reasons, including the disease and its symptoms and any medical, self-prescribed, or dietary treatments. The use of dietary supplements, including tube feedings, herbs, and sports or weight loss products should alert the nurse to the potential for a drug interaction. It is essential that the nurse specifically inquire about dietary supplement use because client self-disclosure about supplement use is the exception rather than the rule (Kennedy, Wang, & Wu, 2008). Practice Pearl: Preoperative Assessment points out the importance of including this assessment when conducting a preoperative evaluation.

The nurse should consider the potential of an adverse drug reaction because of food allergies or insensitivities. Inactive ingredients used as fillers or stabilizers in a medication are referred to as **excipients** and may trigger a reaction that is mistakenly blamed on the active drug ingredient instead (Balbani, Stelzer, & Montovani, 2006). Lactose, gluten, and aspartame are examples of excipients that must be avoided by some individuals. Hot Topic: Drug Excipients and Nutrition Considerations outlines excipients for the nurse to consider when counseling the individual with food allergies or insensitivities. Routine assessment of individuals for nutrition, drug, and medical history is crucial to identify the client at risk for a drug interaction. Box 24-4 outlines risk factors for an interaction between a drug and food or nutrient.

hot Topic

Drug Excipients and Nutrition Considerations

Drug excipients are the inactive ingredients in a medication, whether it is over the counter or a prescription. Inactive ingredients are added for many reasons, including stability, taste, color, or as a preservative. Although these components are therapeutically inactive, they can cause allergic symptoms or intolerances that can be misinterpreted as a drug reaction. The nurse should be aware of the following excipients that can be troublesome to sensitive clients:

Sweeteners
Liquid and chewable medications often have sweeteners added to improve taste. Some manufacturers use sucrose, but sugar-free alternatives are plentiful and can present a problem.
- Sorbitol—a sugar alcohol that exerts a laxative effect.
- Aspartame—a sugar substitute with phenylalanine as part of the ingredients. Clients with the inborn error of metabolism phenylketonuria must limit intake of phenylalanine. Medications containing aspartame are mandated to list phenylalanine content in milligrams/dose.

Dyes
Colorants are added to medications to give them a uniform and identifiable appearance. Some individuals are sensitive to dyes, exhibiting dermatological and gastrointestinal reactions.
- Tartrazine (FD&C yellow #5)—a hypersensitivity to this colorant exists in a small amount of the population, especially clients with salicylate allergy or intolerance because of similar chemical structures. Sensitive individuals develop itching and hives in response to consumption of this dye. Over-the-counter and prescription medications must specify if this dye is used in a product. Most other dyes are designated simply as *artificial color* without specifics.

Preservatives
Preservatives serve an important function in medications, prolonging shelf-life and preventing pathogen growth. The nurse should be alert to any client sensitivity to sulfur salts.
- Sulfites—used as an antioxidant in some drugs and foods. Sensitive individuals tend to be asthmatic. Sensitivity reaction symptoms include wheezing and shortness of breath. The presence of sulfite content must be noted on the label.

Gluten
Gluten is a protein present in wheat, rye, and barley. It can be present in a medication as a filler, presenting a problem for the individual with celiac disease, who must adhere to a lifelong gluten-free diet. This diet is outlined in Chapter 20. Over-the-counter medications can be checked for gluten, looking for words such as wheat extract, starch, or filler. Include dietary supplements such as multivitamins when checking labels because many contain gluten. Consult with a pharmacist about gluten content of prescription medications because this information is not contained on the label.

Lactose
Lactose is used as a filler in capsules and to give substance to pills. It is also found in some dry powder inhalers. Individuals with lactose intolerance will vary in sensitivity to the lactose content of medications, and some must avoid it as an excipient. Individuals with milk allergy may need to avoid this excipient because the amount of protein occurring with it varies and can present a problem to some.

(continued)

Sodium, potassium, calcium, magnesium

A high-mineral content in a medication can be of concern to individuals with some medical conditions (such as sodium and hypertension or potassium and kidney failure). If mineral content exceeds a certain threshold per single dose or maximum daily dose, the amount must be specified on the label of over-the-counter medications.

Label threshold	Single dose (mg)	Maximum dose (mg)
Sodium content	5	140
Calcium content	20	3,200
Potassium content	5	975
Magnesium content	8	600

Over-the-counter medications are mandated to list inactive ingredients on the label for the consumer to review. Prescription medications are exempt from this law with the exception of a requirement to highlight aspartame, sulfites, and tartrazine.

Sources: Adapted from: Food & Drug Administration (FDA), 2004; Plogsted, 2007; Rogkakou, Guerra, Scordamaglia, Canonica, & Passalacqua, 2007; Zarbock, Magnuson, Hoskins, Record, & Smith, 2007.

BOX 24-4	**Risk Factors for Drug Interactions**

- Drugs with narrow therapeutic range
- Underlying medical disease or conditions involving the liver or kidney, which are important sites of drug metabolism
- Conditions associated with use of antiepileptic drugs, chemotherapy, immunosuppressives, or warfarin
- Food allergy, intolerance, or sensitivity
- Excipient content of medication contains allergen or ingredient associated with intolerance
- Malnutrition
- Polypharmacy, including over-the-counter medications
- Pregnant female, child, older adult
- Use of enteral nutrition formula
- Use of herbal medications and other dietary supplements

Medication Classes and Food/Nutrient Interactions

Various classes of drug are more commonly associated with food or nutrient interactions. Some interactions, although theoretically interesting, do not reach clinical significance; others are deserving of careful individual consideration with each client. Table 24-2 outlines by medication class common drug interactions with food or nutrients. Herbal and dietary supplements are considered here and reviewed more fully in Chapter 25.

NURSING CARE PLAN ## Nutrition and Diuretic Use

CASE STUDY

Terence is 62 years old and has hypertension for which he takes a thiazide diuretic twice a day. It was prescribed 6 months ago and he says he has not felt right since that time. He was started on the medication when his blood pressure was consistently higher than 170/94 over several readings during the previous year. He had been reluctant to start taking a medication because he prided himself on his robust health and good physical condition. He had also been worried because he had heard that there were lots of side effects. Now he felt as if his fears were confirmed because he had lost some weight, which he did not feel he needed to lose, and found it hard to drink adequate fluids because he had to go to the bathroom so much. He says that it feels like his heart beats slowly, he feels jittery, thirsty, and weak. He knows he should have returned to the clinic sooner but says it is hard to get away from work and his blood pressure is monitored there. He also knows he got some information about diet when his

medication was first prescribed but cannot recall what it was. He only remembers getting a suggestion to eat lots of bananas, which he dislikes.

Applying the Nursing Process

ASSESSMENT

Height: 5 feet 9 inches Weight: 164 pounds BMI: 24.2
Weight 6 months ago: 169 pounds
BP 148/72 P 62, regular R 14
Skin warm and dry, no edema, dry lips and tongue
Serum potassium 3.5 mEq/L

DIAGNOSES

Fluid volume deficit, risk for related to regular use of diuretic
Knowledge deficit related to the need for dietary sources of potassium

Nutrition and Diuretic Use *(continued)*

NURSING CARE PLAN

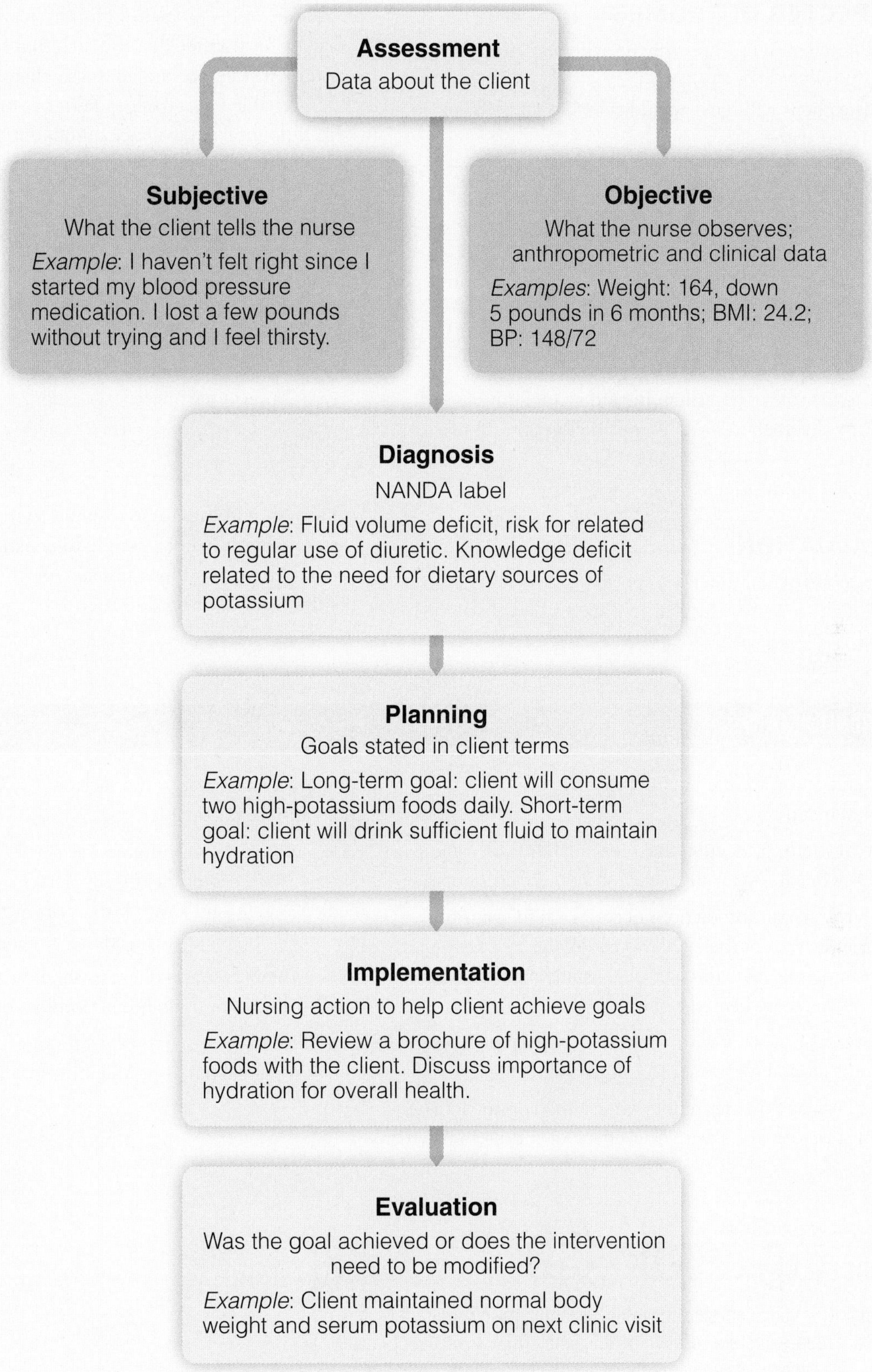

Assessment
Data about the client

Subjective
What the client tells the nurse

Example: I haven't felt right since I started my blood pressure medication. I lost a few pounds without trying and I feel thirsty.

Objective
What the nurse observes; anthropometric and clinical data

Examples: Weight: 164, down 5 pounds in 6 months; BMI: 24.2; BP: 148/72

Diagnosis
NANDA label

Example: Fluid volume deficit, risk for related to regular use of diuretic. Knowledge deficit related to the need for dietary sources of potassium

Planning
Goals stated in client terms

Example: Long-term goal: client will consume two high-potassium foods daily. Short-term goal: client will drink sufficient fluid to maintain hydration

Implementation
Nursing action to help client achieve goals

Example: Review a brochure of high-potassium foods with the client. Discuss importance of hydration for overall health.

Evaluation
Was the goal achieved or does the intervention need to be modified?

Example: Client maintained normal body weight and serum potassium on next clinic visit

■ FIGURE 24-1 **Nursing Care Plan Process: Nutrition and Diuretic Use.**

Nutrition and Diuretic Use *(continued)*

NURSING CARE PLAN

EXPECTED OUTCOMES

The client's lips and tongue will remain moist and pink

The client will have no additional weight loss by (insert date)

The client will state five foods rich in potassium and water-soluble vitamins by (date)

INTERVENTIONS

Provide the client with a 1-week food diary and instruct in its use

Review medication side effects and reinforce reasons for taking medication

Discuss role of potassium in cardiac functioning

Provide brochures about foods rich in potassium

Teach, via demonstration and return demonstration, self-monitoring of blood pressure

EVALUATION

One month later, Terence reported feeling much better and admitted that his earlier inattention had likely caused some of his problems. His physician had adjusted the dose of his thiazide diuretic such that he was taking a larger dose in the morning and a smaller one late in the day. This enabled him to sleep better at night and to adjust his fluid intake to balance output during the day. His mouth did not feel quite as dry and he would suck on lemon drops if it felt dry and he was not thirsty. He was eating more fruit every day. He was relieved that many foods, beside bananas, were rich in potassium. He had gained 2 pounds and felt more secure knowing that he was eating foods that decreased some of the side effects of the diuretic. Figure 24-1 ■ outlines the nursing process for this case.

Critical Thinking in the Nursing Process

1. **How should the nurse respond to the client who states that it is not possible to consume enough potassium from foods to make up the loss that results from taking a diuretic.**

CHAPTER SUMMARY

- Drug interactions can result in alterations in drug effect or nutritional health.

- Food or nutrients can alter the bioavailability of some drugs. Likewise, drugs can alter the absorption of nutrients.

- Some drug–nutrient interactions occur as a result of inhibition or induction of the cytochrome P450 3A4 enzyme system. Grapefruit juice interacts with many medications because of this shared enzyme effect.

- Other interactions occur with altered metabolism of drugs or nutrients after absorption into the bloodstream.

- Altered pharmacokinetics results when a food or nutrient potentiates or competes with the effect of a drug. The competition between the actions of vitamin K and coumadin is an example.

- Risk factors for drug interactions include polypharmacy, malnutrition, use of dietary supplements, and underlying medical conditions. Drugs with a narrow therapeutic range are susceptible to a clinical effect with an interaction.

- Food intolerances and allergies should not be overlooked as contributors to drug interactions or adverse reactions.

- The nurse plays an important role in the assessment and education of clients regarding drug interactions with food or nutrients.

EXPLORE PEARSON **mynursingkit**™

MyNursingKit is your one stop for online chapter review materials and resources. Prepare for success with additional NCLEX®-style practice questions, interactive assignments and activities, web links, animations and videos, and more!

Register your access code from the front of your book at
www.mynursingkit.com.

NCLEX® QUESTIONS

1. A client is taking an MAOI for depression. The nurse knows that teaching about the nutritional interactions has been effective when the client states that which of the following foods should not be eaten?
   1. Pepperoni pizza
   2. Fruit salad
   3. Salsa
   4. Tuna casserole

2. A client is taking warfarin for a coagulation disorder. The nurse knows that teaching about nutritional interactions has been effective when the client states that which of the following foods should be monitored?
   1. Citrus fruits
   2. Pork products
   3. Oatmeal
   4. Spinach salad

3. A client wants to know why tetracycline cannot be taken with milk. The nurse responds that:
   1. "The calcium in milk prevents the absorption of the tetracycline."
   2. "Milk increases the rate of absorption of the tetracycline."
   3. "Tetracycline inhibits the absorption of calcium in milk."
   4. "Milk and tetracycline interact and frequently cause GERD."

REFERENCES

Balbani, A. P. S., Stelzer, L. B., & Montovani, J. C. (2006). Pharmaceutical excipients and the information on drug labels. *Brazilian Journal of Otorhinolaryngology, 72,* 400–406.

British Association for Parenteral and Enteral Nutrition (BAPEN). (2006). *Drug administration via enteral feeding tubes: A guide for general practitioners and community pharmacists.* Retrieved April 25, 2009, from http://www.bapen.org.uk/res_drugs.html

Cohen, K. A., Lautenbach, E., Weiner, M. G., Synnestvedt, M., & Gasink, L. B. (2008). Coadministration of oral levofloxacin with agents that impair absorption: Impact on antibiotic resistance. *Infection Control and Hospital Epidemiology, 29,* 975–977.

Culp, K. R., & Cacchione, P. Z. (2008). Nutrition status and delirium in long-term care elderly individuals. *Applied Nursing Research, 21,* 66–74.

Food and Drug Administration (FDA). (2004). *FDA enhances safeguards for consumers who may have special sensitivities to certain commonly used over-the-counter drug ingredients.* FDA News, PO4-35. Retrieved April 25, 2009, from: http://www.fda.gov/NewsEvents/Newsroom/PressAnnouncements/2004/ucm108269.htm

Gal-Ezer, S., & Shaoul, R. (2006). The safety of mineral oil in the treatment of constipation—a lesson from prolonged use. *Clinical Pediatrics, 45,* 856–858.

Gardiner, P., Phillips, R., & Shaughnessy, A. F. (2008). Herbal and dietary supplement-drug interactions in patients with chronic illnesses. *American Family Physician, 77,* 73–78.

Genser, D. (2008). Food and drug interaction: Consequences for the nutrition/health status. *Annals of Nutrition & Metabolism, 52,* S29–S32.

Hanninen, S. A., Darling, P. B., Sole, M. J., Barr, A., & Keith, M. E. (2006). The prevalence of thiamin deficiency in hospitalized patients with congestive heart failure. *Journal of the American College of Cardiology, 47*(2), 354–361.

Heineck, I., Bueno, D., & Heydrich, J. (2009). Study of the use of drugs in patients with enteral feeding tubes. *Pharmacy World & Science, 31,* 145–148.

Kamali, F. (2009). Novel oral anticoagulants and diet: The potential for infection. *American Journal of Hematology, 84,* 260–261.

Kennedy, J., Wang, C. C., & Wu, C. H. (2008). Patient disclosure about herb and supplement use among adults in the U.S. *Evidence Based Complementary and Alternative Medicine, 5,* 451–456.

Kiani, J., & Imam, S. Z. (2007). Medicinal importance of grapefruit juice and its interaction with various drugs. *Nutrition Journal, 6,* 33.

Kjaer, D., Horvath-Puho, E., Christensen, J., Vestergaard, M., Czeizel, A. E., Sorensen, H. T., et al. (2008). Antiepileptic drug use, folic acid supplementation, and congenital abnormalities: A population-based case-control study. *BJOG, 115,* 98–103.

Koch, K. M., Reddy, N. J., Cohen, R. B., Lewis, N. L., Whitehead, B., Mackay, K., et al. (2009). Effects of food on the relative bioavailability of lapatinib in cancer patients. *Journal of Clinical Oncology, 27,* 1191–1196.

Kumar, N. B., Allen, K., & Bell, H. (2005). Perioperative herbal supplement use in cancer patients: Potential implications and recommendations for presurgical screening. *Cancer Control, 12,* 149–157.

Lentz, K. A. (2008). Current methods for predicting human food effect. *American*

Association of Pharmaceutical Scientists Journal, 10, 282–288.

Lynch, T., & Price, A. (2007). The effect of cytochrome P450 metabolism on drug response, interactions, and adverse effect. *American Family Physician, 76,* 391–396.

Marasanapalle, V. P., Crison, J. R., Ma, J., Li, X., & Jasti, B. R. (2009). Investigation of some factors contributing to negative food effect. *Biopharmaceutics & Drug Disposition, 30,* 71–80.

McCabe-Sellers, B. J., Sharkey, J. R., & Browne, B. A. (2005). Diuretic medication therapy use and low thiamin intake in homebound older adults. *Journal of Nutrition for the Elderly, 24*(4), 57–71.

McColl, K. E. (2009). Effect of proton pump inhibitors on vitamins and iron. *American Journal of Gastroenterology, 104,* S5–S9.

Messina, B. A. (2006). Herbal supplements: Fact and myths—talking to your patients about herbal supplements. *Journal of PeriAnesthesia Nursing, 21,* 268–278.

National Institutes of Health (NIH). (2003a). *Important information to know when you are taking any of the following drugs: Monoamine oxidase inhibitor (MAOI) medications.* Retrieved April 25, 2009, from http://www.cc.nih.gov/ccc/patient_education/drug_nutrient/maoi1.pdf

National Institutes of Health (NIH). (2003b). *Important information to know when you are taking: Coumadin and vitamin K.* Retrieved April 25, 2009, from http://www.ods.od.nih.gov/factsheets/cc/coumadin1.pdf

Nowack, R. (2008). Cytochrome P450 enzyme and transport protein mediated herb-drug interactions in renal transplant patients: Grapefruit juice, St. John's Wort and beyond! *Nephrology, 13,* 337–347.

Pack, A. (2008). Bone health in people with epilepsy: Is it impaired and what are the risk factors? *Seizure, 17,* 181–186.

Phillips, N. M., & Nay, R. (2008). A systematic review of nursing administration of medications via enteral tubes in adults. *Journal of Clinical Nursing, 17,* 2257–2265.

Plogsted, S. (2007). Medication and celiac disease—tips from a pharmacist. *Practical Gastroenterologist,* 58–64.

Rogkakou, A., Guerra, L., Scordamaglia, A., Canonica, G. W., & Passalacqua, G. (2007). Severe skin reaction due to excipients of an oral iron treatment. *Allergy, 62,* 334–335.

Sica, D. A. (2007). Loop diuretic therapy, thiamine balance, and heart failure. *Congestive Heart Failure, 13*(4), 244–247.

Sivas, F., Gunesen, O., Ozoran, K., & Alemdaroglu, E. (2007). Osteomalacia from Mg-containing antacid: A case report of bilateral hip fracture. *Rheumatology International, 27,* 679–681.

Suter, P. M., & Vetter, W. (2000). Diuretics and vitamin B_1: Are diuretics a risk factor for thiamin malnutrition? *Nutrition Reviews, 58*(10), 319–323.

Tanno, F. K., Sakum, S., Masaoka, Y., Kataoka, M., Kozaki, T., Kamaguchi, R., et al. (2008).

Site-specific drug delivery to the middle-to-lower region of the small intestine reduces food-drug interactions that are responsible for low drug absorption in the fed state. *Journal of Pharmaceutical Sciences, 97,* 5341–5353.

Targownik, L. E., Lix, L. M., Metge, C. J., Prior, H. J., Leung, S., & Leslie, W. D. (2008). Use of proton pump inhibitors and risk of osteoporosis-related fractures. *Canadian Medical Association Journal, 179,* 319–326.

Thomsen, K., & Shirley, D. G. (2006). A hypothesis linking sodium and lithium reabsorption in the distal nephron. *Nephrology, Dialysis, Transplantation, 21,* 869–880.

Ulbricht, C., Chao, W., Costa, D., Rusie-Seamon, E., Weissner, W., & Woods, J. (2008). Clinical evidence of herb-drug interactions: A systematic review by the natural standard research collaboration. *Current Drug Metabolism, 9,* 1063–1120.

Wallace, A. W., & Amsden, G. W. (2002). Is it really ok to take this with food? Old interactions with a new twist. *Journal of Clinical Pharmacology, 42,* 437–443.

Williams, N. T. (2008). Medication administration through enteral feeding tubes. *American Journal of Health-System Pharmacy, 65,* 2347–2357.

Wittkowsky, A. K. (2008). Dietary supplements, herbs and oral anticoagulants: The nature of the evidence. *Journal of Thrombosis and Thrombolysis, 25,* 72–77.

Wold, R. S., Lopez, S. T., Yau, L., Butler, L. M., Pareo-Tubbeh, S. L., Waters, D. L., et al. (2005). Increasing trends in elderly persons' use of nonvitamin, nonmineral dietary supplements and concurrent use of medications. *Journal of the American Dietetic Association, 105,* 54–63.

Wooley, J. A. (2008). Characteristics of thiamin and its relevance to the management of heart failure. *Nutrition in Clinical Practice, 23,* 487–493.

Wright, M. J., Proctor, D. D., Insogna, K. L., & Kerstetter, J. E. (2008). Proton pump-inhibiting drugs, calcium, homeostasis, and bone health. *Nutrition Reviews, 66,* 103–108.

Zarbock, S. D., Magnuson, B., Hoskins, L., Record, K. E., & Smith, K. M. (2007). Lactose: The hidden culprit. *Orthopedics, 30,* 615–617.

Zenuk, C., Healey, J., Donnelly, J., Vaillancourt, R., Almalki, Y., & Smith, S. (2003). Thiamine deficiency in congestive heart failure patients receiving long term furosemide therapy. *Canadian Journal of Clinical Pharmacology, 10,* 184–188.

Dietary Supplements in Complementary Care 25

WHAT WILL YOU LEARN?

1. To translate the definition of dietary supplements and illustrate the varied types of these products.
2. To examine the limits of the federal regulations that govern the manufacturing and sale of dietary supplements.
3. To develop appropriate questions to determine dietary supplement use when conducting a nursing assessment.
4. To summarize lifespan specific recommendations regarding dietary supplement use.
5. To assess the effect that limited clinical data on dietary supplements has on the ability to make evidence-based recommendations regarding use.
6. To educate clients about side effects and precautions associated with dietary supplements.

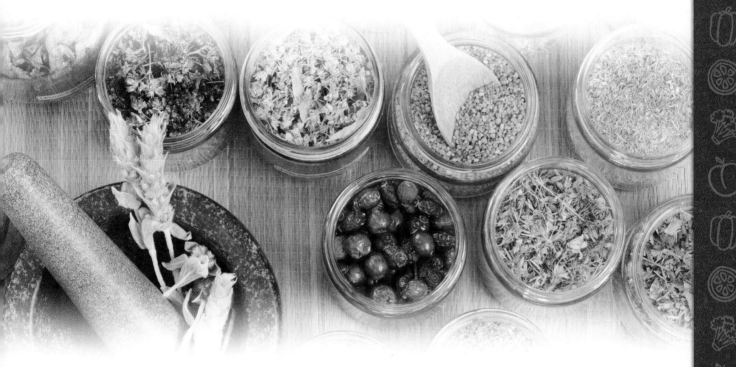

DID YOU KNOW?

▶ Dietary supplements are not evaluated by the Food and Drug Administration (FDA) before being offered for sale to the public.

▶ Case reports exist of dietary supplements that contain substances not listed on the label. Heavy metals, prescription drugs, alternate supplements, and varied botanicals have all been found as contaminants or adulterants.

▶ Bitter orange, or synephrine, is a common ingredient in diet pills and fat-cutting supplements, replacing the banned supplement ephedra. Like ephedra, it is a central nervous system stimulant.

▶ Cranberry juice or extract may help to lower the risk of urinary tract infections in females at risk for these infections.

▶ St. John's Wort, an herb used by some for mild depression, interferes with the effectiveness of oral contraceptives.

KEY TERMS

Nutrition and Complementary Care

Nutrition aspects of complementary care have existed for thousands of years as part of traditional medicine practiced around the world with the use of plant-based treatments. Approximately 25% of modern medicines originated from plants first used in traditional medicine (World Health Organization [WHO], 2008). Although herbal products may come to mind when considering nutritional aspects of complementary care, use of any dietary supplement falls under the umbrella of complementary care. The teen taking amino acid pills in an attempt to build muscle, the overweight adult hoping to lose weight by taking bitter orange "natural" diet pills, and the pregnant female drinking ginger tea for morning sickness are all practicing complementary care. The dietary supplement industry is an ever growing business with over 29,000 products on the market, over 1,000 new products added each year, and yearly sales in excess of $24 billion in the United States (Nutrition Business Journal, 2007; Thurston, 2008). These products include vitamins, minerals, sports nutrition products, weight loss pills and potions, and botanical products, including herbs.

What Is a Dietary Supplement?

The definition of a dietary supplement was formed in 1994 with Congressional passage of the Dietary Supplement Health and Education Act (DSHEA) as outlined in Box 25-1. Examples of products that fall within this definition cover a wide range from cranberry extract pills, whey protein powder, and glucosamine tablets to all herbal supplements and the common multivitamin. Conditions that are among the top reason for using dietary supplements include menopause, insomnia, depression, digestive ailments, and joint pain (Gardiner, Phillips, & Shaughnessy, 2008; Thurston, 2008). The most frequently used supplements by adults in the United States and Canada include multivitamins and minerals, echinacea, fish oils and other omega-3 fats, ginseng, ginkgo, garlic, and glucosamine (NCCAM, 2008a; Singh & Levine, 2006; Wold et al., 2005).

BOX 25-1	Dietary Supplement Definition

What is a dietary supplement?

Congress defined the term "dietary supplement" in the Dietary Supplement Health and Education Act (DSHEA) of 1994. A dietary supplement is a product taken by mouth that contains a "dietary ingredient" intended to supplement the diet. The "dietary ingredients" in these products may include:

- a vitamin,
- a mineral,
- an herb or other botanical,
- an amino acid,
- a dietary substance for use by man to supplement the diet by increasing the total dietary intake (e.g., enzymes or tissues from organs or glands), or
- a concentrate, metabolite, constituent or extract.

   Dietary supplements can also be extracts or concentrates and may be found in many forms such as tablets, capsules, soft gels, gel caps, liquids, or powders. They can also be in other forms, such as a bar, but if they are, information on their label must not represent the product as a conventional food or a sole item of a meal or diet. Whatever their form may be, DSHEA places dietary supplements in a special category under the general umbrella of "foods," not drugs, and requires that every supplement be labeled a dietary supplement.

Source: Food and Drug Administration, 2001.

Botanical supplements are included in the definition of a dietary supplement. **Botanicals** are plants and plant parts, which include herbs. They can be found in many forms, including fresh and dried plants, liquids, and solids. Whole plants, roots, leaves, stems, and flowers can be marketed separately, which makes it difficult to compare between various versions of a plant. The nurse should be aware of the various forms of botanicals that are available and be mindful to determine the part of the plant, the type of preparation, and the amount a client is using. Common preparations include the following (National Institutes of Health [NIH], Office of Dietary Supplements, 2006):

- **Extract.** A liquid extract is made by soaking the plant in liquid that will remove specific components. A dry extract is made by letting a liquid extract evaporate, leaving only dry components that can be made into capsules or tablets.
- Tea or **infusion.** Boiling water is added to fresh or dried botanicals and steeped before drinking hot or cold.
- **Decoction.** Similar to a tea but made by using plant roots, bark, and berries that require longer steeping time in boiling water before they can be consumed.
- **Tincture.** A liquid that is made by soaking the plant in alcohol or water and can be prepared at varying concentrations.

Supplement Facts

Serving Size 1 capsule

Amount Per Capsule	% Daily Value*
Calories 20	
Calories from Fat 20	
Total Fat 2g	3%*
Saturated Fat 0.5g	3%*
Polyunsaturated Fat 1g	†
Monounsaturated Fat 0.5g	†
Vitamin A 4250 IU	85%
Vitamin D 425 IU	106%
Omega-3 fatty acids 0.5g	†

* Percent Daily Values are based on a 2,000 calorie diet.
† Daily Value not established.

Ingredients: Cod liver oil, gelatin, water, and glycerin.

Source: Food and Drug Administration (2005). A dietary supplement labeling guide.

■ FIGURE 25-1 **Supplement Facts Label.**

How Are Supplements Regulated?

Dietary supplements are regulated by the FDA in the United States in accordance with the DSHEA. It is essential that the nurse realize that this law regulates all dietary supplements as food and not as medication. Thus, the rigorous premarket testing to prove safety and efficacy of drugs is not required with dietary supplements. The FDA does not require manufacturers to meet a particular standard of clinical research evidence about supplements, nor is there a requirement to submit any evidence to the government before or while the product is on the market. Should safety concerns arise once a product is on the market, the onus is on the FDA to prove that the supplement caused harm. Criticism exists in the health care industry that a double standard exists for dietary supplements versus medications and that the DSHEA should be revised to better protect consumers from adverse events associated with these drug-like products before they are allowed on the market (DeAngelis & Fontanarosa, 2003).

Labeling and Advertising Requirements

Dietary supplement labels are similar in layout to the nutrition facts found on food labels but have unique requirements. Manufacturers must feature a standardized label as pictured in Figure 25-1 ■. Ingredients are listed and content compared with recommended dietary intake guidelines, if such guidelines exist for the nutrient. Vitamins, minerals, and macronutrients are listed with a comparison to these recommendations. Like medications, a recommended dose for nonnutrient ingredients is listed, but unlike drugs no standard dosage guidelines exist for dietary supplements. The nurse should be aware that dose recommendations vary widely on labels of similar products (Krochmal et al., 2004). Additionally, doses vary between botanical varieties, forms, and preparations. For example, a tea or tablets made from *Echinacea purpurea*, an herb, cannot be compared with *Echinacea augustifolia*, a different variety of the plant species. This variance can make it difficult to assess supplement use and may contribute to a casual attitude toward dose compliance by the consumer. A certain dosage should never be assumed when conducting an assessment. When educating clients about supplement labeling, the nurse should warn that the terms *standardized* and *certified* are used by many supplement manufacturers but have no legal definition in this industry and thus are meaningless. Also, unlike medications there are no required warnings about side effects or interactions with other substances, which may lead some individuals to believe that there are no concerns with supplement use. The FDA does require labels to have a disclaimer that states that product claims have not been evaluated by the agency.

Labeling Claims

Dietary supplement labels cannot make any claims about ability to treat or cure a disease because such claims would qualify the product as a medication. However, supplements are permitted to make three types of claims: health, nutrient, and structure/function. Health claims must be limited to those permitted by the FDA, as outlined in Box 25-2.

BOX 25-2	Permitted Labeling Claims

Labeling claims on dietary supplements are permitted in three categories: structure/function, nutrient content, and health. The FDA requires that claims be truthful and not misleading. The FDA is responsible for regulating package label claims; the FTC regulates claims made in advertising. Premarket review of label claims is *not* done by the government.

Structure/Function Claims

- Link an ingredient in a supplement to the maintenance of general health or the normal function or structure of a body system or part.
- Claims cannot implicitly or explicitly claim to cure, treat, or prevent a disease or condition.
- Words such as *restore, regulate*, and *support* are allowed (for example, *supports* immune health is a permissible claim; *prevents* colds is not allowed and constitutes a claim that is allowed for a medication, not a dietary supplement).
- Structure/function claims are not subject to FDA review and must have a label disclaimer to this effect.

Nutrient Content Claims

- Characterizes the amount of nutrient in the supplement with a percentage or defined words
- Nutrients with established daily value (DV) recommendations can be touted on the label with:
  High in or *excellent source* when 20% or more of the DV of the nutrient is in a dose
  Good source when 10–19% of the DV of the nutrient is in a dose
  High potency when 100% of the DV is in a single nutrient supplement or when 100% of two-thirds of

the nutrients' DV are present in a multivitamin/mineral supplement
- Nutrients without established DVs can have nutrient claims that characterize the percentage of the touted nutrient in the supplement (e.g., contains 40% omega-3 fats)

Health Claims

- Establish a relationship between a disease or condition and the supplement ingredient within parameters permitted by the FDA after careful review of the scientific evidence. For example, claims are allowed that link the decreased risk of neural tube development with adequate folic acid intake. Other health claims allowed are associations between soy protein and coronary heart disease and calcium and osteoporosis. Most dietary supplements do not qualify to make a health claim, yet some make them anyway, chancing FDA monitoring.
- **Qualified Health Claims** are a subset of label claims allowed by the FDA when emerging evidence exists that links an ingredient with health, but the strength of the evidence is limited. Manufacturers petition the FDA to gain approval for this type of claim and are not always successful. Labels must contain qualifying language explaining the limited evidence. Allowed qualified health claims include the association between
  Calcium and colon cancer
  Omega-3 fats and coronary heart disease
  Selenium and cancer
  Vitamins C and E and cancer

Source: FDA, 2003.

Nutrient claims are used to describe the relative amount of nutrient in the product. Structure/function claims allow the product to report helping or strengthening any given structure or function in the body. For example, although a supplement cannot claim to cure osteoporosis, it can claim to "help bone health." Other popular structure/function claims include improving mood, immune status, metabolism, digestion, and sexual health. The FDA is responsible for acting on reports of a product that crosses the line from making structure/function to disease-treating or curing claims on the label. The Federal Trade Commission (FTC) polices the advertising and Internet claims made about products and will issue written warning when it is discovered that improper claims are made. A survey of supplements marketed on the Internet found approximately 55% of the products that made a health claim improperly touted the ability to diagnose, treat, or cure disease and less than half contained the required FDA disclaimer (Morris & Avorn, 2003).

Supplement Safety

The nurse should advise the client who uses dietary supplements that just because a product may be marketed as *natural*,

this term is not synonymous with *safe* or *without harmful effects*. Box 25-3 outlines the varied unsafe side effects of some dietary supplements. Many dietary supplements, and especially herbs, can act in ways that mimic drugs, reinforcing the need to fully assess supplement use by clients. Even dietary supplements that have sound clinical research to support their use can exhibit side effects in some individuals, such as with the negative effects of the herb St. John's Wort on the drug action of oral contraceptives, protease inhibitors used to treat human immunodefi-

BOX 25-3	Potential Safety Concerns with Dietary Supplements

Allergic reaction
Altered blood coagulation or platelet function
Altered effects of anaethesia or analgesia
Enhanced or lessened drug pharmacokinetics/pharmacodynamics
Exposure to contaminants or adulterants (e.g., heavy metals, microorganisms, medications)
Organ or system toxicity (cardiac, liver, neurological, renal)

ciency virus (HIV), and cyclosporines used to prevent organ transplant rejection (Gardiner, Phillips & Shaughnessy, 2008). St. John's Wort has the most known drug interactions of all dietary supplements because it uses a similar drug metabolism pathway common to many medications (Gardiner, Phillips, & Shaughnessy, 2008). Many dietary supplements have the po-

tential to alter platelet aggregation or blood coagulation, a significant concern for those with bleeding disorders, taking anticoagulant medications, undergoing surgery, or combining multiple supplements with the same effect. Supplements with this side effect are noted in Table 25-1. Interaction between sedatives or antidepressants and herbs are another common

Table 25-1 Popular Dietary Supplements**

Supplement	Other Name	Claim	Available Evidence	Reported Side Effects/Warnings
Aloe vera	Burn plant	Wound healer Laxative	Topical use may help heal minor burns/abrasions. Contains strong laxative components.	Do not use on deep wounds. Diarrhea with potassium losses.
ALA	Alpha lipoic acid	↓ Diabetic neuropathy symptoms	Neuropathic symptoms improved vs. placebo.	May ↓ blood glucose.
Artichoke leaf	*Cynara scolymus*	↓ Cholesterol	Insufficient data to draw conclusion.	Case reports of mild bloating.
Bee products	Bee pollen, royal jelly	"Superfood" w/multiple cure-all claims	Significant research lacking. Contain insignificant amount of nutrients.	Allergic reaction in those w/ pollen or bee allergy.
Bitter orange	*Citrus aurantium*, Seville orange, synephrine, zhi shi, sour orange	Weight loss Fat loss	Central nervous system stimulant replacing ephedra in diet pills. Also found in energy drinks. Limited evidence on supplement taken alone.	Case reports of adverse cardiac events, stroke, and hypertensive crisis. Often combined with other stimulants. Avoid use with monoamine oxidase (MAO) inhibitor drugs, heart disease, hypertension.
Black cohosh	*Cimicifuga racemosa*, bugbane, snakeroot	Relief of menopausal symptoms	Inconsistent results, may ↓ hot flashes—requires further study.	Uterine stimulant. Caution w/breast cancer history. Interaction with digitalis. Do not confuse with toxic blue or white cohosh.
Carnitine		Treat carnitine deficiency and cardiac disease ↓ Athletic performance	FDA approved for use in treating mitochondrial disease/carnitine deficiency. No consistent evidence supports use for sport performance. Data still limited on role in cardiac disease.	Gastrointestinal (GI) complaints. Interaction with antibiotic pivampicillin.
Chamomile	*Chamaemelum nobile, Matricaria recutita*	Anti-inflammatory, antispasmodic	Limited human studies insufficient to draw conclusion.	Case report of interaction w/warfarin.
Chasteberry	Vitex agnus, monk's pepper	↓ Menopausal symptoms	Limited data w/lack of evidence of ↓ symptoms.	Avoid w/breast cancer history. May interact with Parkinson's disease drugs.
Chitosan		↓ Absorption of fat	Effects not clinically significant.	Derived from shellfish—caution with this allergy. May ↓ absorption of some nutrients.
Chromium picolinate		↓ Blood glucose ↓ Body fat	No evidence of effect in clients with diabetes w/ normal chromium status. Lack of evidence on body composition effect.	Average American diet contains adequate chromium.

(continued)

Table 25-1 Popular Dietary Supplements** *(continued)*

Supplement	Other Name	Claim	Available Evidence	Reported Side Effects/Warnings
CLA	Conjugated linoleic acid	↓ Weight and body fat	Inconsistent results in humans.	Some studies reporting adverse insulin resistance effect. Fatty liver reported in animal studies.
CoQ-10	Coenzyme Q-10	Treat mitochondrial disease Treat various heart diseases, ↓ risk of myopathy associated with statin drugs	Approved treatment for myopathies from mitochondrial disease. Further study needed on possible adjunctive role in treatment of heart failure and as a supplement in those at risk of myopathy because of statin drugs.	May interfere w/anticoagulant or antiplatelet drugs.
Cranberry	Cranberry juice or extract	↓ Risk of urinary tract infections (UTI) Treat UTIs	Evidence chronic intake may prevent UTIs in females by ↓ adherence of bacteria to bladder wall. Some effect also seen in those w/spinal cord injury. No effect in treating present UTI.	Taste and calorie content of juice often leads to noncompliance with chronic intake. May ↑ risk of oxalate kidney stone. Optimal dose/form of extract not determined.
Danshen	*Salvia miltorrhiza*	Treat cardiovascular disease	Clinical trials of poor quality.	Anticoagulant/antiplatelet effect.
DHEA	Dehydroepiandrosterone	Antiaging Enhance cognitive function, athletic performance, body composition	Limited and conflicting evidence of effect for any claims made.	Risk of reproductive cancers cited w/use.
Dong quai	*Angelica senesis*	↓ Hot flashes and premenstrual syndrome (PMS) symptoms	Clinical studies poor quality w/ no proven affect on hot flashes or PMS symptoms.	Anticoagulant/antiplatelet effect. Uterine stimulant. Avoid use with reproductive cancers.
Echinacea	*Echinacea purpora, E. augustifolia, E. pallida,* coneflower	Immune stimulator, cold treatment/ preventive	Mixed results on cold treatment; may ↓ duration/ symptoms. No effect on cold prevention.	Allergy in those w/allergy to ragweed family. Avoid prolonged continual use and use w/autoimmune disease or immunosuppressant drugs.
Evening primrose	*Oenothera biennis*	Treat PMS	No clinical benefit shown w/large placebo effect in studies	GI complaints, headache.
Feverfew	*Tanacetum parthenium, Chrysanthemum parthenium*	Migraine prevention, pain relief	Mixed results in migraine prevention and relief of mild pain.	Anticoagulant/antiplatelet effect. Oral irritation/sores from chewing leaves. Uterine contractions risk. Avoid w/ allergy to aster/daisy family.
HMB	β-Hydroxy-β-methylbutyrate	↑ Muscle mass	Mixed results w/some evidence of effect in untrained adults.	Reports on side effects lacking.
HCA	Hydroxycitric acid, *Garcinia cambogia*	↓ Weight	Evidence lacking of effect.	GI symptoms, headache, may ↑ blood glucose.
Garlic	*Allium sativum,* allicin, ajo	↓ Cholesterol	Evidence lacking that raw garlic or supplement form significantly ↓ cholesterol.	Anticoagulant/antiplatelet effect. ↓ Concentration of some protease inhibitors.

Table 25-1 Popular Dietary Supplements** *(continued)*

Supplement	Other Name	Claim	Available Evidence	Reported Side Effects/Warnings
Ginger	*Zingiber officinale*	Alleviate nausea, motion sickness	Evidence that may ↓ symptoms of motion sickness vs. conventional medications or placebo. Mixed result in treating nausea in pregnancy, from chemotherapy, or postoperatively.	Anticoagulant/antiplatelet effect.
Ginkgo biloba	Fossil tree, maidenhair tree, yinhsiang, kew tree, baiguo, Japanese silver apricot	Prevent dementia, treat tinnitus and intermittent claudication	No evidence of prevention/delay of cognitive changes in those w/o dementia. Some evidence of mild/modest improvement in cognition in those w/ advanced dementia. Modest effect in ↓ pain from intermittent claudication. Mixed results in treating tinnitus.	Anticoagulant/antiplatelet effect. GI complaints, headache, and dizziness. Uncooked ginkgo seeds are toxic.
Ginseng	Siberian ginseng: *Eleutherococcus ginseng* Korean ginseng: *Panax ginseng* American: *Panax quiquefolius*	"Cure-all" for improving stamina, immunity. ↓ Blood glucose	Unsubstantiated claims as a "cure-all" Claim to ↓ blood glucose unsupported w/only small, short-term studies done.	Anticoagulant/antiplatelet effect. Siberian ginseng interacts with digoxin, monitor for any potentiation of antidiabetic drugs.
Glycerol	Glycerine	↑ Hydration in athletes	Preliminary evidence that high osmolality of glycerol causes fluid shifts to temporarily ↑ cell hydration, but with side effects that can preclude its safe use.	Headache, nausea, blurry vision with cell fluid shifts. Avoid use w/heart failure, kidney disease, and hypertension. May ↑ blood glucose in clients with diabetes.
Glucosamine and Chondroitin	Glucosamine sulfate, glucosamine hydrochloride, chondroitin sulfate	Cartilage repair, arthritis symptoms	Overall mixed results, but evidence of improved symptoms strongest in those w/ moderate/severe knee pain from osteoarthritis. No evidence of improvement in those without osteoarthritis.	Individual trial of glucosamine combined with chondroitin should yield improvement by 3 months or no effect is likely. Side effects rare, but can include dyspepsia.
Goldenseal	*Hydrastastis canadensis*	Anti-inflammatory, antimicrobial	Limited or anecdotal research.	Monitor for interaction w/digoxin and calcium channel blockers.
Guarana	*Paullinia cupana* *Paullinia sorbillis*	Promote weight loss. Provide energy.	Lack of evidence of supplement effect alone. Often combined with other stimulants in weight loss supplements. Found in some energy drinks.	↑ Nervousness, ↑ blood pressure and heart rate as a central nervous system stimulant
Gotu kola	*Centella asiatica*	Antianxiety	Lack of quality studies.	Case reports of hepatotoxicity.
Guggulipid	Guggul gum	↓ Cholesterol	Randomized, controlled trials show mixed or no effect. Claims based on nonrandomized trials done in Asia.	Hypersensitivity rash in some, GI upset, hiccups. May interact with cardiac medications propranolol and diltiazem.
Horse chestnut	*Aesculus hippocastanum*	↓ Venous insufficiency symptoms	Evidence of some effect vs. placebo and equivalent to using elastic stockings for symptom improvement.	Naturally occurring coumarin—caution w/anticoagulant/antiplatelet medication Raw product: toxic. GI irritation, nephropathy.

(continued)

Table 25-1 Popular Dietary Supplements** *(continued)*

Supplement	Other Name	Claim	Available Evidence	Reported Side Effects/Warnings
Kava	Ava, awa, tonga kava pepper, *Piper methysticum*	Antianxiety	Clinical evidence of benefit but with current FDA warning of link to hepatotoxicity.	Hepatotoxicity, platelet disturbances, photosensitivity. Avoid with sedatives, hypnotics, anti-Parkinson drugs.
Licorice	Licorice root, *Glycyrrhiza glabra*	Anti-inflammatory ↓ Hot flashes	No clinical trials on hot flash effect. Preliminary evidence of effect on improvements in liver function tests following hepatitis C.	Excess or long-term use can lead to symptoms of mineralocorticoid excess— ↑ blood pressure, altered fluid and electrolytes w/ ↓ K+. Caution with cardiac medications.
Mangosteen	Mangosteen juice or fruit	"Cure-all"	No clinical trials, only anecdotes.	Reports on side effects lacking.
Melatonin	n-acetyl-5-methotryptamine	Manage sleep disorders, jet lag Treat cancer	Evidence lacking on effectiveness in improving sleep. Preliminary research suggesting role in symptoms of cancer treatment.	Altered drug effects w/ antidepressants, warfarin, nifedipine, sedatives. Daytime sleepiness.
Milk thistle	*Silybum marianum*, Silymarin, holy or Mary thistle	Treat cirrhosis, hepatitis	Mixed results on effect of improving liver function. Animal studies suggestive of some benefit.	Interacts with indinavir. Laxative effect. Allergy in those allergic to plants in aster family.
Noni juice	*Morinda citrifolia*	"Well-being"	Clinical data lacking.	Contains ↑ K+ - caution w/renal disease. Reports of hepatotoxicity unclear.
Omega-3 fats	Fish oils, flaxseed and flaxseed oil, EPA and DHA pills	↓ Triglycerides ↓ Cardiovascular events Improved symptoms of rheumatoid arthritis (RA) and ulcerative colitis	Evidence of ↓ incidence of sudden cardiac death and ↓ triglycerides. Preliminary evidence of improvement of subjective symptoms of rheumatoid arthritis. Not found to prevent relapse of inflammatory bowel disease.	Anticoagulant/antiplatelet effect. Specific dose recommendations should be in consult with primary health care provider. Flaxseeds greater than 45 gm/day w/laxative effect.
Red clover	*Trifolium pratense*	↓ Hot flashes	No evidence of clinically important. ↓ Hot flashes.	Anticoagulant/antiplatelet effect. Consult with oncologist on use in clients with breast cancer history.
Red yeast rice	Xuezhikang, *Monascus purpureus*, Went rice	Alternative to statin drugs for cholesterol reduction	Studies conducted in China report ↓ low-density lipoprotein (LDL) cholesterol.	Case reports of hepatitis associated with use.
SAM-e	s-adenosyl-methionine	Antidepressant	Some clinical evidence of improved symptoms of depression vs. placebo.	Case reports of mania in bipolar disease. Avoid w/ antidepressant drugs or Parkinson's disease.
St. John's Wort	*Hypericum perforatum*, goat weed	Antidepressant	Evidence superior to placebo in ↓ symptoms of mild/moderate depression.	Interacts with large number of medications, including oral contraceptives, cyclosporines, protease inhibitors, statins, verapamil, digoxin, phenytoin, some chemotherapy agents, and more, requiring consultation with pharmacist when considering use. Avoid with antidepressants. Photosensitivity.

MyNursingKit National Center for Complementary and Alternative Medicine (NCCAM), National Institutes for Health

Table 25-1 Popular Dietary Supplements** *(continued)*

Supplement	Other Name	Claim	Available Evidence	Reported Side Effects/Warnings
Saw palmetto	*Serenoa repens*	↓ Symptoms of enlarged prostate	Mixed results with some mild/moderate improvements possible	GI complaints, dizziness. Rule out other causes of symptoms before supplement trial considered.
Senna	*Cassia senna*	Laxative	Evidence as strong stimulant laxative.	Cramping, diarrhea, loss of electroytes. Case reports of liver disease w/ long-term use.
Shark cartilage		Cancer prevention or treatment	Evidence does not support effect based on erroneous belief that sharks do not get cancer.	↓ shark population w/pursuit of false claim.
Valerian	*Valeriana officinalis*, All-heal, garden heliotrope	Enhance sleep Antianxiety	Some evidence may be helpful w/some types of insomnia, but not all. Insufficient evidence for use w/anxiety.	Headache, dizziness, morning tiredness w/ ↑ doses. Avoid w/sedative, antiepileptic drugs. No information on safety of long-term use.
Willow bark	*Salix alba* White willow	Pain relief	Contains precursor to salicylates, salicin. May relieve pain greater than placebo, but data limited.	Anticoagulant/antiplatelet effect. Avoid with aspirin/salicylate allergy or bleeding disorders.

**No dietary supplement is a substitute for medical treatment. Supplements should not be taken/recommended without conferring with the primary health care provider. Dietary supplement use should be avoided by pregnant or lactating females and children unless approved by the primary health care provider.

clinically significant concern (Sood et al., 2008). Other safety issues concern products that can cause allergic reactions, such as the botanicals chamomile and feverfew, which present problems to individuals allergic to ragweed. Chitosan, a supplement erroneously believed by some to foster significant weight loss, is made from shellfish and should be avoided by individuals with that allergy. Dietary supplements were the second most common cause of adverse drug interactions in a 7-year survey done at a poison control center (Vassilev, Chu, Ruck, Adams, & Marcus, 2009).

Practice Pearl: Assessing Dietary Supplement Intake outlines one method of determining the specifics of a client's dietary supplement use. Client Education Checklist: Assessing Supplement Use is an additional tool that can be used to assess supplement intake. The nurse should stress the importance of a client's thorough consideration of available information in consultation with the primary health care provider before the decision to use a supplement is made. A pharmacist can provide

input on potential drug interactions with a supplement and online resources are also available. However, often no medical literature exists on the interaction potential of many supplements (Engdal, Klepp, & Nilsen, 2009). The lack of information about a supplement should not be considered a guarantee of its safety.

Even when best decision-making practices have been used regarding supplement use, the lack of standards and strict regulation of the dietary supplement market can result in a safety risk. Reports have been published outlining cases of supplements that are adulterated or contaminated with microorganisms, heavy metals, and prescription drugs (NCCAM, 2009; Saper et al., 2004). For example, some kelp supplements have been reported to contain arsenic (Amster, Tiwary, & Schenker, 2007) and supplements marketed as aphrodisiacs have been found to contain prescription medications used to treat impotence (Reepmeyer & d'Avignon, 2009). Additionally, actual ingredient and dose content amounts are not always found to match that which is listed on the label (Gilroy, Steiner. Byers, Shapiro, & Georgian, 2003; Harkey, Henderson, Gershwin, Stern, & Hackman, 2001). There is comparatively little clinical research on the safety of nonvitamin/nonmineral dietary supplements contrasted with that available for medications, vitamins, and minerals. Of particular concern is the lack of information on the safe use of dietary supplements by children and pregnant or lactating females. Lifespan Box: Supplement Concerns across the Lifespan outlines supplement safety concerns across the lifespan.

PRACTICE ✦ PEARL

Assessing Dietary Supplement Intake

It can be difficult to assess actual dietary supplement intake when a client cannot recall product ingredients or dosage. Routinely have clients bring any bottles or supplement packages with them to a clinical visit for accurate documentation and assessment of intake.

CLIENT EDUCATION CHECKLIST ✓ **Assessing Supplement Use**

What Dietary Supplements Are You Taking?

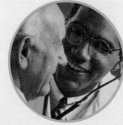

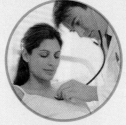

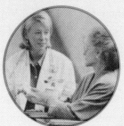

Does Your Health Care Provider Know?

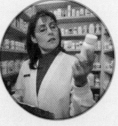

It Matters and Here's Why

This brochure includes three tools to help you and your health care team manage your dietary supplement and medicine intake:

1 Nutrition Assessment
2 Dietary Supplement Diary
3 Medication Diary

First Tool: Nutrition Assessment

Think about the following statements and use this checklist to talk to your health care provider about your nutritional status and whether taking a dietary supplement(s) is right for you.

Nutrition Assessment	Yes/No
I currently take a dietary supplement(s).	
I eat fewer than 2 meals a day.	
My diet is restricted (e.g., don't eat dairy, meat, and/or fewer than 5 servings of fruits and vegetables).	
I eat alone most of the time.	
Without wanting to, I have lost or gained more than 10 pounds in the last 6 months.	
I take 3 or more prescription or OTC medicines a day.	
I have 3 or more drinks of alcohol a day.	

Source: adapted from the Nutrition Screening Initiative.

General Questions About Dietary Supplement Use	Yes/No
Is taking a dietary supplement important to my total diet?	
Are there any precautions or warnings I should know about (e.g., is there an amount or "upper limit" that I should not go above)?	
Are there any known side effects (e.g., loss of appetite, nausea, headaches, etc.)?	
Are there any dietary supplements I should avoid while taking certain medicines (prescription or OTC) or other supplements?	
If I'm scheduled for elective surgery, should I discontinue use of dietary supplements? If so, when?	

Other Questions To Consider…

What is this product for?
What are its intended benefits?
How, when, and for how long should I take it?

Second Tool: Dietary Supplement Diary

To have an accurate record for your health care provider, list all the supplements you take (e.g., multiple, single, or combination vitamins, minerals, or any botanical supplements) and how often. If you are unsure if a product is a dietary supplement, check to see if there is a Supplement Facts Label on the package.

Share this chart with your health care provider so you can discuss what's best for your overall health.

It is very important that you consider your combined intake from all supplements (including multivitamins, single supplements, and combination products) plus fortified foods, like some cereals and drinks. Excess intakes of some supplements may cause health problems.

Supplement	Amount	How Often	Reason
Example: Multivitamin-mineral	I tablet	Once a day	Supplement my diet
Example: Calcium-fortified orange juice	8 oz/ 350 mg	Once a day	Support healthy bones

Refer to "Examples of Products Marketed as Dietary Supplements" in a previous panel for help completing this chart.

Third Tool: Medication Diary

Please complete information about all of the prescription and over-the-counter (OTC) medications that you frequently take or are currently taking (e.g., aspirin, pain reliever, cold medicine, stool softener, etc.). Provide this information to your health care provider so he or she can update your records and better respond to your questions.

	Amount	How Often	Reason
Prescription			
Over-the-Counter			

Health Professionals' Contact List

	Name	Phone #
Hospital		
Doctor Specialty: _____		
Doctor Specialty: _____		
Doctor Specialty: _____		
Doctor Specialty: _____		
Pharmacist		
Dietitian		
Nurse		
Other		

(continued)

CLIENT EDUCATION CHECKLIST **Assessing Supplement Use** *(continued)*

Partners in Health - Working With Your Health Care Providers

With the abundance of conflicting information available about dietary supplements, it is more important than ever to talk with your doctor and other health care providers (dietitian, nurse, pharmacist, etc.) to help you sort the reliable information from the questionable.

Dietary Supplements - More Than Vitamins…

Today's dietary supplements are not only vitamins and minerals. They also include other less familiar substances, such as herbals, botanicals, amino acids, and enzymes. Dietary supplements come in a variety of forms, such as tablets, capsules, powders, energy bars, or drinks.

If you do not consume a variety of foods, as recommended in the Food Guide Pyramid and Dietary Guidelines for Americans, some supplements may help ensure that you get adequate amounts of essential nutrients or help promote optimal health and performance. However, *dietary supplements are not intended to treat, diagnose, mitigate, prevent, or cure diseases*; therefore, manufacturers may not make such claims. In some cases, dietary supplements may have unwanted effects, especially if taken before surgery or with other dietary supplements or medicines, or if you have certain health conditions.

Unlike drugs, but like conventional foods, dietary supplements are not approved by the Food and Drug Administration (FDA) for safety and effectiveness. It is the responsibility of dietary supplement manufacturers/distributors to ensure that their products are safe and that their label claims are accurate and truthful. Once a product enters the marketplace, FDA has the authority to take action against any dietary supplement product that presents a significant or unreasonable risk of illness or injury.

Scientific evidence supporting the benefits of some dietary supplements (e.g., vitamins and minerals) is well established for certain health conditions, but others need further study. Whatever your choice, supplements should not replace prescribed medications or the variety of foods important to a healthful diet.

How To Recognize a Dietary Supplement

At times, it can be confusing to tell the difference between a dietary supplement, a food, or an over-the-counter (OTC) medicine. An easy way to recognize a dietary supplement is to look for the Supplement Facts Panel on the product.

Supplement Facts

Serving Size 1 Packet
Servings Per Container 10

Amount Per Serving	AM Packet	% Daily Value	PM Packet	% Daily Value
Vitamin A	2500 IU	50%	2500 IU	50%
Vitamin C	60 mg	100%	60 mg	100%
Vitamin D	400 IU	100%		
Vitamin E	30 IU	100%		
Thiamin	1.5 mg	100%	1.5 mg	100%
Riboflavin	1.7 mg	100%	1.7 mg	100%
Niacin	20 mg	100%	20 mg	100%
Vitamin B₆	2.0 mg	100%	2.0 mg	100%
Folic Acid	200 mcg	50%	200 mcg	50%
Vitamin B₁₂	3 mcg	50%	3 mcg	50%
Biotin			30 mcg	10%
Pantothenic Acid	5 mg	50%	5 mg	50%

Ingredients: Sodium ascorbate, ascorbic acid, calcium pantothenate, niacinamide, d-alpha tocopheryl acetate, microcrystalline cellulose, artificial flavors, dextrin, starch, mono- and diglycerides, vitamin A acetate, magnesium stearate, gelatin, FD&C Blue #1, FD&C Red #3, artificial colors, thiamin mononitrate, pyridoxine hydrochloride, citric acid, lactose, sorbic acid, tricalcium phosphate, sodium benzoate, sodium caseinate, methylparaben, potassium sorbate, BHA, BHT, ergocalciferol and cyanocobalamin.

Potential Risks of Using Dietary Supplements

Although certain products may be helpful to some people, there may be circumstances when these products can pose unexpected risks. Many supplements contain active ingredients that can have strong effects in the body. Taking a combination of supplements, using these products together with medicine, or substituting them in place of prescribed medicines could lead to harmful, even life-threatening results. Also, some supplements can have unwanted effects before, during, and after surgery. It is important to let your doctor and other health professionals know about the vitamins, minerals, botanicals, and other products you are taking, especially before surgery.

Here a few examples of dietary supplements believed to interact with specific drugs:

- Calcium and heart medicine (e.g., Digoxin), thiazide diuretics (Thiazide), and aluminum and magnesium-containing antacids.
- Magnesium and thiazide and loop diuretics (e.g., Lasix®, etc.), some cancer drugs (e.g., Cisplatin, etc.), and magnesium-containing antacids.
- Vitamin K and a blood thinner (e.g., Coumadin).
- St. John's Wort and selective serotonin reuptake inhibitor (SSRI) drugs (i.e., anti-depressant drugs and birth control pills).

What Should I Know Before Using Dietary Supplements?

Be savvy! Follow these tips before buying a dietary supplement:

- Remember: Safety First. Some supplement ingredients, including nutrients and plant components, can be toxic based on their activity in your body. Do not substitute a dietary supplement for a prescription medicine or therapy.
- Think twice about chasing the latest headline. Sound health advice is generally based on research over time, not a single study touted by the media. Be wary of results claiming a "quick fix" that depart from scientific research and established dietary guidance.
- Learn to Spot False Claims. Remember: "*If something sounds too good to be true, it probably is.*" Some examples of false claims on product labels:
  - Quick and effective "cure-all."
  - Can *treat* or *cure* disease.
  - "Totally safe," "all natural," and has "definitely no side effects."
  - Limited availability, "no-risk, money-back guarantees," or requires advance payment.
- More may not be better. Some products can be harmful when consumed in high amounts, for a long time, or in combination with certain other substances.
- The term "natural" doesn't always mean safe. Do not assume that this term ensures wholesomeness or safety. For some supplements, "natural" ingredients may interact with medicines, be dangerous for people with certain health conditions, or be harmful in high doses. For example, tea made from peppermint leaves is generally considered safe to drink, but peppermint oil (extracted from the leaves) is much more concentrated and can be toxic if used incorrectly.
- Is the product worth the money? Resist the pressure to buy a product or treatment "on the spot." Some supplement products may be expensive or may not provide the benefit you expect. For example, excessive amounts of water-soluble vitamins, like vitamin C and B vitamins, are not used by the body and are eliminated in the urine.

CLIENT EDUCATION CHECKLIST Assessing Supplement Use *(continued)*

Bottom Line

- Do not self diagnose any health condition. Work with your health care providers to determine how best to achieve optimal health.
- Check with your health care providers before taking a supplement, especially when combining or substituting them with other foods or medicine.
- Some supplements can help you meet your daily requirements for certain nutrients, but others may cause health problems.
- Dietary supplements are not intended to treat, diagnose, mitigate, prevent, or cure disease, or to replace the variety of foods important to a healthful diet.

Examples of Products Marketed as Dietary Supplements

Because many products are marketed as dietary supplements, it is important to remember that supplements include vitamins and minerals, as well as botanicals and other substances. The list* below gives some examples of products you may see sold as dietary supplements. It is not possible to list them all here.

Vitamins, Minerals, Nutrients	Botanicals and Other Substances
Multiple Vitamin/Mineral	Acidophilus
Vitamin B Complex	Black Cohosh
Vitamin C	Ginger
Vitamin D	Evening Primrose Oil
Vitamin E	Echinacea
Beta-Carotene	Fiber
Calcium	Garlic
Omega-3 Fatty Acids	Ginkgo Biloba
Folic Acid	Fish Oil
Zinc	Glucosamine and/or Chrondroitin Sulfate
Iron	St. John's Wort
	Saw Palmetto

*Adapted from A Healthcare Professional's Guide to Evaluating Dietary Supplements, the American Dietetic Association & American Pharmaceutical Association Special Report (2000).

Note: the examples provided do not represent an endorsement or approval by any agency or organization that contributed to this material.

FDA MedWatch

If you suspect that you have had a serious reaction to a dietary supplement, you and your doctor should report it to FDA Medwatch:

- Phone: 1-800-FDA-1088
- Fax: 1-800-FDA-0178
- Internet: www.fda.gov/medwatch/how.htm

Dietary Supplement Resources

Federal Government Agencies:

Administration on Aging, DHHS:
http://www.aoa.gov

Food and Drug Administration, DHHS, Center for Food Safety and Applied Nutrition:
http://www.cfsan.fda.gov/~dms/supplmnt.html
http://www.cfsan.fda.gov/~dms/ds-savvy.html
http://www.cfsan.fda.gov/label.html

National Institutes of Health, DHHS:
- Office of Dietary Supplements:
  http://dietary-supplements.info.nih.gov
- National Center for Complementary and Alternative Medicine:
  (http://nccam.nih.gov) and Clearinghouse,
  1-888-624-6226

Office on Women's Health, DHHS:
http://www.4woman.gov/owh/index.htm
or 1-800-994-WOMAN

Federal Trade Commission:
http://www.ftc.gov

U.S. Department of Agriculture, Food and Nutrition Information Center:
http://www.nal.usda.gov/fnic

Others:

American Association of Retired Persons (AARP):
http://www.aarp.org

American Dietetic Association:
http://www.eatright.org

American Pharmacists Association:
http://www.pharmacyandyou.org

Food Marketing Institute:
http://www.fmi.org

National Council on Patient Information and Education (NCPIE):
http://www.talkaboutrx.org

Links to non-Federal government organizations do not represent endorsement of these organizations or their materials.

Organizations that contributed to this educational material are the Administration on Aging (Department of Health and Human Services [DHHS]), American Academy of Family Physicians, American Association of Retired Persons, American Dietetic Association, American Medical Association, American Pharmacists Association, Federal Trade Commission, Food and Drug Administration (DHHS), Food Marketing Institute, International Food Information Council Foundation, National Council on Patient Information and Education, Office of Dietary Supplements (National Institutes of Health, DHHS), and the Office on Women's Health (DHHS).

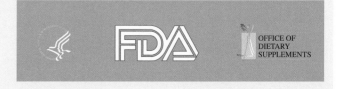

Source: National Institute of Health.

MyNursingKit Food and Drug Administration (FDA) Supplement Warnings

Lifespan

Supplement Concerns across the Lifespan

The limited controlled clinical trials that have been done on dietary supplements primarily were conducted in the adult population. Little to no data exist on supplement use in children, pregnant or lactating females, and the older adult. Even when strong clinical evidence exists for using a dietary supplement in adults, a blanket extension of those recommendations to other populations should not occur. The nurse should be aware of the following concerns:

Children

- Children have larger livers and developing central nervous and immune systems that predispose them to altered absorption, metabolism, and excretion of dietary supplements compared with adults. Developing systems increase risk of supplement side effects (Woolf, 2003). Dosage information is largely based on recommendations for adults, not children.

- Taking multiple dietary supplements increases the risk of side effects. In one survey, some children were reported taking nine or more supplements (Ball, Kertesz, & Moyer-Mileur, 2005).

- Children with chronic conditions, such as cystic fibrosis, cancer, and attention deficit disorder, are more likely to take dietary supplements compared with healthy children. Up to 60% of children with chronic conditions also have nutritional problems (Harris, 2005). This combination along with any use of medications increases the risk of side effects with supplement use.

- Adolescents may use dietary supplements to enhance appearance or sports performance. Teens who have used dietary supplements for sports are more likely to later use anabolic steroids compared with teens who never used supplements marketed to enhance sport performance (Dodge & Jaccard, 2006). Supplement use is highest in adolescents among those who use prescription medications (Gardiner, Buettner, Davis, Phillips, & Kemper, 2008).

- No long-term safety or efficacy clinical data exist for most supplements. Unforeseen side effects may not be attributed to a supplement until it is widely used in a population. Cumulative effects of dietary supplements over the lifetime are not understood.

Pregnant or Lactating Female

- Some botanical supplements are characterized as uterine stimulants or lead to altered blood clotting, both dangerous complications during pregnancy (Dugoua, Mills, Perri, & Koren, 2006).

- Some dietary supplements, especially botanicals, may be teratogens or mutagens (Woolf, 2003).

- Little is understood about whether dietary supplements cross into breast milk or affect milk production (Dugoua et al., 2006).

- Little scientific study has been devoted to the effects of supplements on lactation. The lack of negative data should not be misconstrued as proof of safety.

- Research on supplements and pregnant or lactating females covers small-scale trials, which make it difficult to draw conclusions about effect or safety. Large-scale studies that are needed to give statistical power to any finding are unlikely in this population (Low Dog, 2009).

Older Adult

- Altered pharmacodynamics and pharmacokinetics with aging, along with polypharmacy, predisposes the older adult to potential drug interactions with dietary supplements. In a survey of adults greater than 65 years who use dietary supplements, there was a potential for a drug-supplement interaction with almost half the supplements used (Wold et al., 2005).

- Almost 15% of older adults taking over-the-counter or prescription medications also use herbal supplements. Less than half of those discuss this use with a medical professional (Bruno & Ellis, 2005).

The nurse should ask specifically about dietary supplement use in these populations. Inquiring about lifespan-specific conditions and any self-treatment is an easy way to include the topic in the assessment. Infant colic, nausea and vomiting with pregnancy, desire for improved appearance or athletic performance in adolescence, and attempts to restore skin elasticity with age are examples of lifespan specific motivations to try a supplement.

CT? How might the nurse ask a pregnant female about her supplement use? How could the nurse approach the issue if the client is using herbal supplements that are supported by cultural beliefs?

The FDA has issued alerts and warning about specific dietary supplements when sufficient reports of adverse events have been made. These are outlined in Box 25-4. The nurse should warn clients against using any of these products, because some can still be found on the market.

Who Uses Dietary Supplements?

The use of dietary supplements has been on the rise in all age groups since the passage of the DSHEA in 1994. Estimates range as high as 75% of adults in the United States use dietary supplements at least intermittently when vitamins and minerals are included in the definition. Up to 20% of adults in the United States and Canada reported using nonvitamin/nonmineral types of supplements over a 12-month period (Barnes, Powell-Griner, McFann, & Nahin, 2004; Kelly et al., 2005; Singh & Levine, 2006). Use of nonvitamin/nonmineral supplements by adults over age 65 years doubled between the years 1998 and 2002 (Kelly et al., 2005). Over half of all older adults who take prescription drugs also take at least one dietary supplement (Qato et al., 2008). Over 50% of young children and almost 30% of adolescents are reported to use dietary supplements with vitamins, minerals, and sports nutrition supplements among the most popular (Gardiner, 2005;

BOX 25-4	FDA Supplement Warnings and Alerts

Androstenedione
Aristolochic acid
Chaparral
Comfrey
Ephedra alkaloids
Gamma butyrolactone (GBL)
Gamma hydroxybutyric acid (GHB)
Germander
Jin bu huan
Kava
LipoKinetix
Liqiang 4
Lobelia
PC SPES and SPES
St. John's Wort combined with Indavir
Tiractricol
L-tryptophan
Willow bark
Yohimbe

Source: FDA, 2007.

Gardiner et al., 2008). The nurse should be aware that the prevalence of dietary supplement use is higher among children with a chronic disease or condition. Over 60% of chronically ill children use dietary supplements with almost one-third of those using a supplement that was not recommended by a health care provider (Ball, Kertesz, & Moyer-Mileur, 2005). Further, in 80% of the cases of supplement use, no communication occurred with the health care provider about the supplement, a dismal statistic that has been approximated by other studies in children and adults (Ball et al., 2005; Gardiner et al., 2008; Kemper, Gardiner, Gobble, & Woods, 2006). Males, younger adults, and racial and ethnic minority populations have the lowest rate of disclosure about supplement use (Kennedy, Wang, & Wu, 2008).

Individuals who use dietary supplements do so for a variety of reasons. Some believe that dietary supplements are a safer alternative to over-the-counter or prescription medications (Pilliteri et al., 2008). Others are dissatisfied with traditional medicine or want more personal control over their health (Low Dog, 2009). Supplement use is most prevalent in adults with chronic conditions, especially gastrointestinal complaints; menopausal females; and children with chronic conditions or whose parents use supplements (Gardiner, 2005; Harris, 2005). Clinical studies outlining the health risks of hormone replacement therapy during menopause have caused some women to seek alternative approaches to managing menopausal symptoms, as explained in Hot Topic: Dietary Supplements for Menopausal Symptoms.

hot Topic

Dietary Supplements for Menopausal Symptoms

Reports of adverse outcomes associated with the use of hormone replacement therapy during menopause have led some menopausal females toward a trial of dietary supplements for menopausal symptom relief. The result is an increasing amount of supplements on the market targeted at this population (Low Dog, 2005). Herbal supplements and soy derivatives predominate the offerings found in North America. In particular, relief of vasomotor symptoms, specifically hot flashes, is a popular label claim with these products. The nurse should be aware of the supplements that are available and any recommendations regarding use.

Soy isoflavones: Isoflavones are a component of soy that are felt to have a weak estrogen effect. The theory behind their use in menopause is to offset the diminishing endogenous estrogen production by the body that is felt to be responsible for menopausal symptoms (Carroll, 2006). These plant estrogens, or **phytoestrogens,** can act as an estrogen agonist or antagonist depending on an individual's estrogen environment and the supplement itself (Low Dog, 2005). Use of soy isoflavones to reduce the occurrences of hot flashes has had mixed results in clinical trials, including a substantial placebo effect (Low Dog, 2005; Nelson et al., 2006). Long-term safety is unknown, but some reports exist, warning about endometrial hyperplasia, or thickening of the uterine endometrium, with prolonged use (Nelson et al., 2006). Those who choose to take isoflavones are advised to not exceed 100 mg/day, the amount that mimics that found in a typical Asian diet containing soy (Messina & Wood, 2008).

Red clover: Like soy, red clover contains isoflavones that act as phytoestrogens. Clinical trials using red clover have shown minimal to no effect on the reduction of hot flashes (Low Dog, 2005; Nelson et al., 2006). Based on animal studies with red clover, concern exists that this supplement and others that exert estrogen-like effects may be contraindicated with any estrogen-sensitive conditions, such as reproductive cancers and uterine fibroids (NCCAM, 2008b).

Black cohosh: Black cohosh has the more promising results among dietary supplements marketed to reduce hot flashes, yet clinical evidence is still not definitive (Borelli & Ernst, 2008; NCCAM, 2008b; Reed et al., 2008). Controversy exists about the exact mechanism of action for this herb and whether or not it acts as a phytoestrogen. Better understanding of its action is essential before it can be safely recommended, especially to those with estrogen-sensitive conditions. Reports of hepatotoxicity associated with use of black cohosh exist, but it remains to be proven that black cohosh was directly responsible (Low Dog, 2005; NCCAM, 2008b). It has been recommended that black cohosh products contain a warning label regarding this risk (Mahady et al., 2008).

The nurse should educate clients inquiring about use of dietary supplements for menopause about the limited evidence available on this subject. Additional concerns to relate to the client include:

(continued)

- Labeling laws allow products to make structure/function claims regarding menopause and its symptoms without any premarket scrutiny of research or government approval.
- Limited information is understood about the active substances responsible for symptom relief, making it difficult to make blanket safety recommendations for all females.
- Females with estrogen-sensitive conditions should avoid dietary supplements that are phytoestrogens. Reproductive cancers, endometriosis, and uterine fibroids are examples of diseases affected by estrogen (NCCAM, 2008b).
- Evidence of long-term safety is lacking for these supplements. Cultures that traditionally use these supplements for menopause do not advocate the chronic use as might be seen by those following popular advice and taking them for extended periods and in pill form. For example, studies done on the safety of black cohosh are reported for up to 6 months use only (Low Dog, 2005).

The nurse should also be aware of the use of botanical dietary supplements as a cultural practice by many individuals, as outlined in Cultural Considerations Box: Supplement Use in Traditional Medicine. It is essential that the nurse routinely and specifically ask clients about dietary supplement use. Without integration of information on dietary supplement use into a client's care plan, dangerous interactions with medications or adverse effects on health or treatments could be neglectfully overlooked. For example, use of antioxidant supplements, such as vitamins A and C, may interfere with the intended effects of some cancer treatments and augment the effects of others (Hardy, 2008). The narrow therapeutic window of many anticancer drugs reinforces the

PRACTICE PEARL

Asking about Dietary Supplement Use

Asking about dietary supplement use should be a part of every nursing assessment. Some clients consider only vitamins and minerals when asked about supplement use and need to be prompted with further questions. Caregivers should be asked about supplement use in children. Consider these examples:

- Have you used any dietary supplements in the past year? Tell me about any vitamins, minerals, sports nutrition or weight loss products, and herbs or other natural products you have used.
- Are you taking (or giving your child) any special supplements to prevent or treat a condition?
- Are you using any home remedies for your health (or child's)?
- Are you giving your child any dietary supplements that you take?

Cultural Considerations

Supplement Use in Traditional Medicine

The cutting-edge, mainstream popularity of plant-based dietary supplements, specifically herbs, is long preceded by the use of botanicals in traditional medicine around the globe. Ayurvedic medicine using natural supplements has been practiced in India over many lifetimes. Native American and other Indian cultures use plants for medicinal purposes, many of which have become the base for pharmaceuticals. Traditional Chinese medicine incorporates the use of herbals into the treatment of a vast array of conditions and diseases and accounts for up to 50% of all medicine consumption (WHO, 2008). Folk medicine use of plants is also found in other population groups who have settled in the United States, such as Appalachians (Cavender, 2006). Examples of plants with drug-like actions include foxglove, or digitalis, and valerian, which are the plant-based foundations of digoxin and valium, respectively (Gurib-Fakim, 2006).

Individuals often point to the long-standing use of herbal supplements by these cultures when defending the safety and efficacy of their use in the absence of clinical scientific evidence. It is wise to understand that traditional herbal use in most cultures is not mimicked in the interpretation found in mainstream use, where single herbs are taken instead of the often-used combinations found in traditional medicine (Gurib-Fakim, 2006). Lack of manufacturing or clinical product standardization and conversion of products to manufactured pills versus the use of raw plant parts further alters the translation. Contamination and adulteration of imported and local herbal supplements with heavy metals and drugs has been reported (NCCAM, 2009; Saper et al., 2004). Additionally, varied common names given to herbs can be confusing to the consumer and the health care professional who is trying to assess use. It is recommended that botanical or pharmaceutical names be referenced in an assessment of supplement use to avoid confusion and aid in the prevention of toxic consequences with some products (Wu, Farrelly, Upton, & Chen, 2007).

The nurse should be aware of the influence of cultural beliefs on the use of botanical supplements, often as a first-line of treatment instead of conventional health care, while being mindful of potential side effects and the limited clinical evidence supporting their use.

need to explore the possibility of interactions with dietary supplements. Some individuals may choose to forgo traditional medicine if it appears that dietary supplements work instead. The Evidence-Based Practice Box: Is cinnamon effective at lowering blood glucose levels in individuals with diabetes mellitus? discusses such an example with cinnamon in the treatment of diabetes. Practice Pearl: Asking about Dietary Supplement Use outlines examples of specific questions to ask during an assessment.

EVIDENCE-BASED PRACTICE RESEARCH BOX

Is cinnamon effective at lowering blood glucose levels in individuals with diabetes mellitus?

Clinical Problem: Individuals with diabetes mellitus seek nonpharmacological means of lowering blood glucose levels. Cinnamon has been publicized recently as a readily available supplement that will lower blood glucose.

Research Findings: Several studies on mice and rats were conducted to examine the effect of cinnamon on serum glucose and lipid levels. Researchers followed those early, promising results with studies on adults with type 2 diabetes mellitus. Khan, Safdar, Ali Khan, Khattak, and Anderson (2003) gave 60 subjects capsules of cinnamon (1, 3, or 6 grams) or placebo. Their results showed statistically significant reductions in serum glucose, total cholesterol, LDL cholesterol, and triglycerides.

Several additional studies were conducted to verify those results. A study of 25 postmenopausal women with type 2 diabetes mellitus failed to demonstrate significant reductions in serum glucose or lipid levels (Vanschoonbeek, Thomassen, Senden, Wodzig, & van Loon, 2006). Similar results were obtained by Mang and associates (2006) when examining HbA1c and lipid profiles. Another study examined the effect of cinnamon added to rice pudding on the satiety and postprandial blood glucose of healthy subjects. The researchers found that 6 gm of cinnamon delayed gastric emptying and lowered the postprandial blood glucose.

However, satiety was not affected (Hlebowicz, Darwiche, Bjorgell, & Almer, 2007). In a review of previous studies, Pham, Kourlas, and Pham (2007) noted that cinnamon was well tolerated but that data were insufficient to recommend supplementation. Altschuler, Casella, MacKenzie, and Curtis (2007) extended the previous studies to include adolescents with type 1 diabetes mellitus and determined that cinnamon did not improve glycemic control in that sample. Blevins and associates (2007) conducted a study with adults who were given 1 gram of cinnamon or a placebo daily for 3 months. There were no significant differences in fasting serum glucose, lipid, HbA1c levels, or insulin levels. A follow-up study by the researchers using 6 gm of cinnamon found no effect on blood glucose with 3 gm of cinnamon (Hlebowicz et al., 2009).

Nursing Implications: There is no conclusive evidence that cinnamon is effective in lowering serum glucose in clients with type 2 diabetes.

CRITICAL THINKING QUESTIONS:

1. A client with type 2 diabetes mellitus tells the nurse about reading reports that cinnamon is good for people with diabetes because it lowers blood glucose. What should the nurse tell this client?

2. A client insists that his blood glucose is better now that he is using cinnamon daily. He wants to know if he could discontinue his oral antidiabetic medication if he takes more cinnamon. What is the best response to this client?

Popular Dietary Supplements

Dietary supplements are chosen by some individuals looking to improve overall health, whereas others choose a supplement for a specific purpose, such as enhanced sports performance, weight loss, or to prevent or treat a condition or disease. Table 25-1 outlines a comprehensive overview of the more popular dietary supplements with nursing recommendations.

NURSING CARE PLAN   Nutrition and Dietary Supplements

CASE STUDY

Mahalia, 39, has grown increasingly tired of her 44-year-old sister, Mai. Anytime they get together, Mai eagerly shares the latest information she has learned about supplements or dietary aids. She is a regular customer at a nearby health food store and picks up booklets and fliers with the latest claims of each product. Last month, Mai reported that she had finally gotten her husband started on fish oil capsules as a natural method to lower his cholesterol because the pills that the physician had prescribed were too expensive and would have unpleasant side effects. In the past, Mai had reported treating her self-diagnosed mild depression with St. John's Wort. She said her "maintenance" dose had prevented its recurrence. Anytime Mahalia says she has an ache or pain health concern about herself, her husband, or her children, Mai has a "natural" answer. Because it is time for her annual checkup, she has decided to talk to the nurse and find out the truth about some of Mai's remedies. After all, Mai seems to be the picture of health, although Mahalia knows she does not have as much energy as she used to have. She asks the

(continued)

Nutrition and Dietary Supplements *(continued)*

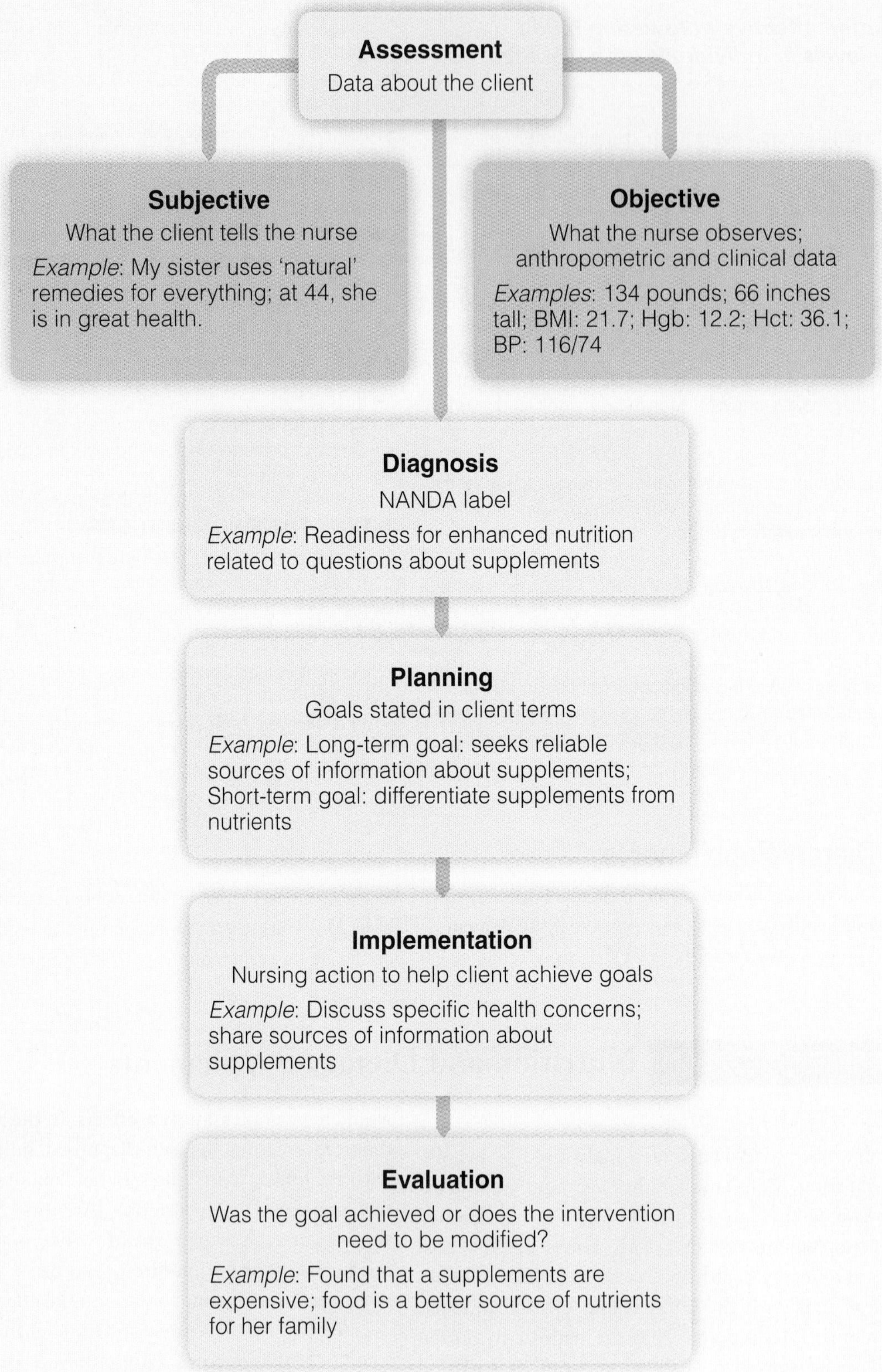

NURSING CARE PLAN

Assessment
Data about the client

Subjective
What the client tells the nurse

Example: My sister uses 'natural' remedies for everything; at 44, she is in great health.

Objective
What the nurse observes; anthropometric and clinical data

Examples: 134 pounds; 66 inches tall; BMI: 21.7; Hgb: 12.2; Hct: 36.1; BP: 116/74

Diagnosis
NANDA label

Example: Readiness for enhanced nutrition related to questions about supplements

Planning
Goals stated in client terms

Example: Long-term goal: seeks reliable sources of information about supplements; Short-term goal: differentiate supplements from nutrients

Implementation
Nursing action to help client achieve goals

Example: Discuss specific health concerns; share sources of information about supplements

Evaluation
Was the goal achieved or does the intervention need to be modified?

Example: Found that a supplements are expensive; food is a better source of nutrients for her family

■ FIGURE 25-2 **Nursing Care Plan Process: Nutrition and Dietary Supplements.**

Nutrition and Dietary Supplements *(continued)*

NURSING CARE PLAN

nurse for some help in figuring out which supplements would be good for her family.

Applying the Nursing Process

ASSESSMENT

Weight: 134 pounds Height: 5 feet 6 inches BMI: 21.7
BP 116/74
Hgb 12.2 Hct 36.1
Occasional headaches; periodic constipation; often tired due to lack of sleep
All body systems normal
Medications: Oral contraceptives

DIAGNOSES

Readiness for enhanced knowledge related to questions about methods to improve health

Readiness for enhanced nutrition related to questions about dietary supplements

EXPECTED OUTCOMES

Plans balanced diet for family

States role of supplements in maintaining and promoting health

Seeks reliable sources of information about dietary supplements

Develops plan for coping with sister's enthusiastic support for supplements

INTERVENTIONS

Family food diary for 1 week

Discuss specific health concerns in the family

Discuss interest in supplement use or if interest is merely because of sister's recommendations

Determine if access to the Internet is available

Share information about balanced diets that incorporate variety and cultural sensitivity

EVALUATION

Mahalia calls the nurse 2 months later to share what she has learned about supplements. She has accessed many of the Internet sources that the nurse shared and has been able to use some of the information. When her sister starts discussing various supplements, Mahalia now knows to ask questions about research that "proves" the claims of the supplement. She has made several visits to health food stores and has found that many supplements are quite expensive. Because the family has no chronic health problems and they eat healthy meals most of the time, she does not feel that supplements are useful for them at this time. She says that they would rather use the money they could spend on supplements for activities the whole family enjoys. Figure 25-2 ■ outlines the nursing process for this case.

Critical Thinking in the Nursing Process

1. **How can the nurse respond to the client who says that supplements are a waste of money?**

CHAPTER SUMMARY

- The nurse plays an important role in the assessment and education of clients regarding dietary supplements.

- Dietary supplements encompass herbal products, vitamins, minerals, sports supplements, amino acids, and any extracted form of these products.

- The Food and Drug Administration regulates dietary supplements as foods and not as medications.

- Dietary supplement labels are allowed to make certain claims as long as the promise of disease prevention or cure is not made.

- Little clinical data are available about the safety and efficacy of many dietary supplements. Long-term data are largely lacking.

- Children, pregnant or lactating females, and the older adult are generally advised to avoid botanical dietary supplements.

EXPLORE **PEARSON mynursingkit™**

MyNursingKit is your one stop for online chapter review materials and resources. Prepare for success with additional NCLEX®-style practice questions, interactive assignments and activities, web links, animations and videos, and more!

Register your access code from the front of your book at
www.mynursingkit.com.

NCLEX® QUESTIONS

1. A client expresses concern about disclosing supplement use to the physician. What should the nurse say to the client?
   1. "It is important to have a trusting relationship with your physician, so disclose what you feel comfortable with at this visit and share more at the next visit."
   2. "Supplements can interact with prescription medications, so it is important that the physician know all supplements you are taking."
   3. "Only the supplements you take regularly need to be disclosed."
   4. "Because most physicians do not approve of clients taking supplements, I will enter them in the record so you do not have to discuss it with the physician."

2. A client wants to use only herbal supplements as a natural means to improve health. How should the nurse respond?
   1. "Herbal supplements rarely have side effects, so it is a safe practice."
   2. "Herbs can be very expensive, so choose them carefully."
   3. "It is important to discuss this issue with your health care provider."
   4. "How will you know which ones to take?"

3. A client is concerned about her menopause symptoms. What supplements might the nurse suggest to ameliorate the symptoms?
   1. Green tea
   2. St. John's Wort
   3. Soy isoflavones
   4. Saw palmetto

4. An elderly client asks the nurse how much of a garlic supplement should be taken to lower the cholesterol level? What response should the nurse make?
   1. "One low-dose capsule a day will be sufficient."
   2. "Eat only fresh garlic, not capsules."
   3. "Research has not determined the best dose."
   4. "Avoid garlic supplements that have not been approved by the FDA."

5. How should the nurse respond to the client who states that a supplement is safe because it was purchased at a reputable health food store?
   1. "A reputable health food store stocks only high-quality products; you have made a good decision."
   2. "The FDA is responsible for safety of supplements, so if 'FDA' is on the label you can be sure it is safe."
   3. "It is better to purchase supplements directly from a supplier to ensure safety."
   4. "The safety or quality of ingredients in supplements often cannot be determined when reading a label."

REFERENCES

Altschuler, J. A., Casella, S. J., MacKenzie, T. A., & Curtis, K. M. (2007). The effect of cinnamon on A1C among adolescents with type 1 diabetes. *Diabetes Care, 30,* 813–816.

Amster, E., Tiwary, A., & Schenker, M. B. (2007). Case report: Potential arsenic toxicosis secondary to herbal kelp supplement. *Environmental Health Perspectives, 115,* 606–608.

Ball, S. D., Kertesz, D., & Moyer-Mileur, L. J. (2005). Dietary supplement use is prevalent among children with a chronic illness. *Journal of the American Dietetic Association, 105,* 78–84.

Barnes, P. M., Powell-Griner, E., McFann, K., & Nahin, R. L. (2004). Complementary and alternative medicine use among adults: United States, 2002. *Advance Data from Vital and Health Statistics, 343.* Hyattsville, MD: National Center for Health Statistics.

Blevins, S. M., Leyva, M. J., Brown, J., Wright, J., Scofield, R. H., & Aston, C. E. (2007). Effect of cinnamon on glucose and lipid levels in non-insulin dependent type 2 diabetes mellitus. *Diabetes Care, 30,* 2236–2237.

Borelli, F., & Ernst, E. (2008). Black cohosh (*Cimicifuga racemosa*): A systematic review of

REFERENCES *(continued)*

adverse events. *American Journal of Obstetrics and Gynecology, 199,* 455–466.

Bruno, J. J., & Ellis, J. J. (2005). Herbal use among U.S. elderly: 2002 National Health Interview Survey. *Annals of Pharmacotherapy, 39,* 643–648.

Carroll, D. G. (2006). Nonhormonal therapies for hot flashes in menopause. *American Family Physician, 73,* 457–464.

Cavender, A. (2006). Folk medicine uses of plant foods in southern Appalachia, United States. *Journal of Ethnopharmacology, 108,* 74–84.

DeAngelis, C. D., & Fontanarosa, P. B. (2003). Drugs alias dietary supplements. *Journal of the American Medical Association, 290,* 1519–1520.

Dodge, K. D., & Jaccard, J. J. (2006). The effect of high school sports participation on the use of performance enhancing substances in young adulthood. *Journal of Adolescent Health, 39,* 367–373.

Dugoua, J., Mills, E., Perri, D., & Koren, G. (2006). Safety and efficacy of St. John's Wort (hypericum) during pregnancy. *Canadian Journal of Clinical Pharmacology, 13,* e268–e276.

Engdal, S., Klepp, O., & Nilsen, O. G. (2009). Identification and exploration of herb-drug combinations used by cancer patients. *Integrative Cancer Therapies, 8,* 29–36.

Food and Drug Administration. (2001). *Overview of dietary supplements.* Retrieved April 27, 2009, from http://www.cfsan.fda .gov/~dms/ds-oview.html#what

Food and Drug Administration (FDA). (2003). *Claims that can be made for conventional foods and dietary supplements.* Retrieved April 27, 2009, from http://www.cfsan.fda.gov/~dms/ hclaims.html

Food and Drug Administration. (2007). *Dietary supplements: Warnings and safety information.* Retrieved April 27, 2009, from www.cfsan .fda.gov/~dms/ds-warn.html

Gardiner, P. (2005). Dietary supplement use in children: Concerns of efficacy and safety. *American Family Physician, 71,* 1068–1071.

Gardiner, P., Buettner, C., Davis, R. B., Phillips, R. S., & Kemper, K. J. (2008). Factors and common conditions associated with adolescent dietary supplement use: An analysis of the National Health and Nutrition Exam Survey (NHANES). *BMC Complementary and Alternative Medicine, 31,* 9.

Gardiner, P., Phillips, R., & Shaughnessy, A. F. (2008). Herbal and dietary supplement-drug interactions in patients with chronic conditions. *American Family Physician, 77,* 73–78.

Gilroy, C. M., Steiner, J. F., Byers, T., Shapiro, H., & Georgian, W. (2003). Echinacea and truth in labeling. *Archives of Internal Medicine, 163,* 699–704.

Gurib-Fakim, A. (2006). Medicinal plants: Traditions of yesterday and drugs of tomorrow. *Molecular Aspects of Medicine, 27,* 1–93.

Hardy, M. L. (2008). Dietary supplement use in cancer care: Help or harm? *Hematology/Oncology Clinics of North America, 22,* 581–617.

Harkey, M. R., Henderson, G. L., Gershwin, M. E., Stern, J. S., & Hackman, R. M. (2001). Variability in commercial ginseng products: An analysis of 25 preparations. *American Journal of Clinical Nutrition, 73,* 1101–1106.

Harris, A. B. (2005). Evidence of increasing dietary supplement use in children with special health care needs: Strategies for improving parent and professional communication. *Journal of the American Dietetic Association, 105,* 34–37.

Hlebowicz, J., Darwiche, G., Bjorgell, O., & Almer, L. O. (2007). Effect of cinnamon on postprandial blood glucose, gastric emptying, and satiety in healthy subjects. *American Journal of Clinical Nutrition, 85(6),* 1552–1556.

Hlebowicz, J., Hlebowicz, A., Lindstedt, S., Bjorgell, O., Hoglund, P., Holst, J. J., et al. (2009). Effects of 1 and 3 g of cinnamon on gastric emptying, satiety, and postprandial glucose, insulin, glucose-dependent insulinotropic polypeptide, glucagons-like peptide 1, and ghrelin concentrations in healthy subjects. *American Journal of Clinical Nutrition, 89,* 815–821.

Kelly, J. P., Kaufman, D. W., Kelley, K., Rosenberg, L., Anderson T. E., & Mitchell, A. A. (2005). Recent trends in use of herbal and other natural products. *Archives of Internal Medicine, 165,* 281–286.

Kemper, K. J., Gardiner, P., Gobble, J., & Woods, C. (2006). Expertise about herbs and dietary supplements among diverse health professionals. *BioMed Central Complementary and Alternative Medicine, 6,* 15.

Kennedy, J., Wang, C. C., & Wu, C. H. (2008). Patient disclosure about herb and supplement use among adults in the U.S. *Evidence-Based Complementary and Alternative Medicine, 5,* 451–456.

Khan, A., Safdar, M., Ali Khan, M. M., Khattak, K. N., & Anderson, R. A. (2003). Cinnamon improves glucose and lipids in people with type 2 diabetes. *Diabetes Care, 26(12),* 3215–3218.

Krochmal, R., Hardy, M., Bowerman, S., Lu, Q., Wang, H., Elashoff, R. M. et al. (2004). Phytochemical assays of commercial botanical dietary supplements. *Evidence-Based Complementary and Alternative Medicine, 1,* 305–313.

Low Dog, T. (2005). Menopause: A review of botanical dietary supplements. *American Journal of Medicine, 118,* 985–1085.

Low Dog, T. (2009). The use of botanicals during pregnancy and lactation. *Alternative Therapies in Health and Medicine, 15,* 54–58.

Mahady, G. B., Low Dog, T., Barrett, M. L., Chavez, M. L., Gardiner, P., Ko, R. et al. (2008). United States Pharmacopeia review of black cohosh case reports of hepatotoxicity. *Menopause, 15,* 628–638.

Mang, B., Wolters, M., Schmitt, B., Kelb, K., Lichtinghagen, R., Stichtenoth, D. O., et al. (2006). Effects of cinnamon extract on plasma glucose, HbA, and serum lipids in diabetes mellitus type 2. *European Journal of Clinical Investigation, 36(5),* 340–344.

Messina, M. J., & Wood, C. E. (2008). Soy isoflavones, estrogen therapy, and breast cancer risk: Analysis and commentary. *Nutrition Journal, 7,* 17.

Morris, C. A., & Avorn, J. (2003). Internet marketing of herbal products. *Journal of the American Medical Association, 290,* 1505–1509.

National Center for Complementary and Alternative (NCCAM), National Institutes of Health. (2008a). *The use of complementary and alternative medicine in the United States.* Retrieved March 1, 2009, from http:// nccam.nih.gov/news/camstats/2007/ camsurvey_fs1.htm

National Center for Complementary and Alternative Medicine (NCCAM), National Institutes of Health. (2008b). *Menopausal symptoms and CAM.* Retrieved March 11, 2009, from http://nccam.nih.gov/health/ menopause/menopausesymptoms.htm

National Center for Complementary and Alternative Medicine (NCCAM), National Institutes of Health. (2009). *Using dietary supplements wisely.* March 11, 2009, from http://nccam.nih.gov/health/supplements/ wiseuse.htm

National Institutes of Health (NIH), Office of Dietary Supplements. (2006). *Botanical dietary supplements: Background information.* Retrieved March 11, 2009, from http://ods .od.nih.gov/factsheets/BotanicalBackground_ pf.asp

Nelson, H. D., Vesco, K. K., Haney, E., Fu, R., Nedow, A., Miller, J., et al. (2006). Nonhormonal therapies for menopausal hot flashes: Systematic review and meta-analysis. *Journal of the American Medical Association, 295,* 2057–2071.

Nutrition Business Journal. (2007). *Nutrition segment sales.* Retrieved April 27, 2009, from http://www.nutritionbusiness.com

Pham, A. Q., Kourlas, H., & Pham, D. Q. (2007). Cinnamon supplementation in patients with type 2 diabetes mellitus. *Pharmacotherapy, 27(4),* 595–599.

Pilliteri, J. L., Shiffman, S., Rohay, J. M., Harkins, A. M., Burton, S. L., & Wadden, T. A. (2008). Use of dietary supplements for

REFERENCES *(continued)*

weight loss in the United States: Results of a national survey. *Obesity, 16,* 790–796.

Qato, D. M., Alexander, G. D., Conti, R. M., Johnson, M., Schumm, P., & Lindau, S. T. (2008). Use of prescription and over-the-counter medications and dietary supplements among older adults in the United States. *Journal of the American Medical Association, 300,* 2867–2878.

Reed, S. D., Newton, K. M., LaCroix, A. Z., Grothaus, L. C., Grieco, V. S., & Ehrlich, K. (2008). Vaginal, endometrial, and reproductive hormone findings: Randomized, placebo-controlled trial of black cohosh, multibotanical herbs, and dietary soy for vasomotor symptoms: The Herbal Alternatives for Menopause (HALT) Study. *Menopause, 15,* 51–58.

Reepmeyer, J. C., & d'Avignon, D. A. (2009). Structure elucidation of thioketone analogues of sildenafil detected as adulterants in herbal aphrodisiacs. *Journal of Pharmaceutical and Biomedical Analysis, 49,* 145–150.

Saper, R. B., Kales, S. N., Paquin, J., Burns, M. J., Eisenburg, D. M., Davis, R. B., et al. (2004). Heavy metal content of Ayurvedic herbal medicine products. *Journal of the American Medical Association, 292,* 2868–2873.

Singh, S. R., & Levine, M. A. (2006). Natural health product use in Canada: Analysis of the National Population Health Survey. *Canadian Journal of Clinical Pharmacology, 13,* e240–e250.

Sood, A., Sood, R., Brinker, F. J., Mann, R., Loehrer, L. L., & Wahner-Roedler, D. L. (2008). Potential for interactions between dietary supplements and prescription medications. *American Journal of Medicine, 121,* 207–211.

Thurston, C. (2008). Dietary supplements: The latest trends & issues. *Nutraceuticals World.* Retrieved March 1, 2009, from http://www .nutraceuticalsworld.com/articles/2008/04/ dietary-supplements-the-latest-trends-issues

Vanschoonbeek, K., Thomassen, B. J., Senden, J. M., Wodzig, W. K., & van Loon, L. J. (2006). Cinnamon supplementation does not improve glycemic control in postmenopausal type 2 diabetes patients. *Journal of Nutrition, 136*(4), 977–980.

Vassilev, Z. P., Chu, A. F., Ruck, B., Adams, E. H., & Marcus, S. M. (2009). Evaluation of adverse drug reactions reported to a poison control center between 2000 and 2007. *American Journal of Health-System Pharmacy, 66,* 481–487.

Wold, R. S., Lopez, S. T., Yau, L., Butler, L. M., Pareo-Tubbeh, S. L., Waters, D. L., et al. (2005). Increasing trends in elderly persons' use of nonvitamin, nonmineral dietary supplements and concurrent use of medications. *Journal of the American Dietetic Association, 105,* 54–63.

Woolf, A. D. (2003). Herbal remedies and children: Do they work? Are they harmful? *Pediatrics, 112,* 240–246.

World Health Organization (WHO). (2008). *Traditional medicine.* Retrieved April 27, 2009, from http://www.who.int/mediacentre/ factsheets/fs134/en

Wu, K. M., Farrelly, J. G., Upton, R., & Chen, J. (2007). Complexities of the herbal nomenclature system in traditional Chinese medicine: Lessons learned from the misuse of Aristolochia-related species and the importance of pharmaceutical name during botanical drug product development. *Phytomedicine, 14,* 273–279.

Appendix A

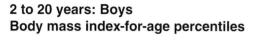

2 to 20 years: Boys
Body mass index-for-age percentiles

NAME _____

RECORD # _____

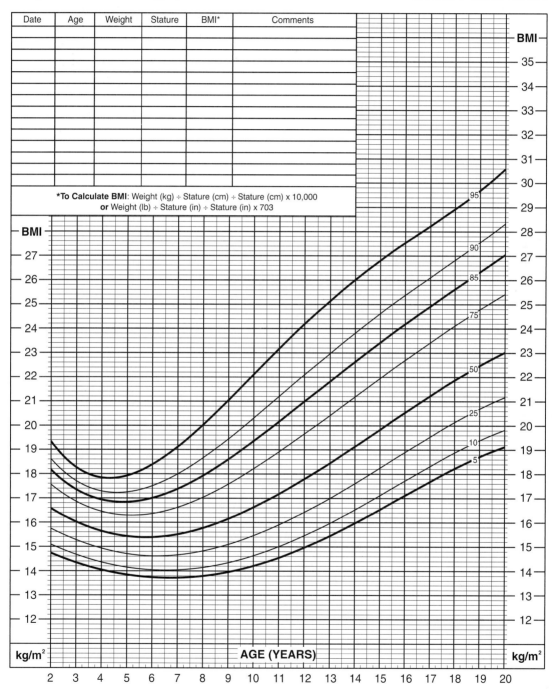

Date	Age	Weight	Stature	BMI*	Comments

*To Calculate BMI: Weight (kg) ÷ Stature (cm) ÷ Stature (cm) x 10,000
or Weight (lb) ÷ Stature (in) ÷ Stature (in) x 703

AGE (YEARS)

Published May 30, 2000 (modified 10/16/00).
SOURCE: Developed by the National Center for Health Statistics in collaboration with
the National Center for Chronic Disease Prevention and Health Promotion (2000).
http://www.cdc.gov/growthcharts

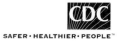

SAFER · HEALTHIER · PEOPLE™

577

2 to 20 years: Girls
Body mass index-for-age percentiles

NAME _____

RECORD # _____

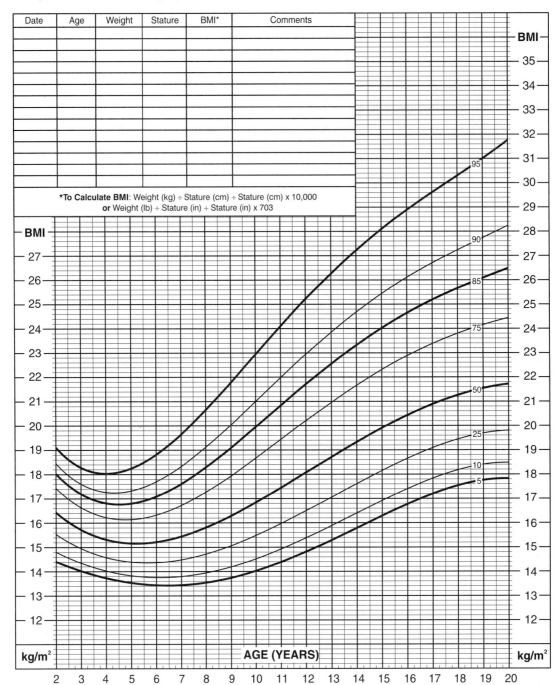

Date	Age	Weight	Stature	BMI*	Comments

*To Calculate BMI: Weight (kg) ÷ Stature (cm) ÷ Stature (cm) x 10,000
or Weight (lb) ÷ Stature (in) ÷ Stature (in) x 703

AGE (YEARS)

Published May 30, 2000 (modified 10/16/00).
SOURCE: Developed by the National Center for Health Statistics in collaboration with
the National Center for Chronic Disease Prevention and Health Promotion (2000).
http://www.cdc.gov/growthcharts

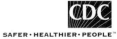

SAFER · HEALTHIER · PEOPLE™

2 to 20 years: Girls
Stature-for-age and Weight-for-age percentiles

NAME _____

RECORD # _____

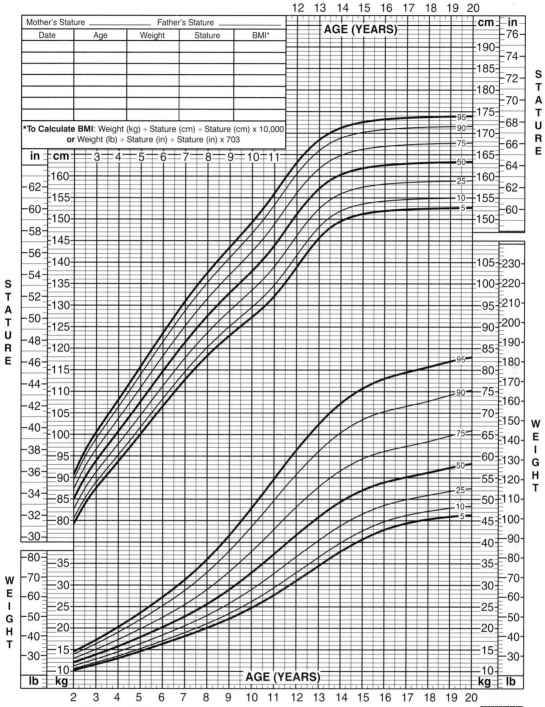

*To Calculate BMI: Weight (kg) ÷ Stature (cm) ÷ Stature (cm) x 10,000
or Weight (lb) ÷ Stature (in) ÷ Stature (in) x 703

Published May 30, 2000 (modified 11/21/00).

SOURCE: Developed by the National Center for Health Statistics in collaboration with
the National Center for Chronic Disease Prevention and Health Promotion (2000).
http://www.cdc.gov/growthcharts

CDC

SAFER · HEALTHIER · PEOPLE™

2 to 20 years: Boys
Stature-for-age and Weight-for-age percentiles

NAME _____

RECORD # _____

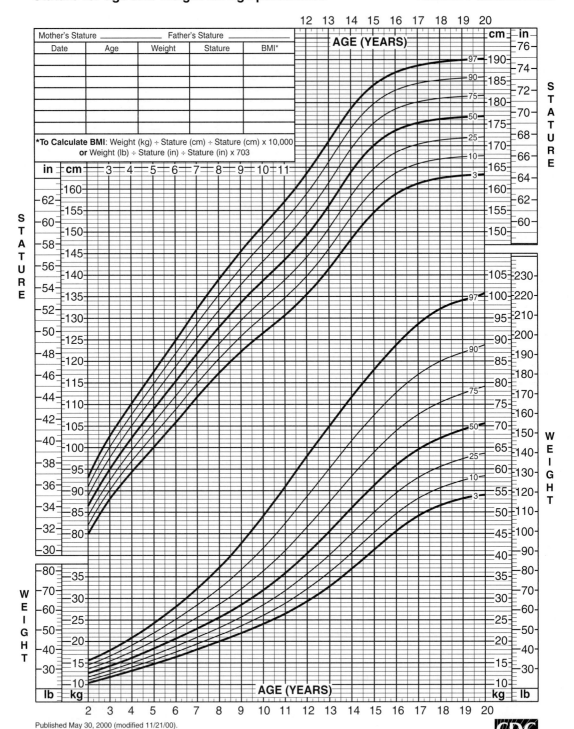

*To Calculate BMI**: Weight (kg) ÷ Stature (cm) ÷ Stature (cm) x 10,000
or Weight (lb) ÷ Stature (in) ÷ Stature (in) x 703

Published May 30, 2000 (modified 11/21/00).
SOURCE: Developed by the National Center for Health Statistics in collaboration with
the National Center for Chronic Disease Prevention and Health Promotion (2000).
http://www.cdc.gov/growthcharts

CDC
SAFER · HEALTHIER · PEOPLE™

Appendix B

Body Mass Index Table

Height (inches)	Normal						Overweight					Obese										Extreme Obesity															
BMI	19	20	21	22	23	24	25	26	27	28	29	30	31	32	33	34	35	36	37	38	39	40	41	42	43	44	45	46	47	48	49	50	51	52	53	54
												Body Weight (pounds)																								
58	91	96	100	105	110	115	119	124	129	134	138	143	148	153	158	162	167	172	177	181	186	191	196	201	205	210	215	220	224	229	234	239	244	248	253	258
59	94	99	104	109	114	119	124	128	133	138	143	148	153	158	163	168	173	178	183	188	193	198	203	208	212	217	222	227	232	237	242	247	252	257	262	267
60	97	102	107	112	118	123	128	133	138	143	148	153	158	163	168	174	179	184	189	194	199	204	209	215	220	225	230	235	240	245	250	255	261	266	271	276
61	100	106	111	116	122	127	132	137	143	148	153	158	164	169	174	180	185	190	195	201	206	211	217	222	227	232	238	243	248	254	259	264	269	275	280	285
62	104	109	115	120	126	131	136	142	147	153	158	164	169	175	180	186	191	196	202	207	213	218	224	229	235	240	246	251	256	262	267	273	278	284	289	295
63	107	113	118	124	130	135	141	146	152	158	163	169	175	180	186	191	197	203	208	214	220	225	231	237	242	248	254	259	265	270	278	282	287	293	299	304
64	110	116	122	128	134	140	145	151	157	163	169	174	180	186	192	197	204	209	215	221	227	232	238	244	250	256	262	267	273	279	285	291	296	302	308	314
65	114	120	126	132	138	144	150	156	162	168	174	180	186	192	198	204	210	216	222	228	234	240	246	252	258	264	270	276	282	288	294	300	306	312	318	324
66	118	124	130	136	142	148	155	161	167	173	179	186	192	198	204	210	216	223	229	235	241	247	253	260	266	272	278	284	291	297	303	309	315	322	328	334
67	121	127	134	140	146	153	159	166	172	178	185	191	198	204	211	217	223	230	236	242	249	255	261	268	274	280	287	293	299	306	312	319	325	331	338	344
68	125	131	138	144	151	158	164	171	177	184	190	197	203	210	216	223	230	236	243	249	256	262	269	276	282	289	295	302	308	315	322	328	335	341	348	354
69	128	135	142	149	155	162	169	176	182	189	196	203	209	216	223	230	236	243	250	257	263	270	277	284	291	297	304	311	318	324	331	338	345	351	358	365
70	132	139	146	153	160	167	174	181	188	195	202	209	216	222	229	236	243	250	257	264	271	278	285	292	299	306	313	320	327	334	341	348	355	362	369	376
71	136	143	150	157	165	172	179	186	193	200	208	215	222	229	236	243	250	257	265	272	279	286	293	301	308	315	322	329	338	343	351	358	365	372	379	386
72	140	147	154	162	169	177	184	191	199	206	213	221	228	235	242	250	258	265	272	279	287	294	302	309	316	324	331	338	346	353	361	368	375	383	390	397
73	144	151	159	166	174	182	189	197	204	212	219	227	235	242	250	257	265	272	280	288	295	302	310	318	325	333	340	348	355	363	371	378	386	393	401	408
74	148	155	163	171	179	186	194	202	210	218	225	233	241	249	256	264	272	280	287	295	303	311	319	326	334	342	350	358	365	373	381	389	396	404	412	420
75	152	160	168	176	184	192	200	208	216	224	232	240	248	256	264	272	279	287	295	303	311	319	327	335	343	351	359	367	375	383	391	399	407	415	423	431
76	156	164	172	180	189	197	205	213	221	230	238	246	254	263	271	279	287	295	304	312	320	328	336	344	353	361	369	377	385	394	402	410	418	426	435	443

Source: Adapted from *Clinical Guidelines on the Identification, Evaluation, and Treatment of Overweight and Obesity in Adults: The Evidence Report.*

Appendix C

Dietary Reference Intakes (DRIs): Recommended Intakes for Individuals, Vitamins
Food and Nutrition Board, Institute of Medicine, National Academies

Life Stage Group	Vit A (µg/d)[a]	Vit C (mg/d)	Vit D (µg/d)[b,c]	Vit E (mg/d)[d]	Vit K (µg/d)	Thiamin (mg/d)	Riboflavin (mg/d)	Niacin (mg/d)[e]	Vit B6 (mg/d)	Folate (µg/d)[f]	Vit B12 (µg/d)	Pantothenic Acid (mg/d)	Biotin (µg/d)	Choline[g] (mg/d)
Infants														
0–6 mo	400*	40*	5*	4*	2.0*	0.2*	0.3*	2*	0.1*	65*	0.4*	1.7*	5*	125*
7–12 mo	500*	50*	5*	5*	2.5*	0.3*	0.4*	4*	0.3*	80*	0.5*	1.8*	6*	150*
Children														
1–3 y	300	15	5*	6	30*	0.5	0.5	6	0.5	150	0.9	2*	8*	200*
4–8 y	400	25	5*	7	55*	0.6	0.6	8	0.6	200	1.2	3*	12*	250*
Males														
9–13 y	600	45	5*	11	60*	0.9	0.9	12	1.0	300	1.8	4*	20*	375*
14–18 y	900	75	5*	15	75*	1.2	1.3	16	1.3	400	2.4	5*	25*	550*
19–30 y	900	90	5*	15	120*	1.2	1.3	16	1.3	400	2.4	5*	30*	550*
31–50 y	900	90	5*	15	120*	1.2	1.3	16	1.3	400	2.4	5*	30*	550*
51–70 y	900	90	10*	15	120*	1.2	1.3	16	1.7	400	2.4[i]	5*	30*	550*
>70 y	900	90	15*	15	120*	1.2	1.3	16	1.7	400	2.4[i]	5*	30*	550*
Females														
9–13 y	600	45	5*	11	60*	0.9	0.9	12	1.0	300	1.8	4*	20*	375*
14–18 y	700	65	5*	15	75*	1.0	1.0	14	1.2	400[i]	2.4	5*	25*	400*
19–30 y	700	75	5*	15	90*	1.1	1.1	14	1.3	400[i]	2.4	5*	30*	425*
31–50 y	700	75	5*	15	90*	1.1	1.1	14	1.3	400[i]	2.4	5*	30*	425*
51–70 y	700	75	10*	15	90*	1.1	1.1	14	1.5	400	2.4[h]	5*	30*	425*
>70 y	700	75	15*	15	90*	1.1	1.1	14	1.5	400	2.4[h]	5*	30*	425*
Pregnancy														
14–18 y	750	80	5*	15	75*	1.4	1.4	18	1.9	600[i]	2.6	6*	30*	450*
19–30 y	770	85	5*	15	90*	1.4	1.4	18	1.9	600[i]	2.6	6*	30*	450*
31–50 y	770	85	5*	15	90*	1.4	1.4	18	1.9	600[i]	2.6	6*	30*	450*
Lactation														
14–18 y	1,200	115	5*	19	75*	1.4	1.6	17	2.0	500	2.8	7*	35*	550*
19–30 y	1,300	120	5*	19	90*	1.4	1.6	17	2.0	500	2.8	7*	35*	550*
31–50 y	1,300	120	5*	19	90*	1.4	1.6	17	2.0	500	2.8	7*	35*	550*

NOTE: This table (taken from the DRI reports, see www.nap.edu) presents Recommended Dietary Allowances (RDAs) in **bold type** and Adequate Intakes (AIs) in ordinary type followed by an asterisk (*). RDAs and AIs may both be used as goals for individual intake. RDAs are set to meet the needs of almost all (97 to 98 percent) individuals in a group. For healthy breastfed infants, the AI is the mean intake. The AI for other life stage and gender groups is believed to cover needs of all individuals in the group, but lack of data or uncertainty in the data prevent being able to specify with confidence the percentage of individuals covered by this intake.

[a] As retinol activity equivalents (RAEs). 1 RAE = 1 µg retinol, 12 µg β-carotene, 24 µg α-carotene, or 24 µg β-cryptoxanthin. The RAE for dietary provitamin A carotenoids is twofold greater than retinol equivalents (RE), whereas the RAE for preformed vitamin A is the same as RE.

[b] As cholecalciferol. 1 µg cholecalciferol = 40 IU vitamin D.

[c] In the absence of adequate exposure to sunlight.

[d] As α-tocopherol. α-Tocopherol includes *RRR*-α-tocopherol, the only form of α-tocopherol that occurs naturally in foods, and the *2R*-stereoisomeric forms of α-tocopherol (*RRR*-, *RSR*-, *RRS*-, and *RSS*-α-tocopherol) that occur in fortified foods and supplements. It does not include the *2S*-stereoisomeric forms of α-tocopherol (*SRR*-, *SSR*-, *SRS*-, and *SSS*-α-tocopherol), also found in fortified foods and supplements.

[e] As niacin equivalents (NE). 1 mg of niacin = 60 mg of tryptophan; 0–6 months = preformed niacin (not NE).

[f] As dietary folate equivalents (DFE). 1 DFE = 1 µg food folate = 0.6 µg of folic acid from fortified food or as a supplement consumed with food = 0.5 µg of a supplement taken on an empty stomach.

[g] Although AIs have been set for choline, there are few data to assess whether a dietary supply of choline is needed at all stages of the life cycle, and it may be that the choline requirement can be met by endogenous synthesis at some of these stages.

[h] Because 10 to 30 percent of older people may malabsorb food-bound B₁₂, it is advisable for those older than 50 years to meet their RDA mainly by consuming foods fortified with B₁₂ or a supplement containing B₁₂.

[i] In view of evidence linking folate intake with neural tube defects in the fetus, it is recommended that all women capable of becoming pregnant consume 400 µg from supplements or fortified foods in addition to intake of food folate from a varied diet.

[j] It is assumed that women will continue consuming 400 µg from supplements or fortified food until their pregnancy is confirmed and they enter prenatal care, which ordinarily occurs after the end of the periconceptional period—the critical time for formation of the neural tube.

Copyright 2004 by the National Academy of Sciences. All rights reserved.

Dietary Reference Intakes (DRIs): Recommended Intakes for Individuals, Elements
Food and Nutrition Board, Institute of Medicine, National Academies

Life Stage Group	Calcium (mg/d)	Chromium (µg/d)	Copper (µg/d)	Fluoride (mg/d)	Iodine (µg/d)	Iron (mg/d)	Magnesium (mg/d)	Manganese (mg/d)	Molybdenum (µg/d)	Phosphorus (mg/d)	Selenium (µg/d)	Zinc (mg/d)	Potassium (g/d)	Sodium (g/d)	Chloride (g/d)
Infants															
0–6 mo	210*	0.2*	200*	0.01*	110*	0.27*	30*	0.003*	2*	100*	15*	2*	0.4*	0.12*	0.18*
7–12 mo	270*	5.5*	220*	0.5*	130*	11	75*	0.6*	3*	275*	20*	3	0.7*	0.37*	0.57*
Children															
1–3 y	500*	11*	340	0.7*	90	7	80	1.2*	17	460	20	3	3.0*	1.0*	1.5*
4–8 y	800*	15*	440	1*	90	10	130	1.5*	22	500	30	5	3.8*	1.2*	1.9*
Males															
9–13 y	1,300*	25*	700	2*	120	8	240	1.9*	34	1,250	40	8	4.5*	1.5*	2.3*
14–18 y	1,300*	35*	890	3*	150	11	410	2.2*	43	1,250	55	11	4.7*	1.5*	2.3*
19–30 y	1,000*	35*	900	4*	150	8	400	2.3*	45	700	55	11	4.7*	1.5*	2.3*
31–50 y	1,000*	35*	900	4*	150	8	420	2.3*	45	700	55	11	4.7*	1.5*	2.3*
51–70 y	1,200*	30*	900	4*	150	8	420	2.3*	45	700	55	11	4.7*	1.3*	2.0*
>70 y	1,200*	30*	900	4*	150	8	420	2.3*	45	700	55	11	4.7*	1.2*	1.8*
Females															
9–13 y	1,300*	21*	700	2*	120	8	240	1.6*	34	1,250	40	8	4.5*	1.5*	2.3*
14–18 y	1,300*	24*	890	3*	150	15	360	1.6*	43	1,250	55	9	4.7*	1.5*	2.3*
19–30 y	1,000*	25*	900	3*	150	18	310	1.8*	45	700	55	8	4.7*	1.5*	2.3*
31–50 y	1,000*	25*	900	3*	150	18	320	1.8*	45	700	55	8	4.7*	1.5*	2.3*
51–70 y	1,200*	20*	900	3*	150	8	320	1.8*	45	700	55	8	4.7*	1.3*	2.0*
>70 y	1,200*	20*	900	3*	150	8	320	1.8*	45	700	55	8	4.7*	1.2*	1.8*
Pregnancy															
14–18 y	1,300*	29*	1,000	3*	220	27	400	2.0*	50	1,250	60	12	4.7*	1.5*	2.3*
19–30 y	1,000*	30*	1,000	3*	220	27	350	2.0*	50	700	60	11	4.7*	1.5*	2.3*
31–50 y	1,000*	30*	1,000	3*	220	27	360	2.0*	50	700	60	11	4.7*	1.5*	2.3*
Lactation															
14–18 y	1,300*	44*	1,300	3*	290	10	360	2.6*	50	1,250	70	13	5.1*	1.5*	2.3*
19–30 y	1,000*	45*	1,300	3*	290	9	310	2.6*	50	700	70	12	5.1*	1.5*	2.3*
31–50 y	1,000*	45*	1,300	3*	290	9	320	2.6*	50	700	70	12	5.1*	1.5*	2.3*

NOTE: This table presents Recommended Dietary Allowances (RDAs) in **bold type** and Adequate Intakes (AIs) in ordinary type followed by an asterisk (*). RDAs and AIs may both be used as goals for individual intake. RDAs are set to meet the needs of almost all (97 to 98 percent) individuals in a group. For healthy breastfed infants, the AI is the mean intake. The AI for other life stage and gender groups is believed to cover needs of all individuals in the group, but lack of data or uncertainty in the data prevent being able to specify with confidence the percentage of individuals covered by this intake.

SOURCES: *Dietary Reference Intakes for Calcium, Phosphorous, Magnesium, Vitamin D, and Fluoride* (1997); *Dietary Reference Intakes for Thiamin, Riboflavin, Niacin, Vitamin B₆, Folate, Vitamin B₁₂, Pantothenic Acid, Biotin, and Choline* (1998); *Dietary Reference Intakes for Vitamin C, Vitamin E, Selenium, and Carotenoids* (2000); *Dietary Reference Intakes for Vitamin A, Vitamin K, Arsenic, Boron, Chromium, Copper, Iodine, Iron, Manganese, Molybdenum, Nickel, Silicon, Vanadium, and Zinc* (2001); and *Dietary Reference Intakes for Water, Potassium, Sodium, Chloride, and Sulfate* (2004). These reports may be accessed via http://www.nap.edu.

Copyright 2004 by the National Academy of Sciences. All rights reserved.

Dietary Reference Intakes (DRIs): Tolerable Upper Intake Levels (UL^a), Vitamins
Food and Nutrition Board, Institute of Medicine, National Academies

Life Stage Group	Vitamin A (μg/d)[b]	Vitamin C (mg/d)	Vitamin D (μg/d)	Vitamin E (mg/d)[c,d]	Vitamin K	Thiamin	Riboflavin	Niacin (mg/d)[d]	Vitamin B_6 (mg/d)	Folate (μg/d)[d]	Vitamin B_{12}	Pantothenic Acid	Biotin	Choline (g/d)	Carotenoids[e]
Infants															
0–6 mo	600	ND[f]	25	ND	ND	ND	ND	ND	ND	ND	ND	ND	ND	ND	ND
7–12 mo	600	ND	25	ND	ND	ND	ND	ND	ND	ND	ND	ND	ND	ND	ND
Children															
1–3 y	600	400	50	200	ND	ND	ND	10	30	300	ND	ND	ND	1.0	ND
4–8 y	900	650	50	300	ND	ND	ND	15	40	400	ND	ND	ND	1.0	ND
Males, Females															
9–13 y	1,700	1,200	50	600	ND	ND	ND	20	60	600	ND	ND	ND	2.0	ND
14–18 y	2,800	1,800	50	800	ND	ND	ND	30	80	800	ND	ND	ND	3.0	ND
19–70 y	3,000	2,000	50	1,000	ND	ND	ND	35	100	1,000	ND	ND	ND	3.5	ND
> 70 y	3,000	2,000	50	1,000	ND	ND	ND	35	100	1,000	ND	ND	ND	3.5	ND
Pregnancy															
14–18 y	2,800	1,800	50	800	ND	ND	ND	30	80	800	ND	ND	ND	3.0	ND
19–50 y	3,000	2,000	50	1,000	ND	ND	ND	35	100	1,000	ND	ND	ND	3.5	ND
Lactation															
14–18 y	2,800	1,800	50	800	ND	ND	ND	30	80	800	ND	ND	ND	3.0	ND
19–50 y	3,000	2,000	50	1,000	ND	ND	ND	35	100	1,000	ND	ND	ND	3.5	ND

[a] UL = The maximum level of daily nutrient intake that is likely to pose no risk of adverse effects. Unless otherwise specified, the UL represents total intake from food, water, and supplements. Due to lack of suitable data, ULs could not be established for vitamin K, thiamin, riboflavin, vitamin B_{12}, pantothenic acid, biotin, carotenoids. In the absence of ULs, extra caution may be warranted in consuming levels above recommended intakes.

[b] As preformed vitamin A only.

[c] As α-tocopherol; applies to any form of supplemental α-tocopherol.

[d] The ULs for vitamin E, niacin, and folate apply to synthetic forms obtained from supplements, fortified foods, or a combination of the two.

[e] β-Carotene supplements are advised only to serve as a provitamin A source for individuals at risk of vitamin A deficiency.

[f] ND = Not determinable due to lack of data of adverse effects in this age group and concern with regard to lack of ability to handle excess amounts. Source of intake should be from food only to prevent high levels of intake.

SOURCES: *Dietary Reference Intakes for Calcium, Phosphorous, Magnesium, Vitamin D, and Fluoride* (1997); *Dietary Reference Intakes for Thiamin, Riboflavin, Niacin, Vitamin B_6, Folate, Vitamin B_{12}, Pantothenic Acid, Biotin, and Choline* (1998); *Dietary Reference Intakes for Vitamin C, Vitamin E, Selenium, and Carotenoids* (2000); and *Dietary Reference Intakes for Vitamin A, Vitamin K, Arsenic, Boron, Chromium, Copper, Iodine, Iron, Manganese, Molybdenum, Nickel, Silicon, Vanadium, and Zinc* (2001). These reports may be accessed via http://www.nap.edu.

Copyright 2004 by the National Academy of Sciences. All rights reserved.

Dietary Reference Intakes (DRIs): Tolerable Upper Intake Levels (UL^a), Elements
Food and Nutrition Board, Institute of Medicine, National Academies

Life Stage Group	Arsenic^b	Boron (mg/d)	Calcium (g/d)	Chromium	Copper (µg/d)	Fluoride (mg/d)	Iodine (µg/d)	Iron (mg/d)	Magnesium (mg/d)^c	Manganese (mg/d)	Molybdenum (µg/d)	Nickel (mg/d)	Phosphorus (g/d)	Potassium	Selenium (µg/d)	Silicon^d	Sulfate	Vanadium (mg/d)^e	Zinc (mg/d)	Sodium (g/d)	Chloride (g/d)
Infants																					
0–6 mo	ND^f	ND	ND	ND	ND	0.7	ND	40	ND	ND	ND	ND	ND	ND	45	ND	ND	ND	4	ND	ND
7–12 mo	ND	ND	ND	ND	ND	0.9	ND	40	ND	ND	ND	ND	ND	ND	60	ND	ND	ND	5	ND	ND
Children																					
1–3 y	ND	3	2.5	ND	1,000	1.3	200	40	65	2	300	0.2	3	ND	90	ND	ND	ND	7	1.5	2.3
4–8 y	ND	6	2.5	ND	3,000	2.2	300	40	110	3	600	0.3	3	ND	150	ND	ND	ND	12	1.9	2.9
Males, Females																					
9–13 y	ND	11	2.5	ND	5,000	10	600	40	350	6	1,100	0.6	4	ND	280	ND	ND	ND	23	2.2	3.4
14–18 y	ND	17	2.5	ND	8,000	10	900	45	350	9	1,700	1.0	4	ND	400	ND	ND	ND	34	2.3	3.6
19–70 y	ND	20	2.5	ND	10,000	10	1,100	45	350	11	2,000	1.0	4	ND	400	ND	ND	1.8	40	2.3	3.6
>70 y	ND	20	2.5	ND	10,000	10	1,100	45	350	11	2,000	1.0	3	ND	400	ND	ND	1.8	40	2.3	3.6
Pregnancy																					
14–18 y	ND	17	2.5	ND	8,000	10	900	45	350	9	1,700	1.0	3.5	ND	400	ND	ND	ND	34	2.3	3.6
19–50 y	ND	20	2.5	ND	10,000	10	1,100	45	350	11	2,000	1.0	3.5	ND	400	ND	ND	ND	40	2.3	3.6
Lactation																					
14–18 y	ND	17	2.5	ND	8,000	10	900	45	350	9	1,700	1.0	4	ND	400	ND	ND	ND	34	2.3	3.6
19–50 y	ND	20	2.5	ND	10,000	10	1,100	45	350	11	2,000	1.0	4	ND	400	ND	ND	ND	40	2.3	3.6

^{a} UL = The maximum level of daily nutrient intake that is likely to pose no risk of adverse effects. Unless otherwise specified, the UL represents total intake from food, water, and supplements. Due to lack of suitable data, ULs could not be established for arsenic, chromium, silicon, potassium, and sulfate. In the absence of ULs, extra caution may be warranted in consuming levels above recommended intakes.

^{b} Although the UL was not determined for arsenic, there is no justification for adding arsenic to food or supplements.

^{c} The ULs for magnesium represent intake from a pharmacological agent only and do not include intake from food and water.

^{d} Although silicon has not been shown to cause adverse effects in humans, there is no justification for adding silicon to supplements.

^{e} Although vanadium in food has not been shown to cause adverse effects in humans, there is no justification for adding vanadium to food and vanadium supplements should be used with caution. The UL is based on adverse effects in laboratory animals and this data could be used to set a UL for adults but not children and adolescents.

^{f} ND = Not determinable due to lack of data of adverse effects in this age group and concern with regard to lack of ability to handle excess amounts. Source of intake should be from food only to prevent high levels of intake.

SOURCES: *Dietary Reference Intakes for Calcium, Phosphorous, Magnesium, Vitamin D, and Fluoride* (1997); *Dietary Reference Intakes for Thiamin, Riboflavin, Niacin, Vitamin B$_6$, Folate, Vitamin B$_{12}$, Pantothenic Acid, Biotin, and Choline* (1998); *Dietary Reference Intakes for Vitamin C, Vitamin E, Selenium, and Carotenoids* (2000); *Dietary Reference Intakes for Vitamin A, Vitamin K, Arsenic, Boron, Chromium, Copper, Iodine, Iron, Manganese, Molybdenum, Nickel, Silicon, Vanadium, and Zinc* (2001); and *Dietary Reference Intakes for Water, Potassium, Sodium, Chloride, and Sulfate* (2004). These reports may be accessed via http://www.nap.edu.

Copyright 2004 by the National Academy of Sciences. All rights reserved.

Dietary Reference Intakes (DRIs): Estimated Average Requirements for Groups
Food and Nutrition Board, Institute of Medicine, National Academies

Life Stage Group	CHO (g/d)a	Protein (g/d)a	Vit A (µg/d)b	Vit C (mg/d)	Vit E (mg/d)c	Thiamin (mg/d)	Riboflavin (mg/d)	Niacin (mg/d)d	Vit B6 (mg/d)	Folate (µg/d)b	Vit B12 (µg/d)	Copper (µg/d)	Iodine (µg/d)	Iron (mg/d)	Magnesium (mg/d)	Molybdenum (µg/d)	Phosphorus (mg/d)	Selenium (µg/d)	Zinc (mg/d)
Infants																			
7–12 mo		9*												6.9					2.5
Children																			
1–3 y	100	11	210	13	5	0.4	0.4	5	0.4	120	0.7	260	65	3.0	65	13	380	17	2.5
4–8 y	100	15	275	22	6	0.5	0.5	6	0.5	160	1.0	340	65	4.1	110	17	405	23	4.0
Males																			
9–13 y	100	27	445	39	9	0.7	0.8	9	0.8	250	1.5	540	73	5.9	200	26	1,055	35	7.0
14–18 y	100	44	630	63	12	1.0	1.1	12	1.1	330	2.0	685	95	7.7	340	33	1,055	45	8.5
19–30 y	100	46	625	75	12	1.0	1.1	12	1.1	320	2.0	700	95	6	330	34	580	45	9.4
31–50 y	100	46	625	75	12	1.0	1.1	12	1.4	320	2.0	700	95	6	350	34	580	45	9.4
51–70 y	100	46	625	75	12	1.0	1.1	12	1.4	320	2.0	700	95	6	350	34	580	45	9.4
>70 y	100	46	625	75	12	1.0	1.1	12	1.4	320	2.0	700	95	6	350	34	580	45	9.4
Females																			
9–13 y	100	28	420	39	9	0.7	0.8	9	0.8	250	1.5	540	73	5.7	200	26	1,055	35	7.0
14–18 y	100	38	485	56	12	0.9	0.9	11	1.0	330	2.0	685	95	7.9	300	33	1,055	45	7.3
19–30 y	100	38	500	60	12	0.9	0.9	11	1.1	320	2.0	700	95	8.1	255	34	580	45	6.8
31–50 y	100	38	500	60	12	0.9	0.9	11	1.1	320	2.0	700	95	8.1	265	34	580	45	6.8
51–70 y	100	38	500	60	12	0.9	0.9	11	1.3	320	2.0	700	95	5	265	34	580	45	6.8
>70 y	100	38	500	60	12	0.9	0.9	11	1.3	320	2.0	700	95	5	265	34	580	45	6.8
Pregnancy																			
14–18 y	135	50	530	66	12	1.2	1.2	14	1.6	520	2.2	785	160	23	335	40	1,055	49	10.5
19–30 y	135	50	550	70	12	1.2	1.2	14	1.6	520	2.2	800	160	22	290	40	580	49	9.5
31–50 y	135	50	550	70	12	1.2	1.2	14	1.6	520	2.2	800	160	22	300	40	580	49	9.5
Lactation																			
14–18 y	160	60	885	96	16	1.2	1.3	13	1.7	450	2.4	985	209	7	300	35	1,055	59	10.9
19–30 y	160	60	900	100	16	1.2	1.3	13	1.7	450	2.4	1,000	209	6.5	255	36	580	59	10.4
31–50 y	160	60	900	100	16	1.2	1.3	13	1.7	450	2.4	1,000	209	6.5	265	36	580	59	10.4

NOTE: This table presents Estimated Average Requirements (EARs), which serve two purposes: for assessing adequacy of population intakes, and as the basis for calculating Recommended Dietary Allowances (RDAs) for individuals for those nutrients. EARs have not been established for vitamin D, vitamin K, pantothenic acid, biotin, choline, calcium, chromium, fluoride, manganese, or other nutrients not yet evaluated via the DRI process.

a For individual at reference weight (Table 1-1). *indicates change from prepublication copy due to calculation error.

b As retinol activity equivalents (RAEs). 1 RAE = 1 µg retinol, 12 µg β-carotene, 24 µg α-carotene, or 24 µg β-cryptoxanthin. The RAE for dietary provitamin A carotenoids is two-fold greater than retinol equivalents (RE), whereas the RAE for preformed vitamin A is the same as RE.

c As α-tocopherol. α-Tocopherol includes RRR-α-tocopherol, the only form of α-tocopherol that occurs naturally in foods, and the 2R-stereoisomeric forms of α-tocopherol (RRR-, RSR-, RRS-, and RSS-α-tocopherol) that occur in fortified foods and supplements. It does not include the 2S-stereoisomeric forms of α-tocopherol (SRR-, SSR-, SRS-, and SSS-α-tocopherol), also found in fortified foods and supplements.

d As niacin equivalents (NE). 1 mg of niacin = 60 mg of tryptophan.

e As dietary folate equivalents (DFE). 1 µg food folate = 0.6 µg of folic acid from fortified food or as a supplement consumed with food = 0.5 µg of a supplement taken on an empty stomach.

SOURCES: *Dietary Reference Intakes for Calcium, Phosphorous, Magnesium, Vitamin D, and Fluoride* (1997); *Dietary Reference Intakes for Thiamin, Riboflavin, Niacin, Vitamin B6, Folate, Vitamin B12, Pantothenic Acid, Biotin, and Choline* (1998); *Dietary Reference Intakes for Vitamin C, Vitamin E, Selenium, and Carotenoids* (2000); *Dietary Reference Intakes for Vitamin A, Vitamin K, Arsenic, Boron, Chromium, Copper, Iodine, Iron, Manganese, Molybdenum, Nickel, Silicon, Vanadium, and Zinc* (2001), and *Dietary Reference Intakes for Energy, Carbohydrate, Fiber, Fat, Fatty Acids, Cholesterol, Protein, and Amino Acids* (2002). These reports may be accessed via www.nap.edu.

Copyright 2002 by the National Academy of Sciences. All rights reserved.

**Dietary Reference Intakes (DRIs): Estimated Energy Requirements (EER) for Men and Women
30 Years of Age[a]**

Food and Nutrition Board, Institute of Medicine, National Academies

Height (m [in])	PAL[b]	Weight for BMI[c] of 18.5 kg/m² (kg [lb])	Weight for BMI of 24.99 kg/m² (kg [lb])	EER, Men[d] (kcal/day)		EER, Women[d] (kcal/day)	
				BMI of 18.5 kg/m²	BMI of 24.99 kg/m²	BMI of 18.5 kg/m²	BMI of 24.99 kg/m²
1.50 (59)	Sedentary	41.6 (92)	56.2 (124)	1,848	2,080	1,625	1,762
	Low active			2,009	2,267	1,803	1,956
	Active			2,215	2,506	2,025	2,198
	Very active			2,554	2,898	2,291	2,489
1.65 (65)	Sedentary	50.4 (111)	68.0 (150)	2,068	2,349	1,816	1,982
	Low active			2,254	2,566	2,016	2,202
	Active			2,490	2,842	2,267	2,477
	Very active			2,880	3,296	2,567	2,807
1.80 (71)	Sedentary	59.9 (132)	81.0 (178)	2,301	2,635	2,015	2,211
	Low active			2,513	2,884	2,239	2,459
	Active			2,782	3,200	2,519	2,769
	Very active			3,225	3,720	2,855	3,141

[a] For each year below 30, add 7 kcal/day for women and 10 kcal /day for men. For each year above 30, subtract 7 kcal/day for women and 10 kcal/day for men.

[b] PAL = physical activity level.

[c] BMI = body mass index.

[d] Derived from the following regression equations based on doubly labeled water data:

Adult man: $EER = 662 - 9.53 \times age\ (y) + PA \times (15.91 \times wt\ [kg] + 539.6 \times ht\ [m])$

Adult woman: $EER = 354 - 6.91 \times age\ (y) + PA \times (9.36 \times wt\ [kg] + 726 \times ht\ [m])$

Where PA refers to coefficient for PAL

PAL = total energy expenditure ÷ basal energy expenditure

$PA = 1.0$ if $PAL \geq 1.0 < 1.4$ (sedentary)

$PA = 1.12$ if $PAL \geq 1.4 < 1.6$ (low active)

$PA = 1.27$ if $PAL \geq 1.6 < 1.9$ (active)

$PA = 1.45$ if $PAL \geq 1.9 < 2.5$ (very active)

Dietary Reference Intakes (DRIs): Acceptable Macronutrient Distribution Ranges

Food and Nutrition Board, Institute of Medicine, National Academies

Macronutrient	Range (percent of energy)		
	Children, 1–3 y	Children, 4–18 y	Adults
Fat	30–40	25–35	20–35
n-6 polyunsaturated fatty acids[a] (linoleic acid)	5–10	5–10	5–10
n-3 polyunsaturated fatty acids[a] (α-linolenic acid)	0.6–1.2	0.6–1.2	0.6–1.2
Carbohydrate	45–65	45–65	45–65
Protein	5–20	10–30	10–35

[a] Approximately 10% of the total can come from longer-chain *n*-3 or *n*-6 fatty acids.

SOURCE: *Dietary Reference Intakes for Energy, Carbohydrate, Fiber, Fat, Fatty Acids, Cholesterol, Protein, and Amino Acids* (2002).

Dietary Reference Intakes (DRIs): Recommended Intakes for Individuals, Macronutrients
Food and Nutrition Board, Institute of Medicine, National Academies

Life Stage Group	Total Water[a] (L/d)	Carbohydrate (g/d)	Total Fiber (g/d)	Fat (g/d)	Linoleic Acid (g/d)	α-Linolenic Acid (g/d)	Protein[b] (g/d)
Infants							
0–6 mo	0.7*	60*	ND	31*	4.4*	0.5*	9.1*
7–12 mo	0.8*	95*	ND	30*	4.6*	0.5*	**11.0**[c]
Children							
1–3 y	1.3*	**130**	19*	ND	7*	0.7*	**13**
4–8 y	1.7*	**130**	25*	ND	10*	0.9*	**19**
Males							
9–13 y	2.4*	**130**	31*	ND	12*	1.2*	**34**
14–18 y	3.3*	**130**	38*	ND	16*	1.6*	**52**
19–30 y	3.7*	**130**	38*	ND	17*	1.6*	**56**
31–50 y	3.7*	**130**	38*	ND	17*	1.6*	**56**
51–70 y	3.7*	**130**	30*	ND	14*	1.6*	**56**
> 70 y	3.7*	**130**	30*	ND	14*	1.6*	**56**
Females							
9–13 y	2.1*	**130**	26*	ND	10*	1.0*	**34**
14–18 y	2.3*	**130**	26*	ND	11*	1.1*	**46**
19–30 y	2.7*	**130**	25*	ND	12*	1.1*	**46**
31–50 y	2.7*	**130**	25*	ND	12*	1.1*	**46**
51–70 y	2.7*	**130**	21*	ND	11*	1.1*	**46**
> 70 y	2.7*	**130**	21*	ND	11*	1.1*	**46**
Pregnancy							
14–18 y	3.0*	**175**	28*	ND	13*	1.4*	**71**
19–30 y	3.0*	**175**	28*	ND	13*	1.4*	**71**
31–50 y	3.0*	**175**	28*	ND	13*	1.4*	**71**
Lactation							
14–18 y	3.8*	**210**	29*	ND	13*	1.3*	**71**
19–30 y	3.8*	**210**	29*	ND	13*	1.3*	**71**
31–50 y	3.8*	**210**	29*	ND	13*	1.3*	**71**

NOTE: This table presents Recommended Dietary Allowances (RDAs) in **bold** type and Adequate Intakes (AIs) in ordinary type followed by an asterisk (*). RDAs and AIs may both be used as goals for individual intake. RDAs are set to meet the needs of almost all (97 to 98 percent) individuals in a group. For healthy infants fed human milk, the AI is the mean intake. The AI for other life stage and gender groups is believed to cover the needs of all individuals in the group, but lack of data or uncertainty in the data prevent being able to specify with confidence the percentage of individuals covered by this intake.

[a] *Total* water includes all water contained in food, beverages, and drinking water.

[b] Based on 0.8 g/kg body weight for the reference body weight.

[c] Change from 13.5 in prepublication copy due to calculation error.

Dietary Reference Intakes (DRIs): Additional Macronutrient Recommendations
Food and Nutrition Board, Institute of Medicine, National Academies

Macronutrient	Recommendation
Dietary cholesterol	As low as possible while consuming a nutritionally adequate diet
Trans fatty acids	As low as possible while consuming a nutritionally adequate diet
Saturated fatty acids	As low as possible while consuming a nutritionally adequate diet
Added sugars	Limit to no more than 25% of total energy

SOURCE: *Dietary Reference Intakes for Energy, Carbohydrate, Fiber, Fat, Fatty Acids, Cholesterol, Protein, and Amino Acids* (2002).

Glossary

abdominal obesity an accumulation of excess fat around the midsection that is considered a risk for cardiovascular disease

acceptable macronutrient distribution range (AMDR) the suggested intake range for a given macronutrient that is sufficient for essential nutrients but not associated with an increased risk of chronic disease

acculturation the adoption of the beliefs, values, attitudes, and practices of a community

acrodermatitis enteropathica a congenital condition that causes zinc deficiency

acute renal failure a rapid decline in kidney function with reduction in glomerular filtration rate and tubular function

acute-phase reactant proteins proteins produced by the liver that participate in the body's response to injury or inflammation during physiological stress

adequate intake (AI) the *recommended* nutrient intake for a group of healthy people when the RDA cannot be determined, usually because of insufficient research data

adipose tissue stored fat in the body that is a source of energy, serves as insulation, and cushions organs

advance directive a legal document that outlines an individual's wishes relating to medical treatment should the individual become unable to communicate

aerobic metabolism that requires oxygen; aerobic exercise is that which requires oxygen and lasts longer than a few minutes

alternate healthy eating index created by researchers at the Harvard School of Public Health to measure compliance with the principles emphasized in the Healthy Living Pyramid

amenorrhea the lack of menstruation

amino acid pool a mix of new and existing amino acids found in the body

amino acids the building block of proteins

amylase an enzyme produced in the saliva and by the pancreas that breaks down carbohydrates for absorption

amylopectine a type of starch that is formed in a branched structure

amylophagia consumption of nonfood starch, such as laundry or corn starch

amylose a type of starch that is formed in a straight chain

anabolism the synthesis of new cellular material, including tissue

anaerobic metabolism that does not require oxygen; anaerobic exercise is that which does not require oxygen and is short-burst and intense in nature

anergy lack of an immune response to an antigen

angular stomatitis fissures at the corners of the mouth

anorexia nervosa a type of eating disorder with strict diagnostic criteria characterized by a refusal to maintain body weight at a minimal weight for height with an intense fear of gaining weight and an altered self-evaluation of personal weight

anorexia of aging diminished appetite that occurs with aging

anthropometric measurements scientific measurements of the body, such as height and weight

antibodies large protein molecules that attack antigens as part of an immune response

antioxidants a substance that functions to neutralize the effects of metabolic and environmental damage to cells caused by oxidation; for example, vitamins A, C, and E

anuria urine volume that is less than 100 mL/day

ariboflavinosis deficiency of the B vitamin riboflavin

aspartame nonnutritive sweetener made with two amino acids, phenylalanine and aspartic acid

ataxia altered gait

atherosclerosis degenerative disease of the lining of the vascular wall leading to narrow, clogged, and hardened arteries

atrophic gastritis diminished gastric acid production by the stomach

baby bottle tooth decay early childhood dental caries caused by sleeping with a bottle containing a carbohydrate source.

bariatric surgery gastrointestinal surgery performed for the purpose of weight loss

beri-beri deficiency of thiamin resulting in muscle wasting and neurological changes

bezoar undigested food mass found in the intestine

binge eating disorder a type of eating disorder consumption of a large amount of food in a short interval of time with an accompanying sense of loss of control, which is not followed by any compensatory measures

bioavailability ability of a substance to be absorbed and used by the body

Bitot's spots foamy spots on the eye because of vitamin A deficiency

body mass index (BMI) an assessment of relative weight for height, expressed as BMI = weight (kg)/height (m)^2

bomb calorimeter a device used to determine the energy content of food by combustion and calculation of water temperature change to indicate heat (energy) release

botanicals plants and plant parts, which include herbs

branched chain amino acids amino acids with a structure that forms a branched chain; includes valine, isoleucine, and leucine

buffers compounds that allow fluids and tissues to keep a constant pH

bulimia nervosa a type of eating disorder characterized by consumption of a large amount of food in a short interval of time with an accompanying sense of loss of control, which is followed by compensatory purging

cachexia weight loss that is comprised of a disproportionate amount of muscle as seen in cancer, HIV infection, and some other chronic diseases; also called *wasting*

cacogeusia a persistent bad or metallic taste in the mouth

carbohydrate a macronutrient containing carbon, hydrogen, and oxygen with 4 kcalories/gm

cardiac cachexia a condition seen in advanced cardiac disease associated with a progressive decline in cardiac performance, resulting in muscle and adipose wasting and undernutrition

catabolism the breaking down of cellular material, including tissue

catalysts substances that alter the rate of a reaction without being changed themselves

chelation a specific type of binding that occurs between a metal ion, such as calcium, magnesium, or other mineral, and another molecule, which results in reduced bioavailability

cholesterol sterol made by the liver and also present in foods of animal origin

chronic kidney disease (CKD) a slow, steady decline in kidney function resulting in reduced glomerular filtration rate and tubular function

colostrum the breast milk produced first after childbirth, which is high in antibodies

community a collection of people with shared characteristics

competitive foods food and beverages available in a school setting that are not part of the government-funded lunch program, including items found in a vending machine, school snack bar, fundraisers, and other food and beverages available in the cafeteria

complementary proteins proteins from different sources that combine to form a complete protein

complete proteins proteins that contain all the essential amino acids

complex carbohydrates a form of carbohydrate that contains more than three sugar molecules

conditionally essential an amino acid that becomes essential under certain physiological conditions

continuous renal replacement therapies (CRRT) slow forms of dialysis used in clients who are medically unstable and unable to tolerate standard dialysis

coronary heart disease also called coronary artery disease; occurs because of narrowed blood vessels that supply the heart

C-reactive protein an acute phase reactant protein that is part of an inflammatory response in the body

culture the way of life of a community at a given time

cyanogens inactive compounds in lima beans and fruit seeds such as apricot pits that can be activated by certain plant enzymes into the poison cyanide

daily value the amount of a nutrient recommended for health, based on current nutritional research

deamination a process that removes nitrogen from a substance

decoction similar to a tea but made by using plantroots, bark, and berries that require longer steeping time in boiling water before they can be consumed

dehydration the loss of solutes and water from the body

denaturation a process that alters proteins by breaking some of the chemical bonds

dialysate the solution used in dialysis to remove solutes from the blood

diet recall a 24-hour history of intake of food, fluids, and dietary supplements

dietary fiber the indigestible carbohydrate found in plant cell walls and woody component

dietary reference intakes (DRIs) national recommendations for daily nutrient intake for well individuals within a population

dipeptide two amino acids

disaccharides a type of simple carbohydrate that contains two sugar molecules

disordered eating a subclinical eating disorder that does not meet the strict diagnostic criteria of anorexia, bulimia, or binge eating

diverticulosis a condition of the large intestine that is characterized by outpouching in the colon wall

dysgeusia altered taste perception

dyslipidemia disorders in lipoprotein metabolism involving high levels of LDL cholesterol, low levels of HDL cholesterol, and high levels of triglycerides

dysphagia difficulty swallowing

dyspnea difficulty breathing

early satiety feeling full quickly when eating

ebb phase the acute phase that immediately follows an injury or other physiological stress

edema fluid accumulation in tissue that causes swelling

edentulism lack of teeth

elemental formulas a type of enteral nutrition product that contains carbohydrate, protein, and fat in a predigested form

empty calorie foods foods that contain kcalories but little nutrients

endogenous insulin insulin produced by the pancreas

energy availability the difference between energy expenditure and energy intake

energy balance the relationship between energy intake and expenditure

energy expenditure the sum of all components of energy used for body processes and physical activity

enriched foods foods that have nutrients replaced that were lost in processing

enrichment replacement of nutrients in a food that were lost during processing

enteral nutrition nutrition that is delivered through the intestinal tract

environmental contaminants harmful substances that are carried in food and water and have the potential to cause acute and chronic disease and to decrease quality of life by their presence

enzymes proteins that are responsible for catalyzing chemical reactions

ergogenic aids anything that helps perform work

essential amino acids amino acids that are not able to be synthesized in the body and are therefore required in the diet

essential fatty acids fatty acids that cannot be synthesized by the body; includes the polyunsaturated fats linoleic and linolenic acids

estimated average requirements (EAR) the average daily nutrient intake value that is estimated to meet the requirements of 50% or more of healthy individuals in a life stage and gender group

estimated energy requirement (EER) the dietary energy intake level predicted to achieve and maintain energy balance in healthy, normal weight individuals of a given age, height and weight, gender, and physical activity level

euglycemia normal blood sugar; 70–110 mg/dL

euhydration the state of water balance where intake and losses are equal

excipients the inactive ingredients in a medication

extract a liquid extract is made by soaking the plant in liquid that will remove specific components; a dry extract is made by letting a liquid extract evaporate, leaving only dry components that can be made into capsules or tablets

exudate the fluid that seeps from an injury site or wound

failure to thrive growth failure in a child

female athlete triad the combination of low-energy availability, diminished bone mineral density, and amenorrhea; may occur along a continuum and progress to an eating disorder, osteoporosis, and amenorrhea

fiber a form of complex carbohydrates that is not digestible

fight-or-flight response a hormonal reaction by the body to physiological stress; leads to release of a cascade of hormones that provide quick energy and central nervous system stimulation

flag sign a horizontal stripe in the hair because of protein malnutrition

flow phase the phase of physiological stress that occurs after the ebb phase until recovery occurs

fluorosis mottled brown teeth from excessive fluoride intake

follicular hyperkeratosis raised bumps around the base of the hair follicle

food allergies a hypersensitive reaction to food involving an immune response

food frequency questionnaire a tool used to assess the quantity of intake of food groups over time

food hypersensitivity an immune reaction triggered by antigens on the food source

food insecurity lack of sufficient food because of financial or access reasons

food intolerances a physical reaction to food that does not involve an immune response; for example, lactose intolerance

food jags repetitive intake of the same foods with little interest in consuming additional foods

food safety prevention of contamination of the food supply from foodborne illnesses, environmental contaminants, naturally occurring toxins, pesticides, and other potentially harmful substances

foodborne illnesses systemic illnesses caused by foodborne infection, caused by a pathogen carried on or in the food source, or food intoxication, caused by a toxin contained by the food source

fortification addition of nutrients to a food that are not naturally occurring in the product

fortified foods foods that have nutrients added that are not naturally present in the food

free radicals by-products of metabolism and the environment that are unstable and cause oxidation in cells

functional fiber the indigestible carbohydrate that also has a physiological function, such as promoting laxation or reducing blood lipids

galactosemia a genetic disorder that causes elevated blood galactose because of an enzyme deficiency

geophagia consumption of dirt, soil, or clay

glossitis magenta tongue with atrophy of the taste buds

glucagon a hormone that signals the breakdown of glycogen

gluconeogenesis the synthesis of glucose from glycogen or protein

gluten a protein found in wheat, rye, and barley

glycemic index (GI) a measure of the rise in blood glucose 2 hours after consuming a portion of food containing 50 gm of carbohydrate

glycogen the storage form of glucose present in the liver and muscle

glycogenolysis the catabolism of glycogen to create glucose

goiter an enlarged thyroid gland because of iodine deficiency

goitrogens a substance contained in brassica family vegetables than can cause a decrease in thyroid function

HAART highly active antiretroviral treatment medications used to treat HIV infection

health claim statement about the hypothesized or proven relationship between a nutrient or substance in a food and a known disease or health-related condition

health prevention actions to avert future disease development

health promotion actions to optimize wellness

healthy eating index a scoring system created by the Department of Agriculture's Center for Nutrition Policy and Promotion to measure the conformance of American diets to the current healthy eating recommendations and federal dietary guidelines

Healthy People 2010 a government health initiative of the Department of Health and Human Services to identify national health priorities and provides guidelines for policies for health promotion and prevention activities

high biological value protein sources of protein that contain all the essential amino acids

high potency when 100% of the daily value (DV) is in a single nutrient supplement or when 100% of two-thirds of the nutrients' DV is present in a multivitamin/mineral supplement

hind milk breast milk that is higher in kcalories and fat and produced toward the end of a feeding

hormones chemicals synthesized in the body that exert an effect elsewhere in the body

hunger-obesity paradox the coexistence of obesity and malnutrition in a person generally because of poverty and food insecurity

hydrogenation the addition of hydrogen to a substance; unsaturated fats are hydrogenated to become more saturated fats or trans fats

hydrophilic that which attracts water

hydrophobic that which repels water

hypercatabolism an increased rate of tissue destruction

hypercholesterolemia elevated blood cholesterol

hyperglycemia high blood sugar; 126 mg/dL or higher

hyperhydration an excess of water in the body

hypermetabolism an increased rate of energy utilization

hypertension high blood pressure defined as blood pressure greater than 140/90 mm Hg

hypertonic a solution with a high concentration or osmolality

hypervitaminosis excess vitamin intake or storage

hypoglycemia low blood sugar; lower than 70 mg/dL

hypohydration a deficit of water in the body

hyponatremia low plasma sodium levels less than 135 mEq/L

hypovitaminosis insufficient vitamin intake or storage

iatrogenic malnutrition the state of poor nutritional health that is caused by health care practices

ileus a lack of intestinal peristalsis

immune response the way in which the body defends against foreign substances, such as with antigens

immunocompetence an assessment of immune status

immunonutrition nutrition therapy using dietary supplementation that targets improvement in immune status

inborn error of metabolism an inherited defect in the way a substrate is metabolized

incomplete proteins proteins that do not contain all the essential amino acids

indirect calorimetry the indirect measurement of energy expenditure by measurement of oxygen consumed and carbon dioxide expired

induction an increase in enzyme action of the cytochrome P450 system that results in a decreased absorption of active drug

infantometer a tool used to measure recumbent length (height) in infants

infusion a drink that is made when boiling water is added to fresh or dried botanicals and steeped before drinking hot or cold

inhibition an decrease in enzyme action of the cytochrome P450 system that results in increased absorption of active drug

insensible water loss water losses that cannot be measured, such as sweat and respiratory losses

insoluble fiber fiber that is insoluble in water, such as cellulose, hemicellulose, and lignin

intradialytic parenteral nutrition (IDPN) the delivery of parenteral nutrition during hemodialysis

isotonic a solution with a concentration that is similar to that of the body

ketone bodies a by-product of incomplete fat metabolism that occurs during excessive fat catabolism because of insufficient carbohydrate availability

kilocalories the amount of energy contained in a food or beverage. Calculated by determining the amount of heat released during combustion of the item in a bomb calorimeter

kilojoule a measure of energy using the metric system and equivalent to 0.239 kilocalorie

koilonychia spoon-shaped fingernails associated with iron deficiency

kwashiorkor malnutrition that occurs because of insufficient protein intake

lacto-ovo vegetarians vegetarians who consume no animal flesh foods but do consume eggs and milk products

lactose intolerance an intestinal condition caused by insufficient synthesis of the intestinal enzyme lactase needed to break down lactose

lanugo a soft downy hair that forms on the body as an attempt to improve altered core temperature regulation because of loss of body fat

laxation bowel movement

limiting amino acid the amino acid present in the least amount in a food

linoleic acid a polyunsaturated omega-6 essential fatty acid

linolenic acid a polyunsaturated omega-3 essential fatty acid

lipoatrophy fat wasting on the body and face associated with HAART

lipodystrophy abnormalities in fat distribution and dyslipidemia associated with HAART

lipoproteins substances consisting of lipids and protein that transport fat-soluble products such as cholesterol, triglycerides, and fat-soluble vitamins in the blood

macronutrients major nutrients, which are carbohydrate, protein, and fat and provide kilocalories

macrophages cells of the immune system capable of taking up cholesterol

macrosomia larger than normal body size in an infant

maintenance hemodialysis (MHD) a type of renal replacement therapy using a venous catheter or arteriovenous fistula

malnutrition imbalance of nutrients from deficiencies or excesses

marasmus malnutrition that occurs because of insufficient energy intake

medical nutrition therapy nutrition care that encompasses the assessment and treatment of any disease, condition, or illness

metabolic acidosis an increase in blood pH because of metabolic changes

metabolic bone disease a complex disorder of poorly mineralized bone because of endocrine changes and alterations in vitamin D, calcium, and phosphorus metabolism

micronutrients minor nutrients, which are vitamins and minerals and do not provide kilocalories

modular formulas a type of enteral nutrition formula that contains simply carbohydrate, protein, or fat

monosaccharides a simple carbohydrate that contains one sugar molecule

monounsaturated fats fats with only one double bond in their carbon chain

morbid obesity obesity characterized as a BMI greater than or equal to 40 and associated with high risk of medical comorbidities

negative food effect a reduction in drug absorption because of the presence of food in the intestine

night eating syndrome (NES) a disordered eating condition characterized by consuming large amounts of food at night, followed by lack of appetite in the morning

nitrogen balance the difference between the amount of nitrogen taken in and that lost

nitrogen equilibrium when nitrogen intake and losses are equal; also called zero nitrogen balance

nonessential amino acids amino acids that the body is able to synthesize and therefore are not required in the diet

nonexercise activity thermogenesis (NEAT) any activity that is associated with muscle contractions as part of the activities of daily living, such as sitting and talking

nonnutritive sweeteners sugar substitutes that contain no kilocalories

nursing process five-step process that includes the systematic gathering of subjective and objective data, analysis of the data for the purpose of establishing nursing diagnoses, planning realistic goals, implementing activities to achieve the goals, and evaluating goal accomplishment

nutrient content claims a statement describing the level of a nutrient or dietary substance in a food product, often comparing that food to a similar food used as a reference; often use terms such as *low, free, reduced,* and *light*

nutrient dense a food containing a significant amount of nutrients for the least amount of calories

nutrition facts food label component of a food label that outlines serving size and nutrient content, comparing nutrient content to recommendations for nutrient intake for the general population

nutritional screening a brief evaluation of risk of malnutrition used to determine if a more thorough nutrition assessment is warranted

nutritive sweeteners sugar substitutes that contain kilocalories

nystagmus altered eye movements that can be a symptom of vitamin deficiency or disease

odynophagia painful swallowing

oliguria urine volume that is less than 500 mL/day

omega-3 fatty acids fatty acids that have the first double bond in the omega-3 position on the carbon chain

omega-6 fatty acids fatty acids that have the first double bond in the omega-6 position on the carbon chain

oncotic pressure the effect of proteins on fluid balance

orthorexia the religious attention to healthy eating at the exclusion of other foods

osmolality the concentration of a solution expressed as the number of dissolved particles with an ionic charge in 1 liter of a solution expressed as a millomoles/liter

osteomalacia a condition that causes soft bones in adults because of vitamin D deficiency

osteopenia low bone mineral density

osteoporosis pronounced loss of bone mass

overnutrition excess intake or stores of nutrients that results in poor nutritional health

pagophagia consumption of ice

palliative nutrition nutrition meant to aid in relief of symptoms or discomfort rather than cure

paralytic ileus lack of bowel sounds or peristalsis

parenteral nutrition nutrition that is delivered intravenously

pellagra deficiency of niacin manifested by dermatitis, diarrhea, depression

peptide bonds bonds between amino acids

peripheral neuropathy tingling in the hands and feet because of neurological changes

peritoneal dialysis (PD) a type of renal replacement therapy that uses the peritoneal cavity as the site to infuse the dialysate and passively diffuse solutes

pernicious anemia autoimmune disease that results in vitamin B_{12} deficiency because of lack of intrinsic factor production by the body

pescatarians vegetarians who consume no animal flesh proteins other than from seafood

pesticides powerful chemical compounds that protect human health by killing insects, animals, and other pests that can cause harm or disease but can also cause harm and death if ingested by humans, pets, and other animals

petechiae pinpoint hemorrhages on the skin

pharmacodynamics the intended action of a medication

pharmacokinetics the absorption, distribution, metabolism, or excretion of drugs

phospholipids a type of lipid comprised of a glycerol molecule, two fatty acids, and a phosphate group that allows some solubility in water; synthesized by the body and not essential in the diet

physiological stress a reaction by the body to injury or inflammation that leads to increased hypercatabolism and hypermetabolism; also called metabolic stress

phytochemicals plant chemicals, including flavonoids and plant pigments

phytoestrogens a weak form of estrogen found in some plants, such as soy and red clover

pica craving for nonfood items

polydipsia excessive thirst

polymeric formula a type of enteral nutrition formula that contains intact proteins, carbohydrate, and fat that require full digestive function

polypeptide Ten or more amino acids bound together

polyphagia excessive hunger

polypharmacy the use of multiple medications, whether prescription or over the counter

polysaccharides a complex carbohydrate with many sugar molecules

polyunsaturated fats fatty acids that have multiple double bonds in the carbon chain

polyuria excessive urine production

positive food effect an increase in drug absorption because of the presence of food in the intestine

preformed vitamins metabolically inactive form of vitamins

primary and secondary prevention primary prevention is the delay or prevention of onset of a disease; secondary prevention is the prevention of disease recurrence

primary structure the specific sequence of amino acids found in a protein

probiotics nonpathogenic bacteria that are found in the intestine

protein digestibility-corrected amino acid (PDCAA) score a method to quantify the quality of a protein based on its composition and digestibility; also called biological value

protein quality the assessment of protein composition and digestibility

protein synthesis the process by which cells build proteins specific to the needs of the body

protein turnover the combined processes of protein synthesis and degradation

protein-energy wasting (PEW) the syndrome of weight loss and malnutrition found in chronic kidney disease because of multiple factors

provitamins metabolically active form of vitamins

qualified health claims a subset of label claims allowed by the FDA when emerging evidence exists that links an ingredient with health, but the strength of the evidence is limited

recombinant human erythropoietin a synthetic form of the hormone erythropoietin that stimulates the bone marrow to produce red blood cells

recommended daily allowance (RDA) the average daily amount of a given nutrient that is sufficient to meet the nutrient requirement of 97% to 98% of healthy individuals in a particular life stage and gender group

refeeding syndrome the metabolic and physical consequences associated with the reintroduction of food following starvation or semi-starvation

renal replacement therapy (RRT) treatment used in renal failure to remove nitrogenous waste products from the blood; also called dialysis

renal threshold the level at which glucose begins appearing in the urine; normally glucose will stay in the blood but between 180 and 240 mg/dL the kidneys are no longer able to retain the excess glucose

respiratory quotient (RQ) the ratio between oxygen intake and carbon dioxide output used to assess the influence of macronutrients on carbon dioxide output; carbohydrate has a higher RQ than does protein or fat

reverse cholesterol transport the process of transport of cholesterol via HDL from cells to the liver for excretion

rickets a condition that causes soft bones and improper mineralization of bones in children from vitamin D deficiency

sarcopenia loss of muscle associated with aging

satiation the process that affects the termination of a meal, a type of fullness

satiety the process that affects the amount of time until the next meal, a type of fullness

saturated fat fatty acids that have no double bonds in the carbon chain

scurvy deficiency of vitamin C that causes altered collagen synthesis and bleeding

selenosis symptoms of selenium toxicity, including hair loss, garlicky breath, fatigue, irritability, gastrointestinal complaints, and nerve damage

semi-vegetarians vegetarians who occasionally eat meat; also called flexitarians

sensible water loss water losses that are measurable, such as urinary output

short bowel syndrome a condition of malabsorption that occurs because of disease or excessive resection of the intestine

simple carbohydrates a form of carbohydrate that contains less than three sugar molecules

solanine a natural poison found in potatoes that causes profound narcotic-like effects

soluble fiber fiber that is soluble in water, such as gums and pectins

solutes particles that are dissolved in a solution

solvent the medium or solution in which solutes are dissolved

somatic protein skeletal protein or muscle mass

starches the storage form of carbohydrate in plants

steatorrhea fatty diarrhea from fat malabsorption

sterols a classification of lipids comprised of large interconnected rings that are synthesized by the body and not essential to the diet; for example, cholesterol

structure/function claims link an ingredient in a supplement or food to the maintenance of general health or the normal function or structure of a body system or part

substrates the substances that act as the reactants in a chemical reaction

sugar alcohols a nutritive sweetener derived from sugar; examples include sorbitol, mannitol, and xylitol

teratogens substances known to be harmful to a developing fetus

tetany physical symptoms from hypocalcemia, including Trousseau's sign and Chvostek's sign

thermic effect of food the energy required to digest and metabolize food

tincture a liquid that is made by soaking the plant in alcohol or water and can be prepared at varying concentrations

tolerable upper intake limit (UL) recommendation under the umbrella of the DRIs that outlines the upper limit of intake of a nutrient for which safety information is available

tongue extrusion reflex tongue thrust, where a baby pushes anything out of the mouth—a sign that needs to be diminished before feeding readiness

total fiber the sum of dietary and functional fibers

trans fats hydrogenated fatty acids with hydrogens on opposite sides of the double bond in the carbon chain (compared with the *cis* formation with hydrogens on the same side)

transamination the transfer of nitrogen from one chemical group to another

triglyceride a type of lipid comprised of a glycerol molecule with three fatty acids attached; the chief form of fat in foods and storage form of fat in the body

tripeptide three amino acids

undernutrition insufficient intake or stores of nutrients that results in poor nutritional health; also called malnutrition

unsaturated fat fatty acids with one or more double bonds in the carbon chain

uremia the buildup of nitrogenous waste products in the blood

vegan a vegetarian who consumes no animal flesh proteins and no foods derived from an animal, such as dairy foods, eggs, and honey

visceral proteins plasma proteins and proteins found in organs

wasting weight loss that is comprised of a disproportioned amount of muscle as seen in cancer, HIV infection, and some other chronic diseases; also called *cachexia*

Wernicke-Korsakoff syndrome a condition that causes neurological changes because of thiamin deficiency

whole grain grains that have not been overly processed and still retain the germ and bran

xerophthalmia alterations in eye health because of vitamin A deficiency that can result in corneal ulcerations, night blindness, and, ultimately, blindness

xerostomia insufficient saliva production

Answers

Chapter 1
Critical Thinking in the Nursing Process

The nurse must always be mindful that clients do not know as much about evidence-based nutrition as the nurse. Many people have misconceptions or questions about the role of nutrition in health, for example, for which the nurse should be able to provide current information. It is important for the nurse to do a nutritional screening using basic anthropometric data coupled with information from a nursing history of the client. Based on client goals, the nurse should focus on education, sharing materials and resources, or referral to a dietitian who can answer more complex questions or develop a focused nutritional plan for the client.

NCLEX® Questions

Answer: 1

Rationale: Anthropometric data are related to the physical characteristics of the body. It includes such things as height, weight, skin fold thickness, and waist measurements. When assessing school-age children, the nurse is primarily concerned with height and weight. Iron and protein status are laboratory data and may be useful in a complete nutritional assessment, but they are not the role of a school nurse. Hip measurements are not appropriate anthropometric measures for school-age children.

Cognitive Level: Application

Nursing Process: Assessment

Category of Client Need: Health Promotion and Health Maintenance

Answer: 1 and 2

Rationale: The ingredients of a food product are listed on the label in descending order by weight, rather than nutritional value. State health departments are not responsible for the content of the labels. The main part of the label is based on 2,000 kcalories, although the fine print includes some information for 2,500-kcalorie diets. The macronutrients (carbohydrates, protein, and fats) and some micronutrients (e.g., sodium and calcium) are included on the label. The calories, grams, and percentages are based on the serving size, so if individuals consume larger or smaller amounts, the calories, grams, and percentages will differ.

Cognitive Level: Analysis

Nursing Process: Evaluation

Category of Client Need: Health Promotion and Health Maintenance

Answer: 3

Rationale: A client with a BMI between 27 and 30 is considered overweight, so the client is consuming nutrients in excess of body requirements. A BMI of 30 or greater is considered obese, and a BMI greater than 40 is considered morbidly obese. There is nothing to indicate that the client has a knowledge deficit or that excess weight is due to fluid retention or impaired metabolism.

Cognitive Level: Application

Nursing Process: Planning

Category of Client Need: Health Promotion and Health Maintenance

Answer: 4

Rationale: All of the data are valuable components of a nutritional assessment; however, the most important factor is to get information about the client's usual nutrient intake. Height and wrist circumference are stable measurements. The nurse may make inferences about socioeconomic level, but none of those are directly related to nutritional status.

Cognitive Level: Analysis

Nursing Process: Assessment

Category of Client Need: Health Promotion and Health Maintenance

Answer: 2

Rationale: Weight can be increased 1 pound per week by increasing caloric consumption of an average of 500 kcalories per day. This is realistic for most clients, depending on other health considerations. Weight gain is promoted by increasing caloric consumption rather than limiting activity in most circumstances. Ten grams of carbohydrates is only equivalent to 40 kcalories, an insufficient amount to promote weight gain. Consumption of organic foods is not related to weight.

Cognitive Level: Application

Nursing Process: Planning

Category of Client Need: Health Promotion and Health Maintenance

Critical Thinking Question

This is a common situation in today's fast-paced society. Eating together as a family is a good habit and one that should be continued as often as possible. Research has shown that TV watching is associated with a greater risk of poor nutrient intake and being overweight. Consider shopping once per week and selecting simple foods that the children can help prepare. This will help with nutrient quality and family time together. Depending on the subjective and objective data gathered, possible nursing diagnoses include: *Knowledge deficit* related to statements regarding television use; *Nutrition, readiness for enhanced* related to expressed desire to improve the nutritional health of the family; *Nutrition, imbalanced, risk of greater than body requirements* related to recent weight gain; *Nutrition, imbalanced, greater than body requirements* related to a BMI exceeding recommended range; and *Sedentary lifestyle* related to excessive television use and no leisure time physical activity.

Answers to Stop and Consider Questions

Box 1-6: Nurse in women's health clinic: assessing nutrition status of pregnant females and providing nutrition education regarding optimal weight gain and nutrition during pregnancy. Educating females about nutrients that are crucial to reproductive health such as iron and folic acid

Box 1-8: Which diagnosis could be used to describe an individual with weight loss because of an eating disorder? *Nutrition, imbalanced, less than body requirements* or *body image, disturbed* How about the client who lacks knowledge about the influence of diet on blood cholesterol? *Knowledge, deficient.*

Chapter 2
Critical Thinking in the Nursing Process

In addition to whole grains, fruits, vegetables, and legumes can be significant sources of fiber. Examples of high-fiber fruit include dried fruits, such as prunes and apricots, and those with edible skins, such as pears and apples. Fruit should be consumed with the skin on rather than peeled. High-fiber vegetables include corn, spinach, and green peas. Legumes include kidney beans, chickpeas, lentils, and soy.

NCLEX® Questions

Answer: 3

Rationale: Very low-carbohydrate diets can induce a state of ketosis in which the body produces ketones as it burns fat for energy. Prolonged ketosis leads to metabolic acidosis, a condition that lowers the pH of blood that may result in extreme muscle weakness, cardiac dysfunction, and eventual death. A very low-carbohydrate diet can result in weight loss but does not usually lead to iron deficiency if the client consumes adequate protein foods that contain iron. Bleeding gums are unrelated to carbohydrate intake. Headaches can result from many causes not related to diet.

Cognitive Level: Application

Nursing Process: Evaluation

Category of Client Need: Physiological Integrity

Answer: 4

Rationale: It is recommended that a minimum of 130 gm of carbohydrate is needed to supply the brain with a needed source of glucose. Carbohydrates should be from a variety of sources.

Cognitive Level: Analysis

Nursing Process: Evaluation

Category of Client Need: Physiological Integrity

Answer: 3

Rationale: Each of the foods listed is a source of carbohydrates. English muffins and whole wheat spaghetti are sources of complex carbohydrates, but the whole wheat spaghetti is the best choice because it is a whole grain.

Cognitive Level: Application

Nursing Process: Implementation

Category of Client Need: Health Promotion and Health Maintenance

Answer: 2

Rationale: Studies have concluded that artificial, or non-nutritive, sweeteners used in appropriate amounts are not harmful. Their approval and use is overseen by the U.S. Food and Drug Administration. However, individuals with phenylketonuria (PKU) should not use aspartame because it contains phenylalanine. Tooth decay is a complex process and the use of artificial sweeteners alone will not prevent dental caries. Most individuals may choose foods with or without artificial sweeteners by preference alone.

Cognitive Level: Analysis

Nursing Process: Evaluation

Category of Client Need: Health Promotion and Health Maintenance

Answer: 3

Rationale: Diverticulosis is a condition in which "pouches" develop in the wall of the large intestine. Foods that are low in fiber pass through the colon more slowly than foods with higher fiber. The result can be increased pressure exerted on the colon wall, causing pouches to develop over time. High-fiber foods decrease the transit time of food through the intestine and prevent constipation. Apples and pears are the highest fiber foods of those listed so they should be promoted for intestinal health.

Cognitive Level: Application

Nursing Process: Implementation

Category of Client Need: Health Promotion and Health Maintenance

Critical Thinking Question

There is no one right or perfect method of losing weight. Each individual needs to find an acceptable, palatable method and then stick to it to achieve weight loss. Maintenance of weight loss requires modification of diet and activity for long-term success. Low-carbohydrate diets have been around for a long time and have been studied extensively.

They can be used successfully by some individuals and have been found to have no adverse effects on lipid levels when used short term. Fiber; calcium; and vitamins A, D, and C intake should be monitored because limited consumption of foods containing these nutrients can occur when carbohydrate intake is low. The nurse can advise the client about good sources of these nutrients to include in the diet. No data are available to guide the client about safety of these diets for long-term use.

Answers to Stop and Consider Questions

Table 2-2: Approximately 25 gm of fiber can be consumed with a breakfast that includes 1 cup of raisin bran and an orange, a lunch that includes two slices of whole grain bread and a pear, and a dinner that includes 1 cup whole wheat spaghetti.

Lifespan Box: Fiber and Dental Issues: The adolescent with orthodontic braces could cut, dice, or shred any fruit or vegetable before eating. For example, a fruit salad can be made with cut apples, peeled oranges, and cut melon. Shredded hard vegetables, such as carrots, can be added to a salad or into a mixed dish. A school-age child who does not like vegetables could be involved in the meal preparation for the whole family, choosing a vegetable and corresponding recipe and assisting with preparation. Vegetables can be added to existing favorite dishes, such as peas added to macaroni and cheese. Raw vegetables such as carrots, broccoli, and celery can be offered with low-fat dressing for fun dipping.

Chapter 3
Critical Thinking in the Nursing Process

The nurse needs to understand that winning may be very important to the teen who is a member of a school team, and that athletes frequently look to peers for information about how to develop a competitive edge. The nurse should use language that the teen understands along with evidence from reputable sources. The nurse should assess and build on the teen's knowledge base, affirming what the teen is doing well and share areas in which he or she could make improvements that will help achieve goals.

Some of the best high-protein, low-fat foods are plant-based proteins such as lentils, black beans, pinto beans, and kidney beans. Some of these beans can be made into salsas or tacos or salads that are nutritious, higher in protein, and lower in fat. Additionally, lean animal-based proteins include fat-free or low-fat dairy foods, such as yogurt, milk, and cheeses; lean cuts of meat; and skinless poultry, such as chicken and turkey.

NCLEX® Questions

Answer: 2

Rationale: Because the client is only expressing interest, the nurse should find out why the client wants to begin this diet. The reasons the client shares will determine how the nurse will proceed with teaching. There is no formula for a high-protein diet, but the nurse could calculate the minimum protein requirement with the client. Protein is typically, but not necessarily, more expensive than foods that contain more carbohydrate or fat. If the protein source is meat, it will be more expensive than if it is legumes. A high-protein diet does not have to be primarily from high biologic value sources.

Cognitive Level: Application

Nursing Process: Planning

Category of Client Need: Health Promotion and Health Maintenance

Answer: 4

Rationale: Complete proteins have all of the essential amino acids needed by humans. They are sometimes called high-quality proteins and come almost exclusively from animal sources. The best sources of protein are those that are acceptable to the client, and they may come from plant sources. There is no minimum amount of complete protein that must be consumed for good health or positive nitrogen balance, although the recommended amount of protein intake from various sources for adults is 0.8 gm/kg/day.

Cognitive Level: Application

Nursing Process: Implementation

Category of Client Need: Health Promotion and Health Maintenance

Answer: 3

Rationale: A variety of incomplete protein sources consumed over the course of a day can ensure adequate protein intake because the incomplete proteins can combine in the body to form complete protein. There is no need to combine proteins in any specific way at each meal. High biologic value protein is complete protein so it does not need to be complemented with other protein sources. A vegetarian diet may contain dairy products and eggs, which are complete proteins, so concern about complementary proteins is not needed.

Cognitive Level: Analysis

Nursing Process: Evaluation

Category of Client Need: Health Promotion and Health Maintenance

Answer: 1

Rationale: A negative nitrogen balance may occur in the individual who has sustained a serious injury or burns or has a wound that is failing to heal. Those individuals need more protein as a source of nitrogen to promote healing. Active teenagers need more calories and more protein, but in a state of good health they are consuming adequate amounts and are not in negative nitrogen balance. The same is true of a preschooler who has a chronic condition. Children have a need for more protein per kilogram than adults, but growth alone does not put a child into a negative nitrogen balance. Vegetarians who are healthy and get adequate protein from a variety of sources will not need extra nitrogen.

Cognitive Level: Analysis

Nursing Process: Evaluation

Category of Client Need: Physiological Integrity

Answer: 2

Rationale: High biologic value proteins have essential amino acids and are more easily digested. The frequency of consuming protein does not increase its biologic value so this client needs additional teaching. Eggs and soy protein are good sources of high biologic value protein. A client with renal disease typically needs to limit intake of protein so should make protein selections that are of high biologic value.

Cognitive Level: Analysis

Nursing Process: Evaluation

Category of Client Need: Physiological Integrity

Critical Thinking Question

Muscle mass is developed by performing strength and resistance training under the direction of athletic trainers in combination with a diet that contains both adequate calories and protein. Eating a diet with protein from a variety of food sources will supply sufficient dietary protein needed for growth and engaging in sports. Chapter 11 discusses protein recommendations for athletes in more detail. Current research has failed to show that protein or amino acid supplements build muscle any more effectively than does consumption of adequate calories and protein.

Answers to Stop and Consider Questions

Box 3-1: A nitrogen balance study is only accurate if all sources of nitrogen intake and output are calculated. Thus, a missed diet recording or lack of collection of a urine void will yield inaccurate information. The result will then lead to improper nutrition advice regarding nutritional status and recommended protein intake. The nurse can explain this to the client when encouraging adherence to a 24-hour urine collection.

Box 3-3: Relying on dairy foods for protein in the diet can lead to insufficient intake of iron because these foods contain no iron. Beans, split peas, and other legumes contain iron. The nurse can assess the reason that plant-based protein sources are not included in the diet and brainstorm ideas with the client on ways to include them where appropriate. For example, a client who eats out often can be encouraged to try a vegetarian burger, bean soup, vegetarian stir-fry with tofu or hummus while dining out rather than first trying to make these foods at home. Beans can be added to a salad. Peanut butter and other nut butters can be used in a sandwich.

Chapter 4
Critical Thinking in the Nursing Process

The nurse should teach the client about the different types of fats found in foods. In addition, the nurse will want to share specific foods that are representative of each category.

Dietary counseling should include emphasis on consuming more monounsaturated fats and less saturated and trans fats. The nurse will also want to teach about the role of soluble fiber in decreasing the cholesterol level as outlined in Chapter 18.

NCLEX® Questions

Answer: 2

Rationale: Cholesterol is found exclusively in animal sources, such as meat and poultry, so the client who is concerned about limiting cholesterol in the diet would limit the intake of these or find low-fat versions that result in lowered cholesterol content; for example, skim or low-fat cheese versus full-fat cheese. The food fact label reports the amount of cholesterol along with the amount of fat, so the client should be instructed to also look at that part of the label. Foods high in cholesterol can be low in fat, such as shellfish, so restricting total fat intake does not always affect cholesterol intake. Eggs have cholesterol, but a low cholesterol diet may also include eggs in moderation. Fried foods are high in fat but may not include cholesterol if the oil used for frying is not animal fat.

Cognitive Level: Application

Nursing Process: Planning

Category of Client Need: Health Promotion and Health Maintenance

Answer: 1

Rationale: Cholesterol is a sterol that is manufactured in the liver and is also found in animal products. Intake should not exceed 300 mg per day, but there is no requirement that it be eliminated from the diet of any age group. Red meat is not the primary source of cholesterol; animal-based foods, including organ meats (chicken or beef liver, for example), eggs, and high-fat dairy products such as cheese have more cholesterol than some types of red meat. Animal foods that contain high amounts of omega-3 fatty acids (deep, cold water fish) have some cholesterol, but the amount is far less than that contained in other sources.

Cognitive Level: Application

Nursing Process: Planning

Category of Client Need: Health Promotion and Health Maintenance

Answer: 1 and 4

Rationale: Omega-3 fatty acids are found in highest concentration in cold water fish. They occur in negligible amounts in grains and poultry.

Cognitive Level: Application

Nursing Process: Implementation

Category of Client Need: Health Promotion and Health Maintenance

Answer: 4

Rationale: Trans-fatty acids are found in processed foods and baked goods like pastries. The client who wants to limit consumption of trans-fatty acids should reduce intake of processed and baked goods unless it is known that unsaturated fats are used in the product. Vegetables do not affect the absorption of trans-fatty acids. Fish does not have trans-fatty acids. Trans fats are manufactured from polyunsaturated fats because those sources have more than one double bond in the carbon chain. Mononunsaturated fats only have one double bond and would not be suitable for hydrogenation to a trans fat.

Cognitive Level: Analysis

Nursing Process: Evaluation

Category of Client Need: Health Promotion and Health Maintenance

Answer: 3

Rationale: White chicken chili has the least amount of total fat in the selections listed. Beef, refried beans, and cheese have higher amounts of fat per serving.

Cognitive Level: Analysis

Nursing Process: Evaluation

Category of Client Need: Health Promotion and Health Maintenance

Critical Thinking Question

It is important to share that fat is an important source of energy and essential fats for young children and that the need for fat as a percentage of total calories in the diet exceeds that of adults. The child's diet should be composed to provide at least 30% of the calories from fat with the remainder of calories coming from proteins and carbohydrates. As the child progresses toward school-age, the amount of fat required is closer to that recommended for adults, 25% to 35% of the total calories in the diet.

Answers to Stop and Consider Questions

Figure 4-11: Olive oil is recommended because it has more unsaturated fat and less saturated fat than does stick margarine or butter.

Box 4-3: The nurse can show Winfred a sample nutrition fact label where total fat, saturated fat, and trans fat are listed. The nurse can advise that Winfred keep his saturated and trans fat intake within recommended levels by comparing product labels in the supermarket and choosing those with less saturated and trans fat.

Lifespan Box: Recommendations for Fat Intake: Infants and Children: The nurse should first assess the reason that a parent is offering skim milk to a toddler; an understanding of parental concerns can serve as a foundation for education. The nurse can then address the parent's concern and provide education about the importance of a full-fat diet for essential neurological development in young children.

Chapter 5
Critical Thinking in the Nursing Process

The nurse could have explored Hilary's spending habits with respect to food, entertainment, coffee, etc. She could also have discussed the possibility of checking with the financial aid office to see if there were aid possibilities that Hilary could explore.

The nurse would emphasize whole grains and legumes along with fruits and vegetables to achieve maximal vitamin intake. Some vitamins, like D, are very difficult on a vegan diet so the nurse may appropriately recommend a supplement that meets but does not exceed the DRI for each vitamin.

Food provides energy in the form of calories; vitamins do not contain or provide energy. Vitamins are necessary for effective and efficient body functions; an excess or deficiency of individual vitamins or combination of vitamins can be detrimental to health. Vitamins that are stored (A, D, E, and K) can be particularly harmful if taken in excess. The ideal source of vitamins is a balanced diet.

NCLEX® Questions

Answer: 2

Rationale: Newborns receive an injection of Aqua-Mephyton (vitamin K) to protect them against hemorrhagic disease of the newborn. Newborns are unable to synthesize vitamin K because their guts are sterile. A single injection is enough to provide protection until the infant is fed. The nurse should know that this practice is standard care and that it would not be necessary "to check" what shot the infant had received. Vitamin C is not used to protect infants from infection, nor are other vitamins given for nutritional purposes to newborns.

Cognitive Level: Application

Nursing Process: Implementation

Category of Client Need: Health Promotion and Health Maintenance

Answer: 1

Rationale: Vitamins are lost from foods during processing; enrichment means adding nutrients back to the foods after processing in completed. The addition of extra vitamins not normally found in foods is fortification. Enriching foods does not add to their safety or mean that individuals should eat more or less of them to meet nutrient needs.

Cognitive Level: Application

Nursing Process: Implementation

Category of Client Need: Physiological Integrity

Answer: 3

Rationale: Rickets is caused by deficiency of vitamin D. In the United States, vitamin D is added to milk so this choice is the best food source of vitamin D. The other foods listed are not sources of vitamin D.

Cognitive Level: Analysis

Nursing Process: Implementation

Category of Client Need: Physiological Integrity

Answer: 1

Rationale: Alcoholics are prone to develop thiamin deficiency because the intestinal absorption of thiamin is disrupted. Thiamin deficiency may cause mental status changes, psychosis, and progress to coma. Folic acid deficiency is associated with anemia, vitamin D deficiency is associated with skeletal changes, and vitamin C deficiency is associated with scurvy.

Cognitive Level: Application

Nursing Process: Planning

Category of Client Need: Physiological Integrity

Answer: 2

Rationale: Increased folic acid is needed prior to pregnancy to prevent neural tube defects and allow normal development of the spinal cord. Folic acid is present naturally in leafy green vegetables, fruit, and liver. Spinach salad is the only food choice listed that reflects understanding of foods that are rich in folic acid; dairy products, meat, fish, and pasta are not significant sources of folic acid.

Cognitive Level: Analysis

Nursing Process: Evaluation

Category of Client Need: Health Promotion and Health Maintenance

Critical Thinking Questions

The precise cause of MS is unknown; however, there is a greater risk of developing MS if a family member has been diagnosed with it. Studies have shown that consumption of vitamin D, particularly at a younger age and in amounts no greater than 200 international units, may have some protective effect.

The nurse could suggest fortified cereals eaten with vitamin D-fortified soy milk as an excellent source of vitamin D. The client should be cautioned that excess vitamin D is toxic, but that a supplement of no more than 200 to 400 international units, coupled with 15 to 20 minutes of sun exposure daily, would be beneficial.

Answers to Stop and Consider Questions

Table 5-5: Green leafy vegetables are a good source of vitamin A. Dark orange vegetables are also good sources.

Table 5-6: It is difficult to meet the 600-international unit recommendation for vitamin D in older adulthood. More than 6 cups of milk would be needed to reach the recommended level. Supplementation is suggested for the older adult because of this difficulty.

Table 5-9: A smoker requires additional vitamin C because of the oxidative stress from smoke. An extra serving of citrus fruit each day provides the needed vitamin C to meet recommended intake.

Table 5-15: Females of childbearing age should consume folic acid from a supplement or fortified food to ensure that needs are met. Folic acid is better absorbed than is folate from food.

Table 5-16: Vegans who consume no animal products must consume vitamin B$_{12}$ from a synthetic source such as a supplement or fortified food.

Chapter 6
Critical Thinking in the Nursing Process

Foods rich in iron are more challenging for vegans, but adequate intake can be achieved with careful planning. Foods containing whole wheat (breads, cereals, pasta) are a good source of iron. Spinach and baked potatoes with skin will also supply iron, along with legumes such as lentils and pinto beans. Tofu can be prepared in many ways and is frequently used by vegans. Dried fruit, such as raisins or apricots, can be added to an iron-fortified cereal as a meal or snack.

Signs of iron deficiency in children are the same as those in adults: pale skin and conjunctiva, listlessness and fatigue, and anemia (low hemoglobin and hematocrit). Inattentiveness and poor school performance can occur. Pica may be present as well as a craving for ice.

NCLEX® Questions

Answer: 3

Rationale: Processed foods have the highest sodium content, so salami should be avoided by a client who needs to reduce dietary sources of sodium. Like most foods, each of the other foods listed contains sodium but significantly less than salami.

Cognitive Level: Analysis

Nursing Process: Evaluation

Category of Client Need: Health Promotion and Health Maintenance

Answer: 2

Rationale: Most public water systems add minute amounts fluoride to the water supply to prevent dental caries. Fluoride supplements should only be used in situations where it is known that fluoride is not added to the water because excess fluoride can cause mottled, discolored teeth in children. Fluoride that is consumed with calcium causes decreased absorption of the fluoride. Adults continue to need fluoride for good dental health.

Cognitive Level: Application

Nursing Process: Implementation

Category of Client Need: Health Promotion and Health Maintenance

Answer: 3

Rationale: Potassium is widely present in unprocessed foods such as fruit, vegetables, meat, and milk. Cottage cheese, as a processed food, has less potassium than the other selections listed. Combined with a pear half, the selection still has less potassium than the other choices. Green leafy vegetables and citrus or tropical fruits contain high amounts of potassium.

Cognitive Level: Analysis

Nursing Process: Evaluation

Category of Client Need: Health Promotion and Health Maintenance

Answer: 4

Rationale: Ascorbic acid, found in orange juice, enhances the absorption of iron. Meat, fish, and poultry, as heme sources of iron, also enhance absorption of supplements. Milk and food with oxalates, such as leafy vegetables, interfere with absorption of iron.

Cognitive Level: Application

Nursing Process: Implementation

Category of Client Need: Physiological Integrity

Answer: 3

Rationale: Clients who consume large amounts of ice or other non-food items like clay often suffer from iron deficiency; the nurse will want to explore the client's dietary intake of iron. Consumption of nonfood items is called pica. Sodium deficiency and dehydration are not likely problems because the amount of ice does not have sufficient fluid volume to cause a decrease in sodium or to satisfy a client who is dehydrated. Potassium deficiency is not associated with pica.

Cognitive Level: Analysis

Nursing Process: Assessment

Category of Client Need: Health Promotion and Health Maintenance

Critical Thinking Question

It is important to consider the overall quality of the diet, but a child needs to consume adequate amounts of calcium. The nurse should explain that milk continues to be the best source of calcium for children and that other beverages should be saved for special occasions or after consumption of milk. Some children also like flavoring added to milk to improve its taste.

The nurse could explain the importance of developing good bone health in childhood as a way to prevent fractures and the development of osteoporosis. Carbonated beverages contain phosphorus regardless of whether they are regular or diet, but colas seem to have more pronounced negative effects on bone than noncola beverages. It would be preferable to reinforce the benefits of milk as part of a quality diet for children and reserve carbonated beverages for special occasions.

Answers to Stop and Consider Questions

Table 6-4: High-protein intake might be found in the diet of someone following a low-carbohydrate diet for weight loss or a high-protein diet to build muscle. The nurse can assess overall calcium intake in the diet to check for sufficient calcium intake. The individual with high protein but inadequate calcium intake can be educated about the increased urinary calcium losses associated with high-protein diets. The nurse can suggest a source of calcium to improve overall intake.

Box 6-2: Multiple factors affect iron status during the lifespan. In infants and children, decreased intake and increased needs for growth are important. During adolescence, poor diet and increased needs for growth occur. For the adolescent female, menstrual losses affect iron status as well. During pregnancy, poor intake and increased needs are risk factors for poor iron status. In the older adult, poor intake and altered absorption from medications and reduced gastric acidity are important to consider.

Lifespan Box: Iron: The pregnant adolescent requires the same iron intake as an older pregnant female but may have more risk factors for poor iron status than the older counterpart. Poor diet and increased needs to meet both the requirements for pregnancy and maternal growth can lead to iron deficiency.

Chapter 7
Critical Thinking in the Nursing Process

The elderly have a diminished sensation of thirst so they may become dehydrated without being aware of it. Dehydration accelerates in the presence of illness or heat. The nurse needs to assess mucous membranes and skin turgor, along with urine output and color.

Healthy elderly individuals can freely select fluids that are not otherwise contraindicated. Water is the fluid of choice, but there is no reason to exclude caffeinated or sweetened beverages as long as there is not a medical condition that precludes them.

NCLEX® Questions

Answer: 2

Rationale: Moderate alcohol consumption has been documented to provide some cardiovascular benefits with the emphasis being placed on moderate. The body metabolizes all alcohol the same way, so the specific kind is not important; quantity is more important. Although the nurse will not want to recommend alcohol to prevent heart disease, it is incorrect to say that alcoholism is a great risk. Likewise, the nurse must give correct information and avoid being judgmental.

Cognitive Level: Synthesis

Nursing Process: Evaluation

Category of Client Need: Health Promotion and Health Maintenance

Answer: 4

Rationale: The first sign of dehydration is dry mucous membranes, most notably the mouth. Skin color is not affected by hydration. The skin may be dry when dehydration is severe, but if early dehydration is because of intense physical activity the individual may still be sweating profusely. Muscle weakness is a sign of advanced dehydration.

Cognitive Level: Synthesis

Nursing Process: Assessment

Category of Client Need: Physiological Integrity

Answer: 2

Rationale: The elderly are more prone to dehydration because of an inability to regulate water balance as effectively as younger adults; therefore, an elderly client with diarrhea may become dehydrated rather quickly. A client who is taking antibiotics does not have an increased need for fluids unless the condition that precipitated the need for antibiotics would make that necessary. A client who is taking diuretics, especially the elderly, should be monitored for signs of dehydration. The client who is experiencing heart failure is more likely to experience fluid overload, so the nurse will monitor for that.

Cognitive Level: Synthesis

Nursing Process: Assessment

Category of Client Need: Physiological Integrity

Answer: 4

Rationale: Coffee is a very mild diuretic, but an individual cannot become dehydrated drinking coffee because the effect is short term and it is made with water. An individual who is bothered by the diuretic effect need only change to drinking decaffeinated coffee. The nurse needs to realize that coffee is a beverage enjoyed by many people, so it is improper to label it as "bad" for any reason. The caffeine in regular coffee acts as a stimulant and may slightly elevate the heart rate, but that generally is not a problem for healthy adults. Coffee does not contain antioxidants, although tea does.

Cognitive Level: Application

Nursing Process: Evaluation

Category of Client Need: Physiological Integrity

Answer: 2

Rationale: Urine that is bright yellow and has a mild odor is indicative of dehydration. The client should increase consumption of fluids for 24 hours to see if the problem resolves. The nurse should not dismiss a client's concern without suggesting further monitoring by the client. Medications may change the color of the urine but do not account for the odor, so the nurse would ask about this finding after having the client first increase fluid intake. This issue is not an emergent problem for the health care provider at this point.

Cognitive Level: Synthesis

Nursing Process: Evaluation

Category of Client Need: Physiological Integrity

Critical Thinking Question

The nurse should remind the individual that it is important to drink fluids even before going outdoors to prevent dehydration. Limit the time outdoors during the warmest part of the day and take frequent drinks of water while outside. Because the elderly can become dehydrated without being aware of thirst, it is important to drink even if not thirsty.

Answers to Stop and Consider Questions

Table 7-4: Boiled coffee is a cultural practice in Turkey, Greece, and Scandinavian countries. Use of a French coffee press also is considered boiling. Individuals with a high blood cholesterol intake who consume boiled coffee can be advised to moderate intake in addition to following a diet that targets reduction in saturated fat intake.

Table 7-7: Moderation is the overall message that the nurse should convey when discussing health and alcohol intake. Even where some health benefits have been reported to exist with alcohol intake, increased amount of alcohol intake is not associated with increased benefit.

Hot Topic: Nutritional Antidotes to Alcohol: The nurse should convey the research findings regarding mixing energy drinks and alcohol. The effects of the energy drink can lead to a false sense of safety that may lead some individuals to drink and drive or drink more alcohol when they are intoxicated. There are no proven antidotes to the effects of excessive alcohol intake.

Chapter 8
Critical Thinking in the Nursing Process

It is important for the nurse to identify specifically what aspect of the diet is a problem for the client. For example, does the client feel like there is insufficient variety, taste, or amount of food? The nurse needs to learn about the client's food preferences or cultural practices that determine the acceptability of certain foods. The nurse should have the dietitian consult with the client to see if there are alternate foods that can be provided to the client. At times, it may be acceptable to have family members or friends bring foods that are part of the diet plan, but it should never be assumed that such practices will completely replace the meals provided by the hospital.

NCLEX® Questions

Answer: 3

Rationale: The metabolic rate is influenced by the activity level, the amount of muscle mass, and body temperature, among other things. Muscle and organ tissue is more metabolically active than fat, so if the person who is overweight has more fat mass, the basal metabolic rate may be slower than someone of the same weight who has more muscle mass. However, the person is not overweight because of the metabolic rate. Increasing physical activity will help develop more muscle mass, which is more metabolically active. No two individuals will have exactly the same metabolic rate.

Cognitive Level: Analysis

Nursing Process: Evaluation

Category of Client Need: Health Promotion and Health Maintenance

Answer: 4

Rationale: The commonly accepted term for the measurement of energy in foods is the *calorie*, even though the more precise term is *kilocalorie*. Grams and ounces refer to weight rather than energy. A kilowatt is a measure of energy but not the energy in food.

Cognitive Level: Application

Nursing Process: Implementation

Category of Client Need: Health Promotion and Health Maintenance

Answer: 1

Rationale: Foods high in protein use the most energy to digest the protein, synthesize amino acids, and metabolize protein into urea and glucose. Alcohol uses the next most amount of energy, followed by the carbohydrates, such as in fruits and vegetables. The overall contribution of these differences to total energy expenditure is minimal.

Cognitive Level: Application

Nursing Process: Implementation

Category of Client Need: Health Promotion and Health Maintenance

Answer: 2

Rationale: A positive energy balance results from caloric intake exceeding energy expenditure, ultimately leading to weight gain. Children who do not engage in much physical activity tend to have a higher weight than those who are active. Impaired glucose tolerance may result when there is excess weight but it tends to develop over a period of years. Children who are physically inactive tend to have greater caloric intake and less expenditure. Resting energy expenditure refers to the energy to rest quietly but awake after a meal.

Cognitive Level: Analysis

Nursing Process: Evaluation

Category of Client Need: Physiological Integrity

Answer: 2

Rationale: One pound is equivalent to approximately 3,500 kcalories of energy. For a client to lose an average of 1 pound per week (3,500 kcalories), the client must consume 500 fewer kcalories or expend 500 more kcalories each day for the 7 days, or some combination of the two alterations in the energy balance equation.

Cognitive Level: Application

Nursing Process: Implementation

Category of Client Need: Health Promotion and Health Maintenance

Critical Thinking Question

A decrease in metabolic rate is associated with aging in general because of loss of skeletal muscle, but weight gain is not inevitable. Menopause and declining estrogen levels may cause some redistribution of body fat, but engaging in regular physical activity and matching nutrient intake to the activity level can prevent weight gain.

Answers to Stop and Consider Questions

Box 8-1: Emma's intake is insufficient to meet her energy expenditure needs. She is in negative energy balance. Addition of a cereal bar with 10 gm of protein and 30 gm of carbohydrate adds 40 and 120 kcalories, respectively, for a total of 160 kcals. Even with this addition, she remains in negative energy balance with 2,130 kcals consumed vs. her need for 2,500 kcals. She needs to consume more energy to meet the metabolic requirements of her physical activity and resting metabolic rate.

Box 8-2: Smoking and a dietary supplement that stimulates the central nervous system both will increase the measurement of energy expenditure, which is why they should be avoided before such a measurement.

Box 8-3: For a 154 lb female (60 kg), the 1 kcal/ kg/hr calculation estimates energy expenditure as 1,680 kcals/day (60 kg × 1 kcal/kg × 24 hr). This is more than that used for the same weight and the WHO formula, 1,525 kcals. Formulas that only use weight overlook the affects that age and height may have on energy needs.

Hot Topic: Is Energy Balance Only About Intake and Expenditure: The nurse can ask the client to recall all liquids consumed as part of a nutrition history. The cumulative energy contribution of the liquids can then be calculated and shared with the client, followed by discussion about alternative beverages that have less energy content. For the client who wishes to maintain intake of caloric beverages, a discussion can include a determination of what foods have the same energy content as the liquids and how liquids do not contribute to fullness for as long as solid food.

Chapter 9
Critical Thinking in the Nursing Process

The "language" of nutrition involves many abbreviations or acronyms, just as in other health disciplines. It is important for the nurse to share current, relevant, and evidence-based information with clients. The information need not focus on details like RDIs or RDA, but rather information that they can use to plan a diet that incorporates principles like nutrient density, variety, balance, and moderation.

NCLEX® Questions

Answer: 3

Rationale: Dietary reference intakes (DRIs) are defined for nutrients, not foods, and include macro- and micronutrients. They include a wide range of recommendations, including the estimated average requirements

(EAR), the recommended daily allowance (RDA), the adequate intake (AI), and the tolerable upper intakes levels (UL) for ages and developmental stages. They are more inclusive than recommendations about caloric intake and do not include tables like the body mass index (BMI) to determine obesity. Dietitians do not use DRIs to plan specific diets for disease. DRIs are intended for the well population.

Cognitive Level: Application

Nursing Process: Implementation

Category of Client Need: Health Promotion and Health Maintenance

Answer: 1

Rationale: The health claim of "low fat" means that each serving of cookies has 3 gm or less of fat. There is no comparison made, so the consumer cannot know how this kind of cookie compares to another kind of cookie. There may be saturated fat in the cookies, even if it is a small amount. Low fat does not mean having fewer calories.

Cognitive Level: Application

Nursing Process: Implementation

Category of Client Need: Health Promotion and Health Maintenance

Answer: 3

Rationale: Nutrient-dense foods contain large amounts of nutrients for the least number of calories, a prime example being fat-free milk containing the same amount of calcium as whole milk but with fewer calories. Therefore, it is nutrient dense for calcium. Density does not refer to the wide availability of a nutrient or to the practice of consuming a variety of foods each day. MyPyramid does not have a specific base, but rather has nutrient-dense foods in each segment.

Cognitive Level: Application

Nursing Process: Implementation

Category of Client Need: Health Promotion and Health Maintenance

Answer: 2

Rationale: Structure-function claims describe a food with regard to a normal structure or function and may not refer to a disease state, which is why it is not a health claim. Milk is a food, not a nutrient.

Cognitive Level: Application

Nursing Process: Implementation

Category of Client Need: Health Promotion and Health Maintenance

Answer: 2

Rationale: Because computers are widely available, the nurse might suggest that a client use the interactive re-

sources at the MyPyramid Web site as a good way to get started on an analysis of the client's current diet prior to determining changes that might be implemented to make the diet healthier. The DRIs are not intended for planning specific individual diets or food intake. The USDA Web site does not provide individual diet planning. The health food section of a grocery store may have pamphlets for specific foods or promote health claims, but the consumer would not expect to find information about diet analysis.

Cognitive Level: Application

Nursing Process: Implementation

Category of Client Need: Health Promotion and Health Maintenance

Answers to Stop and Consider Questions

Box 9-4: First, the nurse should provide positive feedback about the client trying to make dietary changes. It would be important to ask the client about the nutrient content of the potato chips. If the client chose the chips based on the "light" advertising and is unaware of the nutrient content of the snack, advise the client about the meaning of "light" on the label and how the potato chip label should be checked further to see which meaning of "light" is meant. The chips could be light in sodium, fat, or calories or just light in color or texture.

Chapter 10
Critical Thinking in the Nursing Process

There are many things that the nurse can stress to the client, such as wash hands prior to food preparation; thoroughly wash all fresh fruit and vegetables, even those that will be cooked; cook all meats to internal temperatures that will kill any bacteria, preferably using a meat thermometer; wash all food preparation surfaces, counters, and cutting boards with hot, soapy water; and refrigerate all leftovers within 30 minutes of preparation. In addition, check expiration and sell-by dates on purchased foods.

NCLEX® Questions

Answer: 3

Rationale: Primary prevention is aimed at the community level and is designed to reach large groups of people. Teaching high school students about healthy dietary practices is an example of primary prevention. Teaching about specific diets to clients with particular diagnoses is secondary prevention. The nurse would not recommend multivitamin supplements unless the child has a known deficiency.

Cognitive Level: Analysis

Nursing Process: Evaluation

Category of Client Need: Health Promotion and Health Maintenance

Answer: 3

Rationale: The first responsibility of the nurse is to assess the client. The nurse does this by asking about the client's symptoms. The client's response will help the nurse determine what type of foodborne illness might be occurring. The remaining questions would be appropriate after first assessing the client.

Cognitive Level: Application

Nursing Process: Assessment

Category of Client Need: Physiological Integrity

Answer: 2

Rationale: Raw eggs may contain *Salmonella*, which can be deadly, especially in persons with compromised immune systems. Eggs are an excellent source of protein, but they should be used in foods that are thoroughly cooked or baked, and never eaten raw.

Cognitive Level: Application

Nursing Process: Implementation

Category of Client Need: Health Promotion and Health Maintenance

Answer: 4

Rationale: Unpasteurized milk may contain *Salmonella*, a bacterium that is a common cause of foodborne infection. An allergy to a food arises when the body responds systemically to an allergen in the food. Foodborne intoxication occurs when there is a toxin contained by the food, as in home-canned foods. Milk does not cause cancer.

Cognitive Level: Application

Nursing Process: Evaluation

Category of Client Need: Health Promotion and Health Maintenance

Answer: 2

Rationale: Most cultural groups have comfort foods that are served to individuals who are sick; chicken soup is an example of such a food. Comfort foods are usually used in conjunction with other medical, pharmacological, or health practices. Assimilation and acculturation refer to the adoption of the beliefs, attitudes, and practices during the transition to a new community.

Cognitive Level: Analysis

Nursing Process: Assessment

Category of Client Need: Health Promotion and Health Maintenance

Critical Thinking Question

The nurse should be knowledgeable about community resources available to low-income residents and make referrals when appropriate. In addition, the nurse can suggest that families buy more nutrient-dense foods that store well like eggs, canned or dried legumes such as chickpeas and kidney beans, brown rice, peanut butter, whole grain breads that can be frozen, and cheese. High-protein and high-fiber foods are more filling than foods that are high in carbohydrates.

Answers to Stop and Consider Questions

Box 10-4: The nurse should let the client know that the word *natural* on the food label means there are no artificial ingredients. The ingredient listing can be read to check ingredients, such as additives or preservatives, but will not denote whether pesticides were used. Neither natural nor organic labels mean that overall nutritional content of a product can be overlooked.

Chapter 11
Critical Thinking in the Nursing Process

The nurse should be prepared to show clients how to access www.MyPyramid.gov on the computer. The nurse can demonstrate some of the interactive features that enable clients to see how to plan and evaluate food intake. Clients who do not have computer access should be given free materials that are readily available to nurses and other health care providers from the www.MyPyramid.gov Web site or the USDA.

NCLEX® Questions

Answer: 2

Rationale: High glycemic foods may be consumed by the athlete after activity when additional activity is expected to occur in less than 24 hours. High glycemic foods raise the blood glucose level quickly and help restore glycogen levels. Plain bagels are a source of refined carbohydrates, which makes them have a high glycemic index. The other foods listed have less refined carbohydrates in a serving plus more fat, fiber, or protein, all of which contribute to a lower glycemic effect.

Cognitive Level: Application

Nursing Process: Evaluation

Category of Client Need: Health Promotion and Health Maintenance

Answer: 3

Rationale: During a strict training regimen it is safe to increase protein consumption from the usual acceptable range of 0.6 to 0.8 gm/kg to 1.3 to 1.8 gm/kg. The athlete in this case would be consuming about 1.5 gm/kg. Carbohydrate consumption should be increased to provide a ready source of glucose and good glycogen stores. Creatine does not aid protein metabolism. It is important to be aware of fat consumption, but minimizing it at this time will not meet the needs for a training program.

Cognitive Level: Analysis

Nursing Process: Evaluation

Category of Client Need: Health Promotion and Health Maintenance

Answer: 1

Rationale: Creatine aids in the production of adenosine triphosphate (ATP), a source of energy used during muscle-building activity, but has not been tested for safety in those under age 18 years. Creatine is widely available and has been the subject of many studies that demonstrate its effectiveness in limited situations. It does not require physician or health care provider supervision. Side effects, such as weight gain, gastrointestinal (GI) complaints, or bloating, are present in some individuals, but creatine is generally well tolerated. However, there are no long-term clinical studies to demonstrate the effects of prolonged use.

Cognitive Level: Application

Nursing Process: Intervention

Category of Client Need: Health Promotion and Health Maintenance

Answer: 3

Rationale: Female athletes exhibiting any one of the signs of the female athlete triad (amenorrhea, osteoporosis, eating disorder) should be screened for additional signs that might warrant intervention. It is appropriate to drink lots of fluid during a meet and to be tired afterward. The nurse would want to ask about the supplement, but it is not a concern in and of itself.

Cognitive Level: Application

Nursing Process: Assessment

Category of Client Need: Physiological Integrity

Answer: 1

Rationale: A high-carbohydrate diet can be used to achieve maximal glycogen stores that can be used during prolonged exercise. The carbohydrates should be a combination of simple and complex forms. Consuming a high-carbohydrate intake only before planned activity may not provide sufficient amounts to support glycogen stores and blood glucose levels during and following exercise.

Cognitive Level: Application

Nursing Process: Intervention

Category of Client Need: Health Promotion and Health Maintenance

Critical Thinking Questions

Endurance is improved by regular training, which includes attention to diet, the duration and timing of practice, mental preparation, and rest. A diet that includes adequate protein and carbohydrate is important to allow for the growth that is necessary in adolescence and to provide extra nutrients for participation in a strenuous sport. A consultation with a dietitian may help determine the ideal nutrient balance for the individual.

Caffeinated drinks of all kinds have varying amounts of caffeine. Research has shown that caffeine is not beneficial in sports in which endurance is a primary factor. Caffeine will not improve her run time when jogging. If she has concerns about fatigue she might consider making sure that her overall energy and carbohydrate intake are sufficient.

Answers to Stop and Consider Questions

Box 11-2: Consuming whole foods costs less than using protein supplements to meet needs. Whole foods also have the benefit of containing many other important nutrients that would be lacking in supplements of a single nutrient such as amino acid pills or protein powder.

Box 11-3: The nurse can explain to Paul that he is already consuming adequate protein to meet the needs of muscle building provided he consumes adequate energy as well. If he does not consume sufficient calories, some of his protein intake will be sacrificed to meet energy needs instead of being used as a building block for muscle synthesis.

Box 11-6: Michael can assess his own hydration status by making sure that he maintains a urine that is light in color. He can also monitor his weight before and after runs to make sure that he is hydrating adequately and not losing excessive weight nor gaining weight during exercise.

Chapter 12
Critical Thinking in the Nursing Process

The nurse should say that it is important to have data from a balance scale that is regularly calibrated. In addition, adults lose height as they age so it is important to have a measured height. In addition, many medication dosages are calculated based on weight so a correct and current measure is necessary.

The nurse should gather measured height and weight and calculate BMI. Other laboratory and anthropometric data would be part of a more focused health assessment.

NCLEX® Questions

Answer: 2

Rationale: The nomogram represents population data and is a calculation based on height and weight. An athlete with well-developed muscle has greater mass than an individual who is the same height but weighs less. The nomogram does not measure the metabolic rate. The apple or pear shape is determined by actual measurement of waist and hips.

Cognitive Level: Application

Nursing Process: Assessment

Category of Client Need: Physiological Integrity

Answer: 3

Rationale: Underweight is best determined by analysis of the BMI. When it is less than 20 an individual is considered underweight. Waist measurement is based on frame size and fitness and in and of itself is not indicative of being over- or underweight. A hematocrit level of 39 is normal and is not related to weight. Fine wrinkles begin to develop in middle age and are considered a normal finding.

Cognitive Level: Synthesis

Nursing Process: Evaluation

Category of Client Need: Health Promotion and Health Maintenance

Answer: 1

Rationale: A client with a BMI of 33 is considered obese and is at risk for various medical conditions like hypertension or diabetes. The metabolic rate can begin to slow in middle age with any loss of skeletal muscle, but the effect should not be significant at this point. The BMI is not directly affected by deficient knowledge.

Cognitive Level: Application

Nursing Process: Diagnosis

Category of Client Need: Health Promotion and Health Maintenance

Answer: 4

Rationale: The most accurate data should be obtained and recorded by the nurse. Individuals who have difficulty standing but can be assisted should be weighed in a chair scale. An estimation of height can be made from a knee height measurement. Individuals tend to be inaccurate in self-report data, so the nurse should avoid using that unless no alternatives for direct measure are available. A bed scale and supine measurements are not possible in a clinic setting. Unless a client can safely stand long enough to use a balance scale, a chair scale is a safer alternative.

Cognitive Level: Application

Nursing Process: Assessment

Category of Client Need: Health Promotion and Health Maintenance

Answer: 2

Rationale: The albumin level is a routine measure of nutritional status; it declines over time with inadequate protein intake. Fasting blood glucose is not significantly decreased with malnutrition. Decreased serum cholesterol and triglyceride levels are not independent indicators of nutritional status.

Cognitive Level: Application

Nursing Process: Assessment

Category of Client Need: Physiological Integrity

Critical Thinking Questions

The most accurate measure of weight occurs when the individual is consistently weighed on the same scale at about the same time of day. When a client uses a home scale or self-reports weight, the data may not be accurate.

Self-report data from adults and youth tend to be inaccurate with respect to height and weight. If body mass indices are calculated from inaccurate data, the actual prevalence of overweight or obese individuals can be expected to be greater than that reported by the data. If accurate information is required, a sample of the population should be measured for actual height and weight.

Answers to Stop and Consider Questions

Table 12-1: Examples of undernutrition and overnutrition include: an obese child who consumes many high-fat and high-sugar foods but has poor intake of many vitamins and minerals, a female who takes megadoses of vitamins but is deficient in calcium and has osteoporosis, an overweight alcoholic who is deficient in thiamine.

Table 12-6: Relying on BMI as the sole tool to assess weight overlooks the effect of muscle mass and bone mineral density on weight. BMI is not a direct assessment of body composition.

Box 12-5: The client has 14 gm of nitrogen losses per day. In order for this client to be in negative nitrogen balance, intake must be less than 14 gm of nitrogen/day. Intake would need to be less than 87.5 gm of protein for negative nitrogen balance to happen (87.5 gm protein ÷ 6.25 gm nitrogen/gm protein = 14 gm of nitrogen).

Chapter 13
Critical Thinking in the Nursing Process

A woman of average weight should gain 25 to 35 pounds during pregnancy. This weight is distributed to the baby, breasts, amniotic fluid, and increased blood volume, along with increased fat stores to prepare for lactation. This weight gain is necessary for optimum outcomes. It is important to remain physically active during pregnancy, and soon after birth the mother can resume activities. Breastfeeding utilizes many calories and many women slowly lose weight while breastfeeding. Weight loss after pregnancy is enhanced by not gaining excessive weight during pregnancy, returning to a prepregnancy diet, and physical activity.

NCLEX® Questions

Answer: 2

Rationale: Weight gain is critical to a positive pregnancy outcome. The additional weight should come from consuming nutrient-dense foods, and milk is one that is readily available. Skim milk can provide essential nutrients with less fat than whole or 2% milk. The notion that calories can be "saved" from nutrient-dense foods and used on other intake should be dispelled. A calcium supplement may be desirable if a woman is unwilling or unable to drink enough milk to get the recommended amount of calcium on a daily basis. The developing fetus will get adequate calcium, even at the expense of the mother's bones. Milk alone is not responsible for a positive outcome; it must be part of a broader healthy diet.

Cognitive Level: Application

Nursing Process: Evaluation

Category of Client Need: Health Promotion and Health Maintenance

Answer: 3

Rationale: The weight that is gained during pregnancy is distributed to the baby, breast tissue, amniotic fluid, fat stores, and increased blood volume, among other places. Depending on the size of the baby, there is a substantial weight loss in the first few days after birth. The remainder of the weight loss occurs gradually as a result of breastfeeding, if chosen by the mother, decreased caloric intake to prepregnancy levels, and increased physical activity. Achievement of prepregnancy weight often requires discipline on the part of the mother over a period of several months. A mother who is open to weight gain, taking vitamin and mineral supplements, and in general doing what is necessary to have a healthy baby is expressing receptivity to the nurse's teaching.

Cognitive Level: Analysis

Nursing Process: Evaluation

Category of Client Need: Health Promotion and Health Maintenance

Answer: 2

Rationale: A full-term infant has about 6 months of iron stores. Breast milk does not contain iron so the infant does not have additional oxygen carrying capacity. The infant who is exclusively breastfed will need supplemental iron after about 6 months of age. The breastfeeding mother often needs to continue to take iron to replace her body's stores that were transferred to the fetus during pregnancy. Iron does not prevent a fluid volume deficit.

Cognitive Level: Application

Nursing Process: Implementation

Category of Client Need: Health Promotion and Health Maintenance

Answer: 1

Rationale: Successful breastfeeding for the new mother requires adequate nutrition, rest, and a caloric increase of about 500 kcalories per day. Eating 4,000 kcalories per day would lead to substantial weight gain in most females and far exceeds even the amount needed during the last trimester of pregnancy. The nursing mother needs extra fluids throughout the day, not just the morning. Calcium supplements are not intended to fortify breast milk; they are for the mother's needs.

Cognitive Level: Application

Nursing Process: Implementation

Category of Client Need: Health Promotion and Health Maintenance

Answer: 4

Rationale: The nurse needs to complete an assessment prior to developing or implementing a plan of care;

therefore, the nurse needs to determine the dietary habits of the client, regardless of the age. It is important to plan for weight gain, the use of prenatal vitamin and mineral supplements, and the distribution of macronutrients but that cannot be done until after an assessment is completed.

Cognitive Level: Analysis

Nursing Process: Assessment

Category of Client Need: Health Promotion and Health Maintenance

Critical Thinking Question

Research studies have not provided definitive answers to this question. It is important to eat a balanced diet during pregnancy and avoid environmental stressors, like smoke, that are not healthful for anyone. Breastfeeding is ideal for babies, but even that has not been proven to prevent allergies.

Answers to Stop and Consider Questions

Box 13-6: Pharmacists can be consulted about medication safety and breastfeeding.

Chapter 14
Critical Thinking in the Nursing Process

School-age children need to focus on healthy eating and getting adequate activity. Overall, weight loss is not the goal; it is more important to learn good food choices and begin participation in regular physical activity. If weight can be maintained without gains, growth in stature at the time of puberty will alleviate some of the overweight issues.

NCLEX® Questions

Answer: 2

Rationale: Cow's milk should not be introduced until the infant is 1 year old. The renal system is not mature enough until that time, cow's milk may cause gastrointestinal bleeding, and the risk of developing allergies to milk protein increases. When milk is first introduced, it should be whole milk because of the infant's need for fats; however, this should not occur until after the first birthday. The difference in taste is not a significant problem because the infant will have been exposed to many new tastes by the time cow's milk is introduced after the first year.

Nursing Process: Implementation

Cognitive Level: Application

Category of Client Need: Physiological Integrity

Answer: 4

Rationale: The introduction of new foods one at a time allows for detection of allergies, so the infant is not yet ready for multiple foods from the family meal. Cereal should not be put in a bottle because it does not promote the development of muscles used for chewing and is a choking hazard when delivered this way. Fruits are sweet and should not be introduced until the infant is used to cereal and vegetables.

Nursing Process: Evaluation

Cognitive Level: Analysis

Category of Client Need: Health Promotion and Health Maintenance

Answer: 3

Rationale: Children typically enjoy eating foods they help prepare and it serves as a pleasant learning experience. Offering dessert as a bribe for healthy eating does not encourage good food choices and healthy eating habits. Children should play prior to eating so they do not rush through a meal just so they may begin play. Healthy snacks at an appropriate time may help encourage good eating habits.

Nursing Process: Implementation

Cognitive Level: Application

Category of Client Need: Health Promotion and Health Maintenance

Answer: 3

Rationale: Calcium and iron are the nutrients that are most likely to be deficient in an adolescent's diet; therefore, a meal choice that provides iron and calcium helps balance a lunch that is low in those nutrients. Spaghetti and bread contain carbohydrates but are low in iron and calcium; steak and potatoes provide iron but no calcium; the same is true of the chili meal.

Nursing Process: Implementation

Cognitive Level: Application

Category of Client Need: Health Promotion and Health Maintenance

Answer: 4

Rationale: Children who do not drink milk are at risk for developing poor bone mineralization and rickets, which are caused by calcium and vitamin D deficiencies. The nurse will want to assess the child for the presence of these conditions and educate the mother about the importance of incorporating milk and dairy products in the child's diet. Iron, folic acid, vitamin C, and vitamin K are easily consumed from other foods, so the nurse is not concerned about milk as the primary source of those nutrients.

Nursing Process: Assessment

Critical Thinking Question

Breakfast is very important for everyone. Eating breakfast improves the attention span and academic performance of children and lessens the likelihood of becoming overweight. Obesity and weight problems are increasing in children, and skipping breakfast can contribute to that trend. A quick combination of cold cereals or granola-type bars with milk; fruit and fruit juices with yogurt; bagels with peanut butter; or leftovers from another meal require minimal preparation, and everyone can eat something they choose.

Answers to Stop and Consider Questions

Table 14-1: The nurse should first assess the reason that the older baby is being offered pureed food. An understanding of the parents' beliefs can help guide the education needed to explain that progression of food textures is a part of development of both fine-motor and digestive capabilities. Advanced textures are also needed to offer the variety of foods that a child needs.

Box 14-2: The nurse should first assess the reason that the parent is mixing cereal and formula. An understanding of a parent's belief can help guide the education needed to explain that offering cereal before age 4 months is not recommended because of an immature intestinal tract and that mixing cereal and formula does not necessarily help a child sleep longer. Cutting a larger whole in a bottle nipple is a choking hazard and should be discouraged.

Chapter 15
Critical Thinking in the Nursing Process

The nurse would want to do another 24-hour food recall with attention to quantity and quality of foods consumed. The nurse would also want to explore when Laura eats and if she eats with anyone else. As part of the larger assessment, the nurse could ask about the ability to get to a grocery store, problems with food preparation, or dental concerns.

A referral to social service may be necessary to more fully assess her financial resources, access to dental care, or to determine if other issues like depression are present.

When clients have pain that is relieved or diminished, the appetite usually increases. Many pain medications need to be taken with food so the client may need to experiment with the timing and quantity of food to prevent stomach upset. If pain medication is not taken with food, the client may experience nausea and then refuse to eat.

Dehydration is already a risk in the elderly due to diminished thirst. That risk is increased when clients like Laura self-restrict fluids as a means of dealing with incontinence. Incontinence needs to be dealt with as a functional problem, not one that can be managed with fluid restriction.

NCLEX® Questions

Answer: 3

Rationale: Weight loss is the first action to consider in clients with osteoarthritis who are also overweight. Excess weight puts added stress on joints so that even a small weight loss can diminish pain. Calcium and protein do not affect arthritic joints. Foods rich in omega-3 fats may be useful in the inflammation associated with rheumatoid arthritis but have not been demonstrated to relieve symptoms of osteoarthritis.

Cognitive Level: Application

Nursing Process: Implementation

Category of Client Need: Health Promotion and Health Maintenance

Answer: 2

Rationale: Decreased saliva production is a normal age-related change in the elderly that contributes to difficulty swallowing. Periodontal disease may contribute to difficulty chewing, but it is *not* a normal age-related change. Peristalsis may be slowed in aging and there may be slight decrease in bone density in the jaw, but they do not contribute to problems with swallowing.

Cognitive Level: Application

Nursing Process: Evaluation

Category of Client Need: Health Promotion and Health Maintenance

Answer: 1

Rationale: Brown rice and tofu are acceptable to vegetarians and together have a large amount of protein per serving. Cheese crackers and juice smoothies have more carbohydrates than protein, although they are acceptable to lacto-ovo vegetarians. Cream of mushroom soup has protein but not as much per serving as brown rice and tofu.

Cognitive Level: Application

Nursing Process: Implementation

Category of Client Need: Physiological Integrity

Answer: 2

Rationale: Black beans are legumes and have the highest fiber content of any of the other foods.

Cognitive Level: Analysis

Nursing Process: Evaluation

Category of Client Need: Physiologic Integrity

Answer: 4

Rationale: The nurse needs to give fluids to a client with Alzheimer's disease. The client who is forgetful will not take initiative in pouring the water from a pitcher, and a diminished sense of thirst associated with aging may mean that a client will respond negatively to a query about thirst. Congregate eating may increase socialization but will not necessarily affect fluid intake.

Cognitive Level: Application

Nursing Process: Implementation

Category of Client Need: Physiological Integrity

Critical Thinking Question

Dietary sources of calcium and vitamin D are preferable because they provide additional nutrients at the same time. Supplements are acceptable if they are taken in the recommended dosage range. There will be no lasting benefits if they are not taken consistently.

The client could use a pill splitter to cut the large tablets. Another possibility is to take one of the newer reduced size tablets. Depending on other medical contraindications, the client could also take antacid tablets that contain calcium carbonate and are chewable.

Answers to Stop and Consider Questions

Table 15-1: Synthetic vitamin B_{12} is any food fortified with vitamin B_{12}, such as breakfast cereals.

Table 15-4: Effects of aging that cannot be changed include changes in thirst perception, taste, smell, and gastrointestinal function, such as diminished gastric acid production. Medical intervention can improve xerostomia, smell, and taste disorders if they are related to medication side effects if alternative drug choices are available. Strength training may improve age-related loss of muscle. Multidisciplinary collaboration can be implemented for social and financial concerns, medical condition care, hearing, vision, and dental care.

Chapter 16
Critical Thinking in the Nursing Process

The nurse should determine the name of the formula, the length of time the formula is delivered, how the formula is prepared, and how much formula is used in 24 hours.

The health care team will be able to answer any questions. A pump can be programmed to deliver the correct amount of feeding, and home care services will be available if needed. It is important to keep track of the feedings and prepare them according to directions. Keep track of feeding times and any symptoms the client experiences. If a client experiences bloating, choking, vomiting, constipation, or diarrhea it is important to contact the clinic. A fever should also be reported immediately. Many communities have support groups for enteral therapy clients and caregivers.

NCLEX® Questions

Answer: 3

Rationale: The potential for bacterial overgrowth increases with the length of time an enteral feeding is hanging. Enteral feeding solutions are usually infused over 4 to 6 hours before a fresh feeding is hung. A cold feeding may cause gastrointestinal (GI) cramping so it should be avoided. A nurse may flush the tubing at any time but must always do so if the feeding is interrupted to give medications. It is important for the nurse to calculate and monitor the infusion, but that is not why the feeding lasts only 6 hours.

Cognitive Level: Analysis

Nursing Process: Implementation

Category of Client Need: Physiological Integrity

Answer: 4

Rationale: The high dextrose content of TPN means it must not be stopped abruptly, or it may lead to excess circulating insulin and hypoglycemia. As the client begins taking oral feeding, the TPN is gradually reduced over a period of several days. The client may have small frequent meals, but the TPN cannot be safely infused only at night. Ice chips are not an adequate test of the success of oral feeding.

Cognitive Level: Application

Nursing Process: Planning

Category of Client Need: Physiological Integrity

Answer: 1

Rationale: A client on a mechanical soft diet must avoid foods that have casings or peels such as hot dogs or apples. Clients may eat foods that are soft in consistency, ground meats, or boneless fish.

Cognitive Level: Analysis

Nursing Process: Evaluation

Category of Client Need: Health Promotion and Health Maintenance

Answer: 2

Rationale: The client's pancreas may be unable to secrete enough insulin to keep up with the high concentration of dextrose in most TPN solutions; therefore, a small amount of insulin may be added to the TPN, even in clients who are nondiabetic. As the TPN is decreased when the client resumes oral feeding, the insulin is also tapered and eventually discontinued. Blood glucose is monitored and the insulin dosage is adjusted up or down as needed. The nurse monitoring TPN should expect insulin to be added in many cases so does not need to verify it with the physician, although it is important to monitor the blood glucose and report unusual findings to the physician. Insulin is not usually prescribed for type 2 diabetics unless oral medication fails to maintain blood glucose levels.

Cognitive Level: Application

Nursing Process: Implementation

Category of Client Need: Physiological Integrity

Answer: 1

Rationale: A client who is experiencing diarrhea with enteral feeding needs to be assessed for the type of formula and the rate of infusion. A hyperosmolar formula or one that is running too fast can cause diarrhea, so the nurse needs to know the specific formula and rate. It may be important for the nurse to know the reason for the enteral feeding, but the most likely cause of diarrhea is osmolality and rate. Edema, thirst, or consulting the dietitian do not relate to the presence of diarrhea.

Cognitive Level: Analysis

Nursing Process: Assessment

Category of Client Need: Physiological Integrity

Critical Thinking Question

The nurse could offer to work with a colleague to research the practice of using dye as a means of detecting aspiration. The findings could then be shared with the rest of the staff and unit or facility leadership. The nurse could extend the research to consideration of other means to prevent aspiration.

Answers to Stop and Consider Questions

Box 16-4: Continuous delivery of feedings generally has less intestinal side effects and lower risk of aspiration than the other two methods. It does not allow for a period free from feeding. Intermittent feedings utilize less time than continuous feedings but should not be used in those at risk of aspiration. Bolus feedings mimic mealtimes but may cause diarrhea in some and should not be used in those at risk of aspiration.

Box 16-5:

1. $D_{10}W$ = 10% dextrose in water or 10 gm dextrose/100 gm water
2. 10 gm dextrose/100 gm water = 100 gm dextrose in 1,000 gm water (or 1 liter)
3. If 100 gm dextrose in 1 liter, 300 gm dextrose in 3 L
4. 300 gm dextrose/3 L $\times$ 3.4 kcal/gm = 420 kcal in 3 L of 10% dextrose

This amount of energy without any other source of nutrition is insufficient to meet the nutritional needs of any hospitalized client.

Lifespan Box: Malnutrition and the Older Adult: Restrictive diets should be liberalized in the older adult unless there is a strong medical contraindication. The older adult is at risk of malnutrition because of a number of reasons, including possible changes in appetite, intestinal function, mental status, dental health, sensory function, and physical abilities. Psychosocial and economic issues can also be important. Illness can further alter nutrition risk because of symptoms, treatment, and increased metabolic needs that may go unmet.

Chapter 17
Critical Thinking in the Nursing Process

The nurse has a responsibility to respond to client requests and concerns. The nurse would explain that bariatric surgery has certain risks and is used for obese clients who have tried dieting and been unsuccessful at achieving and maintaining weight loss. A complete evaluation for bariatric surgery would include a review of past efforts at weight loss, along with an assessment of the ability to adhere to lifestyle changes that are necessary after surgery.

The nurse would want to emphasize a diet that is composed of a balance of carbohydrates, protein, and fat that emphasizes complex carbohydrates like whole grain breads and cereals. Low-fat or fat-free dairy products should be consumed. Vegetables can be consumed liberally as long as they are not prepared with additional sauces that add calories. Fruits, especially those with edible skins or seeds for added fiber, are included. Any meat should be as lean as possible and chicken or turkey should have the skin removed. Blood glucose levels should lower because of weight loss.

NCLEX® Questions

Answer: 3

Rationale: Assessment data need to be gathered before the nurse can determine if a problem exists. Adolescents do indeed undergo a growth spurt, but an increased appetite accompanies the growth so weight gain may occur. Childhood eating patterns often carry over into adolescence and adulthood so it is important to establish good eating habits at a young age. Until assessment data are gathered, it is inappropriate for the nurse to suggest that overweight or a serious health problem may exist.

Cognitive Level: Application

Nursing Process: Evaluation

Category of Client Need: Health Promotion and Health Maintenance

Answer: 1

Rationale: It is realistic to establish a goal to increase weight by 1 pound a week in the outpatient setting. This approach entails consuming approximately 500 extra kcalories a day along with no increase in physical activity. Initial weight gain may be slow, but it is important to strive for weight gain. Individuals with anorexia nervosa need adequate fluid intake. A maintenance diet is not appropriate for someone with an initial diagnosis of impaired nutrition, nor is it realistic to expect someone with anorexia to begin to request snacks.

Cognitive Level: Application

Nursing Process: Planning

Category of Client Need: Physiological Integrity

Answer: 3

Rationale: Weight cycling or yo-yo dieting is the repeated weight loss followed by weight gain. Successful maintenance of weight loss requires continued vigilance with dietary intake and regular physical activity. Consuming large amounts of fluid may cause weight gain if fluids are high in calories, like sweetened beverages. Weight loss may have been due to a fad diet so the nurse does not want to assume that it is advisable for the client to continue what may be an unhealthy diet. Mere avoidance of simple carbohydrates is not sufficient to maintain weight loss unless it is coupled with an appropriate balance of complex carbohydrates, protein, and fat.

Cognitive Level: Application

Nursing Process: Implementation

Category of Client Need: Physiological Integrity

Answer: 1

Rationale: Orlistat works by promoting excretion, rather than absorption, of fat from meals; therefore, the client needs a multivitamin supplement that contains the fat-soluble vitamins that are being excreted. Loose stools, not constipation, are a common side effect of orlistat.

The type of fat that is absorbed is not affected by the medication. The client needs to have regular medical follow-up at agreed upon intervals, but there is no need to regularly report weight loss.

Cognitive Level: Synthesis

Nursing Process: Evaluation

Category of Client Need: Health Promotion and Health Maintenance

Answer: 4

Rationale: Readiness to change and receptiveness to teaching exist when a client is able to state positive reasons for the change. A client who is focused on what must be given up (ice cream) or doing what someone else (a physician) decides is desirable is not likely to be motivated to learn. Likewise, a negative decision (I won't go) does not enhance readiness to learn.

Cognitive Level: Synthesis

Nursing Process: Evaluation

Category of Client Need: Health Promotion and Health Maintenance

Critical Thinking Questions

The nurse could respond that there is evidence that some individuals do gain weight with stress in the workplace; however, the client can lessen the possibility of weight gain by selecting snacks at work that are lower in empty calories. Foods like grapes or pretzels can be eaten at the desk. It is also important to get up and walk around periodically. The effect of physical activity can be cumulative. In addition, overall diet management outside of work is important.

Many people enjoy chocolate and say they crave it at different times. This type of craving is poorly understood and not associated with any nutritional deficiency. It is not known if the craving is due to any physiological or psychological factors. The nurse can suggest limiting intake to a small piece of chocolate, rather than a whole bar, or substituting for lower-calorie chocolate foods like fat-free pudding or fat-free hot chocolate. The nurse could also suggest a plan for behavior modification using stimulus control or other methods.

Answers to Stop and Consider Questions

Table 17-1: The office and examination room environment should have readily available seating, gowns, blood pressure cuffs, and scales that can accommodate an obese individual without creating an awkward scene. These accommodations are discussed in the section on size acceptance.

Table 17-3: The client can compare product labels and check the nutrition facts panel and serving sizes to make similar product comparisons while shopping.

Box 17-4: The nurse can collaborate with the client to strategize some positive self-talk to practice when challenged with negative self-talk. Assessing the client's motivating factors for weight loss can help determine some ideas for self-talk.

The client without social support can be referred to local weight management classes or groups associated with a clinic, hospital, wellness center, or similar organization.

Box 17-3: The client with hypertension should be educated about the negative effects of stimulants on the cardiovascular system. The nurse can relate case anecdotes of stroke, hypertension, and heart attack occurring with use of these products in some clients.

Box 17-5: Modifiable risks for development of an eating disorder include self-esteem, expression of emotions, chronic dieting, and overvaluation on weight and appearance. The nurse can be engaged in educational programs that target improved self-esteem, appropriate expression of emotions, healthy eating, and challenge environmental influences and thinking that perpetuate the thin ideal.

Lifespan Box: Weight Control in Children, Pregnant Females, and Older Adults: The nurse should educate the client or parent about the importance of adequate nutrition to support growth and development. Restrictive eating during pregnancy can lead to a shortfall in intake of essential nutrients needed for fetal development. Children do not require a structured approach to weight loss unless weight gain surpasses the rate of linear growth, leading to an increasing BMI, or when comorbidities warrant this approach.

Chapter 18
Critical Thinking in the Nursing Process

Some of the first things a nurse can suggest include: eliminate or reduce fried foods and meats high in fat and sodium such as salami, bacon, beef, and hot dogs; increase consumption of whole grains, fruits, and vegetables high in soluble fiber; and eliminate or reduce foods with saturated and trans fats.

Medications that are prescribed to lower cholesterol are designed to be used in conjunction with a low-cholesterol, low-fat diet. In addition, it is important to have a diet that is based on variety, balance, and moderation for weight control (if necessary) and to prevent other conditions like diabetes and high blood pressure from developing.

NCLEX® Questions

Answer: 2

Rationale: Soluble or viscous fiber, which turns into a gel when mixed with liquid, has been shown to lower serum cholesterol levels. Apples are an example of a food that is high in soluble fiber. Other examples are legumes, barley, and flaxseed. Insoluble fiber increases fecal bulk but does not affect cholesterol directly. The other choices are examples of insoluble fiber.

Cognitive Level: Application

Nursing Process: Implementation

Category of Client Need: Health Promotion and Health Maintenance

Correct Answer: 4

Rationale: Roast turkey slices, especially white meat, are low in sodium and fat, making this a good lunch choice. Processed foods and meats, such as salami and ham, are high in sodium content and should be avoided on a low-sodium diet. Shrimp is low in sodium but the salad dressing containing sodium makes this choice incorrect.

Cognitive Level: Analysis

Nursing Process: Evaluation

Category of Client Need: Health Promotion and Health Maintenance

Correct Answer: 2

Rationale: A vegetarian diet may help lower cholesterol, depending on the food choices the vegetarian makes; however, it is possible to consume a low cholesterol and saturated diet without becoming a vegetarian. The human body manufactures cholesterol from saturated fats so even vegetarians can have an elevated serum cholesterol level. Likewise, it is not likely for anyone to consume too little cholesterol.

Cognitive Level: Application

Nursing Process: Planning

Category of Client Need: Physiological Integrity

Correct Answer: 3

Rationale: Desserts are possible for clients on low-fat, low-cholesterol, and low-sodium diets. Besides gingersnaps or fruit, good choices include sherbet, angel food cake, and low-fat frozen yogurts. Some low-fat desserts may be high in calories or carbohydrates so the client needs to understand if that is a factor in food choice. Ice cream, pie crusts, and most cookies contain large amounts of saturated and trans fats so intake should be modified for compliance to a low-fat or low-cholesterol diet.

Cognitive Level: Application

Nursing Process: Implementation

Category of Client Need: Health Promotion and Health Maintenance

Correct Answer: 1

Rationale: Fresh fruit and juices have no fat. Whole wheat cereals combined with low-fat milk offer the client fiber with minimal fat. The other breakfast selections contain items that are higher in fat such as eggs, full-fat yogurt, margarine, and cream cheese. A breakfast that contains these items indicates a need for additional teaching.

Cognitive Level: Analysis

Nursing Process: Implementation

Category of Client Need: Health Promotion and Health Maintenance

Critical Thinking Questions

The nurse should respond that evidence to date consistently shows that low-fat, high-carbohydrate diets reduce LDL cholesterol. Individuals on low-carbohydrate/high-fat diets lose weight over the short term; however, the caloric intake is made up by increased protein and fats. High saturated fat diets increase LDL cholesterol and restrict the healthful foods like fruits and vegetables that provide various nutrient and fiber to the diet. There are no long-term studies that demonstrate the benefits of low-carbohydrate/high-fat diets, but there are known benefits to limiting the intake of fats. Therefore, a diet that provides for restriction of fats and a greater percentage of complex carbohydrates is most likely to lead to long-term reduction in the cholesterol level.

Children are continuing to grow and need nutrient-rich calories from all food groups to provide nutrient balance. Typical low-carbohydrate/high-fat diets do not provide adequate levels of calcium, iron, fiber, or B vitamins. Children need to be carefully assessed for dietary needs according to their ages and developmental stages. A diet that provides for balanced intake along with physical activity is desirable for children. A meal plan that provides weight loss in adults cannot be safely recommended for children.

Answers to Stop and Consider Questions

Table 18-1: Harris Hebrides has three risk factors (age, family history, and hypertension). Because he does not have CHD or CHD risk equivalent status, his LDL goal is less than 130 mg/dL. He is currently not at goal and the nurse should recommend that he schedule an individual visit with a dietitian for dietary management of his cholesterol.

Table 18-5: Instead of salt, suggest adding flavor to foods by using herbs, spices, and salt-free seasoning blends in cooking and at the table. There are low-sodium soup options available in various brands and for almost any type of soup. Turkey and turkey-based products are a good alternative to ham, hot dogs, and bacon. For fruits and vegetables, choose fresh, frozen, or "no added salt" canned varieties. Rinse canned foods to remove excess sodium.

Figure 18-2: When cooking in general, choose oils or fats with high unsaturated fats (monounsaturated and/or polyunsaturated fats) and low saturated and trans fats. When a more solid fat is needed for baking, butter, lard, or margarine are really comparable. Although solid margarine is lower in saturated fat compared to butter or lard, it contains trans fatty acids, which the other two do not. It is best to limit cooking with any of these because of the high saturated fat and/or trans fat content.

For sautéing vegetables or meat, olive oil or canola oil are the better choices due to a low saturated fat-to-unsaturated fat ratio.

Chapter 19
Critical Thinking in the Nursing Process

There are many options for dessert as part of a diabetic meal plan. Carbohydrate content should be considered along with calorie content if weight management is a goal. No specific desserts are prohibited, but choices must be balanced to fit within the dietary prescription. Fresh fruit is a good choice and can be made into a parfait with yogurt. Pudding or ice milk may be selected in place of regular ice cream because they may be lower in calories and fat, but carbohydrate content should still be checked. An occasional special dessert that is high in carbohydrate may be planned as part of a day's meal plan, incorporating its carbohydrate content into the allotment for total daily carbohydrate.

NCLEX® Questions

Answer: 1

Rationale: The typical diet for a person with diabetes should have about 50% to 55% of the calories from carbohydrates. The person with diabetes may have simple and complex carbohydrates, so there is no need to substitute artificial sweeteners when baking. Research has not shown that a low-carbohydrate diet is beneficial for people with diabetes because of the possible deleterious effects of increased fat and protein consumption on cardiovascular and kidney health, respectively. The person with diabetes needs carbohydrates for energy. Carbohydrate counting is only one method of dietary planning and may be too challenging for some people with diabetes to learn.

Cognitive Level: Analysis

Nursing Process: Evaluation

Category of Client Need: Health Promotion and Health Maintenance

Answer: 2

Rationale: Strenuous activity increases the need for carbohydrates because they are the main source of energy for exercising muscle. A client may need to monitor the blood glucose more frequently during an infection, but it is not a reason to increase carbohydrate consumption. Studying, which is a sedentary activity, does not increase the need for carbohydrate any more than eating a large meal does.

Cognitive Level: Application

Nursing Process: Intervention

Category of Client Need: Health Promotion and Health Maintenance

Answer: 4

Rationale: A client with a BMI of 31 is considered obese; a 25-pound weight loss may lessen the risk of complications or eliminate the need for medication, but the presence of the disease and its seriousness will remain a concern. Smaller portions may aid weight loss, but the distribution of nutrients is also important. The client needs to follow the meal plan that considers weight control along with nutrient balance.

Cognitive Level: Analysis

Nursing Process: Evaluation

Category of Client Need: Health Promotion and Health Maintenance

Answer: 2

Rationale: Clients with diabetes mellitus should eat foods with as little trans fat as possible due to the association of trans fat with the development of cardiovascular disease, a condition that is a frequent complication in people with diabetes. The calculation of the amount of fat allowed per meal is based on the total energy needs of the individual, not an absolute number like 10 grams. Eggs can be part of the individual's meal plan. Fish is acceptable as part of the diabetic meal plan depending on the type and method of preparation, so the nurse would want to elaborate on that response.

Cognitive Level: Application

Nursing Process: Intervention

Category of Client Need: Health Promotion and Health Maintenance

Answer: 4

Rationale: An initial teaching session should be focused on assessing the knowledge level of the recipient of the teaching. Once the assessment is completed, the nurse shares relevant information in a manner that is appropriate for the cognitive, developmental, and educational level of the individual(s). For this client, the nurse should give an explanation of the development of diabetes mellitus, the importance of weight control, and work with a dietitian to develop a culturally acceptable meal plan.

Cognitive Level: Application

Nursing Process: Intervention

Category of Client Need: Health Promotion and Health Maintenance

Critical Thinking Question

The nurse should first find out how much regular soda is consumed and how often. An individual with a BMI of 29 should be counseled about weight reduction as part of the diabetic diet plan. Because research has shown that individuals who drink diet beverages with artificial sweeteners do not replace beverage calories with other sources, those who consume regular soda can be counseled about the value of switching to diet soft drinks. This client should be encouraged to try different brands and types (lemon-lime instead of cola, for example) of soda before working on a diet plan that includes regular soda.

Answers to Stop and Consider Questions

Table 19-3. Well-controlled blood glucose levels are needed to determine an accurate carbohydrate-to-insulin ratio. If blood glucose is erratic, no consistent ratio between short-acting insulin and carbohydrate consumed will be apparent. If erroneous ratios are calculated, improper amounts of short-acting insulin will result.

Chapter 20
Critical Thinking in the Nursing Process

The nurse can suggest several interventions that may help. The client can increase fluid consumption, especially water. An increase in activity can also be helpful in those who are sedentary. The client can increase the fiber in the diet by consuming a variety of fruits, vegetables, and whole grains. It is also helpful for the client to plan adequate time for defecation, particularly after meals.

NCLEX® Questions

Answer: 1

Rationale: Smaller, more frequent meals decrease the possibility of stomach distention. The ideal diet should be high in complex carbohydrates, which includes some fibrous foods, and is low in simple sugars. The goal is to prevent rapid emptying of gastric contents.

Cognitive Level: Application

Nursing Process: Intervention

Category of Client Need: Physiological Integrity

Answer: 2

Rationale: When providing liquids to a client with dysphagia, the goal is to prevent choking. Thicker liquids, like fruit nectars, should be tried first with clients under guidance from the speech language pathologist. If they are tolerated well, eventually thinner liquids may be tried.

Cognitive Level: Application

Nursing Process: Implementation

Category of Client Need: Physiological Integrity

Answer: 3

Rationale: During the acute phase, clients take clear liquids until inflammation in the bowel has diminished. The diet is then slowly advanced with increasing amounts of fiber added once inflammation ceases.

Cognitive Level: Application

Nursing Process: Planning

Category of Client Need: Physiological Integrity

Answer: 4

Rationale: Clients with hepatitis need meals and snacks that are high in calories and protein. Eggs are a high-protein food and are easily digested. Fruits and vegetables are good sources of carbohydrates and fiber, but they lack protein. Jell-O and cookies contain simple carbohydrates.

Cognitive Level: Analysis

Nursing Process: Implementation

Category of Client Need: Physiological Integrity

Answer: 2

Rationale: Clients with celiac disease must avoid gluten, which is found in wheat, rye, and barley. The diet must be gluten free and clients are instructed to read labels carefully to minimize the risk of consumption of foods in which wheat products are used as fillers. Other foods may be safely consumed.

Cognitive Level: Application

Nursing Process: Implementation

Category of Client Need: Physiological Integrity

Critical Thinking Question

The nurse should inform the client that nausea and vomiting are common effects of anesthesia. The client should discuss these concerns with the surgeon and anesthesiologist. They may recommend a medication preoperatively or prefer treatment only if nausea and vomiting occur after surgery. The type and duration of anesthesia may affect their occurrence. Frequently, oral medications are prohibited preoperatively, so communication with the surgical team is very important.

Answers to Stop and Consider Questions

Table 20-3: A 50 gm protein diet could include a breakfast with one egg, lunch with ½ cup of milk and 2 oz of meat or chicken, and dinner with 3 oz of meat, fish, or protein. Moderate servings of grains and vegetables could be included. Fruit and fats have negligible protein and need to be included at each meal to supply energy. The diet is extremely limited, making it difficult to meet overall energy needs. Adherence is difficult because of the small portions of protein allowed.

Lifespan Box: Gastroesophageal Reflux in Infants and Children: Caffeine sources in a child's diet could include chocolate, cocoa, and soda. Mints include peppermint and spearmint candies. Fatty foods include fried foods, sauces, and dressings. Acidic foods include oranges, orange juice, and tomato sauce.

Figure 20-3: The loss of villi lessens the surface area for absorption, which results in intestinal discomfort, malabsorption, and diarrhea. The nurse can use the illustration to explain the need for dietary adherence to regenerate the villi to improve nutrient absorption and alleviate symptoms.

Client Education Checklist: Nutrition Intervention in Lactose Intolerance: Food sources of calcium and vitamin D are preferred over dietary supplements because they contain the additional nutrition found in the foods. When intake of calcium and vitamin D-containing foods is insufficient, calcium and vitamin D supplements can be recommended at recommended amounts.

Chapter 21
Critical Thinking in the Nursing Process

Adhering to a potassium and fluid restriction in end-stage renal failure is made more difficult by the presence of diabetes and the need to monitor carbohydrate intake. Some suggestions that the nurse can make to quench thirst while adhering to the diet include drinking low-carbohydrate, tart-tasting fluids within the fluid restriction, such as low sugar or sugar-free versions of cranberry juice cocktail, lemonade, and limeade; freezing these same drinks in ice cube trays and sucking on ice chips made from the juices; using tart-tasting sugar-free hard candies, but being careful of excessive intake of sorbitol contained in them, which can act as a laxative; and good mouth care and oral hygiene practices.

NCLEX® Questions

Answer: 4

Rationale: The nurse should assess the amount of vitamin C supplement consumed by the client. In general, megadoses of vitamin C contribute to the formation of certain types of renal stones that contain oxalate so should be avoided. Modest amounts of vitamin C may be consumed. Vitamin residue does not exist in the bladder; increased fluids are desirable but not for the reason stated.

Cognitive Level: Application

Nursing Process: Implementation

Category of Client Need: Health Promotion and Health Maintenance

Answer: 1, 3, 5

Rationale: A dry mouth is common in clients who have a fluid restriction. Saliva production will be stimulated with tart or frozen items, along with chewing gum that has a tart flavor. Clients may have beverages with caffeine if they wish. One ounce of water per hour will not satisfy thirst and may lead to excessive fluid intake over 24 hours.

Cognitive Level: Application

Nursing Process: Implementation

Category of Client Need: Physiological Integrity

Answer: 1

Rationale: Potassium must be restricted in clients with renal failure because it cannot be readily excreted and when retained can contribute to cardiac irritability. Bananas are high in potassium so must be limited in the diet. The fact that bananas are a source of carbohydrate and low in fiber are not the reason for limiting them in the diet. Bananas do not cause diarrhea.

Cognitive Level: Application

Nursing Proces: Implementation

Category of Client Need: Health Promotion and Health Maintenance

Answer: 2

Rationale: In renal failure, the kidneys lose their ability to excrete protein by-products so protein intake is limited to minimize uremic symptoms. The protein that is consumed should be of high biologic value to ensure that adequate amino acids are available to prevent catabolism. Adequate calories are also needed to accomplish this goal. Fluids are restricted rather than increased. High-sodium foods are restricted as is table salt. Many vegetables are high in potassium so must be limited.

Cognitive Level: Application

Nursing Process: Implementation

Category of Client Need: Health Promotion and Health Maintenance

Answer: 3

Rationale: Research has shown that cranberry juice may help prevent urinary tract infections, especially in women. It is important to drink adequate fluids, but the fluid does not have to be water. The source of protein does not matter, nor must carbonated beverages be avoided.

Cognitive Level: Analysis

Nursing Process: Evaluation

Category of Client Need: Health Promotion and Health Maintenance

Critical Thinking Question

The nurse should tell the client that cranberry juice cannot be used to treat UTIs. The organism that is causing the infection should be identified and appropriate antibiotic therapy initiated. The client should consume adequate fluid, including cranberry juice if desired. The nurse can suggest to the client that she might try drinking a glass of cranberry juice daily to prevent future UTIs, but the effective dose has not been demonstrated in long-term studies.

Answers to Stop and Consider Questions

Hot Topic: Beverage Intake to Prevent Kidney Stone Formation and Recurrence: The nurse should advise the client that staying well hydrated is the most important factor in reducing risk of stone recurrence. It is more difficult for stones to form in a dilute urine than a concentrated one. In clients known to have calcium oxalate stones with low urine citrate levels, inclusion of citrus beverages can be helpful.

Chapter 22
Critical Thinking in the Nursing Process

A client who has had surgery and develops a subsequent infection has increased needs for protein and vitamin C. The metabolic rate is also increased, so the client should have additional calories. The diet should be nutrient dense with high biologic value protein. Eggs, milk, and lean meat should be stressed. If the client has problems with physical mobility, high-fiber protein like legumes should be part of the diet. Citrus fruits are high in vitamin C as are green leafy vegetables.

NCLEX® Questions

Answer: 2

Rationale: Smaller, more frequent meals tend to reduce the energy expenditure required for eating. Clients with COPD typically do not rest well because of the shortness

of breath, so offering a large breakfast is not likely to be tolerated well. Simple carbohydrates lead to greater production of carbon dioxide that is detrimental to these clients. Repair of tissue damage is not a goal in clients with COPD.

Cognitive Level: Application

Nursing Process: Implementation

Category of Client Need: Health Promotion and Health Maintenance

Answer: 3

Rationale: All clients in critical care have regular comprehensive assessments that include vital signs, laboratory data, and physiological changes. A team that includes a dietitian recommends the timing and type of nutritional support that is indicated. A client on ventilator support may be started on enteral feeding if he cannot be weaned from the ventilator. The dextrose supplied by the IV does not have sufficient calories to meet nutritional needs. The nurse must be attentive to the nutritional needs for healing and recovery, so it is incorrect to suggest that a client can go a week without eating or that adequate stores exist within the body to meet nutritional needs.

Cognitive Level: Application

Nursing Process; Implementation

Category of Client Need: Health Promotion and Health Maintenance

Answer: 2

Rationale: Clients with COPD have difficulty getting adequate nutrition due to fatigue that results from experiencing shortness of breath while chewing and swallowing. These clients frequently require nutritional support to meet their metabolic needs. There is nothing to suggest that the young adult with a fracture will be unable to meet nutritional needs for healing. The obese client and the one with an MI may have special diets that are prescribed, but there are no special factors that indicate they are at risk for nutritional problems while in critical care.

Cognitive Level: Analysis

Nursing Process: Evaluation

Category of Client Need: Physiological Integrity

Answer: 3

Rationale: Nutrition care strategies in clients with MODS are dependent on assessment of organ function; serum electrolytes, blood urea nitrogen, creatinine, and liver function tests provide that data. Serum albumin provides some data about protein status only. Vital signs are not sufficient indicators of organ function, nor are age and knowledge of other health problems.

Cognitive Level: Analysis

Nursing Process: Assessment

Category of Client Need: Physiological Integrity

Answer: 4

Rationale: When a client has a functioning gastrointestinal tract, early enteral feeding is less likely to cause complications than parenteral feeding. Liver function test will be performed at least daily but is not an indicator of nutritional status. The client should be started on oral feeding as soon as possible, but those on mechanical ventilation require enteral tube feeding because of the inability to take anything by mouth.

Cognitive Level: Application

Nursing Process: Implementation

Category of Client Need: Physiological Integrity

Critical Thinking Question

There has been a lot of research conducted about preoperative fasting in recent years. The research that has focused on children has led to recommendations that children who receive clear liquids up to 2 hours before surgery arrive at surgery less dehydrated and irritable and have less postoperative pain. Although they may have postoperative nausea and/or vomiting, it is no worse than those who have longer fasts.

Answers to Stop and Consider Questions

Box 22-2: The nurse would want to recommend adequate fluid intake along with good sources of most nutrients, but especially energy, protein, vitamin C, and zinc. Examples of foods to suggest include yogurt mixed with citrus fruit; a smoothie drink made with juice and milk, soy milk, or yogurt; hummus or bean dip with crackers; spaghetti and meatballs with tomato sauce; a stir fry with chicken, beef, or tofu and vegetables.

Box 22-3: Safe food handling practices are covered in Chapter 10. Among the many important points, examples that can be shared with the transplant client include good hand washing before meal preparation and eating; avoidance of cross-contamination of preparation and cooking surfaces used for raw meat, fish, poultry, and eggs with uncooked foods, such as fruits and vegetables; and maintenance of proper temperature for storing and cooking foods.

Chapter 23
Critical Thinking in the Nursing Process

Discuss with the client if there are times of the day when there is greater energy or appetite. Determine if food aversions have developed during treatment. Suggest resting before eating anything. Try small portions of dry or bland foods early in the morning. Ask what foods the client likes and suggest eating them at a time when nausea is not a problem. Suggest trying commercial shakes or drinks that are protein enriched.

NCLEX® Questions

Answer: 4

Rationale: Dysgeusia is an alteration in taste sensation. Many times clients complain of a metallic taste. When glass or ceramic cookware is used in place of metal cookware, it seems to help alleviate the problem. Spices, salt, or carbonated beverages do not have an effect on the condition. Antiemetics are given for nausea and are of no benefit for dysgeusia.

Cognitive Level: Application

Nursing Process: Planning

Category of Client Need: Physiological Integrity

Answer: 2

Rationale: A client with a low neutrophil count is at risk for infection. Bacteria accumulate on cutting boards, which should be washed with warm water and soap between foods, particularly raw meat and poultry. Fresh vegetables can be eaten if they are thoroughly cleaned. Clients with a low neutrophil count may drink fresh, frozen, or bottled juices that are pasteurized. The fiber content of foods does not affect the risk of infection.

Cognitive Level: Analysis

Nursing Process: Implementation

Category of Client Need: Health Promotion and Health Maintenance

Answer: 3

Rationale: The client whose immunity is compromised is subject to a higher incidence of infection; therefore, all hot foods should be thoroughly cooked to ensure that proper temperatures were reached to reduce the risk of food-borne illness. The client has no need for pureed foods or extra water. The blood glucose level may be monitored if the client is taking steroids, but there are no restrictions placed on the client for sugar-sweetened beverages.

Cognitive Level: Application

Nursing Process: Implementation

Category of Client Need: Health Promotion and Health Maintenance

Answer: 2

Rationale: Nausea often accompanies chemotherapy, so antiemetics are prescribed. However, avoidance of foods with a strong odor is very helpful when the symptom is occurring. Clients should eat when they feel able and select foods that they find pleasing. Nutrient-dense foods are desirable, but eating something is more important than quality.

Cognitive Level: Application

Nursing Process: Planning

Category of Client Need: Physiological Integrity

Answer: 2

Rationale: Lipodystrophy that includes abnormal fat distribution does not fully respond to dietary intervention. Exercise may help prevent some accumulation of central fat, but restricting fat or increasing fiber in the diet does not effectively prevent or control this unfortunate side effect of HAART. Lifestyle modifications are recommended for elevated blood lipids that can occur with lipodystrophy but have little effect on the abnormal distribution of body fat that is found. Many of the medications are taken with food, so that advice is already part of the HAART protocol.

Cognitive Level: Application

Nursing Process: Implementation

Category of Client Need: Physiological Integrity

Critical Thinking Question

There are several things the nurse can suggest. The client can be allowed to eat anything that is desired. Small servings in pleasant surrounding may help. Foods that do not have strong odors are usually tolerated better than those that do. Appetite is often better early in the day, so encourage high-quality nutrients at that time. Box 23-11 outlines suggestions for increasing calorie and protein intake.

Answers to Stop and Consider Questions

Box 23-13: When a client is uncertain about the risks and benefits to using any particular type of alternative or complementary medicine, the nurse should further question the client to learn why the therapy is being used. That knowledge can guide the way in which the nurse educates the client about any known risks and benefits.

Box 23-14: Under any circumstance, food insecurity can jeopardize nutritional health even when disease or other conditions are not present. In clients with HIV infection, food insecurity can make it difficult to obtain sufficient food to meet baseline nutritional needs and may also affect availability of safe food that will not contribute to risk of food-borne illness. Nutrition intervention needs to focus first on ways of obtaining adequate safe food.

Chapter 24
Critical Thinking in the Nursing Process

Potassium is one of the most widely available nutrients in foods. As long as a client eats a balanced diet and is willing to eat a few foods that are rich in potassium (potatoes, bananas, citrus fruits), potassium supplements are usually not needed. If a client is unable to eat and is taking a diuretic, then a potassium supplement may be necessary.

NCLEX® Questions

Answer: 1

Rationale: A tyramine-restricted diet is required for all clients taking MAOI medications. Foods containing tyramine affect the MAOI action by blocking a particular enzyme that is responsible for tyramine metabolism. When tyramine builds up, a hypertensive crisis may oc-

cur in the client; therefore, tyramine-rich foods like smoked meats, aged cheeses, soy products, and many beers must be avoided. Pepperoni pizza should not be eaten. Fruits, tomatoes that would be found in most salsa, fish, and pasta may be eaten.

Cognitive Level: Application

Nursing Process: Evaluation

Category of Client Need: Health Promotion and Health Maintenance

Answer: 4

Rationale: A client takes warfarin to minimize clotting; many clients are on long-term therapy with warfarin. Vitamin K is the antidote for warfarin; this means that vitamin K promotes clotting. Therefore, although foods that contain vitamin K can be consumed by clients who are taking warfarin, intake of these should be kept at a steady state so as not to increase or decrease daily vitamin K in the diet. Warfarin doses are managed based on a client's everyday intake of dietary vitamin K; extremes of intake will negatively affect clotting. Examples of these foods are green leafy vegetables, liver, and fortified foods, such as cereals and meal replacement drinks. Citrus fruits, pork, and oatmeal are appropriate foods for someone who is taking warfarin, but spinach intake should be kept consistent.

Cognitive Level: Application

Nursing Process: Evaluation

Category of Client Need: Health Promotion and Health Maintenance

Answer: 1

Rationale: A process called chelation causes reduced bioavailability (absorption) of tetracycline in the presence of calcium ions; therefore, any product that contains calcium should not be taken with tetracycline. The calcium decreases, not increases, the absorption of tetracycline. The interaction of tetracycline and milk do not cause GERD.

Cognitive Level: Application

Nursing Process: Implementation

Category of Client Need: Physiological Integrity

Critical Thinking Question

Lean pork is low in fat; a 4-ounce serving will come close to meeting the RDA. Whole grain and enriched breads and cereals would be good choices for this client. Legumes are low in fat in addition to being a good source of thiamine.

Answers to Stop and Consider Questions

Table 24-2: Medication side effects and dosing guidelines to avoid taking a drug with food can affect nutrition status by fostering reduced dietary intake. For example, nausea or taste changes are side effects of some medications. Drugs that must be taken on an empty stomach can interrupt meal schedule or intake of certain food groups, such as dairy, because of dosing schedule.

Practice Pearl: Mixing Medications with an Enteral Nutrition Formula: The feeding tube needs to be flushed between medication to avoid chelation or a precipitate from forming in the tube and causing a clogged tube.

Hot Topic: Drug Interactions with Fortified Foods and Supplements: Fortified foods that contain calcium, iron, or magnesium include juices and other fortified drinks, hot and cold breakfast cereals, meal replacement drinks and bars, and cereal bars.

Client Education Checklist: Monoamine Oxidase Inhibitors (MAOI) and Tyramine: Tyramine is found in aged and cured foods. Some examples of high-tyramine foods from various cultures include fermented soy products, such as soy sauce, tofu, miso, and kim chee found in Asian cuisines; fava beans and various types of dry hard sausages, and parmesan, romano, and mozzarella cheese found in Mediterranean cuisine; and sauerkraut, pickled herring, and summer sausage found in Eastern European cuisine.

Chapter 25
Critical Thinking in the Nursing Process

Many supplements, especially multivitamins and minerals, may be indicated as part of a treatment plan for a particular condition. Some supplements are of dubious safety and quality, but it would be unfair to say that all supplements are a waste of money.

NCLEX® Questions

Answer: 2

Rationale: It is important to stress to clients that there is a potential interaction between supplements and prescribed medication, so the physician should be informed of all supplements that are used, even if only occasionally. There is no reason to suggest that clients withhold some information for a later visit. It is also inappropriate for the nurse to suggest that by entering the supplements in the medical record the client has no further responsibility to discuss it with the physician.

Cognitive Level: Application

Nursing Process: Evaluation

Category of Client Need: Health Promotion and Health Maintenance

Answer: 3

Rationale: Herbal supplements can have interactions with prescription and nonprescription medications, so the health care provider should be part of the discussion about which supplements are being considered and the reasons for taking them. Herbal supplements can have side effects, so the nurse needs to acknowledge that with clients. Many supplements are not expensive, which is why clients are willing to use them. The nurse needs to avoid the sarcasm that is present in option 4.

Cognitive Level: Application

Nursing Process: Evaluation

Category of Client Need: Health Promotion and Health Maintenance

Answer: 3

Rationale: The nurse must use caution in recommending supplements. Soy isoflavones have been studied and may have a weak effect in diminishing menopausal symptoms. However, women at high risk for breast cancer or with a history of breast cancer are warned to avoid soy supplements because of the potential to further increase cancer risk. The client should discuss the application of this research to her individual circumstances with her health care provider. Green tea has no known effect on menopausal symptoms. St. John's Wort may be used as a mild antidepressant and saw palmetto is claimed to reduce symptoms caused by prostate enlargement.

Cognitive Level: Application

Nursing Process: Implementation

Category of Client Need: Health Promotion and Health Maintenance

Answer: 3

Rationale: The nurse needs to avoid recommending specific dosages of supplements. It is prudent to discuss what has been found in research studies and then recommend that clients discuss potential supplement use with their health care provider. The FDA regulates supplements as food, not medication, so the nurse should not suggest that FDA approval is found on supplement labels.

Cognitive Level: Application

Nursing Process: Implementation

Category of Client Need: Health Promotion and Health Maintenance

Answer: 4

Rationale: A store does not have control over the composition of the supplements it stocks. Many supplements have ingredients of varying quality. The FDA regulates supplements as foods and does not review these products for safety before they go on the market. The FDA does get involved in safety issues with supplements if there is a problem that seems to be caused by the supplement once it is already on the market. A consumer has no more assurance of safety or quality when purchasing supplements directly from a supplier.

Cognitive Level: Application

Nursing Process: Implementation

Category of Client Need: Health Promotion and Health Maintenance

Critical Thinking Questions

There has been only one study that was conducted several years ago that showed cinnamon lowered blood glucose. Several studies that have been conducted since that time failed to obtain similar results; therefore, cinnamon should be used only as a flavoring for foods, not in the hope that blood glucose levels will improve.

The nurse should affirm that studies demonstrated that cinnamon had no harmful effects, but it has not been proven effective at lowering blood glucose. Given that information, he should not discontinue his medication but can continue to enjoy cinnamon with food.

Answers to Stop and Consider Questions

Lifespan Box: Supplement Concerns across the Lifespan: The nurse can use the same type of questions that are used with other clients to determine supplement use. Additional questions can focus on whether the female is using supplements to alleviate any symptoms associated with pregnancy, such as nausea or constipation. When supplement use is influenced by cultural beliefs, the nurse should sensitively explore the reason for their use and any health risks. For example, a conversation with a female taking ginseng for fatigue could be: "I know you have said that you have been feeling tired and that your grandmother took ginseng when she was pregnant and had fatigue. You are taking ginseng capsules and we cannot compare that with the ginseng tea that you mentioned your grandmother used. Did you know that ginseng affects how blood clots and can make it harder to form a blood clot to stop bleeding if excessive amounts are used? I am concerned about the effect that could have on your health and the baby's, especially during delivery."

Index

Page numbers followed by *f* indicate figures and those followed by *t* indicate tables, boxes, or special features. The titles of special features (e.g., Client Education Checklists, Evidence-Based Practice Research, Nursing Care Plans) are capitalized.